S0-AWU-288

Modern Dental Assisting

Hazel O. Torres, CDA, RDA, RDAEF, MA
Ann Ehrlich, CDA, MA
Doni Bird, CDA, RDH, MA
Ellen Dietz, CDA, AAS, BS

W.B. SAUNDERS COMPANY
A Division of Harcourt Brace & Company
Philadelphia London Toronto Montreal Sydney Tokyo

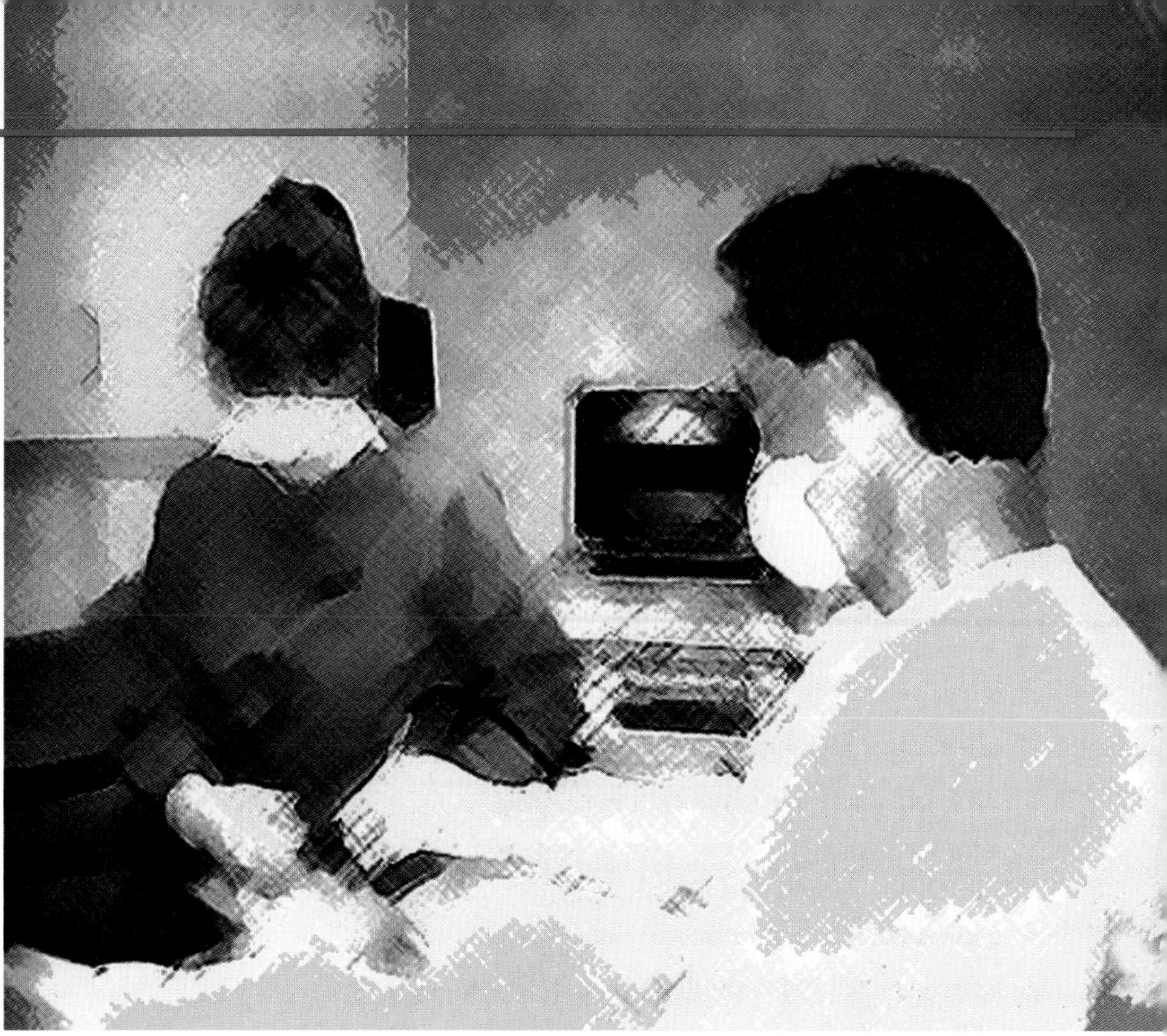

Modern Dental Assisting

fifth edition

W.B. SAUNDERS COMPANY
A Division of
Harcourt Brace & Company

The Curtis Center
Independence Square West
Philadelphia, Pennsylvania 19106

Library of Congress Cataloging-in-Publication Data

Modern dental assisting / Hazel O. Torres . . . [et al.].–5th ed.
p. cm.
Rev. ed. of: Modern dental assisting / Hazel O. Torres, Ann Ehrlich. 4th ed., 1990.
Includes bibliographical references.
ISBN 0-7216-5053-8
1. Dental assistants. I. Torres, Hazel O. Modern dental assisting.
[DNLM: 1.Dental Assistants. 2. Dental Care. WU 90 M689 1995]
RK60.5.T67 1995
617.6′0233—dc20
DNLM/DLC 94-28655

Modern Dental Assisting, 5th Edition ISBN 0-7216-5053-8

Printed in the United States of America

Last digit is the print number: 9 8 7 6 5 4 3

Preface

This is an exciting time to enter a career in dental assisting. New materials and techniques have made dental treatment more comfortable and safer than at any time in the past. Simultaneously, the responsibilities and duties of the assistant are expanding, and new career opportunities are rapidly developing.

Since the first edition, our goal has been to have *Modern Dental Assisting* serve as the comprehensive text for students in formal dental assistant training programs and for those already employed in the field of dentistry who are interested in expanding their knowledge.

The tradition continues in this fifth edition of *Modern Dental Assisting.* This edition provides a comprehensive description of the roles and responsibilities of the dental assistant in a modern dental practice. It contains the information required for students to develop the competencies necessary to meet the demands of dentistry in the late 1990s and on into the 21st century.

This edition also reflects exciting changes for the authors. As new co-authors for this edition, Doni Bird and Ellen Dietz have brought professional expertise plus new ideas, energy, and insights. Their efforts have contributed greatly to determining that this edition covers current techniques in an easy-to-understand format.

An exciting visual change is the use of icons in procedures headings. These icons serve as reminders of protective equipment and commonly used instrumentation required for that procedure.

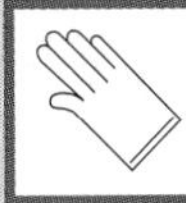

Examination gloves, which are introduced in Chapter 13.

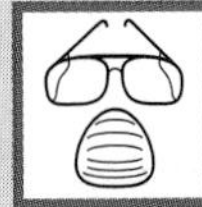

Additional personal protective equipment, which is introduced in Chapter 13.

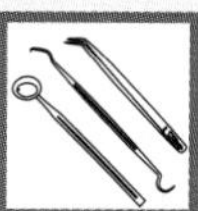

The **basic setup,** which is introduced in Chapter 15.

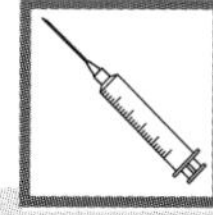

The **local anesthetic setup,** which is introduced in Chapter 20.

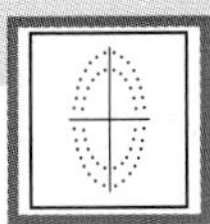

The **dental dam setup,** which is introduced in Chapter 22.

If an item is not required, the icon box is empty.

We wish to make clear that the use of the pronouns "she" and "he" is necessitated by the limitations of the English language. It does not indicate any gender restrictions with regard to the qualifications for employment on the dental health team. However, to simplify identification, the pronoun "he" is used throughout in referring to a patient.

Preclinical topics are covered at the beginning of the book, followed by clinical chapters and then office procedures. Each of the 36 chapters is comprehensive and stands alone. You may study them in any sequence as determined by your instructor, your interest, or your need to know.

There are many topics that apply to several chapters, and cross-references are used throughout to guide you to the appropriate chapter in which the topic is discussed. This will aid you in reviewing information you have already studied or in locating unfamiliar information related to the current topic.

Full color has been added to many photographs and illustrations throughout the text where it is needed to help you fully understand and learn that information.

When an important new term is introduced, it appears in **boldface** and is defined. These are key words that you will want to remember. There is a comprehensive glossary at the end of the book. It includes dental terms that would be difficult to find in a standard dictionary. This is a valuable resource when you need to look up a term quickly. Also at the end of the book there is a comprehensive list of the major references used in the development of this edition.

Many dental procedures are explained in a detailed step-by-step format. Rationales are included with steps for which it is necessary or helpful to understand why that step is performed and why it is important. A special design has been created to make procedures easy to find and use.

A new accompanying workbook has been created for use with this edition, and we strongly recommend using the text and workbook together. The workbook contains **learning objectives** and at least **25 multiple-choice questions** for each chapter. **Competency sheets** are included to test your mastery in performing the skills described in the text.

There is also an Instructor's Manual available for use with this text. It contains the answer keys for the workbook and other helpful information.

All the members of the *Modern Dental Assisting* team wish the reader success in your chosen career in dental assisting.

Hazel O. Torres

Ann Ehrlich

Doni Bird

Ellen Dietz

Acknowledgments

This process of revision and information updating, in-depth research, and incorporation of new techniques has involved many people.

The authors wish to acknowledge the technical assistance, kindness, and support of the following persons: William F. Bird, DDS; Barbara Cancilla, RDAEF; Sharon Collins, RDA; W. Stephen Eakle, DDS; Arnold S. Eilers, AA; Berne J. Holman, DDS; Grace Hom, RDA; Harry Humphreys, DDS; Michael Koffler, DDS; Pamela Landry, RDA; Thomas Mullooly, DDS; John Paul Piro, CDT; Steve Potter, CDT; Melissa Rinck, DDS; Stephen M. Rizzuto, MA; Debbie Robinson, CDA; Phillip Waterman, DDS; Shirley Watt, RDA; and Paul Yeager, DDS.

We also want to thank the many working assistants and instructors who took time to serve as reviewers to provide input on the book during the developmental process. Their insights, suggestions, and questions have greatly strengthened this edition.

Creating a book of this size and scope would not be possible without the excellent professional support we have received from the W.B. Saunders Company staff. We wish to thank the following for their contributions to this edition: Selma Ozmat, Senior Editor, Health-Related Professions; Shirley Kuhn, Senior Developmental Editor; Ellen B. Zanolle, Designer; Anne Ostroff, Copy Editor; Cecilia Roberts, Illustration Specialist; Jacqui Brownstein, Production Manager; Angela Holt, Indexer; and Sandy Won, Editorial Assistant, Health-Related Professions.

Contents

Chapter 26

Periodontics 499

Chapter 27

Pediatric Dentistry 517

Chapter 28

Orthodontics 535

Chapter 29
Endodontics 565

Chapter 30
Oral and Maxillofacial Surgery and Dental Implants 579

Chapter 31
Fixed Prosthodontics........................ 605

Chapter 32
Removable Prosthodontics............... 629

Chapter 1

Introduction to Organized Dentistry

Introduction

This chapter is divided into two sections. First is a brief overview of the history of dentistry, because as dental historian B. W. Weinberger stated, "A profession which is ignorant of its past experiences has lost a valuable asset for it has missed its best guide to the future."

The second part of this chapter is an introduction to the members of a modern dental health team.

The History of Dentistry

"Decay of human teeth has been found in so many places, even from the most ancient times, that it is legitimate to doubt whether there was ever an epoch when the human species was not cursed with toothache" (Bremner, 1939).

For this reason, the history of attempts to relieve the pain of toothache is nearly as old as the human race.

Early Times

EGYPTIANS

The earliest dentist whose name is known was **Hesi-Re,** an Egyptian, who lived about 3000 B.C. At this time, Egyptian physicians specialized in healing specific parts of the body. A monument to Hesi-Re describes him with high regard as "the greatest of the physicians who treat the teeth" (Ring, 1985).

CHINESE

One of the oldest known medical works containing references to dentistry is the Chinese *Canon of Medicine,* which was reputed to have been written by Huang-Ti in about 2700 B.C.

Books on the history of Chinese medicine also mention what is believed to be the earliest record of a cleft lip repair during the Ch'in Dynasty (255–206 B.C.) (Boo-Chai, 1966).

In about the second century A.D., the Chinese developed "silver paste" (amalgam) for fillings. This happened more than a thousand years before dentists in the West discovered the material (Ring, 1985).

PHOENICIANS AND ETRUSCANS

Findings from the fifth and sixth centuries B.C. indicate that the Phoenicians and Etruscans had developed a form of bridgework for the replacement of natural teeth (Weinberger, 1948) (Fig. 1–1).

GREEKS

Hippocrates (460–377 B.C.), the *father of medicine,* was an early advocate of scientific reasoning pertaining to health affairs. He perceived the importance of keep-

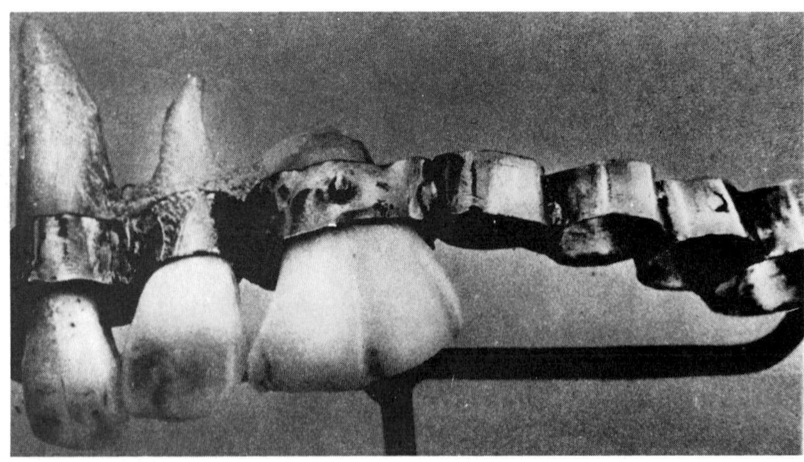

FIGURE 1–1

Ancient Etruscan gold band bridge with a built-in calf's tooth. (From Proskauer, C., and Witt, F.H.: Pictorial History of Dentistry. Cologne, Germany, Verlag M. Dumont Schauberg, 1962.)

ing the teeth in condition and compounded a dentifrice and mouthwash (Hollinshead, 1961).

The famous *Oath of Hippocrates,* a solemn obligation assumed by all who undertook to practice medicine, still serves as the basis of the code of ethics of the medical and dental professions in the United States.

Aristotle (384–322 B.C.) referred to teeth in many of his writings. Unfortunately, he had many curious views on teeth, such as the one stating that men had more teeth than women. These views were held for many centuries, and it was not until the Renaissance that many of these erroneous ideas were corrected (Hollinshead, 1961).

ROMANS

In addition to the treatment of oral diseases and the extraction of teeth, the Romans were skilled in restoring decayed teeth with gold crowns and replacing missing teeth with fixed bridgework.

According to the Roman *Law of the Twelve Tables,* which was written about 450 B.C., the bridge was crafted by a goldsmith and placed by a dentist. This indicates that goldsmiths may have been the earliest dental laboratory technicians.

Cornelius Celsus (25 B.C.–A.D. 50) wrote *De Re Medicina,* a compendium of medical and surgical knowledge. This book contained recommendations on the relief of toothache, ligation (splinting) of loose teeth, and the importance of oral hygiene.

Claudius Galen (A.D. 130–200) is considered to be the greatest physician of ancient times after Hippocrates. In his writings, Galen listed the teeth as bones of the body, and he is credited with being the first author to write about the nerves of the teeth.

He stated, "The teeth are furnished with nerves both because as naked bones they have need of sensibility so that the animal may avoid being injured or destroyed by mechanical or physical agencies, and because the teeth, together with the tongue and other parts of the mouth, are designed for the perception of various flavors" (Guerini, 1909).

Middle Ages and the Renaissance

Scrapion, an Arabian physician who lived in the tenth century, accurately described the numbers of roots of the teeth. He stated that upper molars needed three roots to hold them firm because of their hanging position. He also thought that two roots were sufficient to keep the lower molars in place because they receive support from the jaw.

Although he was Spanish, Albucasis (936–1013) is considered the greatest Arabian surgeon of the Middle Ages. (Writers of this period are referred to as Arabian because they wrote in Arabic.)

In his work, *De Chirurgia,* Albucasis wrote extensively on the scraping of the teeth and is acknowledged as the first author to take into serious consideration dental tartar. He also listed rules for the extraction of a tooth; however, "this was to be attempted only when unavoidable."

Andreas Vesalius (1514–1564) is known as the *founder of modern anatomy.* It was his work that corrected many of the mistaken doctrines of Galen (Weinberger, 1948).

Ambroise Paré (1510–1590), the *founder of modern surgery,* began his career in Paris about 1525 as apprentice to a barber surgeon.

His extensive writings on dentistry include methods for extractions and for the replantation of teeth. He is also credited with being the first to close perforations of the palate with obturators. (An **obturator** is a prosthesis for closing an opening in the palate.)

Later Developments

Pierre Fauchard (1678–1761), the *founder of modern dentistry,* approached dentistry with the training of a scientist and physician. He is credited with being the first to use the term *caries* and to reject the idea that caries was caused by "worms of the teeth" (Fig. 1–2).

Fauchard's book *Le Chirurgien Dentiste,* published in 1728, is considered one of the most important

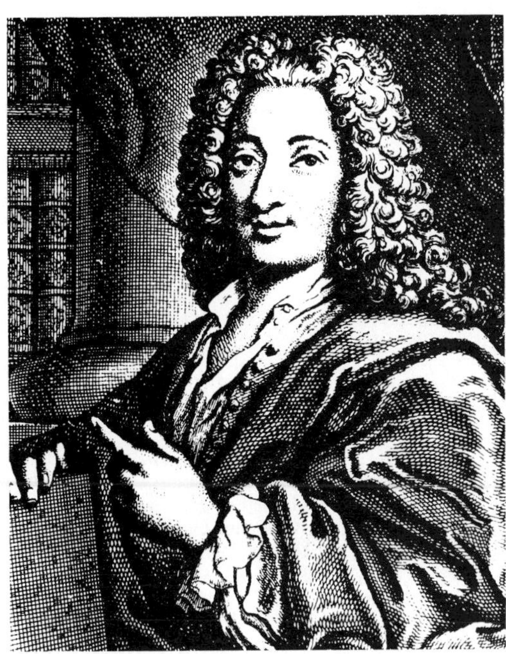

FIGURE 1–2

Pierre Fauchard, the founder of modern dentistry. (From Fauchard, P.: The Surgeon Dentist or Treatise on the Teeth, 2nd ed [Trans: Lindsay, L.]. Pound Ridge, NY, Milford House, 1969.)

books in dental literature. The case records and Fauchard's reflections upon them give the reader an insight into the method of practice, as well as of the standard of dentistry, accepted at the time (Fauchard, 1969).

John Hunter (1728–1793), who is best known as an English anatomist, also made many valuable contributions to dental science. He was the first to make a scientific study of the teeth and to put infection from dental disease upon a sound scientific cause-and-effect basis. He also reformed the classification of the teeth and named the incisors, cuspids, bicuspids, and molars. (Bicuspids are now known as premolars.)

In 1771, Hunter published *Natural History of the Teeth*, a work honored as a milestone in the history of dentistry. In this work, he explained the structure of the teeth and their use, formation, growth, and diseases (Hollinshead, 1961).

In 1895, **Wilhelm Conrad Roentgen** (1845–1923), a German professor of physics, discovered the x-radiation properties of cathode rays, and this led to the development of radiography. By the turn of the century, several Americans had applied x-radiation to dentistry.

The Development of Dentistry in the United States

John Baker, M.D. (1732–1796), was probably one of the first competent dentists to practice in this country. He was born in England, received his medical training there, and came to America in about 1752. He practiced dentistry in Boston, New York, Philadelphia, and many other colonial cities (Hollinshead, 1961).

While Dr. Baker was in Boston, Paul Revere studied with him. When Dr. Baker left Boston in 1768, **Paul Revere** (1735–1818) took over his practice. However, after 6 years of sporadic activity, Revere gave up dentistry.

After the battle of Bunker Hill, the body of Dr. Joseph Warren was hastily buried without being properly identified. Paul Revere is reputed to have later identified Dr. Warren's body by means of a dental appliance. If true, this was the first case in America of identification by means of teeth, and it was an important contribution to forensic dentistry.

At age 14, **John Greenwood** (1760–1819) served in the American Revolutionary army. In 1785 he began the practice of dentistry in New York and in 1789 became dentist to George Washington (Figs. 1–3 and 1–4).

THE AMALGAM WAR

Amalgam was first introduced as "silver paste" in 1826 by M. Taveau of Paris. There was no control of expansion during setting in this early material. This caused major problems after a "silver" restoration was placed.

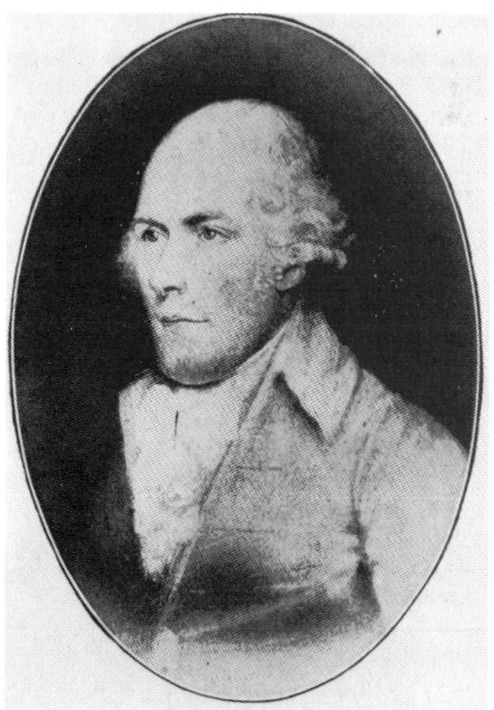

FIGURE 1–3

John Greenwood, dentist to George Washington. (From Koch, C.R.D.: History of Dental Surgery, Vol. III. Fort Wayne, IN, National Art Publishing Co., 1910.)

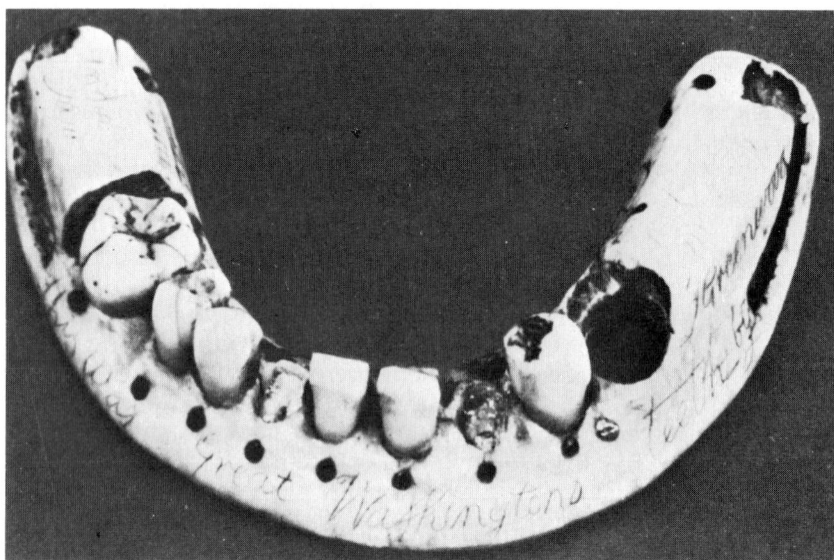

FIGURE 1–4

George Washington's denture. (From Proskauer, C., and Witt, F.H.: Pictorial History of Dentistry. Cologne, Germany, Verlag M. Dumont Schauberg, 1962.)

Amalgam was introduced in New York in 1833 by the Crawcour brothers, who called it "royal mineral succedaneum" (successor to the royal mineral, i.e., gold, which had been used almost exclusively up to that time).

The Crawcour brothers were not qualified as dentists and were prone to unscrupulous methods. Their methods and material created a bitter controversy, which began as an objection to their methods but continued, long after the brothers had left the battle, as a controversy about the material.

This controversy is recorded in the annals of American dental history as the *Amalgam War,* and many early dental societies declared the use of amalgam to be malpractice (Bremner, 1939).

Although these restrictions were later removed, the Amalgam War lasted for nearly two decades, and amalgam was not commonly accepted as a restorative material until significant improvements were made on the basis of the work of Greene Vardiman Black and others.

HORACE WELLS AND WILLIAM MORTON

In 1844, **Horace Wells** (1815–1848), an American dentist, was the first to use nitrous oxide for relief of pain during tooth extraction.

Soon after, **William T. G. Morton** (1819–1868) introduced the use of ether as an anesthetic for dental extractions and later as an adjunct for medical surgical operations.

GREENE VARDIMAN BLACK

Greene Vardiman Black (1836–1915) is referred to as *the grand old man of dentistry.* He was an outstanding scientist of the nineteenth century and made many important contributions to dental science (Figs. 1–5 and 1–6).

In 1891, while a professor of operative dentistry and dental pathology at Northwestern University Dental School, he described the structural elements, characteristics, and physical properties of enamel.

Dr. Black's investigations led to the methods of scientific cavity preparation in teeth and the methods of correctly inserting and making both gold and amalgam fillings. These improvements in cavity preparations were also made possible by introduction of the dental engine (handpiece) in the 1870's.

Dr. Black also made important contributions to dental nomenclature, the improvement of amalgam manufacture, and the standardization of dental instruments.

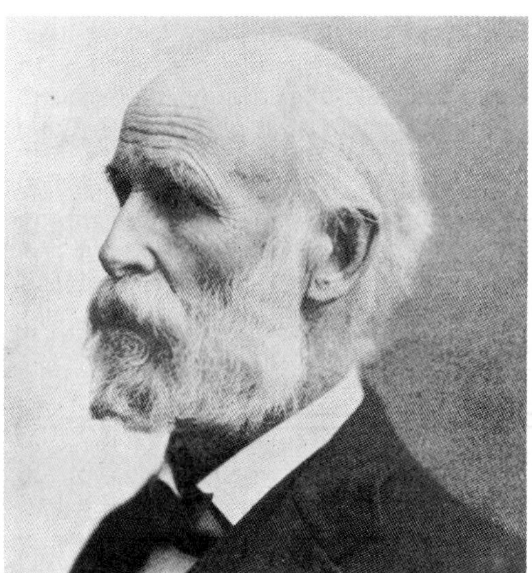

FIGURE 1–5

Greene Vardiman Black, the grand old man of dentistry. (From Koch, C.R.D.: History of Dental Surgery, Vol. I. Chicago, National Art Publishing Co., 1909.)

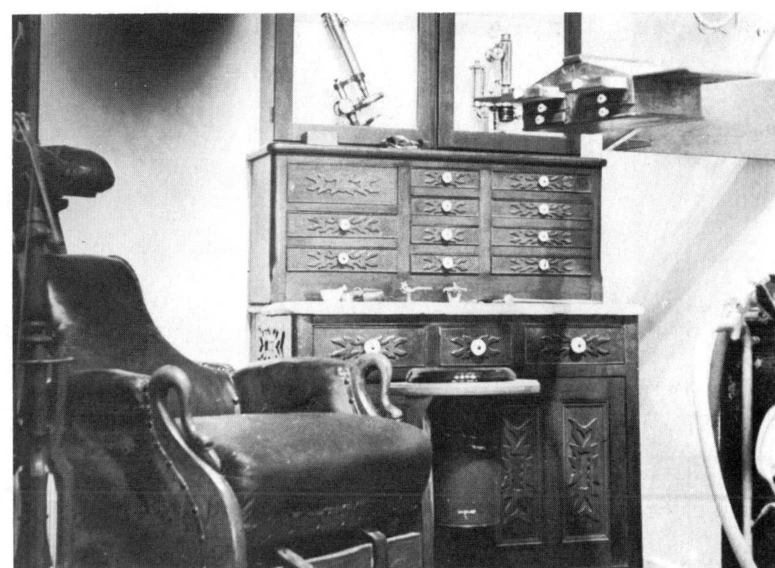

FIGURE 1–6

G. V. Black's dental treatment room, as reconstructed in a Smithsonian Institution exhibit.

DR. C. EDMUND KELLS

Dr. C. Edmund Kells (1856–1928) of New Orleans is usually credited with having hired the first dental assistant, in 1885.

This first "lady assistant" was really a "Lady in Attendance," making it respectable for a woman patient to go into a dental office without being accompanied by her husband or a maiden aunt.

It soon became obvious that the "Lady in Attendance" could be helpful around the office, and by 1900 Dr. Kells was working with both a chairside assistant and a secretarial assistant (Fig. 1–7).

Beginning in 1898, Dr. Kells also worked extensively with x-radiation. Like others of his era, Kells was unaware of the dangers of radiation, and the effects of x-ray exposure ultimately caused his death in 1928.

DENTAL EDUCATION

In 1830 there were approximately 300 dentists in the United States. However, as described by Dr. Chapin Harris, "Of these not more than 40 or 50 had attained much knowledge in any department of the art" (Harris, 1845).

The state of dentistry in the United States soon began to improve, largely through the efforts of Chapin Harris.

In 1840 the Baltimore College of Dentistry, the first dental school in the world, was founded by Chapin

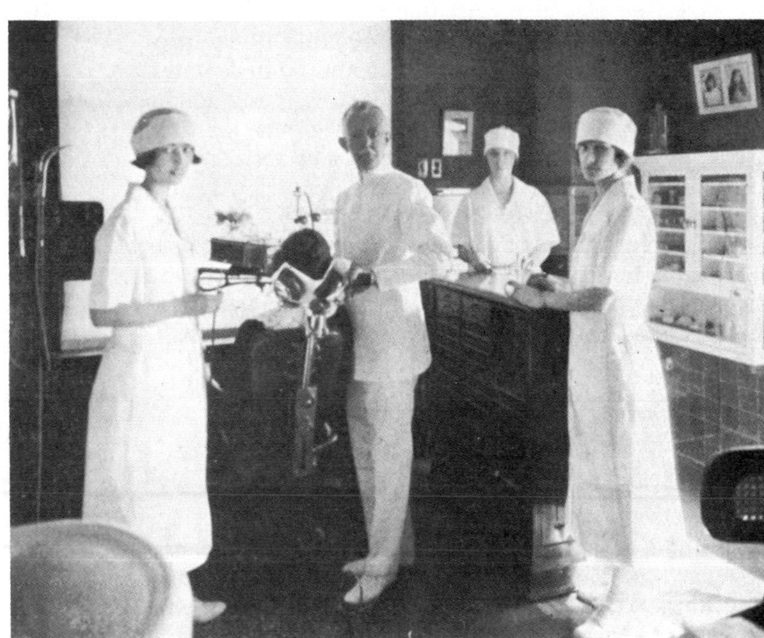

FIGURE 1–7

Dr. C. Edmund Kells and his "working unit." The assistant on the left is keeping cold air on the cavity. The assistant on the right is mixing materials, and the secretary is recording details. Photograph taken about 1900. (From Kells, C.E.: The Dentist's Own Book. St. Louis, C.V. Mosby Co., 1925, p 299.)

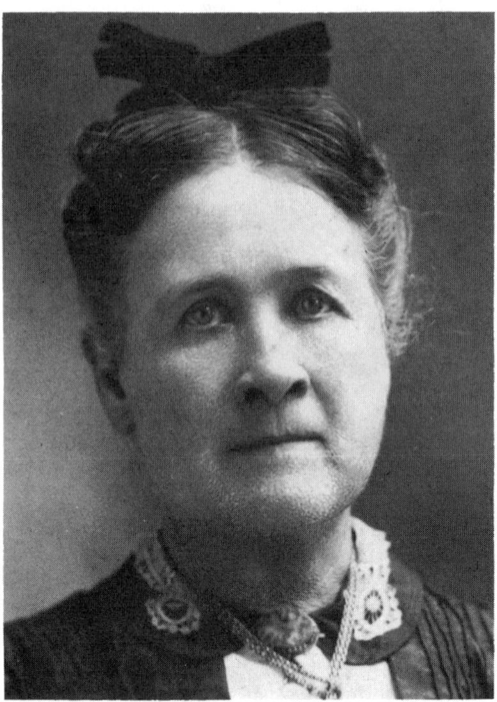

FIGURE 1–8

Lucy B. Hobbs Taylor, the first woman graduate in dentistry. (Courtesy of Kansas State Historical Society.)

Harris and Horace Hayden. This school is now the School of Dentistry at the University of Maryland.

Lucy B. Hobbs Taylor was the first woman graduate in dentistry (Fig. 1–8). She received her diploma in 1866 from the Ohio College of Dental Surgery in Cincinnati and practiced dentistry for nearly 60 years.

Today, the **Commission on Dental Accreditation of the American Dental Association** is responsible for the evaluation and accreditation of all educational programs for the study of dentistry in the United States. These include graduate dental programs, postgraduate specialty programs, and residency programs for dentists. The Commission also regulates and accredits education programs in dental hygiene, dental assisting, and dental laboratory technology.

This accreditation of educational programs provides an assurance of acceptable educational standards on the part of the profession, the educational institution, the students, and the public.

Members of the Dental Health Team

The individuals filling the many roles in a dental practice are referred to collectively as **dental health care workers** (DHCWs). An **auxiliary** is a DHCW who provides direct support services to the dentist. Auxiliaries include dental hygienists, assistants, and laboratory technicians.

Dentist

The dentist is required to have knowledge and proficiency in order to provide total patient care, which includes

- Recognizing the patient's dental needs as they relate to the patient's total physical and emotional well-being
- Applying up-to-date diagnostic skills, with emphasis on conditions relating to the oral cavity
- Utilizing current techniques and skills in all aspects of patient care
- Instructing patients in methods of preventing dental disease

The educational requirements for the dentist trained in the United States include undergraduate education and graduation from a dental school approved by the Commission on Dental Accreditation of the American Dental Association.

The degree granted usually is the DDS (Doctor of Dental Surgery) or the DMD (Doctor of Medical Dentistry). Training for dental specialists includes 2 or more years of postgraduate and graduate education in an approved program in the area of specialization.

All dentists must pass both written and clinical examinations to become licensed in the state in which they practice (see Chapter 2).

Most dentists are members of their professional organization, the American Dental Association (ADA). As a member of the ADA, the dentist must comply with the principles of ethics of the ADA as established by the national, constituent (state), and component (local) societies.

DENTAL SPECIALTIES

Although a general practitioner is trained and legally permitted to perform all dental functions, he or she may elect to refer more difficult cases to specialists who have advanced training in certain areas.

The following are the dental specialties officially recognized by the ADA's Commission on Dental Accreditation.

Dental public health is concerned with preventing and controlling dental diseases and promoting dental health through organized community efforts.

Endodontics is concerned with the etiology, diagnosis, prevention, and treatment of diseases and injuries of the pulp and associated periradicular tissues. (**Etiology** means the study of the cause of a disease. **Periradicular** means surrounding the root of the tooth.)

Oral pathology is concerned with the nature of the diseases affecting the oral structures and adjacent regions.

Oral and maxillofacial surgery is concerned with the diagnosis and surgical and adjunctive treatment of diseases, injuries, and defects of the oral and maxillofacial region.

Orthodontics is concerned with the supervision, guidance, and correction of all forms of malocclusion of the growing or mature dentofacial structures.

Pediatric dentistry is concerned with the preventive and therapeutic oral health care of children from birth through adolescence. It also includes patients beyond adolescence who because of mental, physical, and/or emotional problems need specialized help in receiving dental care.

Periodontics is concerned with the diagnosis and treatment of disease of the supporting and surrounding tissues of the teeth. The scope does not include permanent restorative dentistry.

Prosthodontics is concerned with the restoration and maintenance of oral functions by the restoration of natural teeth and/or the replacement of missing teeth and contiguous oral and maxillofacial tissues with artificial substitutes.

If treatment by the specialist (for example, orthodontics) is lengthy, the patient continues to see the general practitioner for routine care.

Once treatment by the specialist has been completed, the patient usually returns to the general practitioner for continuing care.

Registered Dental Hygienist

The registered dental hygienist (RDH) is an important member of the dental health team, with emphasis in the area of preventive dentistry (Fig. 1–9). The hygienist is trained to

- Record case histories, chart conditions of the oral cavity, and measure the depth of periodontal pockets
- Perform a professional dental prophylaxis, including the removal of stains, plaque, and calculus from crowns and root surfaces
- Expose, process, and evaluate the quality of radiographs
- Provide additional professional services, including scaling and root planing
- Apply sealants and topical fluoride treatments
- Apply and remove periodontal dressings
- Instruct patients in preventive care
- In some states, administer local anesthetics and perform soft tissue curettage
- Perform the tasks of a chairside assistant

The minimal education required for dental hygiene licensure is 2 academic years of college study in an accredited dental hygiene program. Dental hygiene education is also offered in bachelor's and master's degree programs.

The RDH must pass both written national or regional board and clinical state board examinations in order to be licensed by the state in which he or she plans to practice. In most states the hygienist is required to work under the supervision of a licensed dentist.

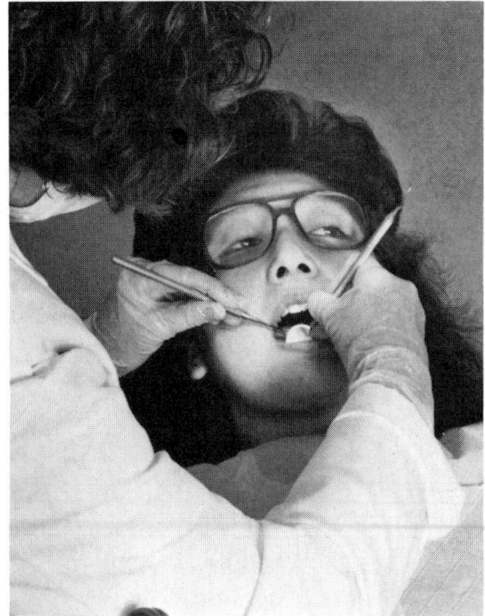

FIGURE 1–9

A dental hygienist is licensed to scale and polish teeth.

Hygienists may be members of their professional organization, the American Dental Hygienists Association (ADHA).

Dental Assistant

An educationally qualified dental assistant is a highly competent individual who may be delegated some of the activities that do not require the dentist's professional skill and judgment.

Although not all states require formal education for dental assistants, minimal standards for the educationally qualified assistant include a program of approximately 1 academic year in length, conducted in a post–high school educational institution accredited by the Commission on Dental Accreditation of the ADA.

Some state boards of dentistry have an additional mechanism whereby they review and evaluate the dental assisting training programs and grant approval if the program meets the state guidelines.

AMERICAN DENTAL ASSISTANTS ASSOCIATION

Dental assistants may be members of their professional organization, the American Dental Assistants Association (ADAA), which has local and state components and a national office maintained in Chicago. **Juliette Southard,** who is considered the founder of this group, was elected the association's first president in 1924 (Fig. 1–10).

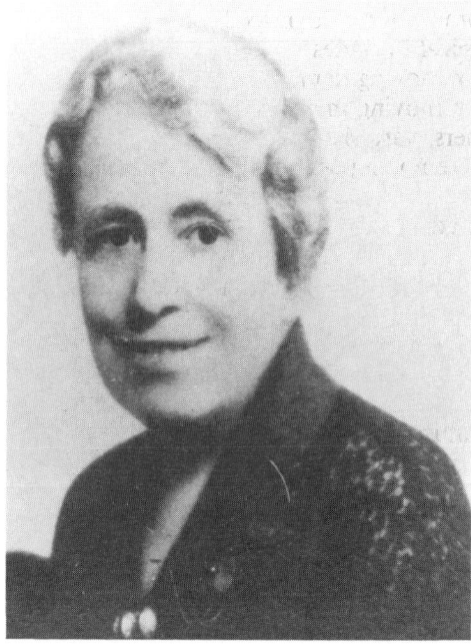

FIGURE 1–10

Juliette Southard, founder and first president of the American Dental Assistants Association. (Courtesy of the American Dental Assistants Association, Chicago, IL.)

Student membership is available for students enrolled in formal training programs. ADAA membership gives the assistant representation and a voice in national affairs, with a far-reaching effect on the career and future of all dental assistants.

The ADAA also provides journals, continuing education opportunities, and group and professional liability insurance plus local, state, and national meetings.

MANY ROLES OF THE DENTAL ASSISTANT

Although each assistant has certain basic skills, there are many specialized roles available within the practice.

Administrative Assistant

The administrative assistant, also known as the **secretarial assistant, business assistant,** or **receptionist,** is responsible for the efficient operation of the business office.

When there are several employees in the business office, each may specialize as **appointments secretary, bookkeeper, patient relations coordinator,** or **insurance clerk** (Fig. 1–11).

An experienced administrative assistant may be promoted to become an **office manager** with responsibility for the smooth functioning of the practice. (These roles are discussed in Chapters 33 and 34.)

Chairside Assistant

The chairside assistant works directly with the dentist in the treatment area. Primary responsibilities in

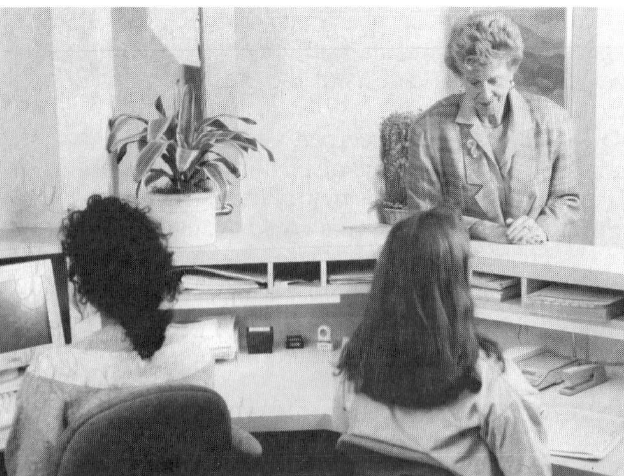

FIGURE 1–11

The business office staff fill many roles. Shown here, the assistant on the left is making a computerized bookkeeping entry. On the right, the assistant is making an appointment for the patient.

this role include but are not limited to

- Seating and preparing patients
- Caring for the treatment room and instruments, including all infection control procedures
- Assisting the dentist at chairside during patient care
- Exposing and processing dental radiographs
- Performing basic laboratory procedures, such as pouring alginate impressions to create diagnostic casts
- Providing patient education

In a practice in which there is a coordinating assistant, the chairside assistant's role is modified to allow more time to assist the dentist at chairside. This is known as **four-handed dentistry,** in which the chairside assistant's responsibilities include oral evacuation, tongue and tissue retraction, and instrument and materials exchange (Fig. 1–12).

Coordinating Assistant

The coordinating assistant's role can best be described as "serving as an extra pair of hands where needed." Primary responsibilities in this role include but are not limited to

- Preparing treatment rooms and caring for instruments
- Seating and dismissing patients
- Exposing, processing, and mounting radiographs
- Providing patient education
- Performing laboratory procedures, including creating temporary coverage and custom impression trays

The coordinating assistant may also work with the dentist and chairside assistant during patient care. This is known as **six-handed dentistry,** and for this the co-

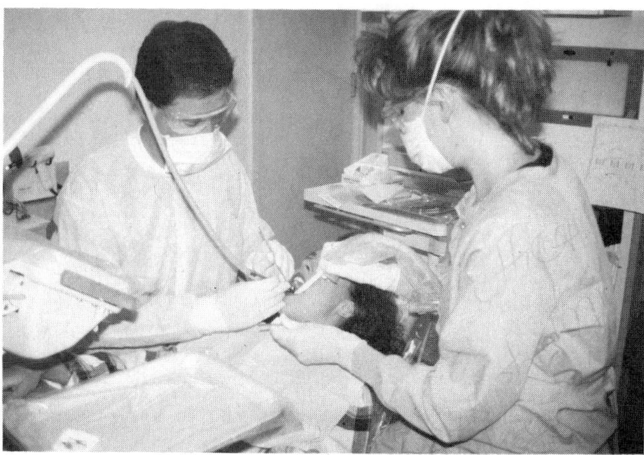

FIGURE 1–12

In four-handed dentistry, the chairside assistant works in close cooperation with the dentist.

ordinating assistant's role includes preparing and passing materials and instruments as needed (Fig. 1–13).

Extended-Functions Dental Assistant

An extended-functions dental assistant (EFDA) is an auxiliary who has been assigned patient care responsibilities beyond the duties traditionally performed by a dental auxiliary.

The requirements for assistants who are qualified to perform these functions usually include certification and/or registration, which are discussed in Chapter 2. The extended functions assigned to qualified dental auxiliaries *may* include the following duties:

- Making radiographic exposures
- Taking impressions for diagnostic casts
- Placing gingival retraction cord
- Applying topical anesthetics
- Polishing coronal surfaces of teeth
- Applying topical fluorides
- Placing and removing dental dam
- Placing and removing matrices and wedges
- Applying liners, varnishes, and bases
- Placing and removing sedative or temporary restorations
- Preparing, placing, and removing temporary coverage
- Placing, carving, and finishing amalgam or composite restorations
- Removing excess cement from coronal surfaces of teeth
- Placing sealants
- Removing sutures
- Placing and removing periodontal dressings
- Performing functions associated with the dental specialties
- Performing additional functions as specified in the Dental Practice Act of the state in which the assistant is employed

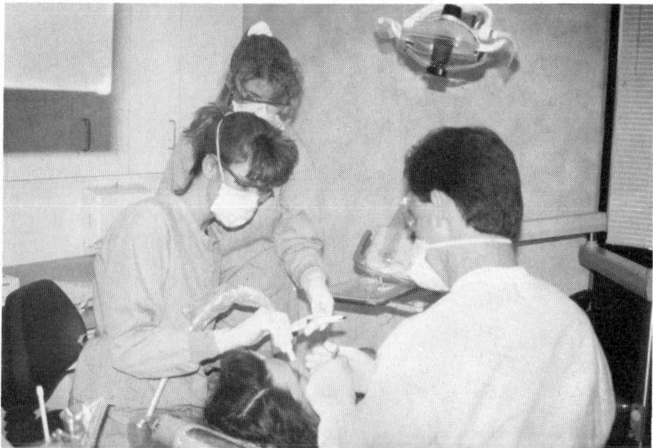

FIGURE 1–13

In six-handed dentistry, the coordinating assistant serves as an extra pair of hands where needed.

Dental Laboratory Technician

The dental laboratory technician may legally perform only the mechanical, technically skilled tasks specified by the written prescription of the dentist.

Many dental laboratory technicians maintain their own laboratories, providing services for many dentists. Others are employed by individual dentists, larger laboratories, or the military services.

Dental laboratory technicians receive their training through apprenticeship, commercial schools, or accredited programs. The **Certified Dental Technician** (CDT) program was established in 1958 by the National Association of Dental Laboratories in cooperation with the ADA.

Programs approved by the ADA are 2 academic years in length and preferably are conducted in an accredited 2- or 4-year college or post–high school institution.

Other Members of the Dental Health Team

A **dental supply salesperson** is a representative from a dental supply house who routinely calls at the dental office. His or her services include taking orders for supplies, providing new product information, and helping to arrange for service and repairs.

A **detail person** is a representative of a specific company, usually a drug or dental product manufacturer, who visits dental offices for the purpose of providing the doctor with information concerning his or her company's products.

A **dental equipment technician** is a specialist who installs and provides service and repairs of dental equipment. This service may be provided under a maintenance contract or on an "as needed" basis.

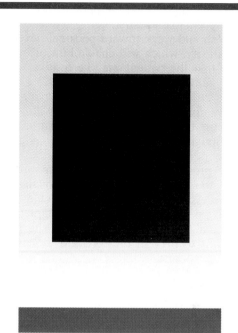

Chapter 2

The Ethical and Legal Aspects of Dentistry

Introduction

The members of the dental team must be committed to fulfilling not only the technical demands of serving patients with quality care but also the moral and legal concerns. In this chapter the ethical and legal aspects of dental practice are addressed.

Although the individual members of the dental health team have specific duties and areas of responsibility, they *all* must work together toward the shared goal of providing the best possible care for their patients.

The composition of the dental health team within an individual office or clinic may vary, yet there is no question that the dentist is the leader of the team. The dentist is in charge and must retain ultimate responsibility for the well-being of the patients and the actions of the employees.

All members of the team must give their complete support and loyalty to the dentist who is the leader of their team. The success of the dental health team, like that of any other team, is dependent upon the attitudes and cooperation of all team members. They must be able to work together in close harmony and be willing to help each other at all times.

Responsibilities of the Dental Assistant

As a member of the dental health team, the assistant has specific obligations and responsibilities to the dentist, the patients, and the other team members (Fig. 2–1).

Responsibilities to the Dentist

- The assistant must give complete and loyal support to the dentist and must at all times treat the dentist with dignity and respect.
- The assistant must be able to accept the dentist's method of practice and share his or her beliefs in the value of preventive dental care.
- The assistant must hold in strictest confidence all things seen or heard in the dental office pertaining to the dentist, the patients, and the other team members.
- The assistant may perform only those duties that are delegated by the dentist and that can be performed in keeping with the assistant's educational qualifications and the state dental practice act.

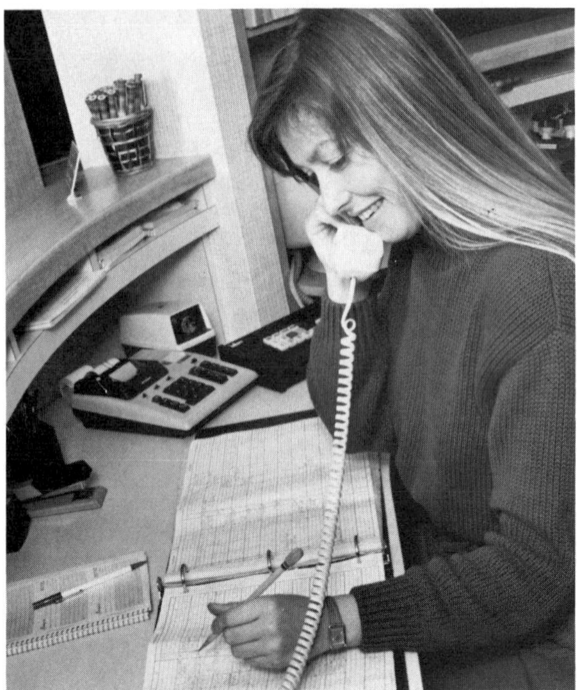

FIGURE 2–1

The assistant has responsibilities to the dentist, the patients, and the other staff members.

- The assistant must at all times carefully follow the instructions given and work to the best of his or her ability.
- The assistant must conduct himself or herself in such a professional manner as to reflect favorably on the dentist, the dental health team, and the dental profession.
- The assistant must maintain a positive attitude in working relationships and not convey personal problems in professional activities.
- The assistant who is not able to accept the responsibilities listed above should give due notice to the employer and seek employment elsewhere.

Responsibilities to the Patients

- The assistant must always perform all duties to the very best of his or her ability, because performance that is less than 100 percent could have disastrous effects for the patient.
- The assistant must demonstrate an attitude of acceptance toward patients from all socioeconomic classes and cultural backgrounds. This includes recognizing that the need for approval and respect is basic to all and that this need may be exaggerated in times of stress.
- The assistant must recognize that the needs of each individual are different. The assistant should make every effort to understand the patient and his needs and should be willing to help the patient meet these needs, in an acceptable manner.
- The assistant should work toward personal development and maturity, which will enable him or her to (1) recognize that the patient may be motivated by factors totally unknown to the assistant, (2) accept the patient as he is, (3) be tolerant of behavior that is not readily understood, and (4) be willing to make the extra effort to be pleasant and understanding although the patient may be irritable, anxious, uncooperative, or demanding.
- The assistant must take necessary steps to protect the health of the patient by carefully following the procedures necessary for maintaining strict asepsis and other practice safety measures (see Chapters 12 and 13). Also, if the assistant is ill, he or she must take precautions to prevent the spread of disease to patients and co-workers.
- The assistant must be neat, clean, properly attired, and professional in appearance, to ensure a favorable impression and inspire patient confidence.
- The assistant must make a positive effort to educate and motivate patients about modern preventive dental care, through enthusiasm and by setting personal examples.
- The assistant's behavior must reflect positively on the dental profession.

Responsibilities to the Other Dental Health Team Members

- The assistant must treat all team members with respect and work with them in a spirit of cooperation.
- The assistant must carefully perform his or her duties and responsibilities and not try to shift these duties onto someone else.
- When not occupied with his or her own duties, the assistant must demonstrate a willingness to help others. In an emergency, the assistant must be prepared to interrupt his or her duties to help other team members.
- The assistant must make every effort to arrive at work on time and to be on duty at all assigned times. This includes guarding his or her health because any absence may cause an unfair hardship to the other team members.
- If, for any reason, the assistant must be absent from work, advance arrangements should be made to ensure that his or her position is covered.
- The assistant must realize that supervision, feedback, and change are occasionally necessary and should accept these in the constructive manner in which they are offered.
- The assistant must at all times maintain current skills and knowledge through active participation in continuing education programs.
- The assistant must handle grievances through the accepted office procedure, such as a staff meeting, before they become major in nature.

Additional Responsibilities

The dental assistant is often required to perform additional duties that may have legal overtones in the practice. These may include but not be limited to

- Never leaving a child patient alone in the treatment room
- Being prepared for emergencies by knowing what to do, how to use emergency equipment and medicaments, and whom to call for help
- Never administering or dispensing medications except on instruction from, and under the direct supervision of, the dentist
- Being careful with oral evacuation procedures to ensure that the patient does not swallow or aspirate any foreign bodies
- Acting as the "third person": as a witness to conversations exchanged and treatment administered
- Not exceeding his or her professional abilities and training
- Refusing any request to perform a procedure that has not been delegated to assistants by the state dental practice act
- Refraining from accepting tips, gratuities, or other inappropriate gifts from patients

The Assistant as a Representative of the Dental Profession

Each dental assistant, in both his or her professional and personal life, acts at all times as a representative of the dental profession. The assistant must realize that although there is much that can be done to promote the cause of dental health through public education, he or she is *not* qualified to make a diagnosis, to establish a fee for a dental service, or to comment on the quality of dental treatment that has been performed.

Dental Ethics

Ethics deals with *moral conduct*, duty, and judgment. It is concerned with standards for determining whether actions are right or wrong. A *code of ethics* is the standard of moral principles and practice to which a profession adheres. These are voluntary controls, not laws, and serve as a method of self-policing within a profession.

American Dental Assistants Association Principles of Ethics

The following are the *Principles of Ethics* as adopted by the American Dental Assistants Association (ADAA). This code of ethics functions as a standard of ethics for all practicing dental assistants (see Principles of Ethics).

Principles of Ethics

- Each individual involved in the practice of dentistry assumes the obligation to maintain and enrich the profession.
- Each member may choose to meet this obligation according to the dictate of personal conscience based on the needs of the human beings the profession of dentistry is committed to serve. The spirit of the Golden Rule is the basic guiding principle of this concept.
- The member must strive to maintain confidentiality and to exhibit respect for the dentist/employer.
- The member shall refrain from performing any professional service that is prohibited by state law and has the obligation to prove competence prior to providing services to any patient.
- The member shall constantly strive to upgrade and expand technical skills for the benefit of the employer and the consumer public.
- The member should additionally seek to sustain and improve the local organization, state association, and the American Dental Assistants Association by active participation and personal commitment.

Note: The format, but not the wording, of these principles has been altered slightly to highlight the content.

Dental Jurisprudence

Dental jurisprudence addresses the *law* as it applies to the practice of dentistry. The term is used to include statutes regulating dental practice, professional liability, professional incorporation, and other legal aspects of the practice of dentistry.

The State Dental Practice Act

Each state has a dental practice act that contains the legal restrictions and controls on the dentist, the dental auxiliaries, and the practice of dentistry. It specifies the requirements for, as well as the restrictions upon, the practice of dentistry within each state.

The act usually creates and designates an administration board, called the Board of Dental Examiners, which interprets and implements these regulations.

The State Board of Dental Examiners

The state Board of Dental Examiners is responsible for the administration of examinations for licensure; for enforcement of statutes, rules, and regulations; and for establishing the requirements for license renewal.

This board adopts rules and regulations that define, interpret, and implement the intent of the dental practice act. The Board of Dental Examiners enforces, supervises and regulates the practice of dentistry within the state.

Licensure (having a license to practice in a specific state) is one mechanism of this supervision. Licensure protects the general public's interest and the interests of the profession, ensures the establishment of standards, aids in keeping incompetent persons out of the field, and assists in the enforcement of the dental practice act.

Certification and Registration

Upon satisfactory completion of an accredited program, or having met the work experience requirements, and holding current cardiopulmonary resuscitation (CPR) certification, the assistant is eligible to sit for the certification examination given by the Dental Assisting National Board, Inc. (DANB). Further information concerning the certification program may be obtained from DANB's Chicago office.

The examination for a certified dental assistant (CDA) covers three areas: chairside assisting, dental radiation health and safety, and infection control.

Certification is a national credential and is also awarded in the following specialty areas: Certified Orthodontic Assistant (COA), Certified Oral and Maxillofacial Surgery Assistant (COMSA), and Certified Dental Practice Management Assistant (CDPMA).

Each year the CDA must complete a minimum of 12 hours of approved continuing education programs, and submit proof of having done so, to remain certified. Assistants who fail to meet these requirements are no longer permitted to use the title Certified Dental Assistant.

Some states require that the Extended Function Dental Auxiliary pass a formal and/or clinical examination to become registered or licensed. Instead of requiring a second examination, some states grant registration to those assistants who have passed the DANB certification examination.

Having met these requirements, the assistant is known as a Registered Dental Assistant (RDA) or Registered Dental Assistant in Extended Functions. Those states that require registration (or licensure) may also require periodic (annual or biannual) renewal of the license.

Even states that do not have registration for extended functions may require registration or licensure for all assistants who expose radiographs. If you work in a state that requires registration of any sort for dental assistants, contact your state board of dentistry for information regarding these requirements.

Direct Supervision

In most states, when the dental practice act assigns extended functions to the auxiliary, it specifies that these functions be performed under the direct supervision of the dentist. Coronal polish and suture removal are examples of procedures usually performed under direct supervision.

Compliance with this requirement is very important! Direct supervision means that the dentist

- Is in the dental office or treatment facility
- Personally authorizes the procedures
- Remains in the office while the procedures are being performed by the auxiliary
- Evaluates the performance of the procedure by the dental auxiliary before the patient is dismissed

General Supervision

The dental practice act may stipulate general supervision for the delegation of certain functions by qualified personnel. Pouring alginate impressions for diagnostic casts is an example of a procedure that might be performed under general supervision.

In most states, general supervision means that the dentist remains responsible for the actions of the auxiliary; however, that procedure may legally be performed without the dentist's being present in the treatment facility.

The Unlicensed Practice of Dentistry

Although assistants may be trained to perform extended functions, legally they may perform only those functions that have been officially delegated to them under the dental practice act of the state in which they are employed.

Performing procedures that have not been delegated is engaging in the unlicensed practice of dentistry, and this is a criminal act. This means that *the assistant who performs "extended functions" that are not legal in his or her state is guilty of the unlicensed practice of dentistry and is committing a criminal act.*

Ignorance of the dental practice act, licensure, or the rules and regulations interpreting the act is no excuse for illegally practicing dentistry.

Legal Recourse

The person practicing dentistry without a license is held responsible for his or her illegal acts. However, under the doctrine of **respondeat superior** ("let the master answer"), the dentist is also held responsible if the illegal acts of his or her employee are committed within the scope of his or her employment. This doctrine holds true even if the employee is specially licensed, such as an RDA or an RDH.

This means that the patient may sue the dentist for an error committed by an employee. However, the employee is still responsible for his or her own actions, and the injured party may also file suit against the auxiliary.

In such an instance, the dentist's liability insurance cannot be counted on to cover the auxiliary. For this reason, the auxiliary providing direct patient care should carry his or her own liability insurance.

The Dentist's Responsibility to the Patient

The Duty of Care

The duty of care owed by a dentist to a patient includes the following: The dentist (1) is licensed; (2) uses reasonable skill, care, and judgment; and (3) uses standard drugs, materials, and techniques.

The dentist may refuse to treat a patient; however, this action must *not* be based on the patient's race, color, or creed. Under the Americans with Disabilities Act, patients with an infectious disease such as HIV disease cannot be refused treatment because of their infection.

In rare cases in which the dentist refuses treatment—for example, if the necessary equipment for such treatment is not in the office, of if the patient requires extensive emergency treatment or general anesthesia—the dentist should refer the patient to a facility where he could receive treatment.

Once a dentist undertakes to render dental care, he or she is expected to charge a reasonable fee and to continue that treatment to completion within a reasonable length of time (usually within 2 years). Otherwise, the dentist may be held liable for **abandonment** (discontinuation of care after treatment has commenced but before it has been completed).

Also, instructions to the patient must be reasonable and be given in a manner and language that the patient can understand. The dentist may not dismiss or abandon the patient without giving written notification of termination. After notification, care must continue for a reasonable length of time (usually 30 days) to allow the patient to secure another dentist's services.

As for the duties of the patient to the dentist, the patient is legally required to pay a reasonable and agreed-upon fee for services rendered, to cooperate, and to follow instructions.

Due Care

The dentist also has a legal obligation to use due care in treating patients. (**Due care** is a legal term meaning just, proper, and sufficient care, or the absence of negligence.) This obligation applies to all treatment procedures, including prescribing, dispensing, or administering drugs and other therapeutic agents.

Due care, as it relates to the administration or prescribing of drugs by the dentist, implies that the dentist is familiar with the drug and with the patient. Thus the dentist must understand the properties of the drug to be prescribed or administered.

The dentist must also have adequate information regarding the health of the patient to know whether the drug that he or she plans to use is suitable for the patient or whether the patient's health record contraindicates its use. This is one of the reasons why a complete, up-to-date health history is essential.

Risk Management

In an age of increasing **litigiousness** (carrying out of lawsuits), the dental team must constantly be aware of the need to avoid unnecessary risks in the dental practice. The major areas of risk management concern are recordkeeping (maintaining of accurate and complete records), gaining informed consent, and doing everything possible to maintain the highest standards of clinical excellence.

Keeping this in mind, legal authorities have noted that the primary factor in avoiding legal entanglements with patients is maintaining a climate of good rapport and open communication with all patients.

Types of Malpractice

Malpractice is professional **negligence** (the failure to use due care, or the lack of due care.) In dentistry, malpractice may be defined in terms of *acts of omission* and *acts of commission.* An act of omission is failure to perform an act that a "reasonable and prudent professional" would perform. An act of commission is an act that a "reasonable and prudent professional" would not perform.

This concept can also be expressed in terms of *reasonable skill, care,* and *judgment.* It is the responsibility of the dentist, *and the auxiliary,* to possess and use that reasonable degree of knowledge and skill that is ordinarily possessed by dentists and auxiliaries practicing in the same community.

Avoidance of Malpractice Litigation

Prevention and communication are the best defenses against malpractice. Patients are least likely to initiate a lawsuit when they have a clear understanding of

- the planned treatment
- reasonable desired results
- their financial obligations

The dental assistant plays an all-important role in the prevention of malpractice litigation.

Silence Is Golden

The assistant must never make critical remarks about dental treatment rendered by the operator or any other dentist. The assistant should never discuss patients and should also avoid discussing the dentist's professional liability insurance.

Under the concept of **res gestae** ("part of the action"), statements made spontaneously by anyone (including the assistant) at the time of an alleged negligent act are admissible as evidence and may be damaging to the dentist.

Consent

When a patient enters a dentist's office, he gives **implied consent,** at least for the dental examination. Provided the patient has the ability to give it, implied consent is given when the patient agrees to treatment.

Unfortunately, implied consent is no longer acceptable in a court of law. **Written consent,** also called *informed consent,* is preferable. Under informed consent, the patient (or guardian) receives an explanation of the diagnostic findings and the prescribed treatment, as well as reasonable expectations as to the results of treatment. The prudent dental practice requires that the patient (or guardian) sign and date an informed consent form before beginning treatment.

A minor or a person who is mentally incompetent cannot give consent. In this situation, consent must be given by the parent or guardian.

When a Patient Refuses Treatment

Radiographs are important diagnostic aids and legal safeguards. If the patient refuses radiographs, a notation of this, signed by the patient, should be included in the patient's record.

Should a patient willfully decline prescribed treatment, the dentist may request that the patient sign a written, dated refusal for treatment. This too is filed with the patient's record.

If the patient discontinues treatment, the records should indicate this decision and the reason given for it. This documentation helps protects the practice from legal recourse should a patient claim negligence against the dentist.

Broken Appointments

The patient's record should include notation of any broken appointments or last-minute cancellations. These changes may be interpreted as contributory negligence on the part of the patient.

Patient Clinical Records

Records regarding patient care are commonly referred to as the **dental chart,** or *patient record.* These records are important legal documents that must be protected and handled with care. This is discussed further in Chapter 33.

All examination records, diagnoses, radiographs, consent forms, updated medical histories, copies of medical and laboratory prescriptions, and correspondence to or about a patient are filed together in that patient's record folder. Financial information is *not* included in the patient chart.

Patient records, which are acceptable in court, clearly show the date and the details of services rendered for each patient. Nothing should be left to memory. See Guidelines for Managing Charting Entries.

Guidelines for Managing Charting Entries

- Keep a separate chart for each patient. Do not use a "group" chart for an entire family.
- Business and financial records are not part of the clinical record. Do not include this information in the chart.
- It is better to chart too much than too little.
- Chart during the examination or patient visit. The longer the time lapse until the charting entry is made, the poorer the records.
- Write legibly and make the entry accurately in ink. Date and initial the entry.
- The chart entry should be complete enough to indicate that nothing was neglected. It should include the reason for the visit, details of the treatment provided, and a record of all instructions to the patient, prescriptions, and referrals.
- Never change the chart after a problem arises. If there is a charting error, correct it properly.

DATE	TOOTH	SERVICE RENDERED
~~2/10/xx~~		~~exam, adult prophy 2/15/xx DDA~~
2/10/xx	3	X-ray, remove amal restoration. Place
		sedative treatment. If pain persists,
		refer to endodontist. 2/15/xx DDA

FIGURE 2–2

These steps must be taken when it is necessary to correct a charting error.

Patient records must never be altered. If an error was made on the patient's chart, it must be corrected through the following procedure. Never paint over or attempt to cover up the entry (Fig. 2–2).

Ownership of Dental Records and Radiographs

The dentist technically "owns" all patient records and radiographs; however, according to some state laws, patients have the rights to access (review) and retrieve (remove) their records and radiographs.

Original records and radiographs are *never* allowed to leave the practice without the dentist's permission. In most situations, duplicate radiographs and a photocopy of the record will satisfy the patient's needs.

If there are any disagreements with the patient on this subject, the assistant should not attempt to make a decision; the matter should be referred to the dentist immediately.

PROCEDURE: **Correcting a Chart Entry**

1. Draw a line through the previous entry. Initial and date this change.
   ☐ *RATIONALE:* The entry must be left so that it is still readable.
2. Make the corrected entry on the first available line.
3. Initial and date the new entry.

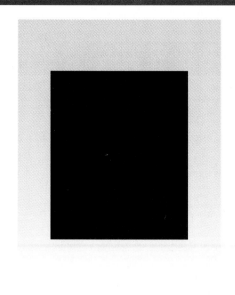

Chapter 3

Head and Neck Anatomy

Introduction

There are many reasons why dental health care personnel must understand the structures of the head and neck and how these structures function together with other body parts and systems. As an example, the structure of bone influences how local anesthetics are administered.

Anatomy is the study of the structure of the body and its parts. **Physiology** is the study of the functions of the body systems. Anatomy and physiology are discussed in this chapter as they relate to the structures of head and neck.

Anatomic Reference Systems

Anatomic reference systems are used to make it easier to describe the body parts in terms of their functions and location. The basic reference systems are structural units and body systems, directions and body planes, and body cavities.

Structural Units and Body Systems

Cells, the basic structural units of the body, are specialized and grouped together to form the tissues and organs of the body.

A **tissue** is a group or layer of similarly specialized cells that join together to form a component of the body and to perform specific functions.

Organs are composed of cells grouped into tissue serving a common function. The tissues and organs of the body are organized into body systems.

Body systems are groups of organs and tissues that perform specialized functions. These systems are outlined in Table 3–1.

Directions and Body Planes

The terms used to describe directions in relation to the whole body are easier to understand when thought of as pairs of opposite directions, such as up and down (Table 3–2).

Planes, which are imaginary lines used to divide the body into sections, are used to describe the location of an organ or problem (Fig. 3–1).

A **sagittal plane** is any vertical plane that divides the body, from top to bottom, into left and right portions.

The **midsagittal plane,** also known as the *midline,* is the vertical plane that divides the body into equal left and right halves (Fig. 3–2).

The **frontal plane,** also known as the *coronal plane,* is any vertical plane, at right angles to the sagittal plane, that divides the body into anterior (front) and posterior (back) portions.

The **horizontal plane,** also known as the *transverse plane,* divides the body into superior (upper) and inferior (lower) portions.

TABLE 3–1

Major Body Systems

BODY SYSTEM	COMPONENTS	MAJOR FUNCTIONS
Skeletal system	206 bones	Protection, support and shape, hematopoietic, storage of certain minerals
Muscular system	Striated muscle Smooth muscle Cardiac muscle	Holding body erect, locomotion, movement of body fluids, production of body heat, communication
Cardiovascular system	Heart Arteries and veins Blood	Respiratory, nutritive, excretory
Lymphatic and immune systems	White blood cells Lymph fluid, vessels, and nodes Spleen and tonsils	Defense against disease, conservation of plasma proteins and fluid, lipid absorption
Nervous system	Central nervous system Peripheral nervous system Special sense organs	Reception of stimuli, transmission of messages, coordinating mechanism
Respiratory system	Nose, paranasal sinuses, pharynx, epiglottis, larynx, trachea, bronchi, and lungs	Transport of oxygen to cells, excretion of carbon dioxide and some water wastes
Digestive system	Mouth, pharynx, esophagus, stomach, intestines, and accessory organs	Digestion of food, absorption of digested food, elimination of solid wastes
Urinary system	Kidneys, ureters, bladder, and urethra	Formation and elimination of urine, maintenance of homeostasis
Integumentary system	Skin, hair, nails, sweat, and sebaceous glands	Protection of body, regulation of body temperature
Endocrine system	Adrenals, gonads, pancreas, parathyroids, pineal, pituitary, thymus, and thyroid	Integrations of body functions, control of growth, maintenance of homeostasis
Reproductive system	Male: testes, penis Female: ovaries, fallopian tubes, uterus, vagina	Production of new life

Major Body Cavities

The **dorsal cavity** contains the structures of the nervous system that coordinate the bodily functions (Fig. 3–3). The dorsal cavity is divided into the **cranial cavity,** which contains the brain, and the **spinal cavity,** which contains the spinal cord.

The **ventral cavity** contains the vital body organs that maintain homeostasis. (**Homeostasis** means maintaining a constant internal environment.)

The ventral cavity is divided into the **thoracic cavity,** which contains the heart and the lungs; the **abdominal cavity,** which contains the major organs of digestion; and the **pelvic cavity,** which contains the organs of the reproductive and excretory systems.

TABLE 3–2

Terms Describing Body Directions

Ventral: Front (belly) surface of the body	*Dorsal:* Back surface of the body
Anterior: Toward the front of the body	*Posterior:* Toward the back of the body
Superior: Uppermost, above or toward the head	*Inferior:* Lowermost, below or toward the feet
Mesial: Toward the midline	*Distal:* Away from the midline
Medial: Toward the midline	*Lateral:* Toward the side or outside

Structures of the Face and Oral Cavity (Figs. 3–4 to 3–6)

LANDMARKS OF THE FACE

- The **outer canthus of the eye** is the fold of tissue at the outer corner of the eyelids.
- The **inner canthus of the eye** is the fold of tissue at the inner corner of the eyelids.
- The **ala of the nose** is the winglike tip of the outer side of each nostril.
- The **philtrum** is the soft vertical groove running from under the nose to the midline of the upper lip.

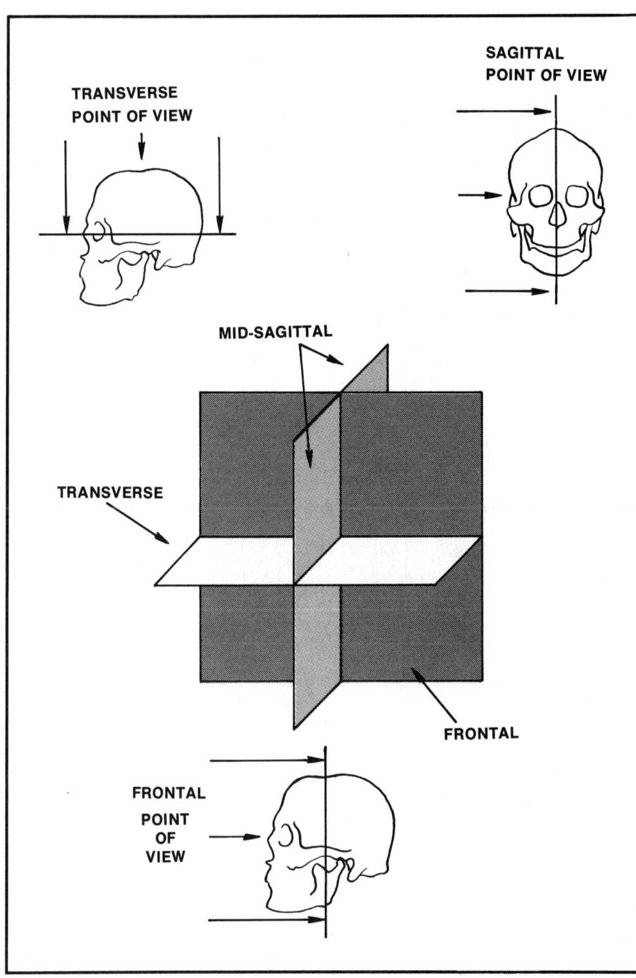

FIGURE 3–1

Planes of the body.

- The **tragus of the ear** is the cartilage projection anterior to the external opening of the ear.
- The **nasion** is the midpoint between the eyes just below the eyebrows. On the skull, this is the point where the two nasal bones and the frontal bone join.

LIPS

The lips, also known as *labia,* form the anterior border of the mouth. They are formed externally by the skin and internally by mucous membrane.

A **commissure** is the angle at the corner of the mouth where the upper and lower lips join.

The red free margins, known as the **vermilion border,** represent a zone of transition from skin, which is normal skin color, to the red mucous membrane portion.

The **labial vestibule** is the area between the lips and the teeth or alveolar ridge.

CHEEKS

The cheeks form the side walls of the oral cavity. The **buccal vestibule** is the area between the cheeks and the teeth or alveolar ridge. (**Buccal** means pertaining to, or directed toward, the cheek.)

FRENUM

A **frenum** is a narrow band of tissue that connects two structures. (*Frenum* is singular; the plural is *frena.*)

The **upper labial frenum** passes from the oral mucosa at the midline of the maxillary arch to the midline of the inner surface of the upper lip.

The **lower labial frenum** passes from the oral mucosa at the midline of the mandibular arch to the midline of the inner surface of the lower lip.

The **lingual frenum** passes from the floor of the mouth to the midline of the ventral surface of the tongue.

In the area of the first maxillary permanent molar, the **buccal frenum** passes from the oral mucosa of the outer surface of the maxillary arch to the inner surface of the cheek.

ORAL MUCOSA

Oral mucosa is the mucous membrane that lines the entire oral cavity. This tissue is highly specialized and adapted to meet the needs of the area it covers (see Chapter 4).

HARD PALATE

The palate serves as the roof of the mouth and separates it from the nasal cavity. The hard palate is the bony anterior portion. It is formed by the inferior (lower) surfaces of the palatine processes of the maxillary bones and the horizontal plates of the palatine bones.

SOFT PALATE

The soft palate forms the flexible posterior portion of the palate. The *uvula* hangs from the free edge of the soft palate. The soft palate can be lifted upward and back to meet the posterior pharyngeal wall. This blocks the entrance to the nasopharynx during swallowing and speech.

PILLARS OF FAUCES

The two arches at the back of the mouth are called the pillars of fauces (Fig. 3–7).

The **anterior pillar of fauces** is also called the *palatoglossal arch* because it is formed by the palatoglossus muscle.

The **posterior pillar of fauces** is also called the *palatopharyngeal arch* because it is formed by the palatopharyngeus muscle.

The opening between the two arches is called the **isthmus of fauces** and contains the palatine tonsil.

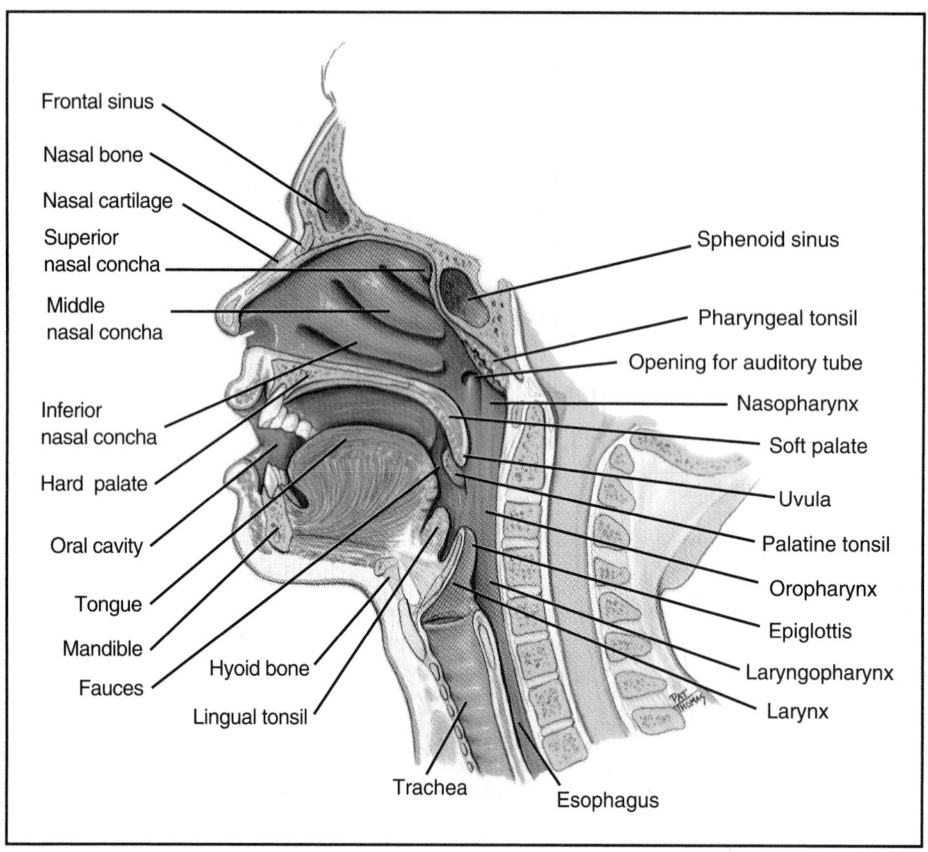

FIGURE 3–2

Midsagittal view of the structures of the head and neck. (From Jarvis, C.: Physical Examination and Health Assessment. Philadelphia, W.B. Saunders Co., 1992, p. 407.)

GAG REFLEX

The gag reflex is a protective mechanism located in the posterior region of the mouth (Fig. 3–8). This very sensitive area includes the

- Soft palate
- Fauces
- Posterior portion of the tongue

Contact of a foreign body with the membranes of this area causes gagging, retching, or vomiting. When working in the patient's mouth, the dental assistant must be very careful not to trigger the gag reflex.

TONGUE

The tongue, which is attached only at its posterior end, consists of a very flexible group of muscles that are arranged to enable it to quickly change size, shape, and position.

The **dorsum** of the tongue, which is the dorsal surface, is covered by a rather thick and highly specialized epithelium. The ventral (underside) surface of the tongue is highly vascular and is covered with very delicate lining mucosa.

Taste

The taste buds, which are the receptor cells for the sense of taste, are located on the dorsum of the tongue (Fig. 3–9). A substance must be mixed with liquid before it can stimulate the taste buds on the tongue.

The taste buds are located on the **fungiform papillae** and in the trough of the large **vallate papillae,** which form a V on the posterior portion of the tongue. The numerous **filiform papillae,** which cover the entire surface of the tongue, provide the sense of touch but do not contain taste receptors. Each taste sensation is received by a specific area of the tongue:

- **Sweet** at the tip
- **Salt** at the anterior sides and tip
- **Sour** at the sides toward the posterior
- **Bitter** in the center of the dorsum toward the posterior

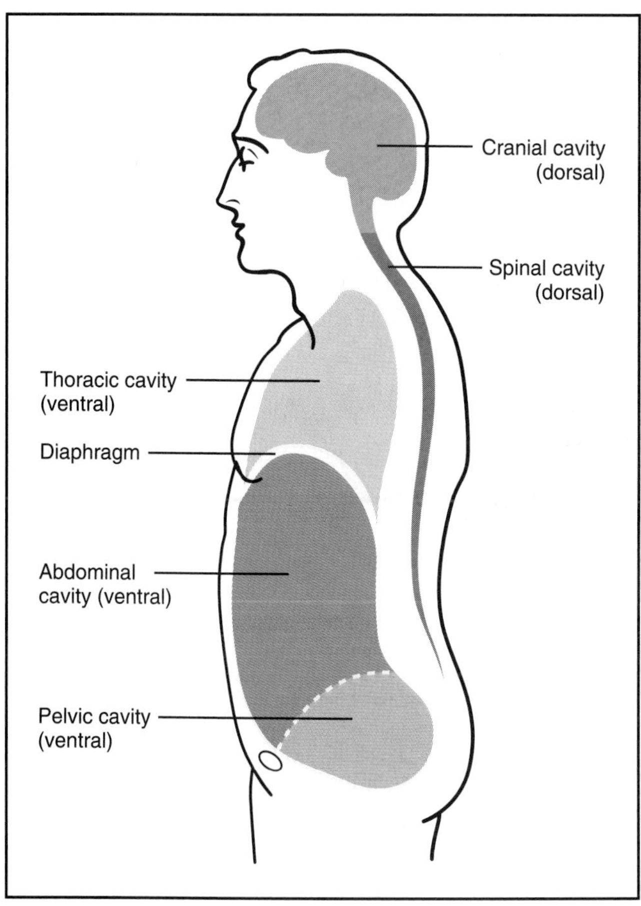

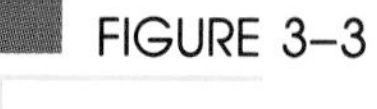
FIGURE 3–3

Major body cavities.

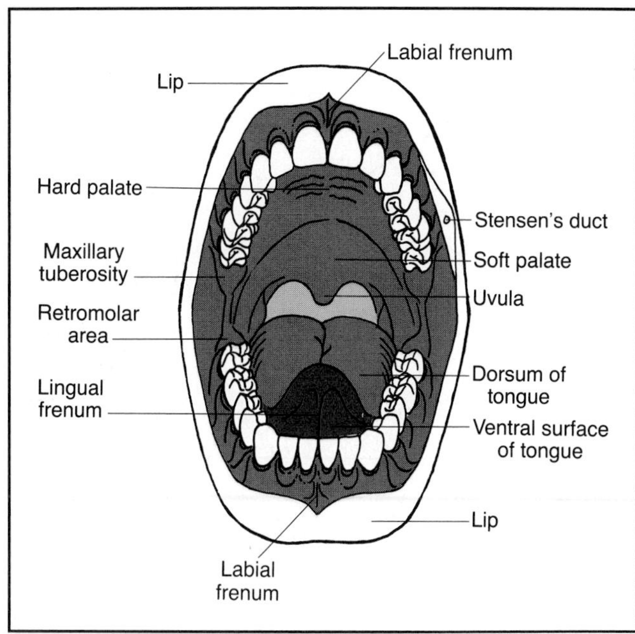

FIGURE 3–5

Structures of the oral cavity.

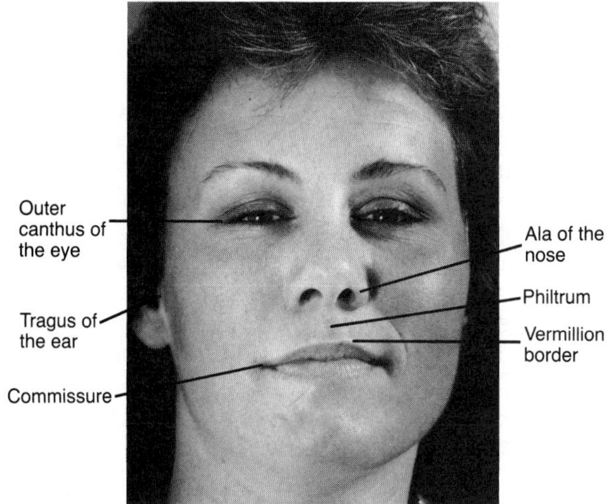

FIGURE 3–4

Landmarks of the face. (From Ehrlich, A., and Torres, H.O.: Essentials of Dental Assisting. Philadelphia, W.B. Saunders Co., 1992, p 42.)

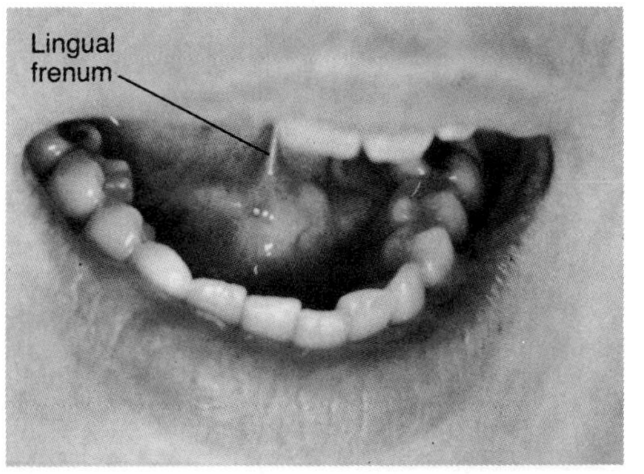

FIGURE 3–6

The lingual frenum and the delicate tissues under the tongue.

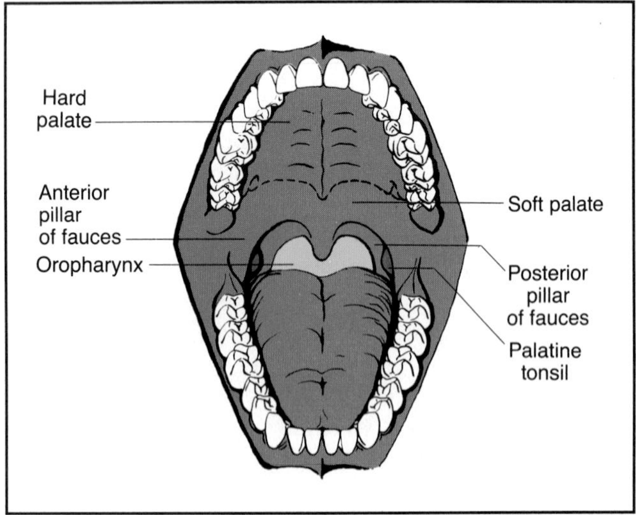

FIGURE 3–7

The pillars of fauces.

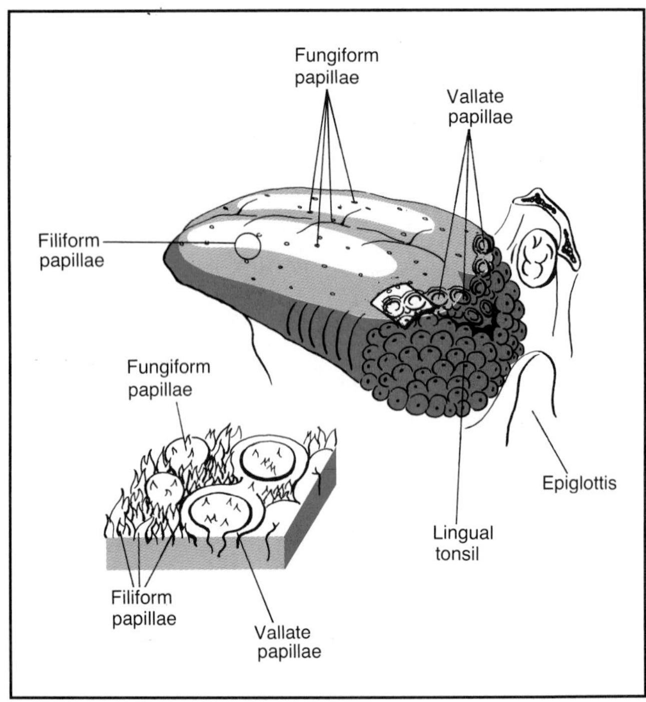

FIGURE 3–9

Schematic of the dorsum of the tongue, showing the types of taste buds.

TEETH

The teeth, which are arranged in the alveolar processes of the maxillary and mandibular arches, are discussed in Chapters 4 and 5.

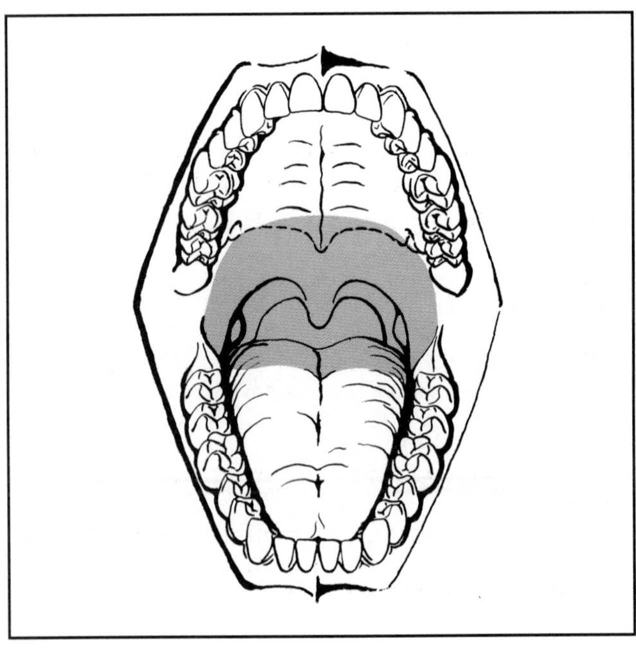

FIGURE 3–8

The gag reflex.

SALIVARY GLANDS

There are three pairs of salivary glands, which produce two to three pints of saliva during a 24-hour period (Fig. 3–10). A lack of an adequate supply of saliva puts the patient at high risk for extensive dental decay. Saliva serves the following five important functions:

1. It acts as a lubricating agent that moistens the mouth and food to make swallowing easier.
2. Salivary amylase, a digestive enzyme found in saliva, begins the breakdown and digestion of carbohydrates (starches).
3. Saliva acts as a cleansing agent that washes away some food particles from the teeth.
4. It acts as a buffer to reduce the pH of acids generated by the bacteria in dental plaque.
5. It serves as the source of fluorides, calcium, and phosphate needed for the remineralization of the teeth (see Chapter 6).

Parotid Glands

The parotid glands are the largest of the salivary glands. One lies subcutaneously just in front of and below each ear. Saliva from the parotid gland is conveyed to the mouth via **Stensen's duct**, which is also known as the *parotid duct*. This duct opens into the mouth from the cheek opposite the maxillary second molar.

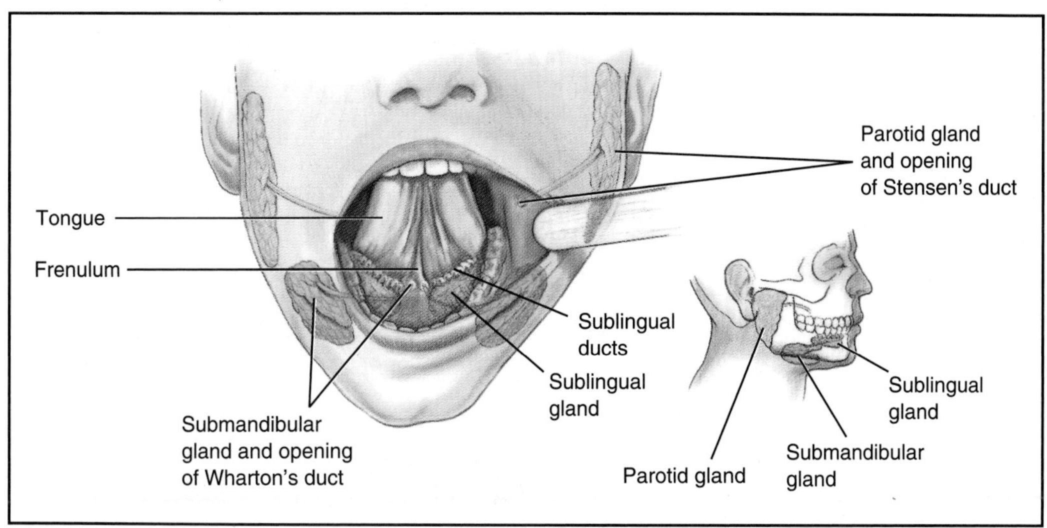

FIGURE 3–10

The salivary glands and ducts. (From Applegate, E.J.: Anatomy and Physiology Learning System Textbook. Philadelphia, W.B. Saunders Co., 1995.)

Submandibular Glands

The submandibular glands are about the size of a walnut and lie on the floor of the mouth beneath the posterior portion of the mandible. Saliva from these glands is conveyed to the mouth by **Wharton's duct,** which opens through the floor of the mouth just lingual to the mandibular incisors.

Sublingual Glands

The sublingual glands are the smallest of the salivary glands. They are located one on either side underneath the tongue. Saliva from these glands is conveyed into the mouth through **Wharton's duct** and the **ducts of Rivinus,** which open under the tongue.

The Skeletal System

There are 206 bones in the human body. For descriptive purposes, the skeleton is divided into the axial and appendicular skeletal systems.

The **axial skeleton** (80 bones) consists of the skull, spinal column, ribs, and sternum. It protects the major organs of the nervous, respiratory, and circulatory systems.

The **appendicular skeleton** (126 bones) consists of the bones of the upper extremities and shoulder girdle plus those of the lower extremities and pelvic girdle. It protects the organs of digestion and reproduction.

The Structure of Bone

Bone is the hard connective tissue that constitutes the majority of the human skeleton. It consists of an organic component (the cells and matrix) and an inorganic (mineral) component.

The minerals, primarily calcium and phosphate, give rigidity to bone. These minerals stored in bones also act as a mineral reservoir to maintain essential blood mineral concentrations in times of an inadequate supply in the body (see Chapter 4).

PERIOSTEUM

The periosteum is a specialized connective tissue covering all bones of the body (Fig. 3–11). It is necessary for bone growth and repair, for nutrition, and for

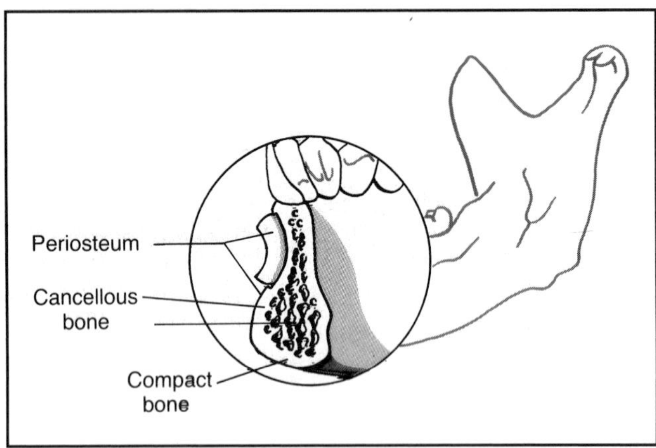

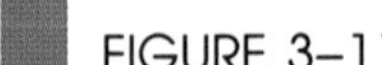

FIGURE 3–11

The structure of bone. A cross-section of the mandible is shown with a portion of the periosteum reflected.

carrying away waste. It is responsible for the life of the bone and is capable of repair.

The outer layer of the periosteum is a network of dense connective tissue containing blood vessels. The inner layer is loose connective tissue containing osteoblasts. (**Osteoblasts** are cells associated with bone formation.)

The periosteum is anchored to bone by **Sharpey's fibers,** which penetrate the underlying bone matrix.

KINDS OF BONE

There are two kinds of bone: compact bone and cancellous bone. **Compact bone,** also known as *cortical bone,* is hard, dense, and very strong. It forms the outer layer of the bones, where it is needed for strength. The **Haversian system** is the internal means by which compact bone receives nourishment.

Cancellous bone, also known as *spongy bone,* is lighter in weight than but not as strong as compact bone, and is found in the interior of bones.

The **trabeculae** of bone are bony spicules in cancellous bone that form a meshwork of intercommunicating spaces that are filled with bone marrow. (*Trabeculae* is plural; the singular is *trabecula.*) The trabeculae appear as a weblike structure in a radiograph (Fig. 3–12).

BONE MARROW

Bone marrow is located within the cancellous bone. **Red bone marrow** is hematopoietic and manufactures red blood cells, hemoglobin, white blood cells, and thrombocytes. (**Hematopoietic** means pertaining to the formation of blood cells.)

Yellow bone marrow is composed chiefly of fat cells and is found primarily in the shafts of long bones.

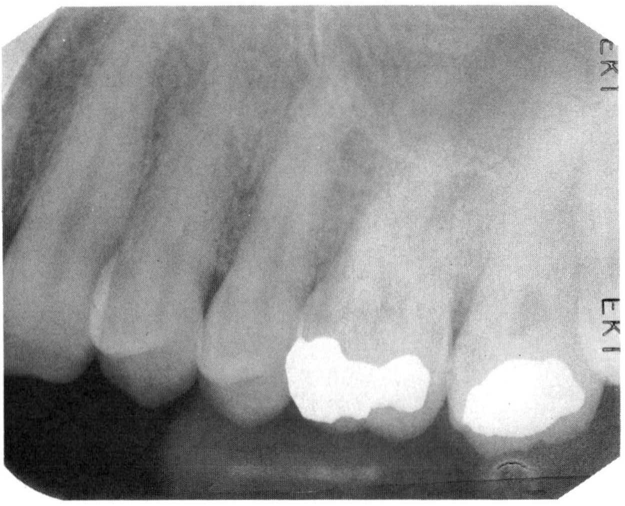

FIGURE 3–12

Radiograph showing trabeculation of the bone. The maxillary sinus can be seen in the upper right corner, and amalgam restorations are present.

CARTILAGE

Cartilage is tough, yet more elastic than bone. It forms structures such as the flexible tip of the nose. Another important function of cartilage is to cover the joint surfaces of bones. Here it is called **articular cartilage** because it protects the ends of the bones as they articulate. (The term **articulate** means to come together or join.)

Joints

Joints, also known as *articulations,* are places where two bones come together.

Fibrous joints, such as the sutures of the skull, do not move. (A **suture** is the jagged line where the bones articulate and form a joint that does not move.)

Cartilaginous joints hold the bones firmly together. Normally, they move only very slightly. The site where these bones come together is called a **symphysis.**

Synovial joints are the movable joints of the body. Some synovial joints are lined with a fibrous sac called a **bursa.** The function of the bursa is to act as a cushion to ease movement. The bursa is lined with **synovial membrane** and filled with **synovial fluid.**

Ball-and-socket joints, such as the hips and shoulders, are a type of synovial joint that allow a wide range of movement.

Hinge joints, such as the knees and elbows, are a type of synovial joint that allow movement in one direction or plane.

Bones of the Skull

The skull is made up of the 28 bones of the cranium, face, and middle ear (Figs. 3–13 to 3–19, Table 3–3). The terms used to describe landmarks on these bones are summarized in Table 3–4.

BONES OF THE CRANIUM

The eight bones of the cranium form a hard protective covering for the brain.

Frontal Bone (1)

The frontal bone forms the forehead, part of the floor of the cranium, and most of the roof of the orbits. (The **orbit** is the bony cavity protecting the eye.) The frontal bone contains the two **frontal sinuses,** one located above each eye.

Parietal Bones (2)

The parietal bones form most of the roof and upper sides of the cranium. The two parietal bones are joined at the **sagittal suture** at the midline. The line of articulation between the frontal bone and the parietal bones is called the **coronal suture.**

In a baby, the **fontanelle** is the soft spot where the sutures between the frontal and parietal bones have not yet closed. It disappears as the child grows and the sutures close.

Occipital Bone (1)

The occipital bone forms the back and base of the cranium. It joins the parietal bones at the **lambdoid suture.** The spinal cord passes through the **foramen magnum** of the occipital bone. (A **foramen** is a natural opening in a bone through which blood vessels, nerves, and ligaments pass. The plural is **foramina.**)

Temporal Bones (2)

The temporal bones form the sides and base of the cranium. Each temporal bone encloses an ear and contains the **external auditory meatus,** which is the bony passage of the outer ear. (A *meatus* is the external opening of a canal.)

The **mastoid process** is a projection on the temporal bone located just behind the ear. (A *process* is a prominence or projection on a bone.)

The lower portion of each temporal bone bears the **glenoid fossa** for articulation with the lower jaw. (A **fossa** is a hollow, groove, or depressed area in a bone.)

The **styloid process** extends from the undersurface of the temporal bone. (A **tuberosity** is a large, rounded process.)

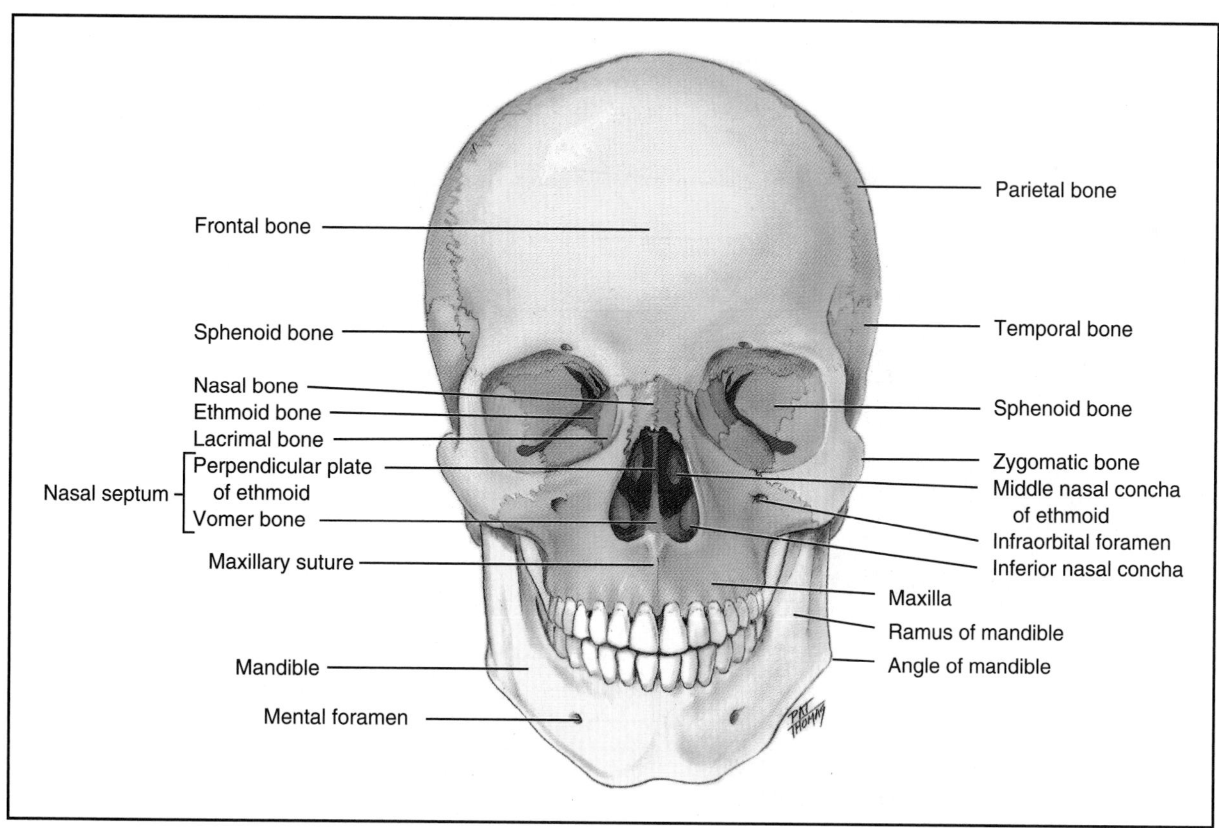

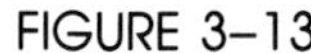

FIGURE 3–13

Frontal view of the skull. (From Applegate, E.J.: Anatomy and Physiology Learning System Textbook. Philadelphia, W.B. Saunders Co., 1995.)

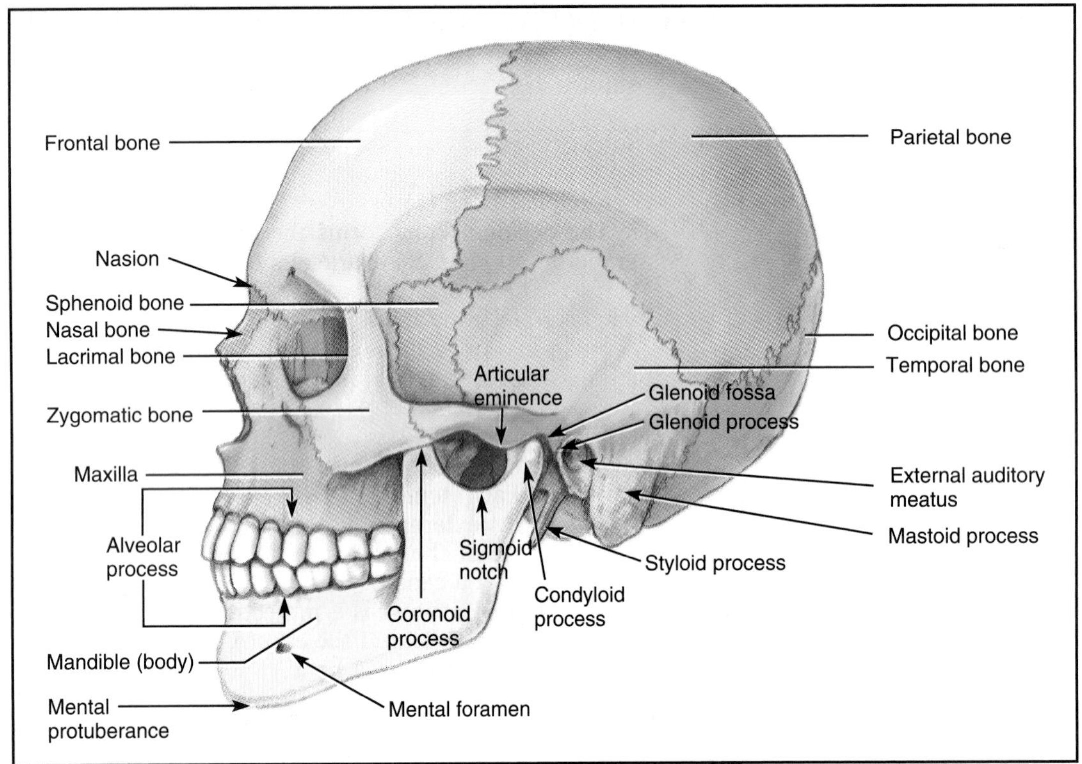

FIGURE 3–14

Lateral view of the skull. (From Applegate, E.J.: Anatomy and Physiology Learning System Textbook. Philadelphia, W.B. Saunders Co., 1995.)

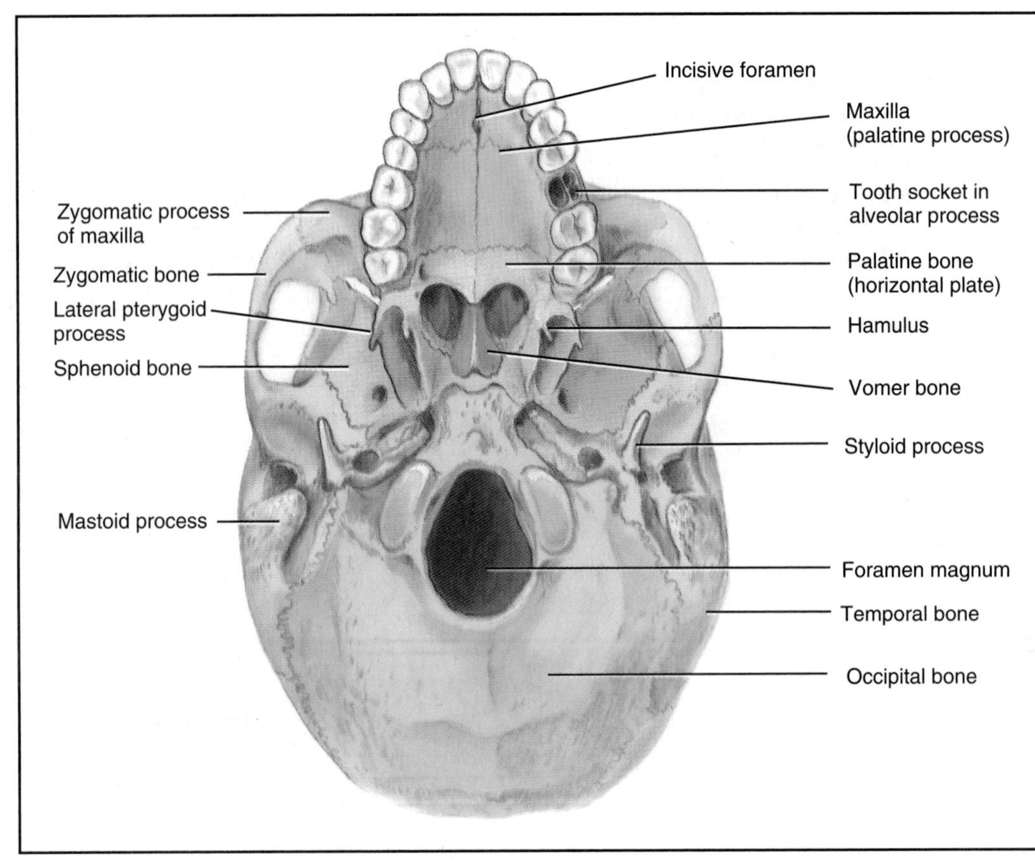

FIGURE 3–15

Base of the skull. (From Applegate, E.J.: Anatomy and Physiology Learning System Textbook. Philadelphia, W.B. Saunders Co., 1995.)

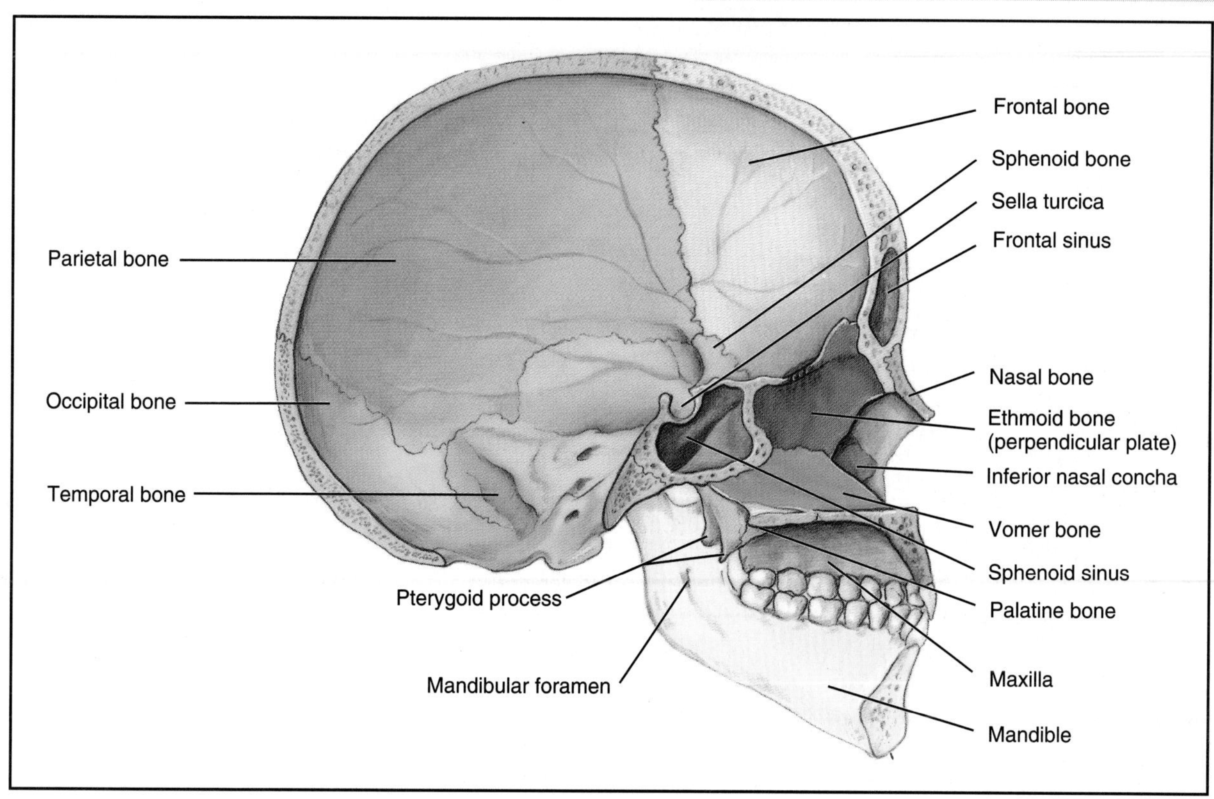

FIGURE 3–16

Midsagittal view of the skull. (From Applegate, E.J.: Anatomy and Physiology Learning System Textbook. Philadelphia, W.B. Saunders Co., 1995.)

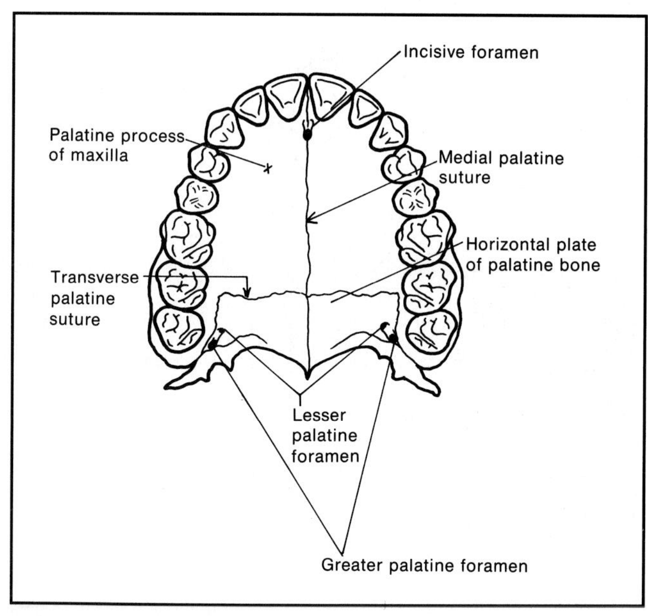

FIGURE 3–17

Bones and landmarks of the hard palate.

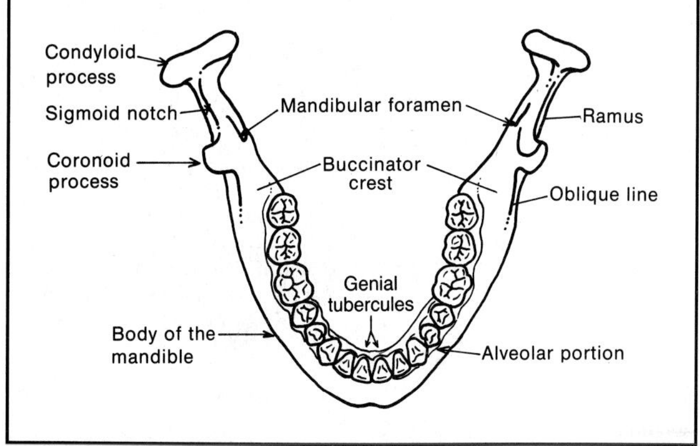

FIGURE 3–18

Topical view of the mandible.

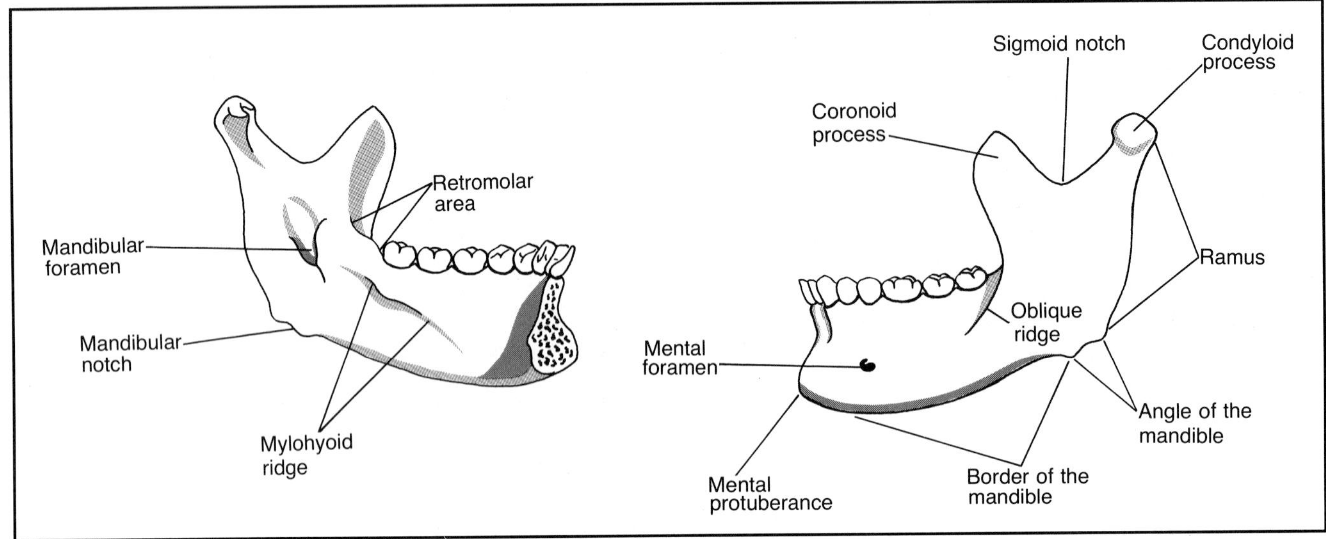

FIGURE 3–19

Medial and lateral views of the mandible.

TABLE 3–3

Bones of the Skull

BONE	NUMBER	LOCATION
8 Bones of the Cranium		
Frontal	1	Forms the forehead, most of the orbital roof, the anterior cranial floor
Parietal	2	Forms most of the roof and upper sides of the cranium
Occipital	1	Forms back and base of the cranium
Temporal	2	Forms the sides and base of the cranium
Sphenoid	1	Forms part of the anterior base of the skull and part of the walls of the orbit
Ethmoid	1	Forms part of the orbit and the floor of the cranium
14 Bones of the Face		
Zygomatic	2	Forms the prominence of the cheeks and part of the orbit
Maxillary	2	Forms the upper jaw
Palatine	2	Forms the posterior part of the hard palate and the floor of the nose
Nasal	2	Forms the bridge of the nose
Lacrimal	2	Forms the part of the orbit at the inner angle of the eye
Vomer	1	Forms the base for the nasal septum
Inferior conchae	2	Forms part of the interior of the nose
Mandible	1	Forms the lower jaw
6 Auditory Ossicles		
Malleus, incus, stapes	6	The bones of the middle ear

Sphenoid Bone (1)

The sphenoid bone is made up of a body and pairs of greater and lesser wings. It forms the anterior part of the base of the skull.

Each **greater wing** articulates with the temporal bone on either side and anteriorly with the frontal and zygomatic bones to form part of the orbit. Each **lesser wing** articulates with the ethmoid and frontal bones and also forms part of the orbit.

The **sphenoid sinuses** are located in the sphenoid bone just posterior to the eye. The **sella turcica** is a depression in the superior surface of the sphenoid bone, which protects the pituitary gland.

The **pterygoid process,** which extends downward from the sphenoid bone, consists of two plates. The

TABLE 3–4

The Terminology of Anatomic Landmarks of Bones

TERM	DEFINITION
Foramen	A natural opening in a bone through which blood vessels, nerves, and ligaments pass
Fossa	A hollow, groove, or depressed area in a bone
Meatus	The external opening of a canal
Process	A prominence or projection on a bone
Suture	The jagged line where the bones articulate and form a joint that does not move
Symphysis	The site where bones come together to form a cartilaginous joint
Tubercle	A small rough projection on a bone
Tuberosity	A large, rounded process on a bone

lateral pterygoid plate is the point of origin for the internal and external pterygoid muscles. The **medial pterygoid plate** ends in the hook-shaped **hamulus** that is visible on some dental radiographs.

Ethmoid Bone (1)

The ethmoid bone forms part of the floor of the cranium, the orbit, and the nasal cavity. This is a complex bone containing honeycomb-like spaces and the **ethmoid sinuses.** The **medial** and **superior conchae,** which are scroll-like structures, extend from the ethmoid bone.

Auditory Ossicles (6)

The auditory ossicles are the bones of the middle ear. In each ear, there are one **malleus,** one **incus,** and one **stapes.**

BONES OF THE FACE

Zygomatic Bones (2)

The zygomatic bones, also known as the *malar bones,* form the prominence of the cheek and the lateral wall and floor of the orbit.

The **frontal process** of the zygomatic bone extends upward to articulate with the frontal bone at the outer edge of the orbit. The zygomatic bones rest upon the maxillary bones and articulate with their zygomatic processes.

The **temporal process** of the zygomatic bone articulates with the zygomatic process of the temporal bone to form the **zygomatic arch,** which creates the prominence of the cheek.

Maxillary Bones (2)

The maxillary bones, also known as the *maxillae* (singular, *maxilla*), form the upper jaw and part of the hard palate.

The maxillary bones are joined together at the midline by the **maxillary suture.** The **zygomatic process** of the maxillary bones extends upward to articulate with the zygomatic bone.

The maxillary bones contain the **maxillary sinuses.** The **alveolar process** of the maxillary bones forms the support for the teeth of the maxillary arch.

The **maxillary tuberosity** is a larger, rounded area on the outer surface of the maxillary bones in the area of the posterior teeth.

Palatine Bones (2)

The horizontal portions of the palatine bones form the posterior part of the hard palate of the mouth and the floor of the nose. Anteriorly, they join with the maxillary bone.

Nasal Bones (2)

The nasal bones join to form the bridge of the nose. Superiorly, they articulate with the frontal bone and constitute a small portion of the nasal septum.

Lacrimal Bones (2)

The lacrimal bones make up part of the orbit at the inner angle of the eye. These small, thin bones lie directly behind the frontal processes of the maxillary bones.

Vomer Bone (1)

The vomer bone is a single, flat bone that forms the base for the nasal septum.

Inferior Conchae (2)

The inferior conchae (singular, *concha*), also known as the *inferior turbinates,* are the thin, scroll-like bones that form the lower part of the interior of the nose. Their function is to increase the interior surface of the nose.

Mandible (1)

The mandible forms the lower jaw and is the only movable bone of the skull. The **alveolar process** of the mandible supports the teeth of the mandibular arch.

The U-shaped mandible, which is the strongest and longest bone of the face, develops prenatally as two parts; however, in early childhood it ossifies (hardens) into a single bone. This symphysis is located at the midline and forms the **mental protuberance,** commonly known as the *chin.*

- A **mental foramen** is located on the facial surface on the left and right in the anterior portions of the mandible.
- The **genial tubercles** are small rounded and raised areas on the inner (medial) surface of the mandible near the symphysis.
- The **mylohyoid ridge** is located on the lingual surface of the body of the mandible.
- The *angle of the mandible* is the area where the mandible meets the ramus.
- The **mandibular notch** is located on the border of the mandible just anterior to the angle of the mandible.
- The **ramus** is the upright portion at each end of the mandible.
- The **coronoid process** is the anterior portion of each ramus.
- The **condyloid process,** also referred to as the *mandibular condyle,* is the posterior process of each ramus.
- The **sigmoid notch** separates the coronoid and condyloid processes.
- The condyloid process articulates with a fossa in the temporal bones to form the **temporomandibular joint.**
- The **mandibular foramen** is located on the lingual surface of each ramus.
- The **oblique ridge** is located on the facial surface of the mandible near the base of the ramus.
- The **retromolar area** is the portion of the mandible directly posterior to the last molar on each side.

Hyoid Bone (1)

The hyoid bone is unique because it does not articulate with any other bone. Instead, it is suspended between the mandible and the larynx, where it functions as a primary support for the tongue and other muscles.

The hyoid bone is shaped like a horseshoe and consists of a central body with two lateral projections. Externally, its position is noted in the neck between the mandible and the larynx. The hyoid is suspended from the styloid process of the temporal bone by the two **stylohyoid ligaments.**

Temporomandibular Joint

The temporomandibular joint (TMJ) receives its name from the two bones that enter into its formation, the temporal bone and the mandible. (Disorders of the temporomandibular joint are discussed in Chapter 11.)

The mandible is attached to the cranium by the ligaments of the temporomandibular joint. It is held in position by the muscles of mastication (Fig. 3–20). (**Mastication** means chewing.) The temporomandibular joint is made up of three bony parts:

1. The **glenoid fossa,** which is lined with fibrous connective tissue, is an oval depression in the temporal bone just anterior to the external auditory meatus.
2. The **articular eminence** is a raised portion of the temporal bone just anterior to the glenoid fossa.
3. The **condyloid process** of the mandible lies in the glenoid fossa.

CAPSULAR LIGAMENT

The capsular ligament is a dense fibrous capsule that completely surrounds the temporomandibular joint. It is attached to the neck of the condyle and to the nearby surfaces of the temporal bone. The ligaments of the temporomandibular joint attach the mandible to the cranium.

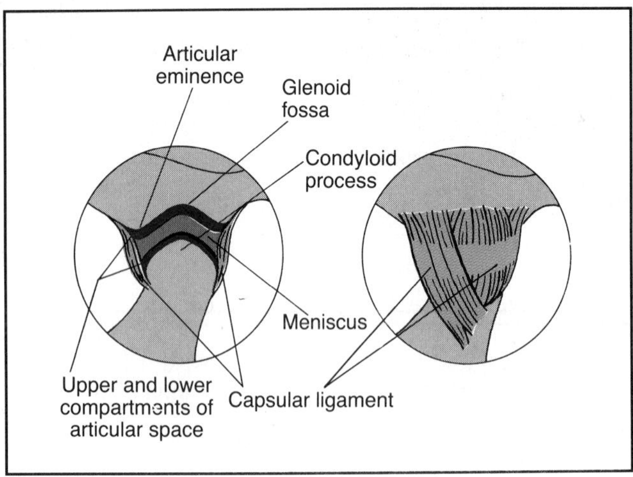

FIGURE 3–20

Parts of the temporomandibular joint.

ARTICULAR SPACE

The articular space is the area between the capsular ligament and between the surfaces of the glenoid fossa and the condyle.

The **articular disc,** also known as the *meniscus,* is a cushion of dense specialized connective tissue that divides the articular space into upper and lower compartments. These compartments are filled with synovial fluid.

MOVEMENTS OF THE TEMPOROMANDIBULAR JOINT

The temporomandibular joints are synovial joints that are constructed to permit specialized hinge and glide movements that permit different degrees of mouth opening (Fig. 3–21).

Hinge Action

The hinge action is the first phase in mouth opening, and only the lower compartment of the joint is used. During hinge action, the condyle head rotates around a point on the undersurface of the articular disc, and the body of the mandible drops almost passively downward and backward.

The jaw is opened by the combined actions of the external pterygoid, digastric, mylohyoid, and geniohyoid muscles. The jaw is closed by the action of the temporal, masseter, and internal pterygoid muscles.

Gliding Action

The gliding action is the second phase in mouth opening and movement. It involves both the lower and the upper compartments of the joint. This phase consists of a gliding movement by the condyle and articular disc forward and downward along the articular eminence.

This movement occurs only during protrusion and lateral movements of the mandible and in combination with the hinge action during the wider opening of the mouth.

Protrusion is the forward movement of the mandible. This happens when the internal and external pterygoid muscles on both sides contract together. The reversal of this forward movement is called **retrusion.**

Lateral movement, the sideways movement, of the mandible occurs when the internal and external pterygoids on the same side contract together.

Side-to-side **grinding movements** are brought about by alternating contractions of the internal and external pterygoid muscles, first on one side and then on the other.

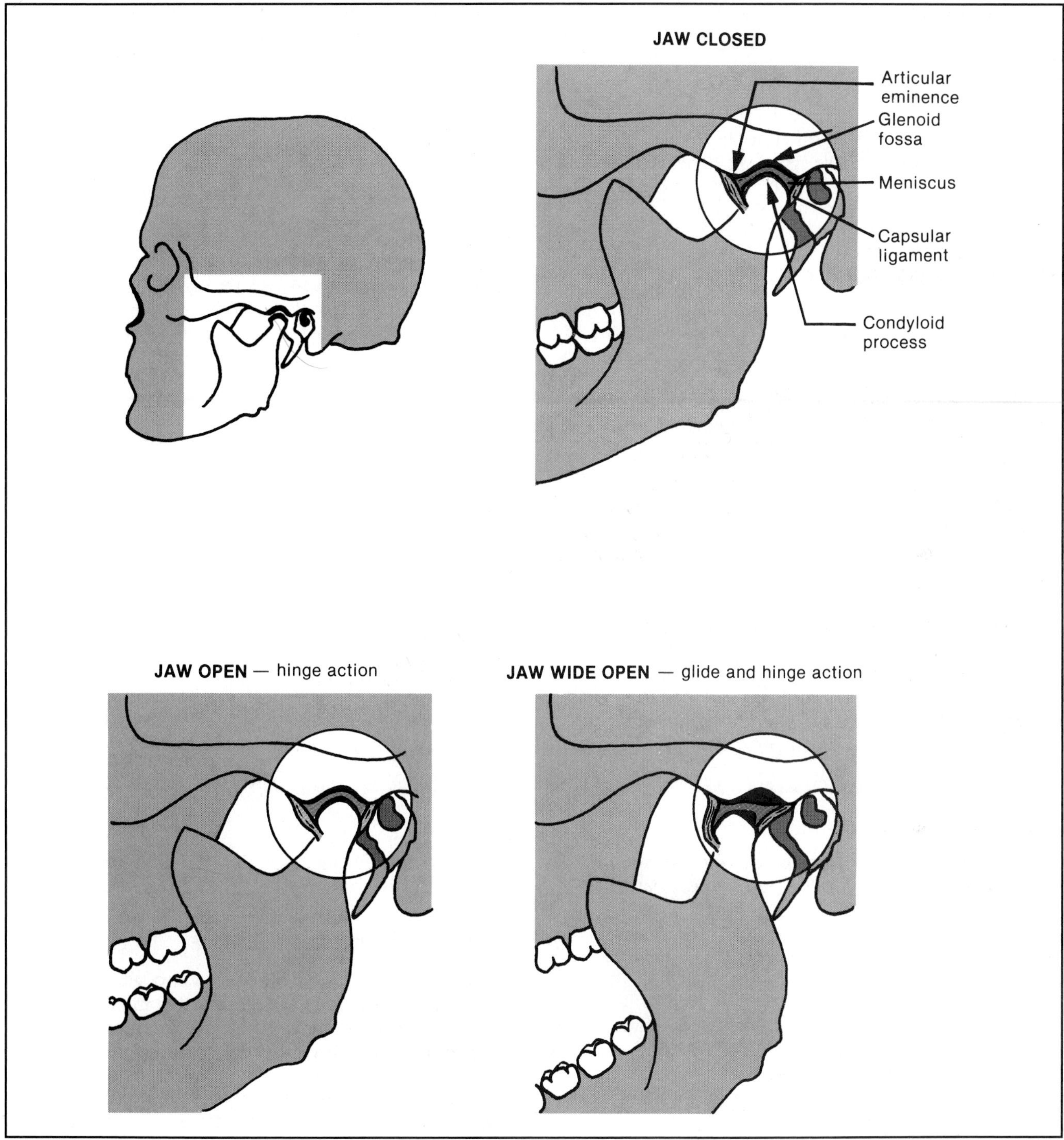

FIGURE 3–21

Hinge and gliding actions of the temporomandibular joint.

The Muscular System

Types of Muscles

There are three types of muscle tissue: striated, smooth, and cardiac. These types are described according to their appearance and their function (Fig. 3–22).

STRIATED MUSCLE

Striated muscles are so named because dark and light bands in the muscle fibers create a striped, or striated, appearance. Striated muscles are also known as the skeletal or voluntary muscles.

Skeletal muscles attach to the bones of the skeleton and make body motion possible. **Voluntary muscles,** such as the muscles of the face and eyes, are so named because we have conscious (voluntary) control over these muscles.

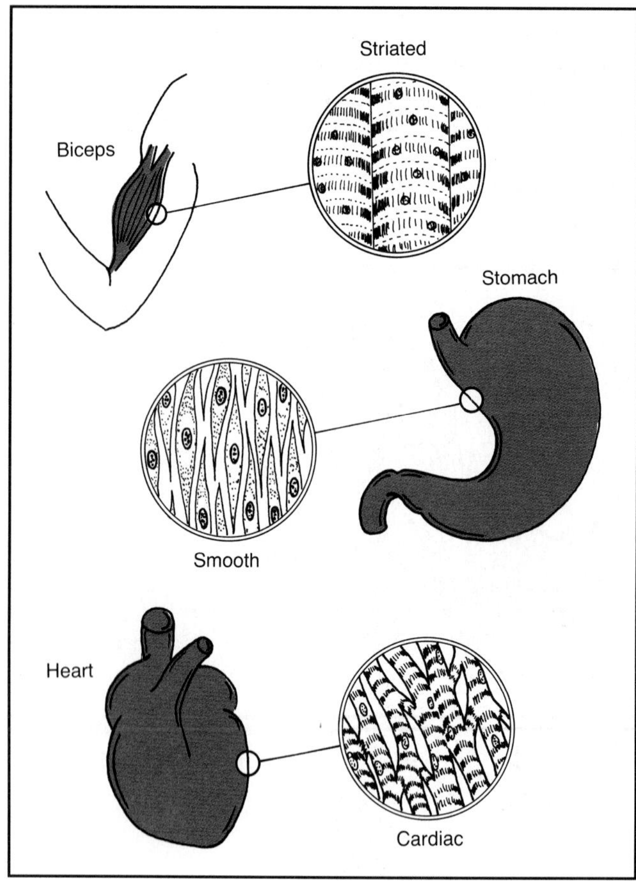

FIGURE 3–22

The types of muscle tissue.

SMOOTH MUSCLE

Smooth muscle fibers move the internal organs, such as the digestive tract, blood vessels, and secretory ducts leading from glands. In contrast to the marked contraction and relaxation of the striated muscles, smooth muscles produce relatively slow contraction.

Smooth muscles are also known as unstriated, involuntary, or visceral muscles. **Unstriated muscles** are so named because they do not have the dark and light bands that produce the striped (striated) appearance seen in striated muscles.

Involuntary muscles are so named because they are under the control of the autonomic nervous system and are not controlled voluntarily. **Visceral muscles** are so named because they are found in the visceral (internal) organs, except the heart. They are also found in hollow structures, such as the digestive and urinary tracts.

CARDIAC MUSCLE

Cardiac muscle is striated in appearance but like smooth muscle in its action. Cardiac muscle forms most of the wall of the heart, and it is the contraction of this muscle that causes the heart to beat.

How Muscles Work

Muscles are the only body tissues with the specialized ability to contract and relax. **Contraction** is the tightening of a muscle, during which it becomes shorter and thicker. **Relaxation** occurs when a muscle returns to its original form or shape.

The muscles of the body are arranged in antagonistic pairs so that when one contracts, the other relaxes. It is these contrasting actions that make motion possible.

PHYSIOLOGIC MUSCLE BALANCE

The teeth are positioned between two sets of muscles (Fig. 3–23). Externally, these are the muscles of the lips and cheeks. Internally, these are the muscles of the tongue. These muscles enclose the **neutral space,** which is occupied by the teeth arranged in the dental arches.

The neutral space is one in which a relative equilibrium of forces is normally maintained through a physiologic muscle balance. The aligning forces of the muscles in this lip-cheek-tongue muscle system are an important factor in maintaining the teeth in a normal lingual (tongue) and buccolabial (cheek and lip) relationship.

As long as the pressure of these muscle sets is in balance, the position of the teeth remains secure. However, imbalance between these sets of muscles can result in abnormal alignment of the dental arches. Such an imbalance could result from an infantile swallow pattern (described later in this chapter) or if part of an important structure (such as the tongue) has been surgically removed in the treatment of cancer.

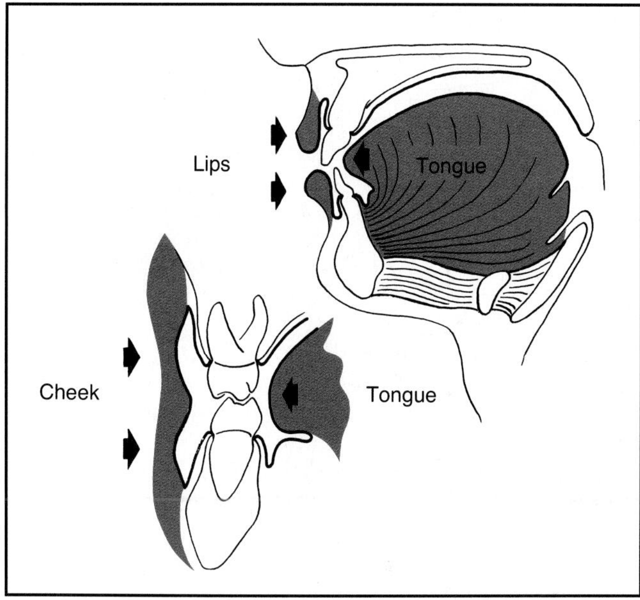

FIGURE 3–23

Physiological muscle balance within the mouth helps to hold the teeth in position in the arches.

MUSCLE ORIGIN AND INSERTION

Muscle origin is the place where the muscle begins (originates). This is the more fixed attachment and/or the end of the muscle that is toward the midline of the body.

Muscle insertion is the place where the muscle ends (inserts). It is the more movable end and/or is the portion of the muscle that is away from the midline of the body.

Some muscles are named for the place of origin and the place of insertion. For example, the origin of the stylohyoid muscle is from the styloid process (of the temporal bone). Its insertion is on the hyoid bone.

Major Muscles of Facial Expression
(Figs. 3–24 and 3–25)

ORBICULARIS ORIS

Function: Closes and puckers the lips. Also aids in chewing and speaking by pressing the lips against the teeth.
Origin: Muscle fibers surrounding the mouth.
Insertion: Into the skin at the angles of the mouth.
Innervation: Facial nerve.

BUCCINATOR

Function: Compresses the cheeks against the teeth and retracts the angle of the mouth.
Origin: Posterior portion of alveolar processes of the maxillary bone and the mandible.
Insertion: Fibers of the orbicularis oris, at the angle of the mouth.
Innervation: Facial nerve.

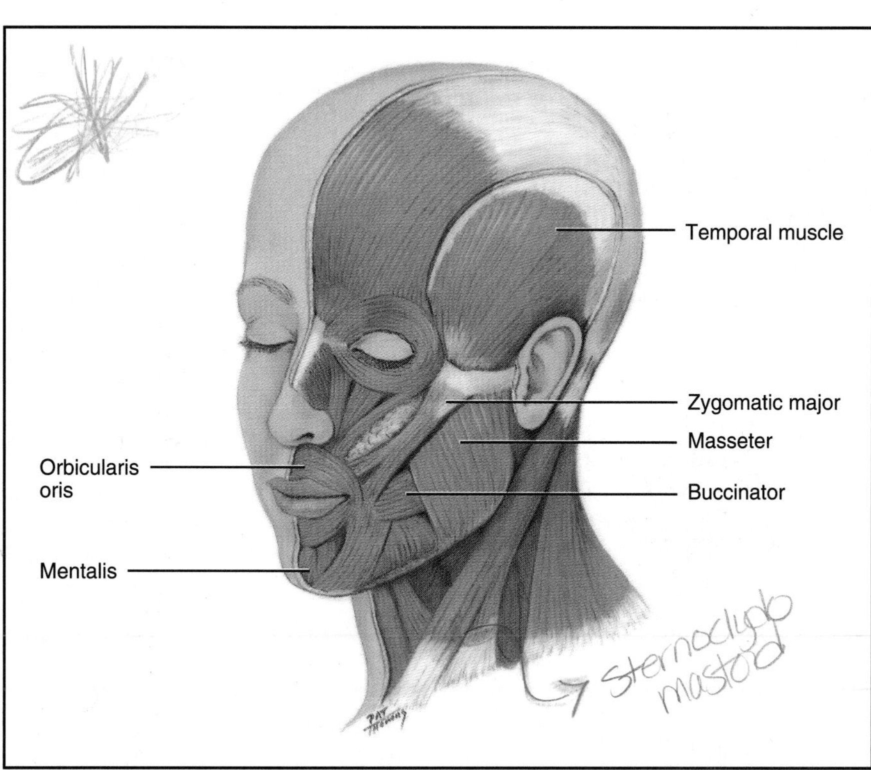

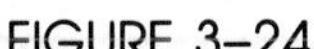
FIGURE 3–24

Major muscles of the face. (From Applegate, E.J.: Anatomy and Physiology Learning System Textbook. Philadelphia, W.B. Saunders Co., 1995.)

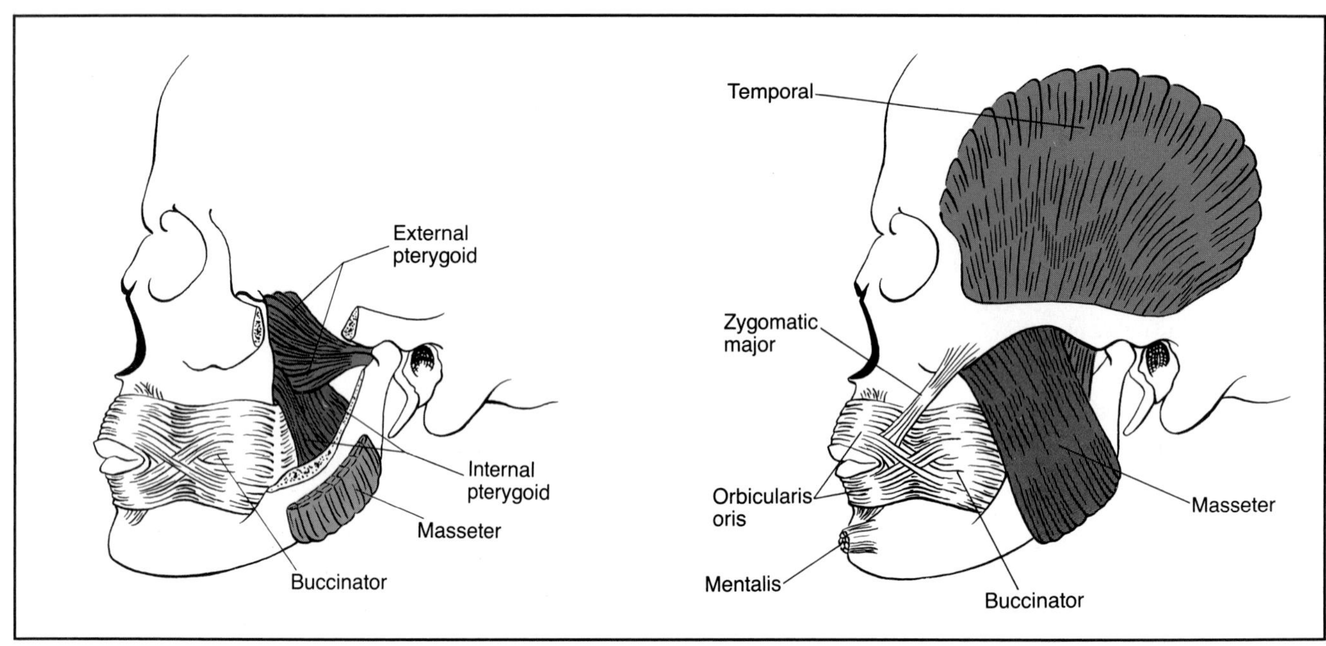

FIGURE 3–25

Muscles of mastication and facial expression (facial and internal views).

MENTALIS

Function: Raises and wrinkles the skin of the chin and pushes up the lower lip.
Origin: Incisive fossa of the mandible.
Insertion: Skin of the chin.
Innervation: Facial nerve.

ZYGOMATIC MAJOR

Function: Draws the angles of the mouth upward and backward, as in laughing.
Origin: Zygomatic bone.
Insertion: Into the fibers of the orbicularis oris.
Innervation: Facial nerve.

Major Muscles of Mastication
(Figs. 3–24 and 3–25)

TEMPORAL

Function: Raises mandible and closes the jaws. Posterior fibers draw protruding mandible backward.
Origin: Temporal fossa of the temporal bone.
Insertion: Coronoid process and the anterior border of the ramus of the mandible.
Innervation: Mandibular division of trigeminal nerve.

MASSETER

Function: Raises the mandible and closes the jaws.
Origin: The superficial part originates from the lower border of the zygomatic arch. The deep part originates from the posterior and medial side of the zygomatic arch.
Insertion: The superficial part inserts on the angle and lower lateral side of the ramus of the mandible. The deep part inserts into the upper lateral ramus and coronoid process of the mandible.
Innervation: Mandibular division of trigeminal nerve.

INTERNAL (MEDIAL) PTERYGOID

Function: Closes jaw. Acting with lateral pterygoid on same side, pulls mandible to one side. The medial and lateral pterygoids on both sides act together to bring lower jaw forward.
Origin: The medial surface of the lateral pterygoid plate of the sphenoid bone, the palatine bone, and the tuberosity of the maxillary bone.
Insertion: Into the inner (medial) surface of the ramus and angle of the mandible.
Innervation: Mandibular division of trigeminal nerve.

EXTERNAL (LATERAL) PTERYGOID

Function: Depresses mandible to open jaws. Also protrudes and moves them from side to side.
Origin: Originates from two heads. The upper head originates from the greater wing of the sphenoid bone. The lower head originates from the lateral surface of the pterygoid plate of the sphenoid bone.
Insertion: Into the neck of the condyle of the mandible and into the articular disc and capsular ligament of the temporomandibular joint.
Innervation: Mandibular division of trigeminal nerve.

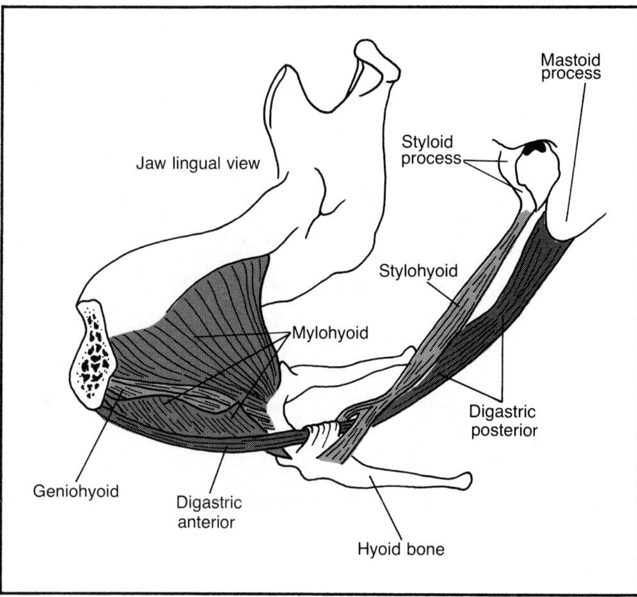

FIGURE 3–26

Muscles of the floor of the mouth.

Major Muscles of the Floor of the Mouth
(Fig. 3–26)

MYLOHYOID

Function: Forms the floor of the mouth. Elevates (raises) the tongue and depresses (lowers) the jaw.
Origin: Is made up of left and right portions, which are joined at the midline. Each portion originates on the mylohyoid line of the mandible.
Insertion: Body of hyoid bone.
Innervation: Trigeminal nerve.

DIGASTRIC

Function: Is composed of two bellies united by a central tendon. The anterior belly opens the jaw and draws the hyoid forward. The posterior belly draws the hyoid back.
Origin: The anterior belly originates from the lower border of the mandible. The posterior belly originates from the mastoid process of the temporal bone.
Insertion: Body and great horn of hyoid bone.
Innervation: Anterior belly, facial nerve; posterior belly, facial nerve.

STYLOHYOID

Function: Draws hyoid up and back.
Origin: Styloid process of the temporal bone.
Insertion: Body of the hyoid bone.
Innervation: Facial nerve.

GENIOHYOID

Function: Draws the tongue and hyoid bone forward.
Origin: The medial (inner) surface of the mandible, near the symphysis.
Insertion: Body of the hyoid.
Innervation: Hypoglossal nerve.

Extrinsic Muscles of the Tongue
(Fig. 3–27)

GENIOGLOSSUS

Function: Depresses and protrudes the tongue.
Origin: Medial (inner) surface of the mandible, near the symphysis.
Insertion: Hyoid bone and the inferior (lower) surface of the tongue.
Innervation: Hypoglossal nerve.

HYPOGLOSSUS

Function: Retracts and pulls down the side of the tongue.
Origin: Body of the hyoid bone.
Insertion: Side of the tongue.
Innervation: Hypoglossal nerve.

STYLOGLOSSUS

Function: Retracts the tongue.
Origin: Styloid process of the temporal bone.
Insertion: Side and undersurface of the tongue.
Innervation: Hypoglossal nerve.

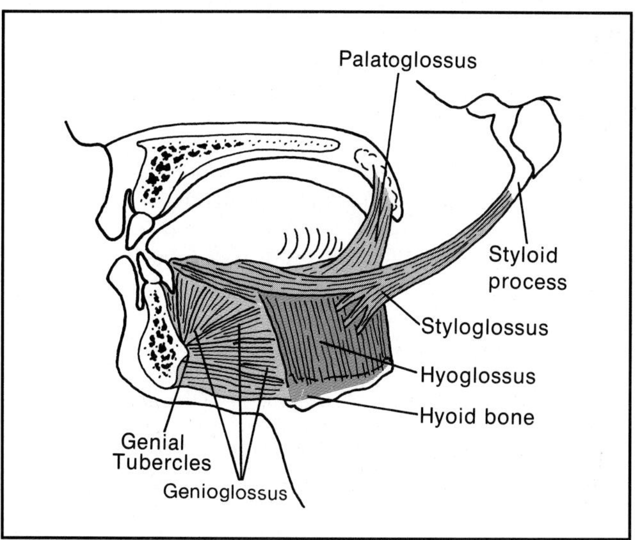

FIGURE 3–27

Extrinsic muscles of the tongue.

Major Muscles of the Posterior of the Mouth

PALATOGLOSSUS

Function: Forms the anterior pillar of fauces. Also raises the back of the tongue and narrows the fauces.
Origin: Soft palate.
Insertion: Side of the tongue.
Innervation: Pharyngeal plexus.

PALATOPHARYNGEUS

Function: Forms the posterior pillar of fauces. Also serves to narrow the fauces and helps shut off the nasopharynx.
Origin: Soft palate.
Insertion: Posterior border of the thyroid cartilage and the aponeurosis of the pharynx.
Innervation: Pharyngeal plexus.

The Cardiovascular System

Structures of the Cardiovascular System

The major structures of the cardiovascular system are the heart, blood vessels, and blood. The circulation of blood within this system is divided into two major subsystems: the pulmonary and the systemic circulations.

Pulmonary circulation includes the flow of blood from the heart, through the lungs (where it receives oxygen), and back to the heart. **Systemic circulation** includes blood flow to all parts of the body except the lungs.

HEART

The heart is a hollow muscular organ that furnishes the power to maintain the circulation of the blood (Fig. 3–28). It acts as a compound pump placed between, and connecting, the pulmonary circulation and systemic circulation. The heart, which is protected by the thoracic cavity, is located between the lungs and above the diaphragm.

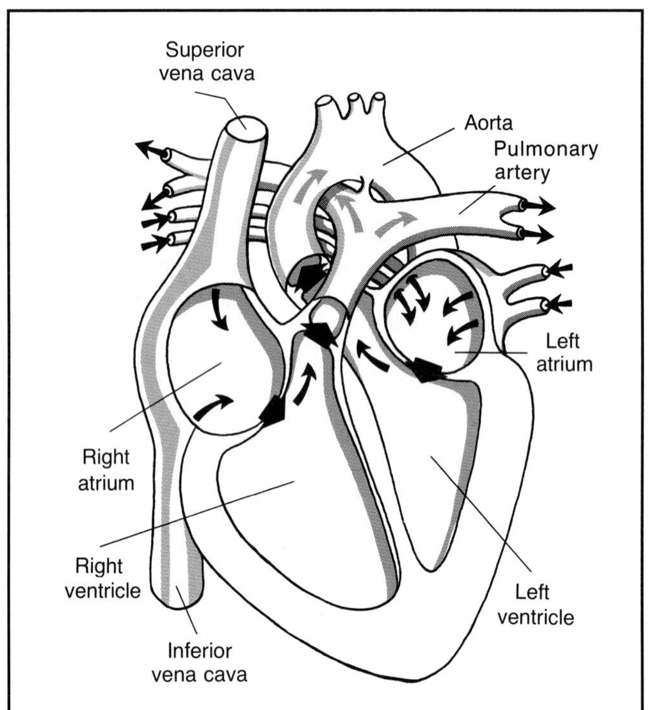

FIGURE 3–28

Structures of the heart.

Pericardium

The heart is enclosed in a double-walled membranous sac known as the pericardium. Pericardial fluid between the layers prevents friction when the heart beats.

Chambers of the Heart

The heart is divided into left and right sides. Each side is subdivided; thus there are a total of four chambers. The two atria, the upper chambers of the heart, are the receiving chambers, and all the vessels coming into the heart enter here. (*Atria* is plural. The singular is *atrium.*)

The two **ventricles,** the lower chambers of the heart, are the pumping chambers, and all vessels leaving the heart emerge from them.

Flow of Blood Through the Heart

The **right atrium** receives blood from the superior and inferior venae cavae, which are the large veins that enter the heart. This blood comes from all tissues except the lungs, contains waste materials, and is oxygen-poor. Blood flows from the right atrium into the right ventricle.

The **right ventricle** receives blood from the right atrium and pumps it out into the pulmonary artery, which carries it to the lungs.

The **left atrium** receives oxygenated blood from the lungs through the four pulmonary veins. (These are the only veins in the body that contain oxygen-rich blood.) Blood flows from here into the left ventricle.

The **left ventricle** receives blood from the left atrium. From here blood goes out into the aorta, which is the largest of the arteries, and is pumped to parts of the body, except the lungs.

BLOOD VESSELS

There are three major types of blood vessels in the body: the arteries, veins, and capillaries.

The **arteries** are the large blood vessels that carry blood away from the heart to all regions of the body (Fig. 3–29). The walls of the arteries are composed of three layers. This structure makes them both muscular and elastic so that they can expand and contract with the pumping beat of the heart.

The **capillaries** are a system of microscopic vessels that connect the arterial and venous systems. Blood flows rapidly along the arteries and veins; however, this flow is much slower through the expanded area provided by the capillaries. This slower flow allows time for the exchange of oxygen, nutrients, and waste materials between the tissue fluids and the surrounding cells.

The **veins** form a low-pressure collecting system to return the waste-filled blood to the heart (Fig. 3–30). Veins have thinner walls than do arteries and are less elastic. The veins have valves that allow blood to flow toward the heart but prevent it from flowing away from the heart.

BLOOD AND BLOOD CELLS

Most of the blood is composed of the liquid plasma. Less than half of the blood's composition is made up of formed elements. The **formed elements,** also known as *blood corpuscles,* include the red blood cells, white blood cells, and platelets.

Plasma is a straw-colored fluid that transports nutrients, hormones, and waste products. Plasma is 91 percent water. The remaining 9 percent consists mainly of the plasma proteins, including **albumin** and **globulin.**

Red blood cells, also known as *erythrocytes,* contain the blood protein **hemoglobin,** which plays an essential role in oxygen transport. Erythrocytes are produced by the red bone marrow. When erythrocytes are no longer useful, they are destroyed by macrophages in the spleen, liver, and bone marrow.

White blood cells, also known as *leukocytes,* have the primary function of fighting disease in the body. There are five major groups of leukocytes:

- **Basophils,** whose exact function is unknown
- **Eosinophils,** which are increased in number in allergic conditions
- **Lymphocytes,** which are important in the process of producing immunity to protect the body
- **Monocytes,** which act as macrophages that dispose of dead and dying cells and other debris
- **Neutrophils,** which fight disease by engulfing and swallowing up germs

Thrombocytes, also known as *platelets,* are the smallest formed elements of the blood. They are manufactured in the bone marrow and play an important role in the clotting of blood.

BLOOD CLOTTING

Hemostasis is the mechanism used by the body to control bleeding, and **coagulation** is the process of blood clot formation. Clotting normally occurs within 4 to 5 minutes of injury to the blood vessel. **Fibrinogen** and **prothrombin** are clotting proteins found in plasma. **Fibrin** is the protein formed by fibrinogen during the normal clotting of blood.

Clot formation involves platelet agglutination (clumping together), the contraction of blood vessels, and coagulation. The clot is a meshwork of fibrin threads that trap blood cells, platelets, and plasma. A few minutes after a clot forms, it begins to contract. This action expels most of the plasma from the clot. As the clot contracts, the edges of the broken blood vessels are pulled together.

BLOOD GROUPS

The safe administration of blood from donor to recipient requires typing and crossmatching. Blood typing, or grouping, is based on the antigens and antibodies found in the blood. The most important classifications are A, AB, B, and O. A patient receiving blood incompatible with his own can experience a serious and possibly fatal reaction.

In addition to matching of these groups, the Rh factor must also be matched according to whether it is positive or negative. The Rh factor is an antigenic substance present in the erythrocytes of most people. A person whose blood contains the factor is **Rh-positive.** A person whose blood does *not* contain the factor is **Rh-negative.**

BLOOD SUPPLY TO THE FACE AND MOUTH

Major Arteries of the Face and Mouth (Fig. 3–31, Table 3–5)

The **aorta** ascends from the left ventricle of the heart. The **common carotid** arises from the aorta and subdivides into the internal and external carotid arteries. The **external carotid** provides the major blood supply for the face and mouth.

The **maxillary artery** is the larger of the two terminal branches of the external carotid. It arises behind the angle of the mandible and supplies the deep structures of the face.

The **facial artery** is another branch of the external carotid. It enters the face at the inferior border of the mandible and can be detected by gently palpating the mandibular notch.

The facial artery passes forward and upward across the cheek toward the angle of the mouth. Then it continues upward along the side of the nose and ends at the medial commissure of the eye.

The **lingual artery** is also a branch of the external carotid. Its distribution is along the surface of the tongue.

The **anterior** and **middle superior alveolar arteries** originate from the infraorbital artery, which is a

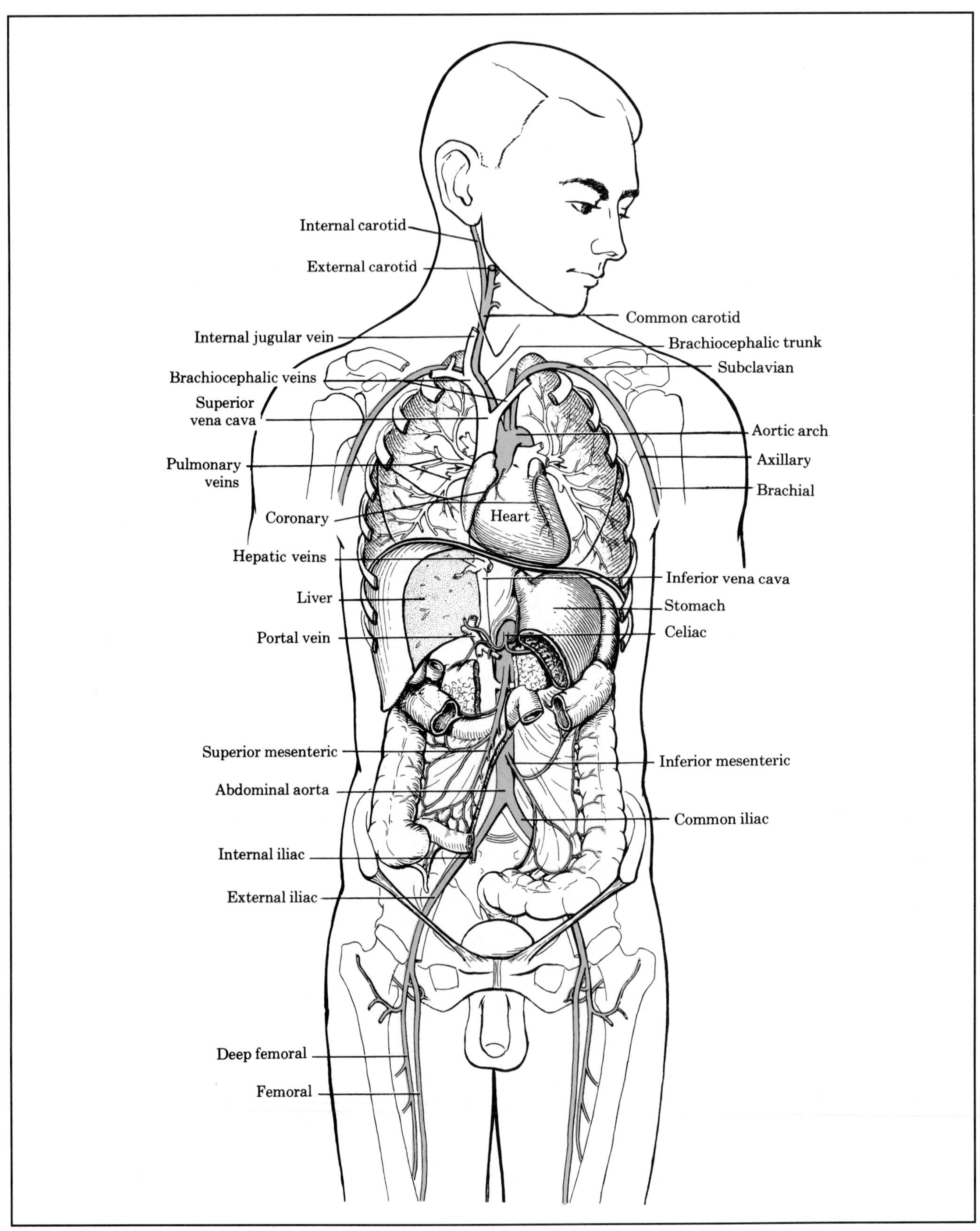

FIGURE 3–29

Principal arteries of the body. (From Dorland's Illustrated Medical Dictionary, 27th ed. Philadelphia, W.B. Saunders Co., 1988.)

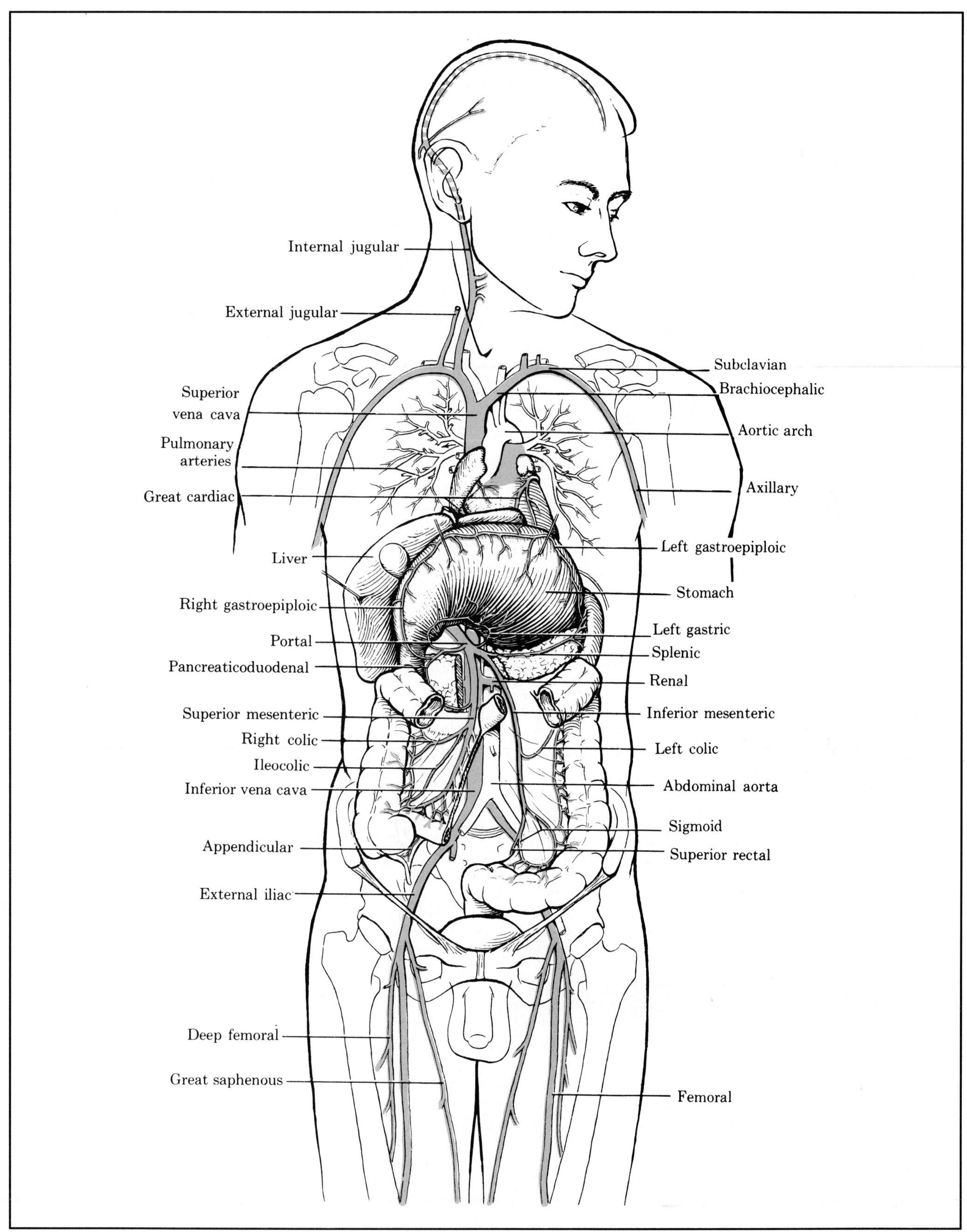

FIGURE 3–30

Principal veins of the body. (From Dorland's Illustrated Medical Dictionary, 27th ed. Philadelphia, W.B. Saunders Co., 1988.)

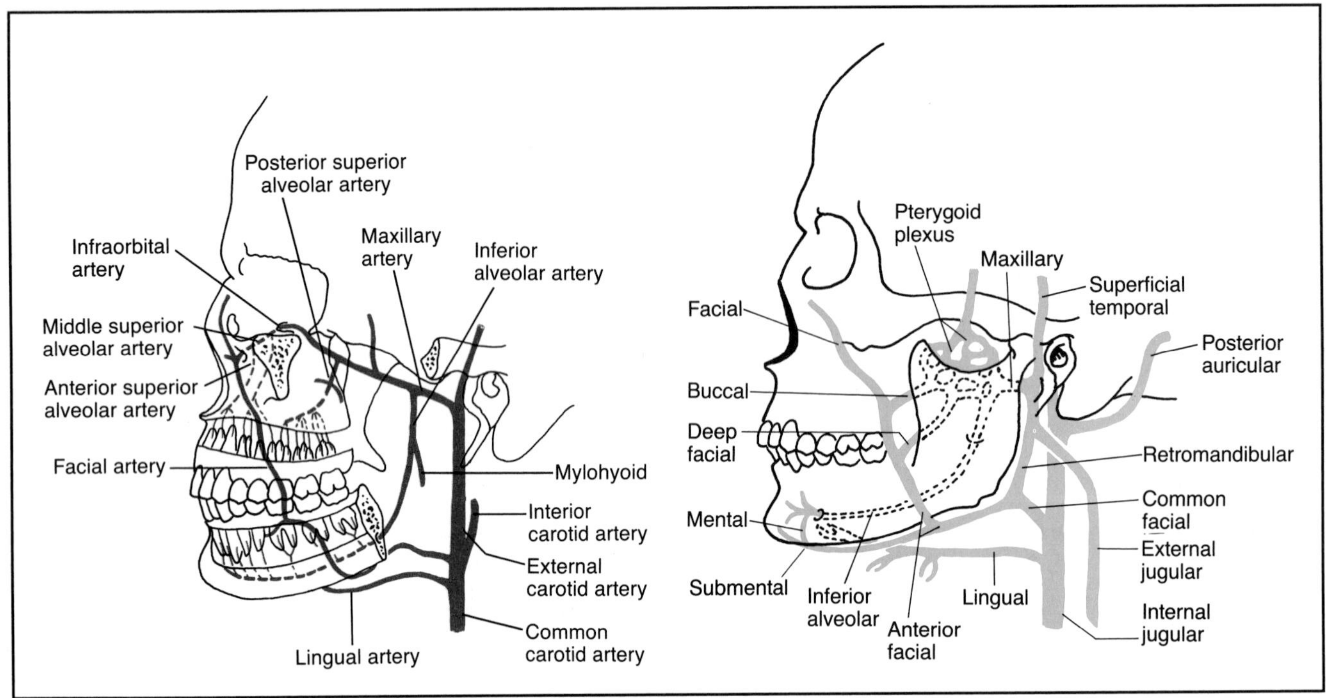

FIGURE 3–31

Major arteries and veins of the face and mouth.

branch of the maxillary artery. Their distribution is to the maxillary incisors and cuspid teeth and to the maxillary sinuses.

The **posterior superior alveolar artery** originates from the maxillary artery, and distribution is to the maxillary molar and premolar teeth and gingiva.

The **inferior alveolar artery** originates from the maxillary artery. It descends close to the medial surface of the mandibular ramus to the mandibular foramen. Before entering the foramen, it gives off the **mylohyoid branch,** which supplies tissues in the floor of the mouth.

The inferior alveolar artery continues along the mandibular canal. Opposite the first premolar it divides into the incisive and mental branches.

- The **incisive branch** continues within the bone to the incisors.
- The **mental branch** passes outward through the mental foramen and anteriorly to supply the chin.

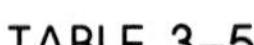

TABLE 3–5

Major Arteries to the Face and Mouth

STRUCTURE	BLOOD SUPPLY
Muscles of facial expression	Branches and small arteries from maxillary, facial, and ophthalmic arteries
Maxillary bones	Anterior, middle, and posterior alveolar arteries
Maxillary teeth	Anterior, middle, and posterior alveolar arteries
Mandible	Inferior alveolar arteries
Mandibular teeth	Inferior alveolar arteries
Tongue	Lingual artery
Muscles of mastication	Facial arteries

Major Veins of the Face and Mouth

(see Fig. 3–31)

The **maxillary vein** receives branches that correspond to those of the maxillary artery. These branches form the **pterygoid plexus.** The trunk of the maxillary vein passes backward behind the neck of the mandible.

The **retromandibular vein** is formed by the union of the temporal and maxillary veins. It descends within the parotid gland and divides into two branches.

- The **anterior branch** passes inward to join the facial vein.
- The **posterior branch** is joined by the posterior auricular vein and becomes the external jugular vein.

The **external jugular vein** empties into the **subclavian vein.** The **facial vein** begins near the side of the nose. It passes downward and crosses over the body of the mandible with the facial artery. It then passes outward and backward to unite with the anterior division of the retromandibular vein to form the **common facial vein,** which enters the internal jugular vein.

The **deep facial vein** goes from the pterygoid plexus to the facial vein. The **lingual veins** begin on the dorsum (top), sides, and undersurface of the tongue. They pass backward, following the course of the lingual artery and its branches, and terminate in the internal jugular vein.

The **internal jugular vein,** which corresponds to the common carotid artery, empties into the **superior vena cava,** which returns blood from the upper portion of the body to the right atrium of the heart.

The Lymphatic System

Structures of the Lymphatic System

The structures of the lymphatic system include the lymph vessels, lymph nodes, lymph fluid, tonsils, and spleen.

LYMPH VESSELS

Lymph capillaries are thin-walled tubes that carry lymph from the tissue spaces to the larger **lymphatic vessels.** Like veins, lymphatic vessels have valves to prevent the backward flow of fluid. Lymph fluid always flows toward the thoracic cavity, where it empties into veins in the upper thoracic region.

Specialized lymph vessels, called **lacteals,** are located in the small intestine. The lacteals aid in the absorption of fats from the small intestine into the blood stream.

LYMPH NODES

Lymph nodes are small round or oval structures located in lymph vessels. They fight disease by producing antibodies, which are part of the immune reaction. In acute infections, the lymph nodes become swollen and tender as a result of the collection of lymphocytes gathered to destroy the invading substances.

The major lymph node sites of the body include **cervical nodes** (in the neck), **axillary nodes** (under the arms), and **inguinal nodes** (in the lower abdomen) (Fig. 3–32).

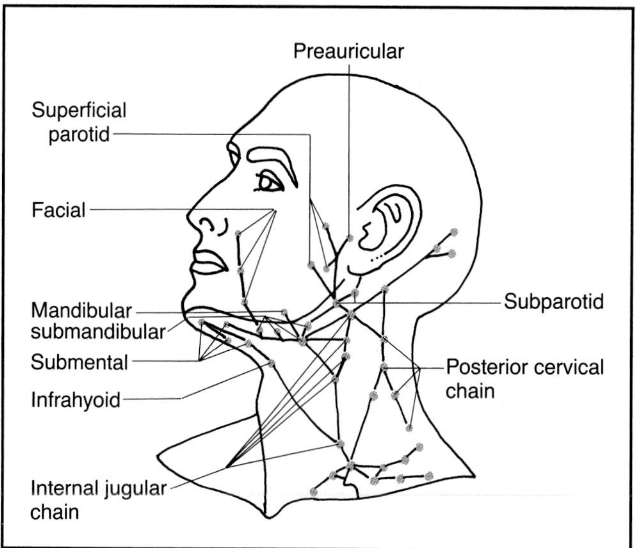

FIGURE 3–32

Major lymph nodes of the face and neck.

LYMPH FLUID

Lymph, also known as **tissue fluid,** is a clear and colorless fluid. Lymph flows in the spaces between the cells and tissues so that it can carry the substances from these tissues back into the blood stream.

LYMPH CELLS

Although the lymphatic system has its own vessels and fluid, it does not have cells or formed elements of its own. Instead, the cellular composition of lymph includes lymphocytes, monocytes, and a few platelets and erythrocytes, all of which are blood cells.

TONSILS

The tonsils are masses of lymphatic tissue located in the upper portions of the nose and throat, where they form a protective ring of lymphatic tissue (Fig. 3–33).

The **nasopharyngeal tonsils,** also known as *adenoids,* are found in the nasopharynx. The **palatine tonsils** are located in the oropharynx between the anterior and posterior pillars of the fauces. They are visible through the mouth. The **lingual tonsils** are located on the back of the tongue.

SPLEEN

The spleen is located in the left upper quadrant of the abdomen, just below the diaphragm and behind the stomach. The spleen produces lymphocytes and monocytes, which are important components of the immune system. It also filters microorganisms and other foreign material from the blood. Other spleen functions include storing red blood cells, maintaining the appropriate balance between cells and plasma in the blood, and removing and destroying worn-out red blood cells.

Specialized Cells of the Lymphatic System

The specialized cells of the lymphatic system play an important part in the immune system. They are described in Chapter 10.

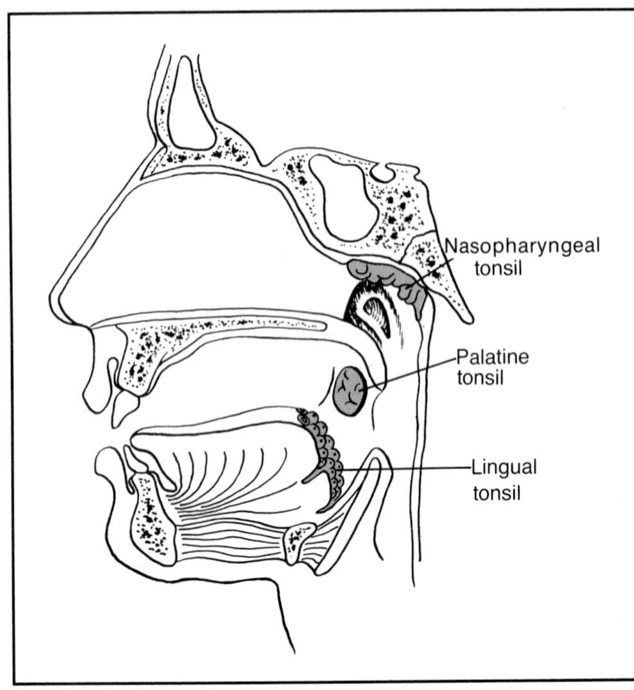

FIGURE 3–33

The tonsils.

The Nervous System

Divisions of the Nervous System

The **central nervous system** consists of the brain and spinal cord. The **peripheral nervous system** consists of the cranial nerves and the spinal nerves. The **autonomic nervous system** consists of ganglia on either side of the spinal cord. (A **ganglion** is a group of nerve cell bodies located outside the central nervous system.)

Structures of the Nervous System

NEURONS

Neurons are the basic cells of the nervous system. The three types of neurons are described according to their functions.

- **Sensory neurons** emerge from the skin or sense organs and carry impulses toward the brain and spinal cord.
- **Motor neurons** carry impulses away from the brain and spinal cord and toward the muscles and glands.
- **Associative neurons** carry impulses from one neuron to another.

A **synapse** is the space between two neurons or between a neuron and a receptor organ. A **neurotransmitter** is a chemical substance that makes it possible for the impulse to jump across the synapse from one neuron to another.

The **myelin sheath** is the white protective covering over some nerves. The nerves covered with myelin are referred to as the *white matter.* Nerves that do not have the protective myelin sheath are gray. They make up the *gray matter* of the brain and spinal cord.

BRAIN AND SPINAL CORD

The brain is the primary center for regulating and coordinating body activities, and each part of the brain controls different aspects of body functions. The brain is organized so that the left side of the brain controls the right side of the body and the right side of the brain controls the left side of the body.

The spinal cord carries all the nerves that affect the limbs and lower part of the body and is the pathway for impulses going to and from the brain. **Cerebrospinal fluid** flows throughout the brain and around the spinal cord. Its primary function is to cushion these organs from shock and injury.

CRANIAL NERVES

The cranial nerves are arranged in 12 pairs, so that both nerves of a pair are identical in function and structure. These nerves serve both sensory and motor functions. The cranial nerves are generally named for the area or function they serve and are identified with Roman numerals (Table 3–6).

SPINAL NERVES

The 31 pairs of spinal nerves are usually named after the arteries that they accompany or the body parts that they innervate.

Innervation of the Oral Cavity

The **trigeminal nerve** is the primary source of innervation for the oral cavity (Figs. 3–34 and 3–35). At the **semilunar ganglion,** the trigeminal nerve subdivides into three main branches: the ophthalmic, the maxillary, and the mandibular.

MAXILLARY DIVISION OF THE TRIGEMINAL NERVE

The maxillary division of the trigeminal nerve supplies the maxillary teeth, periosteum, mucous membrane, maxillary sinuses, and soft palate.

The maxillary division subdivides to provide the following innervation: The **nasopalatine nerve,** which

TABLE 3–6

The Cranial Nerves

NUMBER	NERVE
I	*Olfactory nerves* are sensory for smell
II	*Optic nerves* are sensory for sight
III	*Oculomotor nerves* control muscles of the eyes
IV	*Trochlear nerves* control muscles of the eyes
V	*Trigeminal nerves* each divide into three branches: The *ophthalmic* branches go to the eyes and forehead The *maxillary* branches go to the upper jaw and innervate the teeth and surrounding tissues The *mandibular* branches go to the lower jaw and innervate the teeth and surrounding tissues
VI	*Abducens nerves* control muscles of the eyes
VII	*Facial nerves* innervate the muscles of facial expression, salivary glands, lacrimal glands, and the sensation of taste on the anterior two thirds of the tongue
VIII	*Acoustic nerves* each divide into two branches: The *cochlear* branches, concerned with the sense of hearing The *vestibular* branches, concerned with the sense of balance
IX	*Glossopharyngeal nerves* innervate the parotid glands, the sense of taste on the posterior third of the tongue, and part of the pharynx
X	*Vagus nerves* innervate part of the pharynx, the larynx and vocal cords, and parts of the thoracic and abdominal viscera
XI	*Spinal accessory nerves* innervate the shoulder muscles
XII	*Hypoglossal nerves* innervate the muscles concerned with movements of the tongue

passes through the incisive foramen, supplies the mucoperiosteum palatal to the maxillary anterior teeth. (**Mucoperiosteum** is periosteum having a mucous membrane surface.)

The **anterior palatine nerve,** which passes through the posterior palatine foramen and forward over the palate, supplies the mucoperiosteum intermingling with the nasopalatine nerve.

The **anterior superior alveolar nerve** supplies the maxillary central, lateral, and cuspid teeth, plus their periodontal membrane and gingiva. This nerve also supplies the maxillary sinus.

The **middle superior alveolar nerve** supplies the maxillary first and second premolars, the mesiobuccal root of the maxillary first molar, and the maxillary sinus.

The **posterior superior alveolar nerve** supplies the other roots of the maxillary first molar and the maxillary second and third molars. It also branches forward to serve the lateral wall of the maxillary sinus.

MANDIBULAR DIVISION OF THE TRIGEMINAL NERVE

The mandibular division of the trigeminal nerve subdivides into the (1) buccal, (2) lingual, and (3) inferior alveolar nerves.

The **buccal nerve** supplies branches to the buccal mucous membrane and to the mucoperiosteum of the maxillary and mandibular molar teeth.

The **lingual nerve** supplies the anterior two thirds of the tongue and gives off branches to supply the lingual mucous membrane and mucoperiosteum.

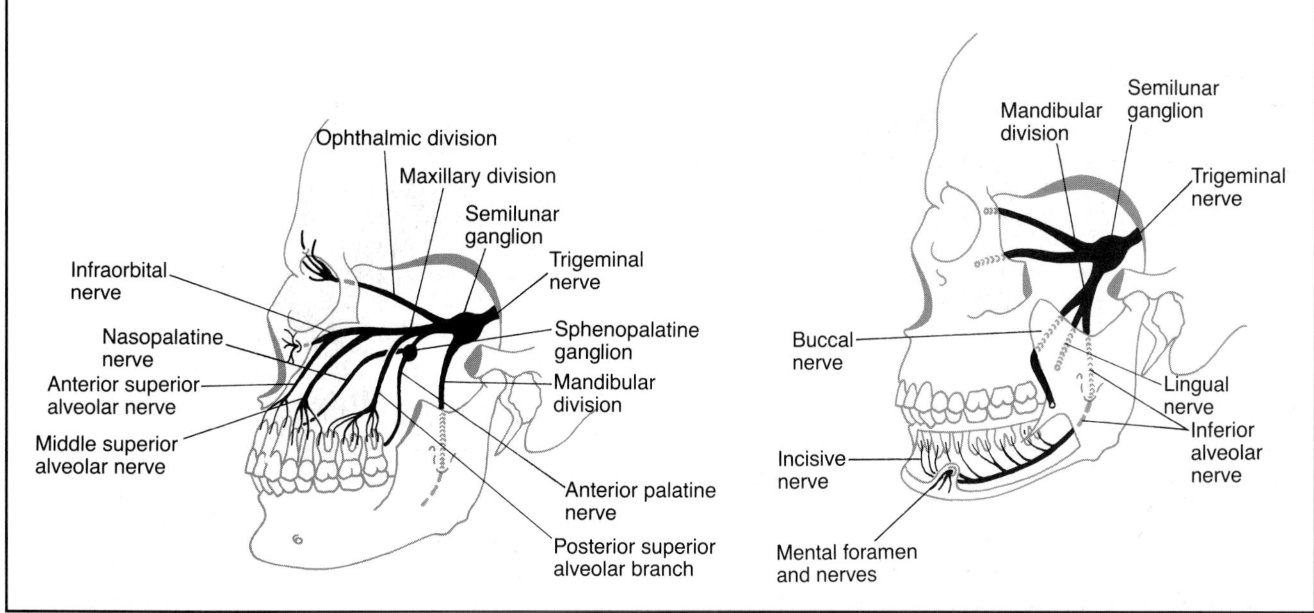

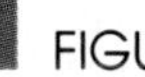
FIGURE 3–34

Maxillary and mandibular innervation.

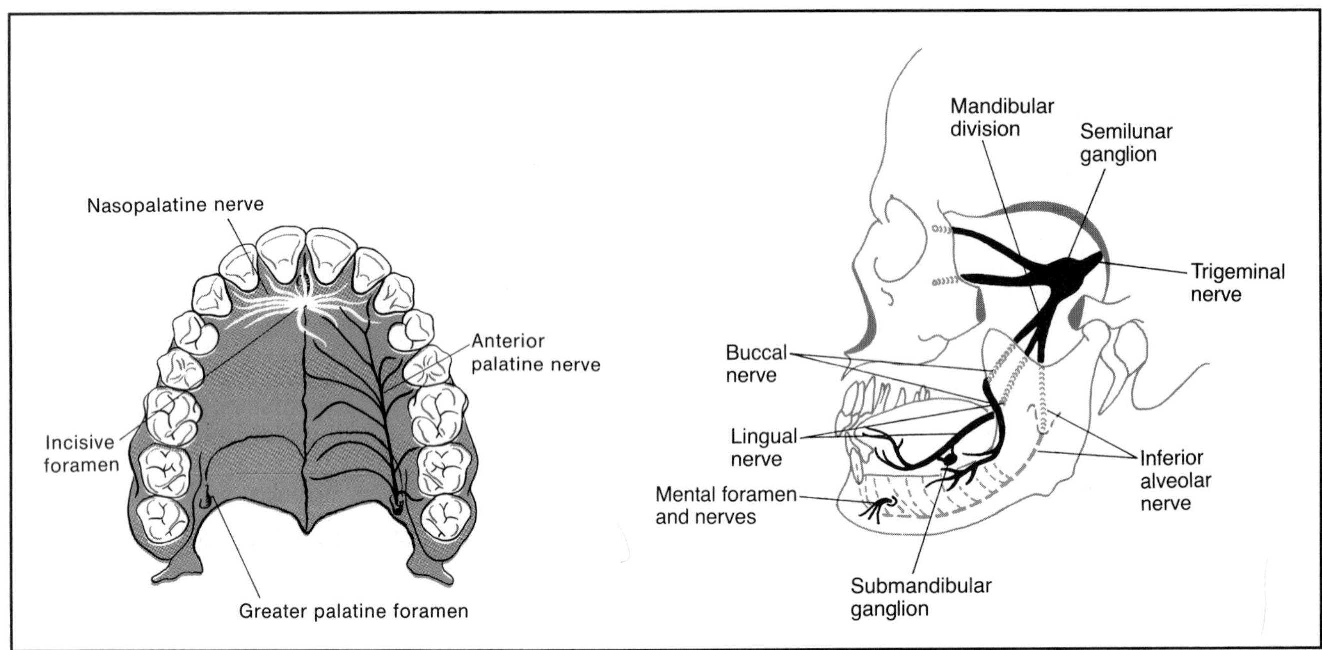

FIGURE 3–35

Palatal, lingual, and buccal innervation.

The **inferior alveolar nerve** subdivides into the following:

- The **mylohyoid nerve,** which supplies the mylohyoid muscles and the anterior belly of the digastric muscle.
- The **small dental nerves,** which supply the molar and premolar teeth, alveolar process, and periosteum.
- The **mental nerve,** which moves outward and anteriorly through the mental foramen and supplies the chin and mucous membrane of the lower lip.
- The **incisive nerve,** which continues anteriorly within the bone and gives off small branches to supply the cuspid, lateral, and central teeth.

The Respiratory System

Structures of the Respiratory System

NOSE

Air enters the body through the nostrils (nares) of the nose and passes through the **nasal cavity.** The nose is divided by a wall of cartilage called the **nasal septum.**

The nose and respiratory system are lined with mucous membrane, which is a specialized form of epithelial tissue. The incoming air is filtered by the **cilia,** which are thin hairs attached to the mucous membrane just inside the nostrils.

Mucus secreted by the mucous membranes helps to moisten and warm the air as it enters the nose. (Notice the difference in spelling between *mucous,* the name of the membrane, and *mucus,* the secretion of the membrane.)

PARANASAL SINUSES

The **paranasal sinuses** are air-containing spaces within the skull that communicate with the nasal cavity (Fig. 3–36). (A **sinus** is an air-filled cavity within a bone.)

The functions of the sinuses include:

- Producing mucus
- Making the bones of the skull lighter
- Providing resonance that helps to produce sound

The sinuses are named for the bones in which they are located:

- The **maxillary sinuses,** the largest of the paranasal sinuses
- The **frontal sinuses,** located within the forehead just above the eyes
- The **ethmoid sinuses,** irregularly shaped air cells separated from the orbital cavity by a very thin layer of bone
- The **sphenoid sinuses,** located close to the optic nerves, where an infection may damage vision

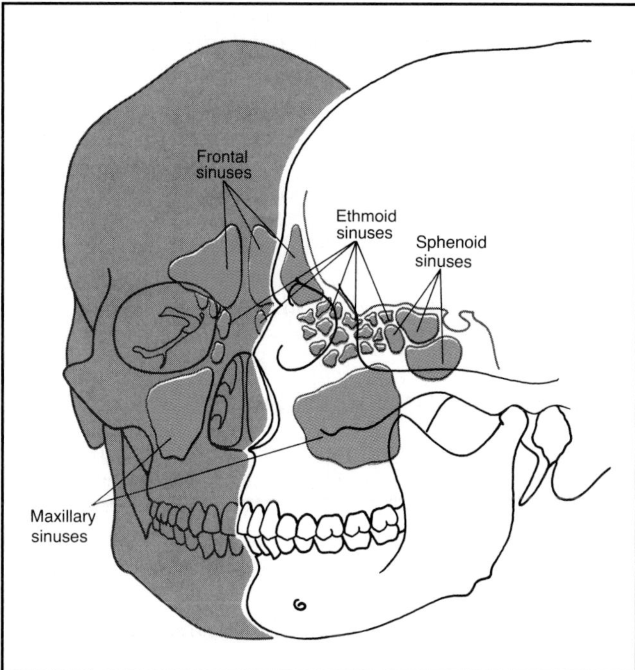

FIGURE 3–36

The paranasal sinuses.

PHARYNX

After passing through the nasal cavity, the air reaches the pharynx, which is commonly known as the *throat.* There are three divisions of the pharynx: the nasopharynx, oropharynx, and laryngopharynx.

- The **nasopharynx** is located behind the nose and above the soft palate. The **eustachian tube,** the narrow tube leading from the middle ear, opens into the nasopharynx.
- The **oropharynx** extends from the soft palate above to the level of the epiglottis below. This is the part of the throat that is visible when one is looking into the mouth.

  This opening leads both to the stomach and to the lungs. Should the patient aspirate anything during treatment, such as a sharp tooth fragment, it could go into either the lung or the digestive system. (As used here, **aspirate** means to accidentally inhale or swallow.)
- The **laryngopharynx** extends from the level of the epiglottis above to the larynx below.

EPIGLOTTIS

The oropharynx and laryngopharynx serve as a common passageway for both food from the mouth and air from the nose. In the act of swallowing, the epiglottis acts as a lid and covers the larynx so that food does not enter the lungs.

LARYNX

The **larynx,** also known as the *voice box,* contains the vocal bands, which make speech possible. The larynx is protected and held open by a series of cartilages. The largest of these and its prominent projection are commonly known as the *Adam's apple.*

TRACHEA

Air passes from the larynx to the trachea. The trachea extends from the neck into the chest, directly in front of the esophagus. It is protected and held open by a series of C-shaped cartilage rings.

LUNGS

The trachea divides into two branches called **bronchi.** Each bronchus leads to a lung, where it divides and subdivides into increasingly smaller branches. The smallest of these branches are called **bronchioles. Alveoli** are the very small grapelike clusters found at the end of each bronchiole. The walls of the alveoli are very thin and are surrounded by a network of capillaries. During respiration the gas exchange between the lungs and blood takes place here.

The Digestive System

Structures of the Digestive System

The major structures of the digestive system are the mouth, pharynx, esophagus, stomach, small intestine, and large intestine (Fig. 3–37).

The **pharynx,** the common passageway for both respiration and digestion, is discussed in the section "The Respiratory System."

The **esophagus** is a collapsible tube that leads from the pharynx to the stomach. The esophagus lies posterior to the trachea and heart and just in front of the spine.

The **stomach** is a saclike organ that lies in the abdominal cavity just under the diaphragm. Glands within the stomach produce the gastric juices that aid in digestion and the mucus that forms the protective coating of the lining of the stomach.

The **small intestine** extends from the stomach to the first part of the large intestine. It consists of three parts: the duodenum, the jejunum, and the ileum.

The **large intestine** extends from the end of the small intestine to the anus. It is divided into four parts: the cecum, the colon, the sigmoid colon, and the rectum and anus.

Swallowing

Swallowing, also known as *deglutition,* is a complex and coordinated activity that moves food and other

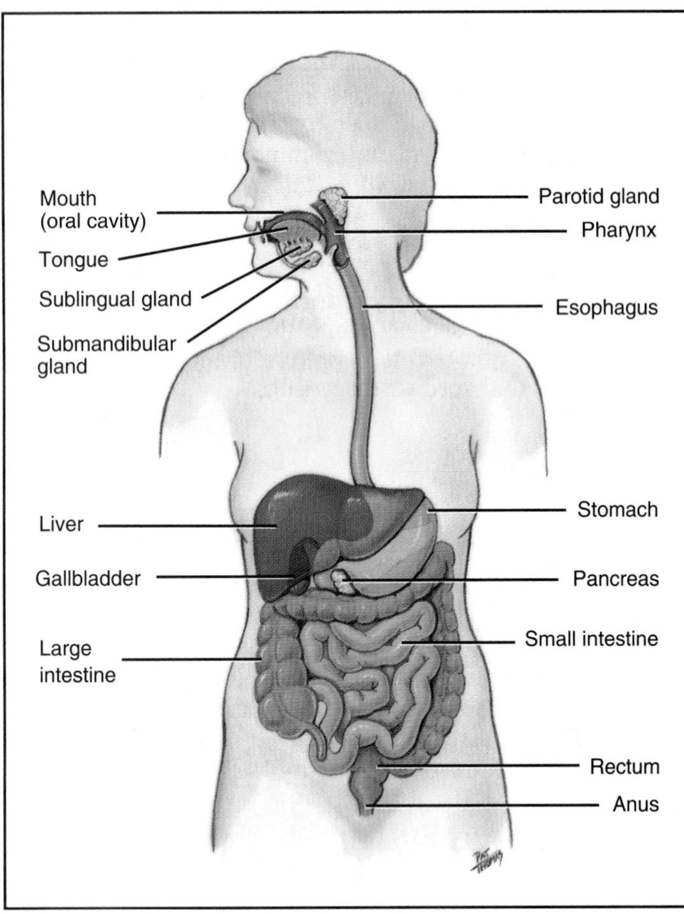

FIGURE 3–37

Major structures of the digestive system. (From Applegate, E.J.: Anatomy and Physiology Learning System Textbook. Philadelphia, W.B. Saunders Co., 1995.)

matter from the mouth to the stomach. For descriptive purposes, it is divided into three phases; however, the act itself is rapid and continuous. Starting to swallow is under voluntary control; however, once it is started, the rest of the swallow is a reflex action.

PHASE ONE

In the adult swallowing pattern, the first phase is collecting the masticated (chewed) food into a mass on the dorsum of the tongue. This mass, called a **bolus,** then passes from the mouth into the pharynx.

During this phase, the lips are closed but relaxed, the teeth are together, and the tongue is wholly contained within the dental arches. The tip of the tongue presses against the hard palate and does not exert active pressure on the anterior teeth.

PHASE TWO

In the second phase, food passes through the pharynx into the beginning of the esophagus. During this time there is a temporary suspension of respiration. The soft palate moves back and upward to close off the nasal passages, and the epiglottis closes off the larynx. This prevents swallowed matter from entering the larynx and, subsequently, the lungs.

PHASE THREE

In the third phase, food passes down the esophagus and into the stomach. As the bolus continues to move downward, the soft palate is lowered, the epiglottis moves out of the way, and the airway is once again available for respiration.

INFANTILE SWALLOW PATTERN

In the infantile swallow pattern, the first phase of swallowing is modified because the infant takes in food by sucking. In the infantile swallow pattern, the tongue in a forward position between the dental arches. This permits the active lip movements that are an important part of the sucking action.

The adult pattern is usually spontaneously adopted soon after the primary teeth come into contact. An infantile swallow pattern that is retained beyond the mixed dentition stage is called **tongue-thrust swallow,** and this is discussed in Chapter 27.

Other Structures of the Digestive System

The **liver** is located in the right upper quadrant of the abdomen. It removes excess **glucose** (sugar) from the blood stream and stores it as **glycogen** (starch). When the blood sugar level is low, the liver converts the glycogen back into glucose and releases it for use by the body.

The liver also destroys old erythrocytes, removes poisons from the blood, and manufactures some blood proteins. In addition, it manufactures bile, which is a digestive juice.

The **gallbladder** is a pear-shaped sac located under the liver. It stores and concentrates the bile for later use. When needed, bile is emptied into the duodenum of the small intestine.

The **pancreas** produces pancreatic juices, which contain digestive enzymes. These juices are emptied into the duodenum of the small intestine.

Digestion

Digestion is the process of breaking down ingested foods into forms that the body can use. Digestion begins in the mouth with mastication (chewing), mixing the food with saliva, and swallowing of food. The digestive enzyme salivary amylase begins the process of breaking down carbohydrates into simpler forms that the body can use.

After the food is swallowed, the churning action of the stomach mixes it with gastric juice. The digestion of carbohydrates continues here, and the digestion of protein begins.

In the small intestine, peristaltic action moves the food along and mixes it with bile and pancreatic juice. (**Peristalsis** is the wavelike muscle action that moves food through the digestive system.) Digestion is completed here, and nutrients are absorbed into the blood stream.

In the large intestine, excess water is absorbed, and the solid waste products are eliminated through the rectum.

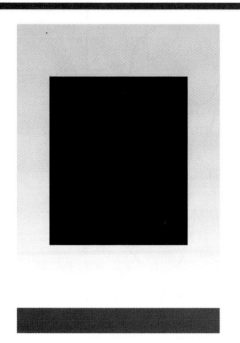

Chapter 4

Oral Embryology and Histology

Introduction

Embryology is the study of the developing individual throughout the stages before birth. The first portion of this chapter covers this development with emphasis on the formation of the teeth and structures of the oral cavity.

Histology is the study of the composition and function of tissues. The second part of the chapter covers the histology of the teeth, their supporting structures, and the oral mucosa that surrounds the teeth and lines the mouth.

Oral Embryology

Pregnancy

Pregnancy begins with **conception,** which is also known as *fertilization.* This occurs when the sperm penetrates and fertilizes the ovum. Conception may occur during the woman's fertile period, which is approximately 2 weeks after the menstrual period.

Birth occurs, on the average, 38 weeks after conception, or 40 weeks after the beginning of the last menstrual period (LMP). A child born at completion of this time period is said to be born *at term.*

The *due date,* or estimated date of birth, may be approximately predicted by adding a year and a week to the date on which the last menstrual period began and then counting back 3 months.

A normal human pregnancy is 9 calendar months. For general descriptive purposes, this is divided into three trimesters of 3 months each.

A physician usually describes prenatal development in weeks on the basis of the date of the last menstrual period. In embryology, developmental age is based on the date of conception, which is assumed to have occurred 2 weeks after the LMP.

The developmental ages noted in this chapter are based on the date of conception.

Prenatal Phases

ZYGOTE PHASE

For the first 2 weeks after conception, the fertilized ovum is known as a **zygote.** This is a time of very rapid change as the cells begin to **proliferate** (increase in number), **differentiate** (change into tissues and organs), and **integrate** (into systems).

EMBRYONIC PHASE

From the end of the zygote phase through the eighth week of pregnancy, the developing individual is known as an **embryo.**

The embryonic phase is a critical time, for it is during these weeks that development begins on all of the major structures of the body. Many of these key

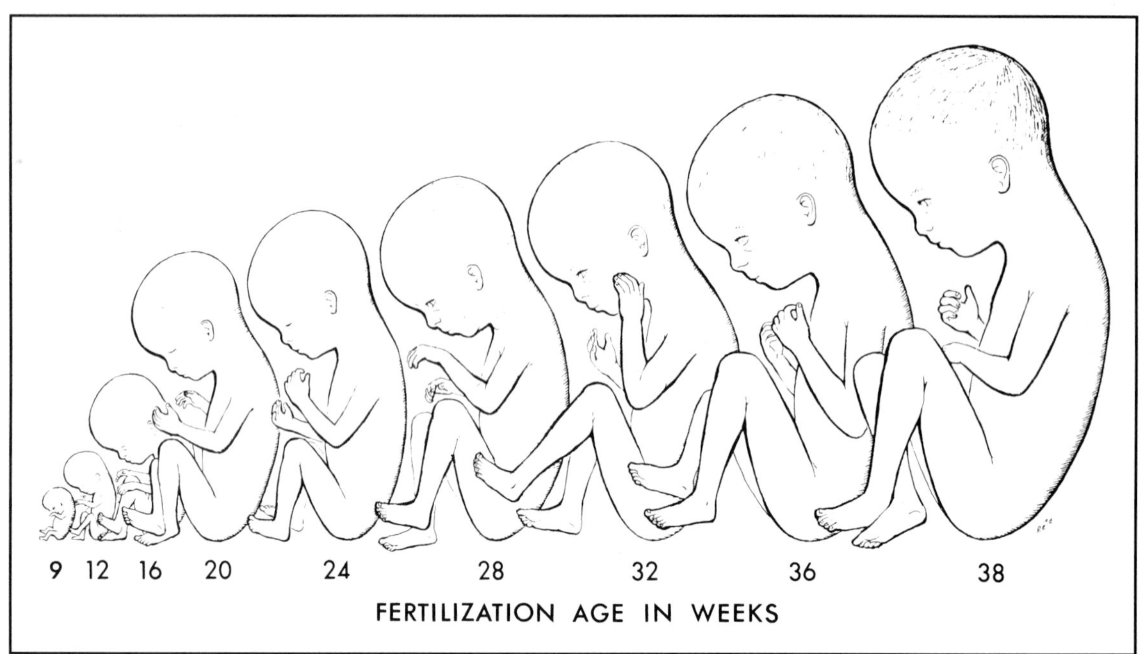

FIGURE 4–1

Diagram of fetuses showing fertilization age in weeks. Drawings are about one-fifth actual size. (From Moore, K.L.: The Developing Human: Clinically Oriented Embryology, 4th ed. Philadelphia, W.B. Saunders Co., 1988, p 87).

developments occur before the mother realizes she is pregnant.

FETAL PHASE

After the embryonic phase, the developing human is called a **fetus.** The fetal phase continues from the ninth week until birth. During the fetal phase, the body systems continue to develop and mature (Fig. 4–1).

Embryonic Development of the Face and Oral Cavity

PRIMARY EMBRYONIC LAYERS

During the third week of development, the cells of the embryo form the three primary embryonic layers: the **ectoderm, mesoderm,** and **endoderm** (Fig. 4–2).

The cells within each of these layers multiply and differentiate into the specialized cells needed to form the organs and tissues of the body.

Ectoderm. The ectoderm differentiates into skin (epidermis) and its accessories (subcutaneous glands, hair, and nails), structures of the nervous system, enamel of the teeth, and lining of the oral cavity. (Both the prefixes *ecto-* and *epi-* mean outside or outer.)

Mesoderm. The mesoderm differentiates into cartilage, bones, muscles, and connective tissues; kidneys and ducts; circulatory and reproductive systems; lining of the abdominal cavity; and the dentin, pulp, and

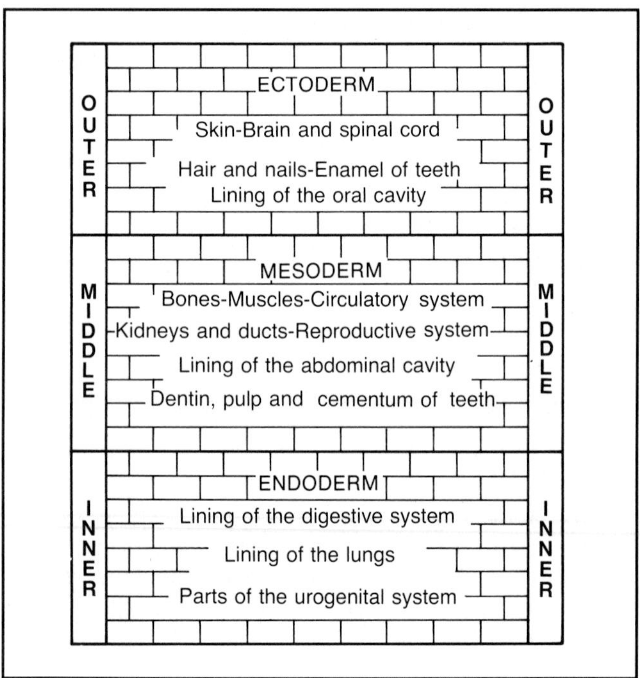

FIGURE 4–2

Schematic representation of the primary embryonic layers.

cementum of the teeth. (The prefix *meso-* means middle.)

Endoderm. The endoderm gives rise to the lining of digestive, respiratory, and urogenital systems. (The prefix *endo-* means inner.)

EARLY DEVELOPMENT OF THE MOUTH

In the fourth week, the **stomodeum,** or primitive mouth, and the primitive pharynx merge, and the stomodeum develops into part of the mouth.

By the beginning of the fifth week, the embryo is approximately 5 mm. in length. The heart is prominent and bulging, and the limbs are indicated (Fig. 4–3).

The site of the face is indicated from above by the region just in front of the bulging forebrain (future forehead) and from below by the first pair of branchial arches (future jaws).

BRANCHIAL ARCHES

By the end of the fourth week, six pairs of branchial arches have formed. The first two of these arches give rise to the structures of the head and neck.

First Branchial Arch. The first branchial arch, also known as the **mandibular arch,** contributes to the formation of the bones, muscles, and nerves of the face. It also forms the lower lip, the muscles of mastication, and the anterior portion of the alveolar process of the mandible.

Second Branchial Arch. The second branchial arch, also known as the **hyoid arch,** forms the styloid process, stapes of the ear, stylohyoid ligament, and a portion of the hyoid bone. It also forms the side and front of the neck, some of the facial muscles of facial expression, and part of the hyoid bone.

Other Branchial Arches. The third branchial arch forms the body of the hyoid and the posterior of the tongue. The fourth, fifth, and sixth arches form the structures of the lower throat, including the thyroid cartilage and muscles and the nerves of the pharynx and larynx.

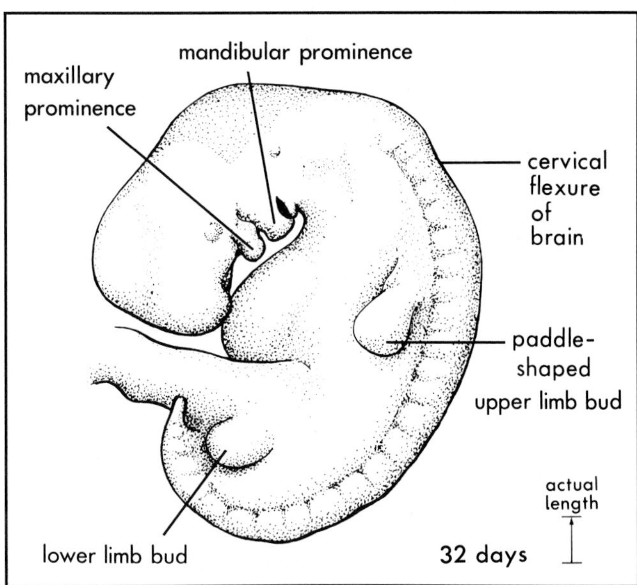

FIGURE 4–3

Diagram of a human embryo during the fifth week. (From Moore, K.L.: The Developing Human: Clinically Oriented Embryology, 4th ed. Philadelphia, W.B. Saunders Co., 1988, p 79).

DEVELOPMENT OF THE HARD AND SOFT PALATES

The hard and soft palates are formed from the union of the primary and secondary palates. Any disruption in the process may result in a cleft lip or cleft palate. These abnormalities and their treatment are discussed in Chapter 8.

Primary Palate. During the fifth and sixth weeks, the primary palate is formed by the union of the **medial nasal process** with the **lateral nasal processes.** The primary palate develops into the portion known as the **premaxilla,** which forms the upper lip and the anterior segment of the hard palate.

Secondary Palate. The secondary palate, which will become most of the hard and soft palates, is formed from folds that develop from the medial edge of the **maxillary processes** at the lateral portions of the oral roof. These folds are known as the **lateral palatine processes.**

Fusion of the Hard and Soft Palates. The **lateral palatine processes** begin to develop at 6 to 7 weeks and grow downward, almost vertically, on either side of the tongue (Fig. 4–4).

As the jaws and the neck develop, the mandible increases in size. This makes it possible for the tongue to move into a lower position below the lateral palatine processes.

During the seventh week, the lateral palatine processes elongate and move to a horizontal position above the tongue.

The processes approach each other and fuse in the midline. They also fuse with the primary palate and the nasal septum. This fusion makes a Y-shaped pattern in the roof of the mouth (Fig. 4–5).

This Y-shaped pattern is visible in the bony hard palate of an infant; however, the bones continue to fuse, and these lines are no longer visible on the adult hard palate.

Fusion usually begins anteriorly during the ninth week. By the twelfth week it is completed posteriorly in the region of the uvula.

In the posterior region, where there is no attachment to the nasal septum, the soft palate and uvula develop.

PRENATAL FACIAL DEVELOPMENT

The development of the human face occurs chiefly between the fifth and eighth weeks. The face develops primarily from the frontonasal process, which covers the forebrain, and the first branchial arch.

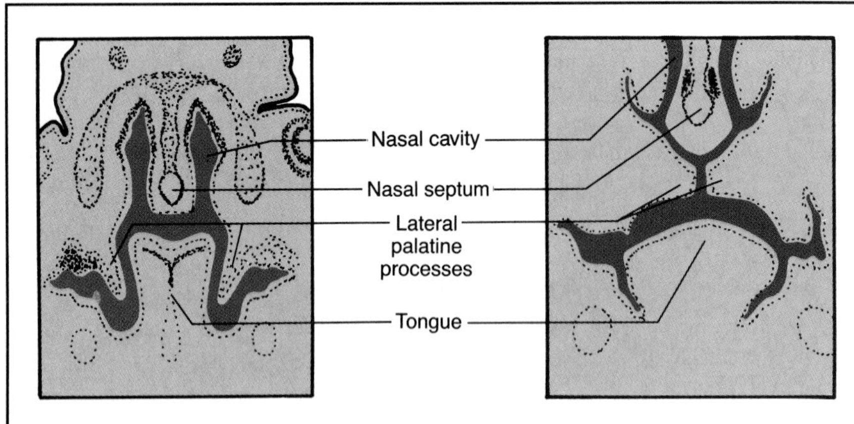

FIGURE 4–4

Formation of the human palate. The figure on the left shows the relationship of the tongue and palatine processes while the tongue is positioned between them. In the figure on the right, the tongue is lower and the palatine processes have moved upward and together to form the secondary palate. (Modified from Arey, L.B.: Developmental Anatomy, rev. 7th ed. Philadelphia, W.B. Saunders Co., 1974.)

The forward growth of the structures of the mouth produces striking age changes in the silhouette of the developing head.

- In the embryo at 1 month, the overhanging forehead is the dominant feature.
- During the second month, there is rapid growth of the nose and upper jaw, whereas the lower jaw appears to lag behind.
- In the third month, the fetus definitely resembles a human being, although the head is still disproportionately large.
- At four months, the face looks human, the hard and soft palates are differentiated, and formation of all the primary dentition has begun.
- During the last trimester, fat is laid down in the cheeks in what is known as "sucking pads." These give a healthy full-term fetus the characteristic rotund contour of the face.

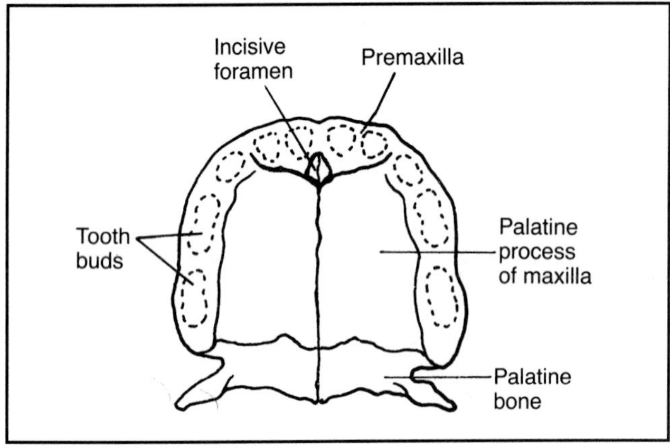

FIGURE 4–5

The bony basis of the hard palate, as shown on the skull of an infant.

PRENATAL DENTAL DEVELOPMENT

The earliest signs of tooth development are found in the anterior mandibular region, when the embryo is 5 to 6 weeks old.

Soon after this, tooth development begins in the anterior maxillary region and the process of tooth development progresses posteriorly in both jaws.

Within a short period of time, the development of all the primary teeth is started. By the seventeenth week, development has begun on the permanent teeth.

At birth, there are normally 44 teeth in various stages of development. Enamel formation is well under way on all primary dentition and may be just beginning on the permanent first molars.

Prenatal Influences on Dental Development

Prenatal dental development is influenced by both genetic and environmental factors.

Genetic Factors. The genetic factor of most common concern is that of tooth and jaw size. It is possible for a child to inherit large teeth from one parent and a small jaw from the other—or to inherit small teeth and a large jaw. A serious discrepancy (difference) in the size relationship of teeth and jaws may cause malocclusion as the child develops.

Less common genetic factors appear in the dentition as anomalies. (**Anomalies** are marked deviations from the normal standards, and these are discussed in Chapter 11.)

Environmental Factors. In the prenatal state, the mother's body provides the environment. Good maternal health and nutrition throughout the pregnancy are essential because those factors that affect the mother's body and health also influence the developing child.

Good nutrition *before* pregnancy helps carry mother and child through the first weeks, which are so critical for the developing child and yet are also the time when morning sickness affects many expectant mothers.

During the pregnancy, fever and disease in the mother will leave their marks in the developing teeth of the fetus.

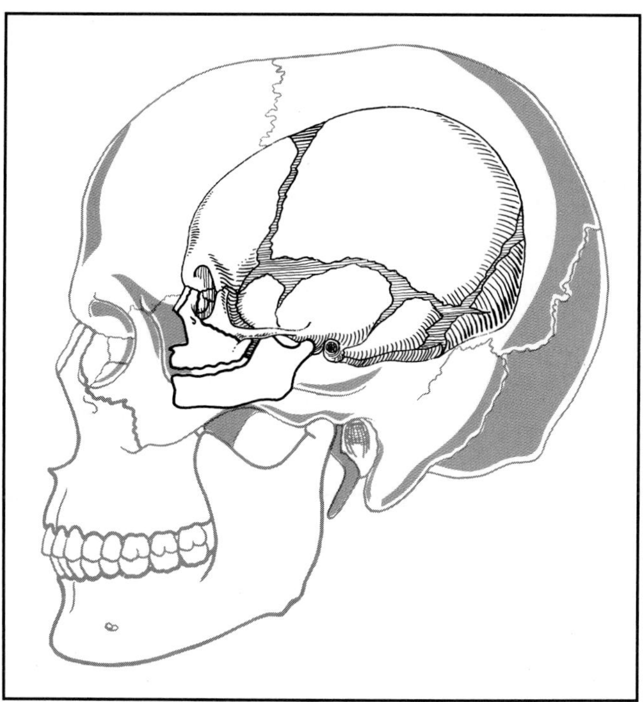

FIGURE 4–6

Growth of the mandible and the maxilla from birth to maturity.

Drugs taken during pregnancy may cause birth defects. Such drugs include prescribed medication, over-the-counter remedies such as aspirin and cold tablets, and abused drugs including alcohol.

Antibiotics, particularly tetracyclines, taken during pregnancy may result in a yellow-gray-brownish stain on the primary teeth. (This is discussed in Chapter 20.)

The mother's dental health is also of concern. Toxins from a dental infection may be dangerous to both mother and child. In addition, a sore mouth limits the nutritional intake of the mother.

Postnatal Facial Development

MODELING AND REMODELING IN FACIAL GROWTH

As shown in Figures 4–6 to 4–8, there is considerable change in the shape of the face from that of the newborn to that of an adult.

After the immediate postnatal period, most facial growth takes place in predictable *growth spurts*, which occur during youth and early adolescence.

It is impossible to derive these "adult bones" by the simple process of uniform, overall growth of the bones present in the face of the newborn. Instead, these bones grow and are reshaped to achieve normal growth and development of the face.

This process involves laying down of new bone in some areas and removal of existing bone from others.

Deposition

Deposition, also known as *apposition,* is the process of laying down new bone. **Osteoblasts** are the cells responsible for new bone formation.

The healing of a fractured bone is one example of new bone formation. Another example is the creation of new bone to fill the socket left after a tooth has been extracted.

Resorption

Resorption is the removal of existing bone by the body. **Osteoclasts** are the cells responsible for this process in which bones cells are resorbed (taken away) by the body.

The loss of the roots of primary teeth is one example of resorption. Another example is the loss of bone from the alveolar ridge after teeth have been extracted.

Modeling

Modeling, which is also known as *displacement,* describes the bone changes that occur along the articulations (joints) of the bones as they increase in size and/or shape to keep up with the growth of the surrounding tissues.

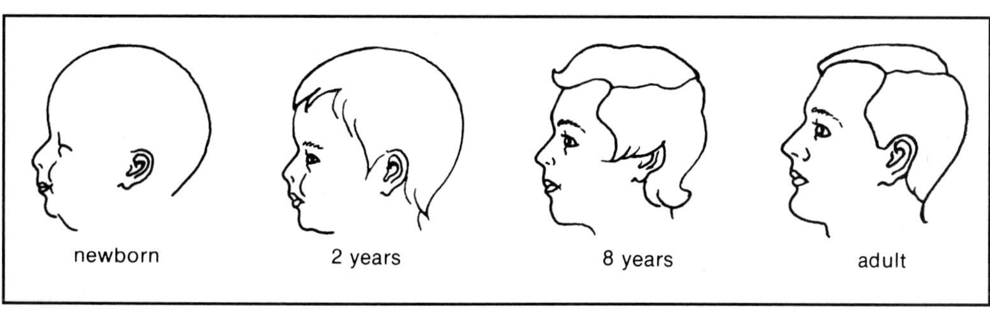

FIGURE 4–7

Age changes in the contours of the face from birth to adulthood.

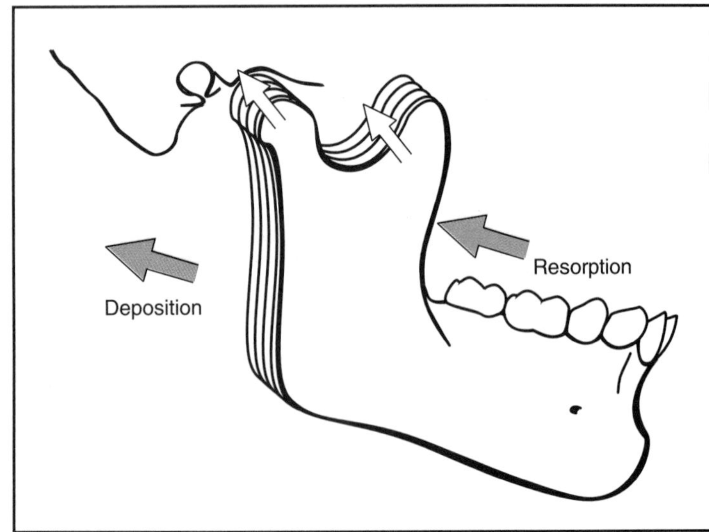

FIGURE 4–8

The mandible grows by displacement, resorption, and deposition. Notice how space is created to accommodate the third molar. (From Sarnat, B.G., and Laskin, D.M.: The Temporomandibular Joint, 4th ed. Philadelphia, W.B. Saunders Co., 1992, p 49.)

Remodeling

Remodeling describes the growth and changes in shape of existing bone. As shown in Figure 4–8, both modeling and remodeling involve the deposition and resorption of bone.

Remodeling in Tooth Movement

Remodeling occurs in response to forces placed on the tooth within its socket. When a missing tooth is not replaced, these forces occur on the adjacent teeth because they have lost part of their support. (This is discussed in Chapter 5.)

These forces are intentionally created as during orthodontic treatment as appliances are used to move the tooth in the desired direction (Fig. 4–9).

When a tooth moves, bone must be resorbed (removed) from the bony socket to make room for the advancing tooth. (As a tooth moves lingually, resorption occurs on the lingual side.)

Deposition takes place on the opposite side of the bony socket, to fill in the space from which the tooth has moved. (As the tooth moves lingually, deposition takes place on the facial side.)

In this way, the width of the space between the socket and the root of the tooth is kept about the same and the tooth remains stable in the jaw. If movement is too rapid, or if resorption and apposition do not occur properly, the tooth becomes loose and may be lost.

POSTNATAL MAXILLARY GROWTH

1. The palate grows downward from its original postnatal position by the deposition and resorption of bone in the nasal area.
2. As the teeth erupt, the height of the alveolar process of the maxilla increases, and this gives added depth to the vault of the palate.
3. Change in the size of the palate is made possible by growth, distally (toward the back) and laterally (toward the side), as it extends toward the pterygoid process.
4. The major growth sites of the maxilla are in the body of the bone itself and at the sutures (frontomaxillary, zygomaticomaxillary, and transverse) and processes (alveolar, orbital, frontal, and palatal).
5. As maturation proceeds, depositional growth continues in the tuberosity area, and general internal reorganization is apparent throughout the maxillary body.
6. During this time, the maxilla and face grow downward and outward. The maxillary sinuses continue to enlarge by resorption.

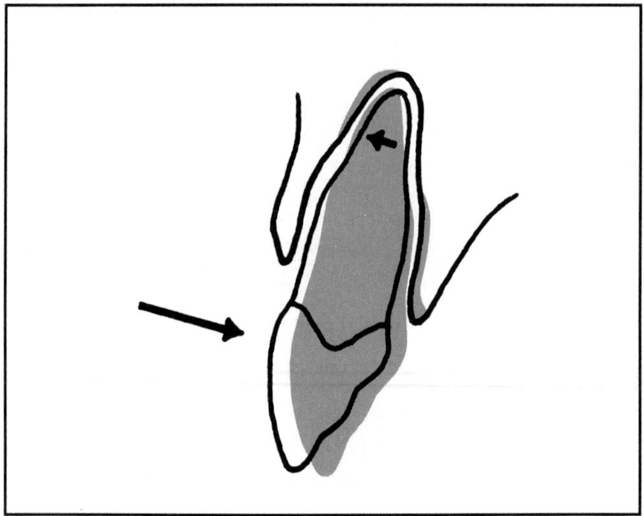

FIGURE 4–9

Movement of a tooth in a lingual direction. The shaded area of bone indicates resportion. The shaded tooth indicates its new position.

POSTNATAL MANDIBULAR GROWTH

1. The mandible grows without adding noticeable width at the anterior border.
2. It develops in a modified V-form by additions on the inner surface and ends of the original bony structure.
3. The angulation of the condyle increases as the newborn grows to adulthood.
4. The alveolus grows upward, outward, and forward as the teeth erupt into their functional positions.
5. There is a slight increase in the size of the inferior border of the mandible in comparison to its increase in height.
6. The ramus grows by deposition of bone on the superior surface and at the condyle.
7. There is slight resorption at the sigmoid notch, the retromolar area, and the internal angle of the ramus.

Life Cycle of a Tooth

During formation, most organs go through one or two developmental processes. For example: the liver grows (one developmental process); bone grows and calcifies (hardens) (two developmental processes).

During **odontogenesis,** which means tooth formation, each tooth must go through three developmental processes. For teaching purposes, these processes are divided into the **growth, calcification,** and **eruption** periods. In reality, these processes overlap considerably and often occur at the same time.

Growth

The growth period may be divided into three stages (Fig. 4–10). These are

- **The bud stage,** also known as *initiation,* in which formation of the tooth begins.
- **The cap stage,** also known as *proliferation,* in which the cells of the developing tooth increase.
- **The bell stage,** also known as *histodifferentiation* and *morphodifferentiation,* in which the different tissues of the tooth form and its shape are established.

BUD STAGE

The bud stage is the beginning of development for each tooth. This stage follows a definite pattern, and it takes place at a different time for each type of tooth.

Initiation starts with the formation of the **dental lamina,** which is a thickened band of oral epithelium that follows the curve of each developing dental arch.

Almost as soon as the dental lamina is formed, it produces 10 enlargements in each arch. These are the **tooth buds** for the primary teeth.

The permanent teeth develop similarly. The dental lamina continues to grow posteriorly to produce tooth buds for the three permanent molars, which will develop distal to the primary teeth on each quadrant.

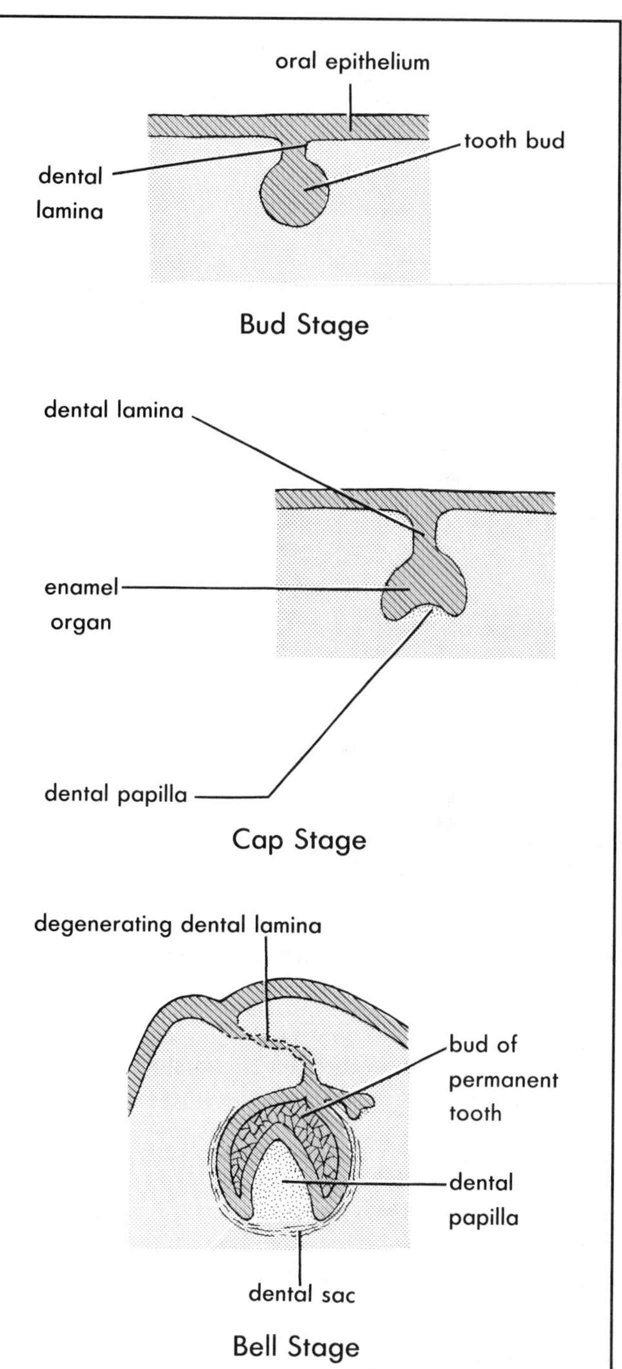

FIGURE 4–10

Schematic representation of the developmental stages of a tooth. (Modified from Moore, K.L.: The Developing Human: Clinically Oriented Embryology, 5th ed. Philadelphia, W.B. Saunders Co., 1993, p 451.)

The tooth bud for the first permanent molar forms at about the seventeenth week of fetal life; the tooth buds for the second molars form about 6 months after birth; and those of the third molars form at about 5 years of age.

The **succedaneous teeth,** which are those permanent teeth that replace the primary teeth, develop from tooth buds in the deep portion of the dental lamina on the lingual side of the primary teeth. These begin to form as early as 24 weeks.

CAP STAGE

During the cap stage, the cells of the tooth grow and increase in number. This growth causes regular changes in size and proportion of the developing tooth, and the solid-looking tooth bud changes into a hollowed caplike shape.

The primary embryonic ectoderm layer, which has differentiated into **oral epithelium,** becomes the **enamel organ,** which will eventually form the enamel of the developing tooth.

The primary embryonic mesoderm layer, now differentiated into connective tissue known as **mesenchyme,** becomes the **dental papilla,** which will form the pulp and dentin of the tooth.

As the enamel organ and dental papilla of the tooth develop, the mesenchyme surrounding them condenses to form a capsule-like structure called the **dental sac.** This will give rise to the cementum and the periodontal ligament.

BELL STAGE

During the bell stage, the cells differentiate and become specialized. This process is called histodifferentiation.

- The epithelial cells become **ameloblasts,** which are the enamel-forming cells.
- The peripheral cells of the dental papilla become **odontoblasts,** which are the dentin-forming cells.
- The inner cells of the dental sac differentiate into **cementoblasts,** which are cementum-forming cells.

As the tooth continues to develop, the dental organ continues to change. It assumes a shape described as resembling a bell. As these developments take place, the dental lamina, which has thus far connected the dental organ to the oral epithelium, breaks up.

The basic shape and relative size of each tooth are established during the process of morphodifferentiation.

Here the dentinoenamel junction and the cementodentinal junction are formed and act as a blueprint for the developing tooth.

In accordance with this pattern, the ameloblasts deposit enamel and the odontoblasts deposit dentin to give the completed tooth its characteristic shape and size.

This process starts at the top of the tooth and moves downward toward the future root. The development of the root, or roots, begins after the enamel and dentin formation have reached the future cementoenamel junction.

As part of this process, the inner cells of the dental sac differentiate into cementoblasts, which produce the cementum to cover the developing root.

Calcification

Calcification is the process by which the structural outline formed during the growth stage is hardened by the deposit of calcium or other mineral salts.

The enamel is built layer by layer by the ameloblasts working outward from the dentinoenamel junction, starting at the top of the crown of each tooth and spreading downward over its sides.

PITS AND FISSURES

If the tooth has several cusps, a cap of enamel forms over each cusp. As growth continues, the cusps eventually coalesce to form a solid enamel covering for the occlusal surface of the tooth. (**Coalesce** means to fuse together.)

Pits and fissures may be formed during this process. A **fissure** is a fault along a developmental groove on the occlusal surface that is caused by incomplete or imperfect joining of the lobes during the formation of the tooth. A **pit** results when two developmental grooves cross each other, forming a deep area that is too small for the bristle of a toothbrush to clean.

The enamel here may be particularly thin, and these areas are often inaccessible for cleaning and are thus sites where decay frequently begins.

Eruption

A tooth may successfully pass through the previous stages and still be unable to function if it is unable to erupt into its normal position.

Eruption is the movement of the tooth into its functional position in the oral cavity. This process can be divided into prefunctional and functional phases.

The **prefunctional phase** of eruption begins with the formation of the root. It involves the journey of the tooth through bone and the oral mucosa as it moves toward its position in the dental arch. The prefunctional phase is completed when the tooth reaches the occlusal plane (Fig. 4–11).

During the **functional phase,** the tooth continues to move into a proper relationship to the jaw and to the other teeth. This is an ongoing process so that the tooth can maintain its position despite attrition (very gradual wearing away of the enamel of the crown) and

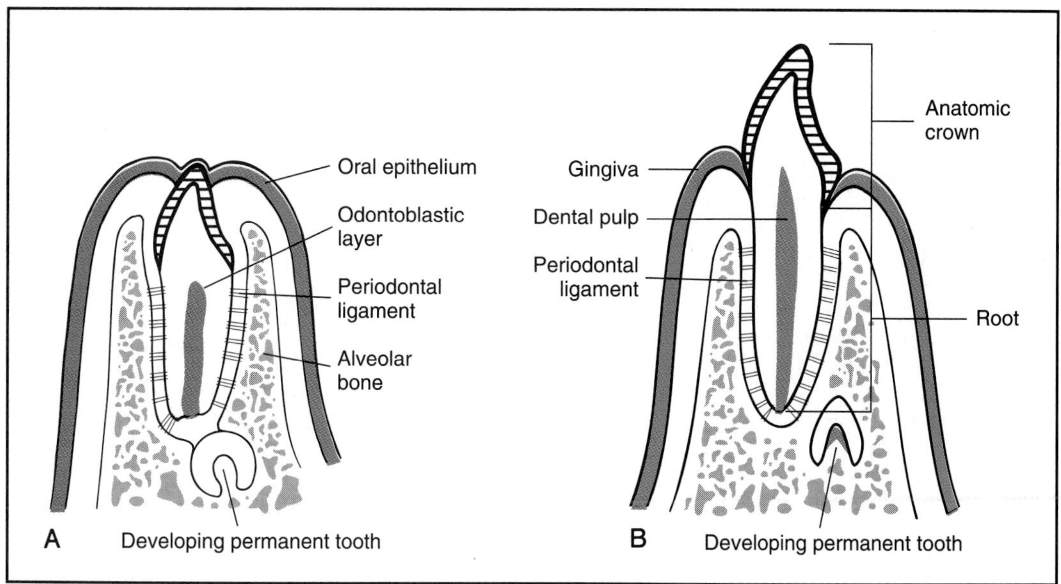

FIGURE 4–11

Eruption of a primary incisor. *A*, The pre-eruption phase; *B*, the functional phases. (Modified from Moore, K.L.: The Developing Human: Clinically Oriented Embryology, 4th ed. Philadelphia, W.B. Saunders Co., 1988, p 429.)

other changes that may occur in the surrounding tissues.

Figures 4–12 and 4–13 show the normal ages for the eruption and exfoliation of the primary and permanent teeth.

EXFOLIATION

Exfoliation is the normal process by which the primary teeth are shed to make way for the permanent dentition.

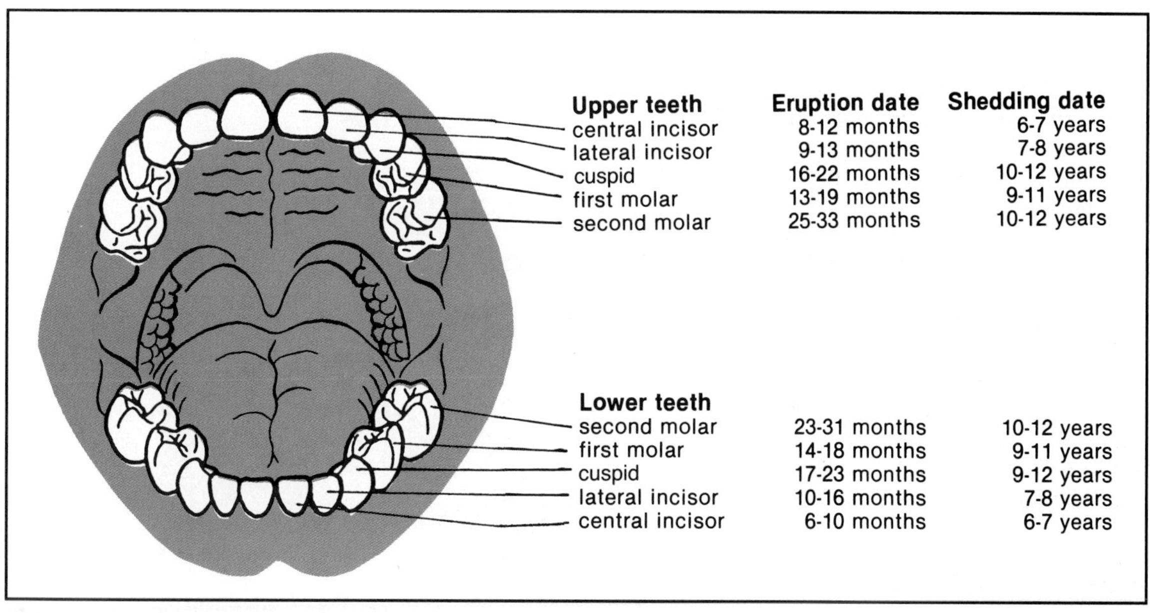

Upper teeth
central incisor
lateral incisor
cuspid
first molar
second molar
Eruption date
8-12 months
9-13 months
16-22 months
13-19 months
25-33 months
Shedding date
6-7 years
7-8 years
10-12 years
9-11 years
10-12 years
Lower teeth
second molar
first molar
cuspid
lateral incisor
central incisor
23-31 months
14-18 months
17-23 months
10-16 months
6-10 months
10-12 years
9-11 years
9-12 years
7-8 years
6-7 years

FIGURE 4–12

Normal eruption and exfoliation ages for the primary teeth.

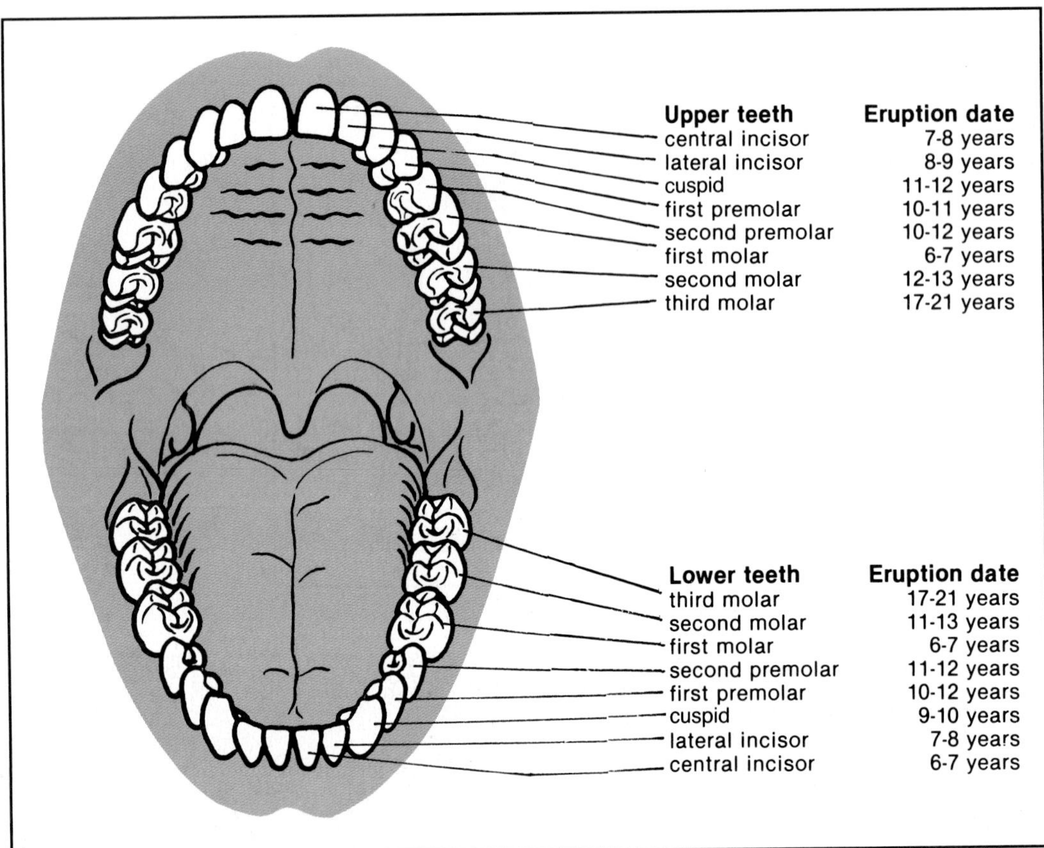

FIGURE 4–13

Normal eruption ages for the permanent teeth.

When it is time for a primary tooth to be lost, osteoclasts cause the resorption of the root, beginning at the apex and continuing in the direction of the crown. Eventually the crown of the tooth is lost because of lack of support.

At first, pressure is directed against the bone separating the primary tooth and its permanent successor. Later, pressure is directed against the root surface of the primary tooth itself. In this manner, the permanent tooth aids in the removal of its predecessor.

The resorption of the roots of the primary incisors and cuspids starts on the lingual surface in the apical third, and the movement of the permanent tooth at this time proceeds in an occlusal and facial direction.

The buds of the developing premolars are located between the roots of the primary molars. Pressure from these developing teeth causes resorption of the roots of the primary molars beginning on the root surfaces nearest the developing teeth.

Throughout this process, the primary tooth serves as a guide for the developing tooth; also, its crown preserves the space needed by the succedaneous permanent tooth (Fig. 4–14).

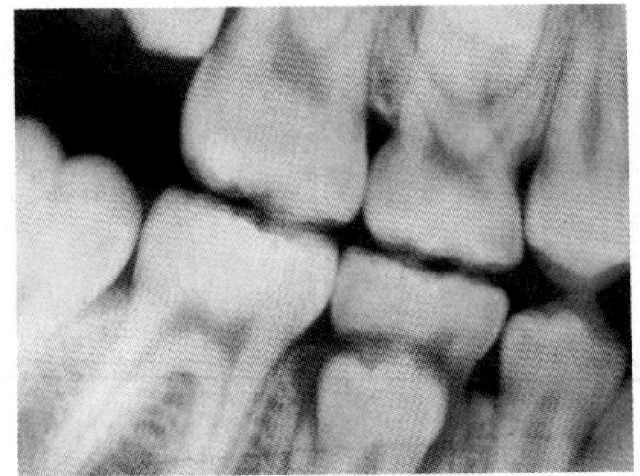

FIGURE 4–14

Radiograph showing normal resorption of the roots of a mandibular primary molar before its being shed. The permanent second premolar is in place waiting to erupt. (From Haring, J.I., and Lind, L.J.: Radiographic Interpretation for the Dental Hygienist. Philadelphia, W.B. Saunders, 1993, p 145.)

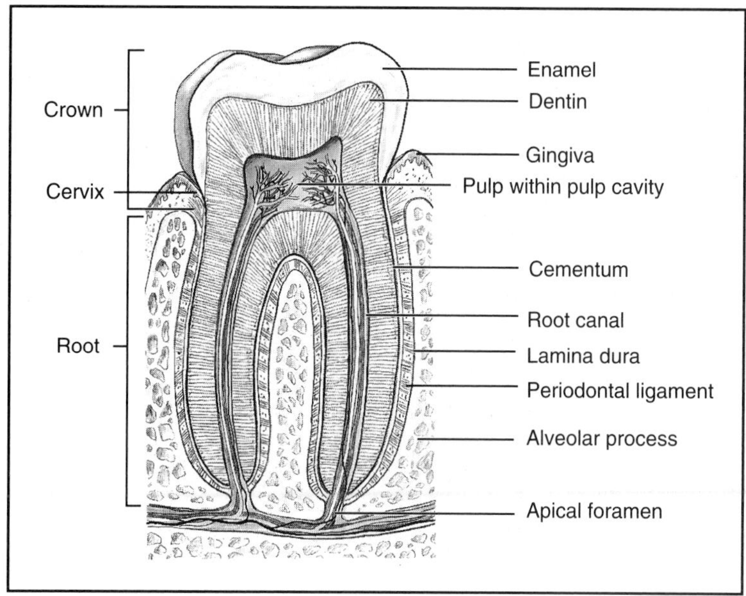

FIGURE 4–15

Tissues of the tooth and surrounding structures. (From Applegate, E.J.: The Anatomy and Physiology Learning System Textbook. Philadelphia, W.B. Saunders Co., 1994.)

Oral Histology

Oral histology includes the study of the tissues of the teeth, the periodontium, and the surrounding oral mucosa (Figs. 4–15 and 4–16).

Anatomic Parts of the Tooth

Each tooth consists of a crown and one or more roots. The size and shape of the crown, and the size and number of roots, vary according to the of type tooth. (The types of teeth are discussed in Chapter 6.)

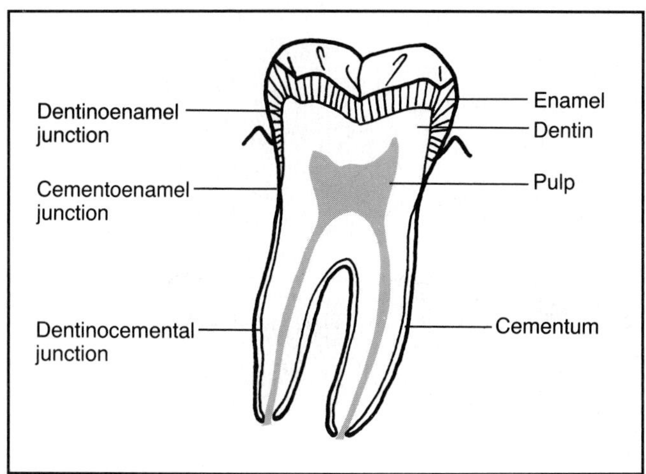

FIGURE 4–16

Tissues of the tooth and their junctions.

CROWN

The **anatomic crown** is that portion of the tooth covered with enamel (Fig. 4–17). The anatomic crown remains constant throughout the life of the tooth.

The **clinical crown** is the portion of the tooth that is visible in the mouth. The clinical crown may vary during the life cycle of the tooth as the tooth erupts into position and again as the surrounding tissues recede.

ROOT

The root of the tooth is that portion normally embedded in the alveolar process and covered with cementum.

Depending upon the type of tooth, the root may have one, two, or three roots. **Bifurcation** means division into two roots. **Trifurcation** means division into three roots.

The tapered end of each root tip is known as the **apex.** Anything that is situated at the apex is said to be **apical.** Anything surrounding the apex is **periapical.**

CERVIX

The cervix is the narrow area of the tooth where the crown and root meet. (The term *cervix* means neck.)

The **cementoenamel junction**, also known as the *cervical line* or the CEJ, is formed by the junction of the enamel of the crown and the cementum of the root.

Tissues of the Tooth

ENAMEL

Enamel, which makes up the anatomic crown of the tooth, is the hardest material of the body. This hard-

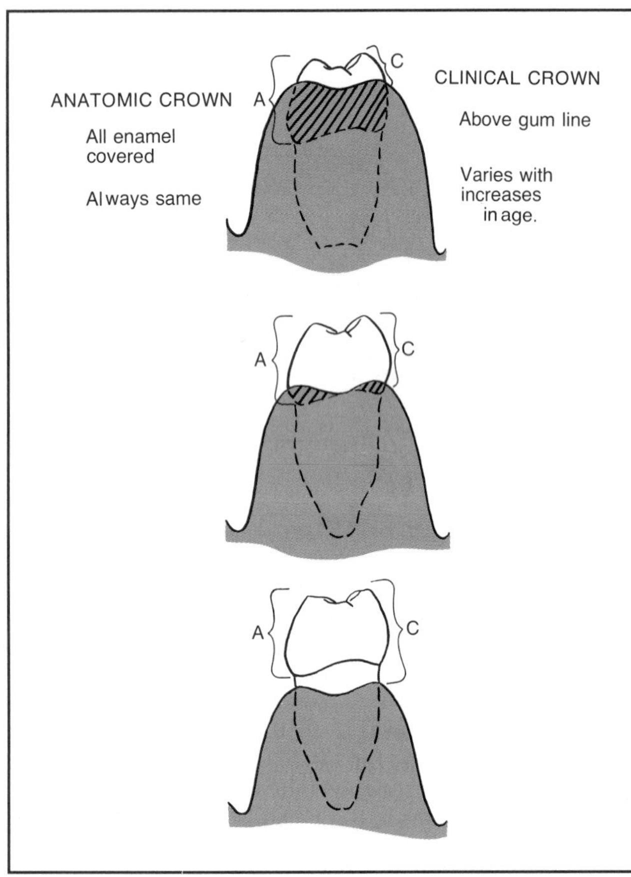

FIGURE 4–17

During the life cycle of the tooth, the anatomic crown remains the same; however, the clinical crown may change at different stages of eruption.

ness is important because enamel forms the protective covering for the softer underlying dentin. It also provides a strong surface for crushing, grinding, and chewing food.

Enamel is able to withstand crushing stresses to about 100,000 pounds per square inch. Although enamel is strong, it is also very brittle, and this brittleness may cause the enamel to fracture or chip. However, the combination of its strength, the cushioning effect of the dentin, and the suspensory action of the periodontium enable enamel to withstand most of the pressures brought against it.

Enamel is translucent and ranges in color from yellowish- to grayish-white. (**Translucent** means that the substance allows some light to pass through it.) These variations in shade are caused by differences in the thickness and translucency of the enamel and in the color of the dentin beneath it.

Structure of Enamel. Enamel, which is formed by ameloblasts, consists of 96 to 99 percent inorganic matter and only 1 to 4 percent organic matrix. **Hydroxyapatite,** which consists primarily of calcium, is the largest mineral component.

Enamel is similar to bone in its hardness and mineral content. However, unlike bone, mature enamel does not contain cells that are capable of remodeling and repair. Nevertheless, some remineralization is possible, and this is discussed in Chapter 6.

Enamel is composed of millions of calcified enamel **prisms,** which are also known as *enamel rods.* These extend from the surface of the tooth to the dentinoenamel junction.

The enamel prisms tend to be grouped into rows organized around the circumference of the long axis of the tooth. The prisms within each row follow a course that is roughly perpendicular to the surface of the tooth.

This organization into rows is clinically important because enamel tends to fracture along the interfacial planes of adjacent groups of prisms.

The diameter of a prism is approximately 5 to 8 microns, depending on its location. In cross-section, the prisms appear to be keyhole-shaped structures consisting of a head and a tail (Fig. 4–18).

Each prism appears to be encased in a **prism sheath,** and the sheathed prisms seem to be held together by an **interprismatic substance,** which is also known as *inter-rod substance.*

All of these structures are hard; of the three, however, the prisms are the hardest and the interprismatic substance is the weakest. These differences make it possible to "acid etch" the teeth for the direct bonding of restorative materials.

Hunter-Schreger bands, which microscopically appear as alternating light and dark bands in the enamel, are caused by the intertwining or changing directions of the enamel prisms.

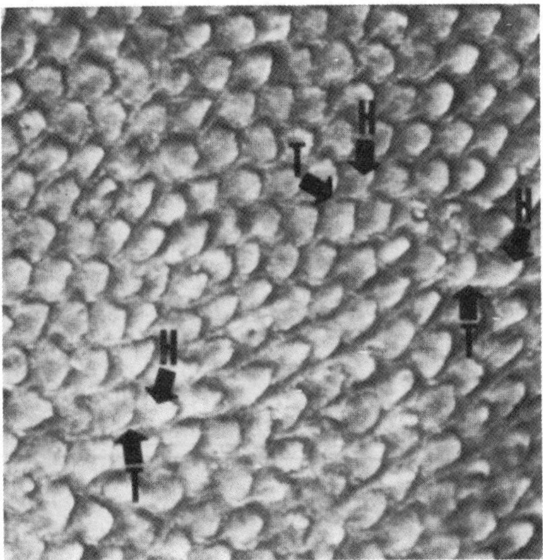

FIGURE 4–18

Scanning electron micrograph of human enamel prisms. Both the head (H) and the tail (T) of the prisms can be seen. (From Davis, W.L.: Oral Histology: Cell Structure and Function. Philadelphia, W.B. Saunders Co., 1986, p 103.)

The **striae of Retzius,** also known as the *strips of Retzius*, are incremental rings, like the growth rings of a tree, representing variations in the deposition of the enamel matrix during the formation of the tooth. Enamel produced prenatally contains only a few of these incremental lines; however, the shock of birth is registered as a ring known as the **neonatal line.**

Enamel tufts start at the dentinoenamel junction and may extend to the inner third of the enamel. They are so named because under a microscope they have the appearance of tufts of grass.

Enamel tufts are the hypocalcified or uncalcified ends of groups of enamel prisms.

Enamel lamellae are thin, leaflike structures that extend from the enamel surface toward the dentinoenamel junction. These consist of organic material with little mineral content. (*Lamellae* is plural. The singular is *lamella.*)

Enamel spindles are the ends of odontoblasts (dentin-forming cells) that extend across the dentinoenamel junction a short distance into the enamel.

DENTIN

Dentin makes up the main portion of the tooth structure and extends almost the entire length of the tooth. It is covered by enamel on the crown and by cementum on the root.

In the primary teeth, dentin is very light yellow. In the permanent teeth, it is light yellow and somewhat transparent. The color may darken with age.

Structure of Dentin. Dentin is a mineralized tissue that is harder than bone and cementum, but not as hard as enamel. Although hard, dentin has elastic properties that are important in the support of enamel, which is brittle.

Dentin is composed of 70 percent inorganic material and 30 percent organic matter and water. The rapid penetration and spreading of the caries in dentin are caused, in part, by its high content of organic substances.

Dentin is formed by the **odontoblasts,** beginning at growth centers along the dentinoenamel junction and proceeding inward toward what will become the pulp chamber of the tooth.

The internal surface of the dentin forms the walls of the pulp cavity. The odontoblasts line these walls, and from here they continue to form and repair the dentin.

Dentin is penetrated through its entire thickness by microscopic canals called **dentinal tubules** (Fig. 4–19). In coronal dentin, these tubules follow an S-shaped curve from the dentinoenamel junction toward the pulp.

Each dentinal tubule contains a **dentinal fiber.** Each fiber, also known as an *odontoblastic process*, is the living filamentous process from an odontoblast in the pulp chamber.

These fibers, which terminate in a branching network at the junction with the enamel or cementum, transmit pain stimuli and make dentin an excellent thermal conductor.

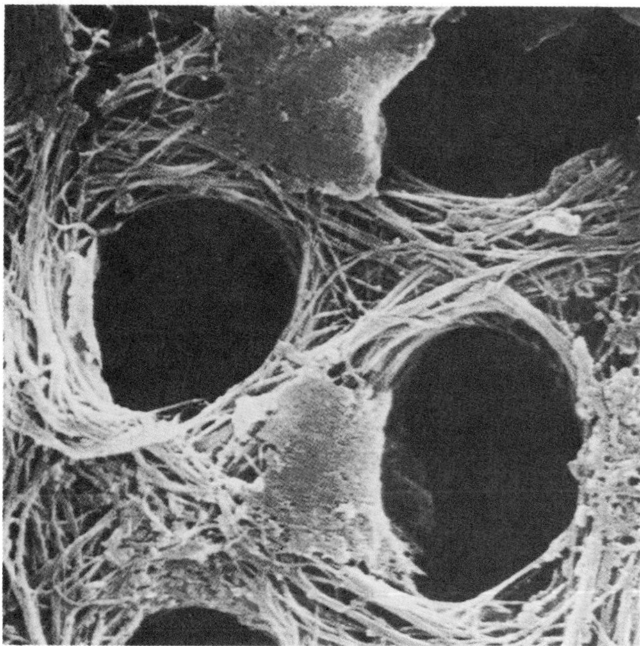

FIGURE 4–19

A micrograph of dentinal tubules (the black areas). This micrograph was produced through the use of a scanning electron microscope. Magnification is 12,000×. (Courtesy of Dr. Donald J. Scales and Anthony J. Piazza, University of Pacific, School of Dentistry, San Francisco.)

Because of the dentinal fibers within the dentin, it is considered to be a living tissue. During operative procedures, dentin must be protected from dehydration and thermal shock. When 1 mm. of dentin is exposed, about 30,000 dentinal fibers are exposed, and thus 30,000 living cells may be damaged.

Because it is capable of continued growth and repair, there are three major types of dentin.

- **Primary dentin,** which is formed before eruption, forms the bulk of the tooth.
- **Secondary dentin** begins formation after eruption and continues at a very slow rate throughout the life of the tooth. This results in the gradual narrowing of the pulp chamber.
- **Tertiary dentin,** also known as *reparative dentin,* is formed in response to irritation and appears as a localized deposit on the wall of the pulp chamber. This may occur in response to attrition, erosion, dental caries, dental treatment, or other irritants.

CEMENTUM

Cementum covers the root of the tooth. It overlies the dentin and joins the enamel at the cementoenamel junction (CEJ).

A primary function of cementum is to anchor the tooth to the bony socket by means of attachment fibers within the periodontium.

Cementum is light yellow and is easily distinguishable from enamel by its lack of luster and its darker hue. It is somewhat lighter in color than dentin.

Structure of Cementum. Cementum, which is formed by **cementoblasts,** is approximately to 50 to 60 percent organic material and is not quite as hard as dentin or bone.

Unlike bone, cementum does not resorb and form again. This difference is important because it makes orthodontic treatment possible. However, cementum is capable of some repair by the deposition of new layers.

As the root develops, **primary cementum,** also known as *acellular cementum,* is formed outward from the cementodentin junction for the full length of the root.

After the tooth has reached functional occlusion, **secondary cementum,** also known as *cellular cementum,* continues to form on the apical half of the root.

As a result, the cervical half of the root is covered with a thin layer of primary cementum and the apical half of the root has a thickened cementum covering.

This continued growth in the apical area aids in maintaining the total length of the tooth by compensating for the enamel lost by attrition.

PULP

The inner aspect of the dentin forms the boundaries of the **pulp chamber** (Fig. 4–20). As with the dentin surrounding it, the contours of the pulp chamber follow the contours of the exterior surface of the tooth.

At the time of eruption, the pulp chamber is large; however, because of the continuous deposition of dentin, it becomes smaller with age.

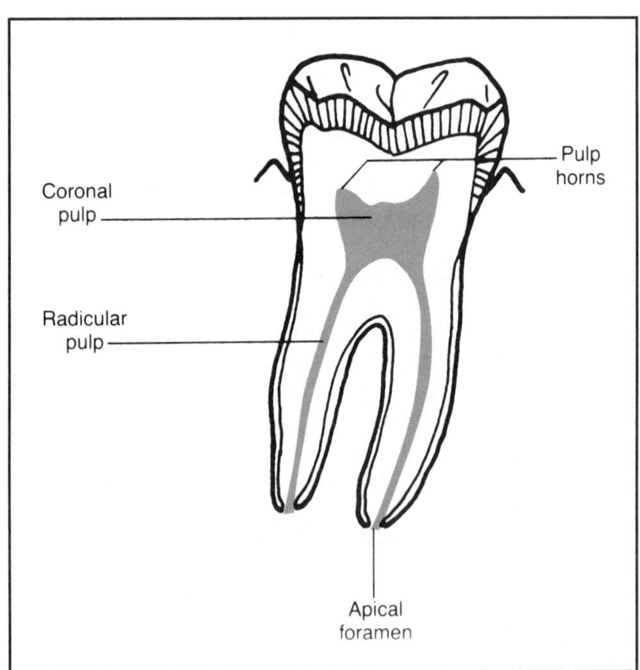

FIGURE 4–20

The dental pulp. (Mandibular first molar in cross-section.)

The part of the pulp that lies within the crown portion of the tooth is called the **coronal pulp.** This includes the **pulp horns,** which are extensions of the pulp that project toward the cusp tips and incisal edges.

The other portion of the pulp is more apically located and is referred to as the **radicular** or **root pulp.** During the development of the root, the continued deposition of dentin causes this area to become longer and narrower.

The radicular pulp of each root is continuous with the tissues of the periapical area via an **apical foramen.**

In young teeth, the apical foramen is not yet fully formed and this opening is wide. However, with increasing age and exposure of the tooth to functional stress, secondary dentin decreases the diameter of the pulp chamber and the apical foramen.

Structure of the Pulp. The pulp is made up of blood vessels and nerves that enter the pulp chamber through the apical foramen. The blood supply is derived from branches of the dental arteries and from the periodontal ligament.

The pulp also contains connective tissue, which consists of cells, intercellular substance, and tissue fluid. **Fibroblasts,** one type of cell contained here, are responsible for the formation of the intercellular substance of the pulp.

The tissue fluid interchange between the pulp and dentin serves the important functions of keeping these tissues supplied with moisture and nutrients.

This generous blood supply also has an important defense function in responding to a bacterial invasion of the tooth.

The nerve supply of the pulp receives and transmits pain stimuli. When the stimulus is weak, the response by the pulpal system is weak, and the interaction goes unnoticed. When the stimulus is great, the reaction is stronger, and pain quickly calls attention to the threatened condition of the tooth.

Periodontium

The periodontium consists of the tissues that surround and support the teeth. These tissues also protect and nourish the teeth. The periodontium is divided into two major units: the **attachment apparatus** and the **gingival unit.**

Attachment Apparatus

The attachment apparatus consists of the **cementum,** the **alveolar process,** and the **periodontal ligament** (Fig. 4–21). These tissues work together to support, maintain, and retain the tooth in its functional position within the jaw.

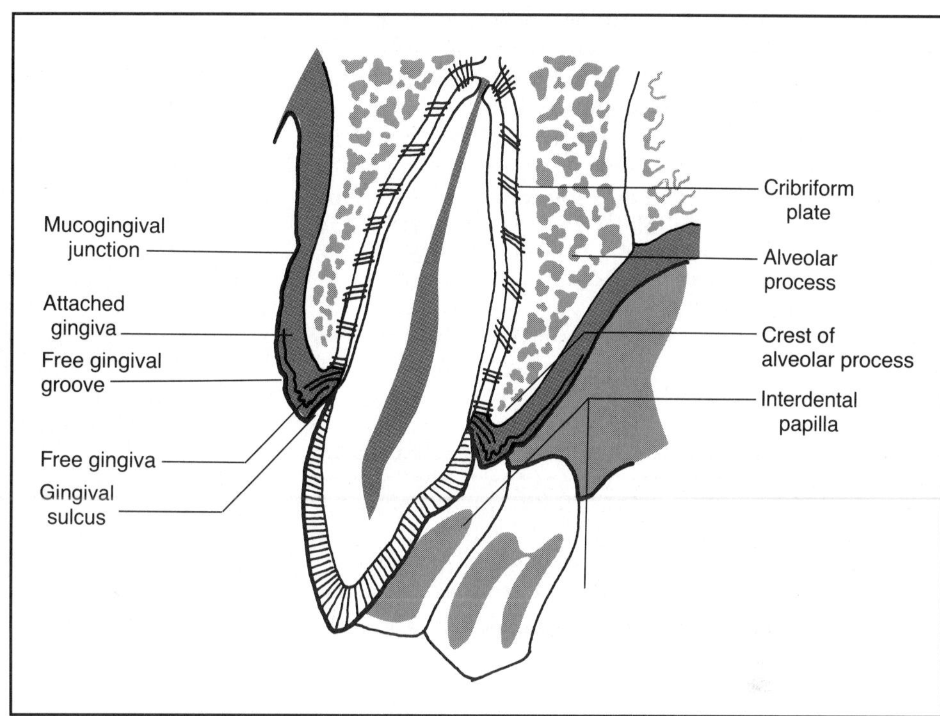

FIGURE 4–21

Anterior teeth and their supporting tissues.

CEMENTUM

Cementum is discussed earlier in the section "Tissues of the Tooth."

ALVEOLAR PROCESS

The alveolar processes are the extensions of the bone of the body of the mandible and the maxilla that support the teeth in their functional positions in the jaws.

Osteoblasts are responsible for the formation of this bone, and **osteoclasts** are responsible for resorption and remodeling of the bone.

The formation and maintenance of the alveolar processes appear to occur in response to the presence or absence of the teeth. The alveolar process develops in response to the growth of the developing teeth. After teeth have been lost, bone of the alveolar process is resorbed, and the ridge decreases in size and changes in shape.

Cortical Plate. The cortical plate of bone is the dense outer covering of the spongy bone that makes up the central part of the alveolar process. The cortical plate provides strength and protection and serves as a site of attachment for skeletal muscles.

The cortical plate of the mandible is denser than that of the maxilla and has fewer openings for the passage of nerves and vessels. This structural difference affects the technique of injection for local anesthetic.

Alveolar Crest. The alveolar crest is the highest point of the alveolar ridge. Here alveolar bone fuses with the cortical plates on the facial and lingual sides of the crest of the alveolar process.

In a healthy mouth, the distance between the cementoenamel junction and the alveolar crest is fairly constant (Fig. 4–22).

Alveolar Socket. The alveolar socket is the cavity within the alveolar process that surrounds the root of a tooth. The tooth does not actually contact the bone here. Instead, it is suspended in place within the socket by the periodontal ligament.

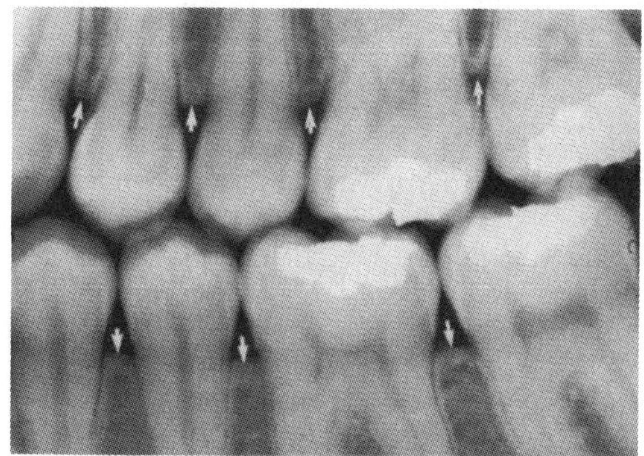

FIGURE 4–22

The alveolar crest as it appears in a radiograph. Arrows indicate the crest. The lamina dura is the white line surrounding the tooth. (From Haring, J.I., and Lind, L.J.: Radiographic Interpretation for the Dental Hygienist. Philadelphia, W.B. Saunders Co., 1993, p 55.)

The bony projection separating one socket from another is called the **interdental septum.**

The bone separating the roots of a multirooted tooth is called the **interradicular septum.**

Lamina Dura. The lamina dura, also known as the *cribriform plate,* is thin, compact bone that lines the alveolar socket. The lamina dura is pierced by many small openings. These allow the blood vessels and nerve fibers in the bone to communicate freely with those in the periodontal ligament.

Periodontal Ligament

The periodontal ligament is dense connective tissue organized into fiber groups that connects the cementum covering the root of the tooth with the alveolar bone of the socket wall.

At one end, the fibers are embedded in cementum; at the other end, they are embedded in bone. These embedded portions become mineralized and are known as **Sharpey's fibers.**

The periodontal ligament ranges in width from 0.1 to 0.38 mm., with the thinnest portion around the middle third of the root. There is a gradual progressive decrease in this width with age.

FUNCTIONS OF THE PERIODONTAL LIGAMENT

Supportive and Protective. The fiber groups are designed to support the tooth in its socket and hold it firmly in normal relationship to the surrounding soft and hard tissues.

This arrangement makes it possible for the tooth to withstand the pressures and forces of mastication.

Sensory. The nerve supply for the ligament is derived from the nerves just before they enter the apical foramen. Innervation is also supplied from nerves in the surrounding alveolar bone.

These nerves provide the tooth with the protective "sense of touch": for example, noticing when a tooth is in premature occlusion because a restoration is too high.

These nerves also act as the sensory receptors necessary for the proper positioning of the jaws during normal function.

Nutritive. The nutritive needs of the ligament are provided by the blood vessels that also supply the tooth and its alveolar bone.

These are derived from the blood vessels that enter the dental pulp through the apical foramen, and from the vessels that supply the surrounding alveolar bone.

Formative and Resorptive. The fibroblasts of the periodontal ligament make possible the continuous and rapid remodeling that is required of these fiber groups.

The cementoblasts and cementoclasts (which form and destroy cementum) are also involved in these remodeling functions. So too are the osteoblasts and osteoclasts (which form and destroy bone).

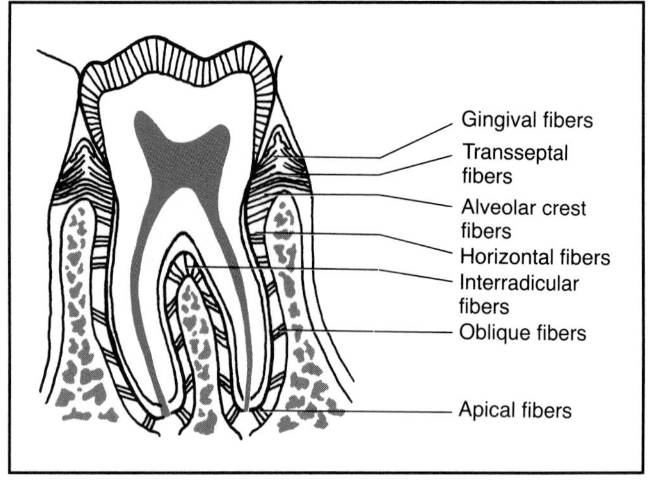

FIGURE 4–23

Periodontal ligament fiber groups.

PERIODONTAL LIGAMENT FIBER GROUPS

The periodontal ligament has three different types of fiber groups (Fig. 4–23). These are the **periodontal fibers,** which support the tooth in its socket; **transseptal fibers,** which support the tooth in relation to the adjacent teeth; and **gingival fibers,** which support the gingiva surrounding the tooth.

Periodontal Fiber Groups

Alveolar crest fibers run from the crest of the alveolar bone to the cementum in region of the cementoenamel junction. Their primary function is to retain the tooth in the socket and to oppose lateral forces.

Horizontal fibers run at right angles to the long axis of the tooth, from the cementum to the bone. Their primary function is to restrain lateral tooth movement.

Oblique fibers run in an upward direction from cementum to the bone. These fiber bundles are most numerous and constitute the main attachment of the tooth. Their primary function is to resist forces placed on the long axis of the tooth.

Apical fibers radiate outward from the apical cementum and insert into the surrounding bone. Their primary functions are to prevent the tooth from tipping; to resist luxation (twisting motion); and to protect the blood, lymph, and nerve supplies.

Interradicular fibers are found only in multirooted teeth. They run from the cementum of the root and insert into the interradicular septum. Their primary function is to aid in resisting tipping and twisting.

Transseptal Fiber Group

The **transseptal fibers,** also known as *interdental fibers,* are located interproximally above the crest of the alveolar bone between the teeth (Fig. 4–24). These fibers originate in the cervical cementum of one tooth

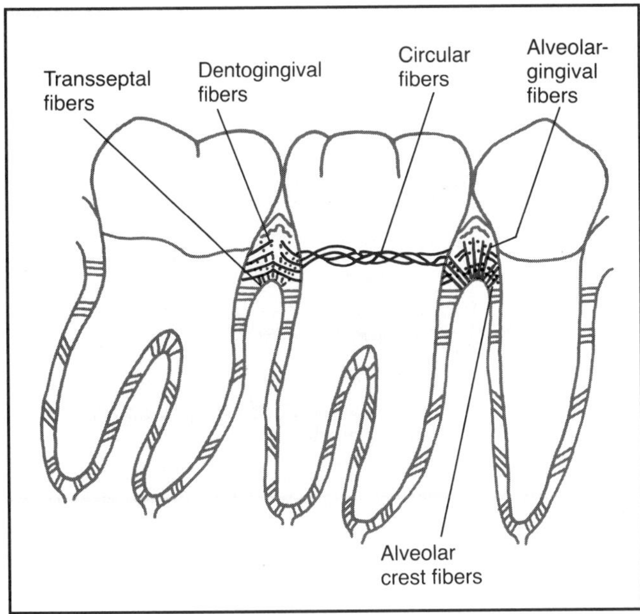

FIGURE 4–24

Transseptal fibers connect one tooth to another.

and insert into the cervical cementum of the adjacent tooth.

Their primary function is to support the interproximal gingiva and to aid in securing the position of the adjacent tooth.

Gingival Fiber Groups

The gingival fibers are located in the lamina propria of the gingiva. (The **lamina propria** is the connective tissue of the gingiva. It lies just *under* the epithelium of the mucous membrane, and just *above* the crest of the alveolar bone.)

These fiber groups serve three specialized functions:

- To hold the marginal gingiva firmly against the tooth
- To provide the firmness necessary to withstand the stress as food moves against it during chewing
- To unite the unattached gingiva with the cementum of the root and the adjacent attached gingiva

The gingival fibers, which do not insert into the alveolar bone, are divided into four groups:

- **Dentogingival fibers** extend from the cervical cementum outward and upward into the lamina propria.
- **Alveologingival fibers** extend upward from the alveolar crest into the lamina propria.
- **Circular fibers** form a band around the neck of the tooth. These fibers are interlaced by other groups of fibers in the unattached gingiva.
- **Dentoperiosteal fibers** extend facially and lingually from the cementum (Fig. 4–25). These fibers pass over the crest of the alveolar bone and then insert into the periosteum of the alveolar process. Their primary function is to support the tooth and gingiva.

Gingival Unit

The gingival unit consists of the specialized epithelial tissues that line the oral cavity and surround the teeth.

Known as the *oral mucosa,* these tissues are divided into two types: lining mucosa and masticatory mucosa.

LINING MUCOSA

Lining mucosa is thin, very delicate tissue that covers the inside of the cheeks, vestibule, lips, soft palate, and ventral surface (underside) of the tongue.

Beneath the lining mucosa is the **submucosa,** which contains blood vessels and nerves. Since lining mucosa is not attached to bone, it moves freely.

The abundant blood supply, and the thinness of the tissue, give lining mucosa a brighter red color than masticatory mucosa.

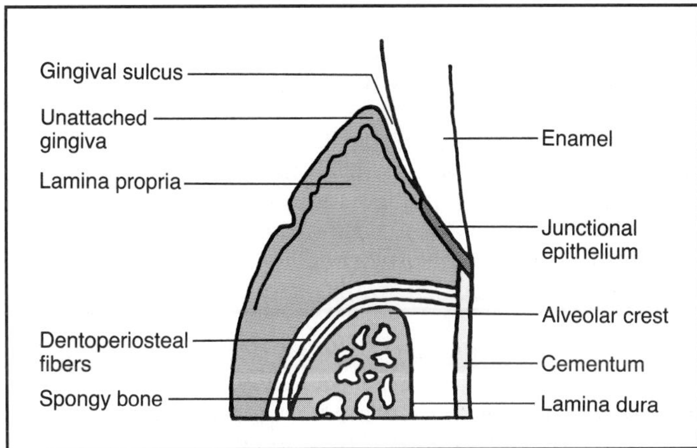

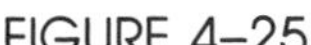

FIGURE 4–25

Dentoperiosteal fibers extend facially and lingually from the cementum.

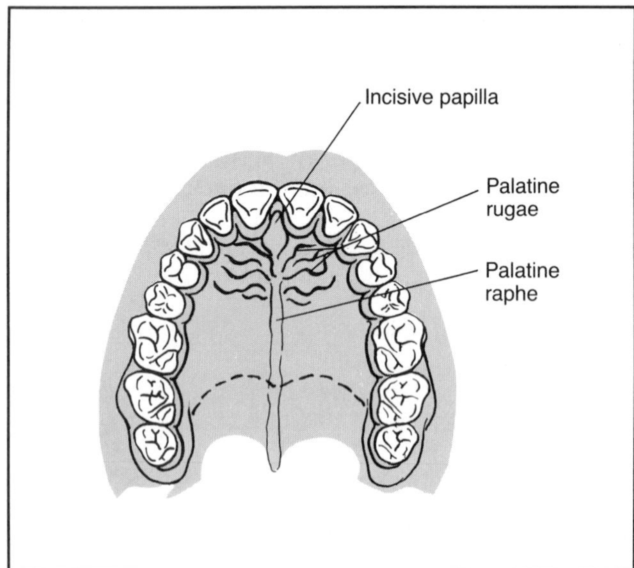

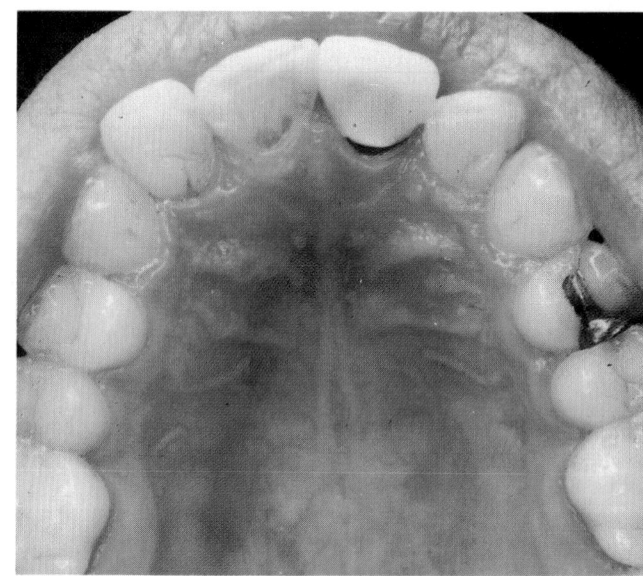

FIGURE 4–26

Tissues of the hard palate shown on a diagram and in a photograph. The patient shown in the photograph also has a porcelain fused-to-metal crown on the left central incisor and a disto-occlusal (DO) amalgam restoration on the left first premolar.

MASTICATORY MUCOSA

Masticatory mucosa covers the hard palate, dorsum (upper surface) of the tongue, and gingiva. (The dorsum of the tongue is discussed in Chapter 4.)

Masticatory mucosa, which is light pink in color, is **keratinized.** This means that it has a horny, tough, protective outer layer. (Lining mucosa is lacking this protective layer.)

There is no submucosa beneath the masticatory mucosa. It is firmly affixed to the bone and does not move. This tissue is a dense, tough covering that is designed to withstand the vigorous activity of chewing and swallowing food.

Covering of the Hard Palate

The masticatory mucosa covering the hard palate is tightly fixed to the underlying bone. It is usually pale pink in color (Fig. 4–26).

The **incisive papilla** is a pear-shaped structure located directly posterior to the maxillary central incisors, at the midline. This is just above the incisive foramen where the nasopalatine nerve enters the mouth. (This is the tissue that may be injured when you bite into something that is too hot.)

The **palatine raphe** is a ridge of masticatory mucosa extending from the incisive papilla posteriorly along the midline. It appears in the mouth as a whitish streak at midline of the palate.

The **palatine rugae** are irregular ridges or folds of masticatory mucosa extending laterally from the incisive papilla and the anterior part of the raphe. (*Rugae* is plural; the singular is *ruga.*)

Gingiva

The gingiva, commonly referred to as **gums,** is masticatory mucosa that covers the alveolar processes of the jaws and surrounds the necks of the teeth (Fig. 4–27). (*Gingiva* is singular; the plural is *gingivae.*)

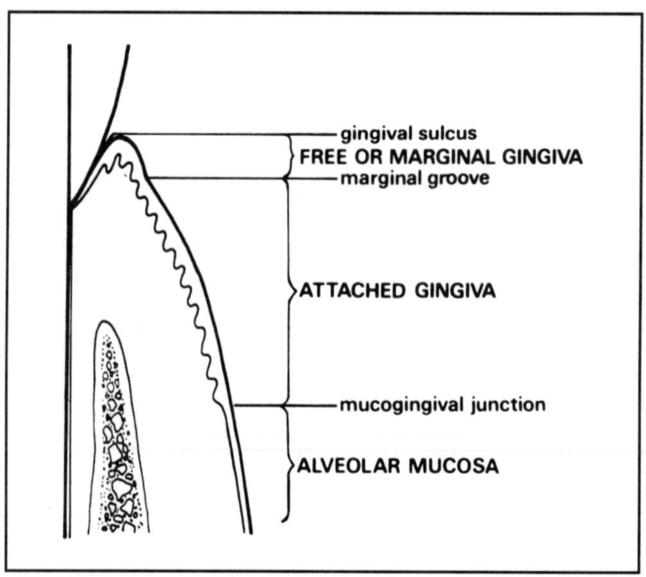

FIGURE 4–27

Structures of the gingiva. (From Carranza, F.A., Jr. [ed]: Glickman's Clinical Periodontology, 7th ed. Philadelphia, W.B. Saunders Co., 1990, p 15.)

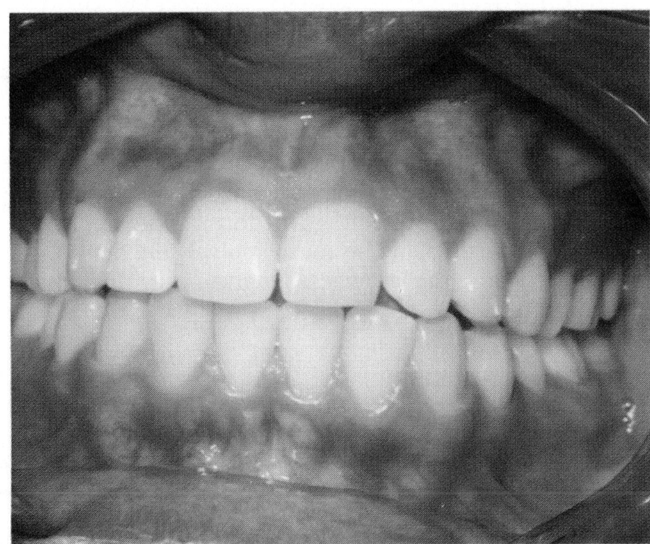

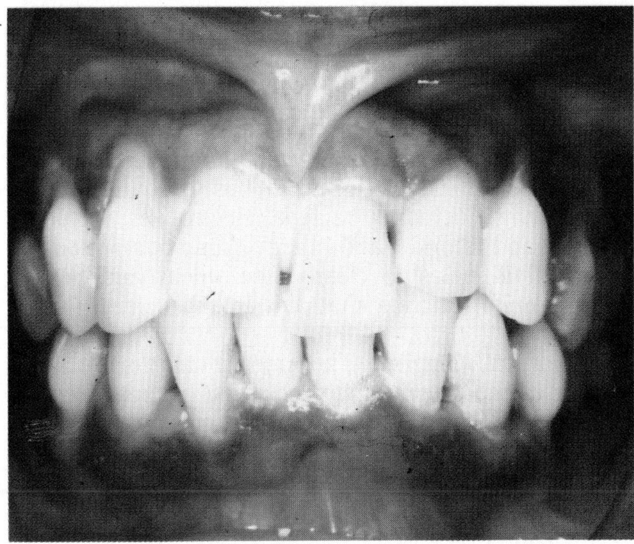

FIGURE 4–28

Gingival pigmentation varies. On the left is healthy gingiva with light pigmentation. On the right is darker pigmentation. This patient has several problems, including gingival recession associated with periodontal disease. In addition, a lateral incisor is missing, and there is a very strong attachment of the maxillary labial frenum.

The gingiva has a rich blood supply derived from three sources: supraperiosteal and periodontal ligament vessels and alveolar vessels, which emerge from the alveolar crest. Innervation is derived from branches of the trigeminal nerve.

Normal gingival tissue has the following characteristics:

- It surrounds the tooth in collar-like fashion and is self-cleansing in form.
- It is firm and resistant and tightly adapted to the tooth and bone.
- The surfaces of the attached gingiva and interdental papillae are stippled and are similar in appearance to the skin of an orange.
- The color of the surface varies according to the individual's pigmentation (Figs. 4–28 and 4–29).

UNATTACHED GINGIVA

Unattached gingiva, also known as **marginal gingiva** or **free gingiva,** is the border of the gingiva surrounding the teeth in collar-like fashion.

The unattached gingiva, which is usually light pink or coral in color, is not bound to the underlying tissue of the tooth. It consists of the tissues from the top of the gingival margin to the base of the gingival sulcus.

The unattached gingiva is usually about 1 mm. wide and forms the soft tissue wall of the gingival sulcus.

Gingival Margin. The gingival margin is the upper edge of the unattached gingiva. This margin appears to form a wavy course as it follows the contour of the cervical line of the tooth.

Gingival Sulcus. The gingival sulcus is the space between the unattached gingiva and the tooth. The normal "probing depth" of a clinically normal gingival sulcus rarely exceeds 2 to 3 mm. (See Chapter 26.)

Epithelial Attachment. In a healthy mouth, the gingiva that lines the gingival sulcus (which is a form of epithelium) attaches to the teeth on the enamel surface just above the cervical line of the tooth. This is known as the **epithelial attachment.**

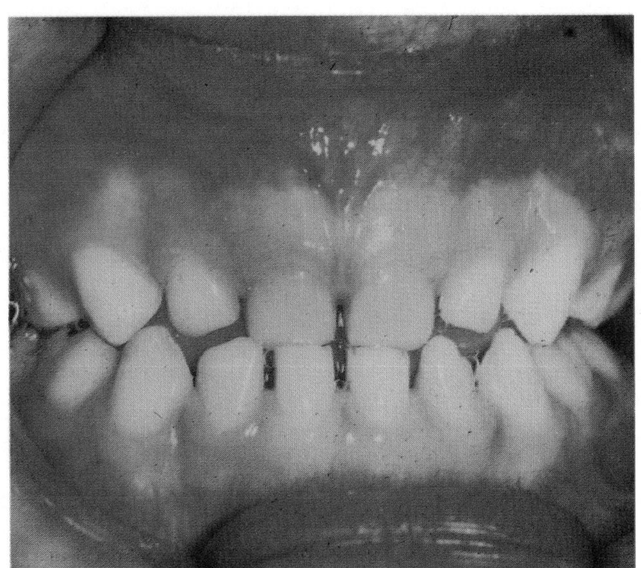

FIGURE 4–29

Healthy gingiva in the primary dentition of a 5-year-old child. The space between teeth, which will increase as the child grows, will create room for the permanent teeth to erupt.

The gingival epithelium, the epithelial attachment, and the dental enamel, which is of epithelial origin, form a continuous epithelial covering for the underlying tissues of the oral cavity.

Sulcular Fluid. Sulcular fluid, also known as *crevicular fluid,* is tissue fluid that seeps into the gingival sulcus through the wall of the sulcus. It contains cellular elements, including bacteria; electrolytes, including calcium and fluoride; and other organic compounds.

This fluid helps to cleanse the sulcus and has an antimicrobial function that aids in the defense of the gingiva.

Interdental Gingiva. The interdental gingiva, also known as the *gingival papilla,* is the extension of the free gingiva that fills the interproximal embrasure between two adjacent teeth. (*Papilla* is singular; the plural is *papillae.*) (This is discussed further in Chapter 5.)

Gingival Groove. The gingival groove, also known as the *free gingival groove,* is a shallow groove that runs parallel to the margin of the unattached gingiva and marks the beginning of the attached gingiva.

ATTACHED GINGIVA

The attached gingiva extends from the base of the sulcus to the mucogingival junction. It is a stippled, dense tissue, self-protecting in form, and is firmly bound and resilient. (The **mucogingival junction** is the point at which the attached gingiva joins the lining mucosa.)

ALVEOLAR MUCOSA

The alveolar mucosa, which is lining mucosa, is found apical to the mucogingival junction and is continuous with the mucous membranes of the cheek, lip, and floor of the oral cavity. It is thin, soft, delicate, and loosely attached.

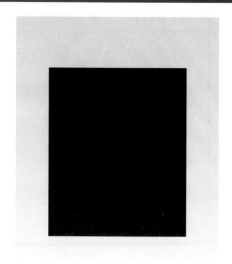

Chapter 5

Tooth Morphology

Introduction

Tooth morphology is the study of the form and structures of the dentition. (**Morphology** is the study of the form of an organ or body part. The term **dentition** refers to the natural teeth in the dental arch.)

Throughout our lifetime, we have two sets of teeth: the primary dentition and the permanent dentition. Except where otherwise indicated, all discussions in this chapter refer to the permanent dentition.

Types of Teeth

We are omnivorous. This means that we eat both meat and plants. To accommodate this variety in diet, our teeth are designed for cutting, tearing, and grinding different types of food.

On the basis of form and function, the teeth of the human permanent dentition are divided into four types: incisors, cuspids, premolars, and molars (Fig. 5–1).

Incisors

Incisors are single-rooted teeth with a relatively sharp and thin edge. Located at the front of the mouth, they are designed to cut food without the application of heavy forces.

Cuspids

The cuspids, also known as *canines*, are located at the "corners" of the arches. They are designed for cutting and tearing foods that require the application of force.

The cuspid crown is thick with one well-developed pointed cusp. The single cuspid root is the longest in the dentition. The bony ridge over the facial portion of the root is known as the **canine eminence.**

Because of its sturdy crown, long root, and location in the arch, the cuspid is referred to as the cornerstone of the dental arch. These teeth are the most stable in the mouth and are usually the last teeth to be lost.

Premolars

The premolars, also known as *bicuspids*, are similar to the cuspids in that they have points and cusps for grasping and tearing. They also have a somewhat broader working surface for chewing food. (There are no premolars in the primary dentition.)

Molars

The molars have more cusps than these other teeth. The shorter, blunter design of these cusps produces a broad working surface that is used for chewing and grinding solid masses of food that require the application of heavy forces.

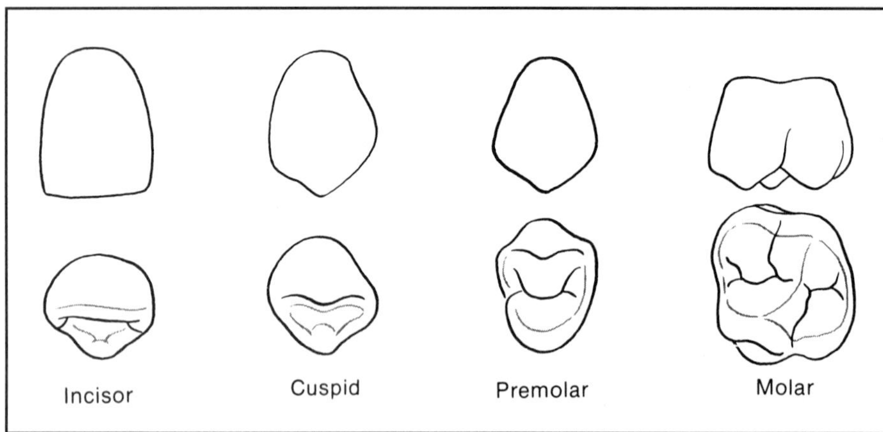

FIGURE 5–1

The types of teeth.

Dental Arches

The teeth are arranged in two dental arches that contain the same number and types of teeth (Fig. 5–2):

- The **mandibular** (lower) arch is capable of movement through the action of the temporomandibular joint.
- The **maxillary** (upper) arch, which is actually part of the skull, is not capable of movement.

As they function, the movable mandibular arch brings the primary forces of occlusion to bear against the immovable maxillary arch. (**Occlusion** is the contact between the maxillary and mandibular teeth in all mandibular positions and movements.)

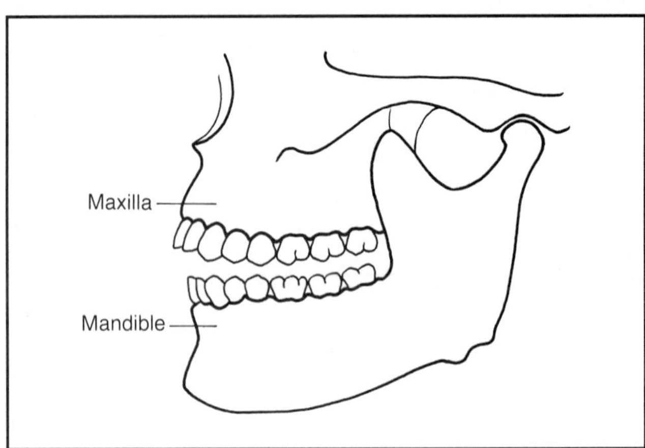

FIGURE 5–2

The dental arches.

Quadrants and Sextants

An imaginary midline divides each arch into mirror-image halves. The two arches, each divided into halves, create four sections, which are called **quadrants** (Fig. 5–3):

- Maxillary right quadrant
- Maxillary left quadrant
- Mandibular left quadrant
- Mandibular right quadrant

In the primary dentition, each quadrant contains two incisors (one central, one lateral), one cuspid, one first molar, and one second molar.

In the permanent dentition, each quadrant contains two incisors (one central, one lateral), one cuspid, two premolars, and three molars.

Sometimes it is necessary to divide the dentition into six parts. Each part is call a sextant. The six sextants are the

- Maxillary right posterior
- Maxillary anterior
- Maxillary left posterior
- Mandibular right posterior
- Mandibular anterior
- Mandibular left posterior

Anterior and Posterior Teeth

As an aid in describing their location and functions, the teeth are classified as being **anterior** (toward the front) or **posterior** (toward the back). In Figure 5–3,

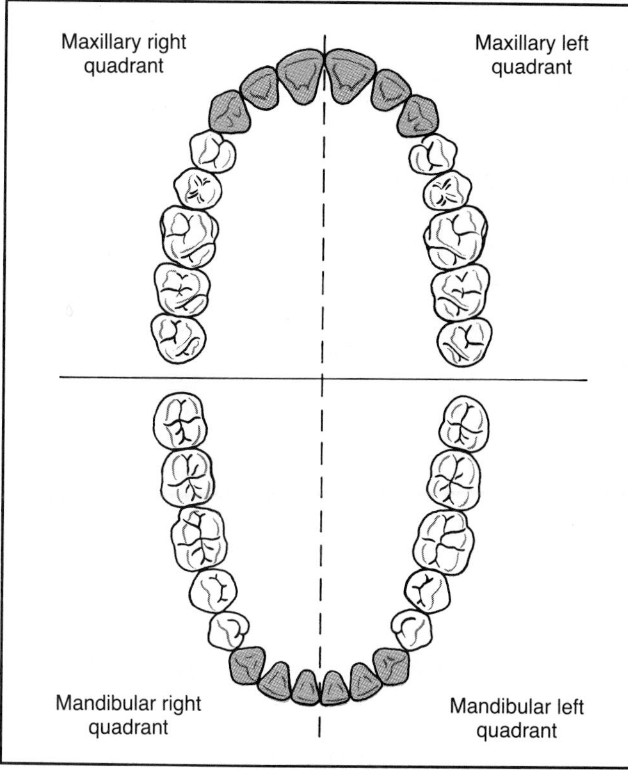

FIGURE 5–3

The dental arches divided into quadrants. This is an occlusal view. The anterior teeth are shaded. The posterior teeth are not shaded.

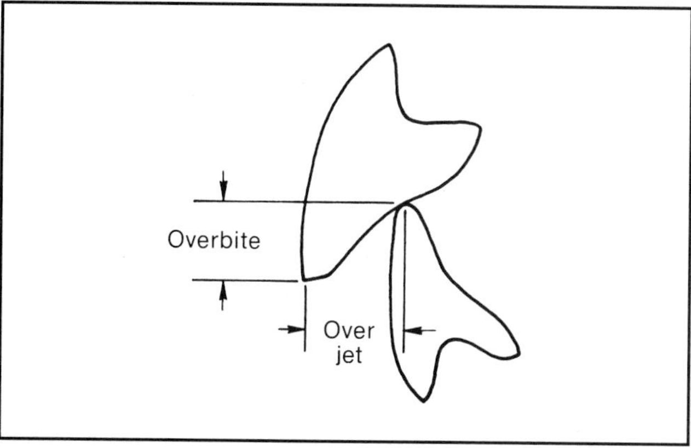

FIGURE 5–4

Overjet is the horizontal overlap of the maxillary teeth. **Overbite** is the vertical overlap of the maxillary teeth.

the anterior teeth are shaded and the posterior teeth are not shaded.

The **anterior teeth** are the incisors and cuspids. They are visible when we smile. These teeth are aligned to form a smooth, curving arc from the distal (back) of the cuspid on one side of the arch to the distal (back) of the cuspid on the opposite side.

The **posterior teeth,** which are the premolars and molars, are aligned with little or no curvature. These teeth appear to be almost in a straight line.

Stabilization of the Arches

Through proper positioning of all its parts, the dental arch is designed to be a unit that remains stable and efficient as long as its normal arrangement is maintained.

However, malocclusion or the loss of one or more teeth may greatly reduce the functioning and stability of the dentition.

OVERJET AND OVERBITE

One adaptation is that the maxillary arch is slightly larger than the mandibular arch, which creates overlapping of the maxillary teeth over the mandibular teeth. This arrangement provides stability and guidance as the jaws come together.

This overlapping is particularly evident in the anterior region, where the larger maxillary anterior teeth create a wider curvature of the arch. The horizontal overlap of the maxillary teeth is called **overjet,** and the vertical overlap of the maxillary teeth is known as **overbite** (Fig. 5–4).

CLOSURE

The anterior teeth are not designed to support fully the occlusal forces on the entire dental arch. Therefore, as the jaws close, the stronger posterior teeth come together first. After they have assumed most of the load, the more delicate anterior teeth come together.

CURVE OF SPEE

The occlusal surfaces of the posterior teeth do not form a flat plane. Those of the mandibular arch form a slightly curved plane, which appears **concave** (curved inward, like the inside of a bowl).

The maxillary arch forms a curved plane that appears **convex** (curved outward, like the outside of a bowl). The curvature formed by the maxillary and mandibular arches in occlusion is known as the curve of Spee (Fig. 5–5).

CURVE OF WILSON

The curve of Wilson is the cross-arch curvature of the posterior occlusal plane. The downward curvature of the arc is defined by a line drawn across the occlusal surface of the left mandibular first molar, extending across the arch and through the occlusal surface of the right mandibular first molar (Fig. 5–6).

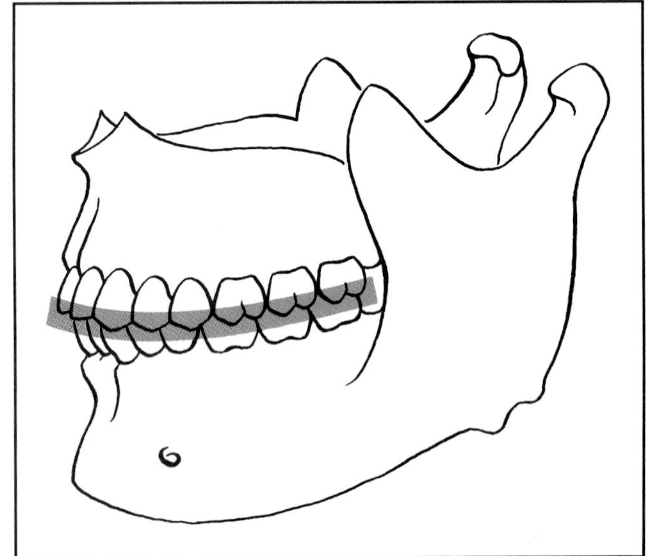

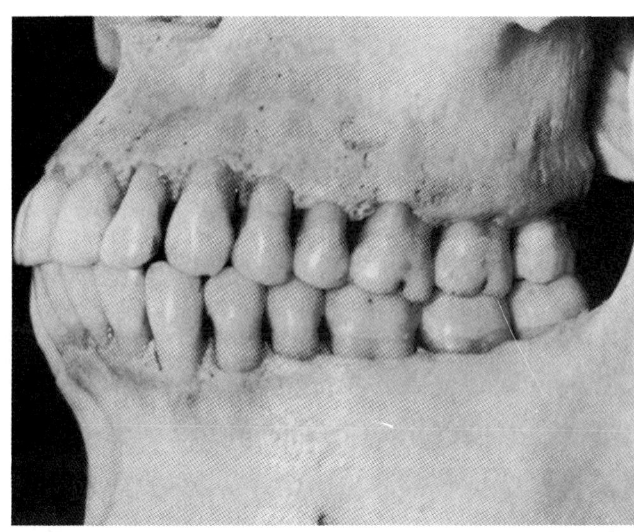

FIGURE 5–5

The curve of Spee is a gentle curvature of the occlusal planes. (Photograph from Ash, M.M. [ed]: Wheeler's Dental Anatomy, Physiology, and Occlusion, 7th ed. Philadelphia, W.B. Saunders Co., 1993, p 422.)

ANTAGONISTS

Each tooth in the dental arch has two antagonists in the opposing arch. These are its class counterpart and the tooth proximal (next) to it (Fig. 5–7). (As used here, the term **antagonists** means teeth in opposing arches that normally contact each other.)

The only exceptions in the permanent dentition are the mandibular central incisors and the maxillary third molars, which have only one antagonist.

The antagonistic relationship of the primary teeth is similar. Here the exceptions are the mandibular central incisors and maxillary secondary molars.

Because each tooth has two antagonists, the loss of one still leaves one remaining antagonist. This helps to keep the tooth in occlusal contact with the opposing arch and in relationship with the surrounding teeth in its own arch.

Should both antagonists be lost, the tooth will become **extruded** (elongated). This happens as the tooth continues to erupt because it no longer has the occlusal contact necessary to maintain its normal position.

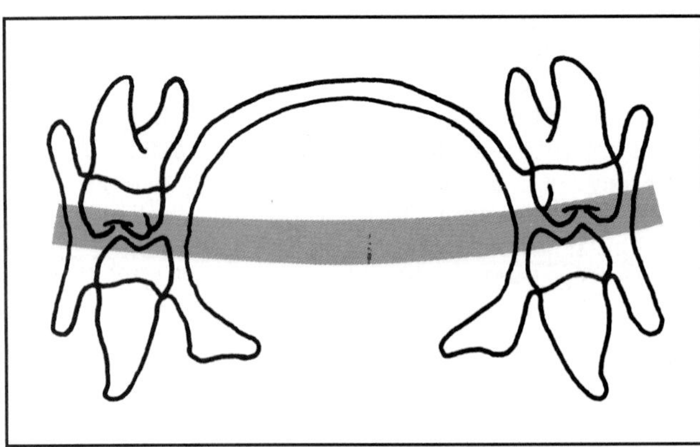

FIGURE 5–6

The curve of Wilson is the cross-arch curvature of the posterior occlusal plane.

ADJACENT TEETH

To increase stability, the teeth in each arch are arranged in contact with adjacent teeth on either side. The exception is the last molar in either arch, which is in contact only with the tooth in front of it.

When a permanent tooth is missing and has not been replaced, the adjacent tooth on either side of the opening **drifts** into the empty space (Fig. 5–8). This lateral shift in position causes the teeth to tilt, and they no longer occlude properly with the teeth in the opposite arch.

OCCLUSAL FORM

The occlusal surfaces of the opposing teeth (antagonists) bear a definite relationship to each other faciolingually (from side to side) and mesiodistally (from front to back).

In normal occlusion, the lingual cusps of the posterior maxillary teeth fit into the central fossae of the occlusal surfaces of the posterior mandibular teeth. This produces a mortar-and-pestle action for effective grinding of food (Fig. 5–9).

This arrangement helps to stabilize the mandible while permitting appropriate movements. It also serves to confine the shock or forces of contact within the root bases of the teeth.

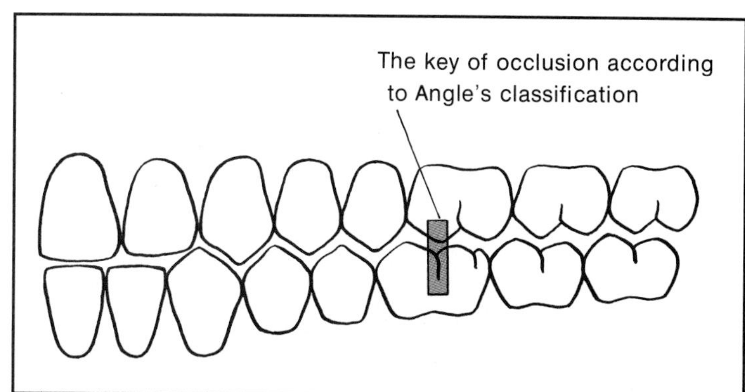
The key of occlusion according to Angle's classification

FIGURE 5–7

The antagonistic relationship of the teeth in the dental arches. In normal occlusion, the mesiobuccal cusp of the maxillary permanent first molar occludes in the buccal groove of the mandibular permanent first molar.

Surfaces of the Teeth

An **axial surface** is a longitudinal surface of the tooth from the occlusal surface, or incisal edge, through the apex of the root. (The term **axial** refers to the long axis, which is an imaginary line passing longitudinally through the center of a tooth.)

Not all tooth surfaces are axial; however, each tooth does have four axial surfaces (Figs. 5–10 to 5–12). The anterior teeth have four axial surfaces plus an incisal edge. The posterior teeth have four axial surfaces plus the occlusal (horizontal) surface.

The surfaces of the teeth are described as follows:

- The **buccal surface** is the axial surface of a posterior tooth that is next to the cheek.
- The **labial surface** is the axial surface of an anterior tooth that is next to the lip.
- **Facial surfaces** is the term used to describe both labial and buccal surfaces. Thus this and the preceding two terms all refer to the surface of a tooth that is next to the cheeks and lips.
- The **lingual surface** is the axial surface of a tooth that is nearest the tongue.
- The **proximal surfaces** are those axial tooth surfaces that are next to each other in the same arch. The mesial and distal surfaces of adjacent teeth are proximal surfaces.
- The **distal surface** is the axial surface of a tooth facing *away from* the midline and toward the back of the mouth.
- The **mesial surface** is the axial surface of a tooth facing in the direction of the midline and toward the front of the mouth.
- The **occlusal surface** is the horizontal chewing surface of the posterior teeth. This is perpendicular to the axial surfaces.

Line and Point Angles

- An **angle** is the junction of two or more surfaces of a tooth (Fig. 5–13).
- A **line angle** is that angle formed by the junction of *two* surfaces of a tooth crown along an imaginary

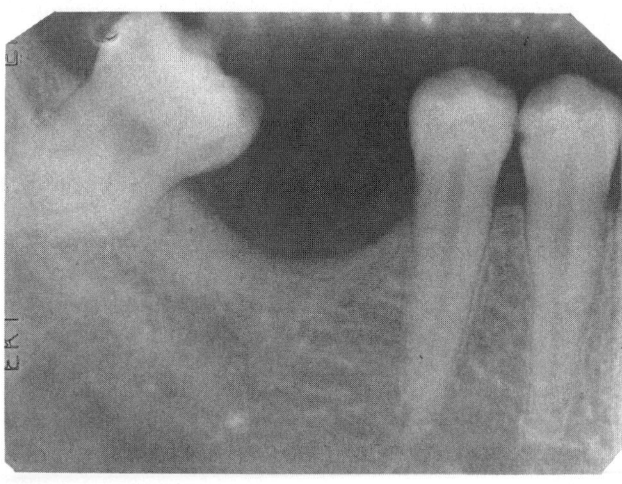

FIGURE 5–8

Radiograph showing the mesial drift of the mandibular second molar after the first molar has been lost.

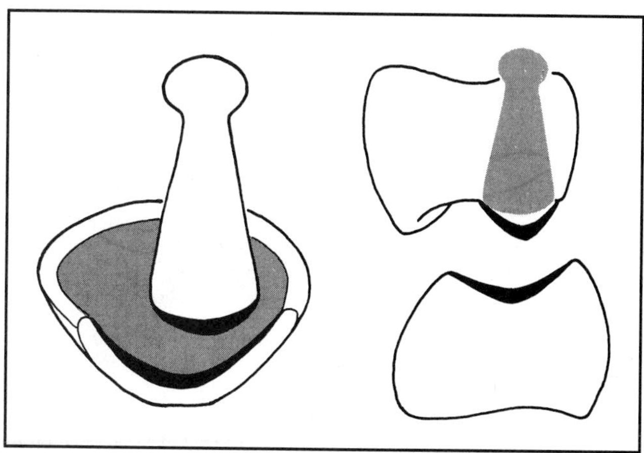

FIGURE 5–9

The occlusal form of the teeth produces a mortar-and-pestle action for the effective grinding of food.

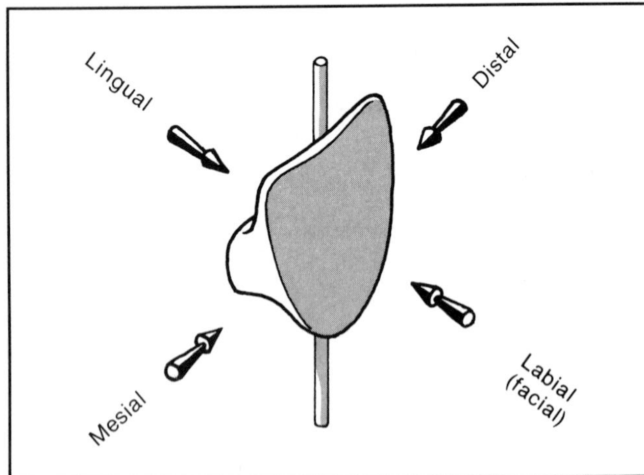

FIGURE 5–10

Axial surfaces of an anterior tooth. (An imaginary long axis is shown through the center of the tooth.)

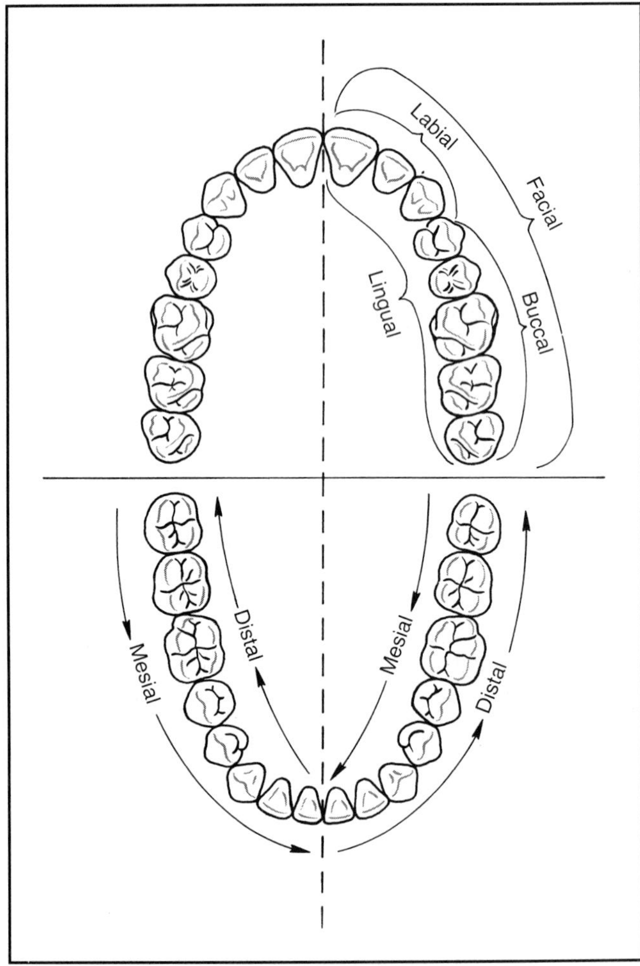

FIGURE 5–12

Axial surfaces of the teeth as they relate to an occlusal view of the dental arches.

line. Its name is derived by combining the names of the two surfaces (for example, *mesiobuccal*).

- A **point angle** is that angle formed by the junction of *three* surfaces at one point. These angles are described by combining the names of the surfaces forming them (for example, *mesiolinguo-occlusal* angle). When combining these words, drop the last two letters of the first word and substitute the letter "o."

Division into Thirds

To make it possible to identify a specific area of the tooth, each surface is divided into imaginary thirds (Fig. 5–14). These thirds are named in accordance with the areas they approximate.

The root of the tooth is divided crosswise into thirds. These are the **apical third** (which is nearest the tip of the root), the **middle third,** and the **cervical third** (which is nearest the neck of the tooth).

The crown of the tooth is divided into thirds in three different directions:

- **Occlusocervical division:** the crosswise division parallel to the occlusal or incisal surface. This division consists of the **occlusal third, middle third,** and **cervical third.**
- **Mesiodistal division:** the lengthwise division in a mesial-distal (front-to-back) direction. This division consists of the **mesial third, middle third,** and **distal third.**
- **Buccolingual division:** the lengthwise division in a labial or buccal-lingual direction. This division consists of the **facial** or **buccal/labial third, middle third,** and **lingual third.**

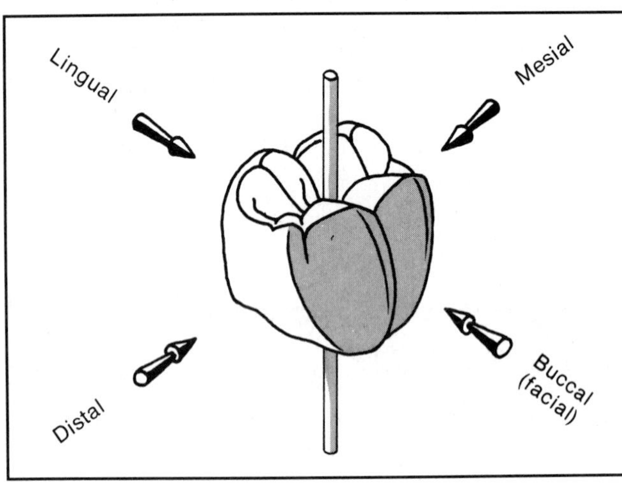

FIGURE 5–11

Axial surfaces of a posterior tooth. (An imaginary long axis is shown through the center of the tooth.)

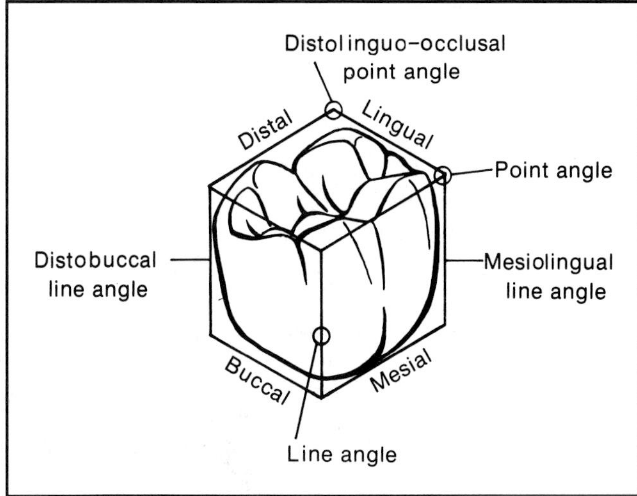

FIGURE 5–13

Line and point angles. A *line angle* is formed by the junction of two surfaces of a tooth crown along an imaginary line. A *point angle* is that angle formed by the junction of three surfaces at one point.

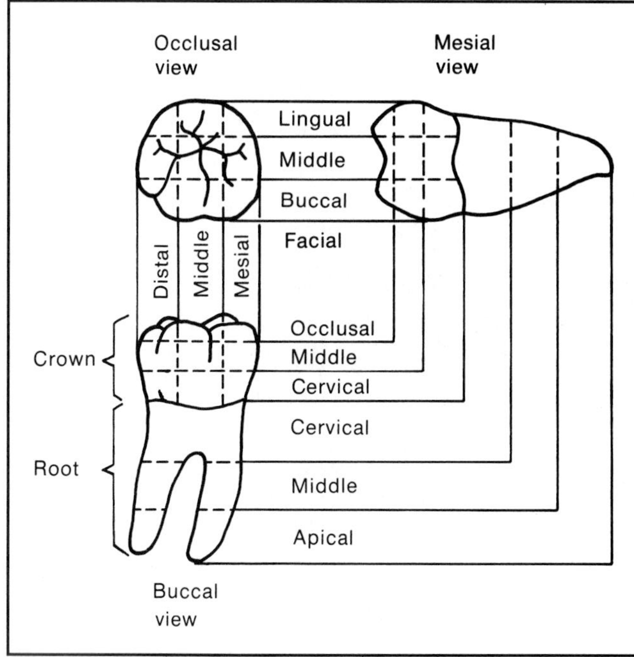

FIGURE 5–14

Division into thirds. For descriptive and comparative purposes, each tooth surface is divided into imaginary thirds.

Anatomic Features of the Teeth

The anatomic features of the teeth help to maintain their positions in the arch and to protect the tissues supporting them. This is accomplished through contours, contacts, embrasures, and occlusal form.

Figure 5–15 is an illustrated glossary of the terms used to describe the anatomic landmarks of individual teeth.

Contours

The contours (shape) of every part of a tooth present curved surfaces except when the tooth is fractured or worn. Some surfaces are convex; others are concave (Fig. 5–16).

Although the general contours vary, the general principle that the crown of the tooth narrows toward the cervical line holds for all types of teeth.

FACIAL AND LINGUAL CONTOURS

The pronounced curvatures found on the facial and lingual surfaces provide natural passageways for food. This action protects the gingiva from the impact of foods during mastication (Fig. 5–17).

The normal contour of a tooth provides the gingiva with adequate stimulation, yet protects it from being damaged by food (Fig. 5–18).

When a tooth is restored, it is important to return it to a normal contour. With **inadequate contour,** the gingiva may be damaged. With **overcontour,** the gingiva will lack adequate stimulation.

MESIAL AND DISTAL CONTOURS

The contours of the mesial and distal surfaces help determine normal contact and embrasure form. These tend to be self-cleansing and further contribute to the tooth's own self-preservation.

Contacts

The **contact area** is the convex region of the mesial or distal surface of a tooth that touches the adjacent tooth in the same arch.

The **contact point** is the exact spot where the teeth actually touch each other. The terms *contact* and *contact area* are frequently used interchangeably to refer to the contact point.

The crown of each tooth in the dental arches should be in contact with its adjacent tooth or teeth. A proper contact relationship between adjacent teeth accomplishes three things:

- It serves to keep food from being trapped between the teeth.

Cingulum—a bulge or prominence of enamel found on the cervical third of the lingual surface of an anterior tooth.

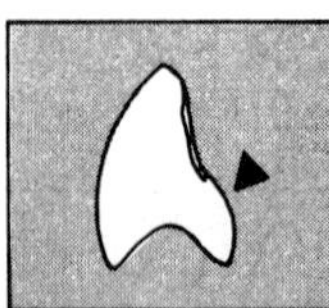

Cusp—(a) a pronounced elevation on the occlusal surface of a tooth terminating in a conical or rounded surface; (b) any crown elevation which begins calcification as an independent center. A cusp is considered to have an apex and four ridges.

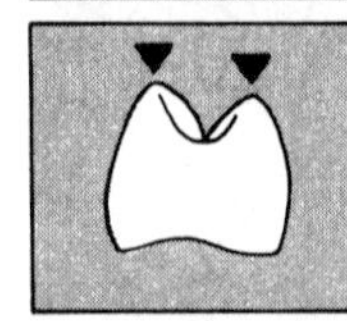

Cusp of Carabelli—the "fifth" cusp located on the lingual surface of many maxillary first molars.

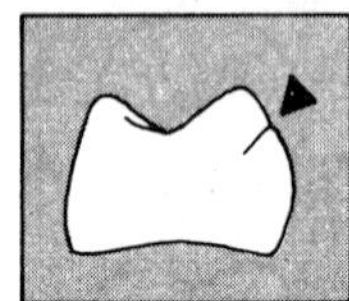

Fissure—a fault occurring along a developmental groove caused by incomplete or imperfect joining of the lobes. When two fissures cross they form a *pit.*

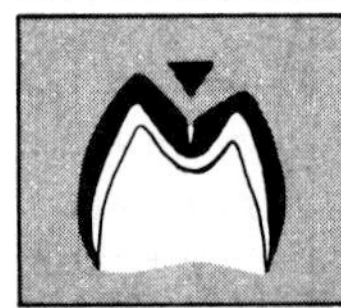

Fossa—a rounded or angular depression of varying size on the surface of a tooth.

Lingual Fossa—a broad, shallow depression on the lingual surface of an incisor or cuspid.

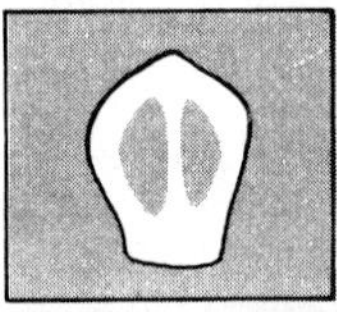

Central Fossa, maxillary molars—a relatively broad, deep angular valley in the central portion of the occlusal surface of a maxillary molar.

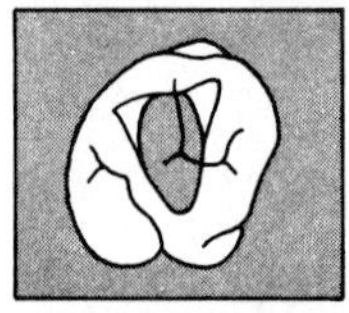

Central Fossa, mandibular molars—a relatively broad, deep angular valley in the central portion of the occlusal surface of a mandibular molar.

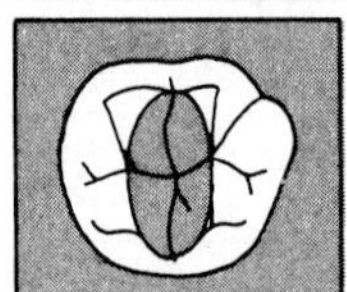

Triangular Fossa—a comparatively shallow pyramid-shaped depression on the occlusal surfaces of the posterior teeth, located just within the confines of the mesial and/or distal marginal ridges.

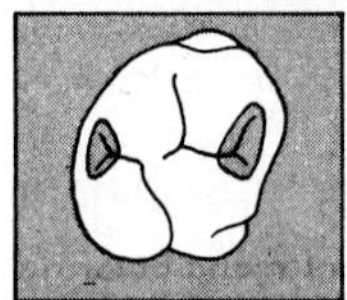

Groove—a small linear depression on the surface of a tooth.

Developmental groove—a groove formed by the union of two lobes during development of the crown.

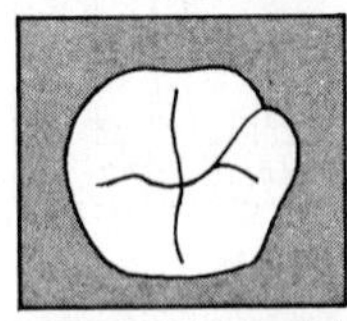

Supplemental Groove—an indistinct linear depression, irregular in extent and direction, which does not demarcate major divisional portions of a tooth. These often give the occlusal surface a wrinkled appearance.

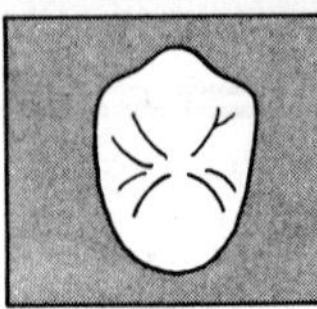

FIGURE 5–15

Illustrated glossary of terms describing anatomic landmarks on individual teeth.

Incisal Edge—formed by the junction of the linguoincisal surfaces of an anterior tooth. This edge does not exist until occlusal wear has created a surface linguoincisally. This surface forms an angle with the labial surface.

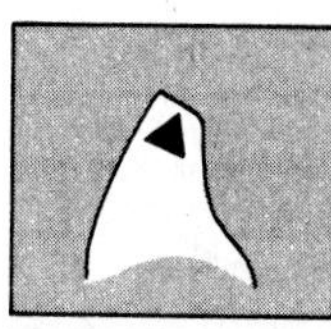

Incisal edge

Lobe—a developmental segment of the tooth. As lobes develop they coalesce to form a single unit.

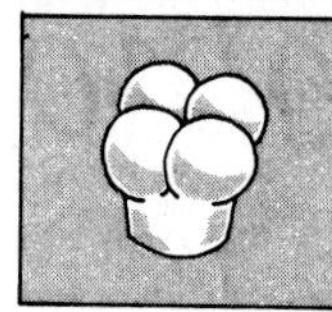

Lobe

Mamelon—a rounded or conical prominence on the incisal ridge of a newly erupted incisor. They are usually three in number, and soon disappear as the result of wear.

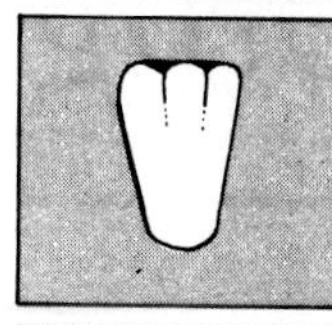

Mamelon

Ridge—a linear elevation on the surface of a tooth. It is named according to its location or form.

Cusp Ridge—an elevation which extends in a mesial and distal direction from the cusp tip. Cusp ridges form the buccal and lingual margins of the occlusal surfaces of the posterior teeth.

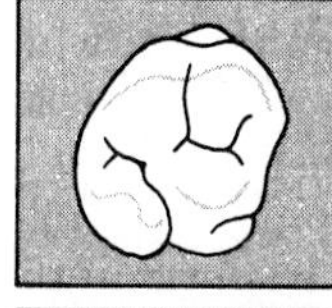

Cusp ridge

Incisal Ridge—the incisal portion of a newly erupted anterior tooth.

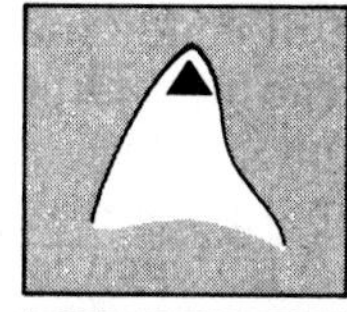

Incisal ridge

Marginal Ridges—elevated crests or rounded folds of enamel which form the mesial and distal margins of the occlusal surfaces of the posterior teeth and the lingual surfaces of the anterior teeth. Marginal ridges on the anterior teeth are less prominent and are linear extensions from the cingulum, forming the lateral borders of the lingual surface.

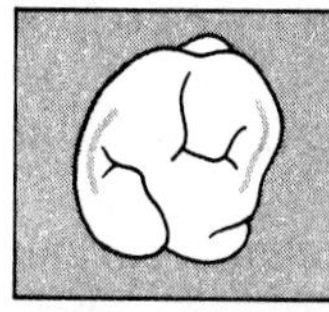

Marginal ridge

Oblique Ridges—elevated prominences on the occlusal surfaces of a maxillary molar extending obliquely from the tips of the mesiolingual cusp to the distobuccal cusp.

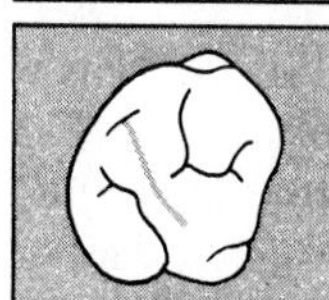

Oblique ridge

Triangular Ridges—prominent elevations, triangular in cross section, which extend from the tip of a cusp toward the central portion of the occlusal surface of a tooth. They are named for the cusp to which they belong. Also described as those ridges which descend from the tip of the cusps and widen toward the central area of the occlusal surface.

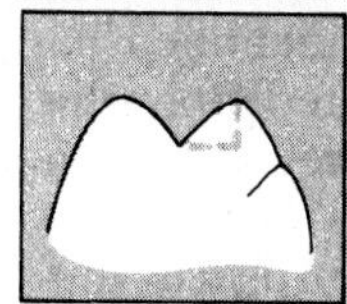

Triangular ridge

Transverse Ridges—made up of the triangular ridges of a buccal and lingual cusp which join to form a more or less continuous elevation extending transversely across the occlusal surface of a posterior tooth.

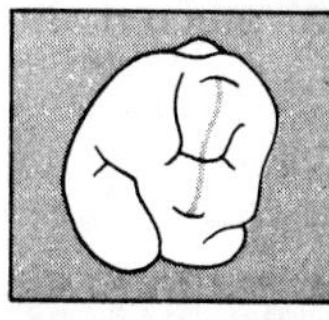

Transverse ridge

Sulcus—an elongated valley in the surface of a tooth formed by the inclines of adjacent cusps or ridges which meet at an angle.

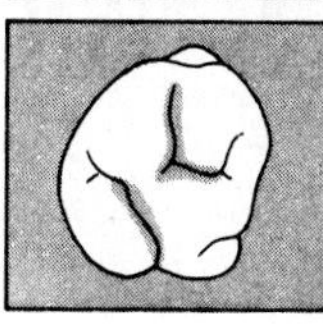

Sulcus

FIGURE 5–15

Continued

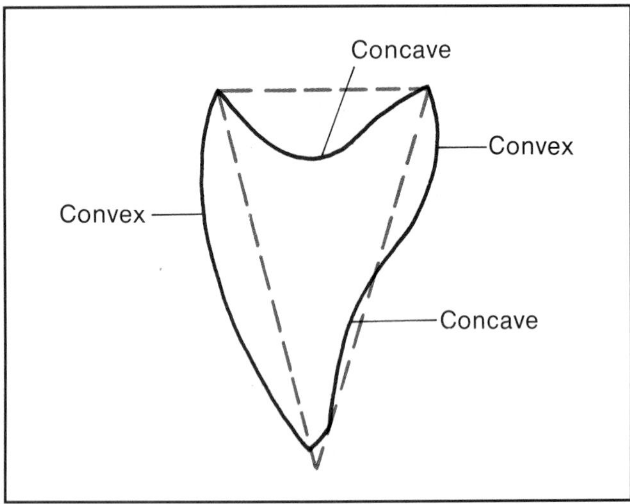

FIGURE 5–16

The surfaces of a single tooth are both convex and concave.

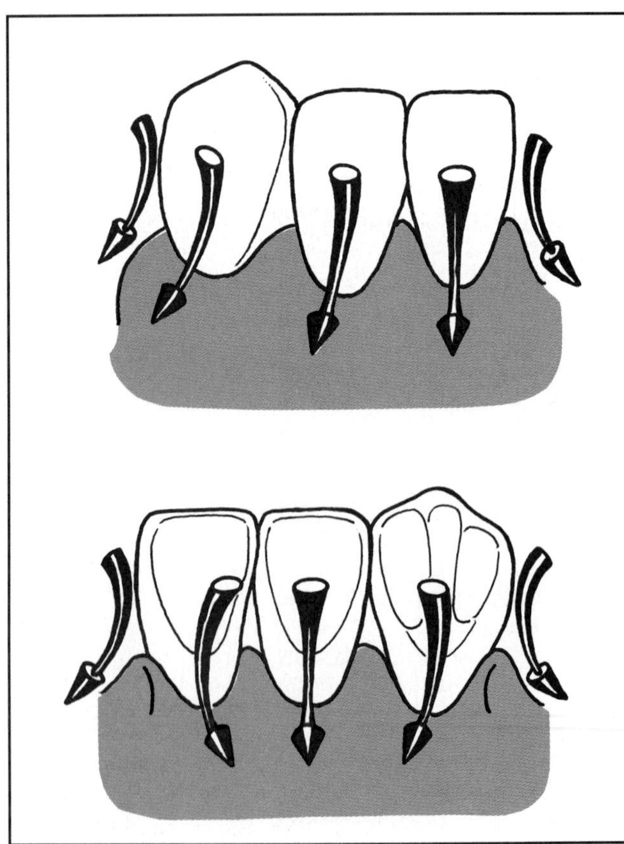

FIGURE 5–17

Pronounced curvatures are found on the facial and lingual surfaces of the tooth. These act to protect the gingiva from the impact of foods during mastication.

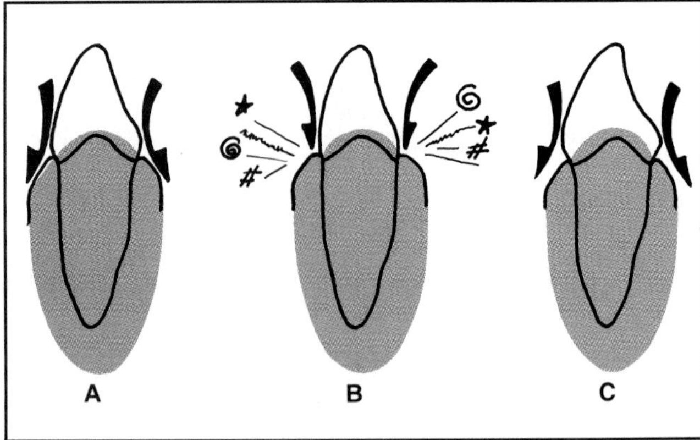

FIGURE 5–18

Tooth contours. *A,* Normal curvature provides the gingiva with adequate stimulation and yet protects it from being damaged by food. *B,* Without adequate contour, the gingiva may be traumatized. *C,* With overcontour, the gingiva will lack adequate stimulation.

- It helps to stabilize the dental arches by the combined anchorage of all the teeth in either arch in positive contact with each other.
- It protects the interproximal gingival tissue from trauma during mastication.

Embrasures

The contact of two teeth at the point of greatest convexity (outward curvature) creates an embrasure. (An **embrasure** is a V-shaped space in a gingival direction between the proximal surfaces of two adjoining teeth in contact.)

The embrasure may diverge in the following directions (Fig. 5–19):

- Facially
- Lingually
- Occlusally
- Apically (normally the interdental papilla of the gingiva fills this embrasure)

Occlusion and Malocclusion

Occlusion is the contact between the maxillary and mandibular teeth in all mandibular positions and movements.

Centric occlusion occurs when the jaws are closed in a position that produces maximal stable contact between the occluding surfaces of the maxillary and mandibular teeth. In this position, the condyles are in the most posterior unstrained position in the glenoid fossae.

Centric occlusion widely distributes the occlusal forces and affords the greatest comfort and stability. It

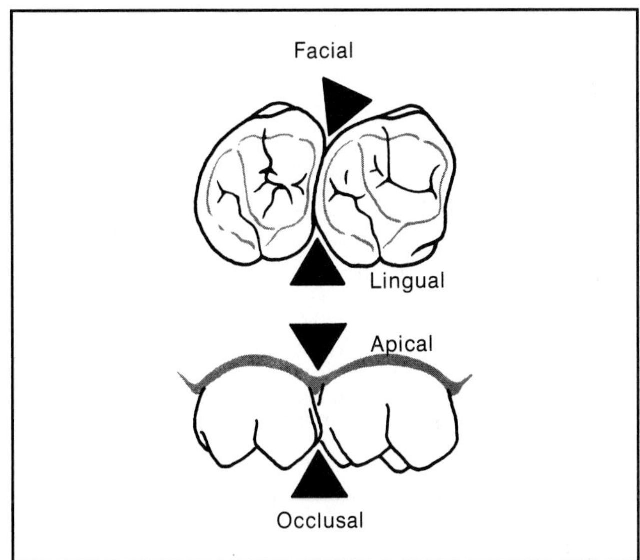

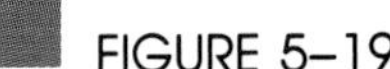

FIGURE 5–19

Embrasures may diverge facially, lingually, occlusally, or apically.

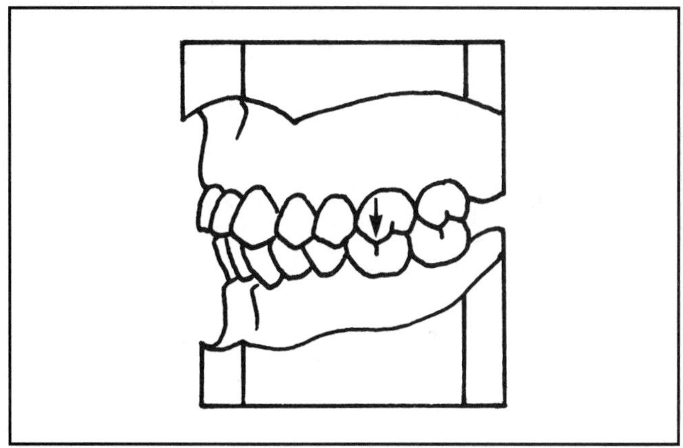

FIGURE 5–20

Class I, or neutroclusion. (From Ehrlich, A., and Torres, H.O.: Essentials of Dental Assisting. Philadelphia, W.B. Saunders Co., 1992, p 67.)

is also the position least likely to cause injury or pain even when heavy muscular forces are used during movement.

Functional occlusion, also known as *physiological occlusion,* is the term used to describe the contact of the teeth during biting and chewing movements.

Malocclusion refers to abnormal or malpositioned relationships of the maxillary teeth to the mandibular teeth when they are in centric occlusion.

Angle's Classification

The system developed by Dr. Edward H. Angle is used to describe and classify occlusion and malocclusion. In this system, the mesial-distal antagonistic relationship of the permanent first molars is considered to be the key of occlusion.

CLASS I (NEUTROCLUSION)

According to Angle's classification, Class I, which is also known as *neutroclusion,* is normal occlusion.

When the jaws are at rest, and the teeth are together in centric occlusion, the mandibular arch and the body of the mandible are in normal mesiodistal relationship to the maxillary arch if the following apply:

- The mesiobuccal (mesiofacial) cusp of the maxillary permanent first molar occludes in the buccal groove of the mandibular first molar (Fig. 5–20).
- The mesiolingual cusp of the maxillary permanent first molar occludes with the occlusal fossa of the mandibular permanent first molar.

Class I may include the situation in which the anteriors or individual teeth are malaligned in their position in the arch; however, it is the relationship of the permanent first molars that determines the classification.

CLASS II (DISTOCLUSION)

In Class II, which is also known as *distoclusion,* the mesiobuccal cusp of the maxillary first molar occludes in the interdental space between the mandibular second premolar and the mesial cusp of the mandibular first molar (Fig. 5–21).

The mandibular dental arch is in a **distal** relationship to the maxillary arch by half the width of the permanent first molar or by the mesiobuccal width of a premolar. This frequently gives the appearance of protrusion of the maxillary anterior teeth over the mandibular anteriors.

Class II, Division 1

The lips are usually flat and parted, with the lower lip tucked behind the upper incisors. The upper lip appears short and drawn up over the protruding anterior teeth of the maxillary arch.

The maxillary incisors are in labioversion. (**Labioversion** is the inclination of the teeth to extend facially beyond the normal overlap of the incisal edge of the maxillary incisors over the mandibular incisors.)

Division 1 Subdivision. The distal relationship of the mandibular dental arch is not in alignment. Instead, it is to one side of the opposing teeth of the maxilla. However, the opposite side of the mandibular arch may be in normal relationship with the opposing maxillary teeth.

Class II, Division 2

This division includes Class II malocclusions in which the maxillary incisors are *not* in labioversion.

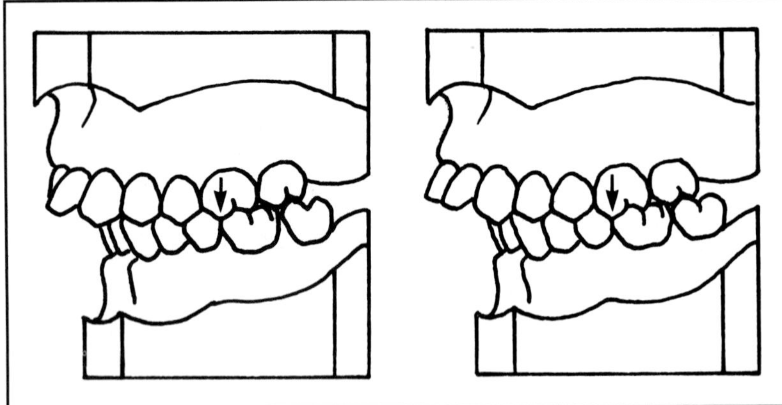

FIGURE 5–21

Class II, or distoclusion. Division 1 is shown on the left. Division 2 is shown on the right. (From Ehrlich, A., and Torres, H.O.: Essentials of Dental Assisting. Philadelphia, W.B. Saunders Co., 1992, p 68.)

The maxillary central incisors are nearly normal anteroposteriorly, and they may be slightly in linguoversion. The maxillary lateral incisors may be tipped labially and mesially.

Linguoversion refers to the position of the maxillary incisors as being in back of the mandibular incisors. (Normally, the maxillary incisors slightly overlap the front of the mandibular incisors.)

Division 2 Subdivision. In this situation, the malocclusion is on one side only (unilateral malocclusion).

CLASS III (MESIOCLUSION)

In a Class III malocclusion, which is also known as *mesioclusion,* the body of the mandible is in an abnormal mesial relationship to the maxilla. This frequently gives the appearance of protrusion of the mandible.

The mesiobuccal cusp of the maxillary first molar occludes in the interdental space between the distal cusp of the mandibular first permanent molar and the mesial cusp of the mandibular second permanent molar (Fig. 5–22).

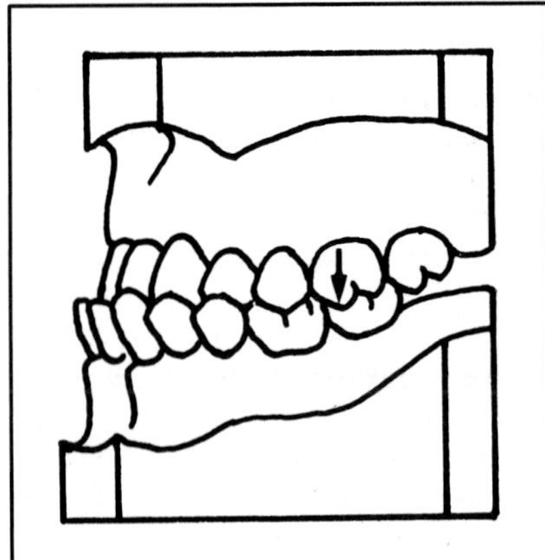

FIGURE 5–22

Class III, or mesioclusion. (From Ehrlich, A., and Torres, H.O.: Essentials of Dental Assisting. Philadelphia, W.B. Saunders Co., 1992, p 69.)

Primary Dentition

The 20 teeth of the primary dentition are also referred to as the *deciduous, baby,* or *milk teeth.* As the term "primary" implies, these teeth will be shed to make way for their permanent successors, which are known as **succedaneous teeth.**

Succedaneous teeth, and the ages at eruption and exfoliation, are discussed in Chapter 4. Diagrams of the primary teeth are shown at the end of the chapter in Figures 5–30 to 5–39.

All the primary teeth should be in normal alignment and occlusion shortly after the age of 2 years. The roots should be fully formed by the time the child is 3 years old.

Between the ages of 4 and 5, the anterior teeth begin to separate and usually show greater separation as time goes on.

After normal jaw growth has resulted in considerable separation, the occlusion is supported and made more efficient by the eruption and coming into occlusion of the first permanent molars immediately distal to the primary second molars. (These are often called the 6-year molars and they do *not* replace a primary tooth.)

The primary teeth serve several important functions:

- They provide adequate chewing surfaces in relationship to the size of the mouth and the strength of muscles of mastication.
- They act as an aid in the acquisition of speech.
- They serve as guides for the developing permanent teeth. Their premature loss can seriously affect the eruption and alignment of the permanent dentition.

Specialized Characteristics of the Primary Dentition

To perform these functions, the primary teeth have the following specialized characteristics:

Number: To accommodate the small jaws of the early years of life, there are fewer teeth in the primary dentition than in the permanent dentition.

Crown size: These teeth are smaller than their counterparts in the permanent dentition. The crowns appear to be short and squat in comparison with the crowns of the permanent teeth. They are milk-white in color, the enamel is thinner, and the pulp chamber is relatively large (Fig. 5–23).

Root design: The roots of the primary molars are long and slender in comparison with those of the permanent molars. The roots flare outward and extend beyond the surfaces of the crown.

This design allows the development of the permanent premolar tooth bud, which occupies the space below and between the roots, while retaining solid support for the primary molars during active function.

PRIMARY MAXILLARY MOLARS

Although there are no premolars in the primary dentition, in some respects the crown of the **primary maxillary first molar** resembles that of a permanent maxillary premolar. However, the divisions of the occlusal surface and the root form with its efficient anchorage make it a molar, in both type and function.

This tooth has four cusps (mesiolingual, mesiobuccal, distolingual, and distobuccal) and three roots (mesiobuccal, distobuccal, and lingual).

The **primary maxillary second molar** resembles the first permanent molar in everything but size. It has four well-developed cusps (mesiobuccal, distobuccal, distolingual, and mesiolingual), one supplemental cusp (the cusp of Carabelli), and three roots (mesiobuccal, distobuccal, and lingual).

PRIMARY MANDIBULAR MOLARS

The **primary mandibular first molar** does not resemble any of the other teeth, primary or permanent. However, it too has four cusps (mesiolingual, mesiobuccal, distolingual, and distobuccal) and two roots (mesial and distal).

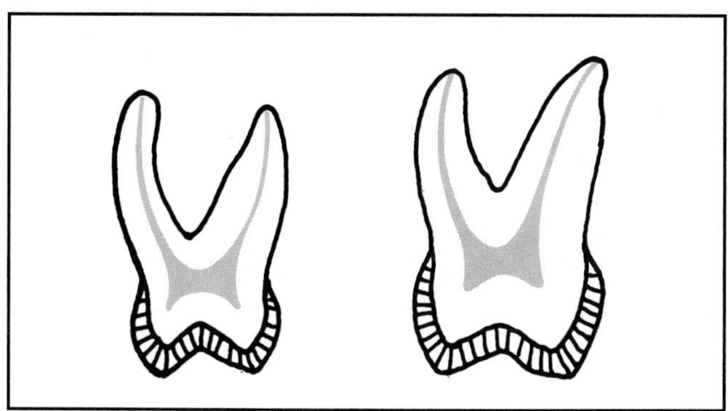

FIGURE 5–23

Cross-sectional comparison of a primary and a permanent molar. In the primary molar, shown on the left, note the differences in shape and pulp size.

The **primary mandibular second molar** resembles the permanent mandibular first molar except in its dimensions. It has five cusps (mesiolingual, mesiobuccal, distolingual, distobuccal, and distal) and two roots (mesial and distal).

Mixed Dentition

When they no longer meet the needs of the growing individual, the primary teeth are lost and are replaced by the permanent teeth, which are larger, stronger, and more numerous.

The exfoliation, or shedding process, of the primary teeth takes place between the fifth and twelfth years. During this mixed dentition stage, the child has some permanent and some primary teeth in position. Figure 5–24 is a radiographic view of the normally developing mixed dentition in a 7-year-old child.

Developing abnormalities often become apparent at this stage. When a potential problem is detected, it is important that the orthodontist examine the child for diagnosis and possible interceptive treatment.

Permanent Dentition

The permanent dentition consists of 32 teeth. Figures 5–25 and 5–26 detail the names of the cusps and roots of each of these teeth. Figures 5–40 to 5–55 at the end of the chapter are diagrams of each of the permanent teeth.

Permanent Incisors

The crowns of the permanent incisors show traces of having developed from four lobes: three facial (labial) and one lingual. The lingual lobe is represented by the **cingulum,** which is located near the middle cervical third of the lingual surface.

Each facial lobe terminates in a rounded eminence known as a **mamelon.** Mamelons are found on newly erupted incisors; however, in normal occlusion, they are soon worn down by use to form the incisal edge.

The **incisal edges** of these teeth are formed at the labioincisal line angle and do not exist until an edge has been created by wear. The incisal edge is also known as the *incisal surface* or *incisal plane.*

The incisal edges of maxillary incisors have a lingual inclination. The incisal edges of the mandibular incisors have a labial inclination. With this arrangement, the incisal planes of the mandibular and maxillary incisors are parallel with each other, fitting together during cutting action like the blades of a pair of scissors.

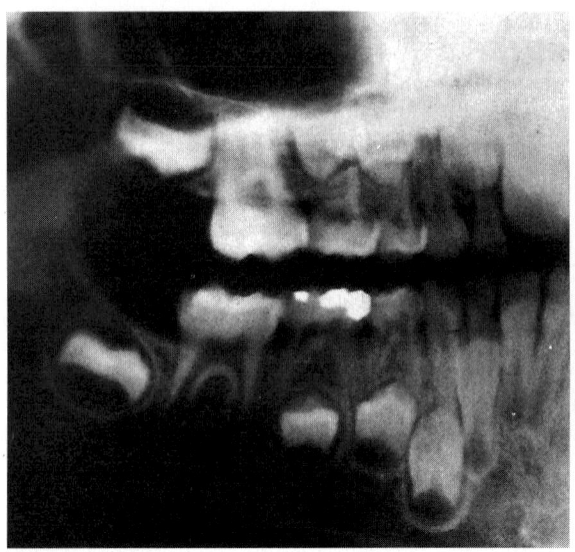
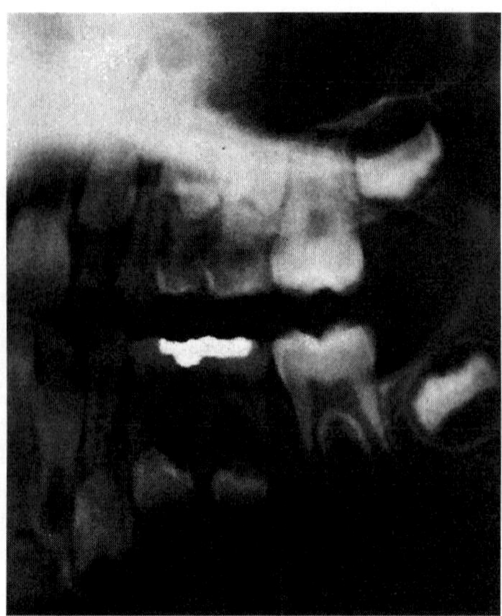

FIGURE 5–24

Panoramic radiograph showing the mixed dentition stage of a 7-year-old boy. (Courtesy of Dr. E. Howden, Chapel Hill, NC.)

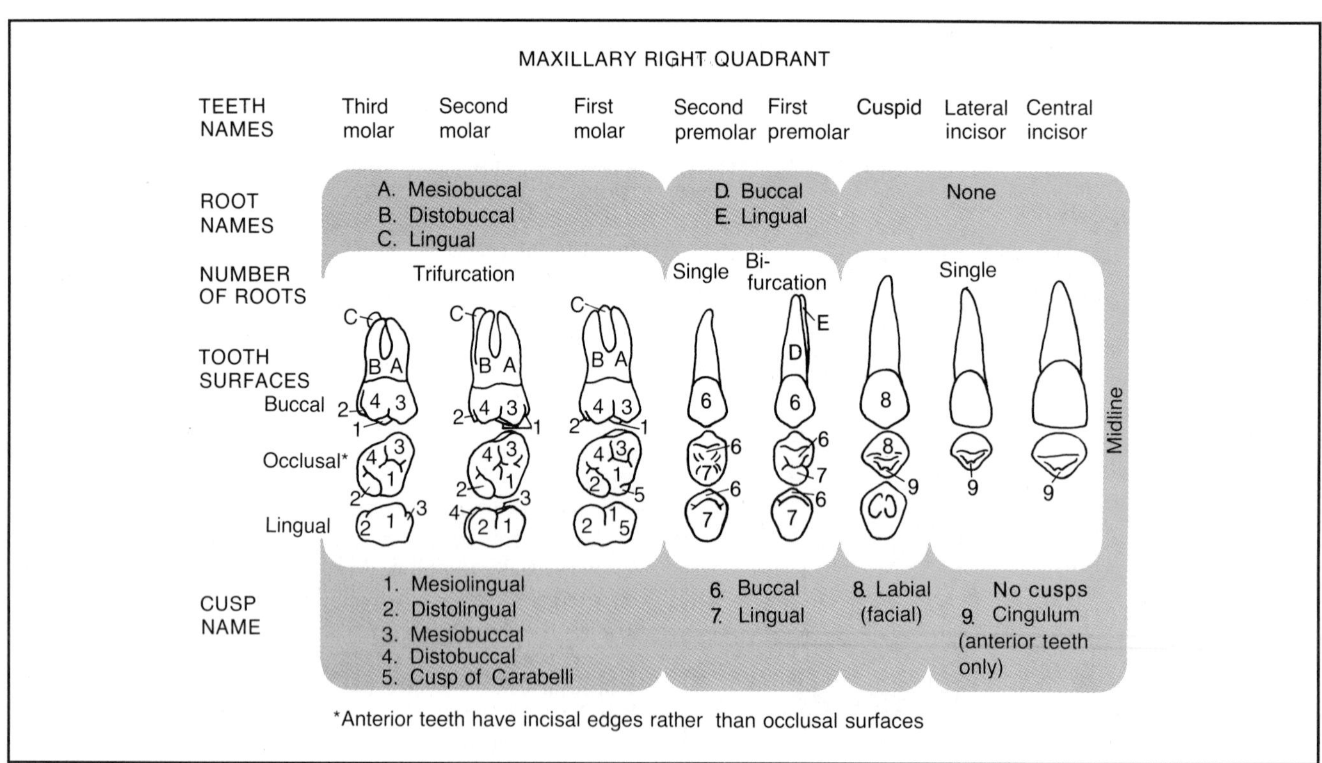

FIGURE 5–25

Names of the cusps and roots of the teeth of the maxillary right quadrant (permanent dentition).

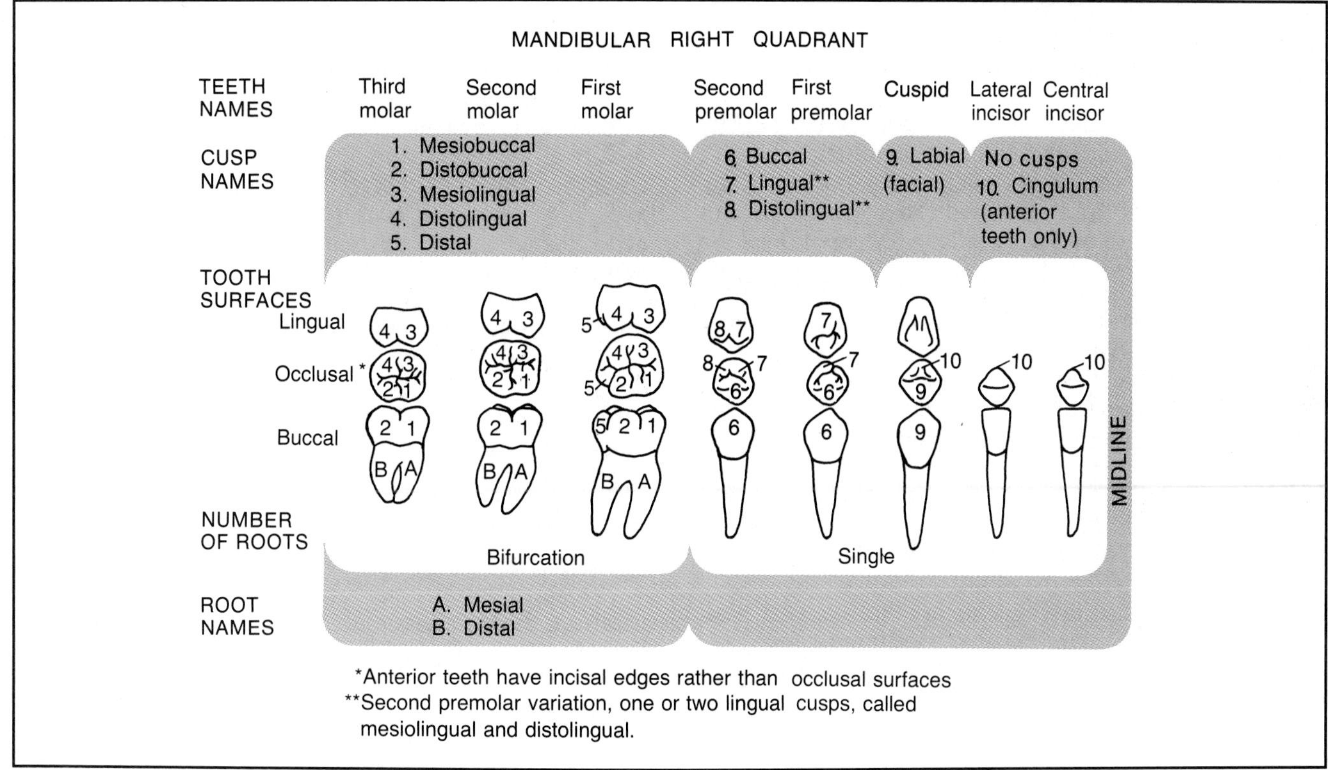

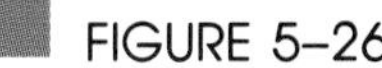
FIGURE 5–26

Names of the cusps and roots of the teeth of the mandibular right quadrant (permanent dentition).

MAXILLARY INCISORS

The **maxillary central incisors** are the widest mesiodistally of any of the anterior teeth and are the most prominent teeth in the mouth. Although they are larger than the maxillary lateral incisors, these teeth are similar anatomically and supplement each other in function.

The **maxillary lateral incisors** are smaller in all dimensions except root length. These incisors vary in form more than any other tooth in the mouth except the third molars and frequently are congenitally missing.

MANDIBULAR INCISORS

The mandibular incisors show uniform development, with few instances of malformations or anomalies. (An **anomaly** is a marked deviation from the normal.)

They have smaller mesiodistal dimensions than any of the other teeth, and the central mandibular incisors are somewhat smaller than the lateral incisors. This is the reverse of the situation found in the maxilla.

Permanent Cuspids

The permanent cuspid crowns are usually as long as those of the maxillary central incisors. The maxillary and mandibular cuspids bear a close resemblance to each other in form and function, with the middle facial lobe of each cuspid highly developed incisally into a strong, well-formed cusp.

Permanent Premolars

The eight premolars of the permanent dentition, two in each quadrant, are located posterior to the cuspids and immediately anterior to the molars. These teeth intercusp with opposing teeth when the jaws are brought together. This makes them efficient as grinding teeth, and they function much like molars.

MAXILLARY PREMOLARS

The maxillary premolars have crowns that are slightly longer than those of the molars. However, the root lengths are similar to those of molars.

- Each **maxillary first premolar** has two cusps (buccal and lingual) and two roots (facial and lingual). The buccal cusp is long and sharp to assist the cuspid with tearing.
- The maxillary first premolars are often slightly larger than the maxillary second premolars.
- The **maxillary second premolar** has two cusps (buccal and lingual) and one root. These cusps are not as sharp as those of the maxillary first premolars.

MANDIBULAR PREMOLARS

- The **mandibular first premolars** are single-rooted and have many of the characteristics of a small cuspid.
- The mandibular first premolar has a long and well-formed buccal cusp and a small, nonfunctioning lingual cusp. (This may be no larger than the cingulum found on some maxillary cuspids.)
- The mandibular first premolars are smaller and shorter than the mandibular second premolars.
- In most instances, the **mandibular second premolars** have three well-formed cusps (one large buccal cusp and the smaller lingual and distolingual cusps). Because of these cusps, these teeth have more of the characteristics of a small molar.

Permanent Molars

There are 12 molars, three in each quadrant, in the permanent dentition. The molar crowns, which have four or five short, blunt cusps, are larger than the crowns of the other teeth. Each molar has two or three roots that help support this larger crown.

MAXILLARY MOLARS

The maxillary molars assist the mandibular molars in performing the major portion of the work of mastication. By virtue both of their size and of their anchorage in the jaws, they are the largest and strongest maxillary teeth.

Each maxillary molar has three well-separated and well-developed roots. A tooth with three roots is said to be **trifurcated,** which means divided into three. A **trifurcation** is the area where the three roots divide.

These roots are the mesiobuccal, distobuccal, and lingual roots. They provide the tooth with maximum anchorage against occlusal forces that would tend to unseat it.

Maxillary First Molar. The maxillary first molar is normally the largest tooth in the maxillary arch. It has four well-developed functioning cusps (mesiolingual, distolingual, mesiobuccal, and distobuccal) and one supplemental cusp of little practical use.

The fifth cusp is called the **cusp of Carabelli.** When present, this cusp is found lingual to the mesiolingual cusp. However, it is often so poorly developed that it is scarcely distinguishable.

Maxillary Second Molar. The maxillary second molar supplements the first molar in function. The crown is somewhat shorter than that of the first molar, and there are four cusps (mesiobuccal, distobuccal, mesiolingual, and distolingual). No fifth cusp is present.

There are three roots (mesiobuccal, distobuccal, and lingual). In general, the roots of this tooth are as long as, if not somewhat longer than, those of the first molar.

Maxillary Third Molar. The maxillary third molar often appears as a developmental anomaly. It differs considerably in size, contour, and relative position from the other teeth. It is seldom as well developed as the maxillary second molar, to which it bears some resemblance.

The third molar supplements the second molar in function. Its fundamental design is similar; however, the crown is smaller, and the roots as a rule are shorter. The roots of this tooth tend to fuse together and the result is a single tapered root.

MANDIBULAR MOLARS

The mandibular molars are the largest and strongest mandibular teeth, both because of their bulk (the crown has four or five cusps) and because of their anchorage in the jaw.

Each mandibular molar has two well-developed roots, one mesial and one distal. A tooth with two roots is said to be **bifurcated,** which means divided into two. A **bifurcation** is the area where the two roots divide.

Mandibular First Molar. The mandibular first molar normally is the largest tooth in the mandibular arch. It has five well-developed cusps (mesiobuccal, distobuccal, mesiolingual, distolingual, and distal).

The two roots (mesial and distal) are very broad buccolingually and are widely separated at the apices. This design gives the tooth firm anchorage in the jaw.

Mandibular Second Molar. The mandibular second molar supplements the first molar in function. Normally the second molar is slightly smaller than the first molar in all directions.

The crown has four well-developed cusps (mesiolingual, distolingual, mesiobuccal, and distobuccal) and two roots (mesial and distal). These roots are not as broad buccolingually as those of the first molar, nor are they as widely separated.

Mandibular Third Molar. Normally the mandibular third molar is similar in design to the other mandibular molars with four cusps and two roots. However, this tooth often presents anomalies in form and in position. A common anomaly is that the multiple roots are fused to form a single root.

TOOTH NUMBERING SYSTEMS

Numbering systems are used as a simplified means of identifying the teeth for charting and descriptive purposes.

The Universal Numbering System

The Universal Numbering System, which is approved by the American Dental Association, is used throughout the United States (Tables 5–1 and 5–2).

In the Universal Numbering System, the permanent teeth are numbered 1 to 32. Numbering begins with the upper right third molar (tooth #1), works around to the upper left third molar (tooth #16), then drops to the lower left third molar (tooth #17), and works around to the lower right third molar (tooth #32).

In the Universal Numbering System, the primary teeth are lettered with capital letters A to T. Lettering begins with the upper right second primary molar (tooth A), works around to the upper left second primary molar (tooth J), then drops to the lower left second primary molar (tooth K), and works around to the lower second third primary molar (tooth T).

TABLE 5–1

Universal Numbering System for Permanent Teeth

NO.	MAXILLARY TEETH	NO.	MANDIBULAR TEETH
1	Maxillary right third molar	32	Mandibular right third molar
2	Maxillary right second molar	31	Mandibular right second molar
3	Maxillary right first molar	30	Mandibular right first molar
4	Maxillary right second premolar	29	Mandibular right second premolar
5	Maxillary right first premolar	28	Mandibular right first premolar
6	Maxillary right cuspid	27	Mandibular right cuspid
7	Maxillary right lateral incisor	26	Mandibular right lateral incisor
8	Maxillary right central incisor	25	Mandibular right central incisor
9	Maxillary left central incisor	24	Mandibular left central incisor
10	Maxillary left lateral incisor	23	Mandibular left lateral incisor
11	Maxillary left cuspid	22	Mandibular left cuspid
12	Maxillary left first premolar	21	Mandibular left first premolar
13	Maxillary left second premolar	20	Mandibular left second premolar
14	Maxillary left first molar	19	Mandibular left first molar
15	Maxillary left second molar	18	Mandibular left second molar
16	Maxillary left third molar	17	Mandibular left third molar

TABLE 5–2

Universal Numbering System for Primary Teeth

NO.	MAXILLARY TEETH	NO.	MANDIBULAR TEETH
A	Maxillary right second molar	T	Mandibular right second molar
B	Maxillary right first molar	S	Mandibular right first molar
C	Maxillary right cuspid	R	Mandibular right cuspid
D	Maxillary right lateral incisor	Q	Mandibular right lateral incisor
E	Maxillary right central incisor	P	Mandibular right central incisor
F	Maxillary left central incisor	O	Mandibular left central incisor
G	Maxillary left lateral incisor	N	Mandibular left lateral incisor
H	Maxillary left cuspid	M	Mandibular left cuspid
I	Maxillary left first molar	L	Mandibular left first molar
J	Maxillary left second molar	K	Mandibular left second molar

Fédération Dentaire Internationale Numbering System

The Fédération Dentaire Internationale (FDI) recommends a *two-digit tooth-recording system.* In this system, the first digit indicates the quadrant and the second indicates the tooth within the quadrant, numbering from the midline toward the posterior. The permanent teeth are numbered as follows:

- The maxillary right quadrant is No. 1 and contains teeth #11 to #18.
- The maxillary left quadrant is No. 2 and contains teeth #21 to #28.
- The mandibular left quadrant is No. 3 and contains teeth #31 to #38.
- The mandibular right quadrant is No. 4 and contains teeth #41 to #48.

The primary teeth are numbered in this manner:

- The maxillary right quadrant is No. 5 and contains teeth #51 to #55.
- The maxillary left quadrant is No. 6 and contains teeth #61 to #65.
- The mandibular left quadrant is No. 7 and contains teeth #71 to #75.
- The mandibular right quadrant is No. 8 and contains teeth #81 to #85.

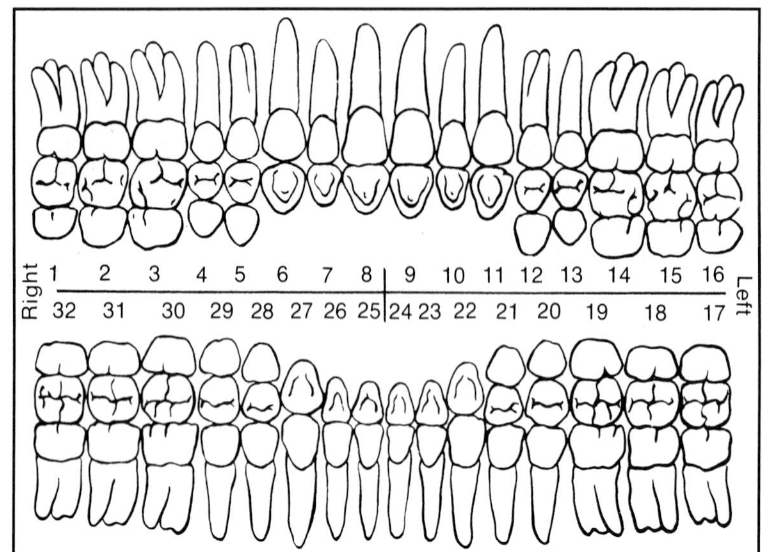

FIGURE 5–27

The permanent teeth as they are represented on a dental chart according to the Universal Numbering System. (Courtesy of Colwell Systems, Champaign, IL.)

It is suggested that the digits be pronounced separately. For example, the permanent cuspids are teeth 1-3, 2-3, 3-3, and 4-3.

Tooth Diagrams

The diagrams used in charting have the teeth arranged so that the right quadrants are on the left side of the page and the left quadrants are on the right side of the page (Figs. 5–27 to 5–29). (Charting is discussed in Chapter 18.)

Radiographs are usually mounted in the same order so that the chart and radiographs are parallel in their representation.

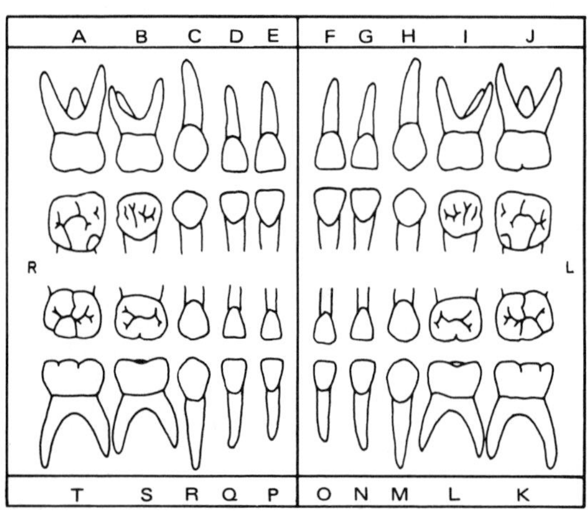

FIGURE 5–28

The primary teeth as they are represented on a dental chart according to the Universal Numbering System. (Courtesy of Colwell Systems, Champaign, IL.)

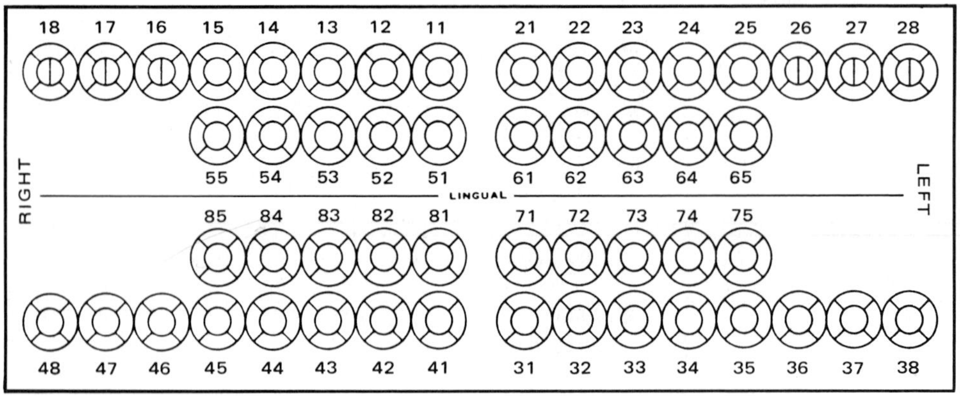

FIGURE 5–29

The Fédération Dentaire Internationale numbering system for both the permanent and primary dentitions. (Courtesy of Colwell Systems, Champaign, IL.)

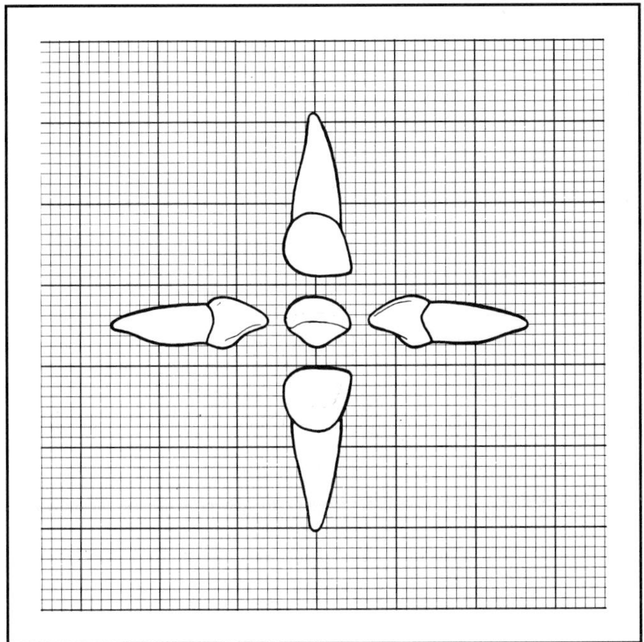

FIGURE 5–30

Primary maxillary left central incisor.

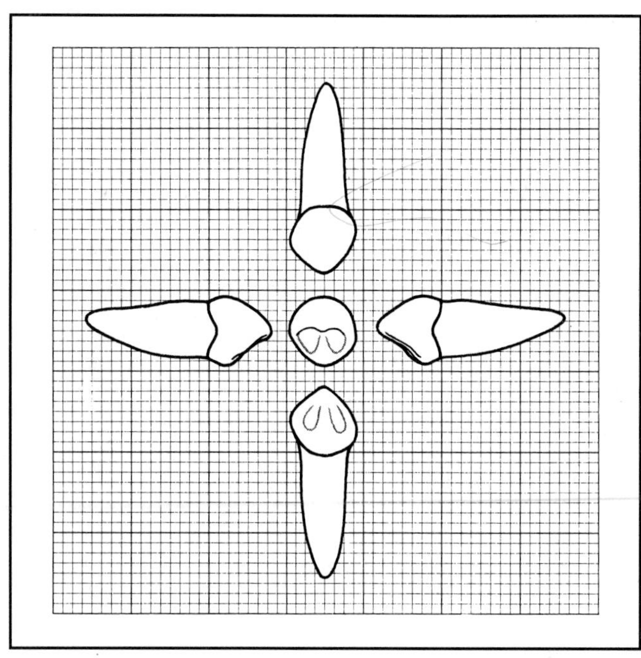

FIGURE 5–32

Primary maxillary left cuspid.

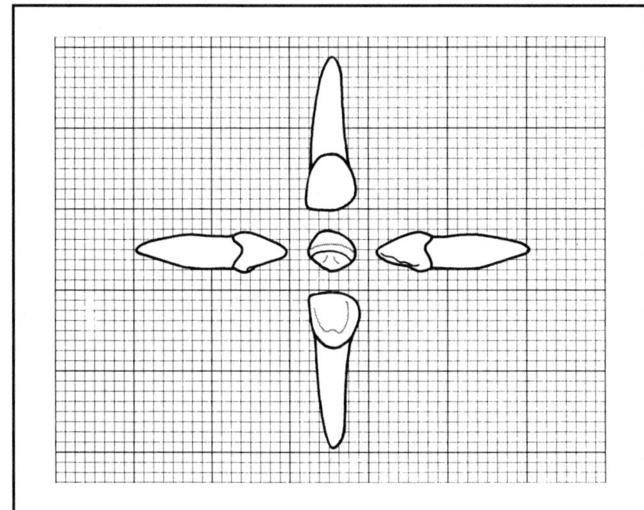

FIGURE 5–31

Primary maxillary left lateral incisor.

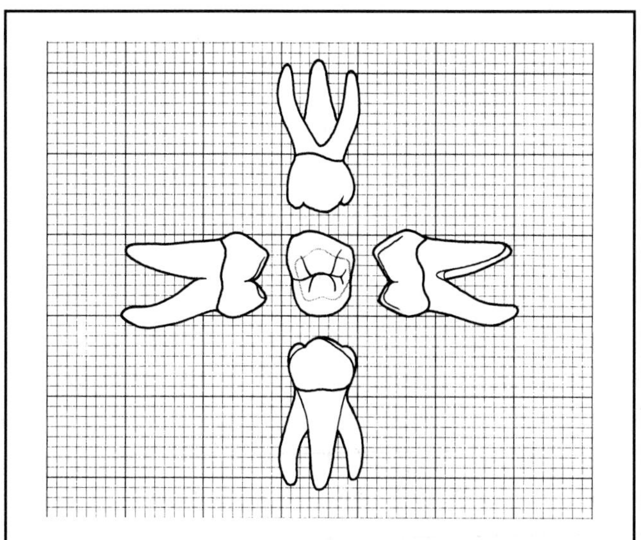

FIGURE 5–33

Primary maxillary left first molar.

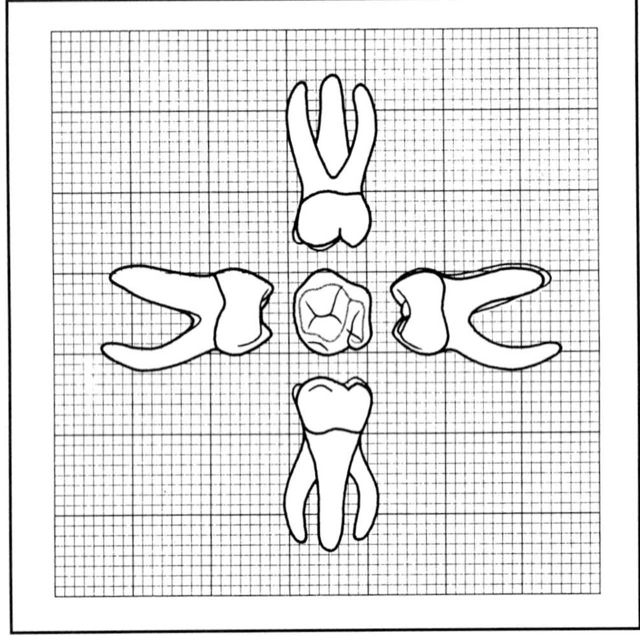

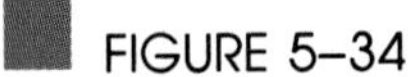

FIGURE 5–34

Primary maxillary left second molar.

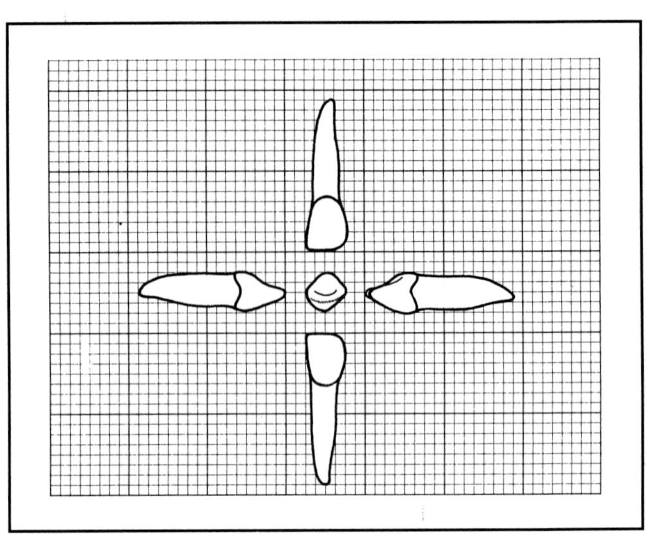

FIGURE 5–36

Primary mandibular left lateral incisor.

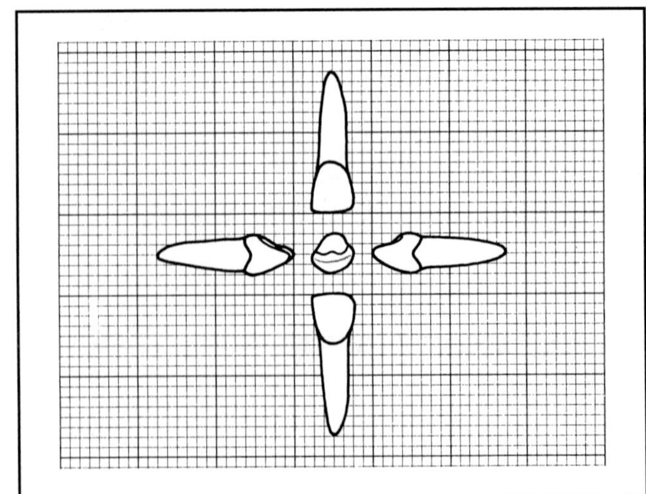

FIGURE 5–35

Primary mandibular left central incisor.

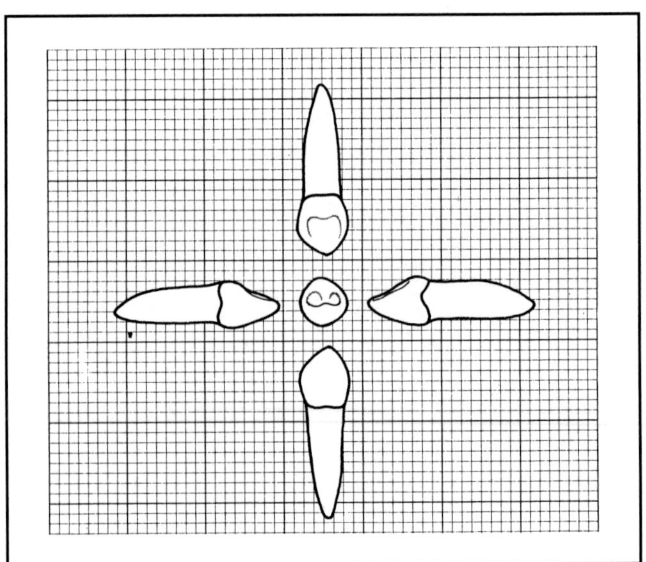

FIGURE 5–37

Primary mandibular left cuspid.

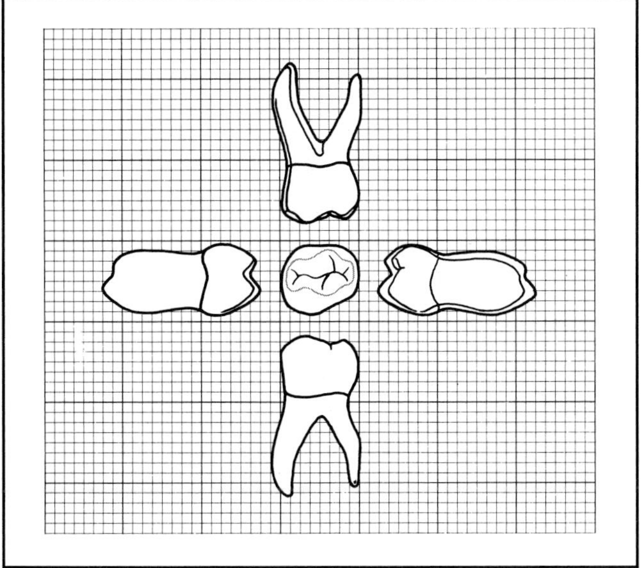

FIGURE 5–38

Primary mandibular left first molar.

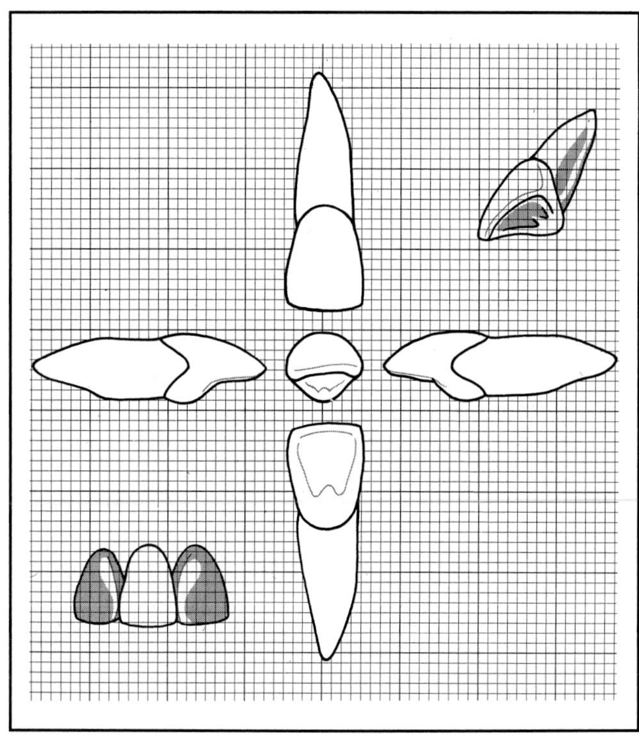

FIGURE 5–40

Permanent maxillary right central incisor.

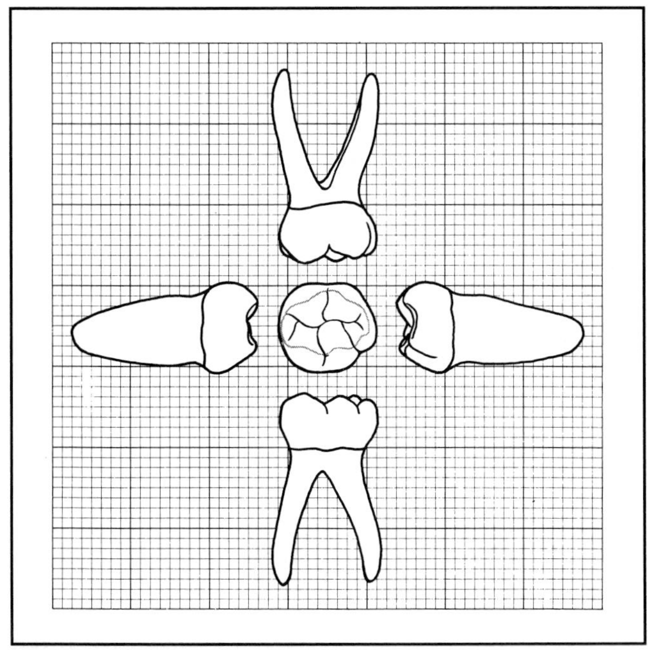

FIGURE 5–39

Primary mandibular left second molar.

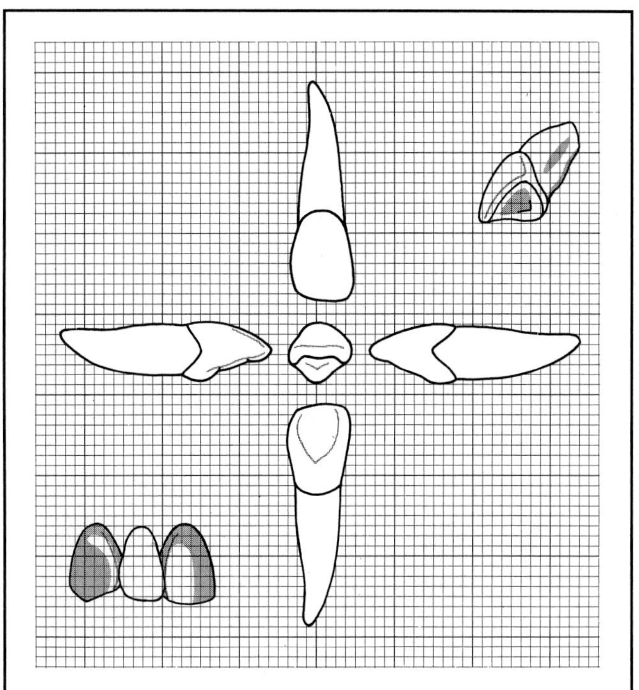

FIGURE 5–41

Permanent maxillary right lateral incisor.

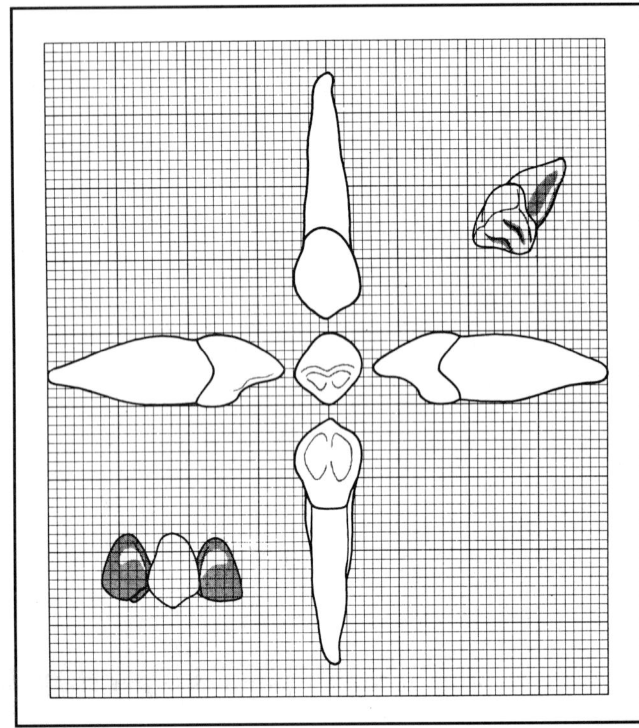

FIGURE 5–42

Permanent maxillary right cuspid.

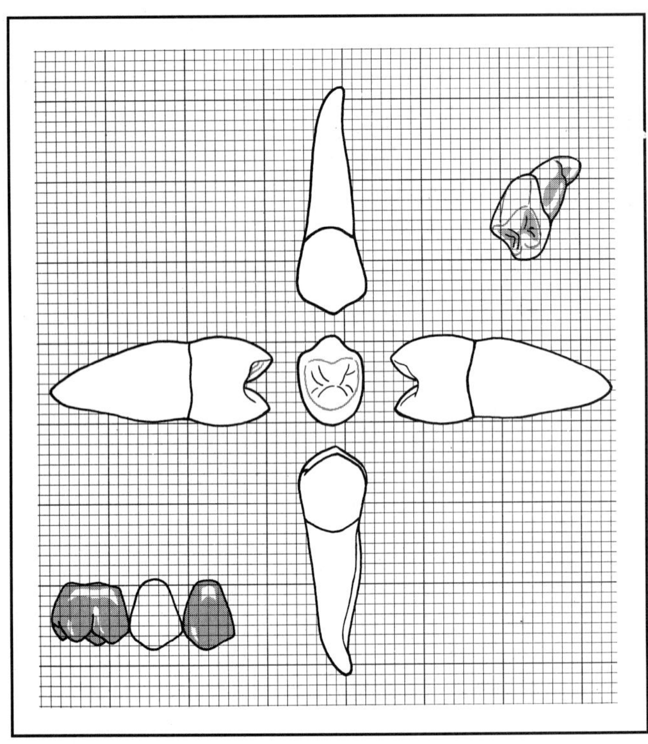

FIGURE 5–44

Permanent maxillary right second premolar.

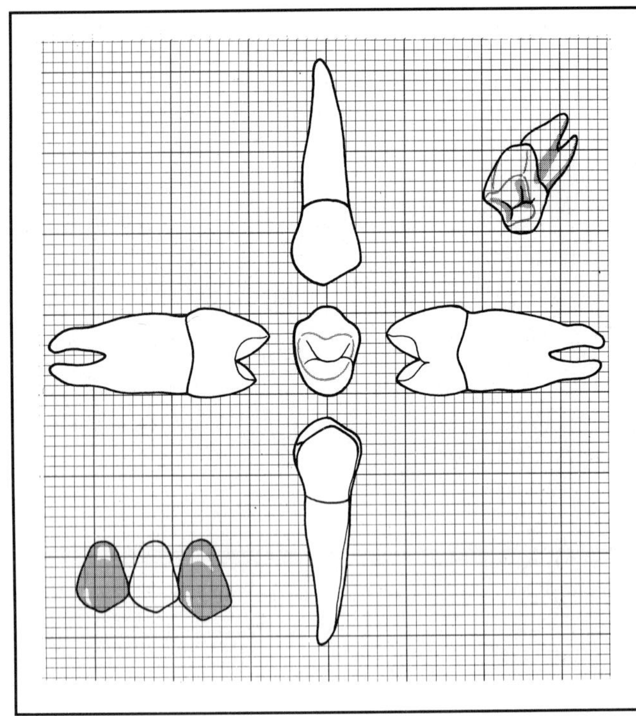

FIGURE 5–43

Permanent maxillary right first premolar.

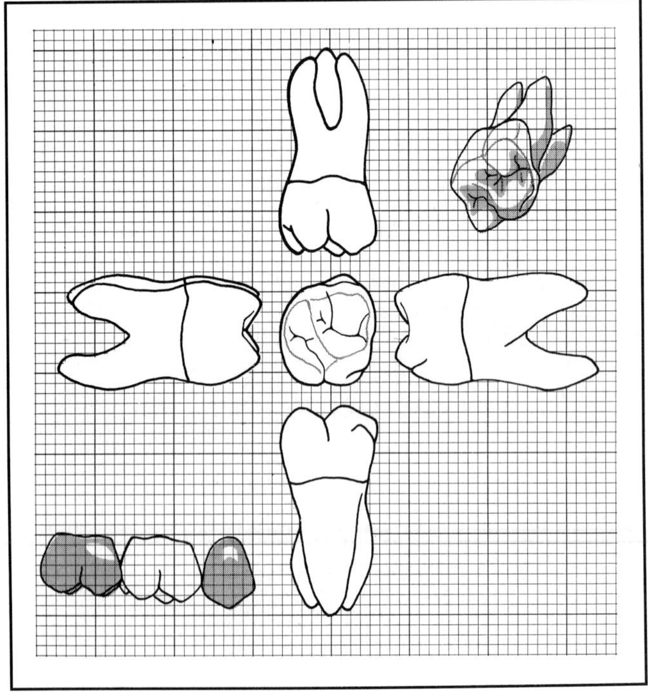

FIGURE 5–45

Permanent maxillary right first molar.

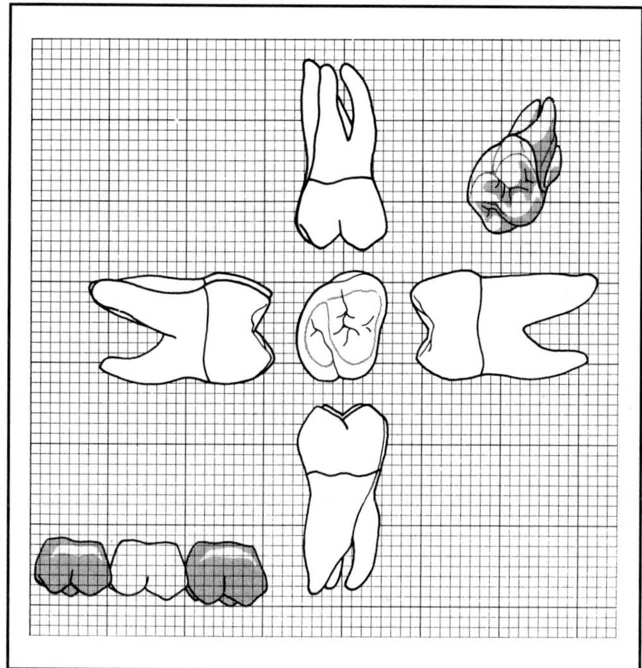

FIGURE 5–46

Permanent maxillary right second molar.

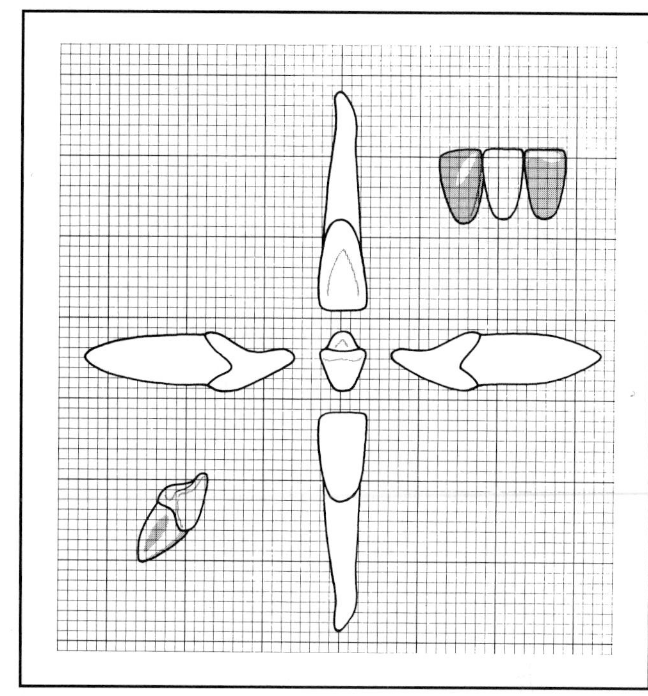

FIGURE 5–48

Permanent mandibular right central inciso

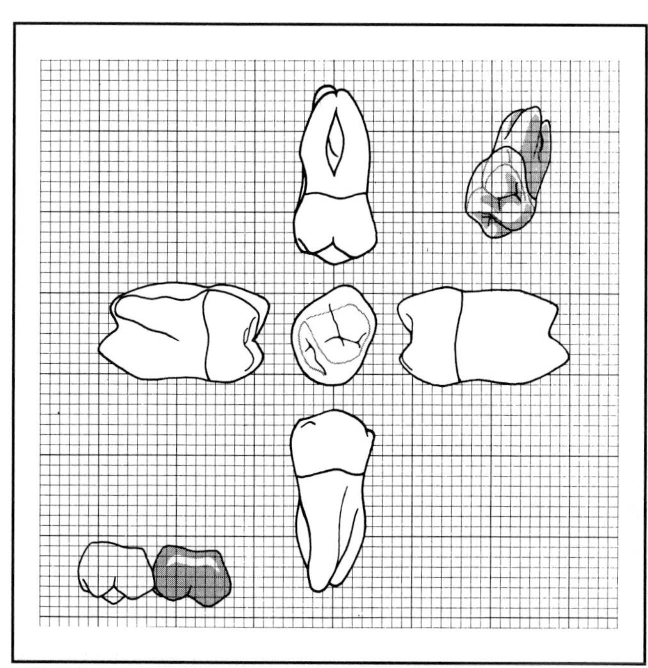

FIGURE 5–47

Permanent maxillary right third molar.

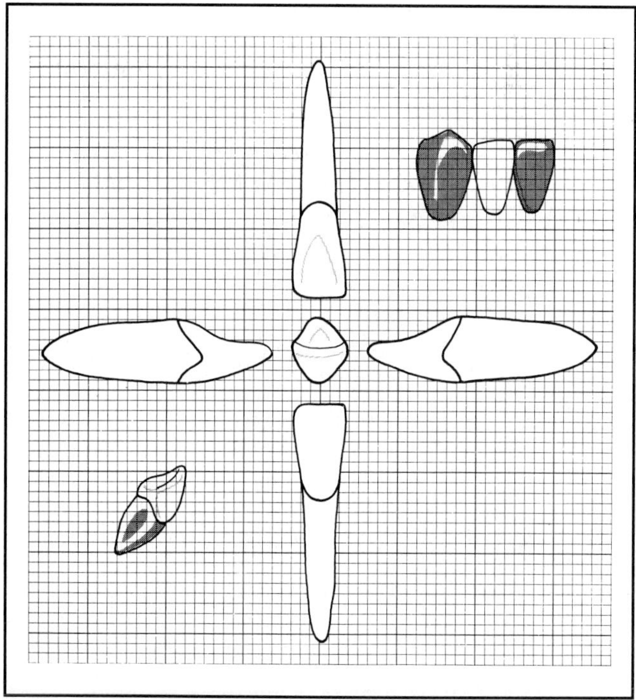

FIGURE 5–49

Permanent mandibular right lateral incisor.

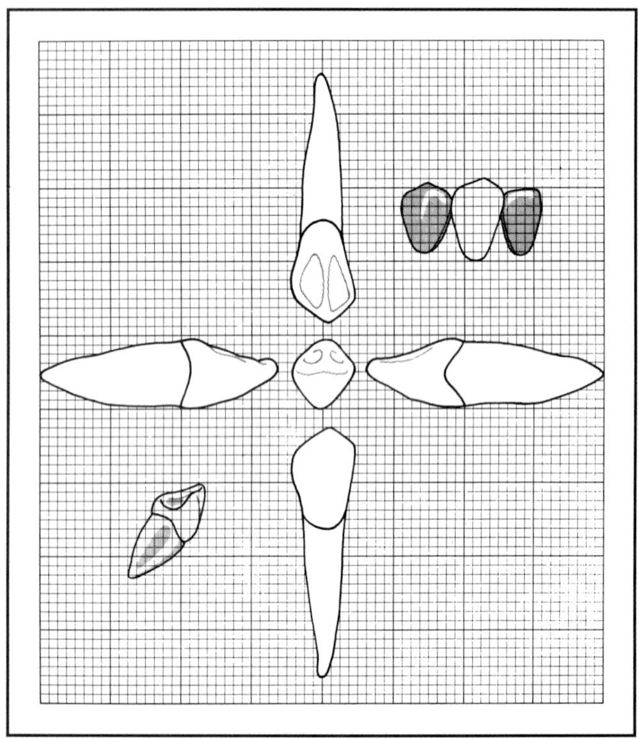

FIGURE 5–50

Permanent mandibular right cuspid.

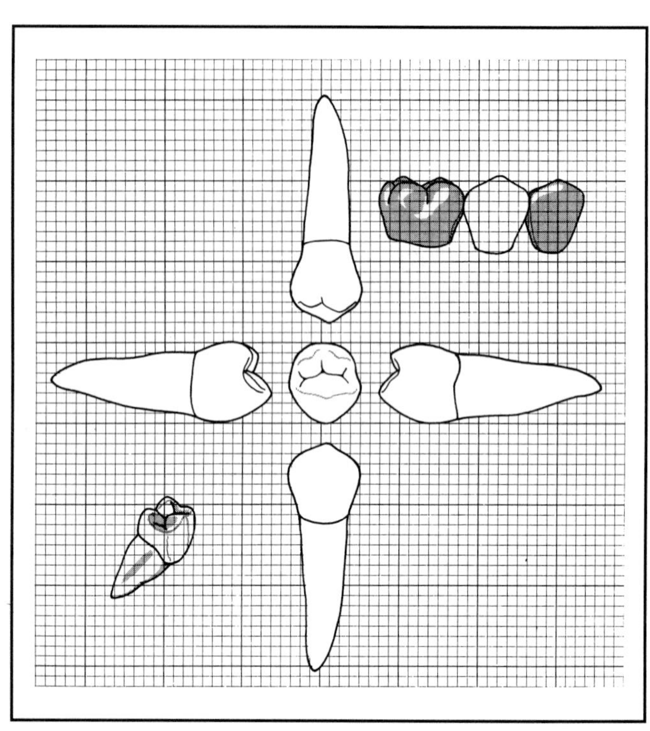

FIGURE 5–52

Permanent mandibular right second premolar.

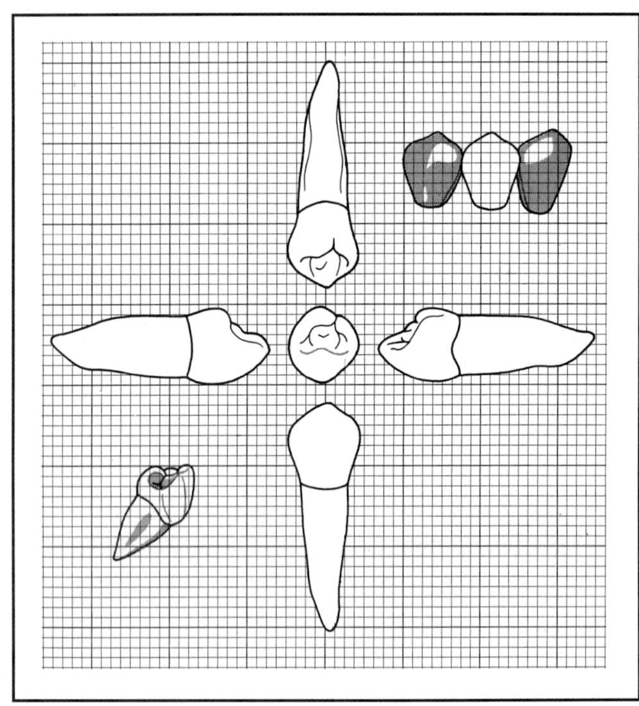

FIGURE 5–51

Permanent mandibular right first premolar.

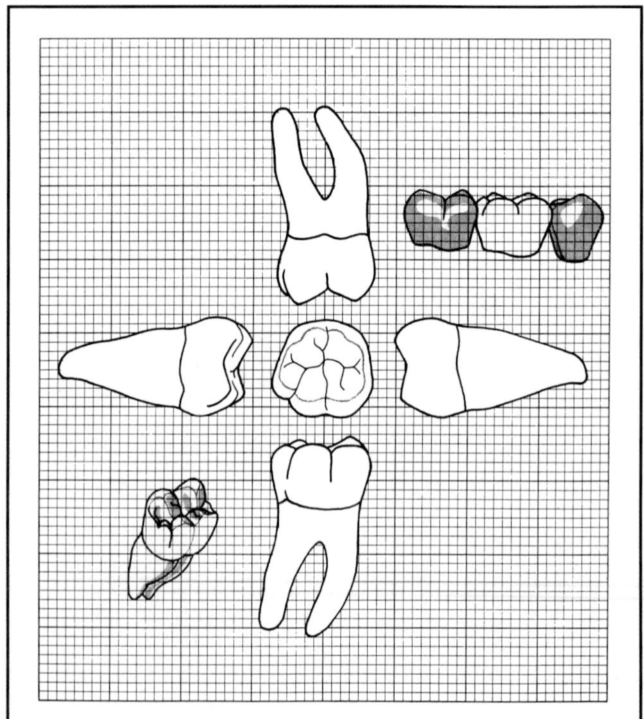

FIGURE 5–53

Permanent mandibular right first molar.

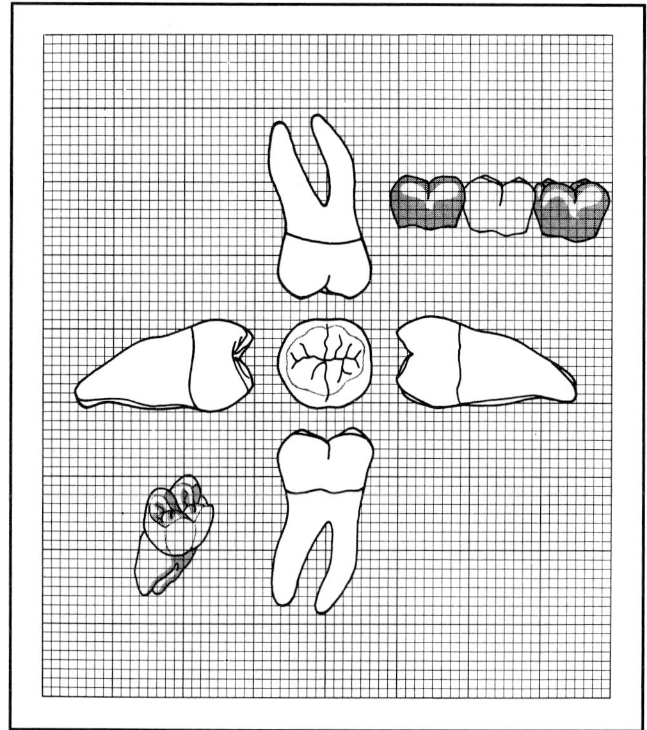

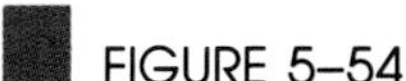

FIGURE 5–54

Permanent mandibular right second molar.

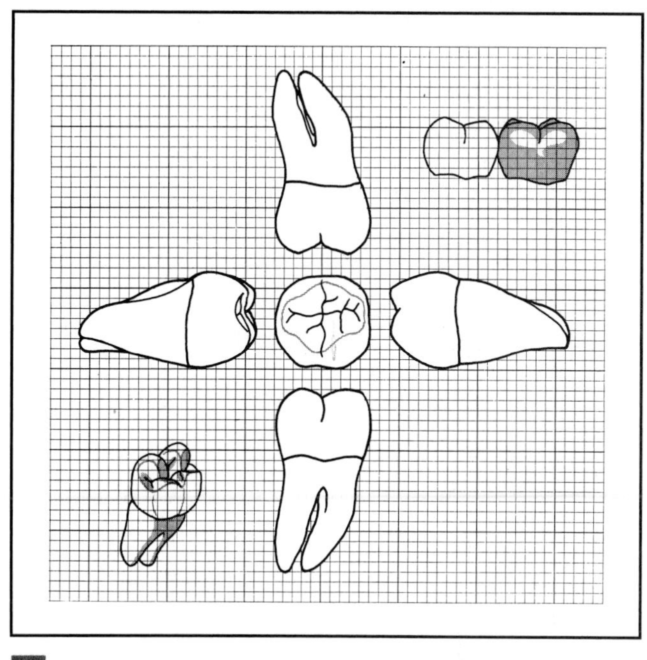

FIGURE 5–55

Permanent mandibular right third molar.

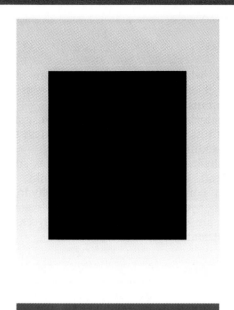

Chapter 6

Preventive Dentistry and Nutrition

Introduction

The goal of preventive dentistry is to achieve and maintain optimum oral health for the longest period of time possible—using the simplest, most universally acceptable methods. Within this broad goal, the primary emphasis is on the prevention of dental decay and periodontal disease.

Dental Health Team Members as Role Models

It is impossible to convince a patient of the value of preventive dentistry if the members of the office team obviously do not believe in, and practice, it. Therefore, it is essential that each team member

- Have all required dental treatment completed
- Maintain good personal oral hygiene
- Follow the guidelines for good nutrition and recommended general healthcare procedures

How Dental Decay Occurs

In order for dental decay to occur, three factors must be present:

- Dental plaque, which contains bacteria
- A nutrient that the bacteria are able to utilize to generate an acid attack
- A susceptible tooth

The bacteria convert the sugar into acid, which attacks the enamel of the teeth. Each time a sugary substance is eaten, this causes a 20-minute **acid attack**. If sugary substances are eaten frequently enough, and if the tooth is unable to resist, these acid attacks cause demineralization of the enamel, which eventually leads to dental decay. (**Demineralization** is the loss of the minerals calcium and phosphorus from the enamel.)

To stop this damage, preventive dentistry includes three steps:

- Removing plaque
- Limiting acid attacks
- Strengthening the resistance of the tooth

Key Components of Preventive Dentistry

This chapter is divided into four sections to reflect the key components of preventive dentistry.

General nutrition is important because being well-nourished throughout life is essential for the development and maintenance of sound teeth and tissues.

Host resistance refers to the ability of the teeth to withstand the acid attacks that damage the enamel. Fluorides play a major role in increasing and maintaining the strength of dental enamel.

Plaque control focuses on the daily removal of all plaque through toothbrushing and other oral hygiene measures.

Patient education is an essential part of preventive dentistry because the patient must learn the new techniques and be motivated to carry through on the necessary steps.

General Nutrition

Good general nutrition depends on an adequate supply of the nutrients that are properly utilized by the body. (**Nutrients** are substances that supply the body with the elements necessary to meet the body's requirements for energy, growth, maintenance, and well-being.)

The key nutrients are carbohydrates, proteins, fats, water, vitamins, and minerals.

- All of these nutrients are available through a well-balanced diet.
- Each has a specific role, and the functions of one nutrient cannot be performed by other nutrients.
- Supplements and vitamin pills cannot make up for eating foods that are not nutritionally adequate.

Energy Needs

Individual energy needs vary widely, depending on age, sex, body weight, level of physical activity, and other specialized demands made upon the body.

If food intake does not meet the body's energy and nutrient needs, changes take place that negatively impact health and well-being. If food intake exceeds the body's energy needs, the excess is stored as fat, and the individual gains weight.

Calories are the basic units used to measure the body's energy needs and use. (A **calorie** is the amount of heat required to raise 1 gram of water by 1° Celsius.) As shown in Table 6–1, each of the key nutrients yields a fixed number of calories per gram.

TABLE 6–1

Calories Per Gram of Nutrient

NUTRIENT	CALORIES PER GRAM
Carbohydrates, which come from plant sources, are our primary energy source.	4
Proteins, which may come from plant or animal sources, are the building blocks of the body. They may also be used for energy.	4
Fats, which are found in many foods, facilitate absorption of the fat-soluble vitamins.	9
Alcohol is not a nutrient. It is a refined substance that the body processes as a carbohydrate. (It is included here to show the caloric content.)	7

Carbohydrates

Carbohydrates, which come primarily from plant sources, are our chief source of energy. They also supply essential vitamins and minerals.

Complex carbohydrates are found mainly in grains, vegetables, and fruits. They are important because they provide energy, additional nutrients, and fiber.

Refined carbohydrates include foods such as sugar, syrup, jelly, bread, cookies, cakes, soft drinks, and other sweets. In contrast to complex carbohydrates, most refined carbohydrates supply only empty calories. (**Empty calories** are calories that provide only energy and no other nutrients.)

CARIOGENIC FOODS

The bacteria in plaque use simple sugars as their food. Refined carbohydrates contain such sugars.

In the mouth the enzyme salivary amylase begins the process of breaking complex carbohydrates down into the simple sugars that the body uses for energy. This process is completed later in the digestive process.

Cariogenic foods are foods that are broken down in the mouth into the simple sugars that can be used by the bacteria in plaque. (**Cariogenic** means decay producing.) There are many variables that affect how harmful these foods may be.

- Refined carbohydrates, such as candy and other sweets, are cariogenic because their sugars are readily available.
- Sugary liquids, such as soft drinks, clear the mouth quickly and are not as cariogenic as sticky sweets, which stay in the mouth longer.
- Foods such as crackers that are not sweet but that stick to the teeth are broken down into sugars in the mouth and can be used by the bacteria.
- Complex carbohydrates, such as fruits and vegetables, are less cariogenic because they clear the mouth before they are converted into simple sugars.
- To reduce the number of acid attacks that the teeth must resist, the frequency of eating sweets should be limited to mealtime.

Proteins

Proteins come from animal (meat and cheese) and plant (legumes and nuts) sources. Their primary functions are to build and repair body tissues, and they are the only nutrients that can carry out these roles. Proteins can also be used to meet energy needs; however, this is not efficient use of these nutrients.

Fats

Fats, which come from both animal and plant sources, provide large amounts of energy in small amounts of food. Fats facilitate absorption of the fat-

TABLE 6–2

Fat-Soluble Vitamins

VITAMIN	IMPORTANT FUNCTIONS	BEST SOURCES	DEFICIENCY SYMPTOMS
Vitamin A	Growth Health of the eyes Structure and functioning of the cells of the skin and mucous membranes Promotes health of the oral structures	Fish liver oils Liver Green and yellow vegetables Fruit (yellow) Butter, milk, cream, cheese Egg yolk	Retarded growth Night blindness Increased susceptibility to infections Changes in skin and mucous membranes
Vitamin D	Helps absorb calcium from digestive tract and build calcium and phosphorus into bones and teeth Growth	Vitamin D–irradiated milk Fish liver oil Sunshine on skin	Rickets Poor tooth development
Vitamin E	Protects vitamin A and essential fatty acids from oxidation Aids in the formation of red blood cells, muscles, and other tissues	Wheat germ oil Vegetable oils Green vegetables Milk fat, butter Egg yolk	Undetermined
Vitamin K	Normal clotting of blood Helps maintain normal liver function	Green leafy vegetables Liver Soybean and other vegetable oils Synthesized by intestinal bacteria	Hemorrhages

soluble vitamins A, D, E, and K. They also provide essential fatty acids. Daily fat requirements are filled by fats contained in the other foods such as meat (in which they occur naturally) and in processed foods such as cookies (in which they were added in processing).

Water

Water is an important part of most body structures. It helps to build tissue and aids in regulating body temperature. An adequate supply is essential daily, for we can live longer without food than we can without water.

Vitamins

Vitamins are organic substances that are necessary in very small amounts for proper growth, development, and optimum health. (**Organic substances** are composed of matter of plant or animal origin.)

The **fat-soluble vitamins** are stored in body fat and are not destroyed by cooking. The functions, sources, and deficiency symptoms of fat-soluble vitamins are described in Table 6–2.

The **water-soluble vitamins**, which are naturally present in food, are easily destroyed during food preparation. These vitamins are not stored in the body and must be consumed each day. The functions, sources, and deficiency symptoms of water-soluble vitamins are described in Table 6–3.

Because of their similar functions, all of the water-soluble vitamins, except vitamin C, are often grouped together and are referred to as the B complex vitamins.

Minerals

Minerals are inorganic substances that are necessary in very small amounts for proper growth, development, and optimum health. (**Inorganic substances** are composed of matter other than that of plant or animal origin.)

Minerals are the components of the bones and teeth that make them rigid and strong. They also play an important part in maintaining other bodily functions. The functions, sources, and deficiency symptoms of minerals are described in Table 6–4.

Food Groups

According to information presented by the United States Department of Agriculture (USDA), there are five recommended food groups. Each group provides some, but not all, of the nutrients needed daily. There is a recommended range of servings for each of the five food groups. Although many servings are recommended for some foods, the portion sizes are small.

- **Bread, cereal, rice, and pasta group:** 6 to 11 servings are recommended daily.
- **Vegetable group:** 3 to 5 servings are recommended daily.

TABLE 6–3

Water-Soluble Vitamins

VITAMIN	IMPORTANT FUNCTIONS	BEST SOURCES	DEFICIENCY SYMPTOMS
Thiamine (B_1)	Growth Promotion of normal appetite and digestion Maintaining good muscle tone and healthy functioning of the heart and nerves	Yeast Wheat germ Organ meats Meat Dried beans and peas Whole grain or enriched products	Beriberi Retarded growth, loss of appetite and weight Nerve disorders Lowered resistance to fatigue Digestive disorders
Riboflavin (B_2)	Helps release energy from carbohydrates, proteins, and fats Growth Health of skin and oral tissues Well-being and vigor	Liver and other organ meats Meat, poultry, fish Milk Eggs Yeast Green vegetables Whole grain or enriched products	Lesions around mouth, particularly at corners Retarded growth
Niacin	Helps other cells use nutrients Necessary to normal function of digestive tract and nervous system	Meat, poultry, fish Milk, butter Whole grain or enriched products The body can convert tryptophan in protein into niacin	Pellagra Glossitis Digestive disturbances Mental disorders
Folic acid (folacin)	Essential to health; found in all body cells Aids in formation of hemoglobin and red blood cells	Liver and organ meats Yeast Dark-green leafy vegetables Dried beans and peas	Digestive disorders Disorders of the hematopoietic system
Pantothenic acid	Aids in the metabolism of carbohydrates, proteins, and fats Aids in the formation of hormones and nerve-regulating substances	Yeast Liver and other organ meats Eggs Whole grain or enriched products	Fatigue, sleep disturbances Headache, malaise Nausea, abdominal distress
Vitamin B_{12}	Aids in the formation of red blood cells and in blood regeneration Used in treatment of pernicious anemia	Liver and other organ meats Muscle meats, fish Milk, cheese Eggs	Not yet known
Biotin	Helps release energy from carbohydrates Aids in the formation of fatty acids	Liver and other organ meats Milk Egg yolk Yeast	Dermatitis, glossitis Loss of appetite, nausea Loss of sleep Muscular pains Hyperesthesia and paresthesia
Vitamin B_6	Aids in absorption and metabolism of proteins and fats Assists in formation of red blood cells	Meat (especially liver), fish Yeast Milk Eggs	Similar to those found in biotin deficiencies
Vitamin C	Essential in the formation and maintenance of the capillary walls, in the strengthening of walls of blood vessels, and in preventing tendency to bleed easily Essential in healing Acts as a detoxifying agent Important to health of gums	Citrus fruits, melons, berries, and other fruits Tomatoes and other raw vegetables	Scurvy Tendency to bruise easily

- **Fruit group:** 2 to 4 servings are recommended daily.
- **Milk, yogurt, and cheese group:** 2 to 3 servings are recommended daily. Children, teenagers, and women up to 25 years of age should have 3 to 4 servings per day.
- **Meat, poultry, fish, dried beans, eggs, and nuts group:** 2 to 3 servings are recommended daily.
- **Fats, oils, and sweets group:** there are no recommended daily servings (this is because the nutrients in this group are readily available in other foods).

TABLE 6–4

Minerals Required for Health

MINERAL	IMPORTANT FUNCTIONS	BEST SOURCES	DEFICIENCY SYMPTOMS
Calcium	Normal development and maintenance of bones and teeth Clotting of the blood Normal muscle activity	Milk and milk products Sardines and other whole canned fish Leafy green vegetables	Retarded growth Poor tooth formation Slow clotting time of blood Increased susceptibility to fractures
Phosphorus	Formation of bones and teeth Release of energy from carbohydrates, proteins, and fats Maintenance of healthy nerve tissue and normal muscle activity	Meat, poultry, fish Milk and milk products Dried beans and peas	Weakness, loss of appetite Retarded growth Porous bones Poor tooth formation
Magnesium	Building bones Release of energy from muscle glycogen Conduction of nerve impulses to muscles	Raw, leafy green vegetables Nuts and seeds Whole grains and soybeans	Muscular twitching and tremors Irregular heart beat Insomnia Leg and foot cramps, shaky hands
Potassium	Muscle contraction Maintenance of fluid and electrolyte balance Release of energy	Oranges, bananas Meats Bran Peanut butter	Abnormal heart rhythm, muscular weakness Lethargy Kidney and lung failure
Chloride	Regulates balance of body fluids Activates enzymes in saliva	Table salt	Very rare Disturbed balance in body fluids
Sodium	Regulates balance of body fluids	Table salt	Difficulty is caused primarily by excess May cause excess fluid retention in body Can lead to high blood pressure
Iron	Formation of hemoglobin	Liver and other organ meats Red meat Egg yolks Green leafy vegetables Dried fruits	Anemia, characterized by: weakness, dizziness, loss of weight, gastric disturbances, and pallor
Copper	Formation of red blood cells	Liver and other organ meats Oysters Dried beans and peas Corn-oil margarine	Anemia Faulty development of bone and nervous tissue
Zinc	Constituent of about 100 enzymes	Meat, especially liver Eggs Seafood	Delayed wound healing Diminished taste sensation
Iodine	Part of thyroid hormones	Seafood Iodized salt	Goiter (enlarged thyroid)
Fluoride	Formation of decay-resistant teeth Maintenance of bone strength	Fluoridated water	Excessive dental decay
Chromium	Metabolism of glucose	Meat Cheese Yeast Whole-grain breads and cereals	Possibly abnormal sugar metabolism
Selenium	Antioxidant, interacts with vitamin E	Meat, poultry, seafood Milk Egg yolk	Not known in humans
Manganese	Functioning of central nervous system Normal bone structure	Nuts and whole grains Vegetables and fruits Tea, instant coffee	Not known in humans
Molybdenum	Part of the enzyme xanthine oxidase	Liver and other organ meats Cereal grains	Not known in humans

Dietary Evaluations

If the patient has any indications of a nutritional disorder, the dentist will refer him to a qualified specialist. However, it may be beneficial for some patients to have a staff member perform a simplified dietary analysis to determine the general adequacy of his diet and the frequency of consuming cariogenic foods.

The patient's cooperation is essential in performing this analysis, for the patient must keep a **diet diary** for about 3 days (Fig. 6–1). In the diet diary, he records each food eaten, including the amount, how it was prepared, and when it was eaten.

The completed diary is reviewed with the use of a **dietary analysis form** (Fig. 6–2). Here the foods are divided into groups and compared with the recommended number of servings per day. Empty calories and the consumption of cariogenic foods are highlighted.

The diary is then reviewed with the patient. Suggestions for modifications that might be beneficial are made in a positive manner. This review is never phrased in critical terms or stated in any way to make the patient uncomfortable.

Oral Manifestations of Nutritional Deficiencies

The tissues of the oral cavity may show early indications of nutritional disorders; however, there are no nutritional deficiencies that by themselves have been demonstrated to cause dental diseases.

Oral disorders of the lips and mouth are generally related to vitamin B complex group deficiency. In addition to generalized inflammation of the oral mucosa, these disorders include the following conditions:

Cheilitis is inflammation affecting the lips. This usually begins as redness and peeling of the skin at the angles of the mouth. Here it is called **angular cheilitis.** As the condition continues, cracks occur in the skin and mucous membranes at the commissure of the lips (Fig. 6–3).

Patient's name ____________________ Date __________

Time	Foods Eaten List each food on a separate line. Note quantity and how prepared
7 am	Orange juice (8 oz.)
7 am	Coffee
7 am	Toast
7 am	Butter
7 am	Jam
12:30	Pizza (1 slice)
12:30	Diet soda (12 oz.)
4 pm	Candy bar
6:30	Chicken, roasted
6:30	Baked potato
6:30	Butter
6:30	Sour cream
6:30	Broccoli
6:30	cheese sauce (on broccoli)
6:30	Ice cream

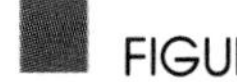

FIGURE 6–1

Sample diet diary. It is important that the patient note everything that was eaten and when it was eaten.

Patient's name ______________________ Date ____________

Food	Veg	Fruit	Meat	Milk	Bread	Other
Orange juice		1				
Coffee						1
Toast					1	
Butter						1
Jam						1
Pizza	1			1	1	
Diet soda						1
Candy bar						1
Chicken, roasted			1			
Baked potato	1					
Butter						1
Sour cream						1
Broccoli	1					
Cheese sauce				1		
Ice cream				1		
Totals	3	1	1	3	2	7

FIGURE 6–2

Sample dietary analysis form. The foods eaten are broken down into groups. Some foods are divided into several groups. For example, a cheese pizza would be divided into bread, vegetable (tomato sauce), and cheese groups.

These symptoms can also be present as a result of other causes, such as a reduction in vertical dimension that results from poorly fitting dentures or marked abrasion of the natural teeth.

Glossitis, an inflammation of the tongue, is characterized by changes in both color and surface of the tongue. The tongue may become fiery red or purplish-red, or it may become smooth and dry in appearance. In other cases it has a pebbly texture. Changes in the tongue may also be due to other causes, and these are discussed in Chapter 11.

Scurvy is the result of a severe vitamin C deficiency. The gingival changes are such that the tissues appear swollen, congested, and tender. The color ranges from bright red to bluish-purple to black, and with even the slightest pressure the diseased tissue will bleed.

Rickets is a disease caused by vitamin D deficiency and occurs mainly in rapidly growing children. Most of the symptoms are manifested in the bones; for example, it produces knock-knees or bow legs. However, there are also dental implications.

Rickets may retard eruption of teeth, cause a change in the order of eruption, and cause the absence of enamel in some areas of some permanent teeth.

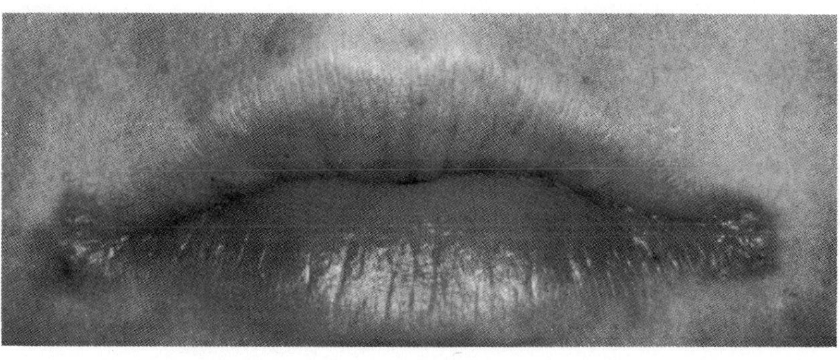

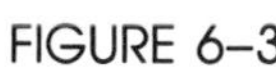

FIGURE 6–3

Angular cheilitis may be an indication of a nutritional deficiency. This may also be caused by other factors. (From Ibsen, O.A., and Phelan, J.A.: Oral Pathology for the Dental Hygienist. Philadelphia, W.B. Saunders Co., 1992, p 38.)

Fluorides

The effectiveness of fluorides in lowering the incidence of dental caries is one of the greatest public health success stories of this century. However, to achieve the maximum benefits, an ongoing supply of both systemic and topical fluorides must be available throughout life.

Systemic Fluorides

Systemic fluorides, which are also known as *dietary fluorides*, are those ingested in water, food, beverages, or supplements. The required amount of fluoride is absorbed through the intestine into the blood stream. This fluoride is taken into the tissues where it is needed, and some is found in saliva. Any excess systemic fluoride is excreted by the body through the skin, kidneys, and feces.

Topical Fluorides

Topical fluorides, which are also known as *nondietary fluorides*, are applied in direct contact with the teeth through mouth rinses, fluoridated toothpaste, and topical fluoride applications. (The application of topical fluorides is discussed in Chapter 27.)

How Fluorides Help the Teeth

DURING DENTAL DEVELOPMENT

In large part, the strength and structure of the teeth depend upon the nutrients available to the developing child. Before birth, all of these must come from the mother's diet. If the mother ingests dietary fluorides, some of these are used by the baby.

Newly erupted teeth are incompletely mineralized. The resistance of these teeth to caries is increased by the continued uptake of minerals and fluoride from systemic and topical sources.

REMINERALIZATION

Research has demonstrated that having ongoing sources of fluoride throughout life further protects the teeth by aiding in the remineralization process.

Acids from plaque attack the enamel surface and cause the minerals calcium and phosphate to be lost. This process is called **demineralization**, and it is the first step toward decay.

The rate of destruction depends upon the abundance of plaque, the type and number of organisms, the amount of carbohydrates available for conversion to acid, and the resistance of the tooth surface.

Remineralization is the process of restoring minerals to a mineralized tissue that has been demineralized. In this damage-control process, the fluorides, calcium, and phosphate found in the saliva work together to replace some of the minerals that have been lost.

Remineralization is able to reverse the damage of early demineralization. However, if the lesion has progressed too far, remineralization cannot halt the process, and it is necessary to repair the tooth with a dental restoration.

HIGH-RISK PATIENTS

For most patients, the combination of fluoridated water and fluoridated toothpaste is effective in preventing dental decay; however, high-risk patients may require additional sources such as topical applications and the use of fluoride rinses. This high-risk category includes patients who

- Have already experienced dental decay
- Live in areas where the public water supply is not fluoridated
- Are prone to root caries
- Have illnesses or are taking medications that slow the flow of saliva
- Are undergoing chemotherapy or radiation treatments that damage the tissues and affect the flow of saliva
- Are anorexic or bulimic
- Have had periodontal surgery that leaves the root surface exposed and sensitive

The Safety and Hazards of Fluorides

Fluorides added to the public water supply and in dental products carry little or no risk when used as directed. The levels of fluoride in controlled water fluoridation are so low that there is little danger of ingesting an acutely toxic quantity of fluoride from fluoridated water.

However, it is important to be aware that fluorides in excessive amounts are poisons. The fatal oral dose of sodium fluoride has been estimated at from 5 to 10 gm.

Lesser amounts may cause accidental poisoning, and even death, in small children. An area of concern is having young children ingest excessive fluorides by eating fluoridated toothpaste or swallowing fluoride rinses or topical gels.

All patients should use fluoride preparations only as recommended by the dentist and should supervise their use by young children.

Fluoridated Water

Approximately 1 part per million (ppm) of fluoride in drinking water has been specified as the safe and recommended concentration to aid in the control of dental decay. This is approximately the equivalent of one drop of fluoride in a bathtub full of water.

Recommended optimum concentrations vary from 0.7 to 1.2 ppm, depending on the climate; lower concentrations are usually recommended in very hot areas where people consume larger quantities of water.

The water in some communities is naturally fluoridated and contains more than twice the optimum level of fluoride. Prolonged exposure to these excessive amounts may cause **dental fluorosis**, which is discussed in Chapter 11.

The maximum benefits from fluoridated water may be expected when these fluorides are available before birth (through the mother's intake) and throughout life.

In areas where fluoridation of the community water supply is not possible, one alternative is the fluoridation of school water. However, since the benefits of fluoride are not available from birth and do not continue throughout life, this is not considered to be a good substitute for community water fluoridation.

IN-HOME WATER FILTERS

Some in-home water filters may remove the fluoride from the water. When this happens, the family will not receive the benefits of the fluoridated water. Fluoride is not removed from the water with ion exchange/softeners, sediment filters, and ultraviolet systems.

BOTTLED WATER

Unless the fluoride content is printed on the label, it is not safe to assume that bottled water contains adequate fluoride to prevent dental decay.

If only bottled water without fluoride is used for drinking and cooking, the family may not receive the full benefits of systemic fluoride.

PRESCRIBED DIETARY FLUORIDE SUPPLEMENTS

Dietary fluoride supplements, in the form of drops or tablets, may be prescribed by the dentist.

A primary use of prescribed dietary fluoride supplements is for patients living in areas where the drinking water contains less than the optimum level of fluoride.

Before prescribing a supplement, the dentist must determine the fluoride level of the family drinking water supply. If the water source is a private well, a water sample can be sent to the local or county health department for a fluoride content analysis.

Prenatal Fluorides. If the expectant mother lives in an area where fluoridated water is not available, the dentist may recommend that she take fluoride supplements as a means of helping the baby develop stronger teeth.

Breast Milk and Formula. Fluoride consumed by the mother does not pass into breast milk. Therefore, a baby who is only breast-fed may not receive enough fluoride.

If a baby is fed only ready-to-use formula that does not contain fluoride, or if the formula is mixed with water that does not contain fluoride, the baby may not receive sufficient fluoride. In these situations, the dentist may prescribe a fluoride supplement for the child.

The effectiveness of these supplements is greater the earlier the child begins to take them. However, their effectiveness also depends upon daily administration over a long period of time, and this requires a very high level of parental motivation.

Dietary supplements of fluoride may be the method of choice for the very young child. For older children, topical fluoride applications or fluoride mouth rinses often may be preferable. Children who are highly susceptible to caries may benefit from receiving both measures.

Cautions. As with all medicines, there is a danger if a child should consume a large quantity. Therefore, as a precautionary measure, the dentist prescribes only a limited amount of fluoride to be dispensed at one time. Each package of fluoride supplement should be labeled *"Caution: Store out of reach of children."*

Topical Fluorides

Topical fluorides come from fluoride applications, fluoridated toothpastes, and rinses.

PROFESSIONAL TOPICAL FLUORIDE APPLICATIONS

Professional topical fluoride applications are recommended for some children soon after the eruption of the permanent teeth and for some high-risk patients. These applications are discussed in Chapter 27.

BRUSH-ON FLUORIDE GEL

A 1.1 percent neutral sodium fluoride brush-on gel is available without prescription. A 2% neutral sodium fluoride brush-on gel is available by prescription.

High-risk patients may use these at home by brushing with them or through home application with a reusable custom tray. Construction of this type of tray is discussed in Chapter 24.

The patient is instructed to use the tray at bedtime. A small amount of the brush-on gel is placed in the tray, and the tray is placed over the teeth for 5 minutes.

If water in the area is fluoridated, the patient is instructed to rinse and spit. (This prevents ingestion of excess fluoride.) If water is the area is not fluoridated, the patient is told not to rinse after the application. (Any fluoride that is swallowed will provide extra dietary fluoride.)

FLUORIDE MOUTH RINSES

Mouth rinses containing fluoride are another way of providing fluorides to persons in areas without fluoridated water and to patients with special needs.

Over-the-counter non-prescription rinses generally contain 0.05 percent sodium fluoride (NaF). They are designed to be used on a daily basis. **Prescription rinses** generally contain 0.2 percent sodium fluoride and are designed to be used once a week.

Because of the danger of ingesting excessive fluoride, the patient must be cautioned not to swallow the mouth rinse.

Fluoride mouth rinses are *not* usually recommended for children under 5 years of age or for some older handicapped children, because they may swallow the rinse rather than spit it out.

FLUORIDE-CONTAINING TOOTHPASTES

Toothpastes containing fluoride are an important ongoing source of topical fluorides. A major benefit of these fluorides is the brushing action that brings them into close contact with all surfaces of the teeth.

However, because of the danger of ingesting excessive fluoride, the patient should be cautioned not to swallow or eat the toothpaste.

Very young children (under 4 years of age) may have difficulty rinsing their mouths and spitting out the excess toothpaste. For these children, particularly those who are receiving fluorides from other sources, the dentist may recommend the following steps:

- Use a child-size toothbrush.
- Use a pea-sized amount of toothpaste on the toothbrush.
- Brush under the supervision of a parent or other responsible person.
- Do not swallow the toothpaste.

Tartar Control Toothpastes. Some toothpastes contain chemicals to slow the build-up of tartar. **Calculus,** which is commonly called *tartar,* is plaque that has hardened and adhered to the teeth. Once calculus has formed on the teeth, the only way to remove it is by professional prophylaxis. This is discussed in Chapter 26.

Plaque Control

Dental Plaque

Dental plaque is a tenacious, soft deposit consisting chiefly of bacteria and bacterial products. Although difficult to see in small quantities, it ranges in color from gray to yellowish-gray to yellow.

Plaque includes specific types of bacterial colonies surrounded by gel-like intercellular substances derived chiefly from the bacteria themselves. It also contains components from saliva and sulcular fluid, leukocytes, epithelial cells, and food debris.

Mutans streptococci (ms), formerly known as *Streptococcus mutans*, are the primary bacterial species associated with plaque and causing dental decay (Fig. 6–4). Lactobacilli are a secondary caries-causing organism. They lack the ability of ms to attach themselves to the tooth and to start the caries process. However, once the environment has become acidic, they become more numerous and active.

These bacteria readily utilize nutrients, such as soluble sugars, which diffuse easily into the plaque. Limiting the supply of these nutrients is one reason why nutrition plays such an important role in preventive dentistry.

Plaque accumulates in sheltered areas between the teeth, within defects in teeth (such as pits and fissures), on calculus, on crowns and bridges, and on full and partial removable dentures.

On the basis of its relationship to the gingival margin, plaque is differentiated primarily as two categories: supragingival and subgingival plaque.

Facultative organisms, those that can thrive in either the presence or the absence of oxygen, dominate the early formation of supragingival plaque.

Anaerobic organisms, those that thrive in the absence of oxygen, dominate in more mature plaque and in subgingival plaque.

SUPRAGINGIVAL PLAQUE

Supragingival plaque is located above the gingival margin. It develops on tooth surfaces, restorations, appliances, and dentures. It also accumulates mostly on the gingival third of the teeth and in surface cracks, defects, rough areas, and overhanging margins of dental restorations.

Significantly more plaque accumulates on the molars than on all other teeth. On the maxillary molars, more plaque is accumulated on the facial surfaces near the parotid glands, whereas on the mandibular molars more plaque tends to accumulate on the lingual surfaces.

Development of Supragingival Plaque

Acquired pellicle is a normal film that forms on a cleaned tooth surface within minutes and is usually from 0.05 to 0.8 microns thick. When stained with

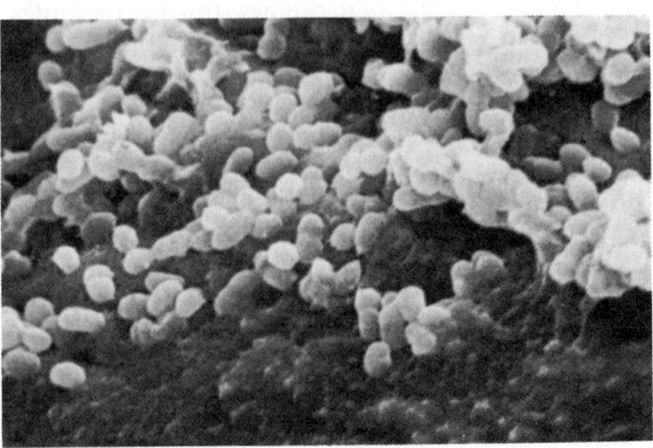

FIGURE 6–4

***Mutans streptococcus* in a lesion on an enamel surface.** (From Nester, E.W., Roberts, C.E., Lidrom, M.E., et al.: Microbiology, 3rd ed. Philadelphia, W.B. Saunders Co., 1983, p 68.)

disclosing solution, the pellicle appears as a pale-stained surface sheen. (**Acquired pellicle** is a colorless, translucent film. It is composed of complex sugar-protein molecules that are a product of the saliva.)

Supragingival plaque formation begins with the adhesion of bacteria on the acquired pellicle. Measurable amounts of supragingival plaque may form within 1 hour after the teeth are thoroughly cleaned, with maximum accumulation reached in 30 days or less.

Plaque mass grows by the

- Addition of new bacteria
- Multiplication of bacteria
- Accumulation of bacterial and host products

Supragingivally, bacteria associated with periodontal health are mainly gram-positive coccal (spherical) and rod-shaped bacteria. These organisms initiate plaque growth by means of their ability to adhere to the pellicle and tooth surface and then to proliferate in that particular ecological niche.

Once supragingival plaque is initiated, secondary bacterial growth and maturation take place. During this phase, bacterial population shifts occur. This is known as **bacterial succession.** In this stage, filamentous organisms and gram-negative bacteria increase.

SUBGINGIVAL PLAQUE

Subgingival plaque is found below the gingiva in the gingival sulcus, where shape of the area makes these structures less subject to natural cleansing activities of the mouth.

In these protected areas, which form a relatively stagnant environment, organisms that cannot readily adhere to a tooth surface may have the opportunity to colonize.

In addition, organisms within these sites have direct access to the nutrients present in sulcular fluid. Also, because of the nature of the gingival sulcus and periodontal pocket, organisms that can exist only in areas of low oxygen concentration can survive in these sites.

The presence of supragingival plaque facilitates the establishment of subgingival plaque by providing sites of attachment and essential growth factors.

Attached Subgingival Plaque

Plaque bacteria are attached to the tooth surface in the gingival sulcus and periodontal pocket. These organisms are thought to be mostly gram-positive rods and cocci, with some gram-negative organisms.

Epithelium-Associated Subgingival Plaque

Epithelium-associated plaque contains predominantly, but not exclusively, motile gram-negative organisms. It does not adhere to the tooth but is in direct association with the subgingival epithelium and extends from the gingival margin to the junctional epithelium.

Because this plaque does not adhere to the tooth, epithelium-associated plaque is not revealed by disclosing solutions.

Personal Oral Hygiene

It has been proved conclusively that plaque is the primary causative factor in caries and is also an important factor in periodontal disease.

Therefore, a primary goal of preventive dentistry is to control plaque by removing it at least once daily. Once plaque has been thoroughly removed, it takes it about 24 hours to form again.

There are many aspects of plaque control and many means and methods of plaque removal. Because all of the activities that are part of plaque removal can be controlled by the individual and must be his responsibility, they are grouped together under the title **personal oral hygiene** (POH).

There is no one right method of plaque removal, and personal oral hygiene must remain personal. Of the many techniques available, the ones selected must be those that are right for the individual patient.

Note: the procedures described here are as the patient would perform them at home. In the office, where the assistant may be exposed to splash contamination, the assistant must wear appropriate personal protective equipment. (See Chapter 13.)

DISCLOSING AGENTS

The thorough removal of dental plaque can be taught more easily when the patient is able to see the plaque. A red disclosing agent is used to temporarily color the plaque to make it visible (Fig. 6–5; see Fig. 21–5).

This disclosing agent is available both as a solution to be painted on the teeth and as artificially sweetened, candy-like tablets.

All ingredients are nontoxic and harmless if swallowed. Before the agent is applied, the patient should be warned that it will color the tongue and gingiva as well as the plaque. However, this stain is soon rinsed away by the saliva.

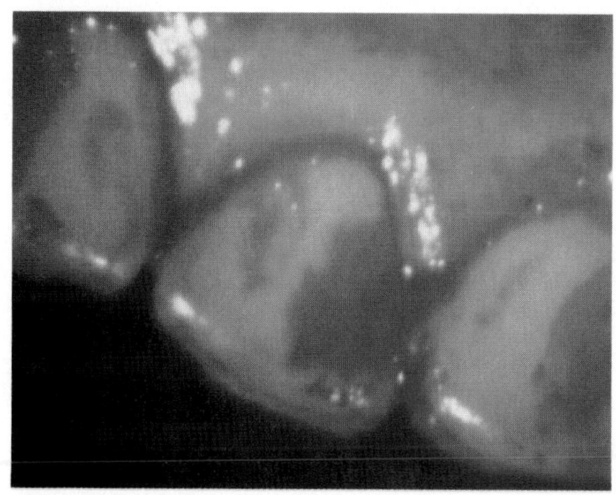

FIGURE 6–5

Disclosing solution on the lingual surface of primary teeth.

Directions for Use of Disclosing Tablets

1. Chew the tablet and swish the resulting solution around in the mouth for at least 30 seconds.
2. Spit the excess liquid into a bowl of running water.
3. Rinse the mouth with plain cool water. The red-colored areas remaining on the teeth indicate plaque, which must be removed. Any pale, filmlike area on the teeth is the acquired pellicle.
4. Disclosing tablets are used daily during the first week or longer. Then they are used on a once-a-week basis and, finally, only as needed to check the effectiveness of the hygiene program.

TOOTHBRUSHES

The primary properties of a toothbrush are flexibility, softness, and diameter of the bristles, as well as strength, rigidity, and lightness of the handle.

The size and style of toothbrush recommended depends largely upon the toothbrushing method employed and the size of the patient's mouth. Toothbrushes should be replaced regularly as the bristles become worn.

A **powered toothbrush** may be useful for physically handicapped individuals who are unable to clean their teeth with a manual brush. They may also be useful for patients with orthodontics bands and brackets and for some patients with periodontal problems.

Toothbrushing Techniques

There are many different toothbrushing techniques, and the one recommended by the dentist depends upon the patient's needs. The system described here is the Bass Method, which was named for Dr. C. C. Bass, an early pioneer in preventive dentistry.

PROCEDURE: Cleaning Facial Surfaces of the Teeth

1. Place the head of the toothbrush horizontally at a 45-degree angle where the gums and teeth meet (Fig. 6–6).
2. Keep the bristles in one place and move the brush gently back and forth, using a vibratory motion, for about 20 strokes.
3. Use light pressure to get the bristles between the teeth, but do not use enough pressure to cause discomfort (Fig. 6–7).
4. Change the position of the head of the toothbrush and repeat this motion as often as necessary to reach and clean all of the outer surfaces of the teeth.

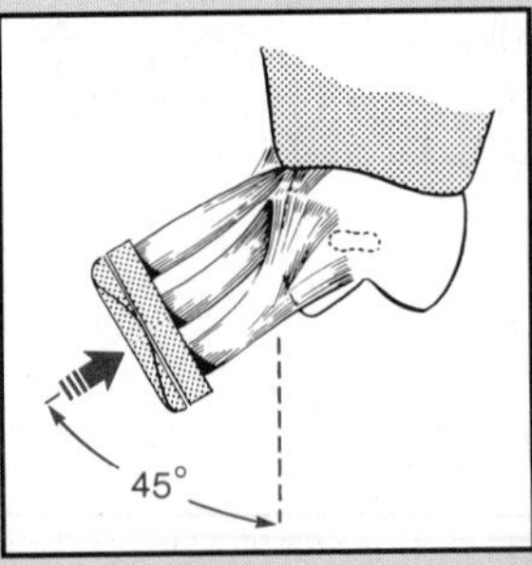

FIGURE 6–6

The toothbrush should be placed at a 45-degree angle to the long axis of the teeth. (From Carranza, F.A., Jr.: Glickman's Clinical Periodontology, 7th ed. Philadelphia, W.B. Saunders Co., 1990, p 689.)

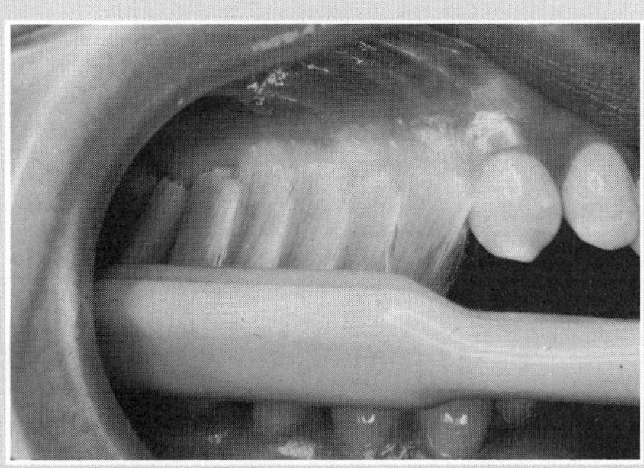

FIGURE 6–7

Application of the toothbrush on the facial surfaces of the maxillary teeth. The gentle pressure from the brush causes blanching of the gingiva. (From Carranza, F.A., Jr.: Glickman's Clinical Periodontology, 7th ed. Philadelphia, W.B. Saunders Co., 1990, p 689.)

PROCEDURE: **Cleaning Lingual Surfaces of the Posterior Teeth**

1. Place the head of the toothbrush horizontally at a 45-degree angle where the gums and teeth meet.
2. Keep the bristles in one place and move the brush gently back and forth, using a vibratory motion, for about 20 strokes (Fig. 6–8).
3. Change the position of the head of the toothbrush and repeat this motion as often as necessary to reach and clean all of the inner surfaces of the upper and lower posterior teeth.

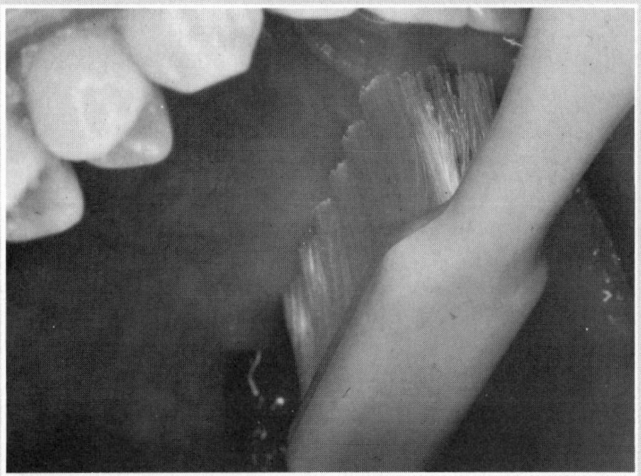

FIGURE 6–8

Placement of the toothbrush on the lingual surfaces of the maxillary molars and premolars. (From Carranza, F.A., Jr.: Glickman's Clinical Periodontology, 7th ed. Philadelphia, W.B. Saunders Co., 1990, p 695.)

PROCEDURE: Cleaning Lingual Surfaces of the Anterior Teeth

1. Hold the head of the toothbrush vertically to clean the inside surfaces of the upper and lower front teeth (Fig. 6–9).
2. Close the lips lightly around the handle of the toothbrush to prevent splattering.
3. Repeatedly make gentle back-and-forth strokes over each tooth and its surrounding gum tissue.
4. Change the position of the head of the toothbrush and repeat this motion as often as necessary to reach and clean all of the inner surfaces of the upper and lower anterior teeth.

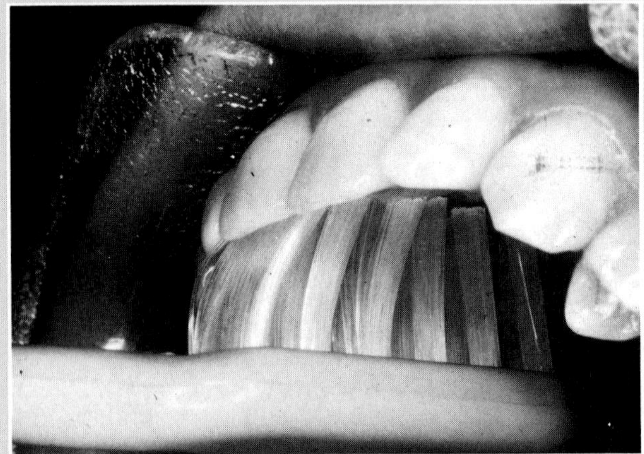

FIGURE 6–9

Placement of the toothbrush on the lingual surfaces of the maxillary incisors. (From Carranza, FA., Jr.: Glickman's Clinical Periodontology, 7th ed. Philadelphia, W.B. Saunders Co., 1990, p 695.)

PROCEDURE: **Cleaning the Occlusal Surfaces**

1. Place the bristles on the chewing surface and move the brush in back-and-forth or small circular motions (Fig. 6–10).
2. Change the position of the head of the toothbrush and repeat this motion as often as necessary to reach and clean all of the occlusal surfaces of the upper and lower teeth.
3. Rinse vigorously to remove loosened plaque and debris.

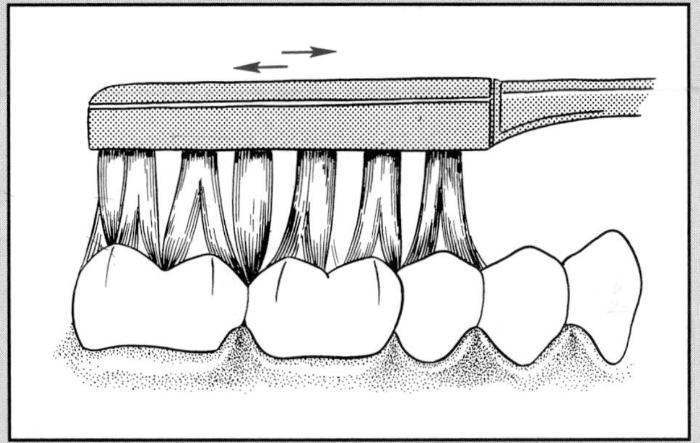

FIGURE 6–10

Placement of the toothbrush on the occlusal surfaces of the mandibular teeth. (From Carranza, FA., Jr.: Glickman's Clinical Periodontology, 7th ed. Philadelphia, W.B. Saunders Co., 1990, p 697.)

Interdental Cleaning Aids

FLOSSING

Dental floss is an effective tool for removing plaque from proximal tooth surfaces. Floss comes in several different styles, primarily waxed or unwaxed, and there are several ways to use dental floss effectively. The dentist may recommend a particular system of flossing. The following is one of the most commonly used methods.

INTERDENTAL AIDS

Special devices are recommended for cleaning between teeth with large or open interdental spaces such as those found in periodontally treated dentition. These devices may be used in addition to dental floss but are not a substitute for it.

Interproximal brushes are small brushes that are available in a variety of shapes. To be most effective, the diameter of the brush should be slightly larger than the gingival embrasure so that the bristles exert pressure on the tooth surfaces.

These small brushes are inserted between the teeth from the facial side and are moved with short back-and-forth strokes in a linguofacial direction.

A tapered **soft wooden tip** that is triangular in cross-section is used to remove interproximal plaque and to stimulate the gingivae. After it is wetted with water, the narrow tip is gently inserted in the interdental

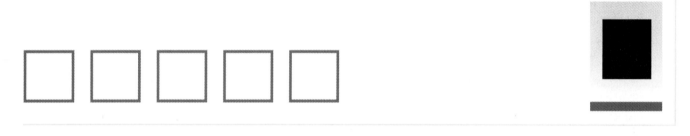

PROCEDURE: Flossing

Preparation

1. Cut a piece of waxed or unwaxed floss about 18 inches long. Wrap the excess floss around the middle or index fingers of both hands and leave a 2- to 3-inch working space exposed.
2. Stretch the floss tightly between the fingers, and use the thumb and index finger to guide the floss into place.

Flossing the Upper Teeth

1. Hold the floss tightly between the thumb and forefinger of each hand. These fingers control the floss, and they should be no more than one-half inch apart.
2. Pass the floss gently between the teeth, using a sawing motion. Do not force or snap the floss past the contact area, for this may injure the interdental gingiva. Guide the floss to the gumline.
3. Curve the floss into a C shape against one tooth. Slide it gently into the space between the gum and the tooth. Using both hands, move the floss up and down on the side of one tooth (Fig. 6–11).

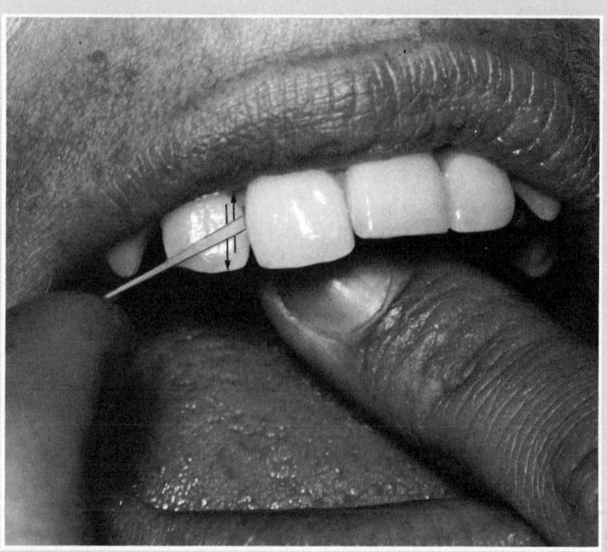

FIGURE 6–11

Flossing. The patient moves the floss along the proximal surface in repeated up-and-down strokes. (From Carranza, FA., Jr.: Glickman's Clinical Periodontology, 7th ed. Philadelphia, W.B. Saunders Co., 1990, p 701.)

4. Repeat these steps on each side of all the upper teeth, including the posterior surface of the last tooth in each quadrant.
5. As the floss becomes frayed or soiled, move a fresh area of floss into the working position.
6. Use a bridge threader to floss under a fixed bridge (Fig. 6–12).

Flossing the Lower Teeth

1. Guide the floss, using the forefingers of both hands.
2. Pass the floss gently between the teeth, using a sawing motion. Do not force or snap it into place. Guide the floss to the gumline.
3. Curve the floss into a C shape against one tooth. Slide it gently into the space between the gum and the tooth.
4. Using both hands, move the floss up and down on the side of one tooth.
5. Repeat these steps on each side of all the lower teeth, including the posterior surface of the last tooth in each quadrant.
6. As the floss becomes frayed or soiled, move a fresh area of floss into the working position.
7. Use a bridge threader to floss under a fixed bridge.

Rinse and Disclose Again

1. Rinse vigorously after flossing.
2. Recheck with disclosing solution to determine that all plaque has been removed.

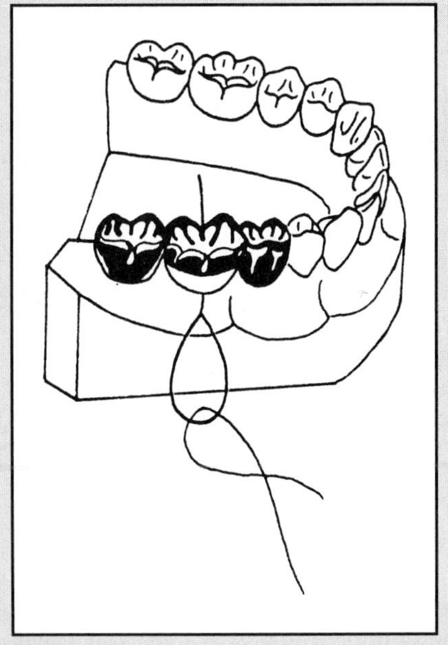

FIGURE 6–12

A bridge threader is used as an aid to clean under a fixed bridge.

space with the base surface of the triangle resting on the interproximal gingiva. The tip is then repeatedly forced gently in and out of the embrasure so that the side of the triangle comes into contact with the proximal tooth surfaces.

Oral Irrigation Devices

Oral irrigators direct water or therapeutic rinse against the teeth and tissues as either a high-pressure steady stream or a pulsating flow. This is known as **supragingival irrigation.** This means that the point of delivery is at or above the gingival margin.

Oral irrigation devices are effective in getting into areas, such as around orthodontic bands, that are not accessible with a toothbrush, and they flush loose debris from the mouth. However, they remove only a very small amount of plaque from tooth surfaces.

Special irrigation attachments allow the irrigation tip to be positioned below the gumline to permit subgingival irrigation with therapeutic solutions. (**Subgingival irrigation** means that the point of delivery is directed below the gingival margin into the gingival crevice or pocket.)

Subgingival irrigation may be recommended to help reduce periodontal pockets or after periodontal surgery. This form of irrigation should be used *only* on the recommendation of the dentist, and it may be provided as an in-office professional service.

Antimicrobial Mouth Rinses

For certain high-risk patients, the dentist may prescribe an antimicrobial mouth rinse containing 0.12% **chlorhexidine** (CHX), which has a broad antimicrobial spectrum effective against gram-positive, gram-negative, and yeast organisms.

The rinse may stain the teeth and oral surfaces. Because the rinse may also affect the taste of certain foods, it is recommended that it be used twice daily after meals. At this time, the patient should brush and use the rinse. However, the patient must be cautioned against swallowing the rinse.

Patient Education in Preventive Dentistry

Patient education is the responsibility of all members of the dental health team as they come into contact with the patient; however, the assistant or hygienist is usually assigned responsibility for providing information, guidance, and motivation.

The major thrusts of patient education in preventive dentistry include

- Presenting a program of personal oral hygiene that the patient will carry out at home on a routine basis
- Counseling to increase the patient's awareness of the role of nutrition in achieving optimum dental and general health
- Creating patient awareness of the need to return regularly for professional prophylaxis, examination, and treatment

In your role as the dental health educator, you must be enthusiastic about helping others learn these skills. You must also be concerned about them as individuals, be sensitive to their needs, and be accepting and tactful in working with them.

A patient education program emphasizes **motivation** and **education.**

Motivation

The dental health team should work to increase the patient's motivational level so he *wants* to learn and apply plaque-control skills. However, ultimately it is the patient who decides what value will be placed on his oral health, and the lower the patient's level of motivation, the less the chance of success for his personal oral hygiene program.

AWARENESS AND INTEREST

The first step must be to make the patient aware that he has a problem that needs to be solved. Then it is necessary to gain the patient's interest and cooperation in solving the problem.

As an example, the patient may not be aware of how much sugar he is consuming each day. Table 6–5 lists the sugar content of popular foods. (Remember, in addition to the amount of sugar present, the frequency of consuming sugar is also important.)

TABLE 6–5

Sugar Content of Popular Foods

FOOD	APPROXIMATE MEASURE	TSP. OF SUGAR
Coca Cola	6 oz.	5
Chocolate milk shake	8 oz.	14
Chocolate ice cream soda	Average size	11
Cinnamon bun with raisins	1 average	8
Jelly doughnut	1 average	7
Iced cupcake	1 medium	9
Peach ice cream	1 cup	15
Orange sherbet	½ cup	19
Apple pie	⅙ of medium pie	14
Chocolate pudding	½ cup	9
Raisins	⅝ cup	17
Candy bar	Average	8
Fudge, plain	1″ square	5
Jelly beans	10	4
Lollipop	1 medium	8

Education

Once the patient is motivated so that he *wants* to learn and use these skills, he must learn how to use them correctly. It is here that the dental health educator can best help the patient.

ACCEPTANCE

The patient can learn more easily when he feels safe, accepted, and respected. In this setting, encouragement is given freely, and correction is structured in a positive manner. Most important, the patient is never scolded, embarrassed, or teased because of his ignorance or errors.

ACTION

The least learning occurs when the patient merely sits and listens, as in a lecture. Far more learning occurs when as many of the senses as possible are involved and the patient is actively participating in the process.

Teaching plaque control is an ideal situation for active learner participation. The following are four educational ideas that combine these factors:

- Present the skills to be learned one at a time and as simply as possible. When possible, use visual aids (such as disclosing tablets) to clarify the point.
- Give the patient an opportunity to practice the new skills. For example, provide a toothbrush and guide the patient as he practices the new brushing technique.
- Provide reinforcement and encouragement until the patient has mastered these skills. For example, a disclosing tablet is used again to demonstrate that all of the plaque has been removed.
- Encourage the patient to continue these new actions at home until the desired habit pattern has been formed.

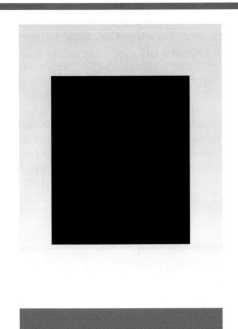

Chapter 7

Psychology and Communication

Introduction

Psychology is the study of behavior and of the functions and process of the mind. Human behavior is usually described in terms of the level of adequacy of social adjustment that the individual is able to achieve.

Good communication, in all forms, is the backbone of any well-run organization, especially the dental office. This chapter is divided into four parts: psychology, communication, written communications, and stress in the dental office.

Psychology

The major divisions and descriptions of psychological terms and disorders are discussed in this section.

Psychosis

A **psychosis** is any major mental disorder in which impairment of mental function has developed to a degree that it seriously interferes with insight, the ability to meet the ordinary demands of life, or the ability to maintain adequate contact with reality. (The term *psychosis* is singular. The plural is *psychoses.*)

A psychosis may be organic (caused by a physical disorder) or functional (caused by a disorder in thinking or reasoning).

Paranoia is an example of a psychosis characterized by delusions of being influenced, persecuted, or treated in some special way. A **delusion** is a false personal belief that is maintained in spite of obvious proof to the contrary.

Schizophrenia is a group of psychoses in which there is a fundamental disturbance of personality. There is also a characteristic distortion of thinking, bizarre delusions, and disturbed perception. (**Perception** means a mental image or the manner in which something is understood.)

Personality Disorders

A personality disorder is any of a large group of mental disorders characterized by rigid, inflexible, and maladaptive behavior patterns that impair a person's ability to function in society.

An **antisocial type** is a personality disorder characterized by repeated behavioral patterns that lack moral and ethical standards and bring a person into continuous conflict with society.

A **compulsive type** is a personality disorder characterized by feelings of personal insecurity, doubt, and incompleteness that lead to excessive conscientiousness, stubbornness, and caution.

A **passive-aggressive type** is a personality disorder characterized by aggressive behavior manifested in passive ways, such as obstructionism, procrastination, and intentional inefficiency.

Neurotic Disorders

A neurotic disorder, also known as a **neurosis,** is a mental disorder with no demonstrable organic basis. The individual may have considerable insight and usually has good contact with reality. Although behavior may be greatly affected, it usually remains within socially acceptable limits.

A neurotic **anxiety state** is a feeling of apprehension, tension, or uneasiness that stems from the anticipation of danger, the source of which is largely unknown or unrecognized. This anxiety may be so severe that the patient is actually panic-stricken.

Hysteria is a neurotic state characterized by disturbances of motor or sensory functions: for example, paralysis resulting from psychological causes rather than from a physical injury.

A **phobia** is a neurotic state characterized by an abnormally intense dread of certain objects or specific situations that would not normally have that effect.

Dental phobias may prevent some patients from seeking or completing necessary care. (The discussion of phobias and treatment follows later in the chapter.)

Normal Behavior

The psychotic finds social adjustment *impossible.* The neurotic is able to make a *moderate* social adjustment; and the so-called normal person is able to make a *better than moderate* social adjustment.

The boundaries between normal and neurotic are unclear. An individual may be considered normal in most aspects of his or her behavior and yet be neurotic in others.

The average "normal" dental patient is likely to be cooperative during treatment, as evidenced by keeping appointments, following through on home care, and meeting financial obligations. Such a patient appears to be relaxed and friendly toward the dental staff and will react to pain but not show *excessive* fear or anxiety.

Understanding Patient Behavior

Psychological reactions are more obvious when the patient appears tense, suspicious, apprehensive, and resistant to suggested treatment. All individuals have emotional needs, and these needs must be considered even when a patient seems confident, comfortable, and agreeable.

BACKGROUND FACTORS

There are many psychological factors that affect the individual's behavior and contribute to his reactions and psychological needs in the dental office.

One factor of major importance is the patient's current life situation. This includes the many stresses, tensions, conflicts, and anxieties that may be present in any part of the patient's life.

Other important factors that influence the patient's reactions to the current situation are his *previous dental experiences* and his *attitudes* and *beliefs* about the importance of his teeth.

These attitudes and beliefs are strongly influenced by the patient's socioeconomic and cultural background, as well as the attitudes of others around him as he was growing up. For example, if a patient grew up in a family for whom going to the dentist was a dreaded experience, he may have difficulty overcoming this attitude.

ANXIETY AND FEAR OF PAIN

The fear of pain is a frequently stated cause of anxiety concerning dental treatment. For many patients, however, it is the *expectation* of pain—not the actual pain—that causes the greatest distress. Unfortunately, the more fearful and anxious the patient becomes, the more sensitive he may be to pain.

Subjective Fears. Subjective fears, also known as *acquired fears,* are based on feelings, attitudes, and concerns that have developed at the suggestions of peers, siblings, or other adults.

Small children, for example, have an intense fear of the unknown. This subjective fear, imaginative as it is, can cause irreparable damage to their composure and conduct during a routine dental visit.

Whether a child or an adult, the patient should be informed in a general and positive way about the dental procedure, the use of equipment, and the sequence of events that can be expected.

Objective Fears. Objective fears, also known as *learned fears,* relate to the patient's experiences and his recall of those experiences. If the experience was **traumatic** (causing mental or physical pain), the patient dreads subsequent treatment. If the experience was a positive one, the patient will not be fearful.

The best way to address objective fear is to be honest when communicating to the patient. Never lie to a patient. For example, it is always best to say, "This will pinch for just a moment," rather than "This won't hurt at all."

Despite their concerns and uneasiness, the majority of patients are able to seek and receive treatment. The dental team can help these patients by seeking to understand patient behavior and actively working to enable the patient to cope with the experience in a positive manner (Table 7–1).

PATIENT RESPONSES

The patient's responses to dental treatment and to the dental team are not limited to what is being said and done at the moment. Rather, responses are influenced by the patient's total personality and his

TABLE 7–1

Helping Patients Deal with Their Fears

PATIENT FEARS	WAYS TO HELP THESE PATIENTS
Fear that the dentist will adopt a negative attitude toward them because they have neglected their teeth	Treat all patients with dignity and respect; provide information about the patient's condition in a manner that is nonthreatening
Fear that the dentist will laugh at them or will think they are cowards or sissies	Reassure the patient in a manner that shows warmth and compassion
Fear of pain associated with dental treatment	Use effective pain control methods; keep the patient informed and warned about any coming discomfort
Fear of loss of control	Help the patient use constructive coping skills

TABLE 7–2

Dental Fears vs. Dental Phobias

DENTAL FEARS	DENTAL PHOBIAS
Fear Level 1 Patients schedule routine dental visits to prevent the consequences of neglect. Most of these patients do not express the need of a fear control program; they may request nitrous oxide sedation.	**Phobia Level 1** Patients do everything to avoid the dental office. They may attempt to obtain relief from pain with home remedies or over-the-counter preparations. Occasionally, they may require hospitalization for dental treatment, depending upon the condition of their mouths.
Fear Level 2 Fear intensifies, and patients may exhibit avoidance behavior. These patients seek dental treatment when they are in pain or have a dental emergency.	**Phobia Level 2** These patients exhibit severe cases of dental neglect. If they seek out dental care for pain, they will rarely return for completion of recommended treatment. They may exhibit irrational and unpredictable behavior. These patients require behavioral modification techniques to learn to control their fear.

background experiences. When working with patients, it is particularly important to remember that

- The patient's response to the situation results primarily from causes that are not part of the present situation.
- These causes are probably not fully understood by the patient and will probably remain largely unknown to the dental team.
- The patient's anxieties concerning treatment may result in hostile, irrational, and inappropriate behavior.
- This hostility is an expression of the patient's anxieties and is not caused by, or directed at, dental personnel.

DENTAL PHOBICS

For some patients, the mere suggestion of a routine dental visit brings overwhelming sensations of panic and terror. These patients are termed **dental phobics.**

The most severely affected dental phobics avoid treatment completely and often seek treatment only under the most aggravated dental symptoms (Table 7–2).

Three techniques have been used successfully to treat phobic dental patients:

Progressive muscle relaxation. During this exercise, the phobic patient is slowly and gradually brought to total body relaxation by alternately tensing and relaxing each major muscle group.

Guided imagery. During this exercise, the patient vividly imagines a tranquil or happy scene, such as a walk along the beach or a calm sunset. By actively imagining a pleasant scene, the patient's mind is distracted from the dental treatment and focuses on relaxation, eliminating the stress/fear response.

Systematic desensitization. The patient is gradually exposed to dental treatment, which ensures that fear can eventually be overcome.

PHARMACOLOGICAL METHODS OF REDUCING PATIENT FEARS

In some cases, it is necessary to treat phobic patients with pharmacological methods to help reduce their fears. These methods, which are discussed in Chapter 20, include analgesia, local anesthesia, and varying levels of sedation.

COPING MECHANISMS

In an attempt to handle the dental situation in a manner that is least stressful to him, the patient uses coping mechanisms. These forms of coping behavior are not neurotic unless carried to extremes. Rather, they are healthy and useful ways of handling a situation in which the patient feels psychologically uncomfortable.

Coping mechanisms become neurotic only when they interfere with action that could avoid danger. For example, it is neurotic behavior when a person uses coping mechanisms to delay treatment until it is too late to save his teeth.

Repression. Repression is the temporary unconscious forgetting of things that produce tension and/or pain. The favorite theory of the individual who uses repression as a coping mechanism is "If I ignore it, it will go away."

This is characterized by the patient who after having a toothache for three weeks finally calls late Friday afternoon for an emergency appointment. He had honestly hoped, as long as he possibly could, that the toothache would "go away by itself."

Rationalization. Rationalization is the process of making plausible excuses or reasons for implausible behavior. It is the "Why I didn't" syndrome. This is characterized by the patient who calls with a highly imaginative reason to explain why he failed to keep his dental appointment.

Procrastination. Procrastination is the process of avoiding an upsetting situation by postponing facing the problem as long as possible. The procrastinator firmly believes that one *should* put off until tomorrow whatever one can get out of doing today!

The procrastinator is often late for this appointment —when he finally does make one. He is also likely to be the patient who has his administrative assistant call at the last minute to cancel the appointment.

Deployment. Deployment is the turning of attention away from an unpleasant stimulus to one that is not tension-producing. It is a coping mechanism that can be used very effectively in the dental setting.

Background music, earphones, video games, relaxation techniques, or even a carefully placed television or a fish tank can be used to divert the patient's attention.

Affiliation. When patients feel threatened, they prefer to be with friends rather than with strangers. All members of the dental team can play an important role by making the patient feel that he is among friends who truly care for him as an individual (and not just a tooth that needs to be filled).

When the patient arrives, he should be greeted promptly, pleasantly, and by name. Name tags should be worn by all personnel so that the patient has the reassurance of knowing the names of those who are treating him. Also, as a matter of routine courtesy, staff members should introduce themselves to the patient as they come into contact with him for the first time.

Control of the Situation. One area in which patients most want to retain control is in communication during treatment. Yet, at the times when the patient most urgently wants to let the dentist know how he is feeling, his mouth is likely to be full of fingers, forceps, and clamps. The use of prearranged hand signals is one way to increase the patient's sense of being "in control" and to allow him to communicate his needs.

Rehearsal. Rehearsal is the act of mentally going through a situation before it actually occurs. It is one of the most important of the normal methods of coping with stress. It is a particularly valuable defense mechanism for children—valuable *if* this mental rehearsal is based on information and not imagination.

Office tours, letting the patient know what to expect at the visit, and keeping the patient informed as treatment progresses are ways in which the dentist and staff can help the patient use rehearsal in a positive manner.

Communication Skills

Effective communication may be one of the most important aspects of the assistant's job, because each of us spends about 90 percent of the working day (and every day) communicating with others (Fig. 7–1).

Communication is the sending of a message by one individual and the receiving of the *same* message by another individual. Every message we send has two parts, which must coincide in time:

- The **statement proper,** or the "This is what I have told you" portion, consists of the words being used.
- The **explanation** is the part of the message that conveys "Now, this is how I expect you to understand it." This part of the message is sent nonverbally.

We communicate with words, facial expressions, appearance, gestures, mannerisms, listening, voice inflection, attitudes, and actions. These may be grouped into the two general categories of verbal and nonverbal communication.

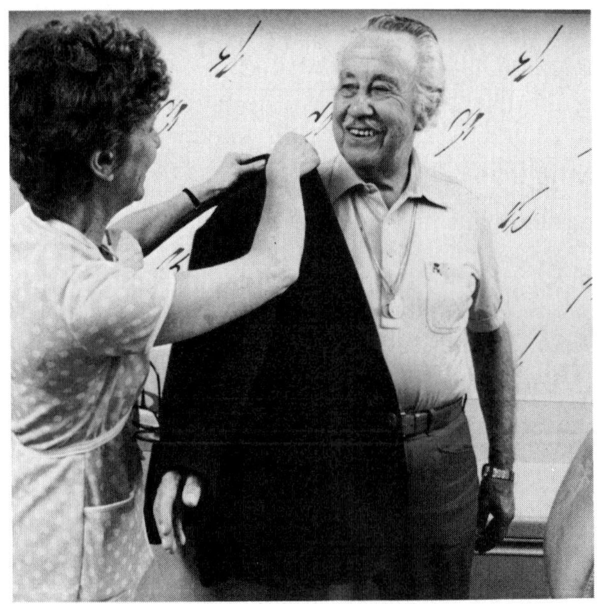

FIGURE 7–1

Communicating effectively with patients is an important part of an assistant's job.

Verbal communication is made up of the words we use, either written or spoken. Most verbal communication is perceived by the ear.

All other forms of communication fall into the category of **nonverbal communication** and are perceived, at an almost subconscious level, through all of the senses.

To communicate with others effectively, you must be sensitive to the messages that are being sent and received through all methods of communication.

Verbal Communication

WORDS ARE IMPORTANT

Words are verbal symbols used to represent an object or a meaning. Unfortunately, these verbal symbols are not repeatedly checked against the things they represent; the result is often confusion, distortion of meaning, or misunderstanding.

Also, words mean different things to different people and may mean different things at different times. Good verbal communication depends upon the foundation of a common language, in which the sender and receiver are using words they both understand to have the same meaning.

In speaking to the dental patient, take care to select words the *patient* understands, rather than confuse him with the technical language and specialized jargon of dentistry. It is also important to select words that will not frighten, intimidate, or upset the patient (see Words Can Hurt!).

VOICE QUALITY

Voice quality makes up more than one-third of the impact of the total message and reveals much about the individual.

You should cultivate a pleasant voice (tonal) quality and should speak slowly, distinctly, and loud enough to be heard easily without being strident or too loud.

In the event of a true emergency in the dental office, it is particularly important that you be extremely careful to keep your voice calm, because it is not *what* is said but *how* it is said that may alarm the patient or the person accompanying the patient.

ASKING QUESTIONS

Questions are used to gather information. Often, the way you phrase a question determines the kind of answer you get. By being aware of this, you can be more effective both in information gathering and in helping patients to feel more at ease.

Closed-Ended Question. A closed-ended question is one that can be answered "yes" or "no." These questions are best used to confirm information, to limit a conversation, or to close a conversation. Closed-ended questions often begin with the words *is, do, has, can, will,* or *shall.* For example, "Mr. Thomas, is next Monday at 9 A.M. convenient for you?" is a closed-ended question that can only be answered "yes" or "no."

Open-Ended Question. An open-ended question is one that requires more than "yes" or "no" for an answer. These questions are best used to obtain information, maintain control of the conversation, or build rapport. (**Rapport** is a feeling of harmony and accord.)

Open-ended questions usually begin with the words *what, when, how, who, where,* or *which.* For example, "Mrs. Jackson, what time of day is best to schedule your appointment?" is an open-ended question.

Words Can Hurt!

INSTEAD OF THIS . . .	TRY THIS . . .
Pain	Discomfort
Shot	Anesthetic
Pull	Remove
Drill	Prepare tooth
Filling	Restoration
False teeth	Denture
Operatory	Treatment area
Waiting room	Reception area

Nonverbal Communication

BODY LANGUAGE

Body language, which is a major part of nonverbal communication, consists of the messages we send by the way we carry ourselves and move about. It also includes our gestures, tone of voice, and facial expressions.

Posture, movements, and attitudes transmit major messages. For example, the person who is depressed moves slowly and with a restrained gait that reflects his mental attitude.

The happy, healthy individual with a bright outlook on life demonstrates this attitude with a free-moving walk that mirrors a sense of well-being.

Hands grasping the chair arms and restless shifting of body position are reliable indicators of inner tension and uneasiness.

Rapid, shallow breathing is also a sign of tension and stress, and you can help the patient relax by encouraging him to breathe slowly and deeply in a more normal pattern.

Facial Expressions. Facial expressions indicate a wide variety of emotional states at which words can only hint. The eyes are particularly expressive of emotion and the patient's mental state of well-being.

Although many patients become adept at hiding their true emotions, you should be aware of the signs of tension, stress, or pain as they are reflected in the patient's expression.

Likewise, you should also be aware of your own facial expression as you interact with the patient, because boredom, lack of interest, and anxiety are all quickly sensed by the patient.

At chairside, you must be particularly careful not to convey a feeling of alarm on your face as a reaction to operative or surgical procedures, because this response could unnecessarily alarm the patient.

Listening Skills

It has been estimated that 90 percent of all spoken words are never heard; yet listening is one of the greatest arts of communication—and one of the most difficult. Good listening requires that you concentrate totally on the patient (see Being a Good Listener).

Relating to the Needs of the Patient

Because no two dental patients are alike, good communication skills between the dental team and the patient are essential. The following section describes ways to help ensure that patient's needs are filled by the dental team.

POSITIVE OFFICE ATMOSPHERE

The physical appearance of the office speaks very loudly to perceptive patients. To ensure that patients feel welcome, the appearance and decor of the practice must reflect a warm, hospitable atmosphere.

Worn or shabby floor covering must be replaced or cleaned when necessary. Plants, magazines, and other reception area amenities must be kept as comfortable and pleasant as one's living room. Plants and fresh floral arrangements reflect a healthy and inviting practice atmosphere.

SINCERITY

Every action and word that takes place in the dental office is a reflection of sincerity. Patients are especially sensitive to verbal intonations and remarks that might otherwise seem comical or humorous. Every member of the dental team must make a conscious effort to think before speaking or acting.

RELATE TO THE PATIENT AS A PERSON

Patients prefer to be treated as "friends of the practice." Every effort should be made to help patients feel welcome and important.

It is advisable to address adults as "Mr.," "Mrs.," or "Miss" at the initial greeting. If, after that time, the patient expresses a desire to be called by a first name or a nickname, then do so. (Make a note of this on the patient's chart for future reference.)

RESPECT THE PATIENT'S TIME

Patients expect the value of their time to be respected and not wasted in unnecessary waiting. Therefore, scheduling appointments and staying on time are two essential components of helping patients feel welcome.

RESOLVE COMPLAINTS AND MISUNDERSTANDINGS PROMPTLY

It has been said that 95 percent of the patients who are dissatisfied never say so; they just leave the practice! Thus, it makes good sense to listen carefully to those few patients who attempt to express dissatisfaction.

One of the best ways to calm an irate patient is to listen silently, using good eye contact, and occasionally nod the head. Do not interrupt. Let the patient finish.

Often this helps the patient calm down slowly. It is then appropriate to say to the patient, "If I hear correctly what you are saying, Mr. Harris, you feel upset about the charge that appeared on last month's statement. Is that right?" This will give the patient a sense of control over the situation.

Make sure that all misunderstandings and concerns are resolved quickly, professionally, and pleasantly. If the patient insists upon speaking with the doctor, instruct the patient that the doctor will call back or speak with him by a specific time that day, and take steps to ensure that this takes place.

Being a Good Listener

Do not let your mind wander. Put aside personal concerns while the patient is talking.

Do not concentrate on formulating your reply. Instead, concentrate on what the patient is actually saying.

Look as well as listen. In this way you can pick up both the verbal and nonverbal information the patient is transmitting.

REMAIN APPROACHABLE

Many patients have a sense of fear about approaching professionals or about asking questions that they may sense are "dumb." One of the best communication techniques the dental office can practice is to display a sense of approachability at all times.

Patients' questions should be encouraged. The dental team should respond with a sense of genuine care and concern to the patient.

If the doctor has a "call-in" or "call-back" time each day for handling phone calls, this time should be used for accessibility to patients. Most patients want to feel reassured that the dental team cares about them.

RESPECT PATIENT CONFIDENTIALITY

In a time of increasing litigiousness, it is more important than ever to keep conversations—and patient records—confidential. If patients feel that their concerns are not taken seriously, or if they detect or sense a lack of confidentiality, the practice-patient relationship may suffer irreparable damage.

Written Communications

Many types of written communications originate from the dental practice. It is important to realize that after telephone communication, written communications are the most important thing that can characterize the practice. Thus the practice image or "perception" is based, to a great degree, upon the type and quality of the printed communications it generates.

Sample letters are shown in Chapters 34 and 36.

Letters to Professional Colleagues

Doctors frequently communicate with other professionals in writing. It is the job of the alert dental assistant to ensure that these communications take place in an expedient and professional-looking manner.

Letters to the doctor's colleagues may include examination findings or referral to specialists. It is important to double-check for spelling accuracy and consistency in sending written communications to other professional practices.

Letters to Insurance Carriers

When completing written correspondence to insurance carriers, make sure that the following are included:

Patient identification information: patient's name, address, contract number or identification number, and social security number

Case information: the nature and extent of the case, as well as any unusual circumstances or conditions, and an estimate of the fees to be incurred

Radiographs: only if required

Letters to Patients

Many practices elect to send letters to their patients for a variety of reasons: welcome, congratulations, acknowledgment of a referral, or completion of an extensive case.

To save valuable time in composing numerous letters, many practices keep on file sample letters under these headings. Some commercially prepared letters are available either in a book or on a computer diskette for use with a word processing program.

The Practice Newsletter

The newsletter represents a valuable communication tool for the practice. Patients enjoy reading about new techniques available, as well as information about the "human" side of the practice. The purposes of a practice newsletter include

- Keeping patients aware of technological and treatment advances
- Keeping patients in touch with the doctor and members of the dental team
- Listing their names as referral sources or contest winners (*note*: names are used here only with the patient's permission)
- Noting changes that have taken place in the practice

Most practices that publish a newsletter for their patients do so on a quarterly basis. A number of professional newsletter preparation organizations are available for producing a quality newsletter, using the doctor's masthead and customizing practice information.

Patient Education Materials

Printed pamphlets, brochures, and statement stuffers are other effective printed communication tools used successfully by many dental practices. When these materials are dispensed, it is essential to include the doctor's name, address, and telephone number on each printed piece.

Another effective marketing mechanism is to write the patient's name on the educational material, as this increases the likelihood that the patient will review the material and refer to it later on.

Stress in the Dental Office

Causes of Stress

Stress is common in the workplace today. Many dental team members feel stressed at times and, therefore, need to find an outlet. Some of the causes of stress in the dental office may include but are not limited to

- Lack of sufficient staff
- Appointment overbooking
- Multiple tasks required simultaneously
- Lack of good communication
- Perceived lack of job advancement

Methods of Stress Reduction

Stress may be reduced by a lifestyle that includes engaging in regular exercise, taking time off, leaving the office behind at the end of the day, and setting realistic expectations. Other methods of handling stress include going for a walk at lunch time, searching out a mentor, and finding a friend in whom to confide.

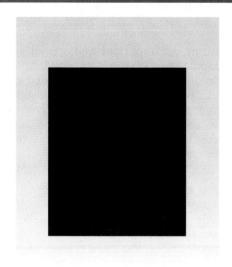

Chapter 8

The Special Patient

Introduction

Each patient who enters the dental office is, in his own way, special. He is an individual with needs and feelings that are unique to him. However, the discussion in this chapter is limited to groups of patients who present special challenges, and rewards, to the dental health team.

The Pregnant Patient

The goal of dental care during pregnancy is to provide dental therapy without undue adverse effects on the mother or the fetus. In general, dental care can be safely and effectively provided to pregnant patients.

There are four general management concepts to consider when treating the pregnant patient:

- Maintain good oral hygiene.
- Provide necessary treatment safely.
- If in doubt about treatment, check first with the patient's obstetrician.
- Keep appointments short.

Maintain Good Oral Hygiene

Pregnancy gingivitis is gingival enlargement that may occur during pregnancy (Fig. 8–1). It may be marginal and generalized, or it may occur as single or multiple tumor-like masses. These masses are called **pregnancy tumors**; however, they are gingival enlargements and not actual tumors.

Pregnancy gingivitis is caused by hormonal changes that increase the tissue response to local irritants, and these conditions usually subside after the mother has given birth.

During the pregnancy, most gingival disease can be controlled or prevented by the removal of local irritants and the maintenance of good oral hygiene.

Provide Necessary Treatment Safely

In most cases, routine dental care can be delivered safely throughout pregnancy, and receiving routine care is far preferable to having to deal with a dental emergency.

A primary precaution is to limit radiographic exposure for women who are known to be pregnant or who might be pregnant. In some practices, all women of childbearing age are asked to "Let us know if you are pregnant."

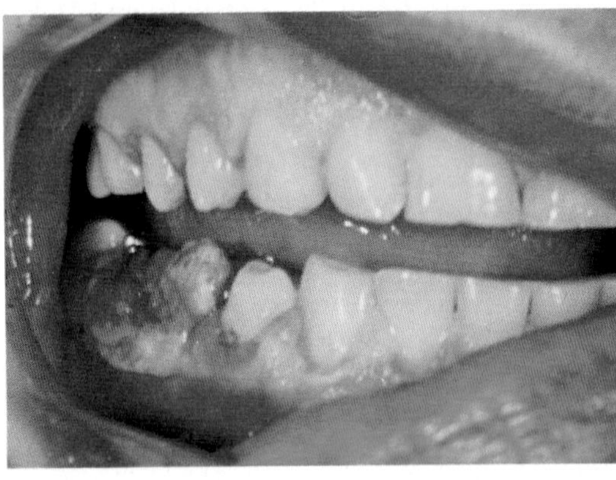

FIGURE 8–1

Localized gingival enlargement in area facial to teeth #28 to #30 in a pregnant patient. (From Carranza, F.A., Jr.: Glickman's Clinical Periodontology, 7th ed. Philadelphia, W.B. Saunders Co., 1990, p 454.)

When a pregnant patient is treated, radiographs should be taken only when necessary. The need should be discussed with the patient so that she can give informed consent. And, of course, a protective lead apron and collar are used on *all* patients.

Check with the Patient's Obstetrician

If possible, any treatment that may cause transient bacteremia is postponed until after the patient has given birth. (**Transient bacteremia** is the temporary presence of bacteria in the blood stream. This is a hazard when the procedure, such as an extraction, causes severe bleeding.)

If the treatment cannot be postponed, the dentist should check with the patient's obstetrician before proceeding. (An **obstetrician** is a physician who specializes in providing care to the pregnant woman before, during, and immediately after birth.)

The dentist may also wish to consult the patient's obstetrician before prescribing medications. This is because most drugs cross the placental barrier and may have possible adverse effects on the developing fetus.

It is also recommended either that nursing mothers avoid the use of drugs during nursing or that nursing be discontinued, if prescription drugs must be taken.

Keep Appointments Short

During the later months of the pregnancy, it is generally not advisable to keep a pregnant patient seated in one position for a long time. If seated in one position too long, the patient may suffer from postural hypotension, which is discussed in Chapter 9.

The Child Patient

Children constitute an important and special group in the dental population. Like adults, children have individual likes and dislikes, as well as fears and complex personalities. The child patient must be treated with the same respect for his dignity and individuality that is afforded to an adult.

The child needs to be understood in terms of his chronological, mental, and emotional age.

- **Chronological age** is the child's actual age in terms of years and months.
- **Mental age** refers to the child's level of intellectual capacity and development.
- **Emotional age** describes the child's level of emotional maturity.

These ages are not necessarily the same. A child at the chronological age of 6 may have a mental age of 8 (mentally he is functioning at the level of the average 8-year-old) and the emotional age of 4 (emotionally he is functioning at the level of the average 4-year-old).

Guidelines, or *norms,* for the average child's development can be used as a crude index to the child's anticipated behavior level at a certain age. A child who differs widely from these norms may have a physical or emotional problem.

However, many children under the stress of a dental appointment may temporarily regress (retreat) to a more immature level of behavior.

The Stages of Childhood

INFANCY (BIRTH TO 2 YEARS)

During this period, the child learns to sit, stand, walk, and run. Vocally, he progresses from meaningless babble to use of simple sentences. Socially, he learns to identify familiar faces and passes through periods of being friendly toward, and then fearful of, strangers.

With the newborn, the parents should wipe the child's gums softly with clean moistened gauze daily. (The gauze is then discarded.) As the teeth begin to erupt, a very small, soft-bristle brush (designed for infants) should be used.

This brush is used without toothpaste until the child is at least 18 months old. Even then, only a very small amount (about pea-size) is used, and the child is not allowed to swallow the toothpaste. When the child is ready, a fluoride-containing toothpaste is desirable; however, caution is necessary because of concern that the child may ingest excessive fluoride by swallowing large quantities of this toothpaste.

EARLY CHILDHOOD (2 TO 4 YEARS)

The 2-year-old child is often referred to as being in the *pre-cooperative stage.* He is too young to form friendships and is not particularly interested in pleasing others. This child is usually shy and still emotionally dependent on his mother or primary caregiver.

He is able to follow simple commands but is not yet sufficiently coordinated to obey commands such as "open your mouth." Often he cannot be reached only by words but must handle and touch objects to fully understand them.

The 2-year-old has all his primary teeth and is ready for his first visit to the dentist. Early dental experiences are extremely important because they shape the future attitude of the individual as a dental patient.

It is preferable that the child make an introductory visit to the dental office before he is in pain or requires emergency treatment.

The 3-year-old is better able to comprehend verbally and tries to please. Children at this age respond positively to praise. They also respond well to word-pictures such as "giant camera" (dental x-ray machine) and "squirt gun" (water syringe).

THE PRESCHOOL CHILD (4 TO 6 YEARS)

This has been described as the "out-of-bounds" age. It is an age of exploration and increasing independence. Behavior patterns are characterized by their wide variation and unpredictability. It is also the beginning of the age of socialization, and most children at this age *want* to cooperate.

The 4-year-old usually listens with interest to explanations and normally is quite responsive to verbal directions. He may also display his independence by refusing to sit in the dental chair or to open his mouth.

Five- and six-year-olds are more self-assured; they love praise and compliments. They are proud of their accomplishments, and this sense of "social pride" can be used in motivating them to keep their teeth clean.

GRADE SCHOOL AGE (6 TO 12 YEARS)

This is the period of socialization: learning to get along with people, learning the rules and regulations of society, and learning to accept them.

It is also the age for mixed dentition, with the loss of the primary teeth and the eruption of the permanent teeth.

The Older Patient

Providing dental care to older patients is called **geriatric dentistry**; however, this is not a recognized dental specialty. Older dental patients are divided into three groups:

- Older individuals aged 65 to 74 are considered to be the "**new-old.**" They are a relatively healthy and active group that is new to retirement and to the term *senior citizen.*
- Those aged 75 to 84 are the "**mid-old.**" They vary from being very active tennis players to individuals with an array of chronic diseases.
- People older than 85 are referred to as the "**oldest-old.**" Individuals in this group usually have more chronic diseases and are increasingly frail.

Oral Health Conditions of the Older Patient

There are certain generalities that describe the oral health conditions that are likely to occur in older patients:

Multiple Health Problems. These patients may have multiple chronic health conditions and may be taking several medications prescribed by different doctors.

Obtaining a current and complete medical and medication history is essential. (Because this is a longer and more complex history, more time should be allowed for this part of the visit.)

Periodontal Disease. This is an increasing problem in the older population. Also, the tissues of older patients may be slower to heal.

Dental Decay. This may increase in the form of coronal and root caries and in recurrent decay around defective restorations.

Dark and Brittle Teeth. The teeth may darken and become more brittle as a result of deposits of secondary dentin that have gradually reduced the size of the pulp chamber. These teeth are more subject to fracture.

Xerostomia. Also known as *dry mouth,* this condition may result from certain disorders and medications that cause a decreased flow of saliva. The saliva that is present may be thick and gummy rather than thin and ropy.

Loss of Vertical Dimension. This may occur because of wearing down of the teeth or because of missing teeth. This contributes to changes in the appearance of the face and wrinkling of the skin around the mouth. (**Vertical dimension** is a measurement of the face at the midline with the teeth in occlusion.)

Bone Resorption. This and loss of the alveolar ridge may be a problem in edentulous patients. (**Edentulous** means without teeth.) This bone loss makes fitting and wearing dentures more difficult.

Ill-Fitting Dentures. These may cause difficulty in chewing or contribute to soft tissue pathology.

Nutritional Status. This contributes to general and dental health problems and may be affected by difficulty in chewing, missing teeth, sores in the mouth, or poorly fitting dentures.

Poor Oral Hygiene. This is due to limited physical mobility, presence of Alzheimer's disease, or other debilitating health problems and may lead to otherwise preventable tooth loss.

Dental Treatment for the Older Patient

The attitudes of the dentist and staff toward the elderly are reflected in their willingness to help the patient feel physically and emotionally comfortable in the dental office.

Positive attitudes start with greeting the patient warmly and respectfully. Although some geriatric patients may have a hearing or memory loss, they resent being treated as if they were stupid or childlike. They should always be addressed directly, and treated with dignity.

Scheduling older patients is dependent upon their health and needs:

- Some retired individuals maintain very busy schedules and want to complete dental care as quickly as possible.
- Other older patients may not be able to tolerate long periods in the dental chair and should be scheduled for short appointments.
- Still other older patients, with few interests and outside contacts, may look forward to social interaction with the dental staff during their dental visits.

The older patient may need more time to walk to the treatment room and may need help getting into and out of the dental chair. The dental chair should be adjusted slowly, and the patient should be asked whether he is comfortable. The patient may not be comfortable in a supine position. If so, it is necessary to modify the normal routine to accommodate these needs.

When the patient is returned to an upright position, he should be encouraged to sit still for a few minutes before he tries to stand. This will help prevent dizziness caused by a rapid change of position.

THE PATIENT WITH A PACEMAKER

If the patient has a pacemaker, this should be highlighted on his chart. (A **pacemaker** is an implanted electronic device to stimulate regular beating of the heart.)

Exposure to electromagnetic interferences can alter pacemaker performance. Therefore, it is advisable to avoid use of the ultrasonic scaler on the patient with a pacemaker. Likewise, the ultrasonic instrument cleaner and microwave oven should not be activated when a patient with a pacemaker is in the office.

WHEN THE PATIENT NEEDS HELP

The older patient may need additional help in understanding directions and in maintaining oral hygiene. An unhurried, detailed, and yet simple explanation of the planned treatment is important. So too is the repetition of key words and phrases. When possible, home care instructions should be provided in writing.

If the patient is unable to understand or remember directions, the dentist and dental team members should be in communication with the caregiver. (A **caregiver** is the person who is responsible for the daily and routine care of the patient. This is often an immediate family member.)

The caregiver may also be helpful in providing supplemental information that the patient may be reluctant to discuss or may simply be unaware of.

The Abused Patient

The Abused Child

Often it is healthcare providers who may detect, or at least suspect, victims of abuse. Because of embarrassment or worse—fear of losing the child or of facing fine or imprisonment—abusive parents tend to make up stories about how the child "fell" or sustained some other injury to the head.

However, child abuse must be suspected as the cause when a child presents with unexplained signs, including

- Injuries in various stages of healing (this indicates injuries that have occurred over a period of time, as opposed to a single accident)
- Repeated injuries
- Chipped or injured teeth
- Scars inside the lips or on the tongue and tears of the labial frena
- Battering or other injuries around the head and neck
- Facial bruises, swelling of the facial structures, or black eyes
- A fractured nose or broken teeth
- Bite marks
- Injuries not consistent with the explanation presented by the parent

By law, in all 50 states, healthcare professionals (physicians, dentists, nurses, social workers) are required to report child abuse cases, and the state or county child protective services *must* be contacted. The name of the person making this report will not be revealed.

Although dental assistants and clerical staff are not legally required to report abuse cases, each member of the dental team has a moral responsibility to report known or suspected abuse cases *to the dentist.*

Reporting of suspected child abuse may be done by telephone, in person, or in writing. Required information necessary to file a report may include

- The name, address, gender, age, height, and weight of the child

- The name and address of the adult having custody of the child
- A description of the current physical and emotional abuse and/or neglect of the child
- Evidence of previous injuries or negligence
- Any information that may assist in establishing the cause of the injuries
- Sketches or photos documenting the nature and location of the injuries

The Abused Spouse

The term **spouse abuse** is defined as violent behavior occurring between partners in an intimate relationship, regardless of marital status. Although this is often referred to as the *battered woman* syndrome, spousal abuse also may be inflicted by women on their male partners.

In the majority of spousal abuse cases, physical injuries occur in the form of punching, kicking, biting, or assault with a weapon. Healthcare providers must also be aware that in addition to physical injuries, psychological abuse and intimidation are integral components of the abuse syndrome.

Unexplained oral and facial trauma (injury) or lesions (sores) *may* indicate that the patient is a victim of domestic violence (see Signs and Symptoms of Domestic Abuse).

Signs and Symptoms of Domestic Abuse

- Facial bruises inconsistent with a typical accident
- Bald or sparse spots on the scalp, possibly indicating hair pulling
- Specific bruise patterns or cuts on the face and ears from punching, slapping, twisting, or pinching
- Unexplained or repeated fractured or avulsed teeth
- Scars or burns on the lips or tongue
- Unexplained broken or bruised jaw or nose
- Oral signs of sexual abuse
- Bruises, rope burns, or finger marks on the neck or submandibular area
- Bilateral eye trauma or injuries around the eyes
- A bite mark on any part of the body

A suspected spouse abuse victim should be interviewed in a private setting. This is because the abuser often tries to remain close to the victim, answering questions directed to the victim.

The Abused Geriatric Patient

Victims of geriatric abuse, also known as *elder abuse*, are usually in poor health and are more likely to be victims of physical violence received from those individuals with whom they live. Most commonly this is a spouse; however, it may be a caregiver or an adult child.

Geriatric abuse may take several forms:

- **Active neglect:** intentionally denying or withholding care.
- **Passive neglect:** unintentionally failing to provide care.
- **Self-neglect:** the patient is no longer willing or able to care for himself.
- **Financial neglect:** the caretaker may withhold care for financial reasons.

Symptoms of geriatric abuse include acute trauma and indicators of prior trauma to the dental and facial structures. These may include eye injuries, fractures of the bones of the cheeks and around the eyes, and bruising of the facial tissues. However, it should be noted that not all facial lesions, mucosal/skin lesions, or discolorations indicate abuse. For example, skin lesions resembling traumatic injuries are sometimes caused by medications, systemic or dermatological diseases, and fungal, bacterial, or viral diseases.

The dental team must be very careful in noting suspicions concerning elder abuse. If elder abuse is definitely suspected, the dentist should report it in the same manner that other abuse is reported.

The Americans with Disabilities Act

The Americans with Disabilities Act (ADA) contains four sections:

- **Title I** eliminates employment discrimination policies.
- **Title II** provides for access to public services by the disabled.
- **Title III** opens public accommodations to the disabled and provides disabled people with access to equal goods and services.
- **Title IV** extends telecommunication services to the hearing and speech impaired.

The ADA provides a national mandate (requirement) for the elimination of discrimination against individuals with disabilities and provides clear, strong, enforceable standards addressing discrimination against disabled people.

Disabilities under this act include, but are not limited to, acquired immunodeficiency syndrome (AIDS) or the human immunodeficiency virus (HIV), cancer, heart disease, diabetes, mental retardation, learning disabilities, and visual and hearing impairment.

The Handicapped Patient

For handicapped persons to function to the best of their ability, they should maintain good dental health because it is an important part of good general health.

The assistant is an important part of the dental health team in providing this care. The role of the assistant caring for the handicapped can be divided into these major areas:

Aiding the Dentist in Providing Treatment. The chairside assistant must be familiar with any specialized techniques and equipment used in treating handicapped patients. The efficiency of all dental team members is important in order to speed and ease treatment.

Providing a Source of Information to the Patient and His Family. Preventive dentistry is particularly important—and may prove difficult—for the handicapped patient.

The assistant may be asked to work with the handicapped patient and his family in developing and implementing a preventive dentistry program tailored to the needs of this patient.

Making the Patient More Comfortable and Reducing Anxiety. The handicapped patient may be particularly apprehensive because of his extensive painful experiences with medical treatment.

He may also be fearful because previous dental treatment has been associated with a toothache or other unpleasant memories. The assistant can best help this patient by a reassuring manner and by learning how to meet the specialized needs of this patient.

When You Meet a Handicapped Person

The following guidelines are provided by the Easter Seals Society on how to enhance your contact with a handicapped person:

1. Do not stop and stare when you see a handicapped person. He deserves the same courtesy that any person should receive.
2. Do not ask embarrassing questions. If the handicapped person wants to tell you about his disability, he will bring up the subject himself.
3. Be yourself when you meet him, and talk about the same things you would with anyone else.
4. Do not be overprotective or oversolicitous. Help him only when he requests it.
5. Do not separate a disabled person from his wheelchair or crutches unless he asks for this. He may want his wheelchair or crutches within reach. Let the handicapped person set his own pace in walking.

Dental Treatment for the Handicapped Patient

The handicapped patient's condition will determine whether treatment is provided in the dental office, the home, or an institutional or a hospital setting.

An evaluation of a patient's medical and social history will help determine necessary modifications of the treatment plan. It may also reveal factors influencing the prognosis. In addition to identifying the handicap, the history can provide information about possible side effects from long-term use of medications and about diet and living conditions that may influence oral health.

Patients with Specific Handicaps

THE BLIND PATIENT

Blind patients have learned to rely on their sense of touch and on verbal communication with others. They may also have an unusually well-developed sense of taste and therefore may find some dental medicaments to be unpleasant.

Once the blind patient is seated, the chair should not be abruptly repositioned without the patient's being informed first. It may also be helpful to touch the patient in a reassuring manner as the chair is positioned.

Care should be taken to explain what is to be done. Blind children may want to touch the instruments to be used.

THE HEARING-IMPAIRED PATIENT

In the dental office, the patient with a suspected hearing loss should be treated with extra care and courtesy. The person with a hearing problem may have no visible evidence of his handicap, and when he does not understand everything said to him, he may well attempt to bluff and give the response that he hopes is appropriate.

If the hearing-impaired patient is accompanied by a hearing interpreter, this is considered acceptable within the description of the law. When talking to this patient, make sure you do the following:

- Stand in front of him so that he can see your face and follow your lip movements.
- Do not shout, but speak slowly and distinctly.
- Keep directions simple and accompany them with a visual demonstration and a written copy of all instructions.

Learning to Speak with a New Denture. Loss of speech acuity may account for some of the difficulty the hard-of-hearing patient may have in adjusting to speaking with a new denture. The hissing sounds, such as *s* and *sh,* are particularly troublesome.

If the patient is willing to cooperate, after the denture is properly adjusted to permit correct sound production, he should be encouraged to practice until he is able to make these sounds correctly.

Because he can no longer count on hearing himself for self-correction of his speech, he must learn to judge his sound production by the placement and "feel" of his tongue.

Some dentists and assistants who specialize in treating hearing-impaired patients learn at least some sign language so that they are better able to communicate with these patients.

THE PATIENT WITH CLEFT PALATE

As discussed in Chapter 4, failure of fusion of the bones and tissues of the hard and soft palates during early prenatal development may result in a cleft lip and/or palate.

This congenital malformation, occurs approximately once in 700 births. (**Congenital** means a condition that is present at birth.)

The defect occurs between 4 and 10 weeks' gestation, often before the woman is aware that she is pregnant. The causes both are *genetic* (clefts tend to "run in families" and are more common in some ethnic groups) and *environmental* (this refers to the mother's health during early pregnancy).

Environmental factors include smoking, alcohol consumption, malnutrition, and substance abuse. Infants of mothers older than 35 are also at increased risk.

A **cleft lip** may occur with or without a cleft palate. The cleft may be *unilateral* (affecting only one side), or it may be *bilateral* (affecting both sides) (Fig. 8–2).

The patient with **cleft palate** may have a cleft only of the hard palate, only of the soft palate, or of both. The normal palate separates the oral cavity and the nasal cavity. With a cleft palate, there is an opening between these two cavities. These children have many problems, including

- The infant cannot nurse properly because he cannot swallow normally and food comes out through the nose.
- Because of the intercommunication between the mouth and nose areas, the child has frequent ear infections and may suffer from a hearing loss.
- As the child develops, the malformation of the mouth makes it very difficult for him to create normal speech sounds.
- Frequently there are dental abnormalities such as missing and malpositioned teeth.

Early Treatment. An **obturator** (an appliance that looks somewhat like a denture without teeth) is fabricated almost immediately for the infant with a cleft palate; the obturator blocks the opening in the palate and is inserted

- To enable the child to nurse
- To prevent collapse of the palatal segments and to stimulate growth of the palatal shelves toward the midline, thereby reducing the size of the cleft

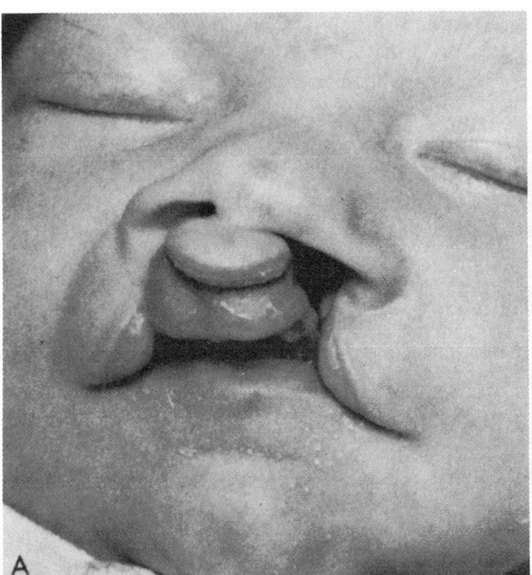

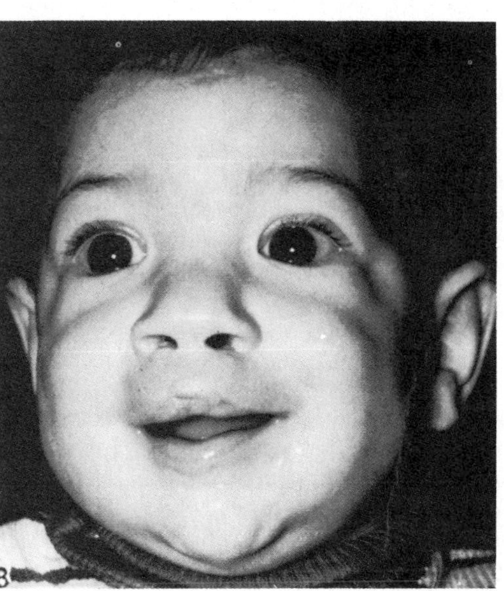

FIGURE 8–2

Bilateral cleft. *A*, Newborn infant with a bilateral cleft. *B*, With the cleft repaired, the growing child has a happy smile. (Photos courtesy of Dr. D. Bradley.)

- To keep the tongue in normal position, thus permitting the tongue to fulfill its role in the development of the jaws and speech
- To reduce nasal irritation and help prevent middle ear infection, which could result in hearing loss

Until the cleft palate opening can be closed surgically, the obturator must be replaced regularly to accommodate the growth of the child.

A cleft lip may be surgically closed when the infant is about 3 months; however, plastic surgery may be required later to correct or improve the appearance of the scar.

The Craniofacial Team. Total treatment for these patients is best handled by a well-organized craniofacial team consisting of the following:

- **Pediatrician:** to evaluate the cleft problem, to refer the patient to the proper specialist for care specific to the problem, and to provide treatment promoting the overall health and development of the child
- **Plastic surgeon:** to evaluate and provide necessary facial surgical procedures and follow-up treatment
- **Social services:** to aid the family with problems related to the care and treatment of the patient with cleft palate
- **Audiology and speech services:** to evaluate speech and hearing and to institute treatment as needed
- **Dental care provider:** to provide preventive, restorative, prosthetic, and orthodontic services

Dental Treatment for the Patient with Cleft Palate. The patient with cleft palate usually requires extensive dental treatment, and he may be a very difficult dental patient. His mouth has been a source of great pain, both physical and psychological.

He may have had repeated oral surgery and may regard any further procedure done in the mouth as a potential source of pain. In addition, this patient may have trouble communicating because of a hearing loss or speech difficulty. Furthermore, he may have been influenced by a natural tendency within the family to pamper a handicapped child.

The patient with cleft palate needs "routine" dental care (as provided by a general practitioner), including dental prophylaxis, preventive treatment, restorative services, and instruction in oral hygiene skills.

MENTAL RETARDATION

Mental retardation refers to subaverage general intelligence functioning, which originates during the developmental period and is associated with impairment in adaptive behavior. For descriptive purposes, the mentally retarded are classified in four groups reflecting the degree of intellectual impairment.

Mild Mental Retardation. Mild mental retardation describes individuals with intelligence quotients (IQs) ranging from 50–55 to 70.

These individuals typically develop social and communication skills during the preschool years, have minimal impairment in sensorimotor areas, and often are not distinguishable from normal children until a later age.

During their adult years, they usually achieve social and vocational skills adequate for minimum self-support but may need guidance and assistance when under unusual social or economic stress.

An individual with mild mental retardation may be capable of receiving dental care in the usual manner. Because his comprehension rate is slow, he may require extra patience, understanding, and reassurance. With help from the dental team, the mildly mentally retarded person can become a good dental patient.

Moderate Mental Retardation. Moderate mental retardation describes individuals with IQs ranging from 35–40 to 50–55. These individuals can talk or learn to communicate during the preschool years.

They may profit from vocational training and, with moderate supervision, can take care of themselves; however, they are unlikely to progress beyond the second grade level in academic subjects. They adapt well to life in the community, but they need supervision and guidance when under stress and generally live in supervised group homes.

A moderately mentally retarded patient will probably require special care in receiving dental treatment. Premedication, restraints, care under general anesthesia, or treatment by a specialist may be required.

Severe Mental Retardation. Severe mental retardation describes individuals with IQs ranging from 20–25 to 35–40. During the preschool period, they display poor motor development and acquire little or no communicative speech. In their adult years, they may be able to perform simple tasks under close supervision. Specialized dental treatment involving the use of general anesthesia is frequently necessary for these individuals.

Profound Mental Retardation. Profound mental retardation describes individuals with IQs ranging from below 20–25. During the early years, these children display minimal capacity for sensorimotor functioning. A highly structured environment, with constant aid and supervision, is necessary throughout life. These individuals require specialized dental care, which is usually provided in an institutional setting.

THE PATIENT WITH DOWN SYNDROME

Patients with Down syndrome, also called *trisomy 21*, have a chromosomal **aberration** (departure from the normal) that usually results in certain abnormal physical characteristics and mental impairment. The mental impairment may range from mild to moderate retardation.

Not all the physical characteristics of Down syndrome are found in all these patients. Commonly, however, the back of the head is flattened, the eyes are slanted and almond-shaped, and the bridge of the nose is slightly depressed. Muscle strength and muscle tone are usually reduced, and one-third of these children have heart problems (Fig. 8–3).

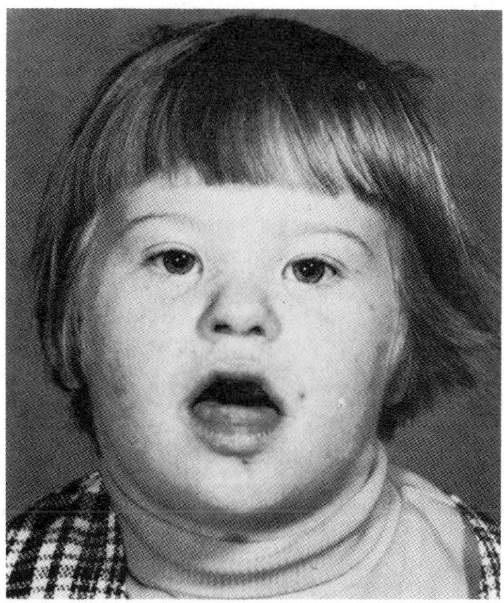

FIGURE 8–3

Three-year-old child with Down syndrome. (Photo courtesy of Dr. E. Howden.)

Frequently there are abnormalities in dental development. Eruption of the teeth may be delayed, with the primary incisors not erupting until after 1 year of age or later.

The teeth may be small and peg-shaped, and malocclusions are common. Periodontal problems are frequent as a result of malaligned teeth, mouth-breathing, or poor home care.

The forward position of the mandible and the underdeveloped nasal and maxillary bones do not provide sufficient space for the tongue. The resulting open-mouth, forward-tongue position gives the appearance of an enlarged tongue.

Dental Treatment for the Patient with Down Syndrome. The type of dental treatment required depends, in large part, upon the mental development and physical problems of the individual. He should be approached in terms of his mental age and abilities and not according to his chronological age.

THE PATIENT WITH CEREBRAL PALSY

Cerebral palsy is a broad term used to describe a group of nonprogressive neural disorders caused by brain damage that occurred prenatally, during birth, or in the postnatal period before the central nervous system reached maturity.

The resultant brain damage is manifested as a malfunction of motor centers and is characterized by paralysis, muscle weakness, lack of coordination, and other disorders of motor function (Fig. 8–4).

In addition to their motor disabilities, many individuals suffering from cerebral palsy have other symptoms of organic brain damage, such as seizure disorders, mental retardation, and sensory and learning disorders, which may be further complicated by behavioral and emotional disorders.

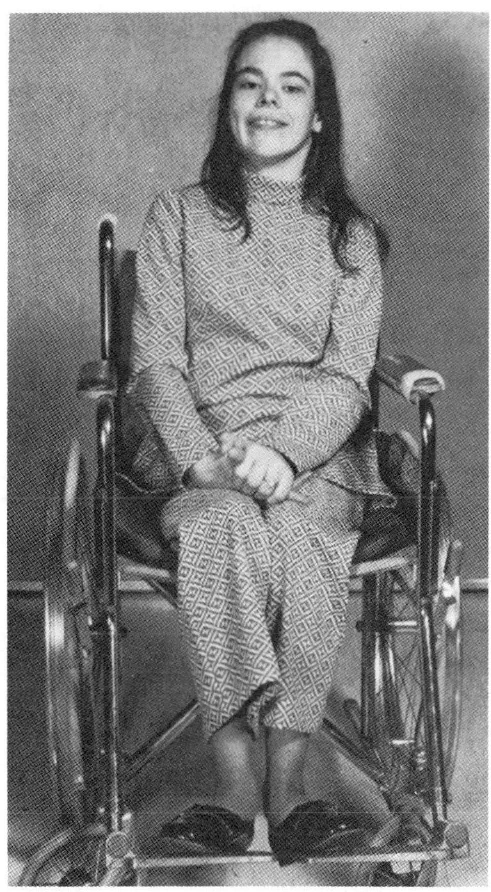

FIGURE 8–4

A 20-year-old cerebral palsy patient. (Photo courtesy of Dr. E. Howden.)

Cerebral palsy is most commonly classified according to the type of motor disturbance. The two most common types are spasticity and athetosis.

- **Spasticity** is characterized by a state of increased muscle tension manifested by an exaggerated stretch reflex.
- **Athetosis** is the type of motor disturbance in which uncontrollable, involuntary, purposeless, and poorly coordinated movements of the body, face, and extremities occur. Grimacing, drooling, and speech defects are present.

Dental Treatment for the Patient with Cerebral Palsy. The contour of the reclined dental chair is excellent for stabilizing many spastic patients. It helps prevent forward motion of the patient and promotes a feeling of security.

If the patient wears leg braces, these should be in an unlocked position during treatment. However, care must be taken that they are locked again at the end of treatment.

Premedication is frequently used to help control and relax the cerebral palsy patient. This, plus patience, understanding, and flexibility by the dental team members, makes routine dental care possible for many of these patients. For some, however, general anesthesia and treatment by a specialist may be necessary.

Restraining straps, or a papoose board that totally immobilizes the patient, should be used only when the patient is physically unable to cooperate in any other way. Mouth stabilization may be maintained with the use of a bite-block or mouth prop with rubber padding.

Oral hygiene in the majority of these patients is unusually poor, owing in part to the nature of their disease and the resulting physical limitations. The patient and the caregiver should receive a thorough orientation to a home care program, with modifications as necessary to meet the patient's special needs.

Frequently a powered toothbrush can be used effectively. Special adaptations of toothbrush handles and other aids to hygiene also may be helpful.

THE PATIENT WITH EPILEPSY

Epilepsy, recurrent convulsive disorders, and **epileptic seizures** are terms that are used interchangeably to designate a symptom complex characterized by recurrent convulsive seizures, resulting in partial or complete loss of consciousness.

If the cause of the seizures is found to be a demonstrable cerebral abnormality, the patient is said to have **organic** or **symptomatic epilepsy.**

In the majority of cases, however, the cause cannot be identified, and these patients are said to have **idiopathic** (of an unknown cause) **epilepsy**. Petit mal and grand mal epileptic seizures are discussed here.

Petit Mal Seizures. Petit mal seizures almost always appear in childhood, diminish after puberty, and rarely persist past the age of 30.

In petit mal seizures, there is a brief loss of consciousness lasting no longer than 30 seconds—more commonly, 5 to 10 seconds. This type of seizure may be manifested in a variety of ways, such as briefly staring into space, a slight quivering of the trunk and limb muscles, drooping or nodding of the head, and upward rolling of the eyes or rapid blinking of the eyelids.

Grand Mal Seizures. Grand mal, or generalized, seizures have many causes and arise in all age groups. They may be preceded by an aura (a brief experience such as an unpleasant odor, visual or aural hallucinations, or strange sensations in the leg or arm) or by localized spasm or twitching of the muscles.

Generalized convulsions of rapid onset may occur simultaneously with the loss of consciousness. The patient collapses, the pupils are dilated, the eyeballs roll upward or to one side, and the face is distorted. Occasionally, the tongue may be severely bitten during a seizure as a result of the rapid contraction of the jaw muscles. (See Chapter 9 on how to care for the patient having a seizure.)

Dental Treatment for Patients with Epilepsy. Phenytoin (Dilantin) is commonly used to control epileptic seizures. A common side effect of this medication is **hyperplasia** (overgrowth) of the gingival tissue (Fig. 8–5).

In most cases, treatment consists of the professional removal of all plaque, followed by a good home care program. In severe cases, the teeth may be completely covered with the hyperplastic tissue. When this happens, surgical or laser removal of the hyperplastic tissue may be necessary.

Because dental treatment may involve the use of drugs that can interact with anticonvulsant medication, the dentist must be aware of the patient's current medication and dosages. The dentist may wish to consult with the patient's physician. Unless contraindicated, epileptic patients undergoing routine dental treatment should be advised to continue their prescribed drug therapy.

Another concern facing the epileptic patient is the danger of injury to hard and soft tissues during a seizure. Dental restorations must be constructed to withstand falls and the strong contraction of the jaw muscles. Thus a strong stainless steel crown is the treatment of choice over a weaker, acrylic-type temporary crown. Fixed prosthetics are preferable to removable ones for epileptic patients; full dentures should be reinforced with mesh to prevent shattering.

THE DIABETES MELLITUS PATIENT

Diabetes mellitus is a metabolic disorder resulting from disturbances in the normal insulin mechanism. There are two types of diabetes, which may occur at any age.

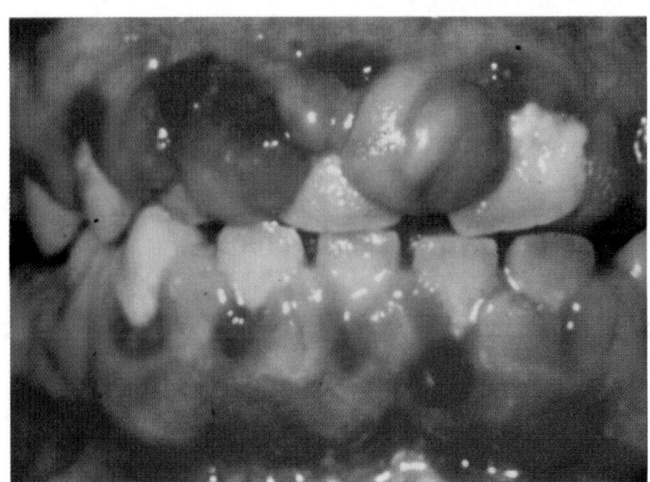

FIGURE 8–5

Gingival enlargement associated with phenytoin (Dilantin) therapy.

Type I Diabetes

Type I diabetes, also known as *insulin-dependent diabetes mellitus* (IDDM), was formerly called *juvenile-onset diabetes.* It is characterized by an absence of insulin secretion, and control of the disease is dependent upon the administration of insulin.

Type II Diabetes

Type II diabetes, also known as *non-insulin-dependent diabetes mellitus* (NIDDM), was formerly called *maturity-onset diabetes.* In most cases it can be controlled through diet and oral medications.

Oral Manifestations of Diabetes

Oral manifestations of diabetes include

Acetone Breath. This has the odor of stale cider or decaying apples.

Dehydration of Oral Soft Tissues. This results from a diminished production of saliva. The "dry mouth" is uncomfortable, and the tongue may have a burning sensation.

Red, Swollen, and Painful Gingiva. As the patient ages, the gingiva becomes fibrous (tougher) and contains a reduced number of blood vessels.

Alveolar Bone Loss. Severe loss of the supporting alveolar bone and the periodontal ligament results in loosening of the teeth (Fig. 8–6).

Toothache. In clinically sound teeth, this is a confusing symptom. The toothache is due to the **arteritis** (inflammation of the arteries) occurring throughout the body. This affects the blood vessels in the dental pulp. Periapical infection, pulpal necrosis, and a periapical abscess may follow.

Delayed Healing. Even diabetic patients whose conditions are controlled show a greater susceptibility to infection and delayed healing. Occasionally, diabetic patients who undergo extractions experience a condition known as a "dry socket." (See Chapter 11.)

Dental Treatment for the Diabetic Patient

As a general rule, diabetics receiving conventional insulin therapy should consume some carbohydrate approximately every 3 hours during their waking hours. Appointment scheduling should be planned around this need.

It is advisable to give diabetics early morning appointments so that they are not kept waiting, because the stress of waiting may result in an adverse reaction.

These patients should also be advised to eat and adjust their insulin intake according to their normal routine before the appointment. (See Chapter 9 for information on how to care for the diabetic patient in distress.)

The diabetic dental patient who wears dentures should never be dismissed without a careful check for pressure points, because any pressure or roughness from the denture can cause gross inflammation. Likewise, after any operative procedure, restorations should be double-checked for roughness and smoothed to prevent irritation.

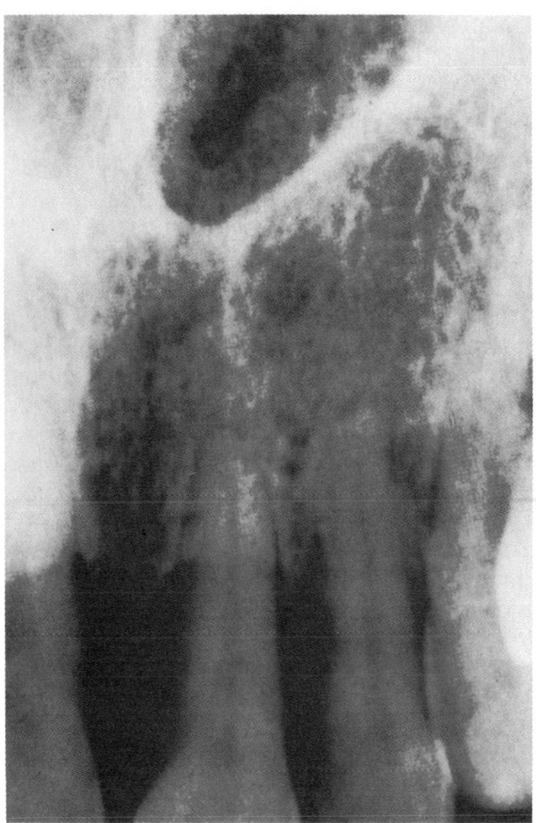

FIGURE 8–6

Periapical radiograph of a patient with diabetes mellitus, showing severe bone loss. (From Ibsen, O.A., and Phelan, J.A.: Oral Pathology for the Dental Hygienist. Philadelphia, W.B. Saunders Co., 1992, p 418).

THE PATIENT WITH ARTHRITIS

Arthritis is an inflammatory condition of one or more joints. There are many forms of arthritis. The most common are rheumatoid arthritis and osteoarthritis.

Rheumatoid arthritis is a chronic systemic disease affecting the connective tissues and joints, in which the joints are swollen, deformed, and painful.

Osteoarthritis is a degenerative joint disease and is the form of arthritis most commonly associated with aging.

The temporomandibular joint may be affected by the arthritis. As a result, the patient may find it extremely difficult to keep his mouth open for a long period of time. The patient may also have a restricted range of jaw motion.

Knowledge of medications taken by this patient is important. For example, regular use of aspirin can increase bleeding time. The arthritic patient may also be taking corticosteroids. In this case the dentist may wish to consult with the patient's physician, before treatment, about any potential interactions between these medications and those to be used in the dental treatment.

Dental appointments for patients with arthritis should be as short as possible and preferably take place during the middle part of the day, when gradual use of the joints and muscles throughout the morning has reduced stiffness.

THE PATIENT WITH A CARDIOVASCULAR DISORDER

Cardiovascular disorders include congenital and acquired heart disease, such as congestive heart failure, rheumatic heart disease, and atherosclerosis.

Patients with heart disease may be taking a wide variety of prescribed drugs, including anticoagulants, which can increase bleeding time. Treatment should be planned in cooperation with the patient's physician.

Patients who are being treated with a monoamine oxidase inhibitor for hypertension (high blood pressure) should *not* receive a local anesthetic containing epinephrine. The use of vasoconstrictors for gingival retraction or hemostasis is also not recommended.

Prophylactic Antibiotics. Patients with cardiovascular disorders, including replacement heart valves, have a marked predisposition to develop subacute bacterial endocarditis. For this reason, the dentist may prescribe prophylactic (preventive) antibiotic therapy before treatment. (**Bacterial endocarditis** is an inflammation of the inner lining of the heart caused by bacteria.)

There is some controversy concerning this use of antibiotics, and some authorities feel that the dangers of a reaction to the antibiotic outweigh the potential benefits of preventing an infection.

THE PATIENT WITH ASTHMA

Asthma is a lung disease that is characterized by airway obstruction that is reversible. During an asthmatic attack, the airways constrict (narrow), and the patient makes a wheezing sound as he breathes.

Attacks range in severity from mild to respiratory failure. In a mild attack, the patient has some difficulty in breathing and is getting adequate air. In respiratory failure, the patient is not getting sufficient air and may die.

Asthma may be caused by allergic reactions. It may also be triggered by stress (such as stress associated with dental treatment).

Dental Treatment for the Patient with Asthma. Asthma should be highlighted on the patient's chart so that the dentist is aware of this condition at each visit. It should also be noted whether or not the patient carries an inhaler containing medication to treat a mild attack.

In the event of a serious attack or an attack that does not respond to this medication, the patient should be transported to a hospital as quickly as possible.

THE PATIENT WITH EMPHYSEMA

Emphysema is a chronic lung disorder in which the patient has ongoing, and increasing, difficulty in breathing. Many of these patients require supplementary oxygen at all times.

Dental Treatment for the Patient with Emphysema. The dentist should check with the patient's physician before treatment. During treatment, the patient will probably be more comfortable seated in an upright position.

THE PATIENT WITH A BLOOD DYSCRASIA

The term **blood dyscrasia** means a pathological condition of the blood, usually referring to the number and types of blood cells. For example, **anemia,** in which the patient has a lower-than-normal number of red blood cells, is a type of dyscrasia.

Table 8–1 shows the normal blood values for adults. A deviation from these norms may indicate a serious problem, for blood dyscrasias can impact the rate at which the patient's blood clots and his ability to heal after treatment.

Dental Treatment for the Patient with a Blood Dyscrasia. If the patient's medical history indicates any type of blood disorder, the dentist may want to check with the patient's physician before proceeding with treatment.

THE PATIENT WITH SEVERE KIDNEY DISEASE

The patient with kidney disease who is on hemodialysis has special problems. (**Hemodialysis** is the use of an artificial kidney machine to filter waste products from the patient's blood.)

TABLE 8–1

Normal Blood Values for Adults

BLOOD TEST	NORMAL VALUES
Hemoglobin	The normal **hemoglobin** for men is 13.5 to 18 grams (gm.) per 100 milliliters (ml.) of blood; for women, it is 12.5 to 16.5 gm. per 100 ml. of blood. A count below 11 indicates a high risk if the patient is to undergo general anesthesia.
Red blood cell count	The normal **red blood cell count** is 4.6 to 6.2 million per cubic millimeter (cu. mm.) of blood for men and 4.2 to 5.4 million per cu. mm. for women.
White blood cell count	The **white blood cell count** is 4500 to 11,000 per cu. mm. for men and women.

The dialysis patient is at high risk for infection. Any dental procedure that causes bleeding may induce bacteremia.

The dialysis patient is usually given anticoagulants both during and after dialysis, and this may result in a tendency to hemorrhage.

Care should be taken not to constrict or disturb the shunt that has been surgically placed in his arm (in some patients, it is implanted in the leg). (A **shunt** is a surgically implanted connective device used for the exchange of fluids during the dialysis process.)

Because of the dialysis patient's impaired kidney function, certain drugs are not excreted normally. Specifically, systemic fluorides are contraindicated. Only topical applications or rinses should be used.

THE PATIENT WITH A STROKE

A **cerebrovascular accident** (CVA), commonly known as a *stroke*, is usually caused by a sudden interruption of the blood supply to the brain that results in damage to part of the brain. Although a stroke can occur at any age, the incidence is highest among adults 60 years of age and older.

There may be no paralysis as a result of such an attack, or there may be partial or complete paralysis on one or both sides of the body. Sometimes the part of the brain that controls the ability to speak is affected.

Facts About the Stroke Patient

The Stroke Patient . . .

- Is *not* mentally disturbed or emotionally ill; however, may suffer temporary personality changes and behavior upsets. These are due to injury to the part of the brain that controls these emotions.
- Is an adult and should be treated as an adult; is often deeply hurt when people treat him like a child or a mentally incompetent individual. Never talk about the patient in his presence as if he were not there.
- Does not necessarily have a hearing impairment. Shouting does not help.
- Tends to tire quickly. May require short appointments and frequent rest periods.

The stroke patient may have difficulty in swallowing. He may drool and find manipulation of his tongue extremely difficult. The pharyngeal muscles may also be involved, and this may affect the patient's ability to chew, wear dentures, and maintain oral hygiene (see Facts About the Stroke Patient).

THE PATIENT WITH MUSCULAR DYSTROPHY

Muscular dystrophy is the term applied to a group of diseases characterized by progressive **atrophy** (wasting away) and weakness of the skeletal muscles and by increasing disability and deformity.

Muscular dystrophy may eventually involve most of the striated muscles in the body. Atrophy of the muscles involved in respiration reduces the vital capacity of the lungs and interferes with the ability to cough.

It is important that the dentist and assistant be aware of the diminished cough reflex of these patients and their inability to clear their throats by coughing. Nitrous oxide sedation and general anesthesia for dental treatment should be avoided for these patients because of their impaired pulmonary (breathing) function.

THE PATIENT WITH ALZHEIMER'S DISEASE

Alzheimer's disease, a type of dementia, is a progressive, chronic degenerative disease of cognitive function of unknown cause. (**Cognition** is the function of the mind that includes all aspects of perceiving, thinking, and remembering.)

Most commonly, the clinical course of Alzheimer's disease is slow deterioration, which can last for 15 years or more. For descriptive purposes, the disease may be divided into three stages:

Stage 1: the early disease, or forgetfulness phase, in which the individual experiences marked changes in mood plus the loss of judgment and memory

Stage 2: the intermediate disease, or confusional phase, in which the individual has increased episodes of extreme irritability and confusion

Stage 3: the late disease, or dementia phase, in which the individual becomes severely disoriented and behavioral problems become quite apparent

The goals of dental care for these patients are to restore and maintain oral health and prevent progression of oral disease.

Because of the degenerative nature of this disease, the behavior of the Alzheimer's patient at his first dental visit may represent his best cognitive functioning level. For this reason, the dental treatment plan should aim to restore oral function quickly and to institute an intensive preventive program.

Dental visits should be scheduled with an awareness of the patient's best time of day. Also, the presence of a familiar caregiver in the treatment room will often allay the patient's fears.

Dentistry for the Confined Patient

Portable equipment that is compact, lightweight, and relatively self-contained is necessary to provide treatment in the home, nursing home, or hospital.

The equipment should include a means of positioning the patient's head, adequate light, handpieces, and other instruments and materials.

Portable radiographic equipment is also available. In some areas, a specially equipped van, usually owned by the dental society or a government agency, may be available for this purpose.

The assistant usually travels with the dentist to provide care for the confined patient. This patient should receive the same consideration and quality of care given to patients in the dental office.

Most operating techniques used in the dental office are adaptable to home care; however, as a general rule, treatment sessions should be shorter than those in an office because the confined patient may tire more easily.

Chapter 9

Medical Emergencies

Introduction

A variety of medical emergencies may occur in the dental office. They may involve a patient; however, it is also possible that a member of the dental staff—or the dentist—might require emergency assistance.

In any of these situations, the dental staff must be capable of providing prompt and appropriate care. As part of their preparedness, all members of the staff should receive annual training in basic life support, including cardiopulmonary resuscitation (CPR).

Protocols for Managing Medical Emergencies

While the patient is in the dental office, the dentist is responsible for that individual's safety. If a medical emergency involving the patient arises during this time, the dentist and staff are responsible for providing prudent emergency care. Therefore, emergency first aid protocols must be established and routinely practiced in the dental office. (As used here, **protocol** means a plan of action or a series of specific steps that must be followed.)

A calm, smoothly functioning staff is capable of handling an emergency in the dental office without compounding the seriousness of the situation by frightening the patient. To prevent panic and complications, every staff member should know, and practice, his or her role in emergency protocols *before* any emergency that may arise.

Because of the suddenness of an emergency, it is not always possible to put on personal protective equipment (PPE) as described in Chapter 13. However, emergency preparedness must include plans to implement the appropriate exposure control measures as quickly as possible.

In some practices, the office manual includes instructions and protocols for use of emergency equipment and administration of medications. It is also imperative that the name and telephone number of nearest emergency medical service (EMS), fire department, and physician be posted by each telephone to contact in case of emergency. In many cities, emergency services are contacted by calling 911. In addition, each patient's medical history must include the name and telephone number of his primary physician.

Documentation of Emergency Treatment

When an emergency arises in the dental office, it is essential that details of the situation be fully documented. After such an emergency, the dentist will make extensive notes in the patient's record explaining exactly what happened, the treatment provided, and the condition of the patient at the time he left the office.

If an emergency is not fully resolved while the patient is in the office, the dentist may phone the patient, his family, or his physician the next day to inquire as to the patient's health.

Diagnostic Vital Signs

Diagnostic vital signs serve as indicators of a patient's health: pulse rate, blood pressure, respiration (breathing) rate, and body temperature.

If it is the office policy to take and record vital signs, these should be taken for each new adult patient and at subsequent recall visits. During an emergency, it is also necessary to monitor the patient's vital signs.

This responsibility usually falls to the assistant, who should monitor the vital signs and record them on the patient's chart next to the date.

Pulse

The pulse is the rhythmical expansion of an artery as the heart beats; it can be felt with the finger. It can readily be detected near the surface of the skin.

The normal pulse rate in resting adults is between 60 and 100 beats per minute (bpm). It is more rapid in a child, ranging from 70 to 110 bpm.

To facilitate taking pulse rates, it is helpful to use a watch that indicates seconds so that these can be observed while the patient's pulse is felt. The pulse is counted for 30 seconds and then doubled to compute the rate for 1 full minute. This rate is then recorded on the patient's chart.

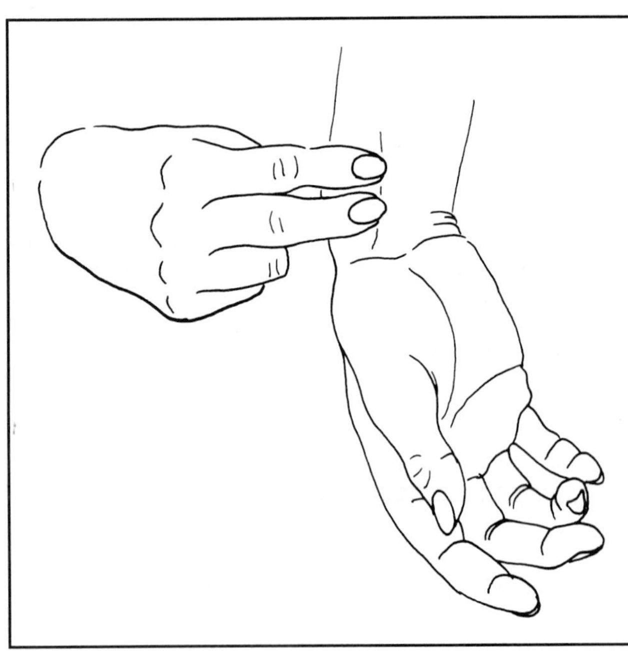

FIGURE 9–1

Taking the patient's pulse in the wrist.

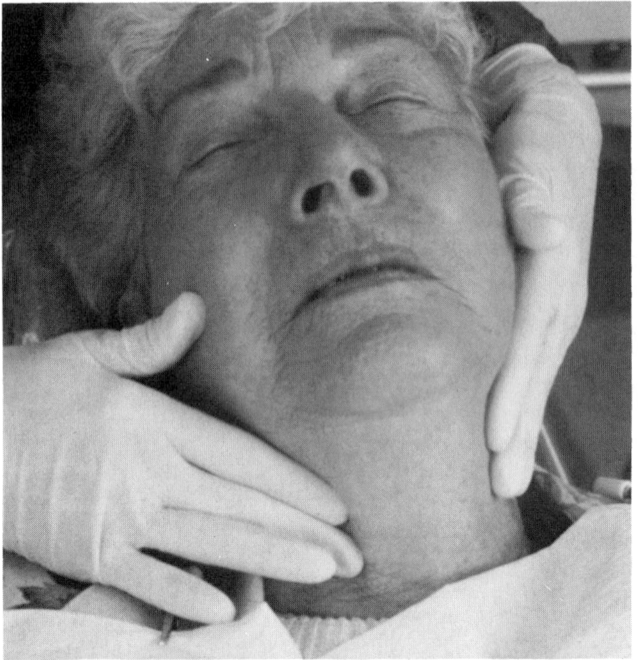

FIGURE 9–2

Checking the carotid pulse on the side of the patient's neck.

PULSE IN WRIST (RADIAL ARTERY)

The radial artery on the inner surface of the wrist (the thumb side) is the most commonly used site for taking the pulse. To take the pulse, place the index and third fingers lightly on the patient's wrist between the radius (bone on the thumb side) and the tendon (Fig. 9–1).

PULSE IN NECK (CAROTID ARTERY)

Detecting the carotid pulse—that is, the pulse in the carotid artery of the neck—is an important part of many emergency procedures. It is important that you know how to do it quickly.

To detect the carotid pulse, place two fingers alongside the patient's larynx (Adam's apple) on the side of the neck nearest you. Move your fingers slowly down this groove to the soft area above the clavicle (collar bone), then palpate this area gently to determine a carotid pulse (Fig. 9–2). (**Palpate** means to feel with the fingers.) Take care not to block the flow of blood in the artery during this procedure.

Blood Pressure

The term **blood pressure** refers to the systolic and diastolic values of arterial pressure. Normal blood pressure ranges are shown in Table 9–1.

Systolic pressure is the highest pressure exerted on the cardiovascular system by the contraction of the left ventricle of the heart. This contraction forces the oxy-

TABLE 9–1

Blood Pressure Classifications for an Adult at Least 18 Years Old

CATEGORY	SYSTOLIC	DIASTOLIC
Normal	less than 130	less than 85
High-normal	130–139	85–90
Hypertension		
Stage 1 (mild)	140–159	90–99
Stage 2 (moderate)	160–179	100–109
Stage 3 (severe)	180–209	110–119
Stage 4 (very severe)	210 or higher	120 or higher

Based on information from the Fifth Report of the Joint National Committee on Detection, Evaluation and Treatment of High Blood Pressure, In *J.A.D.A., 125*:104–106, 1993.

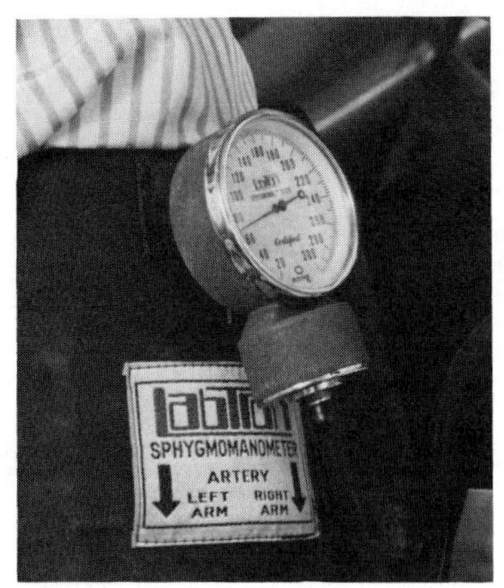

FIGURE 9–3

A blood pressure cuff with an aneroid meter in position.

genated blood out into the blood vessels, causing expansion of the arteries and arterioles and pressure in the tissues.

Diastolic pressure is the lowest pressure of the cardiovascular system. It occurs momentarily when the heart muscle rests and allows the heart to take in more blood before the next contraction.

Systolic and diastolic pressures are measured in millimeters of mercury (mm. Hg) above atmospheric pressure. These are recorded with the systolic value over the diastolic value. For example, 129/78 indicates systolic pressure of 129 and diastolic pressure of 78.

TYPES OF BLOOD PRESSURE METERS

Most commonly, blood pressure is measured by listening to the sounds within the artery. This involves the use of a stethoscope and a sphygmomanometer.

A **sphygmomanometer** is the instrument used to measure blood pressure. It consists of a gauge attached to an inflatable rubber bladder enclosed in a cloth cuff. A rubber bulb with a valve is used to inflate and deflate the bladder. This creates pressure to briefly control the flow of blood in the artery.

A closure, usually nylon tape (Velcro), is used to hold the cuff in place. The pressure readings may be taken with a mercury or aneroid manometer.

A **mercury manometer** provides readings on a column of mercury. The cords lead from the cuff to the manometer in a boxlike frame. This unit needs adequate space and stability on a table or wall for accurate operation.

An **aneroid manometer** provides reading on a dial that is directly attached to the cuff (Fig. 9–3).

A **battery-operated digital manometer** utilizes batteries to provide a digital reading of the pulse rate and blood pressure. The digital manometer may also provide a paper printout of the data. This printout may be given to the patient or placed in the patient's record.

Electronic units provide digital readings or beeping sounds. This type of equipment is used most frequently to monitor the patient's blood pressure when the patient is under general anesthesia.

KOROTKOFF SOUNDS

The sound technique for obtaining a blood pressure reading involves the use of a sphygmomanometer and a stethoscope. Korotkoff sounds are a series of sounds produced as the result of the blood rushing back into the brachial artery that has been collapsed by the pressure of the blood pressure cuff.

As the pressure in the cuff is slowly released, the stethoscope picks up a clear, sharp tapping sound that grows louder and then softens to a murmur as the flow of blood causes the artery to expand to its former shape.

Figure 9–4 is an artist's rendering of the five phases of the brachial artery as Korotkoff sounds are pro-

FIGURE 9–4

Korotkoff sounds are produced during the deflation of the blood pressure cuff. (Modified from Stout, F.W.: The sphygmomanometer: Its development, use, and abuse. *J. Prev. Dent., 6*:169–178, 1980.)

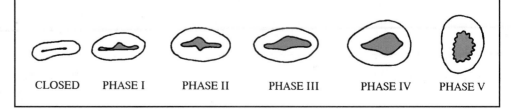

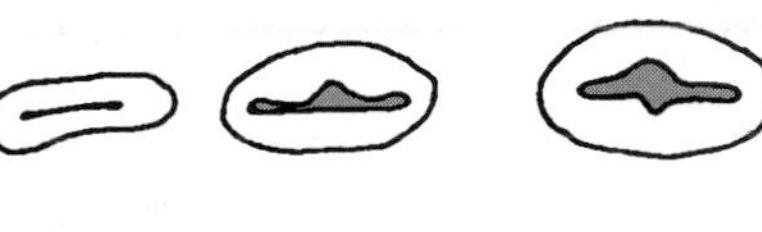
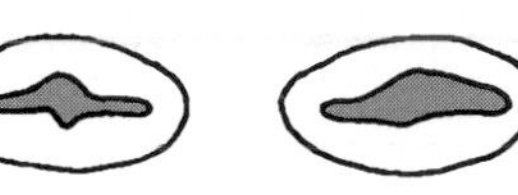

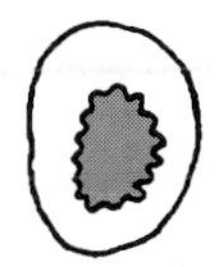

PROCEDURE: **Taking and Recording Blood Pressure**

Instrumentation

Stethoscope
Sphygmomanometer (cuff with pressure meter)
Patient's medical history and chart
Pen and paper

Placing the Blood Pressure Cuff

1. Allow the seated patient to rest quietly for at least 5 minutes before taking his blood pressure. Loosen and move a sleeve that is in the way.
   □ *RATIONALE*: To obtain an accurate reading, blood pressure should *not* be taken through clothing.
2. Extend the patient's arm; support the elbow on the arm of the dental chair or a table. The palm should be facing up.
   □ *RATIONALE*: The patient's arm (at the elbow) should be at the same level as his heart.
3. Place the sphygmomanometer cuff lightly on the patient's arm with the bladder on the inner area of the upper arm near the brachial artery, approximately 2 cm. above the antecubital fossa (Fig. 9–5). (The **antecubital fossa** is the small groove on the inner arm just above the elbow.)
4. Use one hand to stabilize the end of the cuff in this position (just above the elbow). Use the other hand to wrap the cuff around the arm, and use the closure to hold it in place.
   □ *NOTE*: Place the cuff so that the gauge is facing you.
5. Expel all air from the cuff by opening the valve of the bulb and pressing gently on the cuff.
6. Place the earpieces of the stethoscope into your ears so that the earpieces are facing anteriorly.
   □ *RATIONALE*: This position of the earpieces is more comfortable and closes out distracting noises while taking blood pressure.
7. Use your left hand to place and hold the disc (diaphragm) of the stethoscope at the medial side of the tendon and over the brachial artery. This is just below the lower border of the cuff and on the antecubital fossa (see Fig. 9–5; Fig. 9–6).

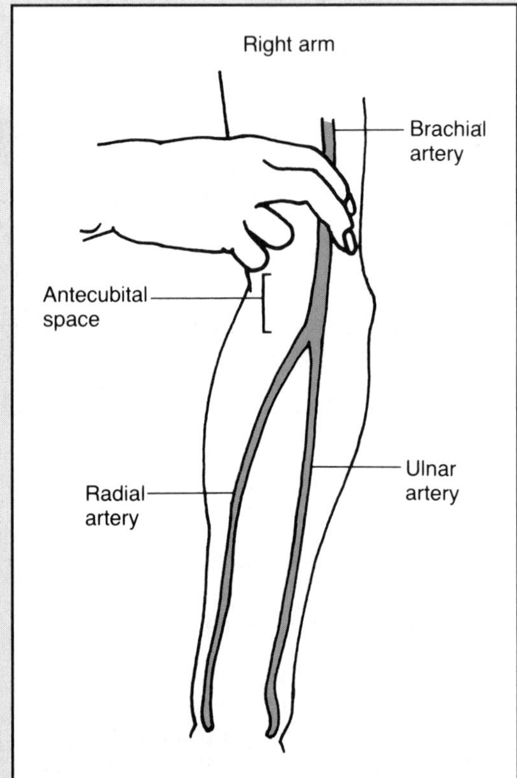

FIGURE 9–5

Locating the antecubital space with the fingers.

□ *RATIONALE*: If the disc is not correctly and firmly placed against the skin, the reading will not be accurate.

Obtaining Blood Pressure Reading

1. Place your right hand, palm down, over the bulb so that the fingers and thumb can be used to rotate the valve and close the opening.
2. Feel the patient's pulse at the wrist or just

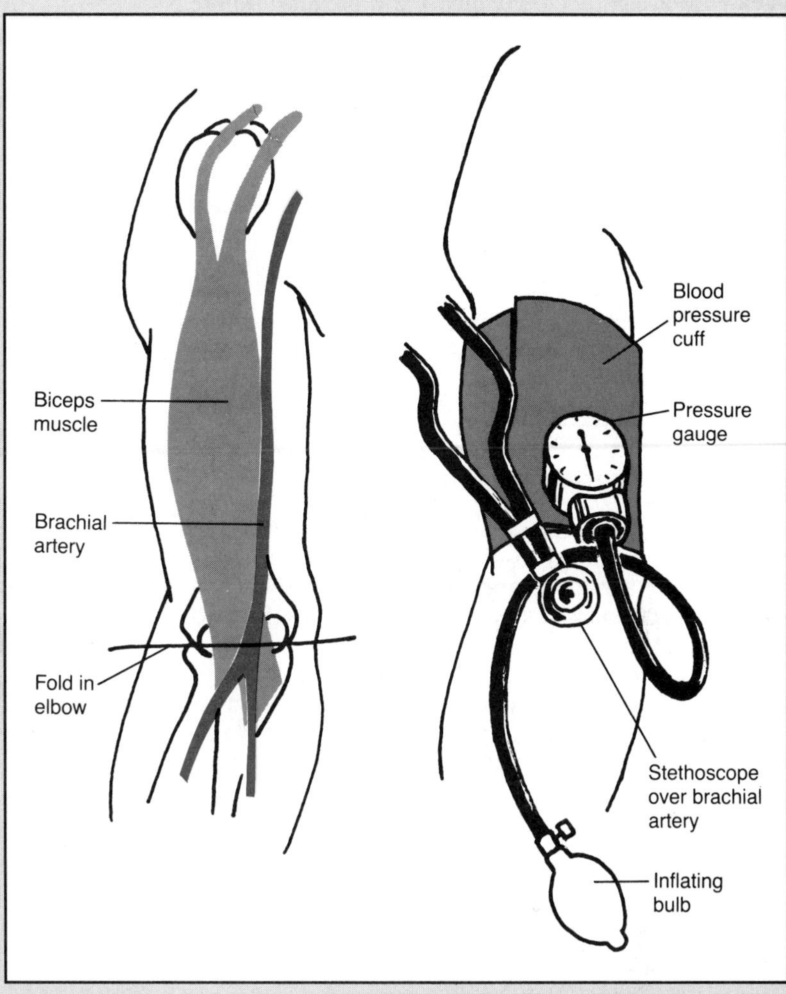

FIGURE 9–6

Positioning the blood pressure cuff and stethoscope.

below the antecubital space; then check to be certain that the stethoscope disc is still accurately placed.

3. Listen for the sound of the pulse. Close the valve and pump the bulb to inflate the cuff until the sound of the pulse can no longer be heard.
   □ *RATIONALE*: This happens when the pressure of the cuff is greater than the patient's systolic pressure.
4. Check the reading on the gauge of the blood pressure apparatus. The reading may be as high as 160 to 170 mm. Hg as the last sound of the pressure is heard.
5. Slowly open the valve and release the air. Permit the mercury to drop in the gauge at 2 mm. Hg per second (2 mm. represents 1 notch on the mercury or aneroid gauge).
6. Close the valve again. While listening with the stethoscope, inflate the cuff by pumping the bulb. The reading on the mercury gauge should be 10 to 20 points above the reading acquired when testing the apparatus (170 to 180).
7. Slowly open the valve and release the pressure on the cuff as you listen with the stethoscope.
8. Note the registration of a sharp, tapping sound as you lower the pressure in the cuff.
   □ *RATIONALE*: This is the registration of the systolic pressure.
9. Slowly continue to release the air from the cuff, deflating the apparatus until you hear the last sound of the heart beat.
   □ *RATIONALE*: This is the registration of the diastolic pressure.
10. Record the reading taken as RAS (right arm seated), or as LAS (left arm seated). Record the pressure as a fraction with the systolic number over the diastolic number.
11. When finished, gently remove the cuff. Disinfect the stethoscope earpieces and diaphragm as recommended by the manufacturer, and return the equipment to its proper place.

duced during the deflation of the blood pressure cuff. At first, the artery is closed off by the pressure of the cuff.

- **Phase I:** There is sudden evidence of a clear, sharp, tapping sound that grows louder.
- **Phase II:** The sound is softened and becomes prolonged into a murmur.
- **Phase III:** The sound again becomes crisper and increases in intensity.
- **Phase IV:** There is a distinct abrupt muffling of the sound.
- **Phase V:** This is the point at which the artery is fully open and the sound disappears.

ABNORMALLY HIGH READINGS

Occasionally, it is necessary to take two or three blood pressure readings to obtain an accurate or average reading. If a patient appears apprehensive during the first reading, wait a few minutes to allow him to relax, and then try again.

If the readings are very high, indicating a problem with hypertension (high blood pressure), the dentist may refer the patient to his physician for further evaluation before continuing with dental treatment.

Respiration Rate

The normal respiration rate for a relaxed adult is 10 to 20 breaths per minute. For a young child, the rate ranges from 20 to 26 breaths per minute.

Respiration in adult males is primarily abdominal, from the diaphragm. The respiration in adult females is primarily from the upper portion of the chest.

When a patient is in shock, has heart disease, or has a partial obstruction of the airway, breathing is rapid, shallow, and labored. If the patient is in respiratory failure (not breathing), there is little or no movement of the chest or the abdomen, and CPR is indicated immediately! (CPR is discussed later in this chapter.)

Body Temperature

The normal oral temperature of a resting person is 37°C (98.6°F). The normal range is 35.8 to 37.3°C (96.4 to 99.1°F). (C stands for Celsius; F, for Fahrenheit.)

Temperature is most commonly taken with a digital (electronic) thermometer that displays the body temperature as numbers in a digital display. The tip (the portion that is placed under the tongue) is protected with a disposable plastic cover, which is discarded after use.

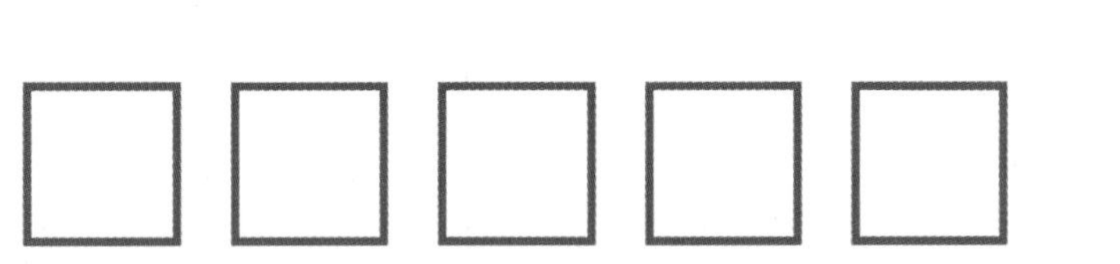

PROCEDURE: **Taking the Patient's Temperature**

Instrumentation

Electronic thermometer
Appropriate protective sheath

Method

1. Turn the thermometer on and place a fresh plastic cover over the tip.
2. When the display indicates that the thermometer is ready, gently place a tip under the patient's tongue.
2. Instruct the patient to close his lips on the thermometer and to refrain from talking or from removing it from his mouth.
3. Leave it in place until the display indicates a final reading.
4. Remove the thermometer from the patient's mouth and record the reading.
5. Turn the thermometer off, remove the plastic cover, and disinfect the thermometer as recommended by the manufacturer.

Observation of the Patient

Ongoing observation of the patient's condition is an important part of emergency preparedness. The alert dental assistant observes the patient's general appearance and gait as he enters the operatory. (**Gait** means manner of walking.)

The patient's response to routine questions should also be noted; slow responses and changes in speech patterns from those of a previous appointment should be noted for the dentist to evaluate.

BREATH ODORS

The assistant should note any unusual breath odors when admitting and seating the patient. These unusual breath odors include

- A **fetid, foul breath,** which may indicate a lung, bronchial, or digestive infection or disorder
- An **acetone (sweet-fruity) breath,** which may indicate diabetes
- The **odor of ammonia,** which may indicate a severe kidney problem
- The **odor of alcohol,** which may indicate that the patient has been drinking or taking unreported medication

Emergency Supplies

In most dental offices, a drawer, tray, or a portable kit is used to store and organize emergency supplies. The assistant may be assigned responsibility for the maintaining and updating of these supplies. Some drugs have expiration dates and must be replaced as necessary. After an emergency, supplies used during the incident must be replenished.

The dentist determines what emergency supplies need to be maintained in the office. A basic emergency kit usually includes the following (Fig. 9–7):

- Ammonia inhalant ampules
- Sugar packets and/or a tube of liquid sugar (decorative icing)
- Nitroglycerin translingual spray
- Preloaded epinephrine syringe
- Disposable plastic syringes
- Ampules of antihistamines and adrenaline
- Bronchodilator inhaler
- Tourniquet
- A pocket mask

The **pocket mask** is designed for mouth-to-mask ventilation of a non-breathing adult, child, or infant. It is an alternative to mouth-to-mouth or mouth-to-nose breathing, which are described later in this chapter.

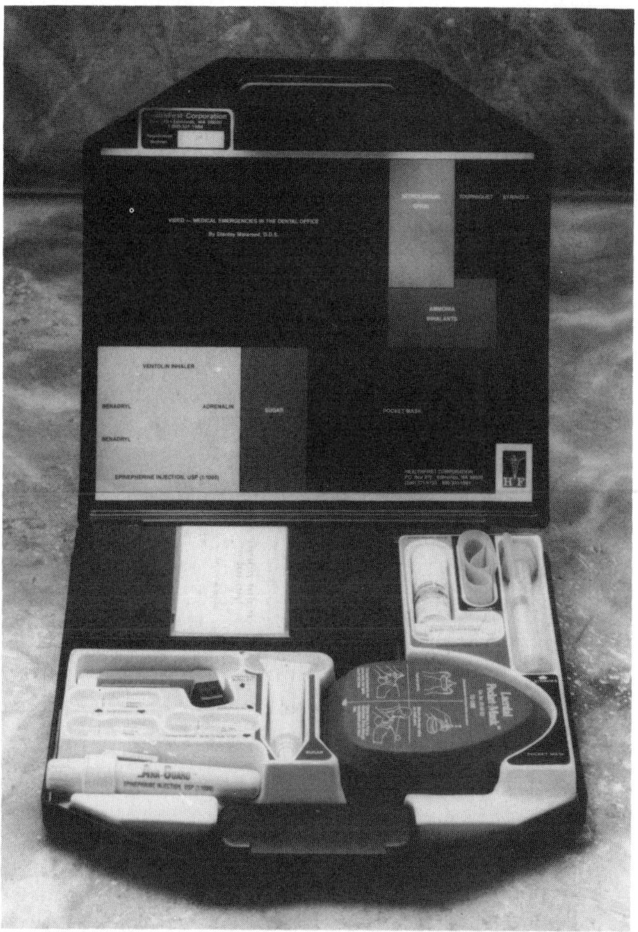

FIGURE 9–7

Basic emergency kit. On the right, from top to bottom, are syringes (for use with the ampules of Benadryl or adrenalin); a tourniquet; nitrolingual spray (a translingual nitroglycerin spray); ammonia inhalants; and a pocket mask. On the left, from top to bottom, are a training video; Ventolin (a bronchodilator); an ampule of Benadryl (an antihistamine); an ampule of adrenalin (also known as epinephrine); liquid sugar; and a preloaded epinephrine syringe. (Courtesy of Healthfirst Corp, Edmonds, WA.)

Directions for use of the mask are on the container. The mask is reusable; however, the one-way valve (which goes in the rescuer's mouth) should be discarded after a single use.

Oxygen

One hundred percent oxygen (O_2) is the ideal agent for resuscitation of a patient who is unconscious but still breathing. However, if the patient is not breathing, air must be forced into his lungs through rescue breathing or similar emergency measures.

A portable unit with two tanks of oxygen may be stored where it can be moved quickly into a treatment room if needed. An "E"-size cylinder provides approximately 78 liters of oxygen per minute for one-half hour. A reserve tank of oxygen should also be available for the treatment of emergency situations. *Note*: The oxygen cylinder is always green.

If the dentist administers nitrous oxide–oxygen sedation to patients, the oxygen from these units may be used for emergency situations (Fig. 9–8). (See Chapter 20.)

RESUSCITATION MASKS

Sterile resuscitation masks in adult and child sizes should be stored in each operatory so that a mask can be placed quickly on the oxygen unit. (These are *not* the same masks that are used to administer nitrous oxide–oxygen sedation.)

The masks should be constructed of clear plastic, edged in a rubber rim that seals the mask around the patient's mouth and nose. The clear plastic enables the operator to observe the patient's mouth and nostrils.

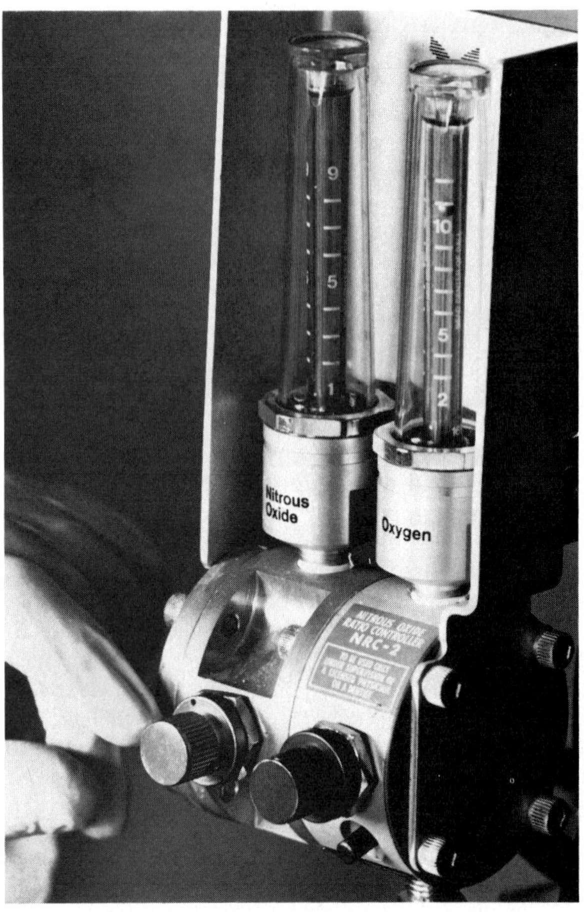

FIGURE 9–8

To provide emergency oxygen, the nitrous oxide–oxygen flow meter is set to 100 percent oxygen.

Cardiopulmonary Resuscitation (CPR)

In an emergency in which the patient is not breathing and the heart is not beating, CPR must be started immediately. CPR combines rescue breathing, to ensure adequate air to the lungs, with external cardiac compression to stimulate the heart (Fig. 9–9).

This emergency support system must be enacted immediately so that the flow of oxygen-carrying blood quickly reaches the brain. The cells of the brain, the most sensitive tissue in the body, are irreversibly damaged after 4 to 6 minutes without oxygen.

Possible CPR Complications

There are always dangers in applying CPR; however, these must be weighed against the possibility of saving a life. The complications include

- Broken ribs or sternum (breastbone)
- Pneumothorax (a broken rib puncturing the lung)
- Laceration of the liver, spleen, lungs, or heart by the broken ribs. (This is a serious complication and can usually be avoided if CPR is properly performed.)

Because of these risks, it is *most* important that the persons applying CPR be properly trained and that they retain their proficiency in CPR by updating their skills periodically.

Before proceeding, study the diagram of the ribs, sternum, and xiphoid process (Fig. 9–10). (The **xiphoid process,** which is made of cartilage, forms the lower tip of the sternum.)

The ABCs of Life Support

In all emergency situations, the rescuers must promptly initiate the ABCs of basic life support: **a**irway, **b**reathing, and **c**irculation.

The **airway** must be opened and maintained. To establish an airway, tilt the patient's head back by pressing on the forehead while using the other hand to lift the chin. (This is known as the *tilt-lift* method.)

Performing a *finger-sweep* is an important part of establishing an airway; however, it is performed *only* on an unconscious patient. If the patient is conscious, the rescuer may be bitten or trigger the gag reflex.

In a finger-sweep, the index finger is used in a hooking motion to sweep across the inside of the mouth from one side to the other (Fig. 9–11).

Breathing must be evaluated to determine whether the patient is breathing. If the patient is not breathing, the Heimlich maneuver or rescue breathing must be started immediately.

Circulation must be monitored to determine whether the heart is beating. If the heart is not beating, external cardiac compression is started immediately to restore circulation.

Cardiopulmonary Resuscitation (CPR)

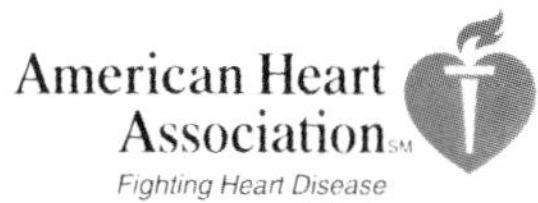

AIRWAY

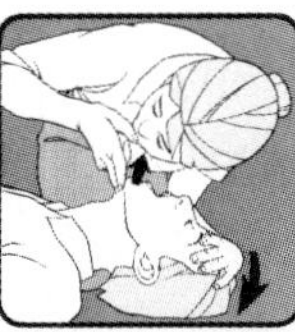

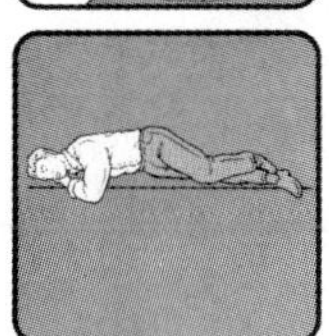

Establish unresponsiveness. If victim is unresponsive, call EMS (Emergency Medical Services — 911 in many areas), turn victim on back, and then open airway using head tilt–chin lift.

Check breathing (look, listen, feel).

If victim is unresponsive and breathing and has no evidence of trauma, place on his or her side in recovery position.

BREATHING

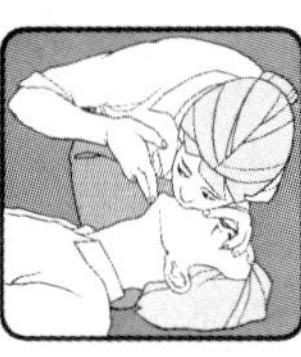

If victim is not breathing, begin rescue breathing.

Give 2 slow breaths. If airway is blocked, reposition head and try again to give breaths. If still blocked, perform the Heimlich maneuver.

CIRCULATION

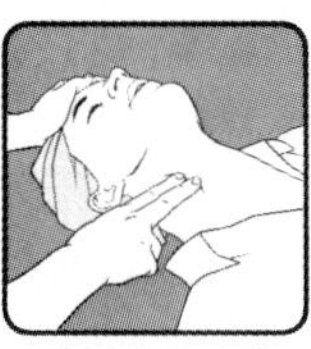

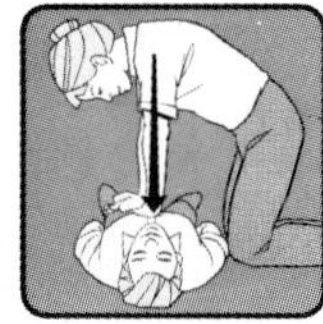

Check carotid pulse.

If victim has no pulse, begin chest compressions.

Depress sternum 1½ to 2 inches.
Perform 15 compressions (rate: 80–100 per minute) followed by 2 slow breaths.

After 4 cycles check pulse. If there is no pulse, continue cycles beginning with chest compressions.

Continue uninterrupted until advanced life support is available.

FIGURE 9–9

Procedure for cardiopulmonary resuscitation (CPR) in basic life support emergency. (Courtesy of American Heart Association, Cardiopulmonary Wall Chart, Dallas, TX.)

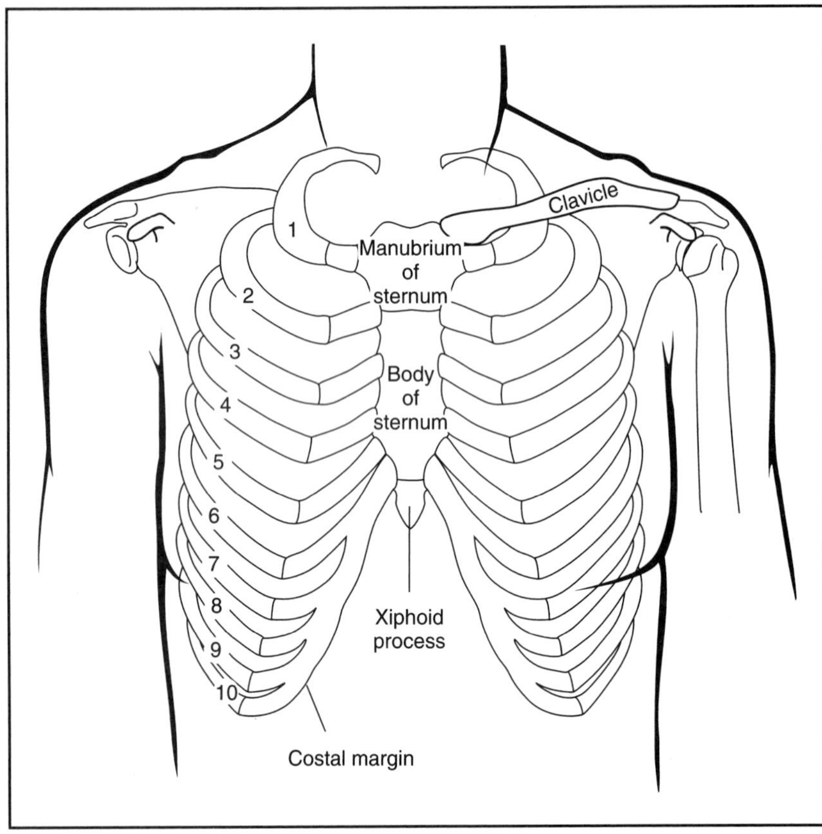

FIGURE 9–10

Anterior view of the rib cage. (From Jacob, S.W., and Francone, C.A.: Elements of Anatomy and Physiology, 2nd ed. Philadelphia, W.B. Saunders Co., 1989, p 57.)

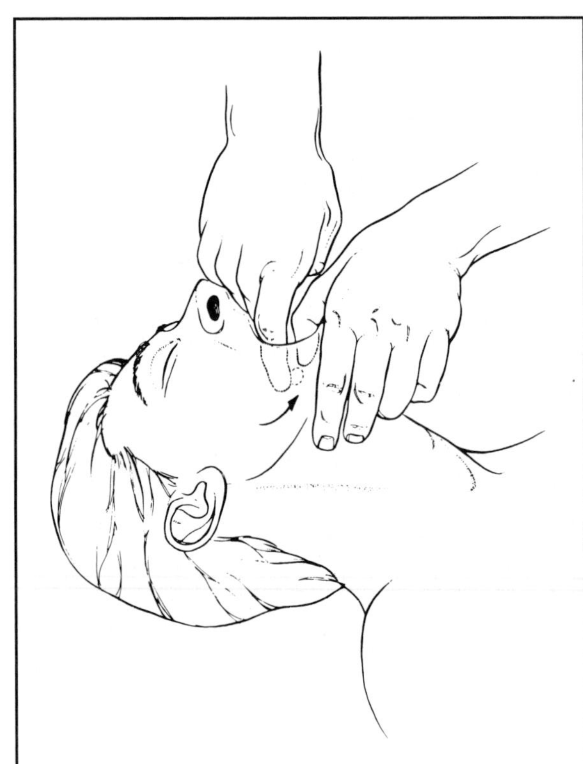

FIGURE 9–11

Finger-sweep. Place your index finger along the side of the mouth, sweep across with the finger, and pull the foreign material up and out of the oral cavity. (From Henry, M., and Stapleton, E.: EMT Prehospital Care. Philadelphia, W.B. Saunders Co., 1992, p 133.)

Rescue Breathing

Rescue breathing, which is also known as *artificial ventilation*, is breathing that is artificially maintained by one individual for another through the forced exchange of air in the lungs.

The rescuer's exhaled air provides approximately 16 percent oxygen. This is sufficient to sustain life if the patient's other vital systems are functioning.

CHILD OR INFANT RESCUE BREATHING

If the patient is a child or infant, the force of air should be lessened, and the inflation rate should be increased to 20 times per minute (once every 3 seconds).

Your mouth can be placed over the nose and mouth of a child. If the position of the child's mandible is difficult to maintain, use the hand to move the mandible forward.

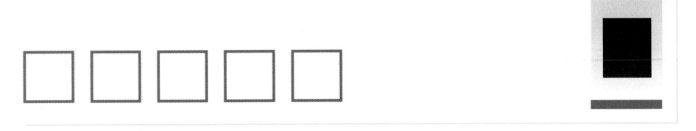

PROCEDURE: **Preparing for Rescue Breathing**

1. Determine that the patient is unconscious and not breathing.
2. Check for obvious injuries and call for help.
3. Place the patient in a supine position on a hard surface such as the floor.
4. Use the tilt-lift method to establish an airway (Fig. 9–12).
5. With your ear close to the patient's mouth, listen for 5 seconds for breathing. Observe the patient's chest for rise and fall.
   □ *RATIONALE*: If the patient has started breathing on his own, do not start rescue breathing.
6. Use a finger-sweep to clear any foreign material in the mouth or throat.
7. Remove any dental prosthesis the patient is wearing if it is likely to drop free of the dental arch. Otherwise, leave the prosthesis in place to effect a seal with the patient's lips during resuscitation.
8. Use one of the following methods to start rescue breathing:

   - Mouth-to-mouth
   - Mouth-to-nose
   - Artificial airway

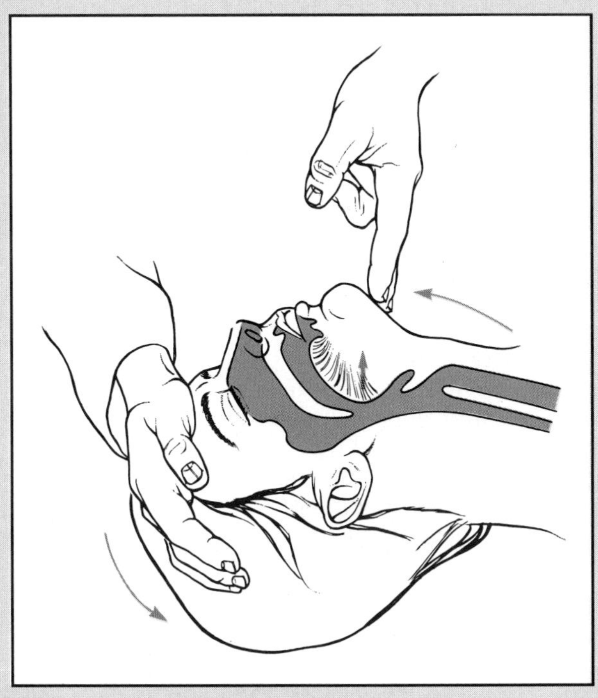

FIGURE 9–12

Tilt the victim's head back, and lift the chin. Then pinch the nose shut. (From Henry, M., and Stapleton, E.: EMT Prehospital Care. Philadelphia, W.B. Saunders Co., 1992, p 51.)

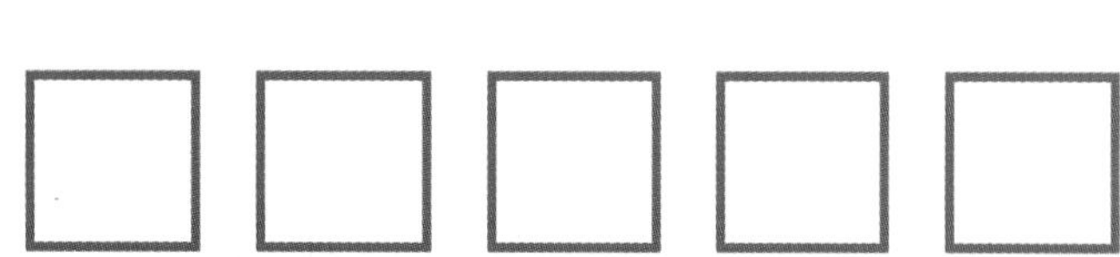

PROCEDURE: **Performing Adult Mouth-to-Mouth Technique**

1. Kneel at the patient's side near his head. If the patient is in the dental chair, lower position of the chair to enable the operator to use the operator's stool.
2. Establish an airway by placing one hand on the patient's forehead and tilting the head back. Place the fingers of other hand under the border of the mandible and lift the chin upward and forward (see Fig. 9–12).
   □ *RATIONALE*: This position opens the airway by causing the tongue to drop to the floor of the mouth so that it does not obstruct the passage of air into the throat.
3. Place your ear by the patient's mouth to detect breathing. Note the rise and fall of the chest during this procedure. Hold this position for 3 to 5 seconds. If the patient is *not* breathing, begin rescue breathing immediately.
4. Use the palm of the hand placed on the forehead to support position of tilted head. Use the fingers of that hand to pinch closed the patient's nose.
5. Take a deep breath. Make a tight seal by placing your mouth completely around patient's mouth and deliver two full, slow breaths (Fig. 9–13).
   □ *RATIONALE*: This inflates the lungs. Pause before proceeding, to allow the patient's lungs to deflate.
6. Keep the patient's head tilted and check the carotid artery for a pulse for 5 seconds.
7. If the patient is *not* breathing but has a pulse, continue rescue breathing. If the patient's chest rises rapidly, stop inflation and permit the patient to exhale. Repeat the cycle 12 times per minute (once every 5 seconds). The rising of the chest is more important than rhythm.
8. Check for the carotid pulse. Continue rescue breathing if the patient is not breathing on his own.

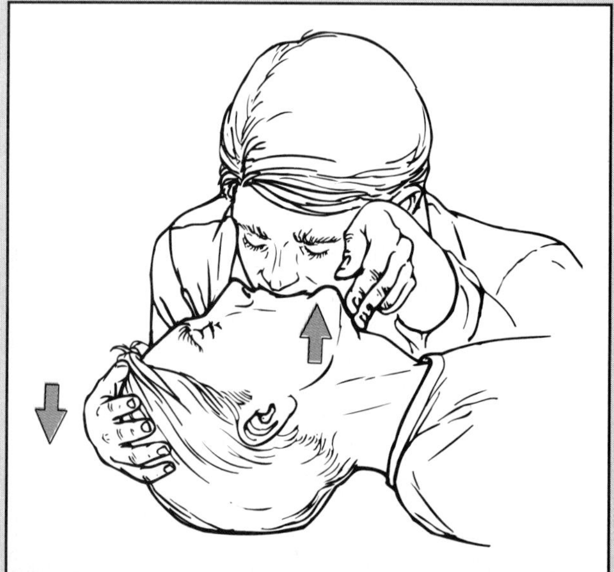

FIGURE 9–13

Give two slow, deep breaths. Watch for the patient's chest to rise.

PROCEDURE: **Performing Mouth-to-Nose Technique**

1. If the patient's mouth is severely injured or the teeth are missing, use the mouth-to-nose technique.
2. Close the patient's mouth with one hand, holding the lips sealed.
3. Take a deep breath, and seal your lips over the nose.
4. Blow air into the nose until the chest rises (Fig. 9–14). Give one breath every 5 seconds.
5. Stop to allow the patient's mouth to open and exhale the air.
6. Turn your head toward the patient's chest, and check for rise and fall to determine whether the patient is breathing on his own.
7. Check the patient's carotid pulse once every minute. Continue mouth-to-nose ventilation as needed or until an ambulance arrives.

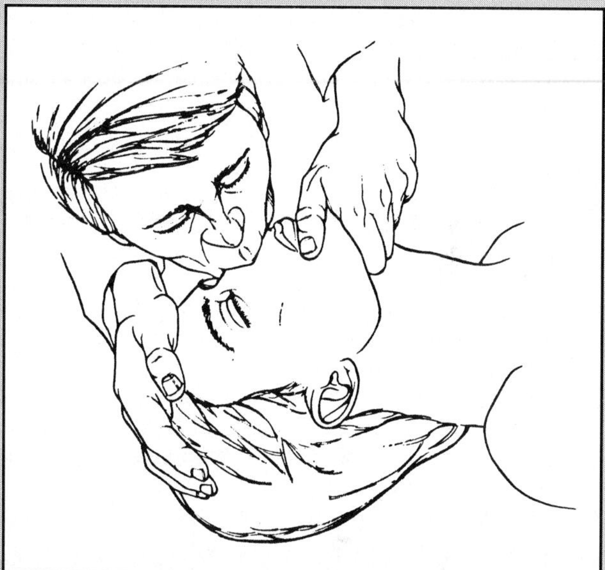

FIGURE 9–14

Maintain a head tilt–chin lift, and seal your mouth around the patient's nose while closing the patient's mouth to prevent air leakage during ventilation. (From Henry, M., and Stapleton, E.: EMT Prehospital Care. Philadelphia, W.B. Saunders Co., 1992, p 113.)

PROCEDURE: **Positioning for External Cardiac Compression**

1. To find the proper position, using the hand nearest the patient's legs, run your fingers around the rib cage from the opposite side of the chest to the *center* of the sternum. Place the index and middle fingers of this hand over the notch just above the xiphoid process.
2. Place the heel of the opposite hand above the width of the fingers. This hand is placed approximately 1½ to 2 inches *above* the tip of the sternum (Fig. 9–15).
   □ *IMPORTANT*: Do not place the heel of the hand on the xiphoid process. This could cause it to fracture and possibly puncture the lung.
3. Move the other hand so that the heel of this hand is directly over the one that is already in place. Keep your fingers off the chest by lacing them together.
4. Position your body so that your shoulders are directly over the patient's chest. Your hips become a fulcrum for pivoting your upper body weight directly over the patient so that as the compressions are given in a straight downward motion, the weight of your upper body creates the force.
5. Compress the chest by pressing down and then releasing (Fig. 9–16). Each compression should push the chest down about 2 inches.
6. As you perform chest compressions, it may be helpful to think to yourself "One and two and three and..." and so on. This helps keep the rhythm of the compressions.

FIGURE 9–15.

Find hand position on the sternum.

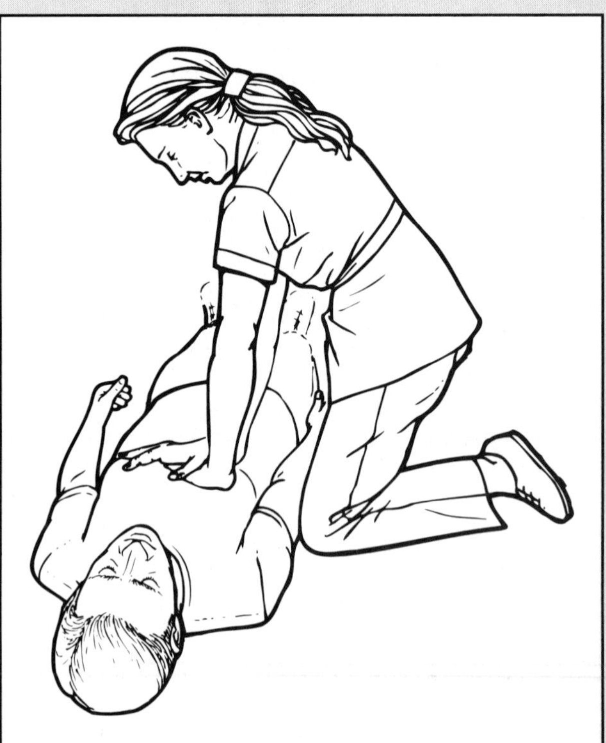

FIGURE 9–16

Position shoulders over hands. Compress chest 15 times.

ARTIFICIAL AIRWAY DEVICES

Disposable S-shaped devices designed to fit the curvature of the oropharynx may be used. They are available in sizes for adults and children. Caution is needed when the artificial airway devices are used, to prevent rupture of the tracheal tissues.

Artificial airway devices are used when a patient has serious mouth injuries or is unconscious. They are *not* usually used on conscious patients because the extension of the device into the posterior of the throat causes a gag reflex.

External Cardiac Compression

In external cardiac compression, the rescuer's hands must be positioned properly on the patient's chest. If the hands are not positioned properly, the patient may be injured.

ADMINISTERING CPR TO A CHILD

The rescuer must use restraint in administering external cardiac compressions to the small child or infant.

In a child 8 years old or younger, only the heel of one hand is placed on the sternum for chest compression.

In an infant, only the tips of the index and middle fingers are used to compress the sternum, while the infant is held in the lap of the rescuer. *Caution:* Heavy compressions can cause injury to the liver or spleen.

Inflation of the lungs should be applied, with the same ratios to external cardiac compressions (5:1 for two rescuers, or 15:2 for one rescuer). Compressions are maintained at 80 to 100 per minute.

When providing rescue breaths to a child, the rescuer's lips seal both the patient's mouth and nose. For the small child and infant, a lesser volume of air is indicated in order to avoid damage to the lungs.

PROCEDURE: **Performing One-Rescuer CPR**

1. Double-check that the patient is not breathing and does not have a pulse.
2. Call for help.
3. Place the patient in a supine position, kneel down beside him and artificially ventilate with two full rescue breaths.
4. Check for a carotid pulse for 5 seconds.
5. If the patient does not start breathing spontaneously after the first inflation and there is no pulse, begin CPR immediately.
6. Position your hands on the patient's chest to begin compressions. Give 15 compressions.
7. For one rescuer administering CPR, continue the ratio of compressions to inflations on a 15:2 cycle (15 chest compressions to 2 lung inflations). Deliver four complete cycles per minute, which equals 80 chest compressions per minute. Then recheck the pulse.
8. Continue CPR until the patient resumes breathing on his own, until an ambulance arrives, or until you are physically no longer able to administer CPR.

PROCEDURE: **Performing Two-Rescuer CPR**

1. The first rescuer provides rescue breathing and the second rescuer provides cardiac compressions. The second rescuer takes directions from the first rescuer as to when to assist. The members of the team may periodically alternate positions to avoid fatigue.
2. The patient is placed in a supine position on a flat, hard surface such as the floor.
3. The first rescuer kneels closely at the patient's side near the shoulders. He or she opens the airway and quickly inflates the patient's lungs by delivering two long breaths, using the mouth-to-mouth technique.
4. The second rescuer kneels facing the patient's chest, at the patient's shoulder on the opposite side, and checks for the carotid pulse. If there is no pulse or breathing, CPR is begun immediately.
5. The second rescuer moves into position with hands on the patient's sternum ready to begin external cardiac compressions.
6. The first rescuer takes a deep breath, carefully positions his or her mouth, and inflates the patient's lungs.

   □ *RATIONALE*: For the action to be effective, the rescuer's lips must completely seal the patient's mouth.
7. The first rescuer turns his or her head toward the patient's chest to observe rise of the patient's chest as the air enters the lungs.
8. The second rescuer is in position at the other side of the patient's upper chest with his or her hands positioned to begin the external cardiac compressions.
9. The second rescuer compresses the chest at a rate of 80 to 100 compressions per minute. The chest of an adult should be compressed 2 inches each time.
10. The first rescuer ventilates the patient slowly (on the upstroke between compressions) at the ratio of 5:1 (five chest compressions to one lung inflation).
11. The patient's breathing is checked every few minutes.
12. Two-rescuer CPR is continued until the patient breathes on his own, until a professional emergency team arrives, or until both rescuers are physically unable to continue.

Obstruction of an Airway by a Foreign Body

A sudden coughing spasm or movement by the patient during a dental procedure may cause the accidental aspiration (inhaling or swallowing) of a foreign object. The patient's discomfort is immediate; his hands go to his throat as spasms of coughing or choking occur.

- If the patient cannot speak, cough, or breathe, the airway is completely blocked.
- If the airway is not completely blocked, high-pitched noises and wheezing will occur as he inhales.
- If the object is not dislodged, it may shift, and complete blockage of the airway could then occur.
- First aid is the same for both a completely blocked and a partially blocked airway.

Rescuing the Patient with a Blocked Airway

When a patient grasps at his throat (the universal sign for choking), turns pale, and is not coughing, ask "Are you choking?" or "Can you speak?" A person getting enough air to cough or speak is getting enough air to breathe.

If the patient is coughing forcefully or can speak, do *not* administer treatment for a blocked airway. Instead, let him try to cough up the object by himself. Stay with the patient and encourage him to cough up the object.

If the patient continues to cough without dislodging the object, or if he stops coughing and cannot breathe or speak, call for help (an ambulance). Then you must begin the abdominal thrusts immediately.

Abdominal thrusts, also known as the *Heimlich maneuver*, are an external compression method in which the rescuer utilizes the air in the patient's lungs as an aid in expelling the foreign object lodged in the trachea or bronchi.

(text continued on page 157)

PROCEDURE: **Performing Abdominal Thrusts**

On a Conscious Standing Patient

1. Call for help. Assist the patient to stand alongside the dental chair.
2. Supporting the patient, go quickly to the back of the patient while briefly explaining the procedure. Instruct the patient to keep his mouth open during the procedure.
3. Place your arm around the waist of the patient and position your fist so that the thumb side is against the midline of the patient's abdomen slightly above the navel and well below the rib cage. Instruct the patient to lean slightly forward over your hand and arm.
4. Grasp your fist with the other hand and, pressing into the patient's abdomen (at the diaphragm) give quick, *inward* and *upward* thrusts with a slight pause between the thrusts. Deliver thrusts 6 to 10 times, or as needed (Fig. 9–17).
   □ *RATIONALE:* The purpose of this maneuver is to forcefully expel air from the lungs so that the object is dislodged.
5. Repeat this procedure several times, if necessary, until the object is dislodged or other help is required. When the object is removed, the patient will resume breathing freely again.

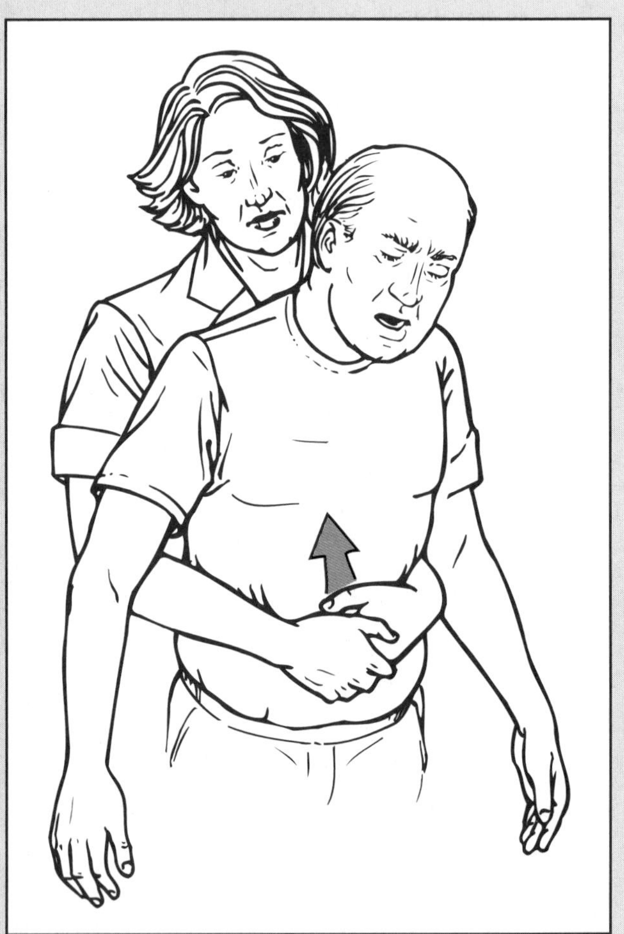

FIGURE 9–17

Rescuing the patient with a blocked airway. Place the thumb side of your fist against the middle of the patient's abdomen just above the navel. Grasp your fist with the other hand. Give quick, upward thrusts. Repeat until object is coughed up or person becomes unconscious.

On a Conscious Seated Patient

1. Quickly position yourself behind the patient and chair.
2. Squat, kneel, or stoop so that you can wrap your arms around the patient from behind.
3. Instruct the patient to lean forward slightly on your hands and to keep his mouth open.
4. Using the same technique as for a standing patient, apply short inward and upward thrusts, and repeat as needed.

On a Patient on the Floor

1. If the patient is unconscious or extremely obese, assist him to the floor and place him in a supine position.
2. Lift the patient's head and chin, then do a finger-sweep of the oral cavity to remove the foreign object if possible.
3. If unsuccessful, position yourself close to the patient's torso and straddle one of his legs.
4. Place the heel of one hand at the patient's abdomen above the navel and well below the xiphoid process.
5. Place your other hand directly over the first hand. Administer a firm, quick, upward thrust to the patient's diaphragm. Repeat this maneuver 6 to 10 times as needed.

On an Unconscious Patient with Complete Obstruction

1. Place the patient in a supine position.
2. Open the airway, using the tilt-lift method.
3. Attempt to ventilate, using mouth-to-mouth technique.
4. If unable to get air into the patient's lungs, reopen the airway, and then attempt again to ventilate.
5. If the airway is still blocked, administer abdominal thrusts and rescue breaths alternately.
6. Between thrusts, grasp both the patient's tongue and chin; then lift the mandible and gently draw the tongue away from the back of the patient's throat.
7. With your index finger, sweep the patient's oral cavity from cheek to cheek, reaching back near the oropharynx.
8. A dislodged object found in the oral cavity should be carefully lifted out to avoid letting the object fall back into the patient's throat.

Chest thrusts, *not* abdominal thrusts, are used if the patient is in advanced pregnancy (6 to 9 months) or is so obese that the rescuer cannot reach around or find the waist.

1. Standing behind the patient, reach up and place your arms directly under the patient's armpits.
2. Place the thumb of one fist on the middle of the patient's sternum level with the armpits.

3. With the other hand grasping the fist, apply a quick backward and upward thrust (Fig. 9–18).
4. Continue the quick backward and upward thrusts until the foreign object is dislodged.

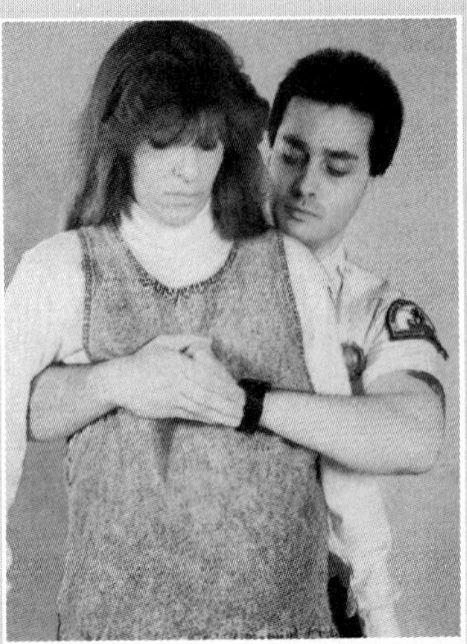

FIGURE 9–18

In a pregnant patient, pressure is applied to the sternum approximately at the level of the armpits. (From Henry, M., and Stapleton, E.: EMT Prehospital Care. Philadelphia, W.B. Saunders Co., 1992.)

Life-Threatening Emergencies

Most life-threatening emergencies in the dental office occur during or immediately after the administration of local anesthesia or during the ensuing treatment.

The types of procedures during which medical emergencies most commonly arise in the dental office are tooth extraction and endodontic treatment. These are two procedures in which adequate pain control may be difficult to achieve and patient anxiety is high. In fact, stress may be a significant factor in the majority of medical emergencies sustained in the dental office.

Regardless of the causes, it is essential that dentist and staff be trained to recognize and respond to any medical emergencies that may arise.

The six most common medical emergencies occurring in the dental office are

- Unconsciousness
- Altered consciousness
- Convulsions (seizures)
- Respiratory distress
- Drug-related crises
- Chest pain

Unconsciousness

SYNCOPE

Syncope, commonly known as *fainting*, is a transient loss of consciousness, and it is by far the most common medical emergency in the dental office. (**Transient** means passing or temporary. **Unconsciousness** is a lack of response to sensory stimulation.)

When a patient is in a stressful situation, experiencing the "fight or flight" syndrome, and seated upright, cerebral blood flow is diminished. The brain cannot function properly without adequate blood flow, and the patient's ability to respond is diminished.

Patients about to go into syncope become pale and sweaty. They may complain of nausea, of feeling faint, or of dizziness. They may actually lose consciousness.

PROCEDURE: **Treating a Patient with Syncope**

1. Place the patient in a supine position with the feet elevated to a position higher than his head (10 to 15 degrees).
   ☐ *RATIONALE*: This position causes the blood to flow away from the stomach and back toward the brain and is frequently enough to revive the patient.
2. After tipping the chair back, establish an airway by tilting the patient's head back while lifting the chin. Also loosen any constricting garments, such as a necktie or tight collar.
3. Syncope patients usually resume breathing spontaneously within 10 seconds. Oxygen should be administered, however, as a precaution.
4. Monitor and record the patient's blood pressure and other vital signs.
   ☐ *RATIONALE*: The patient in syncope has a diminished heart rate (about 30 beats per minute) and has a detectable pulse. The blood pressure is low but gradually increases as the patient recovers.
5. If the patient has not revived within 10 to 15 seconds, remove the oxygen mask. Fracture an ampule of spirits of ammonia in a gauze sponge and waft it gently under the patient's nostrils.
   ☐ *RATIONALE*: The pungent odor causes the patient to inhale quickly and thus receive additional oxygen. However, do not hold spirits of ammonia directly under the nostrils, because the ammonia vapors may cause irritation to the membranes of the nasal passages.
6. Usually the patient revives fully in 1 to 2 minutes. Dental treatment should be postponed, and another adult should be contacted to drive the patient home.

PROCEDURE: Treating a Conscious Patient with Hypoglycemia

1. Place the patient in the position most comfortable for him.
2. Offer 4 oz. of orange juice or a sweetened soft drink. Continue this every 5 to 10 minutes for 30 minutes.
   ☐ *RATIONALE:* This raises his blood sugar level.
3. If the patient feels comfortable and vital signs are normal, dental treatment may be resumed.

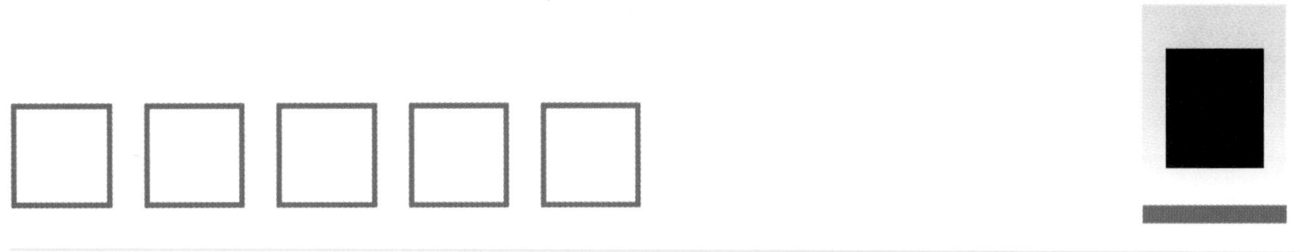

PROCEDURE: Treating an Unconscious Patient with Hypoglycemia

1. If the patient is unconscious, place him in a supine position, with the feet elevated.
   ☐ *RATIONALE:* Hypoglycemic patients usually maintain adequate breathing and circulation on their own.
2. Smear liquid sugar on the patient's oral mucosa for rapid absorption into the blood stream.
3. If the patient does not regain consciousness within 10 seconds, call the EMS.
4. Check vital signs, and begin life support measures as indicated.
5. Should the unconscious patient convulse, treat the seizures first, then the hypoglycemia.
6. Never administer oral liquids to an unconscious patient.
   ☐ *RATIONALE:* This may cause choking.
7. If the patient is unconscious and you are not sure whether he is suffering from diabetic coma or insulin shock, place a sugar cube under his tongue, or smear liquid sugar on his oral mucosa for rapid absorption into the blood stream.
   ☐ *RATIONALE:* If the condition is insulin shock, there will be less chance of brain cell damage. (Diabetic coma is discussed later in this chapter.)
8. If vital signs return to normal and the patient feels well, dental treatment may continue.
9. If there is any doubt as to the patient's ability to leave the office unescorted, arrangements should be made for someone to drive him home.

SHOCK

Shock is a state in which blood flow to peripheral tissues (including the brain) is inadequate to sustain life. An early symptom of shock is the loss of consciousness. The three most common types of shock are hypovolemic, cardiogenic, and vasodilation shock.

Hypovolemic shock is caused by a lower-than-normal volume of blood. This is the result of bleeding.

Cardiogenic shock is caused by abnormal function of the heart.

Vasodilation shock is caused by the dilation of blood vessels. This allows blood to remain in the tissues and prevents the normal flow of blood throughout the cardiovascular system. Syncope is the most common form of this type of shock.

Stimuli that can cause vasodilation shock include fright, extreme heat or cold, extreme fatigue, and, in times of stress (such as during surgery), an increased need of the body organs for oxygen.

Altered Consciousness

The conscious patient who begins acting strangely may be experiencing altered consciousness. There are many causes of altered consciousness, and in the dental office, hypoglycemia is one of the most common.

HYPOGLYCEMIA

Hypoglycemia, also known as *insulin shock*, is abnormally low blood sugar. Although it can happen to anyone, it happens most frequently in insulin-dependent diabetics when a high level of insulin causes a decrease in blood sugar to the brain.

The hypoglycemic patient may seem confused and even appear drunk. He may also exhibit cool moist skin, a mild tremor, and headache, and he may complain of hunger. Unconsciousness may follow. Hypoglycemia is associated with a rapid heart rate, but blood pressure should not be affected.

POSTURAL HYPOTENSION

Postural hypotension, also known as *orthostatic hypotension*, is altered consciousness due to reduced circulation. It may occur after a long appointment, when the patient has been in a supine position for 2 hours or more in a lounge-type dental chair. (**Hypotension** means reduced circulation, lower-than-normal blood pressure.)

The patient's blood pressure drops, and a sudden change in position may cause light-headedness and fainting. To avoid adverse reactions, the patient should be positioned upright very slowly.

Individuals who are predisposed to postural hypotension include elderly persons with high blood pres-

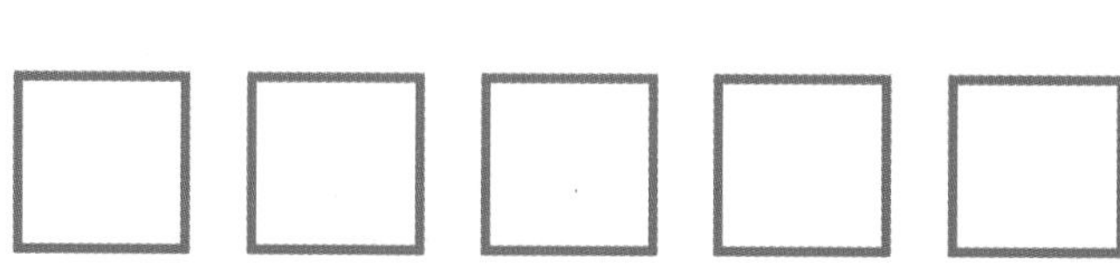

PROCEDURE: Treating a Patient with Postural Hypotension

1. Immediately reposition the patient in a supine position.
2. If the patient is unconscious and does not revive upon reassuming the supine position, check his breathing.
3. If breathing is not normal, call for help and begin emergency procedures immediately.
4. If breathing is normal, slowly return the patient to an upright position. If he still feels dizzy and faint, lower him to the supine position once again. Oxygen may be administered.
5. Check the patient's blood pressure before dismissing him. If he is taking antihypertensive drugs, he should be accompanied by another adult when dismissed and advised to see a physician.

   □ *NOTE:* The patient's physician should be advised if the patient has had difficulty regaining normal vital signs.

sure and patients taking antihypertensive drugs (for high blood pressure), tricyclic antidepressants, narcotics, or drugs for Parkinson's disease.

Postural Hypotension in the Pregnant Patient. While in a supine position, the pregnant patient may feel dizzy or light-headed and may faint. This is caused by the pressure of the enlarged uterus on the abdominal veins. This pressure reduces venous return to the heart and results in decreased cardiac output and cerebral anoxia (lack of oxygen to the brain).

Contrary to the usual treatment for fainting or postural hypotension, the patient should be turned onto her left side or moved into an upright sitting position. The change of position relieves the pressure on the involved blood vessels.

Convulsions

Convulsions, also known as *seizures*, may produce generalized skeletal muscle contractions. Convulsions occurring in the dental office most often involve epileptic patients with poorly controlled seizures or patients with well-controlled seizures who are fearful of receiving dental treatment.

Local anesthetic overdose may also be associated with seizures. This is discussed later in this chapter.

EPILEPTIC SEIZURES

The vast majority (90 percent) of epileptic patients experience grand mal seizures, or *generalized tonic-clonic seizures* (GTCS). (**Tonic** means the muscles are contracted; **clonic** refers to muscle spasms.) Epilepsy is discussed in Chapter 8.

Before a grand mal seizure, the patient may experience a warning aura such as a peculiar smell, taste, vision, or sound. This may last several seconds or several hours.

In the second phase (the tonic phase), the patient loses consciousness and experiences a brief (10- to 20-second) period of generalized rigidity of the muscles. During this phase, the patient may arch his back and emit a strange sound as air is expelled from the lungs. This is followed by generalized skeletal-muscle contractions and relaxations that may last from 2 to 5 minutes.

During the third phase (the clonic phase), muscle contractions may be violent or barely detectable. The respiratory, cardiovascular, and central nervous systems are stimulated simultaneously. In the final phase, muscle contraction ends with these systems depressed. This phase lasts from 10 to 30 minutes, and during this time the patient sleeps deeply and may be difficult to arouse.

Respiratory Distress

A conscious patient who experiences breathing difficulty is in respiratory distress.

BRONCHOSPASM

A bronchospasm is the partial obstruction of the airway. In most cases it can easily be managed; sometimes, however, it can progress to an asthmatic attack that is life-threatening. (The patient with asthma is discussed in Chapter 8.)

Asthmatic patients should bring their bronchodilator aerosol medication to every appointment. The office emergency kit should include a bronchodilator, preferably albuterol. (Albuterol is preferable to epinephrine because it does not stimulate the cardiovascular system.)

The patient experiencing a bronchospasm breathes in short, gasping inspirations with long, wheezing expirations. Other symptoms may include sweating and flushing of the face and upper torso.

Local Anesthetic Overdose

Local anesthetic overdose most often involves patients who are physically small. Most anesthetic blood levels peak about 5 to 10 minutes after injection.

Signs and symptoms of anesthetic overdose include

- Twitches (resulting from central nervous system stimulation)
- Talkativeness
- Increased apprehension
- Slurred speech, and stuttering

As the local anesthetic blood level increases, muscular twitching may progress to generalized convulsions. These seizures continue until the blood level of local anesthetic drops *below* the seizure threshold for that drug. (The **seizure threshold** is that level of the drug in the body at which it causes convulsions.)

Allergic Reactions

An **allergy** is an altered state of reactivity in body tissues, or a state of hypersensitivity to specific antigens. An **antigen** is a substance that causes an immune response through the production of antibodies. An antigen that can trigger the allergic state is known as an **allergen.**

The allergen may be a drug, a food, latex protein, or the venom from an insect sting. Sensitivity to a specific allergen may be immediate or delayed, and sensitivity may be built up over a period of time, as with repeated small doses of antibiotics.

Histamine is normally found in all tissues of the body; however, when the body comes into contact with certain substances to which it is sensitive, an excess of histamine is released. It is this excess histamine that causes the physical symptoms of an allergic reaction. **Antihistamines** are drugs that are antagonistic to histamine and are used to counteract its effect.

Allergic Reactions Involving the Skin. Most allergic reactions are relatively mild and involve only the skin. This type of reaction causes **urticaria** (swollen areas), **wheals** (very large hives), and possibly a rash and severe itching.

PROCEDURE: **Treating a Patient Having an Epileptic Seizure**

1. As with other types of unconscious patients, a convulsing patient should be placed in a supine position, but foot elevation is not critical.
   □ *RATIONALE:* Because blood pressure usually increases during a seizure, it is not necessary to elevate the patient's feet.
2. Check for airway, breathing, and circulation. Basic life support becomes most critical when a seizure patient is unconscious.
3. Never leave an unconscious patient alone.
4. Contact the EMS as soon as the seizure begins.
   □ *RATIONALE:* More severe seizures may require intravenous anticonvulsant drugs such as diazepam or midazolam. These should be administered only by trained professionals.
5. If the seizure occurs while the patient is seated in the dental chair, leave the patient in the chair. Remove all materials from the patient's mouth as quickly as possible.
6. During the seizure, protect the patient from sustaining injury. Cushion the head, if necessary. Gently hold the patient's arms or legs, but do not attempt to completely immobilize the seizure patient.
   □ *IMPORTANT:* Do not put anything in the convulsive patient's mouth!
7. Talk to the patient and explain what is happening. Explain that he or she has had a seizure and give reassurance.
8. If a family member has accompanied the patient, this person may be most helpful during the seizure recovery phase in giving reassurance.
9. In most seizure cases, the patient recovers on his own.
10. Allow him to rest until he feels sufficiently recovered. Reschedule his appointment and have an adult drive him home.

PROCEDURE: **Treating a Patient with Bronchospasm**

1. Position the patient as comfortably as possible. Patients who experience difficulty in breathing usually prefer to sit up.
2. If available, administer a bronchodilator. Usually, the asthmatic can medicate himself.
3. The spasm usually subsides within minutes of one or two doses of bronchodilator medication.
4. If a bronchodilator is not available, if the patient has no history of asthma, or if the episode continues, call the EMS.
5. If the patient becomes unconscious, or if the lips or nail beds turn blue, administer oxygen immediately.
6. Once the episode is over, treatment may be resumed if both the dental team and the patient are comfortable.

PROCEDURE: Treating a Patient with a Local Anesthetic Overdose

1. Immediately call the EMS for help.
2. Place patient in a supine position.
3. Maintain airway, using the tilt-lift method. Administer oxygen, if necessary.
   □ *RATIONALE:* Maintenance of the airway is the most important step in management of local anesthetic overdose because oxygenation helps the body eliminate the local anesthetic from the blood.
4. If the patient is having seizures, protect the patient as you would for epileptic seizures.
5. Continue to monitor vital signs until the ambulance arrives.

PROCEDURE: Treating a Patient Experiencing Anaphylaxis

1. Call the EMS immediately.
   □ *RATIONALE:* Immediate treatment is imperative. This is a life-threatening condition.
2. Recline the patient to a supine position with the feet elevated.
   □ *RATIONALE:* The patient has shocklike symptoms, and this is the position of choice for treating shock.
3. Ensure an open airway. If the patient is having respiratory difficulty, administer oxygen.
4. Epinephrine (1:1000), in a dosage of 0.3 to 0.5 mg., may be administered subcutaneously. If the reaction is severe, an additional dose may be administered in another 10 minutes.
   □ *RATIONALE:* Epinephrine is a vasoconstrictor that counteracts the vasodilation action of the histamine.
5. Antihistamines (diphenhydramine or chlorpheniramine) may also be administered.
   □ *NOTE:* If antihistamines are administered, their use orally is usually continued for several days after the incident.
6. As the patient responds, breathing becomes more normal and relaxed. The heart rate remains elevated, but the strength of the pulse improves. Blood pressure increases.
7. Continue to monitor vital signs until help arrives.

However, even a mild allergic reaction can develop into a life-threatening, systemic reaction. The patient undergoing an allergic reaction involving only the skin should be kept under observation. If indicated, antihistamines are administered to relieve the swelling and alleviate the itching.

Anaphylaxis. Anaphylaxis, formerly referred to as *anaphylactic shock,* is a systemic allergic reaction that may be immediate, severe, and fatal, running its course within seconds or minutes.

In general, the more rapidly the symptoms of an allergic reaction develop, the more likely they are to become serious.

This reaction occurs with a sudden release of histamines, causing capillary dilation that results in generalized edema and an accompanying drop in blood pressure. It is the drop in blood pressure that causes the shocklike symptoms, including loss of consciousness and a weak pulse.

Obstruction of the airway and trachea, due to swollen tissues, may cause wheezing and labored breathing. The patient may also show signs of choking, nausea, coughing, cyanosis, and loss of consciousness. (**Cyanosis** is a bluish tinge to the skin that is caused by a lack of oxygen.)

Sensitivity to any medication that might cause this kind of reaction must be posted in red on the patient's chart. Also, many patients wear a "Medic Alert" necklace or a bracelet (or carry a card in their wallet) to alert first aid personnel to the nature of the allergy or special medical condition.

Chest Pain

ANGINA PECTORIS

Angina pectoris, commonly referred to just as *angina,* is the result of narrowing of the coronary arteries and decreased blood flow to the heart. It may be caused by extreme physical exertion or by emotional stress such as pending dental treatment. It is usually relieved by rest or by the administration of nitroglycerin.

Angina pectoris is characterized by a substernal pain (pain under the sternum), feeling of heavy pressure or weight on the chest, or a constricting feeling or burning between the shoulder blades. The constriction of blood flow causes pain similar to that of a heart attack, with radiating pain located in the arm and chest. Cyanosis, shortness of breath, and a feeling of anxiety may also be present.

Nitroglycerin is administered to relieve the pain of angina pectoris. It may be administered sublingually by placing a tablet under the tongue as needed. (**Sublingual** means under the tongue.) Patients who require nitroglycerin tablets usually carry a supply with them at all times.

An alternative is a translingual aerosol, which is sprayed in a metered dose onto or under the tongue. (**Translingual** means through the tongue.) The nitroglycerin is quickly absorbed through the mucous membranes lining the underside of the tongue and the floor of the mouth.

PROCEDURE: Treating a Patient with Angina Pectoris

1. Position the patient at a 45-degree angle.
   □ *RATIONALE*: Angina patients are more comfortable in this position.
2. The pain may be relieved by administering 100 percent oxygen and nitroglycerin. One sublingual nitroglycerin tablet or translingual spray dose may be followed in 20 minutes by at least a second dose.
   □ *IMPORTANT:* If the patient wears a transdermal form of nitroglycerin, the administration of additional nitroglycerin is *not* usually recommended.
3. If there is no history of angina or chest pain, or if severe pain continues, call EMS immediately.

Instead of using tablets, some angina patients wear a transdermal patch, which provides a constant ongoing supply of nitroglycerin. (**Transdermal** means through the skin.)

ACUTE MYOCARDIAL INFARCTION

An acute myocardial infarction (AMI), commonly known as a *heart attack*, occurs when one or more of the coronary arteries that supply blood to the heart muscle becomes blocked. This blockage may result in the destruction of that portion of the heart muscle. Immediate treatment is essential to prevent further damage and possible death. Symptoms of a heart attack include

- A feeling of apprehension
- Severe pain in the chest
- Shortness of breath
- Nausea
- Perspiration
- Ashen-gray color of the skin
- Cyanosis of mucous membranes

At the onset, pain usually is located at the sternum and the left arm and radiates to the neck and the left side of the chest. It may remain in the chest or the back or may even travel up to the mandible.

The patient may also complain of feeling as though he were being held in a vise pressing on his chest and impeding his breathing. Although the pain associated with an AMI is very similar to that of angina at the onset, an AMI lasts longer, is more severe, and does not respond well to nitroglycerin.

If a patient experiences any combination of these symptoms, it is imperative that he receive emergency treatment as quickly as possible.

Cardiac Arrest

In cardiac arrest, the heart has stopped beating and the patient has stopped breathing. There is no pulse or respiration, and oxygen is not being taken into the tissues.

Cardiac arrest can happen at any time, anywhere, and at any age. It may be caused by a heart attack, by a reaction to medication, or by other factors. The heart may stop beating completely, or it may fibrillate. (**Fibrillation** is when the heart beats too rapidly, randomly, or ineffectively to maintain circulation.)

Death occurs when the heart stops pumping blood. However, if the heart can be forced to beat and the patient forced to breathe, the blood will be oxygenated and will circulate so that the brain and other tissues will receive the necessary supply of blood. This emergency care may keep the patient alive until the heart can be restarted and is beating on its own.

DIAGNOSTIC SIGNS OF CARDIAC ARREST

- Loss of consciousness, no responsiveness
- No perceptible breathing
- No heart beat or pulse
- Dilated pupils (the pupils begin to dilate 30 to 40

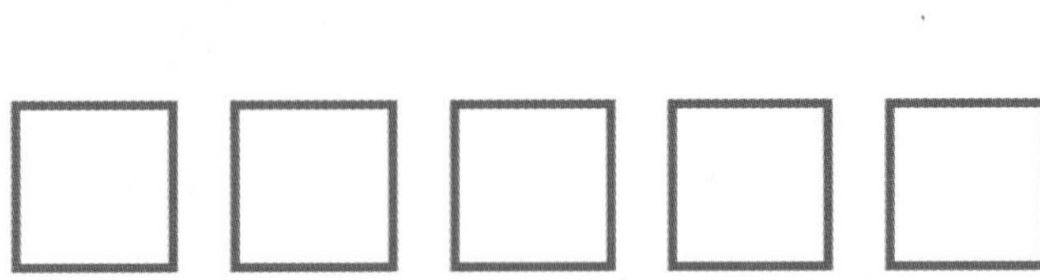

PROCEDURE: **Treating a Patient with Acute Myocardial Infarction**

1. Call the EMS immediately.
2. Reassure the patient in quiet tones and keep him quiet. Do not allow the patient to attempt to move himself.
3. Keep the conscious patient in a sitting position. If blood pressure drops, or if the patient loses consciousness, move him to a supine position and elevate the feet slightly.
4. Administer oxygen via nasal cannula or nasal hood at a 4- to 6-liters-per-minute flow rate.
5. Administer two doses of either translingual or sublingual nitroglycerin.
6. Loosen tight clothing such as a collar and tie.
7. The dentist may administer nitrous oxide and oxygen to relieve chest pain that does not subside after nitroglycerin is given.
8. Stay with the patient until help arrives.

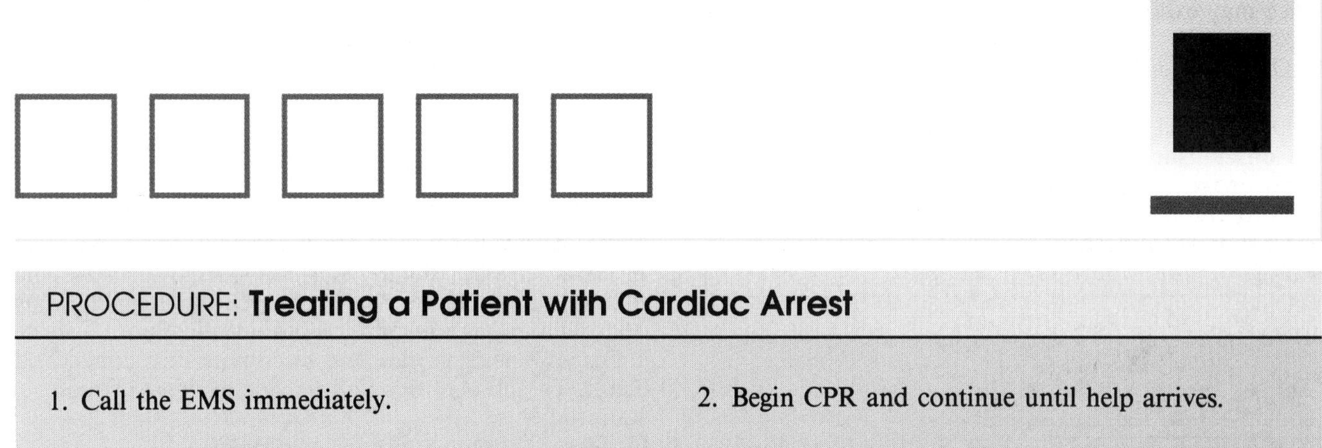

PROCEDURE: Treating a Patient with Cardiac Arrest

1. Call the EMS immediately.
2. Begin CPR and continue until help arrives.

seconds after an adverse effect on circulation of the blood to the brain; complete dilation occurs within 1 minute of cardiac arrest)
- Cyanosis

Other Medical Emergencies

Hemorrhage

During dental treatment, the tissues of the oral cavity may be traumatized, causing **hemorrhaging** (excessive bleeding). One important function of the patient's medical history is to identify patients with bleeding problems before any treatment is provided. When excessive bleeding occurs, it may be controlled mechanically or with hemostatic drugs.

MECHANICAL CONTROL OF HEMORRHAGING

Blood oozing from an open tooth socket after extraction can be controlled by the application of a folded sterile gauze sponge compress over the wound.

The patient is requested to bite firmly, and the compress may remain in place for 20 to 30 minutes. It is replaced as necessary with a fresh compress until bleeding is controlled.

If the wound cannot be controlled with the application of a compress, the operator may suture the wound closed. Another alternative is to cauterize the area with the electric cautery.

If a severed blood vessel is the cause of the hemorrhage, the dentist may ligate the vessel. (As used here, **ligate** means to tie closed.) If the injury to the tissue is more complex, the dentist may request that a physician be called to attend to the patient.

HEMOSTATIC DRUGS

To control bleeding, a number of hemostatic drugs are available. The dentist determines the choice of medicament by the type of hemorrhage and by the patient's medical history.

- A **coagulant** is an agent that promotes the clotting of blood.
- An **astringent** is an agent that is applied topically to control bleeding by causing capillaries to contract.
- A **vasoconstrictor**, such as epinephrine, is used to control minor gingival bleeding. This is discussed in Chapter 20.

Clotting Aids

Gelfoam is a gelatin-based sponge material that is placed into an open socket or wound. Gelfoam disturbs the blood platelets and establishes the framework for fibrin to form a clot.

Oxycel is an oxidized cellulose that releases cellulosic acid, which has an affinity for hemoglobin, thus forming a clot. Oxycel may be placed dry into the wound.

Surgicel is oxidized regenerated cellulose applied as a gauze square. It is highly resistant to displacement and is effective when placed on bleeding surface tissues.

Tannic Acid. Tannic acid, which is found in tea, aids in causing formation of a clot. This is particularly helpful for controlling bleeding until a patient with a bleeding problem can return to the office.

The patient is instructed to moisten the tea bag in a sterile surgical gauze sponge and place it over the surgical site. The patient should bite firmly to apply adequate pressure. This usually stops hemorrhaging and helps form a clot.

Cerebrovascular Accident

A cerebrovascular accident (CVA), commonly known as a *stroke*, is a sudden interruption of the blood supply to the brain. (CVA's are discussed in Chapter 8.)

The patient experiencing a stroke while in the dental office may exhibit the following symptoms:

- Dizziness and confusion as to his surroundings
- Numbness or paralysis
- Difficulty in speaking and swallowing
- Consciousness and awareness of his surroundings but inability to talk
- Convulsions
- Loss of consciousness
- Loss of control of body functions

Diabetes Mellitus

Diabetes mellitus is discussed in Chapter 8. However in the diabetic patient, medical complications necessitating emergency care may occur if the prescribed routine for diabetes is not followed. Two of the most common complications are hypoglycemia and hyperglycemia.

Hypoglycemia, also known as *insulin shock*, is abnormally low levels of blood sugar. (This was discussed earlier in this chapter.) **Hyperglycemia**, more commonly known as *diabetic acidosis*, is abnormally high levels of blood sugar.

DIABETIC ACIDOSIS

Diabetic acidosis, also known as *hyperglycemic coma*, occurs because of an abnormally *increased* level of sugar in the blood. This may occur because the patient has eaten too much sugar-containing food, has not taken enough insulin, or has an infection.

Diabetic acidosis can lead to convulsions, coma, and death. The clinical signs of diabetic acidosis include

- Acetone breath (smelling like fruit)
- Warm, dry skin and dry mouth
- Rapid and weak pulse
- Air hunger, rapid deep breathing
- Unresponsiveness to questioning
- Loss of consciousness

PROCEDURE: **Treating a Patient Experiencing CVA**

1. Alert the dentist and call for emergency help immediately.
2. Remain calm, reassure the patient, and make him comfortable.
3. Administer oxygen if indicated.
4. Monitor vital signs.
5. Remain with the patient until help arrives.

PROCEDURE: **Treating a Patient Experiencing Diabetic Acidosis**

1. If the patient is conscious, ask when he ate last and whether he has taken his insulin.
   □ *RATIONALE*: He has probably eaten but has not taken his insulin.
2. Call the patient's physician or an EMS immediately.
   □ *RATIONALE*: In diabetic acidosis, the patient needs insulin and other medication promptly.

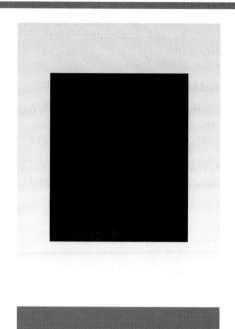

Chapter 10

Microbiology and Disease Transmission

Introduction

This chapter is divided into five major sections: microbiology, disease transmission, body defenses, diseases of major concern to dental personnel, and preventing disease transmission.

Microbiology

Microbiology is the study of microorganisms, which are living organisms that are so small they are visible only with a microscope. Large numbers of microorganisms are always present in every human environment. Most live in warm, moist, and dark areas where there is an adequate food supply.

The mouth is an ideal breeding area for many microorganisms, and nearly every microorganism that has been identified has, at one time or another, been isolated from the oral cavity.

Another ideal breeding area is on a gloved hand. Here too the environment is warm, moist, and dark.

Most microorganisms do *not* produce human illness. In fact, they are valuable allies in many ways. For example, bacteria normally found in the intestinal tract aid in the digestion of food.

Pathogens

A **pathogen** is a microorganism that is capable of causing disease. (Pathology, the study of diseases, is discussed in Chapter 11.) **Etiology** is the study of the factors that cause disease and the method of their introduction (transmission) to the host. (The **host** is the individual who is ill because of a pathogen.)

There are three factors that influence the disease-producing capability of a pathogenic organism:

- Host resistance
- Virulence
- Concentration

Host resistance is the ability of the body to resist the pathogen. The healthier you are, the better is your resistance to disease. Resistance is increased through appropriate immunizations and by maintaining good health habits.

The state of lowered resistance can result from fatigue, physical or emotional strain, poor nutrition, injury, surgery, or the presence of other diseases.

Virulence, which is also known as *infectivity*, describes the ability of the pathogen to overcome the body's defenses and cause disease. A highly virulent pathogen is able to overcome the body's defenses—even in healthy individuals who are able to resist other diseases.

If the patient's immune system is compromised (damaged), he is less able to withstand pathogens that do not make others sick. The immune system may be damaged by disease such as the human immunodeficiency virus (HIV), immunosuppression therapy (to prevent rejection of a transplanted organ), by radiation, by chemotherapy, or in the elderly.

Concentration refers to the number of the pathogens that are present. The more pathogens that are present, the better are their chances of overwhelming the host and producing disease.

The exposure control (also known as *infection control*) activities in the dental office are aimed at preventing the transmission of disease-producing organisms by reducing the number of pathogens that are present.

The major types of pathogenic microorganisms are bacteria, rickettsiae, viruses, protozoa, and fungi.

Bacteria

Bacteria are one-celled microorganisms that are described or identified in several different ways. (*Bacteria* is plural. The singular is *bacterium.*) (The bacteria associated with dental plaque are discussed in Chapter 6.)

GRAM-POSITIVE AND GRAM-NEGATIVE BACTERIA

A cell wall encloses the contents of each bacterium. One system of describing bacteria is based on the reaction of the cell wall to a dye called Gram's stain.

- Those bacteria that are stained by the dye are classified as **gram-positive**. (They appear dark purple under the microscope.)
- Those bacteria that do not hold the stain are classified as **gram-negative**. (They are almost colorless and nearly invisible under the microscope.)

SHAPES OF BACTERIA

When viewed under a microscope, bacteria have three shapes: spheres, rods, and spirals (Fig. 10–1).

Bacteria that are spherical are called **cocci,** and they reproduce by dividing into two. Those cocci that form chains as they divide are called **streptococci**. Examples of infections caused by streptococci include pharyngitis (a severe sore throat commonly known as "strep throat"), tonsillitis, pneumonia, and endocarditis.

Those cocci that form irregular groups or clusters are called **staphylococci**. Examples of infections caused by staphylococci include boils and other skin infections, endocarditis, and pneumonia.

Rod-shaped bacteria are called **bacilli**. (The singular is *bacillus*). Tuberculosis is an example of a disease caused by a bacillus.

Spiral-shaped bacteria are called **spirochetes**. These bacteria have flexible cell walls and are capable of movement. Lyme disease, which is transmitted to humans through the bite of an infected deer tick, is caused by a spirochete. So is syphilis, which is discussed later in this chapter.

AEROBES AND ANAEROBES

- **Aerobes** are a variety of bacteria that require oxygen in order to grow.
- **Anaerobes** are bacteria that grow in the absence of oxygen and are actually destroyed by oxygen.
- **Facultative anaerobes** are organisms that can grow in either the presence or the absence of oxygen.

CAPSULES

Some types of bacteria form a capsule that forms a protective layer covering the cell wall. *Streptococcus mutans*, which is a causative factor in dental caries, forms such a capsule.

Bacteria with this protective coating are generally virulent. This is because the capsule increases their ability to resist the body's defense mechanisms. The capsule may also prevent antibiotics from working on the bacteria.

SPORES

Under unfavorable conditions, some bacteria change into a highly resistant form called spores. Tetanus, which is discussed later in this chapter, is an example of a spore-forming bacillus.

Bacteria remain alive in the spore form but are inactive. As spores, they cannot reproduce or cause disease. However, when conditions are favorable again, the bacteria once more become active and capable of causing disease.

Spores represent the most resistant form of life known. They can survive extremes of heat and dryness even in the presence of disinfectants and radiation. Because of this resistance, harmless spores are used to test the effectiveness of the techniques used to sterilize dental instruments. (This is discussed in Chapter 13.)

Rickettsiae

The rickettsiae (singular, *rickettsia*) are short, nonmotile rods that normally live in the intestinal tract of insects such as lice, fleas, ticks, and mosquitoes.

The diseases caused by rickettsiae are typhus and Rocky Mountain spotted fever. These diseases are transmitted to humans by the bite of an infected insect.

Viruses

Viruses are infectious agents that are so small they can be seen only with electron microscopes. Despite their minute size, many viruses cause fatal diseases.

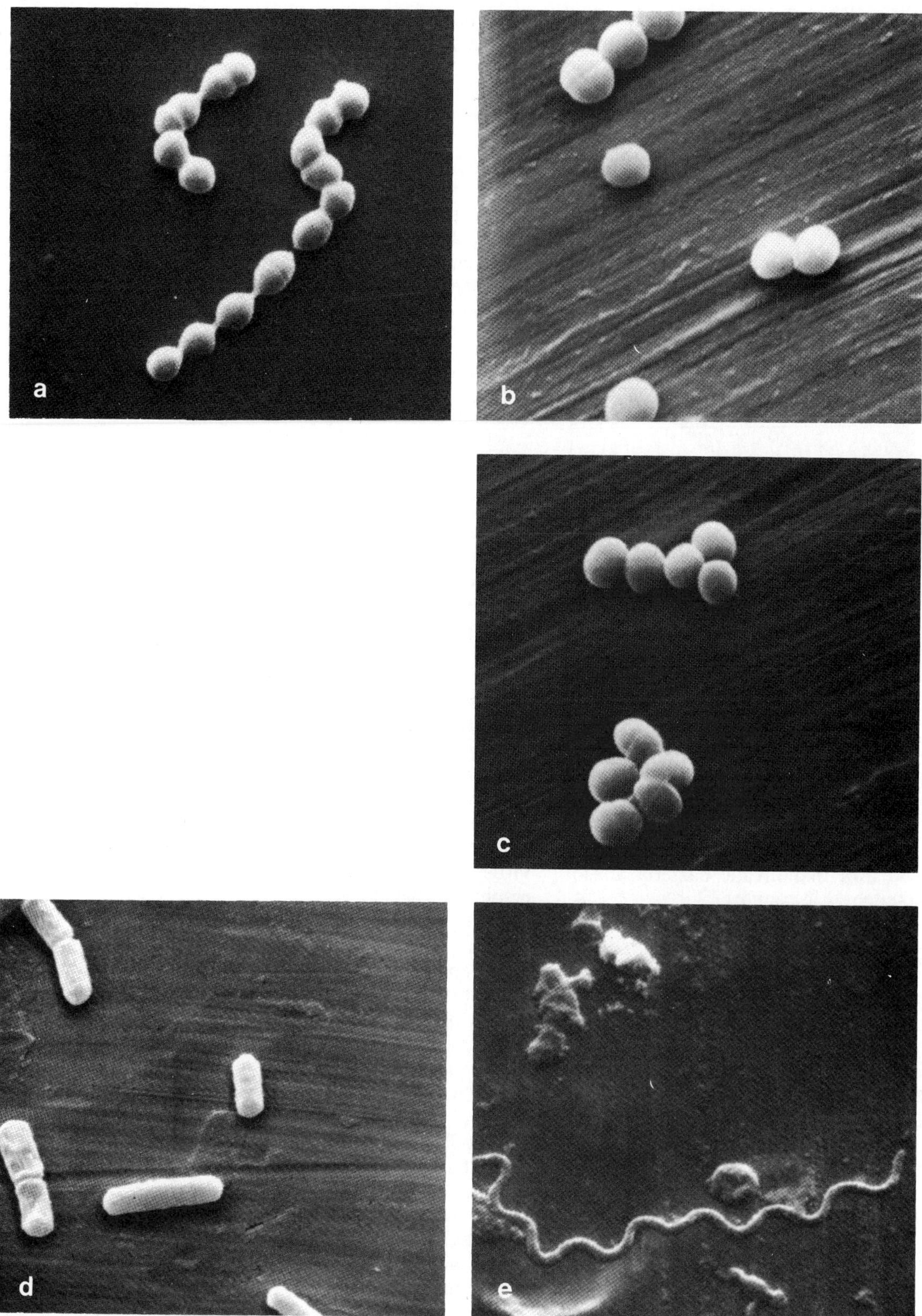

FIGURE 10–1

Scanning electromicrographs showing the shapes of bacterial cells. *a,* Pneumococci in short chains. *b,* Streptococci: a single, a pair, and a short chain. *c,* Clumps of cocci. *d,* Rod-shaped bacilli: a single cell and pairs. *e,* A spirochete, *Treponema pallidum.* (From Ackerman, V., and Dunk-Richards, G.: Microbiology. Philadelphia, W.B. Saunders Co., 1991, p 12.)

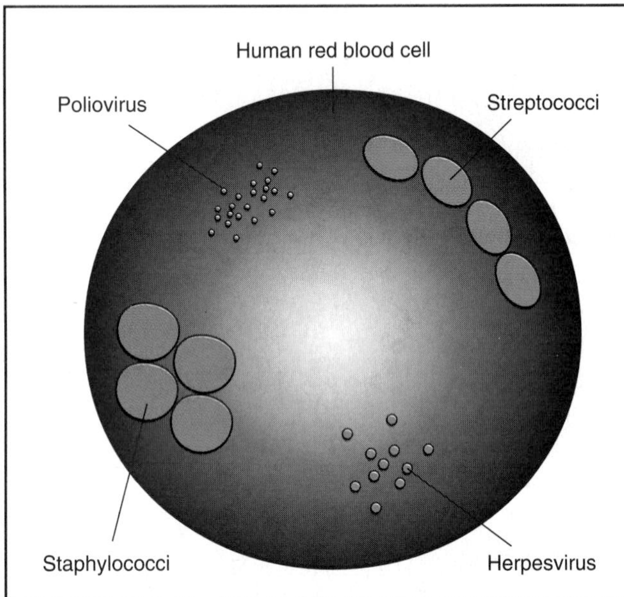

FIGURE 10–2

Relative sizes of pathogens shown in comparison with the size of a single human red blood cell. Seven hundred of these red blood cells side by side would cover the period at the end of this sentence. (Modified from Ackerman, V., and Dunk-Richards, G.: Microbiology. Philadelphia, W.B. Saunders Co., 1991, p 9.)

Figure 10–2 illustrates the comparative sizes of several types of bacteria and viruses.

Viruses can live and multiply only *inside* an appropriate host cell. The host cells may be human, animal, plant, or bacteria. Viruses that invade bacteria do so within another host (such as a human).

A virus invades a host cell, replicates (produces copies of itself), and then destroys the host cell, so the viruses are released into the body.

Viruses are extremely resistant to efforts to kill them with heat or chemicals. They are also capable of mutation. This means that viruses are able to change their genetic pattern, so they are better suited to survive current conditions and to resist efforts to kill them.

Examples of diseases caused by viruses include colds, influenza, smallpox, measles, chickenpox, herpes, hepatitis, acquired immunodeficiency syndrome (AIDS), and poliomyelitis.

Protozoa

Protozoa (singular, *protozoon*) are single-celled microscopic animals without a rigid cell wall. Although some protozoa cause parasitic diseases, not all are pathogens.

Those protozoa that are pathogens cannot survive freely in nature and must be spread by vector transmission. Diseases caused by protozoa include malaria, amebic dysentery, and African sleeping sickness. (Vector transmission is described later in this chapter.)

Fungi

Fungi are plants, such as mushrooms, yeasts, and molds, that lack chlorophyll. (Chlorophyll is the substance that makes plants green, and fungi are *not* green.) Athlete's foot, ringworm (which is not a worm), and candidiasis are examples of diseases caused by fungi. (*Fungi* is plural; the singular is *fungus.*)

Candidiasis is part of the normal flora of the skin, mouth, intestinal tract, and vagina. However, when a person is ill or the immune system is compromised, it is also capable of causing disease. (Candidiasis is discussed in Chapter 11.)

Disease Transmission

The term **disease** describes a state in which there is a sufficient departure from the normal so that symptoms or signs or both are produced.

A **symptom** is subjective evidence of a disease, such as a toothache that is observed by the patient. A **sign** is objective evidence of disease, such as a cavity that can be observed by someone other than the patient.

An **infectious disease** is one that is *communicable* or *contagious.* All of these terms mean that the disease can be transmitted (spread) in some way from one person to another.

The infectious diseases of primary concern in the dental practice are hepatitis, human immunodeficiency virus (HIV), tuberculosis, herpesviruses, and infectious respiratory agents.

Infection control procedures, discussed in Chapter 13, are designed to prevent disease transmission in the dental practice. However, before it is possible to prevent this transmission, it is important to understand how it takes place.

Bloodborne Transmission

Bloodborne diseases include, but are not limited to, hepatitis B virus (HBV) and HIV.

Bloodborne transmission, also known as *direct transmission,* occurs through contact with blood and potentially with other body fluids that are contaminated with blood. (**Borne** means carried by. **Contaminated** means not sterile and potentially capable of spreading disease.)

Saliva is of particular concern during dental treatment because frequently it is contaminated with blood. Although blood is not visible in the saliva, it may be present.

Because dental treatment often involves contact with blood and always with saliva, bloodborne diseases are of major concern in the dental office.

SPLASH

Bloodborne diseases may be transmitted during a dental procedure by splashing the mucosa or nonintact skin with blood or blood-contaminated saliva. (Intact skin, which is not broken in any way, acts as a natural protective barrier. Nonintact skin, in which there is a cut, scrape, or needlestick injury, does not protect against pathogens entering the body.)

PARENTERAL TRANSMISSION

Parenteral means through the skin, and the term is commonly associated with injections. However, parenteral disease transmission also means piercing the mucous membranes or skin barrier.

Parenteral transmission of bloodborne pathogens can occur through needlestick injuries, human bites, cuts, abrasions, or any break in the skin.

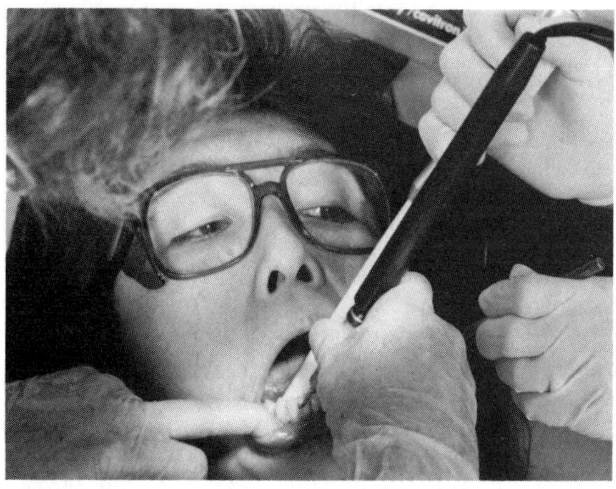

FIGURE 10–3

Spatter during dental procedures is of special concern to the dentist, chairside assistant, and hygienist.

Airborne Transmission

Airborne transmission, also known as *droplet infection*, is the spread of disease by droplets of moisture containing bacteria or viruses. These droplets are spread as people cough, talk, breathe, sing, or sneeze. (When someone sneezes, he sprays contaminated particles out about 8 feet and up about 4 feet.)

Diseases such as tuberculosis, measles, and the common cold are transmitted in this manner.

AEROSOL SPRAY

The high-speed handpiece and the ultrasonic scaler create an aerosol spray that is an airborne infection hazard for the dentist, hygienist, and assistant (Fig. 10–3). The primary concern with these mists is the hazard of inhaling them.

Inhaling the bacteria and debris in this aerosol mist is approximately the equivalent of having someone sneeze in your face twice per minute—at a distance of 1 foot!

MISTS

Mists are droplet particles larger than those generated by the aerosol spray. Mists, like those from coughing, can transmit respiratory infections; however, they do not appear to transmit hepatitis B or HIV despite being inhaled.

SPATTER

Spatter consists of large droplet particles contaminated with blood, saliva, and other debris. Spatter is created during all restorative and hygiene procedures utilizing rotary and ultrasonic dental instruments. It may be also created by the use of the air-water syringe. (See Chapters 14 and 15.)

Spatter droplets travel further than the aerosol mist and tend to land on the upper surfaces of the wrist and forearms, upper arms, and chest and may reach the necktie-collar area of the dentist, assistant, and/or hygienist. HIV, tuberculosis, hepatitis, the herpesvirus, and respiratory illnesses may all be transmitted in this manner.

Cross-Contamination

Disease transmission by cross-contamination, which is also known as the *indirect mode* of transmission, involves coming into contact with a contaminated surface, instrument, or substance.

Food Transmission. Many diseases are transmitted by contaminated food that has not been cooked or refrigerated properly. For example, the hepatitis A (HAV) and hepatitis E (HEV) viruses are spread by contaminated food or water.

Fecal/Oral Transmission. Many pathogens are present in fecal matter. If proper sanitation procedures, such as handwashing after use of the toilet, are not followed, these pathogens may be transmitted directly by touching another person or transmitted indirectly by contact with contaminated surfaces or food.

This form of transmission occurs most commonly among healthcare and daycare workers (who frequently change diapers) and by food handlers.

In the Dental Office. Diseases may be indirectly transmitted by soiled hands and towels, dirty instruments, and even dust. Also, anything that is touched during patient care is considered contaminated and potentially capable of spreading disease.

This includes faucet handles, switches, handpieces, instruments, drawer handles, materials, dressings, the patient's chart, protective eyewear, and even the pen used to make the chart entry.

Sexually Transmitted Diseases

Sexually transmitted diseases (STDs), also known as *venereal diseases* (VD), requires direct person-to-person contact, as in sexual activity. STDs include HIV, gonorrhea, syphilis, herpes, chlamydia, and hepatitis B.

These diseases, which may produce lesions in the oral cavity, can also be transmitted in a dental setting through contact with contaminated blood, saliva, or sores on the mucous membranes of the mouth.

Carrier Transmission

A **carrier** is an individual who harbors, in his body, the specific organisms of a disease without obvious symptoms and is capable of transmitting this disease to others. Among carrier-transmitted diseases are hepatitis B, herpesvirus, tuberculosis, typhoid fever, and HIV.

- A carrier may have had the disease and recovered.
- A carrier may have been exposed to the disease and may be coming down with it but may not yet have obvious symptoms.
- A carrier may have been exposed to the disease but will never be sick with it.

Having a complete, up-to-date medical history on each patient is helpful in detecting someone who might be a carrier, but this is not 100 percent reliable. Therefore, it is always necessary to assume that every patient is a potential carrier.

Autogenous Infection

Pathogenic microorganisms present in the patient's mouth do not normally cause an infection because they are not able to enter the blood stream. However, when there is bleeding, these pathogens are able to enter the blood stream and may cause infection in some individuals. In dentistry this is of concern because procedures such as extractions and periodontal surgery do cause bleeding in the mouth.

Bleeding occurs when there is a break in a blood vessel. Usually this is a very small capillary; however, even the smallest opening allows blood to escape. It also allows microorganisms that are present in the mouth to enter the blood stream.

In this way the patient may actually infect himself with bacteria that are present in his own mouth. This is known as autogenous or self-infection. (**Autogenous** means self-produced.)

TRANSIENT BACTEREMIA

When bacteria enter the blood stream this causes the temporary presence of bacteria in the blood. This is called **transient bacteremia.** (**Transient** means temporary or moving, and **bacteremia** means the presence of bacteria in the blood.)

For most healthy patients, this is not a problem since the body is able to quickly destroy the bacteria. However, this is dangerous for high-risk patients such as those with a history of congenital heart disease, rheumatic fever, open-heart surgery, pacemakers, and certain other forms of heart disease and those with an artificial joint such as a hip replacement or with a dental implant.

For these patients, there is danger of **bacterial endocarditis** (bacterial infection of the lining of the heart) or a bacterial infection at the site of the implant. Prophylactic antibiotic administration for these patients is discussed in Chapter 20.

Vector Transmission

A **vector** is an animal or insect that transfers an infective agent from one host to another. In vector transmission there is no direct human-to-human transmission. Instead, a vector is required in order to spread the disease.

Malaria is an excellent example of vector transmission. The disease is spread when an infected human is bitten by a specific type of mosquito. The infected mosquito then spreads the disease when it bites another human. There is no direct person-to-person transmission of malaria.

Ways in Which Disease Can Be Transmitted in the Dental Office

STAFF-TO-PATIENT TRANSMISSION

Infection from a staff member's nose, mouth, or hands may be spread to the patient via airborne transmission or by cross-contamination during treatment.

PATIENT-TO-STAFF TRANSMISSION

Infectious organisms, either airborne or bloodborne, that are sprayed from the patient's mouth can be transmitted to the dentist, hygienist, or assistant through his or her own nose or mouth or through a break in the skin.

PATIENT-TO-PATIENT TRANSMISSION

Patient-to-patient transmission occurs through cross-contamination. This may happen when instruments or materials contaminated during the treatment of one patient are not sterilized or disinfected properly before use in the treatment of another patient.

Body Defenses Against Disease Transmission

Natural Barriers

Intact skin and mucous membranes are the first natural barriers that keep bacteria from entering the body. As long as the skin remains intact, only rare types of bacteria can pass through it.

Bacteria and other particulate material present in the air as it is inhaled are rapidly removed as the air travels through the nasal passages.

Any foreign matter clings to the moist surfaces and minute hairs of the mucous membrane that lines these passages. The mucus of the posterior two-thirds of the nose is replaced every 10 to 15 minutes.

Bacteria and dust particles settling in the eyes are removed by the mechanical flushing effect of tears. Many of the bacteria that enter through the mouth are swallowed and destroyed by the acid environment of the stomach.

The Immune System

The immune system plays an extremely important role in the body's ability to resist pathogens. There are no specialized organs of the immune system; however, specialized cells from the lymphatic system, the thymus, and other body parts all help to provide this protection.

The **thymus** is an endocrine gland that is located just above the heart. It plays roles in both the lymphatic and endocrine systems.

ANTIGEN-ANTIBODY REACTIONS

An **antigen** is a substance such as a virus, bacterium, or other toxic substance that induces (causes) an immune response through the production of antibodies. (A **toxic** substance is a poison.)

Antibodies are substances developed by the body in response to the presence of a specific antigen.

The **antigen-antibody reaction,** also known as the *immune reaction,* involves the binding of antigens to antibodies to form antigen-antibody complexes that may render the toxic antigen harmless.

SPECIALIZED CELLS ASSOCIATED WITH THE IMMUNE REACTION

Lymphocytes

Lymphocytes, which are a type of white blood cell, serve specialized functions in immune responses.

Monocytes, which are lymphocytes that are formed in the bone marrow, are transported to other parts of the body, where they become macrophages. **Macrophages** protect the body by destroying invading bacteria and by interacting with the other cells of the immune system.

B-Lymphocytes. B-lymphocytes, also known as *B-cells,* are also produced in the bone marrow. When confronted with a specific type of antigen, they are transformed into plasma cells.

Plasma cells produce and secrete antibodies. Each antibody is specifically coded to match one antigen. The antibodies made by plasma cells are called **immunoglobulins**.

T-Lymphocytes. T-lymphocytes, also known as *T-cells,* are small lymphocytes that are produced in the bone marrow. They mature in the thymus or as a result of exposure to thymosin, which is secreted by the thymus.

The primary function of T-cells is to indirectly aid cellular immune responses. **Helper T-cells** are a type of T-cell that stimulates the production of antibodies by B-cells. **Suppressor T-cells** are a type of T-cell that suppresses B-cell activity.

The quantities and types of T-cells present in the blood is an important measure of the health of the immune system.

Lymphokines

Lymphokines, which are produced by the T-cells, are molecules other than antibodies that are involved in signaling between the cells of the immune system. The role of lymphokines is to attract macrophages to the site of infection or inflammation and then to prepare them for attack.

Interferon

Interferon, which is also produced by the T-cells, is released by cells that have been invaded by a virus. Interferon induces noninfected cells to form an antiviral protein that inhibits viral multiplication. It also enhances antiviral immunity and is capable of modifying immune responses.

Complement

Complement is a protein substance occurring in normal blood serum. In an antigen-antibody reaction, complement brings about the destruction of a cell by penetrating the cell wall, allowing fluid to fill the cell, and causing the cell to rupture.

THE IMMUNE SYSTEM IN ACTION

The action of the immune system can be described as being in four stages.

Stage One

- Viruses invade the body and seek cells in which they can reproduce.
- Macrophages consume some of the invading viruses.
- Helper T-cells are activated.

Stage Two

- Helper T-cells begin to multiply.
- They attract complement to the area.
- They also stimulate the multiplication of B-cells sensitive to the virus.
- B-cells start producing antibodies.

Stage Three

- Complement proteins break open cells invaded by the virus and spill the viral contents.
- Antibodies produced by the B-cells inactivate the viruses by binding with them.

Stage Four

- As the infection is contained, suppressor T-cells halt the immune response.
- B-cells remain ready in case the same virus invades again.

Immunity

Immunity is a condition of an organism that allows it successfully to resist a specific infection. An individual who produces a large number of antibodies against a bacterium is said to be *resistant*, or *immune*, to infection from that bacterium.

There are two main categories of immunity: natural and acquired.

Natural immunity is immunity with which a person is born: that is, natural antibodies.

Acquired immunity is subdivided into two groups: *naturally acquired immunity* is obtained naturally through having had a disease; *artificially acquired immunity* is obtained through vaccination.

Vaccinations, which are also referred to as *immunizations,* are a major factor in disease prevention. It is extremely important that dental healthcare workers (DHCW) be immunized against vaccine-preventable diseases, including hepatitis B, influenza, measles, mumps, rubella, and tetanus.

Diseases of Major Concern to Dental Healthcare Workers

Hepatitis

Hepatitis, which is an inflammation of the liver, varies in seriousness from a minor flu-like illness to a fatal liver disease. The severity of the disease depends upon the type of hepatitis virus involved and the ability of the host to resist the disease.

Early symptoms of hepatitis often include loss of appetite, nausea and vomiting, jaundice, and fever. (**Jaundice** is yellowish discoloration of the skin and eyes.)

There are at least five types of hepatitis, each of which is caused by a different virus: hepatitis A virus (HAV), hepatitis B virus (HBV), hepatitis C virus (HCV), hepatitis D virus (HDV), and hepatitis E virus (HEV).

HEPATITIS A

Hepatitis A is *not* a bloodborne infection. It is spread via the fecal/oral route, most commonly through contaminated food and water. This is one of the less serious forms of hepatitis.

HEPATITIS B

Hepatitis B is a serious disease that may result in prolonged illness, destruction of liver cells, cirrhosis, and death. It is a bloodborne disease that may also be transmitted by other body fluids, including saliva.

Anyone who has ever had the disease, and some persons who have been exposed but have not been actively ill, may be carriers of the hepatitis B virus. This means that even patients who appear to be healthy and have no history of the disease may be a source of infection. This presents a high risk for dental personnel because dental treatment brings them into contact with saliva and blood.

Also, dental healthcare workers may unknowingly be carriers of the disease. In this situation there is always the risk of transmitting the infection to the patient during treatment.

Hepatitis B Immunization

All dental personnel with occupational exposure should be immunized against the hepatitis B virus. (Determining occupational exposure is described further in Chapter 12.)

Occupational Safety and Health Administration (OSHA) regulations require that the employer offer hepatitis B vaccination, at no cost to the employee, to new employees within 10 days of initial assignment. (This applies only for employees who have occupational exposure.)

A new employee who has been vaccinated must show proof of vaccination. An employee who refuses vaccination must sign a release. There are two hepatitis B vaccines that are widely used: Recombivax HB and Engerix-B.

For long-term protection, a regimen of three doses given at the ages of 0, 1, and 6 months is recommended. To be most effective, the injections should be given in the arm and not in fatty tissue (such as the buttocks).

Post-vaccination testing for the anti–hepatitis B antibodies is recommended and should be performed 1 to 6 months after the third injection. Formation of these antibodies indicates that the individual has developed immunity. Individuals who have been vaccinated but do not develop these antibodies are known as **nonresponders**.

Nonresponders should be given a fourth vaccine dose and retested after 1 month. Should antibodies still not be present, the three-dose series should be repeated; the dose given the previous month is considered the initial dose of the series.

These vaccines are considered safe for pregnant women. Currently there are no recommendations for booster injections; however, this may change.

HEPATITIS C

Hepatitis C is similar to hepatitis B in that the virus is bloodborne and may be present in the carrier state. Transmission is frequently through blood transfusions; however, it can also be transmitted by contact with contaminated blood. At this time, there is no vaccine against hepatitis C.

HEPATITIS D

Hepatitis D is also spread by bloodborne transmission. It can only be present as a co-infection with hepatitis B. Successful vaccination for hepatitis B and use of the other measures to prevent hepatitis B transmission are also successful in preventing a co-infection with hepatitis B.

HEPATITIS E

The hepatitis E virus, which is not bloodborne, is most frequently transmitted in fecal/oral routes through contaminated food or water. The disease occurs most frequently as epidemics in developing countries, and transmission is not a major concern in a standard dental setting.

Human Immunodeficiency Virus Infection

The human immunodeficiency virus is bloodborne. The virus attacks and weakens or destroys the immune system. A blood test can be used to determine the presence of antibodies to HIV before symptoms appear.

A **positive result**, also known as a *seropositive result*, indicates that the individual is infected with HIV, is a carrier, and is capable of transmitting it to others. (As used here, "sero-" refers to serum, which is the liquid portion of blood.)

A **negative result**, also known as a *seronegative result*, means that no infection was present at the time of the test. This does not suggest immunity against the virus.

A dental healthcare worker who becomes HIV positive should notify the dentist/employer immediately so that a decision can be made regarding having this individual continue in providing direct patient care. Currently decisions are made on the basis of a case-by-case evaluation of the circumstances.

HIV AND AIDS

A person may be HIV positive and be asymptomatic. (**Asymptomatic** means not showing any clinical indications.) At this time, there are medical therapies that may delay the progression of the disease; however, they cannot cure it.

As the infection progresses, HIV slowly damages the immune system and weakens the body's defenses against other diseases such as tuberculosis, hepatitis, cancers, and opportunistic diseases.

Later the HIV-positive individual becomes symptomatic (has clinically defined symptoms) and is classified as having AIDS. AIDS is the clinical end point of the HIV infection and results in death. AIDS is discussed in Chapter 11.

ROUTES OF HIV TRANSMISSION

- HIV is transmitted most easily through blood, semen, and vaginal secretions during sexual intercourse. (This is a particular threat to women, who are 10 times more likely than men to become infected in this manner.)
- HIV is transmitted through exposure to shared needles (for drug use) and through tattoo needles.
- HIV is transmitted through accidental exposure to blood that occurs in occupational settings.
- HIV can be transmitted through organ donation, transfusion of contaminated blood or blood products, and commingling of blood in rituals such as becoming "blood brothers."
- HIV can be transmitted by the infected mother to her child during birth or through breast-feeding.

Transmission of HIV itself is a concern, but not a major threat, in the dental setting. However, patients who are HIV-positive often have other diseases that can be transmitted more easily through dental treatment. Transmission of these diseases, particularly tuberculosis and hepatitis B, is a major threat to dental personnel.

TUBERCULOSIS

Tuberculosis, which is caused by the bacterium *Mycobacterium tuberculosis*, is the leading cause of death from infectious diseases worldwide. Although it involves primarily the lungs, it can affect any organ or tissue, including the mouth.

Because HIV-infected patients have a weakened immune system, they are highly susceptible to tuberculosis. Therefore, HIV and tuberculosis are often present together. However, of the two, tuberculosis is a greater health risk for healthcare workers. One reason for this is that the rod-shaped tubercle bacillus is able to withstand disinfectants that kill many other bacteria.

Signs of Tuberculosis

If any of the following signs are present, the dentist should be notified immediately, for it may be necessary to refer the patient for diagnosis and treatment before providing dental care.

- A productive cough lasting more than 3 weeks (in a productive cough, sputum comes up into the mouth; **sputum** is thick mucus from the lungs that is ejected through the mouth)
- Unexplained fever, fatigue, or night sweats
- Unexplained weight loss and anorexia (loss of appetite)
- Being a member of a high-risk group

High-risk group factors include

- Close contact with individuals who have active tuberculosis
- Infections, such as HIV, that weaken the immune system
- Drugs, such as immunosuppressant drugs, that suppress the immune system
- Age (the very young and the very old are less resistant to disease)
- Living in closely confined quarters such as a nursing home or prison
- Other high-risk health factors and behaviors

The Transmission of Tuberculosis

Infected with Active Disease. A patient with the signs described above who is diagnosed with tuberculosis is in the active stage. This patient may easily spread the disease through close contact.

Tuberculosis is spread primarily when the individual coughs and the tubercle bacilli, which are present in the sputum, are expelled through the mouth.

These bacteria are inhaled by other persons and are carried to the lungs. A healthy individual is usually able to fight off the infection; however, someone who is already weakened may become infected.

Infection without Active Disease. Ninety percent of all people who are exposed to tuberculosis belong to this group. They carry the virus but *never* have active symptoms. They do not transmit the disease at this stage; however, if resistance is weakened, the tuberculosis may become active.

After the patient has had the active disease and seems to be well, he will always be a carrier for the disease.

Skin Tests

The tuberculin skin test may be indicated annually for clinical personnel who risk exposure to this disease. However, the test results are not always accurate. When there is any doubt concerning these test results, x-rays and laboratory tests are necessary to establish a more definitive diagnosis.

A **negative** result indicates that the individual has not been exposed to the disease; however, this may be a false negative result. A **positive** result indicates exposure to the disease but does not necessarily always indicate infection with it.

There is no effective form of protective immunization against tuberculosis. There are drugs used to treat the disease; however, these medications are not effective against the newer drug-resistant strains of tuberculosis.

Providing Dental Treatment

Providing dental treatment for patients with active tuberculosis presents special risks, and the dentist will consult with the patient's physician before proceeding with treatment. If possible, dental treatment will be postponed until the patient no longer has symptoms of active tuberculosis.

Of special concern to the dental team is the use of the dental handpiece or an ultrasonic scaler, which will result in airborne particles in the treatment room.

To minimize the risk, the use of the ultrasonic scalers and high-speed handpieces is contraindicated or severely limited. Dental dam is used to isolate the area, and the high-volume oral evacuation (HVE) system is used to reduce the flow of airborne particles.

Herpesvirus Infections

There are four major herpesviruses that affect humans:

- **Herpes simplex virus** (HSV), which is divided into two types: **herpes simplex virus type 1** (HSV1), which causes primarily oral lesions, and **herpes simplex virus type 2** (HSV2), which causes primarily genital lesions
- **Herpes zoster** or **varicella-zoster virus** (HZV), which causes herpes zoster, shingles, and chickenpox
- The **cytomegalovirus** (CMV), which is normally latent (does not produce disease) but may become active when the immune system is damaged (once active, it is highly contagious and is transmitted by most body fluids)
- The **Epstein-Barr virus** (EBV), which causes infectious mononucleosis and Burkitt's lymphoma, which is a malignant neoplasm involving lymphatic tissues

HERPES SIMPLEX VIRUS, TYPE 1

Herpes simplex virus type 1 is a viral infection that causes recurrent sores on lips. Because these sores frequently develop when the patient has a cold or a fever of other origin, the disease has become commonly known as *fever blisters* or *cold sores.*

Primary Herpes

The disease, which is highly contagious, makes its first appearance in very young children, 1 to 3 years of age, and is known as primary herpes.

The child may have a slight fever, pain in the mouth, increased salivation, bad breath, and a general feeling of illness. The inside of the mouth becomes swollen, and the gums are inflamed.

Many lesions appear simultaneously on the lips, inside the cheeks, and on the tongue and gums. These sores are yellow and irregularly shaped. Later in the course of the disease, a red ring of inflammation forms around them.

Only during the first attack of herpes simplex do the sores occur over a widespread area within the mouth, and this attack is also known as **herpetic stomatitis**.

Healing begins naturally within 3 days, and the illness is usually over in 7 to 14 days. During this time, supportive measures can be taken to make the child more comfortable, to relieve the pain, and to prevent secondary infection.

Recurrent Herpes Labialis

After this initial childhood infection, the virus of herpes simplex lies dormant, to reappear later in life as the familiar recurring fever blister or cold sore (Fig. 10–4).

In this second stage of the disease, the characteristic sore usually appears on the *outside* of the patient's lip, at the vermilion border (where the red part of the lip meets the adjoining skin). This manifestation is known as recurrent herpes labialis. A peculiarity of the disease is that in each succeeding attack, the sore always develops in the same place.

A burning sensation, itching, or a feeling of fullness usually is noted about 24 hours before the sore actually appears. The lip becomes swollen and red, and the sore of the herpes is small and covered with a yellow scab.

Recurrences tend to take place when the patient's general resistance is lowered as a result of stress, fever,

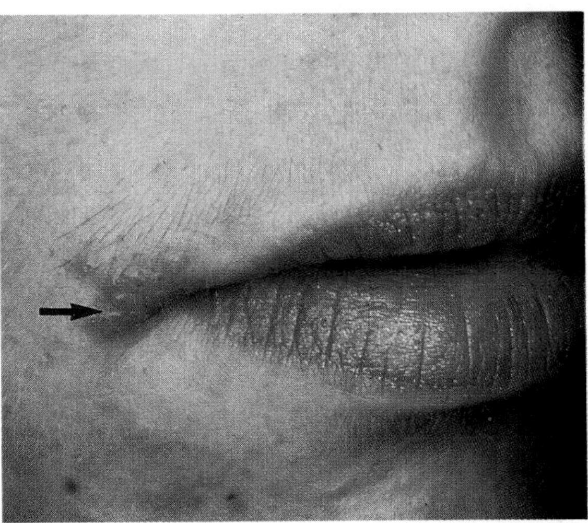

FIGURE 10–4

Herpes labialis of the right commissure. (From Ibsen, O.A., and Phelan, J.A.: Oral Pathology for the Dental Hygienist. Philadelphia, W.B. Saunders Co., 1992, color plate 3.)

illness, injury, and exposure to the sun. The use of sunscreen with a sun protective factor of 15 helps to prevent sun-induced recurrences of herpes.

Attacks may recur as infrequently as once a year or as often as weekly or even daily. As in the case of primary herpes, recurrent herpes labialis sores heal by themselves in 7 to 10 days, leaving no scar.

HERPES SIMPLEX VIRUS, TYPE 2

Herpes simplex virus type 2, also known as *genital herpes*, is one of the most common sexually transmitted diseases in the United States. Initial symptoms, which generally appear 2 to 10 days after infection, include tingling, itching, and a burning sensation during urination.

Within a week, clusters of painful blisters develop on the mucosal tissue of the genital area. These sores eventually become crusty and usually heal without scarring. Once a person is infected, outbreaks will recur even without reinfection. The disease can be transmitted only during these recurrences.

A mother with active vaginal or cervical herpetic lesions at the time of delivery can pass the virus to her newborn. About 50 percent of such newborns are infected as they pass through the birth canal. Of those infants infected, at least 85 percent are severely damaged or killed by the virus.

HERPES TRANSMISSION

The major transmission route for the herpesvirus is through direct contact with lesions. When oral lesions are present, the patient may be asked to reschedule his appointment for a time after the lesions have healed. Even when there are no active lesions, there is still the possibility of transmission through saliva or the aerosol spray from the dental handpiece.

Because there is no preventive vaccine to protect against herpes, it is essential that precautions be taken to prevent exposure.

Protective eyewear is particularly important because a herpes infection in the eye may cause blindness. Gloves protect against infection through lesions or abrasions on the hands.

Tetanus

Tetanus, also known as *lockjaw*, is an extremely dangerous and often fatal disease that is caused by a spore-forming bacillus found in soil, dust, or animal or human feces.

This microbe is usually introduced into the body through a wound or break in the skin (as in a puncture wound from a soiled instrument).

The organism causing tetanus produces severe muscle spasms and rigidity that give the disease its popular name, lockjaw. The disease can be prevented by the administration of a vaccine; however, immunity must be kept current through booster doses. (It is important that dental personnel keep all of the immunizations current.)

Measles

Measles, which may be prevented by the administration of a vaccine, is a potentially serious viral disease.

It is easily spread by airborne transmission and has an incubation period of 10 to 12 days. The disease is characterized by a rash; however, the first symptoms are a cough and fever.

Three to four days before the appearance of the rash, patches called **Koplik's spots** may appear in the oral cavity. These patches are small, irregular in shape, and red with bluish-white specks and are located on the mucosa of the cheeks and lips. The disease is highly contagious at this stage.

Rubella

Rubella, known as *German measles* or *3-day measles*, is a mild form of measles usually characterized by a slight rash and swollen glands. Rubella may be prevented by the administration of a vaccine.

The danger from rubella is to women, particularly during the first trimester of pregnancy. If the mother has rubella, she runs the risk of giving birth to a child who is severely deformed, mentally retarded, deaf, blind, or stillborn.

Mumps

Mumps is a viral infection that causes inflammation and swelling of the parotid glands and sometimes the submandibular salivary glands. It is accompanied by headache, chills, fever, and swelling of the neck and cheek.

The swelling starts below the lobe of the ear and may involve the entire cheek as it spreads from the angle of the jaw to the corner of the eye. There is usually pain when the patient attempts to open his mouth. Mumps can be prevented by the administration of a vaccine.

Syphilis

Syphilis, a sexually transmitted disease, is caused by *Treponema pallidum* spirochetes. Although these are quite fragile outside of the body, there is danger of direct cross-infection in the dental operatory, through contact with oral lesions.

The **first stage** of syphilis is the presence of a painless ulcerating sore, known as a **chancre**, which is infectious *on contact*. When it occurs on the lip, it may resemble herpes, but the crusting is darker.

A person may contract syphilis and, at first, be unaware that he has the disease. Also, because the primary lesions heal by themselves, he may believe he is cured.

The **second stage** is also infectious, and immediate infection may occur through contact with an open sore. Signs of special interest to dental personnel are

- Split papules at the corners of the mouth
- Grayish-white, moist, so-called mucous patches on the tongue, roof of the mouth, tonsils, or inner surfaces of the lips (these are *highly infectious*)
- Generalized measles-type rash, poxlike pustules, oozing sores, and falling out of hair

The **third stage**, known as *latent syphilis,* is usually fatal, and it may occur after the disease has been dormant for 20 years. In this stage, **gumma** nodules may form on the tongue or palate. A pattern of ulceration and healing of the hard palate may eventually lead to perforation.

Preventing Disease Transmission

The prevention of disease transmission is of utmost importance in the dental office. To do this, it is necessary to break the chain of infection, which consists of four parts: (1) virulence, (2) numbers, (3) a susceptible host, and (4) a portal of entry (Fig. 10–5).

Virulence

The goal is to prevent coming into contact with these virulent pathogens. One step is to have a complete and up-to-date medical history on each patient. Another step is to always follow the infection control protocols, which are discussed in Chapter 13.

Numbers

These pathogens must be present is quantities sufficient to overwhelm most body defenses. The number

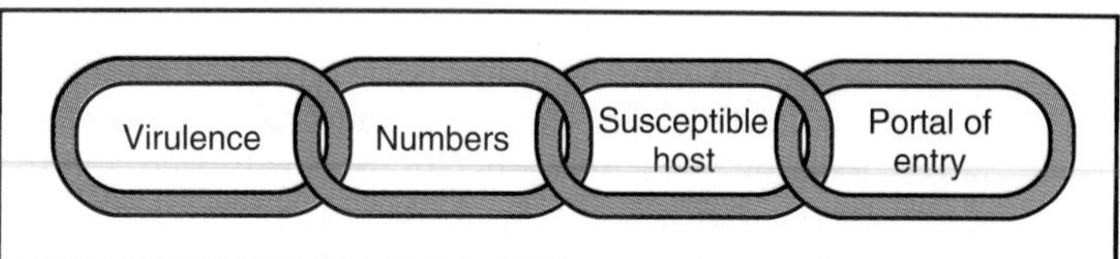

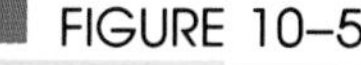

FIGURE 10–5

To break the chain of infection, at least one part must be removed.

of pathogens may be directly related to the bioburden present. (**Bioburden** refers to organic by-products that may contaminate the surface of an object.)

Sterilization of all dental instruments used in the patient's mouth and the disinfection of all materials or surfaces contaminated during treatment help to reduce these numbers.

Also, dental dam and the high-volume oral evacuation (HVE) system are used to minimize and control the blood-contaminated aerosol created by the high-speed handpiece during treatment.

Before treatment, some dentists have a patient rinse his mouth with an antiseptic mouth rinse. The purpose of this is to reduce the number of microorganisms present in the patient's mouth.

Susceptible Host

A susceptible host is one who is unable to resist infection by the pathogen. An individual who is in poor health, is chronically fatigued and under extreme stress, or has a compromised immune system as a result of other causes is likely to be susceptible to disease.

Staying healthy, frequent handwashing, and keeping immunizations up-to-date improve the possibility of resisting infection.

Portal of Entry

The pathogens must find an appropriate portal of entry into the body. (**Portal** means door or means of entering.) The portals of entry for airborne pathogens are the nose and mouth.

Bloodborne pathogens must have access to the blood supply. Their portal of entry may be through a disruption of the blood stream (when there is bleeding). More commonly, access may be through a break in the skin via a cut, a sore, an abrasion, or an accidental injection (such as a needlestick injury).

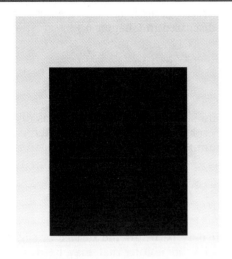

Chapter 11

Oral Pathology

Introduction

Pathology is the study of disease. It is important that dental personnel be able to recognize pathological conditions in the mouth, realize how they impact the patient's general health and dental treatment, and understand how to prevent their transmission. (Modes of disease transmission are discussed in Chapter 10. Infection control measures, to prevent disease transmission, are discussed in Chapter 13.)

Inflammation and Healing

Inflammation

Acute inflammation is the immediate and localized protective response of the body to physical injury or to the invasion of pathogenic organisms. In contrast, **chronic inflammation** is a slow, ongoing process that may result in permanent tissue damage.

The four cardinal signs of inflammation, which are caused primarily by the increased amount of blood in the affected area, are (1) redness, (2) edema (swelling), (3) heat, and (4) pain. Purposes of inflammation are as follows:

- The initial purpose of inflammation is to destroy the irritating or injurious agent and to remove it and its by-products from the body.
- If this is not possible, the inflammatory process limits the spread of the causative agent and its harmful effects throughout the body.
- Finally, inflammation is the mechanism for the repair or replacement of tissues damaged or destroyed by the offending agent.

Healing and Repair

Healing is the body's process of repairing or replacing the injured tissues. This process begins with inflammation.

The site of inflammation is quickly filled and surrounded by a continuous network of fibrin fibers, which are formed by fibrinogen during the normal clotting of blood. At the edges of the infected area, the fibroblasts (connective tissue cells) begin to grow among these fibers. (Clotting is discussed in Chapter 3.)

Soon the entire inflammatory area is surrounded by a wall or sac of fibrin and fibrous connective tissues that tends to confine the inflammatory process and to prevent its spread.

HEALING AFTER ORAL SURGERY

With a complex injury, such as the extraction of a tooth, several steps are required before the healing process is complete; however, the healing process begins immediately after surgery.

The first stage is the formation of a clot in the tooth socket to control bleeding and protect the exposed bone. If the process is not disturbed, this occurs within a few minutes.

If infection or uncontrolled bleeding is present initially, the normal mechanism of post-surgical healing will be out of balance. As a result, the clot may fail to form normally and healing may take longer.

The clot normally remains in place for 6 to 7 days and then is naturally sloughed away. By the seventh day, granulation tissue, which is newly formed soft tissue, replaces the clot. In time, tough connective tissue replaces the granulation tissue.

The trabeculae of new bone are formed in the socket in approximately 37 to 38 days. The complete regeneration of bone at the site of the surgery takes several months.

Types of Oral Lesions

Lesions are observable variations from the normal. **Lesion** is a broad term that includes wounds, sores, and any other tissue damage caused by either injury or disease. Characterizing the type of lesion present in a disease is one of the earliest steps in formulating a differential diagnosis.

Lesions of the oral mucosa may be classified as to whether they extend *below* the surface, extend *above* the surface, or are *flat* or *even* with the surface.

Lesions Extending Below the Surface

An **ulcer** is a defect or break in continuity of the mucosa so that a punched-out area similar to a crater exists. An ulcer may be small (2 mm.) or quite large (several centimeters).

An **erosion** of the soft tissue is a shallow defect in the mucosa caused by mechanical trauma, such as in chewing. (**Trauma** means wound or injury.) The margins may be ragged and red and quite painful.

An **abscess** is a localized collection of pus in a circumscribed area. (**Circumscribed** means within a limited area.) Periapical and periodontal abscesses are discussed later in this chapter.

A **cyst** is a closed sac or pouch lined with epithelium that contains fluid or semisolid material. The material within the cyst is not always infectious. In dentistry, a cyst may contain the crown of an unerupted tooth.

Lesions Above the Surface

Blisters, also known as *vesicles*, are sharply circumscribed lesions filled with a watery fluid. They are rarely seen in the oral cavity because they tend to rupture, leaving ulcers with ragged edges.

A **pustule** is similar to a blister but contains pus. A **hematoma** is similar to a blister but contains blood.

A **plaque** is any patch or flat area that is slightly raised from the surface. (This is *not* the same as dental plaque, which is discussed in Chapter 6.)

Lesions That Are Flat or Even with the Surface

These lesions are sharply circumscribed areas of discoloration. An **ecchymosis**, the technical term for bruising, is an example of this type of lesion.

Lesions That May Be Either Raised or Flat

Nodules, which may be below the surface or slightly elevated, are small solid lesions that may be detected by touch.

Granuloma is a term with many meanings. In dentistry, it is commonly used to describe a type of nodule that contains granulation tissue. (The suffix *-oma* means tumor or neoplasm.)

A granuloma may appear on the gingival surface as a swollen mass, or it may be located within the bone as a periapical granuloma at the apex of a nonvital tooth.

Tumors, also known as *neoplasms*, are defined as any growth of tissue that exceeds the normal form, is uncoordinated with the other body processes, and serves no useful purpose to the host.

A tumor may be **benign** (not life-threatening) or **malignant** (life-threatening). These are discussed further in the section "Oral Cancer."

Disturbances in Development of the Jaws

Macrognathia and Micrognathia

Macrognathia is a condition characterized by abnormally large jaws. (The prefix *macro-* means abnormally large. The word part *gnathia* means jaw.) Most commonly this occurs in the mandible, and the result is a Class III malocclusion.

Micrognathia is a condition characterized by abnormally small jaws. (The prefix *micro-* means abnormally small.) Most commonly this occurs in the mandible, and the result is a Class II malocclusion.

Exostoses

An exostosis is a benign bony growth projecting outward from the surface of a bone. (*Exostosis* is singular. The plural is *exostoses.*) An exostosis may also be referred to as a torus. (A **torus** is a bulging projection. The plural is *tori.*)

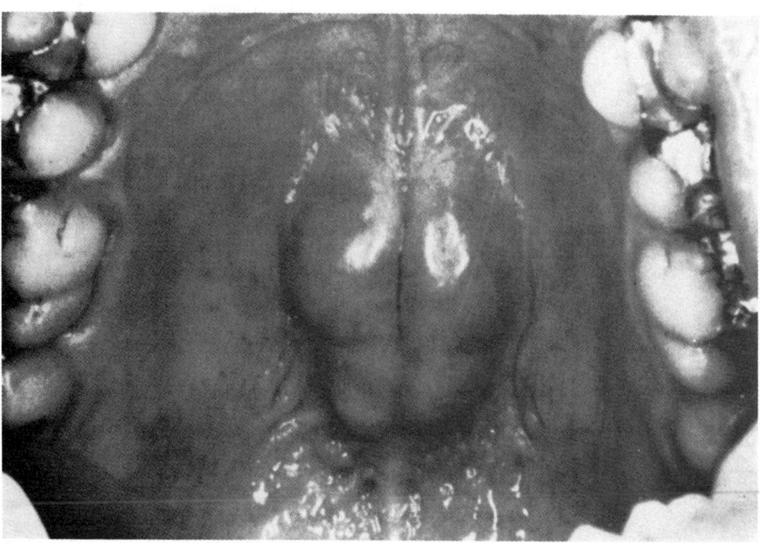

FIGURE 11–1

Torus palatinus. (From Regezi, J.A., and Sciubba, J.J.: Oral Pathology. Philadelphia, W.B. Saunders Co., 1989, p 387.)

A **torus palatinus** is a bony overgrowth in the midline of the hard palate (Fig. 11–1). A **torus mandibularis** is a bony overgrowth on the lingual aspect of the mandible near the premolar and molar areas (Fig. 11–2).

These growths are not harmful; however, it may be necessary to remove them so that a full or partial denture may be placed and comfortably retained.

Disturbances in Dental Development

Disturbances in any stage of dental development may cause a wide variety of anomalies. (An **anomaly** is an abnormality or marked deviation from the normal.)

Normal dental development is discussed in Chapter 4. Cleft palate, which is a disturbance in the development of the hard and soft palates, is discussed in Chapter 8.

An **ameloblastoma** is a tumor made up of remnants of the dental lamina that failed to disintegrate after the tooth buds were formed.

Anodontia is the congenital absence of teeth. It may be partial or total and may affect the primary or the permanent dentition or both. This classification includes congenitally missing teeth. Most commonly involved are third molars, followed by maxillary lateral incisors and second premolars (Fig. 11–3).

Patterns of anodontia tend to be hereditary and may be associated with ectodermal dysplasia (Fig. 11–4). (**Ectodermal dysplasia** is a group of hereditary disorders involving tissues, such as enamel, that are derived from the embryonic ectoderm layer.)

Supernumerary teeth are any teeth in excess of the 32 normal permanent teeth. These teeth may be normal in size and shape; however, they are most frequently small and poorly developed (Fig. 11–5).

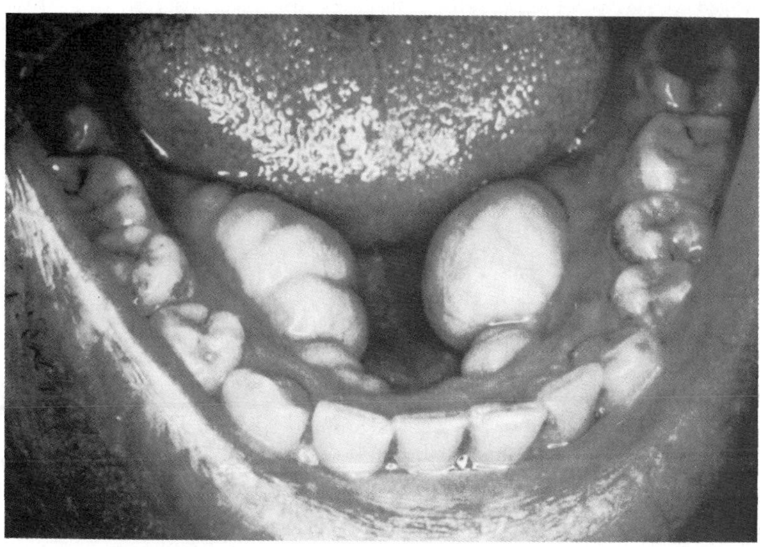

FIGURE 11–2

Torus mandibularis. (From Regezi, J.A., and Sciubba, J.J.: Oral Pathology. Philadelphia, W.B. Saunders Co., 1989, p 388.)

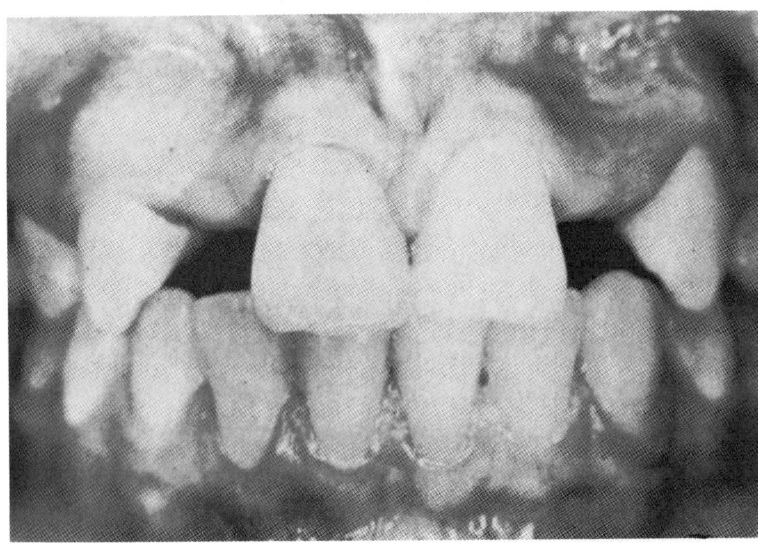

FIGURE 11–3

Congenitally missing maxillary lateral incisors. (From Regezi, J.A., and Sciubba, J.J.: Oral Pathology. Philadelphia, W.B. Saunders Co., 1989, p 469.)

Macrodontia is the term used to describe abnormally large teeth. It may affect the entire dentition or may be manifested in only two teeth such as the maxillary central incisors.

Microdontia is the term used to describe abnormally small teeth. When microdontia affects an entire dentition, it is frequently associated with other defects, such as congenital heart disease or Down syndrome.

Dens in dente, also known as *a tooth within a tooth,* is a developmental anomaly that results in the formation of a small toothlike mass of enamel and dentin within the pulp. Radiographically, this resembles a tooth within a tooth.

Variation in form may include extra, missing, or fused cusps or anomalies of roots; however, the most common variations are in the form of peg-shaped teeth.

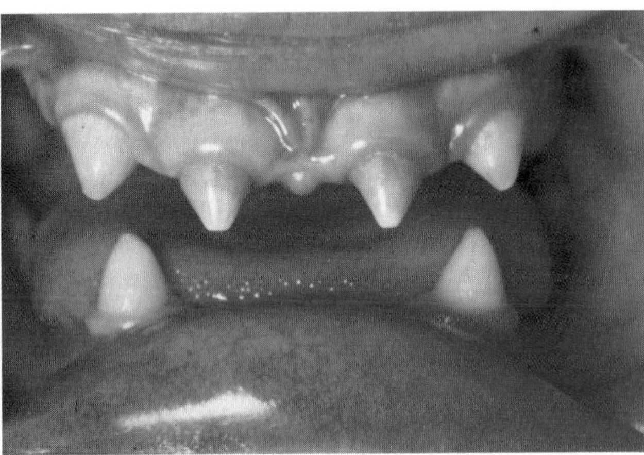

FIGURE 11–4

Partial anodontia in a patient with hereditary ectodermal dysplasia.

Hutchinson's incisors, a variety of peg-shaped teeth, are usually associated with maternal syphilis (Fig. 11–6).

Fusion is the joining together of the dentin and enamel of two or more separate developing teeth. Fusion of teeth leads to a reduced number of teeth in the dental arch (Fig. 11–7).

Gemination is an attempt by the tooth bud to divide. When this attempt is not successful, it is indicated by an incisal notch.

Twinning means that the tooth bud division is complete, and the result is the formation of an extra tooth. This tooth is usually a mirror image of its adjacent partner in the dental arch.

Defects in Enamel Formation

Amelogenesis imperfecta is a hereditary abnormality in which there are hypoplasia-type defects in the enamel formation, hypocalcification-type defects in enamel calcification, or both. (The prefix *hypo-* means decreased or deficient. **Hypoplasia** is the incomplete or deficient development of an organ or tissue. **Hypocalcification** is the incomplete calcification or hardening of a tissue such as the enamel of a tooth.)

Hereditary enamel hypoplasia is a type of amelogenesis imperfecta that is characterized by teeth with crowns that are hard and glossy, yellow, and cone-shaped or cylindrical. However, the enamel of these teeth fails to harden properly. Instead, it remains soft and is soon lost because of mechanical stresses.

In contrast, **environmental hypoplasia** is caused by injury to the ameloblasts during development. It is characterized by pitting or grooving of the enamel at the same levels on all teeth forming at that time.

This may be caused by fever, illness, or trauma to the individual (or to the mother if the damage occurred during prenatal development). The scarring of the enamel is permanent, easily recognized clinically,

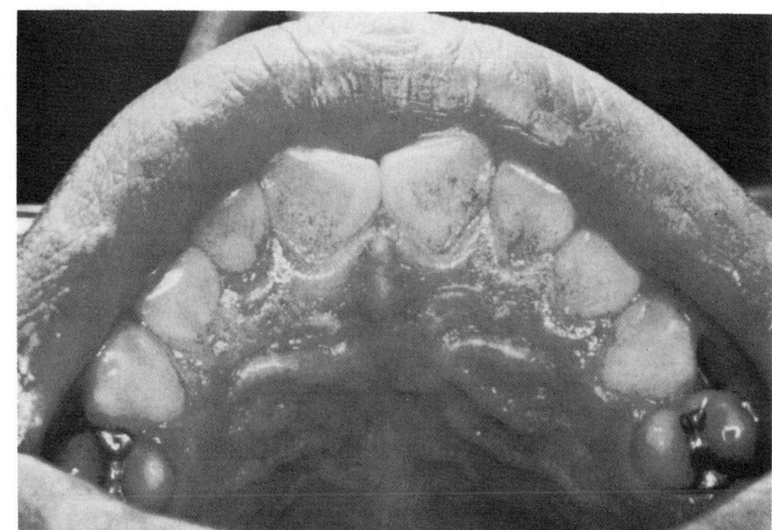

FIGURE 11–5

Supernumerary incisor teeth. (From Regezi, J.A., and Sciubba, J.J.: Oral Pathology. Philadelphia, W.B. Saunders Co., 1989, p 471.)

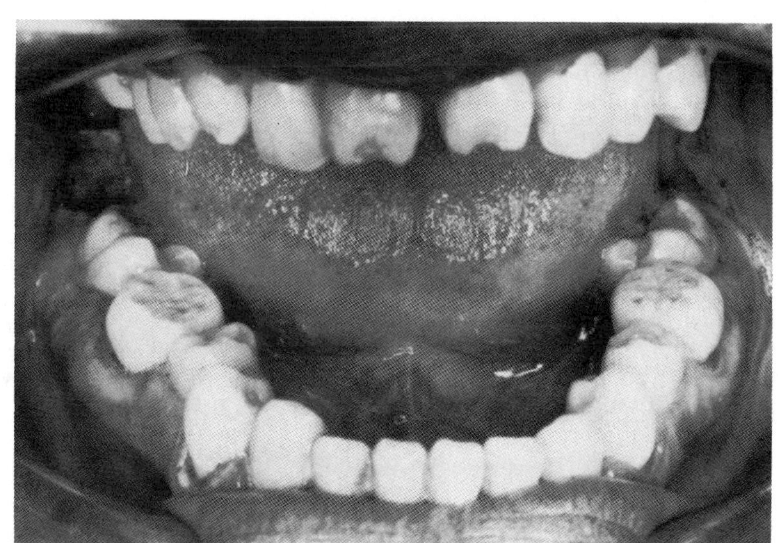

FIGURE 11–6

Notched "Hutchinson" incisors. (From Regezi, J.A., and Sciubba, J.J.: Oral Pathology. Philadelphia, W.B. Saunders Co., 1989, p 36.)

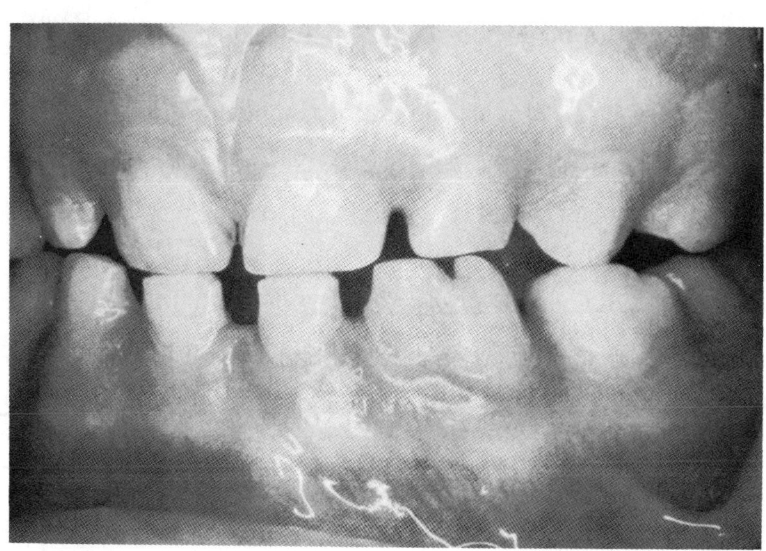

FIGURE 11–7

Fusion of primary incisor and cuspid. (From Regezi, J.A., and Sciubba, J.J.: Oral Pathology. Philadelphia, W.B. Saunders Co., 1989, p 463.)

and readily assessed chronologically (on the basis of the age at which the damage occurred).

Defects in Dentin Formation

Dentinogenesis imperfecta is a hereditary condition that affects dentin formation and is found in both the primary and permanent dentition.

Clinically, it is characterized by opalescent, almost amber teeth that have a normal contour upon eruption; however, very soon the enamel tends to chip away from the dentin and the teeth become worn down.

Abnormal Eruption of the Teeth

PREMATURE ERUPTION

Natal teeth are those teeth present at birth. **Neonatal teeth** are those that erupt within the first 30 days of life. The teeth most commonly involved are the mandibular incisors. Because of the lack of root formation, these teeth are soon shed if they are not removed.

ANKYLOSIS

Ankylosis of a tooth is the abnormal fusion (joining together) of cementum or dentin with the alveolar bone. When an ankylosis has been established between tooth and bone, the growth in height of the alveolar process stops in the affected area. Also, the tooth does not continue to erupt and move occlusally.

However, alveolar growth and movement toward occlusion continue for the neighboring teeth. This causes the ankylosed tooth to have a submerged appearance so that it seems to be "pressed down" into the jaw. As growth continues, the neighboring teeth will tilt over the ankylosed tooth.

IMPACTIONS

Impaction is the term used to describe any tooth that remains unerupted in the jaws beyond the time at which it should normally be erupted (Fig. 11–8). Impaction may be caused by

- Premature loss of primary teeth
- Shifting of the developing tooth into a horizontal or other abnormal position
- Shifting of the developing tooth into a position from which it cannot erupt because of the presence of other teeth, lack of jaw space, or abnormally large tooth crowns

Impactions and their treatment are discussed further in Chapter 30.

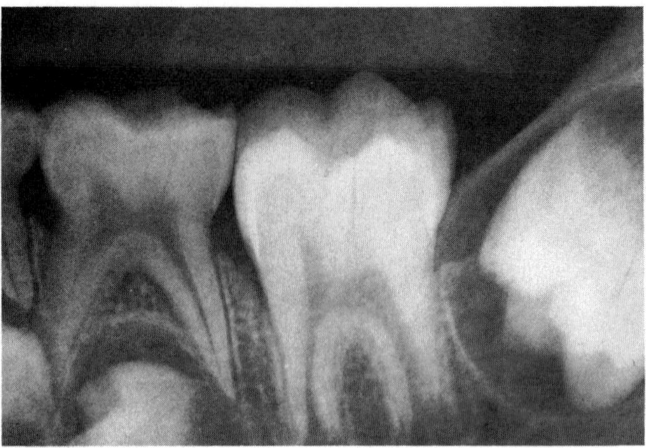

FIGURE 11–8

Impactions in mixed dentition. The primary second molar is still in place and the permanent first molar has erupted. The permanent second premolar and the permanent second molar are impacted.

Abnormal Wear of the Teeth

ATTRITION

Physiological attrition is the gradual and regular wearing away of tooth substance as a result of chewing. It affects the incisal, occlusal, and interproximal surfaces.

Pathological attrition is abnormal wear that is confined to a single tooth or a group of teeth and is caused by abnormal function or position of teeth. Excessive attrition of the chewing surfaces may result from bruxism, from excessive chewing of tobacco or gum, or from other oral habits.

ABRASION

Abrasion, which is not caused by chewing, is the pathological wearing away of dental hard tissue substance by the friction of a foreign body. The most prevalent type of abrasion is caused by improper toothbrushing.

Abrasion may also be caused by habits such as opening hairpins with the teeth, excessive pipe smoking (with the pipe clenched between the teeth), or the mechanical action of the clasps of ill-fitting partial dentures.

EROSION

Dental erosion is the superficial loss of dental hard tissue by a chemical process that does not involve bacteria. Erosions are usually located in the gingival third of the facial surfaces of the teeth, especially the maxillary incisors.

Erosions may be idiopathic (of unknown origin) or may be caused by a known acid source, such as that seen in bulimic individuals (who vomit frequently).

Cementoclasia is the erosion of cementum caused by excessive trauma of faulty occlusion, by excessive pressure during orthodontic treatment, and by diseases.

Hypercementosis, or abnormal thickening of the cementum, may be local or general and may result from chronic inflammation or lack of an antagonist. (The prefix *hyper-* means increased or excessive.)

ABNORMAL RESORPTION

Absorption is the body's process of removing existing bone or hard tissue tooth structure. The resorption of the roots in primary teeth occurs naturally and is considered normal. All other types of resorption are abnormal.

The traumatic causes of resorption are of a mechanical, chemical, or thermal nature, and resorption is often found in impacted teeth.

The replantation of avulsed teeth is also often complicated by their subsequent root resorption (Fig. 11–9). (An **avulsed** tooth is one that has been torn or knocked out of its socket. This is discussed further in Chapter 27.)

Inflammation of the pulp can cause **internal resorption** of the internal hard structures of the tooth. The tooth with internal resorption is usually asymptomatic, but may have a "pink" appearance, which is caused by the decomposition of the pulp tissue within the tooth. (**Asymptomatic** means without symptoms.)

Abnormal resorption is most frequently diagnosed by radiographs, because dental resorption rarely causes disturbing symptoms; however, immediate endodontic treatment is required in order to stop the progression of the internal resorption.

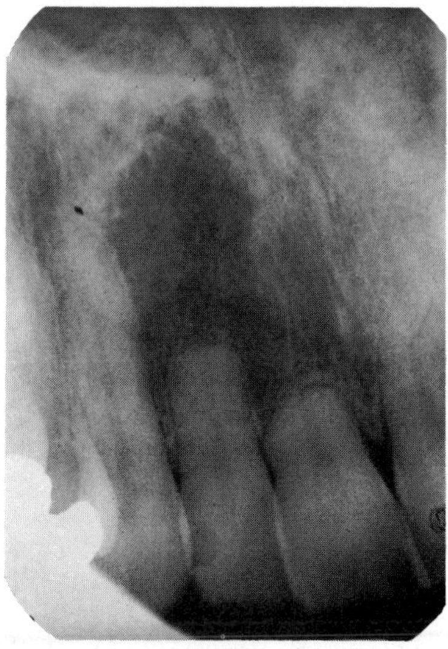

FIGURE 11–9

Abnormal resorption of the maxillary right central and lateral incisors. (Radiograph courtesy of Dr. Stephen N. Bender.)

Diseases of the Teeth

Fluorosis

Fluorosis, which is also known as *mottled enamel,* is caused by the ingestion of excessive amounts of fluorides. Fluorosis is most likely to occur in areas where the water is naturally fluoridated and contains amounts of fluoride that far exceed the recommended fluoride level for water, of 1 part per million (ppm).

However, it may be caused by excessive fluorides from other sources such as repeatedly eating fluoridated toothpaste or swallowing topical fluoride solutions.

Fluorosis is most common among children who ingest excessive amounts of fluoride during enamel formation and calcification. This is during the period from the third month of gestation through the eighth year of life.

The severity in the appearance of teeth discolored by fluorosis may range from minor to severe involvement. Severe involvement may appear as a pitted, brown-stained surface (Fig. 11–10). Minor involvement is characterized by discoloration or intermittent white flecking or spotting on the enamel (Fig. 11–11).

Dental Caries

Dental caries is a disease caused by the activity of bacteria and their by-products in dental plaque. The bacteria involved are *Streptococcus mutans* and lactobacilli. This destructive process, which is commonly referred to as **decay**, involves the hard structures of the teeth that are exposed in the oral cavity.

As with other forms of infection control, steps to control caries include reducing the number of bacteria (through plaque removal and by limiting the food supply) and increasing host resistance (strengthening the tooth with fluorides). These control steps are discussed further in Chapter 6.

Caries is characterized by the disintegration of enamel, dentin, and cementum, leading to the formation of open lesions, which are commonly known as **cavities**.

When the decay process reaches the dentin, it spreads rapidly in all directions and may widely undermine the enamel. This often occurs without any visible changes until extensive destruction has taken place. Unless arrested, the caries continues to spread through the dentin into the pulp of the tooth.

INCIPIENT CARIES

Incipient caries, also known as *white lesions,* is the beginning stage of dental decay, and it affects only the enamel of the tooth. (**Incipient** means beginning.)

Incipient caries develops as decalcification (the loss of minerals in the enamel) progresses. If that process is halted at this point, the tooth can repair itself through

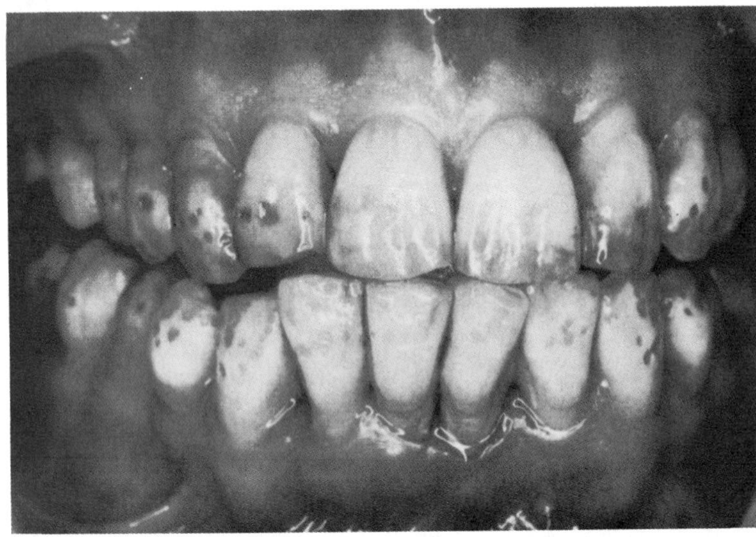

FIGURE 11–10

Enamel hypoplasia resulting from excessive levels of fluoride in drinking water. (From Regezi, J.A., and Sciubba, J.J.: Oral Pathology. Philadelphia, W.B. Saunders Co., 1989, p 475.)

remineralization (the replacement of these minerals by the body). The processes of decalcification and remineralization are described in Chapter 6.

ARRESTED CARIES

Arrested caries is a carious lesion that does not show any marked tendency for further progression. However, once enamel is lost to this extent, it can never form again.

Thus the manifestation of caries persists throughout the life of the affected tooth and may require repair through restorative dentistry.

ROOT CARIES

Gingival recession, particularly in older patients, may expose the cementoenamel junction (CEJ) and the cementum of the root. This exposed area is susceptible to decay. These lesions are known as *root caries* (Fig. 11–12). A lesion in this area that is not caused by decay is referred to as a **cervical abrasion** or **cervical erosion.**

RAMPANT CARIES

Rampant caries is the term used to describe a mouth in which there is widespread decay. This is usually found in high-risk patients. (This is discussed in Chapter 6.)

Baby Bottle Mouth. Rampant dental decay in a baby or toddler, known as baby bottle mouth (BBM) or *nursing bottle syndrome* (NBS), occurs when a bottle containing sweetened liquid is given to the infant frequently, especially before sleep.

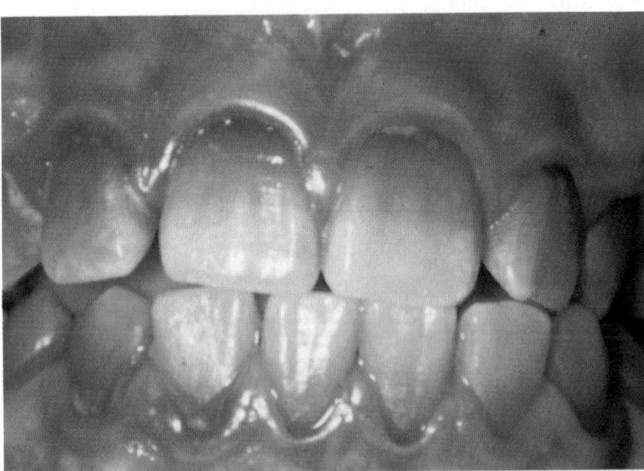

FIGURE 11–11

Discoloration of the teeth caused by the intake of excessive fluorides. (This patient also has poor oral hygiene and a periodontal problem.)

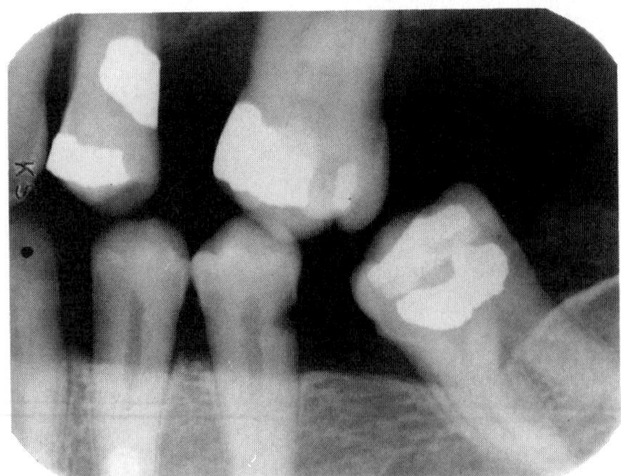

FIGURE 11–12

Root caries appears as a crater-shaped radiolucency just below the cementoenamel junction on the mandibular second premolar. As a result of the loss of the first molar, the second molar is drifting mesially and the maxillary molar has extruded. (From Haring, J.I., and Lind, L.J.: Radiographic Interpretation for the Dental Hygienist. Philadelphia, W.B. Saunders, 1993, p 115.)

Sugar in the liquid mixes with bacteria in dental plaque to form acid, which attacks the enamel. When children are awake, the action of saliva tends to carry away the liquid. During sleep, however, little saliva is produced, and the acid remains in contact with tooth enamel because the liquid tends to pool around the infant's teeth.

If a child must have a bedtime bottle for comfort, the bottle should be filled with cool water. The parents may want to consider a pacifier instead. However, the pacifier should never be dipped in honey or other sweets, for this sugar can be just as damaging as that in the nursing bottle.

RECURRENT CARIES

Recurrent caries is decay occurring beneath the margin of an existing dental restoration. This is caused most frequently by wear of the restoration or microleakage between the restoration and the tooth. (**Microleakage** is a microscopically small opening between the tooth and restoration that allows fluids and debris to seep downward into the tooth and cause recurrent decay.)

Dentin Hypersensitivity

Dentin hypersensitivity is a common intermittent sensation that affects many people when they eat, drink, or touch their teeth.

The pain can be caused by mechanical, chemical, thermal, or bacterial stimuli. The tooth can become sensitive after enamel loss that follows occlusal wear, toothbrush abrasion, or chemical erosion. Sensitivity also results from exposure of the root surface, which is caused by gingival recession.

Home treatments for dentin hypersensitivity include the use of a desensitizing toothpaste containing potassium nitrate. Topical fluoride rinses are also recommended.

If these steps fail, the dentist may apply a desensitizing agent to occlude (seal) the open ends of the exposed dentinal tubules. In severe cases, the dentist may place a composite restoration with a glass ionomer base.

Diseases of the Dental Pulp

Despite being protected by the dentin that completely surrounds it, the delicate tissue of dental pulp is subject to irritation or injury in several ways:

- **Deep carious lesions** that expose the pulp to the invasion of microorganisms
- **Trauma** (injury) such as a blow to the tooth or improper occlusion
- **Deep cavity or crown preparations** that may injure the pulp through exposure, drying, or irritation caused by the action of the handpiece
- **Chemical irritation** from chemicals found in cavity cleaners, acid etching agents, cements, and filling materials, which can cause pulpal inflammation
- **Thermal damage** such as excessive heat during a cavity preparation

The pulpal reaction to injury depends on the nature of the injury, the degree of pulpal damage, and the vitality of the pulp.

Hyperemia

The initial response of the pulp to shock or irritation is **hyperemia,** which is an increase of blood in the small arteries of the pulp. The presence of larger-than-normal amounts of blood within the pulp chamber creates pressure on the nerve fibers that is often severe enough to produce pain.

Hyperemia is usually temporary, and the pulp returns to normal if the irritation is removed as quickly as possible. However, if the irritation remains, progressive destructive changes take place, and permanent damage may result. Hyperemia may be caused by

- Cold, such as when very cold food or air comes in contact with the tooth
- Galvanic shock, which happens when two dissimilar metals come into contact in the mouth
- Injury due to biting on something hard
- Decay or fracture of the tooth
- The irritation that may accompany preparation or treatment of the tooth
- The trauma of occluding with a restoration that is not carved properly (too high)

Pulpitis

Pulpitis is an inflammation of the pulp, which is usually accompanied by pain. It may have many causes; however, not all toothache is the result of pulpitis. (The differential diagnostic tests used by the dentist are discussed in Chapter 29.)

Pulpitis may be divided into two general groups: **reversible pulpitis**, in which the pulp will recover, and **irreversible pulpitis**, in which the pulp will not recover.

REVERSIBLE PULPITIS

Reversible pulpitis occurs when the pulp becomes slightly inflamed as the result of a temporary irritation of the dentinal tubules. This may be caused by restorative procedures, periodontal curettage, or cervical erosion.

The patient experiences sharp pain when the tooth is exposed to hot or cold liquids or to air. When the stimulus is removed, the patient experiences immediate relief.

The pulp usually heals itself once the cause of the irritation has been removed or corrected.

IRREVERSIBLE PULPITIS

Irreversible pulpitis occurs when the pulp cannot heal itself or when the irritation continues or becomes more severe. The degree of pulpal inflammation can range from mild to severe, which results in irreversible pulpal damage and eventually necrosis of the pulp (pulp death).

Most commonly this occurs when bacteria from a carious lesion pass through the dentinal tubules and enter the pulp. The active growth of these microorganisms in the pulp produces rapid destructive changes and a build-up of pressure.

Irreversible pulpitis can be asymptomatic (without pain); however, when there is pain, it may take many different forms. The pain may be sharp or dull, pulsating or constant, and localized or diffuse, and it may last only minutes or for hours.

The application of cold to the tooth with irreversible pulpitis often brings relief from the pain. After the diagnosis of irreversible pulpitis has been made, the only choice for treatment is endodontic therapy or extraction.

HYPERPLASTIC PULPITIS

Hyperplastic pulpitis is a form of irreversible pulpitis that may occur in a young tooth that has severe caries (Fig. 11–13.) Here the chronically inflamed pulp becomes hyperplastic (overgrown) and forms a bulbous mass, called a **pulp polyp**, that looks like reddish cauliflower-like growths within the decayed crown.

Hyperplastic pulpitis is usually painless and may be discovered during the clinical examination. It may be treated with either a pulpotomy (Chapter 27) or endodontic therapy (Chapter 29).

NECROTIC PULP

Necrotic pulp refers to the death of a dental pulp. (**Necrosis** means the death of tissue in a localized area.) The pulp may die because of bacterial invasion, or death may be caused by a blow to the tooth that disrupts the nerve and blood supply.

APICAL PERIODONTITIS

Apical periodontitis is an inflammation of the periodontal tissues at the apex of a non-vital (dead) tooth, and the patient experiences pain from the slightest pressure on the tooth.

Apical periodontitis is caused by the contaminants from the diseased pulp that have spread down the pulp canal, out through the apex of the tooth, and into the hard and soft tissues of the jaw.

PERIAPICAL ABSCESS

A periapical abscess, which occurs when apical periodontitis is left untreated, is a circumscribed (localized) collection of pus surrounding the apex of the root tip. (This is not the same as a periodontal abscess, which is discussed later in this chapter.)

As the abscess forms, pressure from the swelling and pus at the root end pushes the tooth upward in its socket, making it feel high and sensitive to touch. The abscess in this acute stage is marked by local bone and soft tissue destruction, which appears as a radiolucency on a radiograph (Fig. 11–14).

If the accumulated pus at the end of the tooth finds no pathway for immediate drainage, the jaw may swell, and the patient will have extreme pain.

Over time, if the tooth has not been treated, spontaneous drainage may occur through the bone and mucosa adjacent to the root end of the abscessed tooth. The pathway through which the pus has burrowed through the alveolus in order to drain into the mouth is called a **fistula**.

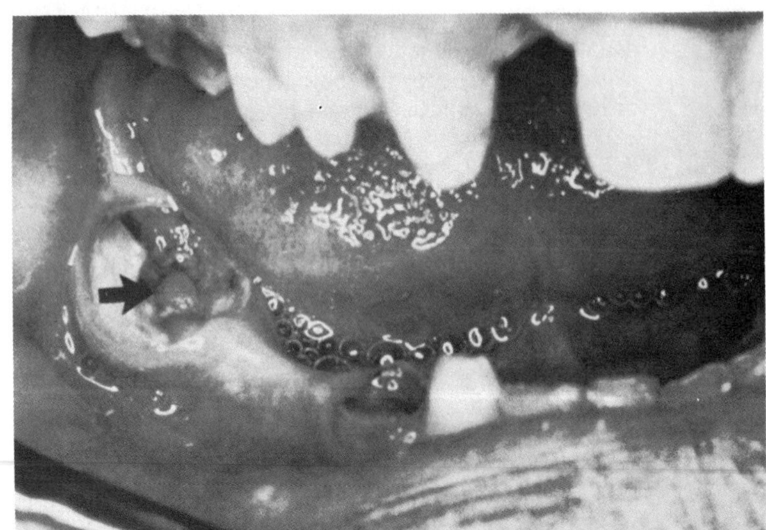

FIGURE 11–13

Hyperplastic pulpitis of first permanent molar. (From Regezi, J.A., and Sciubba, J.J.: Oral Pathology. Philadelphia, W.B. Saunders Co., 1989, p 392.)

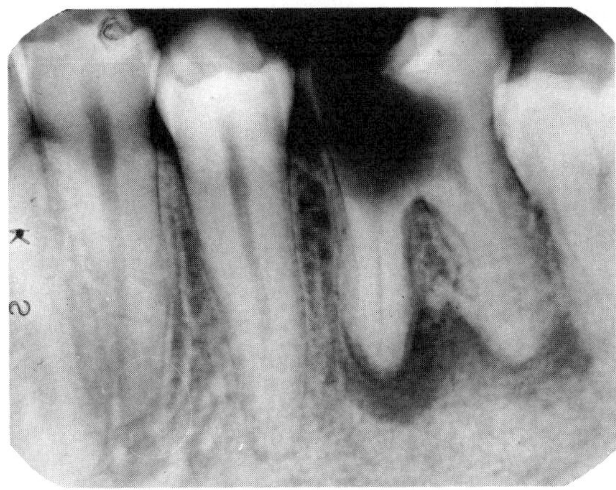

FIGURE 11–14

Radiograph showing a large periapical abscess at the tip of the mesial root of a badly decayed mandibular first molar. (From Haring, J.I., and Lind, L.J.: Radiographic Interpretation for the Dental Hygienist. Philadelphia, W.B. Saunders Co., 1993, p 152.)

The gingival tissue into which the pus finally drains may swell, causing an abscess of the gum, These **gum abscesses**, which are commonly known as *gum boils*, are seen more frequently in children than in adults.

Periodontal Diseases

Periodontal diseases involve pathological changes in the soft and hard tissues that support the teeth. Treatment of these diseases is discussed in Chapter 26.

The majority of periodontal diseases are bacterially induced inflammatory conditions. (This means that they are caused by the bacteria in dental plaque, which is discussed in Chapter 6.) However, they may also be affected by other conditions in the mouth and systemic causes such as endocrine disturbances.

Case Types of Periodontal Disease

Periodontal diseases are identified by five case types according to the severity of the disease and the amount of tissue destruction that has occurred at the time of the examination.

Case Type I. Gingivitis is inflammation of the gingivae. It is characterized clinically by the red and puffy appearance of the tissues.

The gingival surface appearance is no longer stippled, and the tissues bleed easily. The periodontal probe reading is less than 4 mm., and there is *no* bone loss.

This group includes *plaque-associated gingivitis*, which is initiated by the accumulation of supragingival bacterial plaque next to the gingival tissues, and acute necrotizing ulcerative gingivitis (which is discussed later in this chapter).

Case Type II. Early periodontitis is the progression of gingival inflammation into the alveolar bone crest (Fig. 11–15). There is early bone loss and the formation of periodontal pockets of 4 to 6 mm. in depth.

Case Type III. Moderate periodontitis is a more advanced stage of early periodontitis. There is increased destruction of the periodontal structures, and the periodontal pockets become deeper. The teeth begin to become mobile as a result of noticeable bone loss. There may be furcation involvement in multi-rooted teeth.

Case Type IV. Advanced periodontitis is still further progression of periodontitis. There is severe destruction of periodontal structures. The mobility increases, and the teeth become very loose. In multi-rooted teeth, the furcations are involved.

Case Type V. Refractory periodontitis is the continued progression of periodontal disease *after treatment*. For unknown reasons, these cases do not respond to therapy and usually end with the loss of the teeth.

Periodontal Pocket

A periodontal pocket, which is caused by local irritation such as microorganisms and their products, is a pathologically deepened portion of the gingival sulcus. Such pockets are important clinical features of periodontal disease.

Pocket formation starts as an inflammatory change in the connective tissue wall. If left untreated, progressive pocket formation leads to destruction of the supporting periodontal tissues.

The outer appearance of a periodontal pocket may be misleading because it is not necessarily a true indication of what is taking place throughout the pocket wall.

Periodontal pockets may be detected along the mesial, lingual, distal, and/or facial surfaces of the tooth.

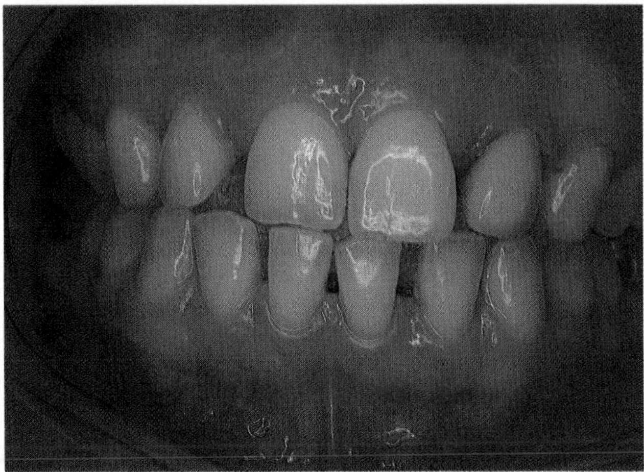

FIGURE 11–15

Case type II periodontitis. Notice the lack of normal stippling on the gingival tissue.

Pockets of different depths and types may also occur on different surfaces of the same tooth and on approximating surfaces of the same interdental space.

The zones of pocket involvement are **supra-bony**, which is coronal involvement above the level of the bone, and **infra-bony,** which is involvement when the walls of the pocket areas are at the level of the alveolar bone.

Periodontal Abscess

A periodontal abscess forms in the soft tissues of a periodontal pocket. It is not directly related to the condition of the dental pulp, and the vitality of the tooth is not usually affected by its formation.

Early-Onset Periodontitis

Periodontitis, which includes case types II to V, usually occurs in older individuals and may be referred to as *adult-onset periodontitis*. Periodontitis is, however, also found in children.

Early-onset periodontitis, formerly known as *juvenile periodontitis*, is periodontal disease occurring in otherwise healthy adolescents and young adults. There are two general groups of early-onset periodontitis: *localized* and *generalized,* which is a rapidly advancing form of periodontal disease.

Prepubertal periodontitis is localized periodontal disease occurring in children that may occur at the time of or shortly after the eruption of the primary teeth.

Pubertal gingivitis is the increasing severity of gingivitis that occurs during puberty. Although this is believed to be associated with increases in female sex hormone secretions during this time, the success of treatment depends upon excellent oral hygiene.

Bone Loss Associated with Periodontal Disease

Changes in other tissues of the periodontium are important, but it is the destruction of bone that eventually is responsible for loss of the teeth.

The height of the alveolar bone is normally maintained by a constant equilibrium between bone formation and bone resorption. When resorption exceeds formation,

- Bone height is reduced.
- Support is lost, and the tooth becomes mobile. (**Mobile** means able to move in its socket.)
- When enough bone support is gone, the tooth is lost.

Bone destruction in periodontal disease results primarily from the local factors that cause gingival inflammation and trauma from occlusion. It may also be caused by systemic factors, but their role has not been defined.

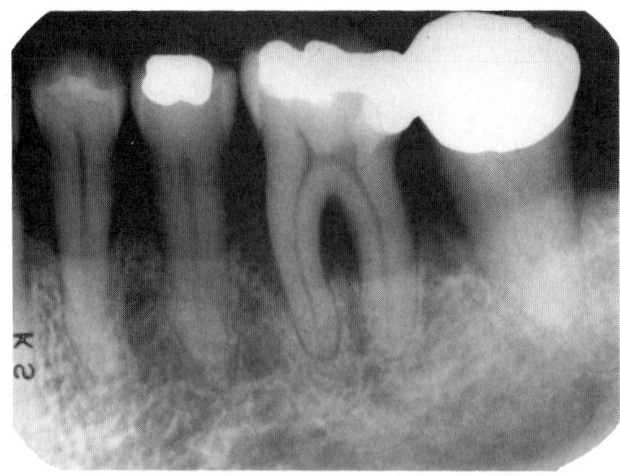

FIGURE 11–16

Radiograph showing the furcation area of the mandibular first molar. (From Haring, J.I., and Lind, L.J.: Radiographic Interpretation for the Dental Hygienist. Philadelphia, W.B. Saunders Co., 1993, p 131.)

FURCATION INVOLVEMENT

Furcation involvement refers to conditions of bone loss in which the bifurcation and trifurcation of multirooted teeth are denuded by periodontal disease (Fig. 11–16). (**Bifurcation** is the division into two roots. **Trifurcation** is the division into three roots.)

Dehiscence is a condition in which there is exposure of the root of the tooth as a result of localized bone loss of the cortical plate extending the full length of the tooth root.

Fenestrations occur when only isolated areas along the root are involved and the marginal bone is intact.

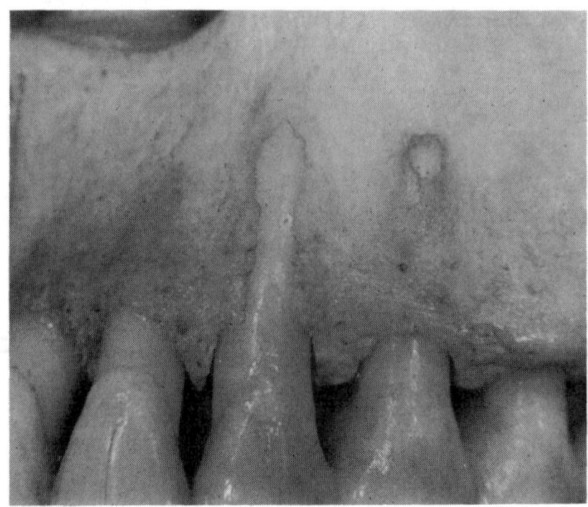

FIGURE 11–17

Dehiscence on the cuspid and fenestration of the first premolar. (From Carranza, F.A., Jr.: Glickman's Clinical Periodontology, 7th ed. Philadelphia, W.B. Saunders Co., 1990, p 70.)

These areas are usually covered by periosteum and overlying gingiva (Fig. 11–17).

Other Diseases of the Oral Soft Tissues

Acute Necrotizing Ulcerative Gingivitis

Acute necrotizing ulcerative gingivitis (ANUG), a painful, progressive bacterial infection, is classified as a form of gingivitis. It is associated with decreased resistance to infection under conditions such as poor nutrition, extreme stress, or lack of adequate rest. Patients who are HIV-positive may present with a particularly virulent form of ANUG.

ANUG is characterized by malaise, severely bad breath, and the appearance of grayish or yellowish-gray ulcers, which are most commonly found on the marginal and interproximal gingivae. (**Malaise** is a vague feeling of physical discomfort.)

The thin, grayish-white pseudomembrane covering the ulcers may be easily wiped off, exposing a highly inflamed area that bleeds very easily. These tissues are so painful that it is difficult to chew or to brush the teeth.

Gingival Hyperplasia

Gingival hyperplasia, also known as *gingival overgrowth,* is the generalized enlargement of the gingiva. (**Hyperplasia** means an abnormal increase in the number of normal cells, in normal arrangement, in a tissue.)

In severe hyperplasia, the gingiva may cover the crowns of the teeth. It is essential that patients with hyperplasia maintain excellent oral hygiene. Periodontal treatment, such as root planing and scaling or a gingivectomy, may be required. (See Chapter 26.)

Hormonal imbalances, as in puberty and pregnancy, may temporarily cause generalized gingival enlargement (see Fig. 8–2).

It may also be due to hereditary factors. These symptoms usually appear before age 20. When no known cause can be established, it is said to be **idiopathic hyperplasia**. (**Idiopathic** means without known cause.)

Drug therapy is also a major cause. Drugs known to cause gingival hyperplasia include

- Anticonvulsants such as phenytoin (Dilantin) that are used to control the convulsions of epilepsy (see Fig. 8–6)
- Drugs such as cyclosporine that are used to prevent organ transplant rejections
- Some medications, such as nifedipine (Procardia) and diltiazem (Cardizem), used to treat hypertension and other heart disorders

Pericoronitis

Pericoronitis is an inflammatory process occurring in a "gingival flap" of tissue found over the crown of a partially erupted tooth. The condition may be chronic, acute, or subacute.

The most frequent site is around the lower second or third molar region. The heavy flap of gingival tissue covering portions of the crown of the partially erupted tooth makes an ideal pocket for debris accumulation and bacterial incubation. Also, tissues may be traumatized during chewing. This may result in pain, swelling, and/or infection.

In the acute phase, pain and swelling in the area are prominent features. Symptoms of a sore throat and difficulty in swallowing or opening the mouth may also be present. When the area is infected, there may also be symptoms of general malaise and rise in temperature. Treatment is discussed in Chapter 26.

Leukoplakia

Leukoplakia is a general term meaning "white patch." It may occur anywhere in the mouth. Very little pain is associated with leukoplakia unless ulceration and secondary infection have developed.

The lesions vary in appearance and texture from a fine white transparency to a heavy, thick, warty plaque. To be classified as leukoplakia, the lesion should be firmly attached to the underlying tissue, and rubbing or scraping with an instrument should not remove it.

The cause of leukoplakia is unknown, but presence of the disease is commonly linked to chronic irritation or trauma, such as might result from smoking, cheek-biting, or ill-fitting dentures.

The condition very often precedes development of a malignant tumor. For that reason, early diagnosis and treatment are important. (Hairy leukoplakia is discussed later in this chapter in the section "Acquired Immunodeficiency Syndrome.")

Lichen Planus

Lichen planus is a chronic mucocutaneous disease affecting the skin and oral mucosa. (**Mucocutaneous** means occurring on the mucous membrane of the lip and on the adjoining skin.)

On the oral mucosa, the patchy white lesions have a characteristic pattern of circles and interconnecting lines called Wickham's striae (Fig. 11–18).

Candidiasis

Candidiasis is a superficial infection caused by the yeastlike fungus *Candida albicans*. It is the most common oral fungal infection; however, it does not commonly occur in the healthy general population.

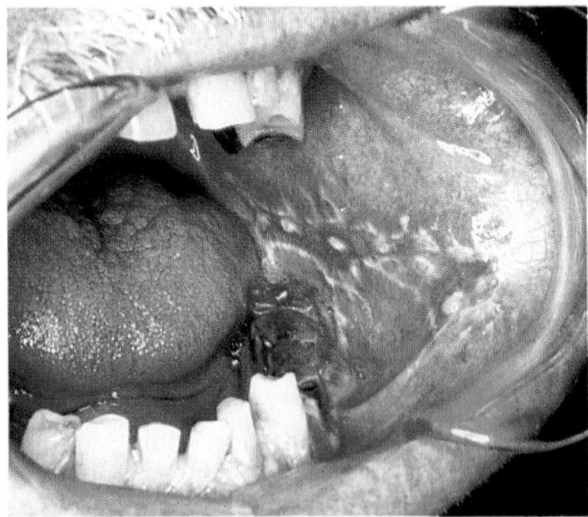

FIGURE 11–18

Lichen planus on the buccal mucosa. (From Ibsen, O.A., and Phelan, J.A.: Oral Pathology for the Dental Hygienist. Philadelphia, W.B. Saunders Co., 1992, plate 20.)

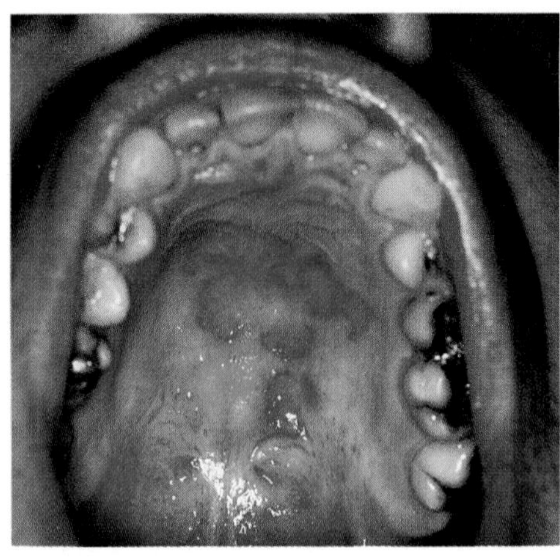

FIGURE 11–19

Erythematous candidiasis. (From Ibsen, O.A., and Phelan, J.A.: Oral Pathology for the Dental Hygienist. Philadelphia, W.B. Saunders Co., 1992, plate 31.)

Candidiasis does occur under such conditions as antibiotic therapy, diabetes, xerostomia (dry mouth), and weakened immunological reactions. It can be the initial clinical manifestation for patients with acquired immunodeficiency syndrome (AIDS). (This is discussed later in this chapter.)

Candidiasis is accompanied by discomfort or pain, halitosis (offensive breath odors), and dysgeusia (a distorted sense of taste). The clinical signs of oral candidiasis depend on the site of involvement and the manner in which the organism interacts with the host tissue.

PSEUDOMEMBRANOUS CANDIDIASIS

In pseudomembranous candidiasis, also known as *thrush*, creamy white plaques (resembling cottage cheese or curdled milk) form in the mouth. The patient frequently complains of a burning sensation, an unpleasant taste, or the feeling of "blisters" forming in the mouth. These "blisters" generally prove to be the pseudomembranous plaques. (**Pseudomembranous** means pertaining to a false membrane or tissue.)

These plaques can be scraped off, and removing them rarely causes bleeding. When bleeding is present, it is likely that the patient has an additional mucosal problem.

HYPERPLASTIC CANDIDIASIS

Hyperplastic candidiasis appears as white plaques that cannot be removed by scraping. This form is most commonly found on the buccal mucosa in HIV-infected patients.

ATROPHIC CANDIDIASIS

In atrophic candidiasis, which is also known as *erythematous candidiasis*, "bald" red patches may appear on areas of the dorsum of the tongue and on the palate (Fig. 11–19).

This form of candidiasis usually follows exposure to a broad-spectrum antibiotic, and the patient complains that his mouth feels scalded or burned (as if he had swallowed something too hot).

In most patients, antifungal therapy begins to resolve the infection within 2 to 3 days, with complete clearing after 10 to 14 days.

If the lesions are still present after this time or recur quickly, further investigation is necessary to rule out endocrine disturbances or immunological deficiencies.

Aphthous Ulceration

Aphthous ulceration, also known as *aphthous stomatitis* or *canker sores*, is a common form of oral mucosal ulceration.

Recurrent aphthous ulceration (RAU) is a disease that causes recurring outbreaks of blister-like sores inside the mouth and on the lips (Fig. 11–20). These sores appear on the non-keratinized movable parts of the mouth (the lining mucosa of the cheeks, edge of the tongue, floor of the mouth, palates, and the soft red part of the lip).

In the early stages of an outbreak of the disease, the patient experiences a burning sensation followed by the formation of small blisters. When the blister breaks, the typical ulcer forms. It is small and oval, and the center is yellow to gray and is surrounded by a red margin.

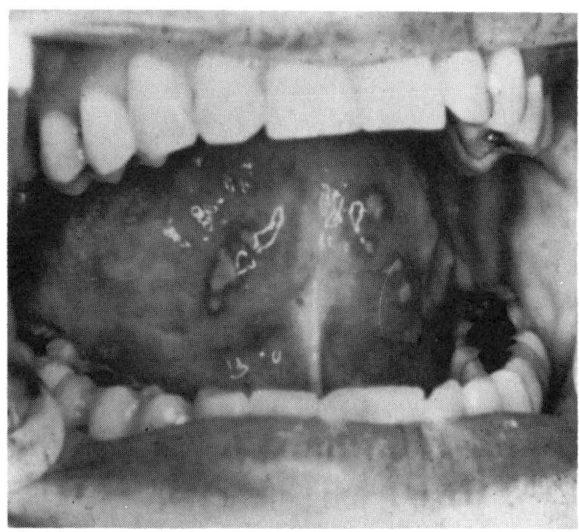

FIGURE 11–20

Aphthous stomatitis. (Courtesy of National Institute of Dental Research, Bethesda, MD.)

Minor RAU is the mildest form of involvement and represents 90% of all cases. Patients experience recurring episodes fewer than six times a year, and the lesions usually heal within 7 to 10 days.

Major RAU, which occurs in only about 10% of the cases, is characterized by more frequent outbreaks of larger, deeper ulcers that take longer to heal. This is found most often in patients with a compromised immune system.

The patient with RAU is often debilitated (weakened), for these sores make eating and drinking quite difficult. Various agents, such as topical anesthetics for pain control and drugs to promote healing, may be prescribed.

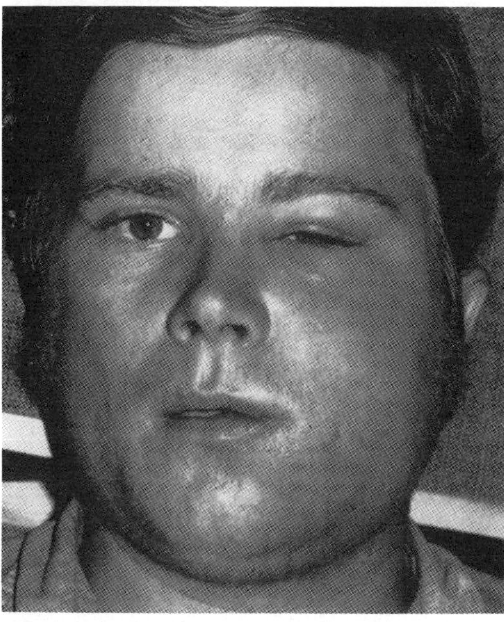

FIGURE 11–21

Acute facial cellulitis. (From Pedersen, G.W.: Oral Surgery. Philadelphia, W.B. Saunders Co., 1988, p 196.)

Cellulitis

Cellulitis is a condition in which an inflammation is *not* controlled and contained within a localized area. Instead, it spreads through the substance of the soft tissue or organ (Fig. 11–21).

In cellulitis, swelling usually develops rapidly, with high fever. The skin usually becomes very red, and the area is characterized by severe throbbing pain as the inflammation localizes.

Cellulitis associated with oral infections is potentially dangerous, for it can travel quickly to sensitive tissues such as the eye or brain.

Conditions of the Tongue

Glossitis is the general term used to describe inflammation and changes in the topography of the tongue. (**Topography** means features of the surface of the tongue.)

In **black hairy tongue,** which may be caused by the oral flora imbalance after the administration of antibiotics, the filiform papillae are so greatly elongated that they resemble hairs. These elongated papillae become stained by food and tobacco, hence the name *black hairy tongue.*

In **geographic tongue**, the surface of the tongue becomes the seat of multiple zones of desquamation (loss) of the filiform papillae in several irregularly shaped but well-demarcated areas. Over a period of days or weeks, the bald spots and the whitish margins seem to migrate across the surface of the tongue by healing on one border and extending on another (Fig. 11–22).

Bruxism

Bruxism is an oral habit consisting of involuntary gnashing, grinding, and clenching of the teeth in other than chewing movements. It is usually performed during sleep and is commonly associated with stress or tension.

Bruxism causes abnormal wear of the teeth. It also damages the periodontal ligament and associated supporting structures and is a major factor contributing to temporomandibular disorders.

In addition to stress-reduction techniques, a night guard or removable splint is a frequently used temporary aid in the treatment of bruxism. The purpose of this splint appliance is to reduce the damage caused by the grinding while the patient is asleep (Fig. 11–23).

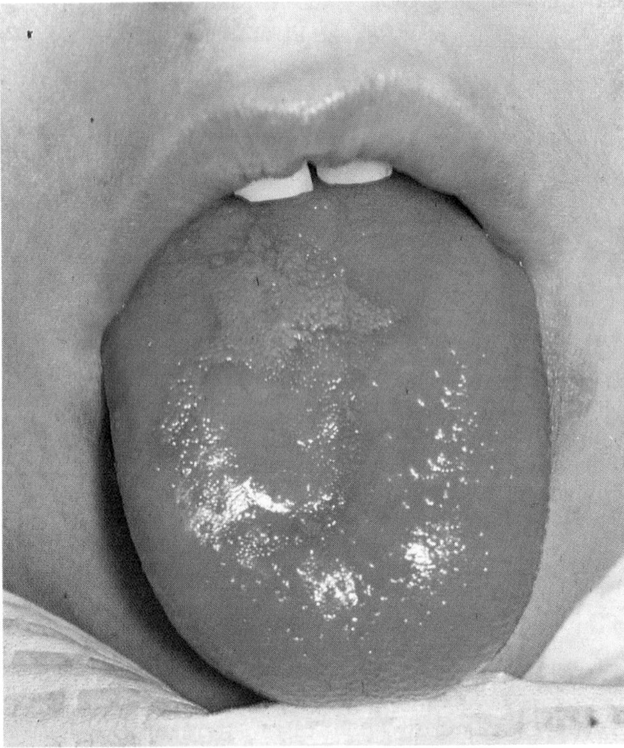

FIGURE 11–22

Geographic tongue.

Temporomandibular Disorders

The structure of the temporomandibular joint (TMJ) is described in Chapter 4. Problems that prevent the joint from functioning normally are known as **temporomandibular disorders** (TMD) or *myofascial pain dysfunction* (MPD).

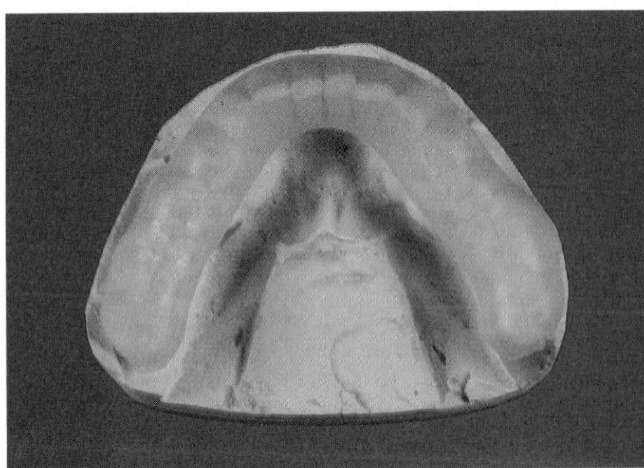

FIGURE 11–23

An acrylic bite plate used to limit the damage caused by bruxism. (Shown here on a diagnostic cast.)

The diagnosis and treatment of these disorders are among the most perplexing problems confronting the clinician in dentistry and medicine. Frequently, diagnosis is multidisciplinary in scope, requiring contributions from dentists, physicians, psychiatrists, psychologists, neurologists, neurosurgeons, and others for complete analysis of the patient's condition.

Symptoms

One of the reasons that TMJ disorders are so difficult to diagnose is that the symptoms are so varied. They most frequently include pain, joint sounds, and limitations of movement.

PAIN

Patients with temporomandibular disorders may report a wide range of types of pain. These include headaches, pain in and around the ear (when no infection is present), pain on chewing, and pain in the face, head, and neck.

Also included are tenderness and spasms (cramps) of the muscles of mastication. These spasms can become part of a cycle that results in tissue damage, increased pain, muscle tenderness, and more spasms.

JOINT SOUNDS

Clicking, popping, or crepitus may be heard when opening the mouth. (**Crepitus** is the grating sounds that may be heard in a damaged joint.) The dentist may use a stethoscope to listen for these sounds.

LIMITATIONS OF MOVEMENT

Limitations of movement lead to difficulty and pain on chewing, yawning, or wide opening of the mouth. Trismus, the most common cause of restricted mandibular movement, may severely limit the patient's degree of mouth opening. (**Trismus** is a spasm of the muscles of mastication.)

Other limitations of jaw movement include "getting stuck," "locking," or "going out."

Causes of Temporomandibular Disorders

Temporomandibular disorders are considered stress-related, and oral habits such as clenching the teeth or bruxism frequently are very important contributing factors. These disorders have many other causes, which include

- Accidents involving injuries to the jaw, head, or neck

- Diseases of the joint, including several varieties of arthritis
- Malocclusion, in which the teeth come together in a manner that produces abnormal strain on the joint and surrounding tissues

Categories of Temporomandibular Disorders

The following are the major categories of TMJ disorders, with examples:

Acute Masticatory Muscle Complaints. These are characterized by muscle inflammation, muscle spasms, and protective muscle splinting (the muscle limits the movement of the mandible in order to limit the pain caused by such motions).

Articular Disc Derangement. The disc, which allows smooth movement of the joint, may be displaced or damaged. This may cause clicking sounds, limited ability to open the mouth and many of the other symptoms associated with TMJ disorders.

Problems Resulting from Extrinsic Trauma. These injuries from external causes may be dislocation of the joint, fracture of the bones, and internal derangement of the joint.

Joint Diseases. Degenerative and inflammatory forms of arthritis may severely damage the joint.

Chronic Mandibular Hypomobility. (Hypomobility means a limited ability to move.) In the mandible this may be influenced by damage to the joint (either the bony portions or the articular capsule), contracture (shortening) of muscles of mastication, or damage to the articular disc.

Baseline Records

The following baseline records are normally obtained from patients suspected of having a TMJ disorder:

Complete Medical and Dental Histories. A thorough history may be the most important means of diagnosing TMJ disorders. This may take an hour or more of in-depth questioning and probing.

Clinical Examination. A thorough clinical evaluation normally includes evaluation of mandibular movements, examination of the oral cavity, the TMJ, the muscles of the head and neck, and an analysis of the occlusion.

Mounted Diagnostic Casts. The casts, with a bite registration, are used to detect abnormalities that may interfere with the patient's occlusion.

Radiographic Examinations. These may include intraoral radiographs of the teeth and extraoral films of the joint.

Additional Diagnostic Techniques. As necessary, these may include blood tests, electromyography (to evaluate muscle function), and specialized imaging techniques.

Treatment of Temporomandibular Disorders

INITIAL TREATMENT, PHASE 1, REVERSIBLE

Initial treatment is directed at managing symptoms and may include the following:

- A soft **diet** to limit pain from chewing
- **Medication** such as analgesics, tranquilizers, and anti-inflammatory agents to relieve the muscle spasms and pain
- **Physical therapy,** including heat, massage, and therapeutic muscle exercise
- **Behavior modification** and psychological counseling to relieve the stress that may be causing bruxism
- **Removable appliance therapy** to limit the damage caused by bruxism

SUBSEQUENT TREATMENT, PHASE 2, IRREVERSIBLE

Additional forms of treatment may be necessary. These are designed primarily to effect a permanent alteration of the occlusion and may include

- **Occlusal adjustment**, also known as equilibration, to remove occlusal interferences that may be causing problems
- **Restorative and prosthodontic treatment** to restore the mouth to optimal health
- **Orthodontic treatment** to achieve normal occlusion
- **Surgery,** which is performed only after all other treatments have failed

Arthroscopy

Diagnostic arthroscopy is a surgical procedure in which an arthroscope is inserted into the capsule of the TMJ to allow the doctor direct visual examination of a joint. These images, which are projected on a video screen, may be magnified one to 10 times.

In **surgical arthroscopy**, also known as *arthroscopic surgery*, the arthroscope and very small surgical instruments are also inserted into the joint to allow the surgeon to perform the necessary procedures.

Surgical arthroscopy is considered as an alternative only when nonsurgical treatment has failed to relieve symptoms that cause severe pain and interfere with activities of daily living, such as talking.

Neurological Involvements

Trigeminal Neuralgia

Trigeminal neuralgia, also known as **tic douloureux**, is severe pain caused by inflammation of the trigeminal (fifth cranial) nerve. This pain, which has been described as excruciating, stabbing, and searing, may last a few seconds. However, the initial incident is usually followed by additional episodes, often of increasing severity.

The disorder is particularly difficult to diagnose because the pain could be coming from a toothache, a TMJ disorder, or another neurological problem.

Bell's Palsy

Bell's palsy is paralysis of the facial (seventh cranial) nerve that causes distortion on the affected side of the face.

Oral Cancer

Oral cancer is one of the 10 most frequently occurring cancers in the world; however, the incidence, as well as the site, of the cancer varies greatly from country to country. In the Western countries, the site most often affected is the vermilion border of the lip.

Most oral cancers do not cause pain in the early stages, and the dentist is most likely to be the first to detect them. These cancers will kill if not detected early enough or if left untreated, yet many can be cured if detected and treated early in their development.

Carcinomas

A **carcinoma** is a malignant neoplasm (growth) of the epithelium (tissue lining the mouth) that tends to invade surrounding tissue (bone and connective tissue) and to spread (metastasize) to other regions of the body (usually to the neck and cervical lymph nodes).

Carcinomas are found on the soft tissues of the mouth, including the lips, tongue, cheeks, and floor of the mouth, and they usually appear first as an ulcerated area (Fig. 11–24).

An **adenocarcinoma** is a malignant tumor that arises from the submucous glands underlying the oral mucosa. (The prefix *adeno-* means gland.) This tumor first appears clinically as a lump or bulge beneath overlying normal mucosa.

A **sarcoma** is a malignant neoplasm arising from supportive and connective tissue such as bone. An **osteosarcoma** is a malignant tumor involving the bone. In the mouth, the affected bones are the bones of the jaws. Although the cancer may start in the bone, it may spread and involve the surrounding soft tissues.

Leukemia

Leukemia is a malignant disease (cancer) of the blood-forming organs that is characterized by proliferation of immature leukocytes (white blood cells).

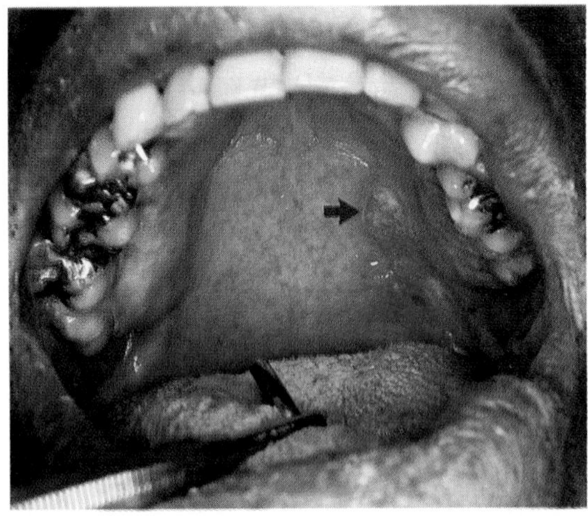

FIGURE 11–24

Squamous cell carcinoma. (From Ibsen, O.A., and Phelan, J.A.: Oral Pathology for the Dental Hygienist. Philadelphia, W.B. Saunders Co., 1992, plate 33.)

Oral symptoms of leukemia may be some of the first indications of the disease. These symptoms include hemorrhage, ulceration, enlargement, spongy texture, and magenta coloration of the gingiva.

Enlargement of lymph nodes, symptoms of anemia, and general hemorrhagic (bleeding) tendencies are also typical.

Smokeless Tobacco

Smokeless tobacco, as chewing tobacco or snuff, presents a serious health hazard. It is a major concern because of the high rates of precancerous leukoplakia and oral cancer occurring among users of smokeless tobacco. Also, cancers of the pharynx, larynx, and esophagus occur 400 to 500 times more frequently among users than among nonusers.

Smokeless tobacco is also linked to serious irritation of the oral mucosa and increased incidence of tooth loss from periodontal disease (Fig. 11–25).

Because 90 percent of the nicotine in smokeless tobacco is absorbed through the mucous membrane and directly into the blood stream, the medical hazards of smokeless tobacco are directly linked to nicotine. These include heart disease, elevated blood pressure, aggravated diabetic conditions, and gastric and duodenal ulcers.

Warning Signs of Oral Cancer

The following are warning signs of oral cancer:

- White, smooth, or scaly patches in the mouth or on the lips

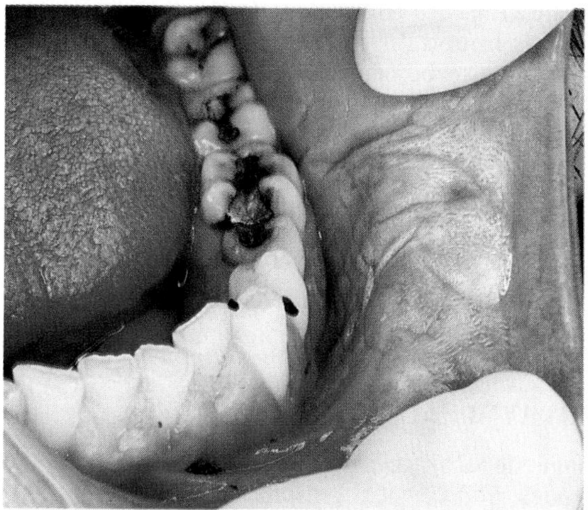

FIGURE 11–25

White corrugated lesion caused by patient's repeatedly placing smokeless tobacco in this area. (From Ibsen, O.A., and Phelan, J.A.: Oral Pathology for the Dental Hygienist. Philadelphia, W.B. Saunders Co., 1992, plate 18.)

- Swelling or lumps in the mouth or on the neck, lips, or tongue
- Numbness, burning sensation, feeling of dryness, or pain in the mouth without apparent cause
- A red spot or sore on the lips or gums or inside the mouth that does not heal within 2 to 3 weeks
- Repeated bleeding in the mouth without apparent cause
- Difficulty or abnormality in speaking or swallowing

The Prevention of Oral Cancer

Oral cancer is most often seen in association with the use of tobacco, excessive alcohol intake, poor oral hygiene, neglected teeth, and factors that chronically irritate the tissues.

The following steps are helpful in preventing oral cancer and should be taken by *everyone*:

- Avoid prolonged exposure to strong direct sunlight (this is a contributing cause of cancer of the lips).
- Don't smoke or use smokeless tobacco.
- If a denture or tooth irritates the surrounding tissue, have the dentist correct it.
- Any lump, scaly area, or white spot on the lips or mouth that lasts longer than 2 weeks should be seen by a dentist or physician.
- Eat a balanced diet to maintain optimal health.
- Maintain good oral hygiene.
- See your dentist regularly for a thorough examination (the steps in a cancer examination are described in Chapter 18).

Dental Implications of Radiation Treatment

Because radiation for treatment of head and neck cancer affects the salivary glands, the blood vessels, and the bones of the jaws, patients receiving this treatment can be expected to develop specific dental problems.

In **xerostomia**, there is not a total absence of saliva, but what is present is of a very creamy, thick, ropy nature.

Radiation caries, which is caused by the lack of saliva, usually appears first in the cervical areas of the teeth. The teeth may also become extremely sensitive to hot and cold stimuli.

A program of good oral hygiene and daily application of a sodium fluoride gel may be used to help control radiation caries.

This lack of adequate saliva and the reduced blood supply to the tissues can also precipitate oral infection, delay healing, and make it very difficult to wear dentures.

Osteoradionecrosis is the necrosis (death) of bone after radiation treatment. This tissue death increases the risks associated with a dental extraction, including the possibility of fracturing the jaw, fracturing the tooth, and failure to heal.

For these reasons, patients should not have teeth extracted after they have been treated with head and/or neck radiation. To avoid this problem, it is necessary in some cases to extract the patient's teeth before the radiation treatment.

Dental Implications of Chemotherapy

The following are direct oral effects of chemotherapy:

Mucositis. This is an inflammatory change in the oral mucosa in which the mucosa takes on a whitish appearance.

Aphthous Ulceration. This is a common side effect of most antineoplastic agents.

Transient Reactions. Cheilitis (inflammation of the lips), **glossitis** (inflammation of the tongue), and **paresthesia** (an abnormal burning or tingling sensation, or the loss of sensation) are less common and transient reactions. (**Transient** means that they will go away without additional treatment.)

Xerostomia. This dryness of the mouth, caused by the lack of normal salivary secretions, is another transient phenomenon in chemotherapy. Recovery usually occurs within 10 days.

Delayed Healing. Because antineoplastic drugs act nonselectively on all dividing cells, interference with healing may be anticipated when the drug is administered during the healing period.

Dentinal Malformation. Chemotherapy in children during dentinal development can be expected to produce dental defects.

Other Disorders with Oral Manifestations

Many systemic diseases may produce manifestations in the oral cavity, sometimes before they are evident in any other part of the body.

Eating Disorders

ANOREXIA NERVOSA AND BULIMIA

Anorexia nervosa, usually referred to simply as *anorexia*, is a personality disorder manifested by extreme aversion to food, abnormal behavior directed toward losing weight, and an intense fear of gaining weight.

The disease occurs primarily in young females, with the average age at onset between 17 and 20 years. Anorexia deprives the body of the nutrients necessary to maintain life, health, and maturation. The anorexic may suffer from amenorrhea (lack of menstruation), chronic heart disorders, kidney impairment, and death due to cardiac failure caused by electrolyte imbalances.

Bulimia nervosa, usually referred to simply as *bulimia*, is a personality disorder in which the symptoms are an irresistible urge to overeat with avoidance of fattening effects by vomiting, abusing purgatives (laxatives), or both. Bulimia also has serious physical consequences, including death due to heart failure, because the electrolyte balance within the body is disrupted.

There are also dental problems associated with these disorders. First, there is decalcification and erosion of the enamel caused by stomach acids during vomiting activity.

There may also be enlargement of the parotid and occasionally the submandibular salivary glands. Although this is not painful, it may result in a temporary decrease in the production of saliva.

Rampant caries is a major concern. This may be caused by the weakened enamel, the lack of adequate salivary protection, and the high carbohydrate intake that is part of the bulimic activity.

Acquired Immunodeficiency Syndrome

Acquired immunodeficiency syndrome (AIDS) is the end-stage disease for an individual infected with HIV. HIV is discussed in Chapter 10. The complications of AIDS are discussed here.

OPPORTUNISTIC INFECTIONS

Because the patient's immune system is damaged, death is usually caused by an opportunistic disease. (An **opportunistic infection** is one that normally would be controlled by the immune system but that cannot be controlled because the system is not functioning properly.)

The following are important oral manifestations; however, it is important to remember that these manifestations may also be caused by other disorders.

CANDIDIASIS

Candidiasis, which was previously discussed, may be the initial presenting sign of the progression from HIV-positive to AIDS status. In a patient with a compromised immune system, candidiasis can be a very debilitating and serious disorder.

CERVICAL LYMPHADENOPATHY

Lymphadenopathy means disease or swelling of the lymph nodes, and cervical lymphadenopathy is the enlargement of the cervical (neck) nodes. Lymphadenopathy, which is indicative of a systemic problem, is frequently seen in association with AIDS.

LYMPHOMA

Lymphoma is the general term used to describe malignant disorders of the lymphoid tissue. In the immunocompromised individual, it may occur as a solitary lump or nodule, a swelling, or a nonhealing ulcer that occurs anywhere in the oral cavity.

The swelling may be ulcerated or may be covered with intact, normal-appearing mucosa. Usually painful, the lesion grows rapidly in size and may be the first evidence of lymphoma.

Diagnosis is made from a biopsy because this phenomenon closely resembles other oral diseases.

HAIRY LEUKOPLAKIA

Most individuals having hairy leukoplakia (HL) are HIV-positive, and it can be an important early manifestation of AIDS status.

Hairy leukoplakia is a filamentous white plaque usually found unilaterally or bilaterally on the lateral borders (sides) in the anterior portion of the tongue (Fig. 11–26).

It may spread to cover the entire dorsal surface of the tongue. It can also appear on the buccal mucosa, where it generally has a flat appearance.

KAPOSI'S SARCOMA

Kaposi's sarcoma (KS) is a form of cancer that usually begins with skin lesions. In the mouth, Kaposi's sarcoma may appear as multiple bluish, blackish, or reddish blotches that are usually flat in early stages. Squamous cell carcinoma and non-Hodgkin's lymphoma may also appear in the mouth.

HERPES SIMPLEX

Herpes simplex lesions usually occur on the lip. However, in immunocompromised patients, the lesions

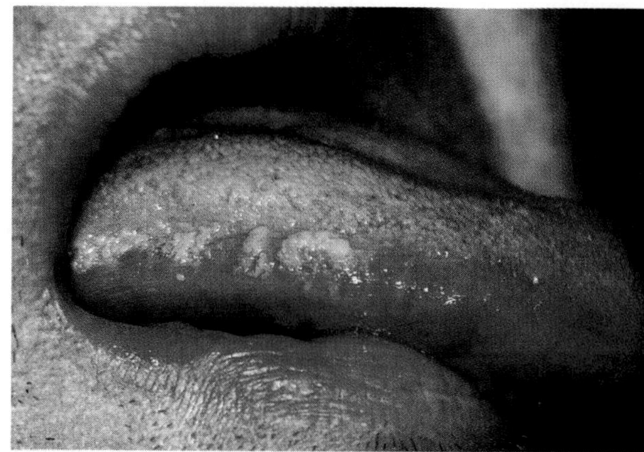

FIGURE 11–26

Hairy leukoplakia on the lateral borders of the tongue. (From Ibsen, O.A., and Phelan, J.A.: Oral Pathology for the Dental Hygienist. Philadelphia, W.B. Saunders Co., 1992, plate 13.)

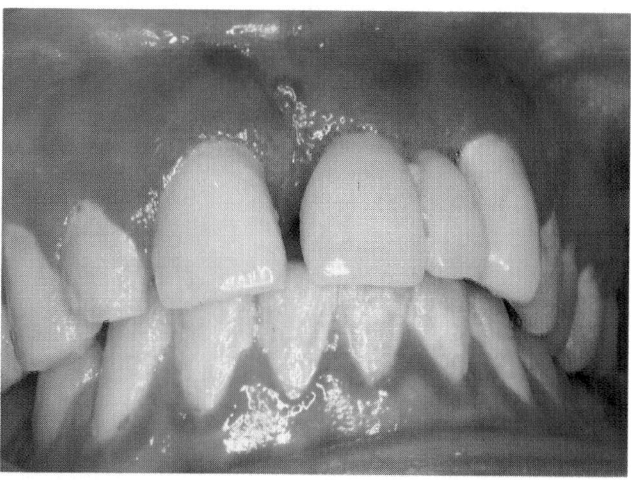

FIGURE 11–27

HIV-associated periodontitis.

may occur throughout the mouth. (Herpes is also discussed in Chapter 10.)

A mucocutaneous ulcer caused by the herpes virus that persists longer than 1 month is particularly significant as an indicator of AIDS.

HERPES ZOSTER

In the immunocompromised patient the latent herpes zoster virus, also known as varicella zoster or shingles, may cause intraoral manifestations in the form of blisters following the course of some branches of the trigeminal nerve. The blisters break and form ulcers.

These lesions are generally unilateral (on one side of the mouth) and are very painful. Complaints of pain coming from the teeth, without apparent dental cause, may be an early symptom of herpes zoster.

HUMAN PAPILLOMAVIRUSES

Human papillomaviruses (HPVs) are responsible for warts such as oral papillomas. These appear most commonly in immunocompromised individuals. Diagnosis is made based on history, clinical appearance, and biopsy.

These warts appear spiky, and some have a raised, cauliflower-like appearance; others are well-defined, have a flat surface, and all but disappear when the mucosa is stretched.

Although these warts can be removed by surgery or carbon dioxide laser excision, they frequently recur after removal.

HIV GINGIVITIS

HIV gingivitis (HIV-G), also known as **atypical gingivitis** (ATYP), is characterized by a bright red line along the border of the free gingival margin.

In some cases, there may be progression of the bright red line from the free gingival margin over the attached gingival and alveolar mucosa. In other cases, there are petechia-like patches over the gingiva. (**Petechiae** are small pinpoint bruises.)

HIV PERIODONTITIS

The periodontal lesions of HIV periodontitis (HIV-P), also known as **AIDS virus–associated periodontitis** (AVAP), resemble those observed in acute necrotizing gingivitis superimposed upon a rapidly progressive periodontitis (Fig. 11–27).

Other symptoms include interproximal necrosis and cratering; marked swelling and intense erythema over the free and attached gingiva; intense pain; spontaneous bleeding; and bad breath.

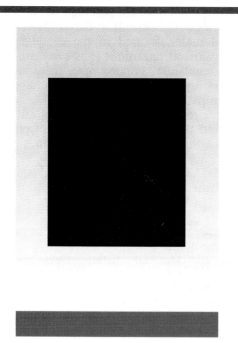

Chapter 12

Hazard Communication Management

Introduction

Hazard communication management, an Occupational Safety and Health Administration (OSHA) requirement, is one of many government regulations that apply to the dental practice.

This chapter discusses the following regulations affecting the dental practice: **state and federal agencies**, the **OSHA Hazard Communication Standard**, the **OSHA Bloodborne Pathogen Standard**, and **Medical Waste Management**.

Although compliance with these regulations is the dentist/employer's responsibility, a staff member may be designated as the **office safety coordinator** or supervisor.

In this role, he or she is responsible for following the dentist's instructions to ensure that the practice is in compliance with regulations, that necessary training takes place in a timely manner, and that the appropriate records are maintained.

State and Federal Agencies

The guidelines and requirements discussed in this chapter are established and/or enforced primarily by three federal agencies. These agencies are OSHA, the Centers for Disease Control and Prevention (CDC), and the Environmental Protection Agency (EPA).

Many states and some communities have similar regulations and requirements. When the state or local regulation is more stringent (stricter) than the federal requirement, that law applies.

The dentist and staff must be aware of and comply with the federal, state, and local regulations.

The Occupational Safety and Health Administration

The Occupational Health and Safety Administration of the U.S. Department of Labor issues and enforces regulations pertaining to employee safety in the workplace.

OSHA POLICIES

OSHA requires that employers (dentists) maintain certain safe work practices to ensure that employees are protected from potential hazards in the dental office.

OSHA requires that certain of these policies or standards be kept on file, be posted in full view of employees, or be readily accessible to employees. This may be either in easy-to-understand written form or available on computer for review by employees.

One such requirement is that the "*OSHA Workplace Poster*" be displayed in a prominent location where all employees can see it. Another is that a "*Caution: Radiation in Use*" sign be posted at the entrance to each treatment room where x-rays are used to produce radiographs.

OSHA INSPECTIONS

OSHA has the authority to conduct unannounced inspections of all workplaces, including dental offices, on the basis of complaints from patients or from current or former employees, or in such instances in which suspected health and safety violations may be present.

Occasionally, OSHA may conduct random unannounced investigations of healthcare practices. In general, random OSHA investigations are conducted only in practices with 11 or more employees.

Upon completion of the investigation, OSHA examiners will make specific violations (if any exist) known to the employer in writing. The employer has 15 working days to make the necessary changes or to show a "good faith" attempt to comply.

Should the employer not make the necessary changes, citations may be issued, for which the employer is held liable.

The Centers for Disease Control and Prevention

The primary mission of the CDC is to track, investigate, and report the spread, virulence (strength), and incidence of specific diseases affecting the U.S. population.

The CDC also has a significant role in controlling diseases by establishing exposure control guidelines for the prevention of cross-contamination. These guidelines, which are also known as *infection control guidelines,* are designed to safeguard both healthcare personnel *and* their patients.

Although the CDC establishes these guidelines, it is *not* an official regulatory agency and lacks the power to enforce these standards.

Guidelines that protect the well-being of *employees* are enforced by OSHA. Guidelines that protect the well-being of *patients* are enforced under state laws.

The Environmental Protection Agency

The EPA, or a similar state agency, deals with issues of concern to the environment or public safety, such as air and water pollution and waste management. Of particular concern to the dental practice is the disposal of infectious waste. (Waste management is discussed later in this chapter.)

OSHA Hazard Communication Standard

The OSHA Hazard Communication Standard, often called the *Employee Right to Know Law,* covers the rights of employees to know the potential dangers associated with hazardous chemicals in the workplace.

Products and materials used in the dental office that are not classified as hazardous substances are not covered by this regulation. For example, medications (such as pills and injectable drugs), which are directly administered to a patient, are not included.

The goal of this regulation is to ensure that all employees understand the dangers of, and correct procedures for, handling hazardous chemicals that they may be exposed to during their employment.

Under this OSHA regulation, the dentist is required to develop, implement, and maintain a four-part Hazard Communication Program:

1. Labeling of potentially hazardous products or materials used in the dental office
2. Maintaining of Material Safety Data Sheets (MSDSs)
3. Training employees in safe handling of hazardous chemicals
4. Maintaining a written Hazard Communication Program

Product Labeling

Dental products that contain any ingredient that is considered hazardous must come from the supplier or manufacturer with a label identifying the chemical or chemicals and containing an appropriate hazard warning (Fig. 12–1).

It is very important that the dental assistant read the labels of all materials used in the dental office and follow the warning recommendations for cleaning up spills and proper disposal, as well as the directions for use and storage.

TRANSFER TO A SECONDARY CONTAINER

If a hazardous substance is transferred to a secondary container, the new container must be labeled with either a photocopy of the original label or a new label, which includes all of the manufacturer's information stated on the original label (Fig. 12–2).

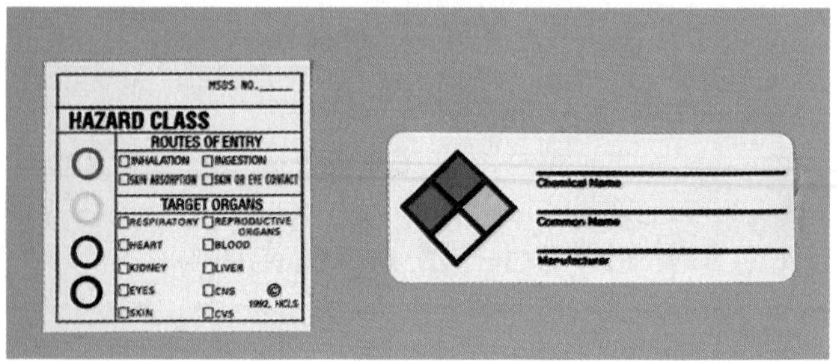

FIGURE 12–1

Hazardous substances must be clearly labeled.

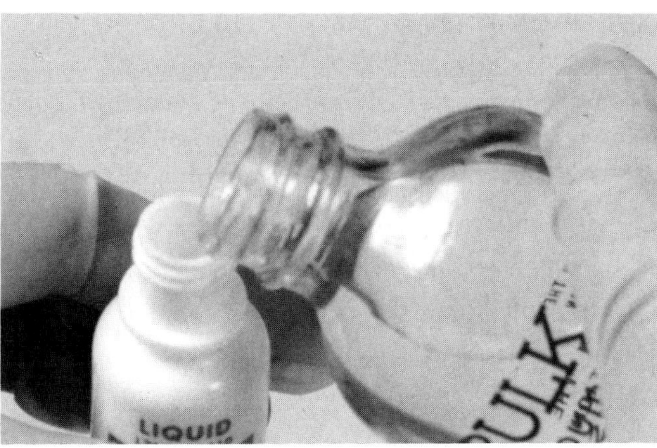

FIGURE 12–2

When a substance is transferred to a secondary container, that container must be labeled properly.

The exceptions to this requirement are those products identified as being for immediate use by the employee who transfers the product. (**Immediate use** means within the 8 hours of a work shift.)

However, if the product is transferred for later use, or for use by another employee, the new container must be properly labeled with the hazardous substance information. For example, when disinfection solutions are mixed for use and/or are transferred to smaller spray bottles, these containers must be properly labeled.

X-ray tanks or automatic processors must also be labeled with the information included on the manufacturer's containers of fixer and developer.

Material Safety Data Sheets (MSDSs)

Material Safety Data Sheets are detailed information bulletins prepared by the manufacturer or supplier of any product that contains a chemical considered to be hazardous.

OSHA requires the dentist to maintain an up-to-date file of MSDSs for each product used in the practice that contains a potentially hazardous chemical or chemicals. The dentist/employer must also train employees in how to read these information sheets.

These MSDSs must be readily available for employee use. New or revised MSDSs must be made available within 5 days of receipt, and employees must be notified.

Also, if the dental office changes or substitutes brands of a specific product, a new MSDS must be secured, even though the chemical composition may be identical.

MSDS INFORMATION

The dental assistant should take time to study these MSDSs because they contain valuable information about precautions and safe handling of each product. Each MSDS must contain the following information:

- Identification: the chemical and common (generic) names
- Hazardous ingredient or ingredients
- Physical and chemical characteristics
- Fire and explosion hazard data
- Health hazard data
- Reactivity data
- Spill and disposal procedures
- Protection information
- Handling and storage precautions, including proper waste disposal
- Emergency and first-aid procedures
- Date of preparation of the MSDS
- Name and address of the manufacturer or supplier

MAINTAINING A HAZARDOUS MATERIALS LOG

The Hazardous Materials Log is a list of all of the potential hazardous substances present in the dental office, including information as to where the substance is found. For example, zinc is a hazardous substance that is found in the alloy used in amalgam restorations.

There must be an MSDS on file for each substance. If the MSDS is available, the manufacturer or distributor should be contacted immediately to obtain it.

Responsibility for creating this log, and regularly updating it, is usually assigned to the office safety coordinator or to the assistant responsible for ordering supplies.

Employee Training

Dentists must provide training for employees (1) at the time of their initial assignment, (2) whenever a new hazardous material is introduced into the workplace, and (3) whenever procedures for safe handling and emergencies are modified.

Records must be kept of each training session, and these records are to be retained for at least 5 years. The employee may be asked to sign the record to indicate that the training was conducted.

Although the dentist is responsible for providing the training, the dental assistant is responsible for routinely following these safety precautions.

Maintaining a Written Hazard Communication Program

The employer/dentist is responsible for maintaining a written hazard communication program and for keeping required records related to this program. This must include the following:

A List of Hazardous Chemicals. This list includes chemicals used in the practice and where they are found. It is organized in the Hazardous Materials Log and must be available to employees. This list must be updated when new products are introduced into the practice.

Material Safety Data Sheets. The file must be kept up to date and be available to all employees.

Labels and Other Forms of Warning. This includes the protocol (instructions) to be certain that all employees read and understand the labels on containers.

It also includes specific instructions on how to prepare labels when transferring substances into secondary containers.

Training. Details concerning training materials and records regarding training sessions are included here.

Guidelines for Minimizing Hazards in the Dental Office

- Keep a minimum of hazardous chemicals in the office.
- Read the labels and use only as directed.
- Store chemicals only in their original, properly labeled containers.
- Store according to the manufacturer's directions.
- Keep containers tightly covered.
- Avoid mixing chemicals unless consequences are known.
- Wear appropriate personal protective equipment (PPE) when handling hazardous substances. (**Personal protective equipment** is barrier clothing required by OSHA for the protection of the healthcare worker.)
- Wash hands immediately after removing gloves.
- Avoid skin contact with chemical; immediately wash skin that has come in contact with chemicals.
- Maintain good ventilation.
- Do not eat, drink, smoke, apply lip balm, or insert contact lenses in areas where chemicals are used.
- Keep chemicals away from open flames and heat sources.
- Always have an operational fire extinguisher handy.
- Know and use proper cleanup procedures.
- Keep neutralizing agents available for strong acid and alkaline solutions.
- Dispose of all hazardous chemicals according to MSDS instructions.

Precautions for Handling Hazardous Materials

PERSONAL PROTECTIVE EQUIPMENT

Appropriate PPE must be worn when handling hazardous materials. This is not necessarily the same equipment that is worn during patient care, which is discussed in Chapter 13.

Depending upon the material being used, this equipment may include safety goggles, industrial-grade nitrile gloves, and National Institute for Occupational Safety and Health (NIOSH)–approved masks.

ACID ETCH SOLUTIONS AND GELS

Examples include solutions and gels for acid etch techniques associated with placement of composite restorations, sealants, and orthodontic brackets. (These solutions contain phosphoric acid.)

Hazards include acid burns with possible sloughing of tissue and eye damage.

Precautions

- Handle acid-soaked materials with forceps or gloves.
- Clean spills with a commercial acid spill cleanup kit.
- Avoid skin or soft tissue contact.
- In case of eye or skin contact, rinse with a large amount of running water.

FLAMMABLE GASES

Examples include liquid petroleum gas (LPG), nitrous oxide, and oxygen. (Although nitrous oxide and oxygen are not flammable by definition, they do support and accelerate the combustion of flammable gases.)

Hazards include fire and explosion of pressurized gas tanks. Chronic exposure to nitrous oxide may cause spontaneous miscarriage and other physical problems, including damage to the liver and central nervous system. (Nitrous oxide safety precautions are discussed further in Chapter 20.)

The NIOSH has established a maximum exposure level of 25 parts per million (ppm) of ambient gases. (The term **ambient** refers to gases that have escaped into the air.)

Precautions

- Secure gas cylinders with heavy chains to prevent accidental tipping.
- Avoid having sparks or flames near flammable gases.
- Periodically test the entire system for leaks. This includes tanks, lines, nitrous oxide unit, hoses, and masks.
- The rubber bag may be checked for leaks by putting air in it and then submerging the bag in soapy water. (Escaping air bubbles indicate a leak.)
- If there is any question of a leak, monitoring equipment is used to test the level of ambient nitrous oxide in the air.
- In the treatment room, use a scavenging system to remove excess gases exhaled by the patient.
- When placing the mask on the patient, take care to fit it carefully and snugly over the patient's nose to avoid leakage.
- Maintain adequate ventilation in the dental office.
- Make certain that tanks are properly labeled.
- Close off valves before moving a cylinder or when a cylinder becomes empty.

FLAMMABLE LIQUIDS

Examples include solvents such as acetone and alcohol.

Hazards include fire or explosion.

Precautions

- Store flammable liquids in tightly covered containers.
- Provide adequate ventilation.
- Have fire extinguishers available at locations where flammable liquids are used.
- Avoid sparks and flames in areas where flammable liquids are used.

ORGANIC MATERIALS

Examples include alcohols, ketones, esters, solvents, and monomers such as methylmethacrylate and dimethacrylate, which are used with self-curing resins.

Hazards include fire, allergic manifestations (such as contact dermatitis), possible mutagenesis, irritation to mucous membranes, respiratory problems, nausea, liver and kidney damage, central nervous system depression, headache, drowsiness, and loss of consciousness. (**Contact dermatitis** is a skin rash caused by an allergic reaction to a substance.)

Precautions

- Avoid skin contact.
- Avoid excessive inhalation of vapors.
- Work in well-ventilated areas.
- Use forceps or utility gloves when handling contaminated gauze or brushes.
- Keep containers tightly closed when not in use.
- Store containers on flat, sturdy surfaces.
- Clean outside surfaces of containers after use to prevent contamination by residual materials during the next use.
- Use a commercially available, flammable solvent cleanup kit in case of spill.

GYPSUM PRODUCTS

Examples include dental plaster and stone.

Hazards include irritation and impairment of respiratory system, silicosis (a lung disease), and irritation of the eyes.

Precautions

- Use plaster and other gypsum products in areas equipped with an exhaust system.
- Wear the prescribed protective accessories while handling powders or trimming diagnostic casts.
- Minimize exposure to powder during handling.
- Avoid inhaling gypsum powder.

FORMALDEHYDE

Examples include a component of solutions used in chemical vapor sterilizers.

Hazards include formaldehyde's property as a human **carcinogen** (a cancer-causing agent); routes of entry are through inhalation, ingestion, and skin contact.

Precautions

- Use only in well-ventilated area.
- Wear nitrile gloves when handling solutions (such as pouring solutions into sterilizer).
- Follow the manufacturer's directions carefully.
- If skin contact occurs, immediately wash with soap and water.

MERCURY

Examples include mixing mercury with an alloy to prepare amalgam for use in posterior restorations.

Hazards include nausea, loss of appetite, diarrhea, tremors, depression, fatigue, increased irritability, headache, insomnia, allergic manifestations (such as contact dermatitis), pneumonia, nephritis, dark pigmentation of marginal gingiva, and loosening of the teeth.

Precautions

- Work in a well-ventilated space.
- Avoid direct skin contact with mercury.
- Avoid inhaling mercury vapor.
- Store mercury in unbreakable, tightly sealed containers away from heat.
- When preparing amalgam for restorations, use preloaded capsules. (This avoids exposure while measuring mercury.)
- When mixing amalgam, always close the cover before starting the amalgamator.
- Reassemble amalgam capsules immediately after dispensing the amalgam mass. (The used amalgam capsule is highly contaminated with mercury and is a significant source of mercury vapor if left open.)
- Leftover scrap amalgam (that was not used) is stored under water in a tightly closed container.
- Scrap amalgam (that has been retrieved from dental unit traps) is disinfected in a solution of bleach and water.
- Clean spills, using appropriate procedures and equipment; do not use a household vacuum cleaner.
- Place contaminated disposable materials in polyethylene bags and seal.

Special Mercury Considerations

Mercury may be absorbed directly through skin contact or from the inhalation of mercury vapors. According to OSHA regulations, the safe mercury vapor level is 0.05 mg. in the breathing zone for 8 hours per day, 40 hours per week. Any office that exceeds this limit is considered contaminated.

Urinalysis (laboratory testing of the urine) may be performed to measure the mercury level in the body. The normal level is about 0.015 mg. of mercury per liter of urine. The maximum allowable level according to OSHA is 0.15 mg. of mercury per liter.

When working with mercury, perform all procedures over a confined work area, such as a small tray, that will not absorb mercury and will limit any mercury or amalgam spill. In case of an accident, a "Mercury Spill Kit" is used to clean up the spill immediately by following the directions on the kit.

PHOTOGRAPHIC CHEMICALS

Examples include chemicals used to process radiographs.

Hazards include contact dermatitis and irritation of eyes, nose, throat, and respiratory system from vapors and fine particles of chemicals.

Precautions

- Wear appropriate protective clothing and equipment.
- Minimize exposure to dry powder during mixing of solutions.
- Work in well-ventilated areas.
- Clean up spilled chemicals immediately.
- If contact occurs, wash off chemicals with large amounts of water and a pH-balanced soap.
- Regularly launder clothing that comes in contact with photographic solutions, following OSHA guidelines.
- Store photographic solutions and chemicals in tightly covered containers in a cool, dark place.

PICKLING SOLUTIONS

Examples include acids used for surface cleaning (pickling) a cast restoration.

Hazards include burning of the skin, irritation of the skin and mucous membranes, damage to eyes, and irritation to the respiratory system.

Precautions

- Wear appropriate protective clothing and equipment.
- Use forceps with rubber covers on the tips to hold the object being pickled.
- Use pickling solutions in well-ventilated areas.
- Minimize the formation of airborne droplets.
- Avoid splattering of solution and putting hot objects into the solution.
- Store pickling solutions in covered glass containers.
- Keep soda lime or a commercial acid spill cleanup kit available in case of spills.
- In case of eye or skin contact, rinse with a large amount of running water.
- Seek medical attention as necessary.

VISIBLE LIGHT-CURED MATERIALS

Examples include light-cured restorative materials.

Hazards include the fact that without protective shielding repeated exposure to the curing light used to polymerize these materials can cause retinal damage to the eyes.

Precautions

- Be certain that the curing light is properly equipped with a protective shield (see Fig. 27–3).
- Avoid looking directly at the light when applying it to the tooth surface.

General Precautions for Storing Dental Materials

The careful use and storage of dental materials is important to ensure that these preparations retain their therapeutic activity and identity.

Changes in composition of materials can occur for many reasons, and when changes take place, the product may no longer retain its effectiveness.

A basic "safe" policy for the storage of dental medications and materials is to keep them in a dry, cool, dark place where they are not exposed to direct sunlight.

Follow Instructions. The best methods of packaging and storage have most likely been determined by the manufacturer. The manufacturer's instructions for storage should be followed.

Light. This is the prime factor in the deterioration of sodium hypochlorite (household bleach), epinephrine, and hydrogen peroxide. Change in color is one of the most common signs of deterioration.

Expiration Date. The expiration date that may be listed on the substances should always be noted. Also, fresh supplies should always be stocked behind the current inventory so that the oldest product is used first.

The Bloodborne Pathogens Standard

According to the OSHA definition, "**Bloodborne pathogens** are pathogenic microorganisms that are present in human blood and can cause disease in humans. These pathogens include, but are not limited to, hepatitis B virus (HBV), and human immunodeficiency virus (HIV)." (Bloodborne pathogens are discussed in Chapter 10.)

The Bloodborne Pathogens Standard sets forth the specific requirements that OSHA believes will prevent the transmission of bloodborne diseases to employees.

Specifically, the scope and application of the Standard covers all persons occupationally exposed to blood or other **potentially infectious materials** (PIMs) as defined in the Standard.

Many states have similar regulations, and whichever requirement is more stringent (stricter) applies. The description here is based on the OSHA standard.

Compliance

To comply with this standard, the dentist/employer must take the following steps:

1. Read the OSHA standard.
2. Perform the occupational exposure determinations.
3. Establish a written exposure control plan and implement the plan.
4. Institute a training and education program.
5. Maintain certain records.

Occupational Exposure Determination

The OSHA guidelines state that tasks in the dental office should be evaluated according to the *degree of risk involved* and classified in either of the following categories. These classifications are *not* rigid and may cross over, depending upon the job performed.

CATEGORY I

Category I tasks include all procedures or other job-related tasks that involve an inherent potential for mucous membrane or skin contact with blood, body fluids, or body tissues or a potential for spills or splashes of them. (In dentistry, saliva is *always* considered to be contaminated with blood.)

Most, although not necessarily all, tasks performed by the dentist, dental hygienist, chairside dental assistant, and laboratory technician belong to this category. The use of all appropriate protective measures is required for every employee engaged in Category I tasks.

CATEGORY II

Category II tasks include the normal work routines that do *not* involve exposure to blood or to body fluids or tissues; however, exposure or potential exposure *may* be required as a condition of employment.

Clerical or nonprofessional workers who, as part of their duties, may assist in cleaning the treatment rooms, who handle instruments or impression materials, or who send dental cases to laboratories, are classified as Category II employees.

Appropriate protective measures should be readily available to *every* employee engaged in Category II tasks.

Establish a Written Exposure Control Plan

The purpose of a written exposure control plan is to eliminate or minimize employee exposure. The plan must be specific to the employee's workplace and must be accessible to employees. It must also be available to OSHA on request.

The plan includes the use of engineering and work practice controls, PPE, housekeeping practices, and other aspects of the exposure control. The plan must be reviewed and updated at least annually, or whenever new tasks and procedures affect occupational exposure.

UNIVERSAL PRECAUTIONS

Universal precautions are important exposure control procedures that are used in the treatment of all patients. These precautions are discussed in Chapter 13.

The use of **PPE**, which includes protective clothing, gloves, masks, and protective eyewear during patient care, is also discussed in Chapter 13.

Engineering and Work Practice Controls

Engineering controls involve the use of equipment or devices to prevent exposures. **Work practice controls** involve altering the way procedures are performed to prevent exposures.

ENGINEERING CONTROLS

- Handwashing facilities must be readily available to all dental staff.
- Contaminated needles and other sharp implements must be handled in accordance with OSHA regulations.
- Contaminated reusable sharps containers must be puncture-resistant, labeled or color-coded, and leakproof.
- OSHA also requires that dental offices have at least one eyewash station that is capable of completely flushing both eyes continuously (Fig. 12–3).

WORK PRACTICE CONTROLS

Eating, drinking, smoking, application of cosmetics or lip balm, and handling of contact lenses are prohibited in work areas of the dental office where there is *reasonable* likelihood of occupational exposure. This includes all treatment areas, the laboratory, the darkroom, and sterilization areas.

Furthermore, all food substances and beverages must be stored *away from* refrigerators, cabinets, or countertops where blood or other potentially infectious materials are present.

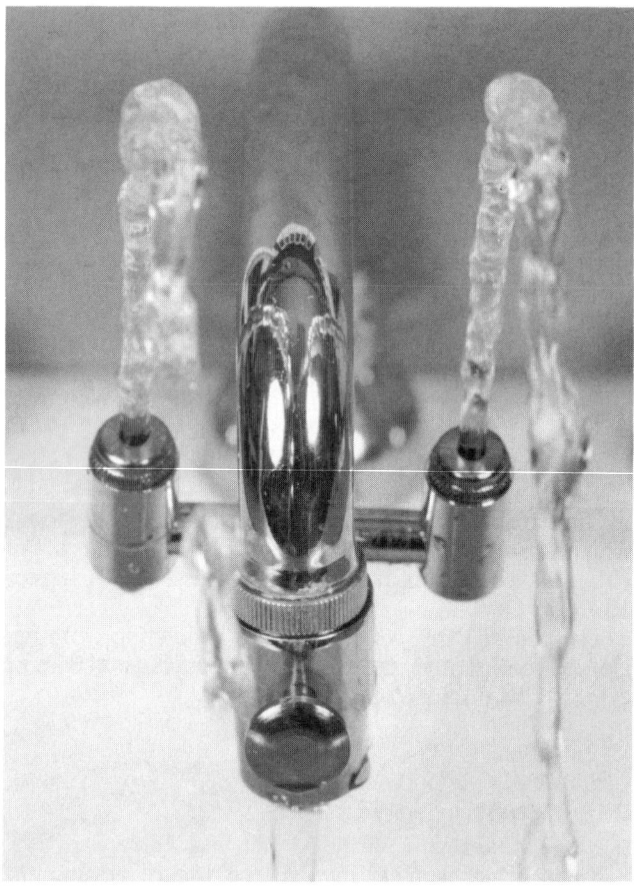

FIGURE 12–3

OSHA requires that dental offices have eyewash stations capable of continuous flushing of both eyes simultaneously.

Every effort must be made to minimize splashing, spraying, or spattering of blood or other potentially infectious materials during all work procedures.

Blood, saliva, or other infectious materials must be placed in approved containers for collection, handling, storage, shipping, and disposal.

Housekeeping Requirements

The Housekeeping section of the Bloodborne Pathogens Standard requires that employers maintain a safe and sanitary work environment. This includes provisions for handling contaminated sharps, spills, and broken contaminated glassware and regulated waste.

SHARPS

The term **sharps** means any sharp or pointed object that can penetrate the skin or oral mucosa. In dentistry the most common types of sharps are

- Needles
- Scalpel blades and disposable scalpels
- Exposed ends of dental arch wires
- Broken glass
- Burs and endodontic instruments

OSHA regulates *contaminated* sharps only. EPA and state waste disposal regulations may cover both contaminated *and* unused or uncontaminated sharps.

A **sharps container** must be closable, puncture resistant, leakproof on sides and bottom, and marked with the biohazard label or color-coded red to identify it as a hazard (Fig. 12–4).

A sharps container should be located as close as practical to the area in which the sharps are used. Preferably one sharps container is placed in each treatment room and possibly an additional one in the sterilization area.

Guidelines for Handling Sharps

- Sharp items should be considered as potentially infectious materials and thus handled with *extraordinary* care to prevent accidental injuries.
- Sharps must be disposed of by placing them into a sharps container located as close as practical to the area in which they are used.
- Contaminated sharps are never touched with bare hands. (Wear appropriate gloves or use transfer forceps.)
- Keeps the sharps disposal system securely in place, away from the edge of the countertop.
- Never attempt to transfer contaminated sharps from one container to another.
- Never tip the sharps container while the top is open.

Guidelines for Sharps Disposal

- Place materials to be disposed of as near to the container as possible.
- Pull back the spring-loaded cover located on the top of the container.
- Place the contaminated objects inside the box.
- Release the top to its original closed position.

Recapping a Used Syringe

A used needle must be recapped before it is removed from the syringe. Safely recapping the needle, also known as *resheathing*, is a major concern in reducing the hazard associated with handling sharps.

To reduce the danger of accidental needlestick injury, the used needle is never bent or broken before disposal. Also, when a used needle is recapped, the syringe is *never* held in one hand while the needle cap is replaced with the other hand.

Instead, a "hands-free" or "one-hand" technique must be used. A **hands-free technique** involves the use of a recapping device, such as the one shown in Figure 12–5. This allows the assistant to slip the needle into the cap without touching it.

In a **one-hand technique**, the needle guard is placed on the tray, and the used needle is wiggled into the

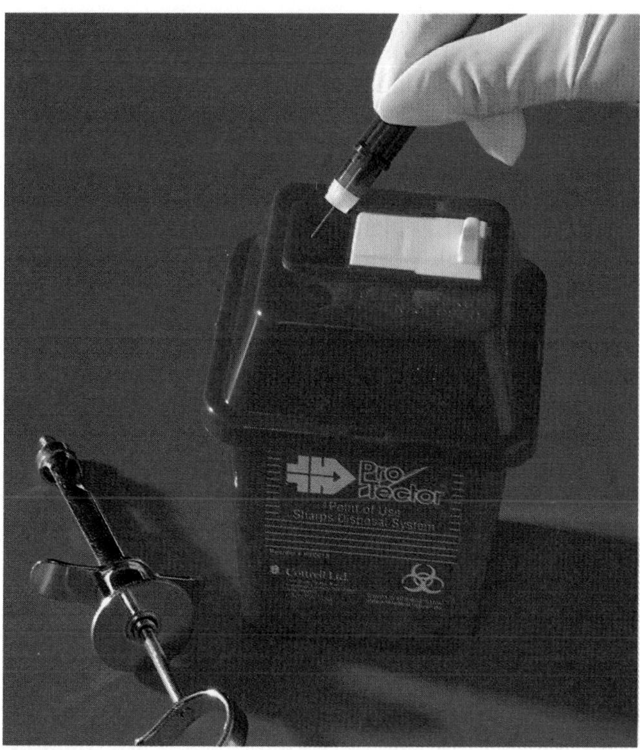

FIGURE 12–4

A puncture-resistant sharps disposal container should be located as close as practical to the area in which the sharps are used.

cover (Fig. 12–6). Once the end of the needle is covered, it may safely be brought into position.

TREATMENT ROOM CARE

OSHA requires that the employer develop and implement a written cleaning schedule. It should include the following procedures:

1. Clean and decontaminate all equipment and environmental and work surfaces that have been contaminated with blood or other potentially infectious materials.
2. Remove and replace contaminated protective coverings such as plastic wrap.
3. Inspect and decontaminate, on a regular basis, reusable receptacles such as bins, pails, and cans that are likely to become contaminated.
4. Implement a procedure to use mechanical means to pick up broken glass.
5. Store or process reusable sharps safely.
6. Place regulated waste in a closable and labeled or color-coded container.
7. Keep sharps containers upright, within easy access to personnel; replace routinely, keep closed when moving, and do not allow to be overfilled.
8. Discard all regulated waste according to federal, state, and local regulation.
9. Use appropriate PPE when handling contaminated laundry.

The details of treatment room care before and after a patient visit are discussed in Chapter 14.

Infectious Materials Spills

Spilled or dropped potentially infectious materials, such as gauze saturated with blood, must be cleaned up immediately.

Utility gloves and protective barrier clothing are worn. (Examination gloves are not adequate.) On a smooth, hard surface—for example, the floor—wet the area with a suitable disinfectant such as a 1:10 sodium hypochlorite solution.

Use a large wad of paper towels so that the gloves do not contact the liquid. Discard the towels after use.

Apply the disinfectant again. Leave the area wet for 10 minutes and then dry it with fresh paper towels.

Remove gloves carefully to avoid touching the contaminated outside, and wash hands immediately. Wash, dry, and autoclave gloves before reuse.

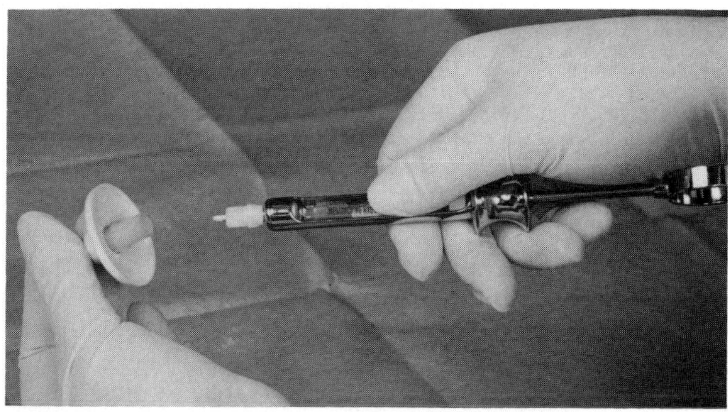

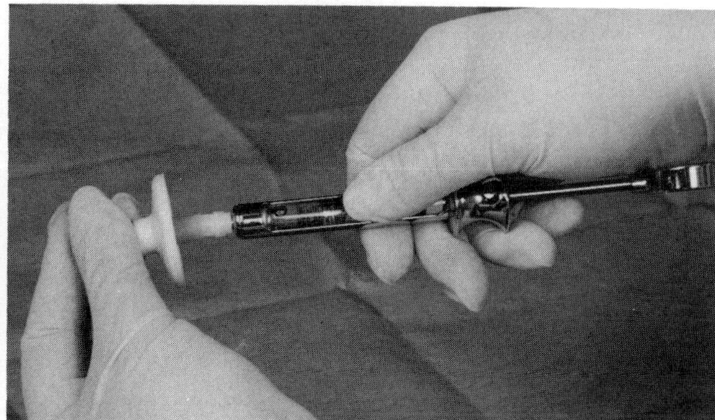

FIGURE 12–5

Needle recapping with a needleguard. *Left,* The needle cap is placed in the holder. *Right,* The holder is grasped securely below the shield while the needle is recapped.

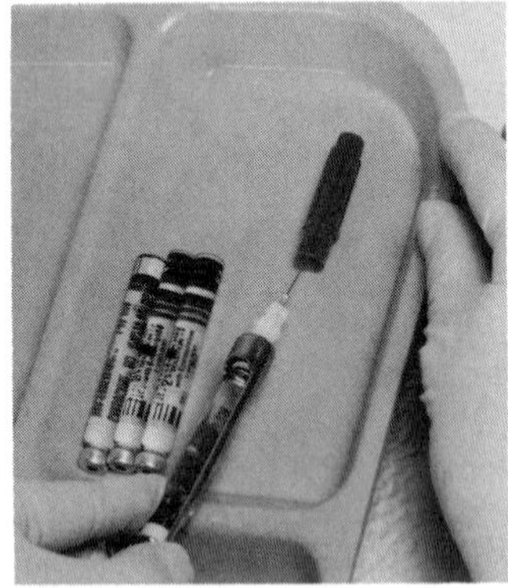
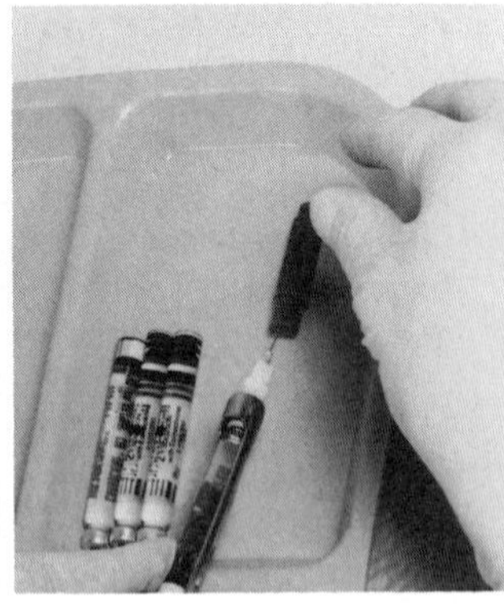

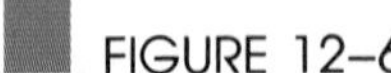
FIGURE 12–6

One-handed needle recapping. *Left,* Place cap on flat, stable surface. Using one hand, insert needle into cap. *Right,* Once the tip of the needle is safely covered, the other hand may be used to complete positioning it.

Broken Glass

If contaminated broken glass or something sharp drops, do *not* pick it up with the hands. Instead use tongs, forceps, or a dust pan and brush. Discard, clean and disinfect, or sterilize items used for this purpose.

Broken glass or dropped sharps are discarded in the sharps container. After the sharp material has been removed, disinfect the area as after a spill.

Discarding Local Anesthetic Cartridges

Local anesthetic solution is supplied in a glass cartridge that is discarded after a single use. It is necessary to review state and OSHA regulations to determine how this must be discarded.

In some states, this is always disposed of as a sharp. In others, where it is discarded depends upon the condition of the cartridge. In these situations,

- If the glass anesthetic cartridge is broken, pick up the broken glass as previously described and discard the broken glass with the sharps.
- If the glass anesthetic cartridge is not broken and not visibly contaminated with blood, discard it with other nonhazardous waste.
- If the glass anesthetic cartridge is visibly contaminated with blood, discard it with regulated waste. (This could occur if blood is aspirated into the solution during the injection. This is discussed in Chapter 20.)

Laboratory Specimens

Medical laboratory specimens, such as biopsy samples of suspected oral cancerous lesions, to be transported outside of the office for evaluation must be placed in leakproof bags and labeled appropriately.

Dental impressions must also be placed in leakproof bags and labeled appropriately.

Contaminated Laundry

It is the responsibility of the employer either to provide disposable clothing for staff or to assume responsibility for laundering or professional cleaning of protective clothing. Staff members may *not* take this laundry home for processing.

A commercial laundry or dry cleaning service may be used. In this situation the laundry bag, which should be red, must be clearly labeled with a biohazard symbol.

Many offices have in-house laundry facilities. If reusable uniforms are worn, they may be washed in hot water with a 1:100 bleach-to-water concentration, followed by machine drying.

If a staff member or janitorial person is designated to care for the office laundry, this person must receive special training in this role and wear PPE when handling soiled or contaminated clothing. This includes protective gloves, a mask, and eyewear.

Employee Information and Training

Every occupationally exposed member of the dental team must be provided with information and training at the time of initial employment or assignment (within 10 days) and at least once each year thereafter. The training must be conducted during regular office (working) hours and at no cost to the employee.

The method of training may be accomplished by direct instruction by the employer or office safety supervisor, by attending seminars and continuing education programs, by having outside professionals come to the office to conduct the training, or by a combination of any of these methods.

MAINTAINING TRAINING RECORDS

The dentist as employer is required to maintain records of all training sessions. The recordkeeping requirements are similar to those training in hazard communication management.

TRAINING SPECIFICS

Employee training must include the following:

1. How to obtain a copy of the Code of Federal Regulations and an explanation of its contents
2. Information on the epidemiology and symptoms of bloodborne diseases and on the modes of transmission of bloodborne pathogens
3. An explanation of the exposure control plan and how to obtain a copy
4. Information on how to recognize tasks that might result in occupational exposure
5. Explanations on uses and limitations of work practice and engineering controls, as well as PPE
6. Information on the proper use, location, removal, handling, decontamination, and disposal of PPE

7. Information and availability of hepatitis B vaccinations
8. Emergency information such as the fire evacuation plan
9. Information on reporting an exposure incident and post-exposure follow-up
10. Information on warning labels, signs, and color-coding

Hepatitis B Vaccination

Under the OSHA ruling, the dentist as an employer must educate the employee about the risks of acquiring the hepatitis B virus in the workplace and the benefits of vaccination. (Hepatitis B vaccination is discussed further in Chapter 10.)

The employer *must* provide hepatitis B vaccinations free of charge to all employees who have direct or indirect contact with the patient's blood or saliva. However, the employee may either consent to or decline vaccination.

If a staff member who has already received the inoculations is hired, this person may be required to show proof of immunization as a condition of employment. A copy of this document is retained with the employee's medical record.

Exposure Incidents

An **exposure incident** means a specific eye, mouth, other mucous membrane, non-intact skin, or parenteral contact with blood or other potentially infectious material (including saliva) that results from the performance of an employee's duties.

(**Parenteral** means piercing mucous membranes or the skin barrier through needlesticks, human bites, cuts, abrasions, or injection.)

Although this definition covers a wide range of potential incidents, they are commonly referred to as *needlestick injuries.*

MANAGING AN EXPOSURE INCIDENT

Should such an injury occur, it must be reported to the dentist immediately.

What the Employee Must Do

1. Stop operations immediately.
2. Report the exposure incident to the employer.
3. Remove gloves.
4. If the area of broken skin is bleeding, gently squeeze the site to express a small amount of visible blood.
5. Wash hands thoroughly, using antimicrobial soap and warm to hot water.
6. Dry the hands.
7. Apply a small amount of antiseptic to the affected area.
8. Apply an adhesive bandage to the area.

What the Employer Must Do

After the report of an exposure incident, the employer must make immediately available, at no cost to the employee, a confidential medical evaluation and follow-up that includes the following steps:

1. Document the route or routes of exposure and the circumstances in which the incident occurred.
2. Identify and document the source individual unless the employer can establish that identification is infeasible or prohibited by state or local law. (**Source individual** means any individual whose blood or other potentially infectious materials may be a source of occupational exposure.)
3. Obtain results of testing of the source individual's blood, if they are available.
4. Collect and test the employee's blood after consent is obtained. By law, the results of the employee's serum (blood) testing are held confidential from the employer.
5. Administer medically indicated prophylaxis such as necessary injections of gamma globulin, hepatitis B vaccine booster, and/or tetanus booster.
6. Provide appropriate counseling.
7. Evaluate reported illnesses in weeks after the incident.

POST-EXPOSURE FOLLOW-UP

The exposed worker must be offered medical counseling and human immunovirus (HIV) testing, as well as follow-up HIV testing at 6-week, 12-week, and 6-month intervals after exposure.

The exposed worker is offered hepatitis B immune globulin and hepatitis vaccine; a tetanus booster may also be recommended.

No adverse action can be taken against workers who are exposed but who choose not to be tested or not to participate in post-exposure follow-up. Any employee refusing the follow-up procedures must sign a written "informed refusal" form. These factors must be recorded on an *OSHA 200* log form.

Recordkeeping

EMPLOYEE MEDICAL RECORDS

The Employee Medical Record is an accurate confidential record that the dentist must establish and maintain for each employee covered by the OSHA standard. These records, which must be retained for at least the duration of employment plus 30 years, should include

- The name and social security number of the employee
- A copy of the employee's hepatitis B vaccination records and medical records relative to the employee's ability to receive vaccination

- The circumstances of any exposure incident (such as a needlestick) and name of the source individual
- A copy of follow-up procedures as they relate to the employee's ability to receive vaccination or to post-exposure evaluation after an exposure incident

Medical Waste Management

Waste Defined

Although the term "medical waste" is commonly used, the more accurate terms are *regulated waste* and *infectious waste.*

REGULATED WASTE

Regulated waste, according to the OSHA definition, is liquid or semi-liquid blood or other potentially infectious materials and items that would release blood or other potentially infectious materials if compressed. (A cotton roll, dripping wet with saliva, is an example of such an item.)

Other potentially infectious materials are body fluids that are visibly contaminated by blood.

While this waste is in the dental office and a potential hazard to employees, it is covered by OSHA regulations.

INFECTIOUS WASTE

When applied to dentistry, the EPA definition of infectious waste is contaminated sharps, teeth, pathological waste, and blood-soaked items. Commonly referred to as *hazardous waste,* such waste comes under EPA regulations when it leaves the dental office.

Disposal of Medical Waste

Once contaminated waste leaves the office, it is regulated by the EPA, as well as by state and local laws.

The dental team must be aware of, and comply with, the specific waste regulations affecting the state and community where the practice is located.

When covered by more than one regulation, the dental practice must comply with the strictest law.

Identifying Medical Waste

In the dental office, the following items are designated as medical waste and are subject to regulation:

- Sharps
- Body tissues and extracted teeth (if the extracted tooth is given to the patient it is not considered to be medical waste)
- Blood and other bioburden-soaked items such as bloody cotton rolls and gauze squares. (**Bioburden** is any visible organic debris.)

Under most regulations, the manner of disposal is determined by the amount (weight) of infectious materials to be disposed of.

The average dental practice, which produces about 1 pound of needles and 1 pound of blood-soaked articles in a 20-day work month, is in the category of being a "small producer" of infectious waste, and disposal is regulated accordingly.

The law requires that the dentist maintain records of the final disposal of this medical waste. This includes documentation of how, when, and where it was disposed of.

Handling Dental Office Waste

The dental assistant must take extra precautions not to contact contaminated waste. During waste handling, PPE must be worn, including nitrile utility gloves.

Waste must be handled depending upon whether it is considered *nonhazardous* (not contaminated) or *hazardous* (visibly contaminated with bioburden, such as blood or excess saliva).

NONHAZARDOUS WASTE

Nonhazardous waste should be discarded in covered containers made of durable material such as plastic or metal receptacles (Fig. 12–7). For ease in handling,

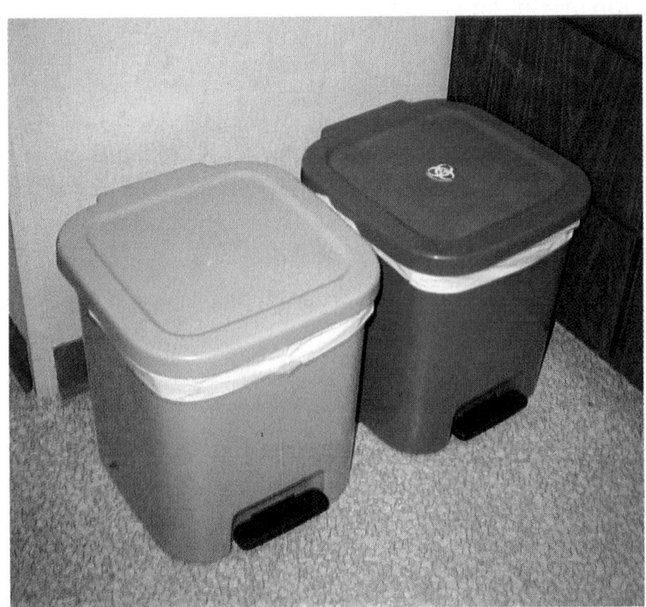

FIGURE 12–7

Waste is separated in clearly marked containers. Unregulated waste is on the left; regulated waste is on the right.

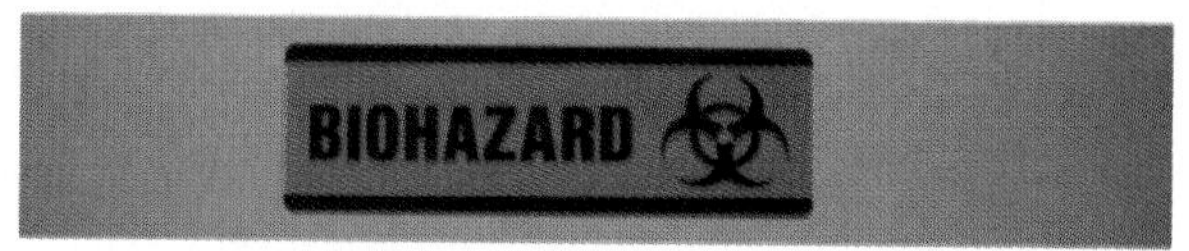

FIGURE 12–8

Hazardous waste must be labeled with the universal biohazard symbol.

nonhazardous waste receptacles should be lined with plastic bags. Nonhazardous waste includes disposable paper towels and paper mixing pads.

HAZARDOUS WASTE

Hazardous waste must be routinely separated from nonhazardous waste. It must also be properly covered and labeled with a *universal biohazard* sticker, label, or tag, legible from a distance of 6 feet (Fig. 12–8).

Receptacles for hazardous medical waste must be covered with a properly fitted lid that can be opened with a foot pedal. Keeping the lid closed prevents air movement, as well as the spreading of contaminants.

A receptacle such as a bin positioned beneath a cabinet top or flush with the counter surface, hidden from view, is also desirable.

Waste receptacles are lined with sturdy plastic bags that can be removed without touching the interior of the liner. Do not overfill the container; take this waste out a minimum of once daily.

Double-bagging of liners is recommended with hazardous waste receptacles, to eliminate accidental exposure should one of the bags rip or tear. Many practices use red plastic bags to readily identify them as medical waste.

Discard medical waste in a leak-resistant package that is impervious to moisture. The bag should be strong enough to prevent tearing or breaking under normal handling conditions.

Seal the bag to prevent leakage during transportation to the final dump site. If hazardous waste is shipped, store the containers in a safe place (a spare refrigerator used only for that purpose) to maintain the integrity of the contents and to control odor until the pick-up date.

Fire and Other Emergency Evacuation Policies

OSHA regulations state that the employer must maintain a written fire-safety policy. This includes the maintenance of fire extinguishers and training employees how to use them.

A diagram of the office layout, including emergency exits and locations of fire extinguishers, should be posted. The employer should also have emergency numbers for police, fire, and ambulance response posted.

If the practice is located in a geographical area subject to earthquakes, tornadoes, hurricanes, and other natural disasters, appropriate written procedures and evacuation plans must also be provided and made available to employees.

Other Signage Requirements

All exits from buildings and areas of potential exposure (x-rays, microwaves, biohazards, and other harmful substances) must be posted with appropriate signage.

All exits must be marked with an illuminated exit sign with the word "exit" in lettering at least 5 inches high. The stroke of the lettering must be at least ½-inch wide.

When directions to exits are not immediately apparent, signs of explanation or direction must be posted. For example, doors, passages, or stairways that are not exits, but could be mistaken for exits, must be appropriately marked "not an exit," "storeroom," and so forth.

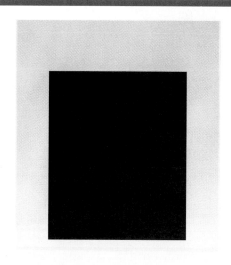

Chapter 13

Infection Control

Introduction

The Occupational Safety and Health Administration (OSHA) Bloodborne Pathogens Standard is discussed in Chapter 12. The modes of disease transmission are discussed in Chapter 10. You should review both before continuing with this chapter.

The goal of the infection control program is the 100 percent prevention of disease transmission throughout the dental practice both for the patient and the dental team.

The term **sepsis** means the presence of disease-producing microorganisms. **Asepsis** means the condition of being free from pathogenic microorganisms. It also includes the steps taken to prevent contact with pathogens.

Because of the sensitive tissues involved, asepsis cannot be achieved within the oral cavity; however, the use of an antiseptic mouth rinse by the patient just before treatment temporarily reduces the number of pathogens by up to 50 percent. In addition, other steps must be taken to reduce the number of pathogens present there and to limit their spread.

Infection Control Guidelines

The terms **infection control** and **exposure control,** which are used interchangeably, include the precautions necessary to protect the dentist, employees, and patients from the spread of infectious diseases through the dental practice.

Infection control within the dental office is accomplished (1) through compliance with the OSHA regulations and guidelines established by the Centers for Disease Control and Prevention (CDC); (2) by having a complete medical history for each patient; and (3) by employing Universal precautions in the treatment of *all* patients. (**Universal precautions** are designed to prevent disease transmission in a healthcare setting.)

Infection Control Protocols

OSHA requires that the dentist, as the employer, provide written exposure protocols to be in place and that these be readily accessible to the employee. (A **protocol** is a series of specific steps that must be followed.) These protocols include

- Exposure determination (see Chapter 12)
- Hepatitis B vaccination (see Chapters 10 and 12)
- Standard operating procedures (SOPs)
- Documented staff training
- Universal precautions
- Documentation of employee exposure incidents

STANDARD OPERATING PROCEDURES

According to the OSHA regulations, the dentist must establish SOPs regarding infection control for the tasks in every occupational exposure risk category (see Chapter 12).

These SOPs should include both the use of **personal protective equipment** (PPE) and **mandatory work practices** necessary to prevent the transmission of disease. (Work practices are discussed in Chapter 12.)

The dentist is responsible for ensuring staff compliance with these SOPs. However, all members of the dental team also have a responsibility to follow these regulations carefully at all times.

STAFF TRAINING

According to the OSHA regulations, the dentist is required to provide an in-office staff training program that includes information regarding modes of bloodborne infections and methods of infection control to prevent the spread of an infectious disease.

This training must be provided within 10 days for new employees and annually for all other staff members.

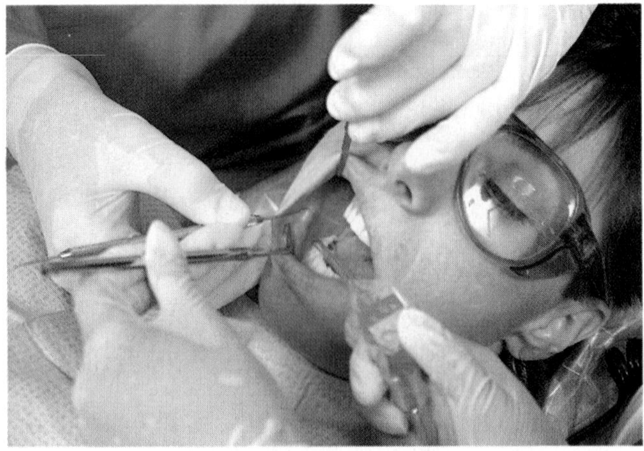

FIGURE 13–1

Semicritical items. Instruments used in the patient's mouth that *do not penetrate soft tissue or bone* are classified as semicritical items.

Classifications of Instruments, Equipment, and Surfaces

According to CDC guidelines, all instruments, equipment, and surfaces used during patient care are divided into three classifications: critical, semicritical, and noncritical clinical items. The infection control steps necessary in the care for these items depend upon their classification.

CRITICAL ITEMS

Critical items are those surgical and other instruments used to penetrate soft tissue or bone. These devices include forceps, scalpels, bone chisels, scalers, and burs. These devices *must* be sterilized before reuse.

SEMICRITICAL ITEMS

Semicritical items are instruments such as mouth mirrors and amalgam condensers that *do not* penetrate soft tissue or bone but do contact oral tissues (Fig. 13.1). These items should be sterilized before reuse. If this is not possible (because the instrument will be damaged by heat), the instrument should receive, at a minimum, high-level disinfection.

NONCRITICAL CLINICAL ITEMS

Noncritical clinical items are devices, such as the position-indicator device (PID) of the x-ray head, that come into contact only with intact skin. They may be processed between patients with intermediate-level or low-level disinfection.

Universal Precautions

The term **universal precautions** refers to a set of precautions designed to prevent the transmission of human immunodeficiency virus (HIV), hepatitis B virus (HBV), and other bloodborne pathogens in a healthcare setting.

In dentistry, according to these universal precautions, the blood and saliva of all patients are considered *potentially infectious* for HIV, HBV, and other bloodborne diseases.

Universal precautions means that the same infection control procedures must be used for *all* patients for *all* dental procedures. Simply stated, each patient is treated as if he or she were infected with a potentially fatal disease!

Importance of the Patient's Medical History

Although universal precautions are routinely followed for every patient, the dentist must be aware when there are special risks involved. An example of such a risk would be planning treatment for a patient with a highly infectious disease, such as the early stages of active tuberculosis.

A written medical history plays an essential part in preventing disease transmission by alerting the dentist to patients with special conditions or high-risk profiles.

The CDC recommends that a comprehensive medical history be obtained on each patient and that it be reviewed and updated at subsequent recall visits. Specific questions should be asked with regard to

- Medications taken
- Current and recurrent illnesses
- Unintentional or unexplained weight loss
- Lymphadenopathy (disease involving the lymph nodes)
- Oral soft tissue lesions

- Other unusual infections
- Symptoms of early active tuberculosis (see Chapter 10)
- History of previous diseases such as hepatitis, tuberculosis, and sexually transmissible diseases
- Allergic reactions, including those associated with latex

Protective Barrier Techniques

The purpose of protective barriers is to prevent dental personnel and patients from coming into contact with infectious or hazardous materials.

Barrier techniques include the routine use of dental dam, placing protective barriers on treatment room equipment, and wearing PPE.

Dental Dam

The dental dam, which is discussed in Chapter 22, is an important protective barrier because it reduces the amount of contamination in the aerosol spray generated during use of the handpiece.

The high-volume oral evacuation (HVE) system, which is discussed in Chapter 16, is used in conjunction with the dental dam to reduce the amount of aerosol spray that is released into the air.

Treatment Room Barriers

All environmental surfaces likely to be touched during a dental procedure must be *either* covered with protective barriers or cleaned and disinfected after use with a high-level surface disinfectant. When planning barrier placement and work procedures, remember the less you touch, the less you have to worry about.

The use of effective barriers permits more efficient treatment room preparation between patients. However, barriers must be waterproof and large enough to completely cover the surface being protected (Fig. 13–2). Items covered by protective barriers do not require surface disinfection after treatment *unless* the barrier comes off or tears.

Disposable covers for the **handles of the operating light** may be made of clear plastic, aluminum foil, or a plastic-backed towel. An alternative is to use removable handle covers that are sterilized and reused.

The head and upper portion of the **patient chair** are usually protected with a lightweight plastic cover, similar to a dry-cleaning bag.

A similar covering is used on the **x-ray head and arm**. The controls for the x-ray machine are protected by taping a sheet of lightweight plastic over them.

Controls on office signaling systems (in which a button is pushed to indicate a response) are also protected by taping a sheet of lightweight plastic over them.

Dental hoses, handpiece tubing, and the **handle of the air-water syringe** and the **HVE tip holder** should be covered with clear plastic film or tubing (sometimes referred to as a "sox").

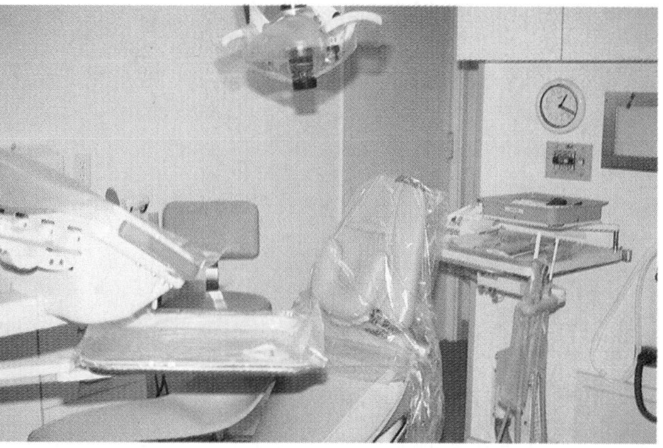

FIGURE 13–2

Surfaces touched during patient care should be covered by protective barriers. If not protected, they *must be* cleaned and surface disinfected at the end of the procedure.

Countertops, the patient tray, and other work surfaces may be covered with a plastic-backed paper or other fluid-resistant barrier.

Personal Protective Equipment (PPE)

In general, PPE for dental healthcare workers (DHCW) includes **protective clothing, gloves, masks,** and **protective eyewear** (Fig. 13–3).

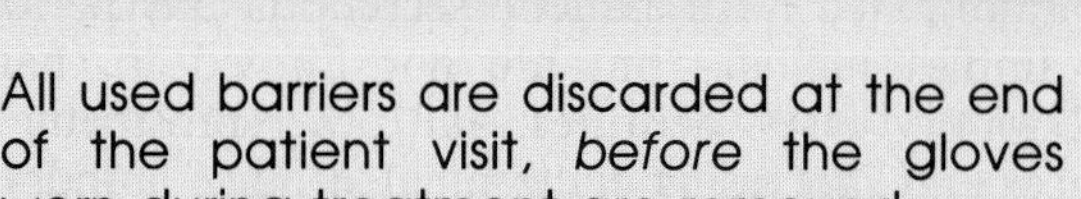

Guidelines for Use of Protective Barriers

- All used barriers are discarded at the end of the patient visit, *before* the gloves worn during treatment are removed.
- Clean protective barriers are placed *after* the treatment room has been cleaned and disinfected and *after* the utility gloves have been removed. Further detailed steps in placing and removing these barriers are discussed later in this chapter.

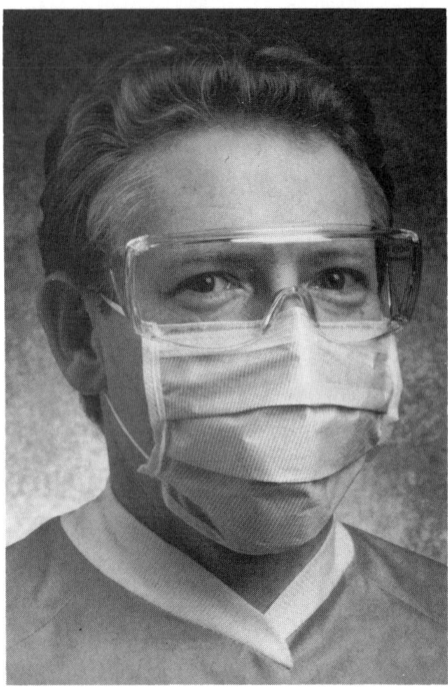

FIGURE 13–3

Protective clothing, eyewear, and masks. Gloves, which must also be worn, are not visible in this photo. (Courtesy of Johnson and Johnson Dental Division, Arlington, TX.)

Category I and II personnel *must* wear PPE when performing procedures capable of causing splash, spatter, or contact with body fluids or with mucous membranes or when touching items or surfaces that may be contaminated with these fluids.

Category I personnel routinely perform tasks that involve exposure to blood or other potentially infectious materials. **Category II personnel** may on occasion perform tasks that involve exposure to blood or other potentially infectious materials.

The term **spatter** describes larger droplets in an aerosol spray. **Splatter** describes larger droplets formed when a fluid splashes. However, these terms are commonly used interchangeably to describe droplets of potentially infectious material.

Appropriate PPE must also be worn when other clinically related activities that require handling items contaminated with patient secretions are performed. Examples include, but are not limited to, handling laboratory cases, dentures, and other prosthetic appliances and processing contaminated office laundry.

Protective Clothing

The primary purpose of protective clothing is to protect the worker from exposure to contaminated material. Protective clothing can include smocks, slacks, split skirts, laboratory coats, surgical scrubs (hospital operating room clothing), scrub (surgical) hats, pants, and shoe covers. Technically, clinic shoes and hosiery are also part of PPE. (The care of protective clothing is discussed in Chapter 12.)

The decision as to the type of protective clothing to be worn is based on the degree of anticipated exposure to infectious materials. For example, there is a high risk of exposure to contaminated aerosol when the high-speed handpiece is being used during a cavity preparation.

There is a lesser risk of exposure while an examination is being charted because that procedure does not involve use of equipment that creates contaminated aerosol.

PROTECTIVE CLOTHING REQUIREMENTS

- Protective clothing should be made of fluid-resistant material.
- To minimize the amount of uncovered skin, clothing should have long sleeves and a high neckline.
- The cuff of the sleeve must be tucked inside the band of the glove.
- During high-risk procedures, protective clothing must cover dental personnel at least to the knees when seated.
- Buttons, trim, zippers, and other ornamentation (which may harbor pathogens) should be kept to a minimum.

The use of disposable outer clothing is an option. These must be made of fluid-resistant material, must meet the other criteria for protective garments, and are discarded after use.

Guidelines for Use of Protective Clothing

- Because protective clothing can spread contamination, it is *not* worn out of the office for any reason, including travel to and from the office.
- Protective clothing should be changed at least daily.
- If a protective garment becomes visibly soiled or saturated with chemicals or body fluids, it should be changed immediately.
- Protective clothing must not be worn in staff lounge areas or when workers are eating or consuming beverages.

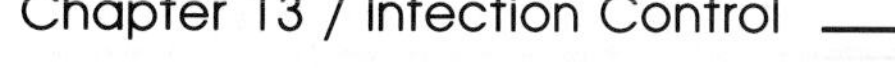

Protective Masks

A mask is worn over the nose and mouth to protect the wearer from inhaling possible infectious organisms spread by the aerosol spray of the handpiece or air-water syringe and by accidental splashes.

The two most commonly used types of masks are the *dome-shaped* and the *flat types.* The dome-shaped type is preferable, particularly during lengthy procedures, because it conforms more effectively to the face and creates an air space between the mask and the wearer.

Protective Eyewear

The universal precautions include the use of protective eyewear as part of PPE. Its purpose is to protect against the potential danger of eye damage resulting from aerosolized pathogens (especially herpes) and from debris such as flying scrap amalgam or tooth fragments.

Protective eyewear also prevents splattered solutions or caustic chemicals from injuring the eyes. Such damage may be irreparable and lead to permanent visual impairment or blindness.

There are two types of protective eyewear used during patient care: (1) glasses with protective side shields and (2) clear face shields. Protective goggles are worn when laboratory tasks such as using the lathe or model trimmer are performed.

If prescription glasses are worn, protective side shields must be added. Contact lens wearers *must* wear protective eyewear with side shields or a face shield.

Guidelines for Use of Protective Masks

- A fresh mask is worn when the DCHW is treating each patient.
- The mask *must* fit snugly to the face, particularly around the nose and mouth.
- A wet mask is *not* an effective mask.
- When a mask becomes damp, visibly soiled, or spattered, it is replaced with a fresh one.
- A mask should not be worn for more than 1 hour.
- The mask is discarded after a single use.

After each treatment or patient visit, protective eyewear should be cleaned and disinfected according to the manufacturer's instructions.

FACE SHIELDS

A chin-length plastic face shield may be worn as an alternative to protective eyewear; however, a shield does not replace the use of a face mask as protection against inhaling contaminated aerosols.

When splashing or spattering of blood or other body fluids is likely during a procedure (such as surgery), a face shield may be worn *in addition to* a protective mask.

PROTECTIVE EYEWEAR FOR PATIENTS

Patients should be provided with protective eyewear because they also may be subject to eye damage during the procedure. This may result from (1) handpiece spatter; (2) spilled or splashed dental materials, including caustic chemical agents; and (3) airborne bits of acrylic or tooth fragments (see Fig. 13–1).

In cases in which specific types of laser treatment are performed, patients must be supplied with special filtering lens glasses.

Gloves

Gloves must be worn by the dentist, assistant, and hygienist during *all* patient treatment in which there is the possibility of contact with the patient's blood, saliva, or mucous membranes.

All gloves used in patient care *must be* discarded after single use. This is because washing gloves may cause **wicking** (penetration of liquids through undetected holes in the gloves). Deterioration of gloves may also be caused by disinfecting agents, oils, oil-based lotions, and the heat of sterilization.

Before gloves are put on, the hands must be thoroughly washed and dried. (Handwashing instructions follow later in the chapter.)

EXAMINATION GLOVES

Examination gloves, which are usually made of latex and are often referred to as *latex gloves* or *exam gloves,* are the type most commonly worn by dental personnel during patient care. These gloves are *not* sterile and serve strictly as a protective barrier for the wearer.

Examination gloves are selected by hand size and may be supplied as ambidextrous (fitting either hand) or fitted specifically to either the left or right hand.

Gloves Damaged During Treatment

Gloves are effective only when they are intact. (**Intact** means not damaged, torn, ripped, or punctured.)

Guidelines for Use of Examination Gloves

- Wear a pair of gloves for only one patient.
- Discard gloves after a single use. (They are *not* washed and reused.)
- Do not wear jewelry under gloves. (Rings harbor pathogens and may tear the glove.)
- Change gloves frequently. (If the procedure is a long one, change gloves about once each hour.)
- If gloves are torn or damaged, change them immediately.
- Use overgloves as necessary.

If gloves are damaged during treatment, they must be changed immediately. The procedure for regloving is as follows:

1. Excuse yourself and leave chairside.
2. Remove and discard the damaged gloves.
3. Wash hands thoroughly.
4. Reglove before returning to the dental procedure.

Hypoallergenic Gloves

Occasionally healthcare providers or patients may experience serious allergic reactions to latex, specifically to the proteins in the latex examination gloves or dental dam.

Most commonly, this reaction, which is known as **latex sensitivity**, is one of contact dermatitis, which may take the form of blisters, swelling, or a rash. In some cases, wheezing, coughing, or sneezing also occurs.

In the event of an allergic reaction or suspected latex allergy, hypoallergenic gloves, made of an alternative material such as vinyl, are worn instead of latex examination gloves. (**Hypoallergenic** means designed to reduce the signs and symptoms associated with an allergic reaction.)

STERILE SURGICAL GLOVES

Sterile gloves, the type used in hospital operating rooms, should be worn for invasive procedures involving significant amounts of blood or saliva, such as oral surgery or periodontal treatment.

Sterile gloves are supplied in prepackaged units to maintain sterility before use. They are provided in specific sizes and are fitted to the left or right hand. Hand preparation and the use of surgical gloves are discussed in Chapter 30.

GLOVE LINERS

Glove liners, also known as *undergloves*, may be worn under examination or surgical gloves for the comfort of the wearer. Glove liners are put on immediately *after* the hands are washed and dried and *before* examination or surgical gloves are put on.

Glove liners are lightweight and made of soft white cotton. Because they never come into contact with the patient's body fluids, glove liners may be laundered and reused.

OVERGLOVES

Overgloves, which are also known as "food handler" gloves, are made of lightweight, inexpensive, clear plastic. These gloves are put on over examination or sterile gloves for brief, single-use occasions.

Appropriate uses of overgloves also include pouring impressions, handling laboratory cases, developing x-rays, answering the telephone, or making a chart entry.

If you leave the chair for any reason during treatment of a patient, overgloves should be used. If overgloves are not used, contaminated examination gloves should be removed and your hands washed *before* you leave chairside. Upon returning, you should wash and dry your hands and use fresh examination gloves.

MAINTAINING INFECTION CONTROL WHILE GLOVED

During a dental procedure, it may be necessary to touch surfaces or objects such as drawer handles or materials containers. If these are touched with a gloved hand, both the surface and glove are contaminated. One option to minimize the possibility of cross-conta-

Guidelines for Use Of Overgloves

- Overgloves are *not* an acceptable alternative to examination gloves.
- Overgloves are placed before the secondary procedure is performed and are removed *before* the patient treatment that was in progress is resumed.
- Overgloves are discarded after a single use.

mination is the use of an overglove when it is necessary to touch a surface.

Another alternative is to keep a supply of individual paper towels within reach at chairside. These are individual towels rather than a continuous roll and would not become contaminated when a towel is removed. Each towel is discarded after a single use.

Infection control procedures for use in mixing and passing dental materials are discussed in Chapter 23.

Opening Drawers and Cabinets

With proper planning before a procedure is begun, it is not necessary to stop during treatment to take supplies out of a drawer or cabinet; however, should it be unavoidable, do *not* use a contaminated gloved hand for this purpose.

Instead, pick up a paper towel by touching only one side of the paper towel. Use the other side of the paper towel to open the drawer or cabinet and to remove containers. Discard the used towel immediately.

Opening Containers

During the procedure, it may become necessary to open containers of materials or supplies. When opening a container, use overgloves, a paper towel, or a sterile gauze sponge to remove the lid or cap. In doing this, take care not to touch any surface of the container.

Use sterile cotton pliers to remove an item from the container. If the container or bottle is touched, it is contaminated and must be disinfected at the end of the procedure.

UTILITY GLOVES

Utility gloves are *not* used during direct patient care. Instead, they are worn when the treatment room is cleaned and disinfected between patients and while contaminated instruments are handled. Utility gloves may be washed, sterilized, and reused.

Utility gloves are made from a puncture-resistant, heavy nitrile (industrial-strength) material. Each staff member responsible for cleanup procedures must have his or her own designated pair of utility gloves.

Handwashing

The environment between the hand and inner surface of the glove is warm, dark, and moist. These are ideal conditions for bacteria and other microbes to thrive! Therefore, thorough and frequent handwashing is essential.

Hands should be washed thoroughly at the beginning and end of the day. In addition, they must be washed each time before gloves are put on and immediately after gloves are removed.

Liquid soap is always used during handwashing. Bar soap is never used because it may transmit contamination. For many routine dental procedures, such as examinations and nonsurgical techniques, handwashing with a plain soap is adequate. An antimicrobial soap, which helps to reduce the microbes on the skin, should be used before surgical procedures.

Healthy skin is better able to withstand the damaging effects of repeated washing and of wearing gloves. Hand lotion or a protective skin barrier cream should be used to help keep skin healthy.

Keep nails short and clean. Long nails are likely to harbor pathogens, puncture examination gloves, or accidentally poke a patient. Also, microorganisms thrive around rough cuticles and can enter the body through any break in the skin.

An orangewood stick and a nail brush should be used to clean soiled areas of the skin and to clean under the fingernails. The orangewood stick may be discarded after a single use or autoclaved and reused. The nail brush may be disinfected and reused or may be purchased as a prepackaged disposable with an orangewood stick.

To minimize cross-contamination, it is preferable that treatment room sinks be equipped with "hands-free" faucets that are activated electronically or with foot pedals.

Sterilization

Sterilization is the process by which *all* forms of life are completely destroyed in a specified area. These forms include all forms of microbial life, such as bacteria, fungi, viruses, and bacterial spores.

Sterile is an absolute term! There is no such thing as "partially sterile" or "almost sterile." *All* instruments used in intraoral treatment must be sterilized.

Forms of sterilization involve the use of heat above the temperature of boiling water. The three accepted forms of sterilization most commonly used in the dental office are (1) **autoclaving**, (2) **chemical vapor sterilization**, and (3) **dry heat sterilization.**

All reusable items that come in contact with the patient's blood, saliva, or mucous membranes must be sterilized through one of these three methods before reuse.

Ethylene oxide gas sterilization is an accepted form of sterilization; however, because of the time involved (8 to 10 hours per load or overnight) and the toxicity of the fumes, it is more appropriate for a hospital setting and is not commonly used in dental offices.

Flash sterilization, a shortcut method of sterilization, is *not* recommended for routine instrument sterilization in the dental office. Also, although heat is involved, boiling water is *not* an accepted form of sterilization.

Maintaining Sterility

It is not possible to maintain the sterility of unwrapped instruments. For this reason, instruments must be wrapped before sterilization and kept wrapped

PROCEDURE: **Handwashing Before Gloving**

Instrumentation

Liquid soap (dispensed with a foot-activated or electronic device)
Orangewood stick
Nail brush
Paper towels

Handwashing

1. Remove all jewelry, including watch and rings.
   ☐ *RATIONALE:* Jewelry is difficult to clean, can harbor microbes, and can puncture the gloves.
2. Use the foot or electronic control to regulate the flow of water. If this is not available, use a paper towel to grasp the faucets to turn them on and off. Discard the towel after use.
   ☐ *RATIONALE:* Faucets may have been contaminated by being touched with soiled or contaminated gloved hands.
3. Use a liquid soap, dispensed with a foot-activated or electronic device.
   ☐ *RATIONALE:* Bar soap transmits microorganisms. So does touching a dispenser that may be contaminated.
4. Scrub the hands vigorously with warm water to remove surface debris.
   ☐ *RATIONALE:* Scrubbing the first time removes gross debris. Warm water is less drying to the skin than hot water.
5. Scrub again.
   ☐ *RATIONALE:* Secondary scrubbing removes residual debris and tenacious microorganisms more effectively.
6. Get soap under the nails. At the beginning of the day (and more often if necessary), use an orangewood stick and a nail brush to clean soiled areas of the skin and to clean under the fingernails.
   ☐ *RATIONALE:* Microorganisms thrive beneath the free edges of the finger nails.
7. Rinse the hands with cool water.
   ☐ *RATIONALE:* Cool water closes the pores.
8. Use a paper towel to dry the hands and then the forearms.
   ☐ *RATIONALE:* Reusable cloth towels remain moist, contribute to microbial growth, and spread contamination.

until ready to be used. The type of wrap used depends upon the sterilization method.

Preset trays and cassettes are used to organize instruments and supplies according to procedure. For example, a practice would have trays for examinations, composite restorations, amalgam restorations, and other commonly performed procedures (see Chapter 15).

The instruments for each of these trays or cassettes are kept together during cleaning. These are wrapped, labeled, sterilized, and stored together. They are not unwrapped until just before use in patient care. (Their preparation is discussed later in this chapter.)

Each package must be clearly labeled with the contents and the date of sterilization. Sealed nylon tubing, plastic bags, and biofilm/paper bags remain sterile for 1 year. (These bags are a combination of biofilm, a strong clear plastic, on one side and paper on the other.) Paper-bagged or cloth pack–wrapped instruments should be resterilized after 1 month if not used.

Autoclaving

Autoclaving, which is sterilization by superheated steam under pressure, is the preferred method of instrument sterilization (Fig. 13–4).

The advantages are that the results are consistently good and that instruments may be wrapped before sterilization. Although stainless steel instruments may be autoclaved without damage, the disadvantage of autoclaving is that the steam will rust, dull, or corrode other metals, especially carbon steel.

Glass slabs and dishes, rubber items, and stones can be autoclaved but must be dry before sterilization.

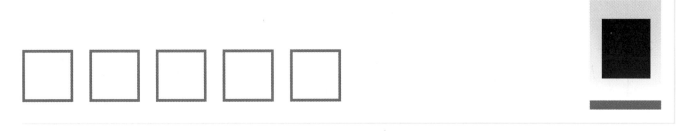

PROCEDURE: **Handwashing After Removing Gloves**

1. Repeat the steps for handwashing before gloving.
   □ *RATIONALE:* Bacteria can grow in gloves or enter gloves through even a pinhole opening.
2. Apply a hand lotion or a protective skin barrier cream.
   □ *RATIONALE:* This helps to protect hands and keep skin healthy.

PRESSURE, TEMPERATURE, AND TIME

There are three major factors required for autoclaving: pressure, temperature, and time.

Pressure. The amount of pressure used during autoclaving is expressed in terms of *psi* (pounds per square inch) or *kPa* (kilopascals) (1 kPa = 0.145 psi). Most dental autoclaves operate effectively at 15 to 20 psi.

Temperature. To achieve proper pressure, the temperature must reach and be maintained at 121°C (250°F). As the temperature and pressure increase, superheated steam is formed. It is exposure to this superheated steam that brings about sterilization.

Superheated steam, which is lighter than air, rises to the top of the autoclave chamber. As more superheated steam is formed, it eliminates air from the autoclave, and the steam penetrates the materials in a top-to-bottom flow.

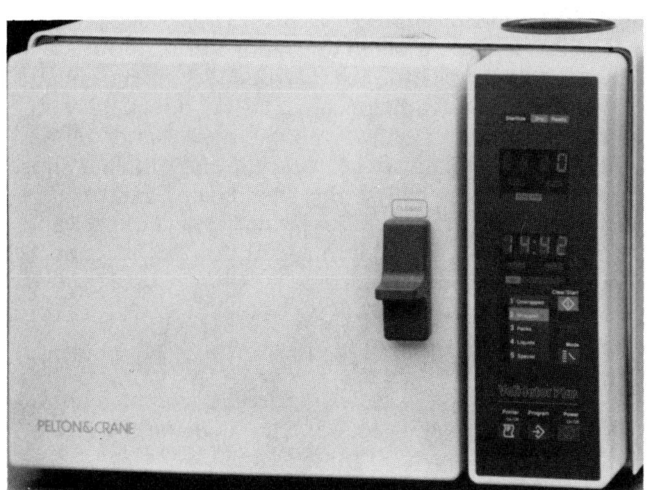

FIGURE 13–4

An autoclave sterilizes through a combination of time, temperature, and pressure. (Courtesy of Pelton & Crane Co., Charlotte, NC.)

The air must be eliminated so all of the load in the autoclave is exposed to the superheated steam for the appropriate length of time.

Time. Wrapped loads take a minimum of 20 minutes *after* full pressure and temperature have been achieved within the chamber of the autoclave.

WRAPPING INSTRUMENTS FOR AUTOCLAVING

Instruments must be clean, but not necessarily dry, before wrapping for autoclaving. Non–stainless steel instruments and burs may be dipped in a corrosion-inhibitor solution (1 percent sodium nitrate) before being wrapped. (An alternative for these instruments is sterilization by dry heat.)

Nonperforated closed containers (solid closed metal trays, capped glass vials) or aluminum foil cannot be used in an autoclave because they prevent the steam from reaching the inner sections of the pack. Cassettes, with openings on all sides, may be successfully autoclaved.

Packaging used for autoclaving must be porous enough to permit the steam to penetrate to the instruments. This packaging could be a fabric; however, most commonly it is sealed biofilm/paper pouches, nylon tubing, sterilization wrap, and paper-wrapped cassettes.

The bag or wrap is heat-sealed or sealed with tape because pins, staples, and paperclips make holes in the wrap that allow microorganisms to pass through.

THE AUTOCLAVE IN OPERATION

Distilled water is used in most autoclaves. Tap water often contains minerals that may damage the autoclave by building up as deposits on the inner surfaces. Dis-

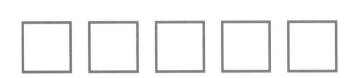

PROCEDURE: Loading the Autoclave

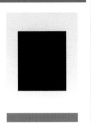

1. Prepare packs with a suitable wrapping material.
   □ *RATIONALE:* The steam must be able to penetrate the pack. (Preparation of these packs is discussed later in this chapter.)
2. Arrange autoclave contents to facilitate the top-to-bottom flow of steam.
   □ *RATIONALE:* Objects not reached by steam will not be sterilized.
3. Separate articles and packs from each other by a reasonable space. Glass or metal canisters should be tilted at an angle.
   □ *RATIONALE:* This permits a free flow of steam in and around all instrument packs.
4. Place larger packs, which might block the flow of steam, at the bottom of the chamber.
   □ *RATIONALE:* Trapped air in the autoclave will inhibit the top-to-bottom flow of steam.
5. Never overload the autoclave.
   □ *RATIONALE:* Large loads prevent the autoclave from reaching the correct temperature and pressure and make it difficult for the steam to flow properly.

tilled water is preferred because it has been treated to remove these minerals.

Before operation, always check to be certain that an adequate supply of water is present. For this and other steps in operating the autoclave, it is important that the manufacturer's directions be followed exactly.

Sterilization will not occur unless the autoclave is operated at the appropriate pressure and temperature for an adequate length of time. The pressure and temperature must be reached before timing begins. The length of this warm-up time depends upon the autoclave and the size of the load.

Many autoclaves are equipped with automatic controls that start the timing process only when the proper temperature and pressure have been achieved.

If the autoclave must be manually timed, *before* starting to time the sterilization cycle, check the gauges to determine that the heat and pressure conditions have been reached.

Venting and Drying. At the end of the sterilization cycle, the steam is vented into the atmosphere, and the contents of the autoclave are allowed to dry and cool. With newer models, this should occur automatically.

If the machine is not equipped to do this, open the door of the autoclave slightly after the pressure has dropped within the chamber. Do this with *extreme caution* because the contents and remaining steam are very hot! The contents should be allowed to dry and cool before they are removed.

Monthly examine the door gasket on the autoclave to determine that is not leaking or defective. A worn or damaged gasket does not permit the autoclave to function properly, and the gasket must be replaced immediately.

Chemical Vapor Sterilization

Chemical vapor sterilization is very similar to autoclaving except a chemical is used instead of water to create a vapor for sterilizing (Fig. 13–5).

The advantage of chemical vapor sterilization is that it does not rust, dull, or corrode dry metal instruments. The disadvantages are that (1) adequate ventilation is essential because the chemicals used give off unpleasant and harmful fumes, (2) instruments must be absolutely dry before they are placed in the sterilizer (if not dry, they will rust), and (3) chemical vapor sterilization is not recommended for large loads or tightly wrapped instruments.

PRESSURE, TEMPERATURE, AND TIME

The three major factors in chemical vapor sterilization are **pressure** (20 to 40 psi), **temperature** (132°C [270°F]), and **time** (20 minutes).

WRAPPING INSTRUMENTS FOR CHEMICAL VAPOR STERILIZATION

Instruments must be clean and dry before they are wrapped and placed in the chemical vapor sterilizer.

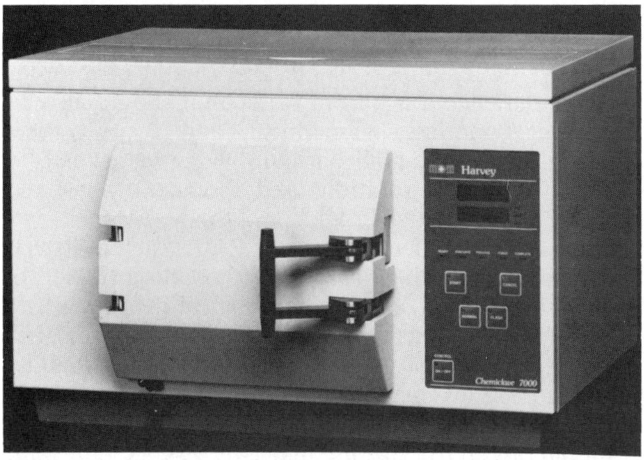

FIGURE 13–5

A chemical vapor sterilizer uses a chemical vapor instead of water. (Courtesy of MDT, Torrance, CA.)

Also, care must be taken not to create packs that are too large to be sterilized throughout.

Standard packaging for chemical vapor sterilization includes biofilm/paper bags, nylon see-through tubing, sterilization wrap, and wrapped cassettes.

Nonperforated closed containers (solid metal trays, capped glass vials) and aluminum foil cannot be used in a chemical vapor sterilizer because they prevent the sterilizing agent from reaching the instruments inside.

THE CHEMICAL VAPOR STERILIZATION IN OPERATION

Operation of a chemical vapor sterilizer is very similar to that of an autoclave. However, there are important differences, and the manufacturer's directions must be followed exactly.

Packs for this form of sterilization should be kept small and loosely wrapped. Also, instruments *must be dry* when they are placed in the chemical vapor sterilizer because any moisture increases the amount of water present during operation, and the instruments may rust.

The assistant should refer to the Material Safety Data Sheet (MSDS) for chemical vapor solutions to determine the proper steps and precautions for working with the chemical vapor sterilizer.

Dry Heat Sterilization

Dry heat sterilization is an alternative method for sterilizing instruments that will rust in an autoclave. The advantage is that the instruments will not rust *if* they are thoroughly dry before being placed in the sterilizer. The disadvantages are that the sterilization process is time consuming and may not be effective because of operator errors in calculating the correct time.

TEMPERATURE AND TIME

Dry heat sterilization depends completely on a combination of time and temperature. For sterilization to occur, both time and temperature must be correct throughout the load. The following time and temperature combinations are used:

160°C (320°F): 120 minutes
170°C (340°F): 60 minutes

WRAPPING INSTRUMENTS FOR DRY HEAT STERILIZATION

Instruments must be clean and dry before being wrapped for dry heat sterilization. The wrapping material *must* be heat resistant. Aluminum foil, metal, and glass containers may be used in the dry heat oven.

The instruments should not be wrapped too tightly because they may puncture the wrapping. Paper and cloth packs should be avoided because they may char.

THE DRY HEAT STERILIZER IN OPERATION

The manufacturer's directions are followed in loading and operating the dry heat sterilizer.

Instruments must be thoroughly dried and wrapped before being placed into the dry heat sterilizer. If wet, they may rust.

Sterilization does not occur unless heat reaches all areas of all instruments. Therefore, when the dry heat chamber is loaded, care must be taken to permit adequate circulation of air around the articles. This includes having hinged instruments, such as surgical forceps, hemostats, and scissors, with their hinges opened during sterilization.

Timing does not start until the desired temperature has been reached throughout the load—and this can be difficult to judge. Use of an oven thermometer helps; however, dry heat sterilization cannot readily be controlled as accurately as other forms of sterilization.

Once the sterilization cycle has started, additional instruments may *not* be added to the load. This is because the cooler instruments lower the temperature of the oven significantly.

At the end of the cycle, packs are very hot and must be allowed to cool before they are handled.

Monitoring Sterilization

The CDC guidelines recommend that steps be taken to determine that sterilization has actually occurred throughout the load during sterilization. This requirement is met only through biological monitoring.

BIOLOGICAL MONITORING

Biological indicators involve the use of spores that are harmless (but highly resistant to heat) to prove that sterilization has taken place.

Weekly monitoring through biological indicators for

each sterilizer in the office is recommended by the CDC guidelines, and in some states this is mandated by law.

Biological indicators for steam autoclave or chemical vapor sterilization contain spores of *Bacillus stearothermophilus*. Indicators for dry heat or ethylene oxide sterilization contain spores of *Bacillus subtilis*.

Each type of biological indicator should be used to verify *only* the sterilization method for which it is designed.

One common form of biological indicator test consists of three strips of special paper impregnated with the appropriate spores. Two of the strips are placed inside instrument packs in the test load, and the sterilizer is operated under normal conditions. The third strip is retained as a control.

After the load has been sterilized, all three strips are cultured. This is usually done by an outside laboratory. (It may be done in the dental office if the appropriate incubation equipment is available.) The laboratory sends a report to document that cultures were read at 24, 48, and 72 hours.

- A **negative report** indicates sterilization did occur.
- A **positive report** indicates corrective procedures must be taken immediately.

These reports must be kept on file as part of the documentation requirements of the exposure control program.

PROCESS INDICATORS

Process indicators, which change color when exposed to heat, are incorporated into tapes, bags, and wrapping materials used in packaging instruments for sterilization.

These indicators are useful within the practice to identify those instrument packs that have been processed through the sterilizer. Because they do not indicate that heat and other conditions were maintained for the appropriate *length* of time for sterilization to have occurred, they do not replace the use of biological indicators to monitor sterilization.

DISINFECTION

Disinfection is the killing of pathogenic agents by chemical or physical means. It does *not* include the destruction of spores and resistant viruses. The purpose of disinfection is to reduce the microbial population when sterilization is not possible.

The terms "disinfectants" and "antiseptics" are *not* used interchangeably. **Disinfectants** are applied to inanimate objects such as countertops or equipment. **Antiseptics** prevent the growth or action of microorganisms and are applied on living tissue.

When working with any disinfection solution, it is necessary to wear appropriate PPE to prevent skin, nose, or eye irritation. It is also essential that the manufacturer's instructions be followed exactly.

Ideally, the chemical disinfectant should offer residual biocidal effect on treated surfaces; it should also be fast-acting, odorless, economical, and easy to use. (**Biocidal** means the ability to kill living organisms.)

The disinfecting solution used should be registered by the Environmental Protection Agency (EPA).

High-level disinfectants are EPA-registered "sterilant/disinfectant" chemicals used to obtain a high-level disinfection of heat-sensitive semicritical instruments.

The EPA classification as a "sterilant/disinfectant" must be shown on the product label. The manufacturer's directions regarding appropriate concentration and exposure must be followed exactly.

Liquid chemical agents that are less potent than those in the "sterilant/disinfectant" category are *not* appropriate for processing critical or semicritical dental instruments.

Intermediate-level disinfectants, which are EPA registered as *hospital disinfectants*, are labeled for tuberculocidal activity. This means they are capable of killing the mycobacteria that cause tuberculosis. Mycobacteria are among the most resistant groups of microorganisms. A germicide that is effective against them should also be effective against many other pathogens.

These disinfectants should be used on countertops and dental unit surfaces that may have become contaminated with patient material.

Low-level disinfectants, which are *not* labeled for "tuberculocidal activity," are acceptable only for general housekeeping purposes such as cleaning floors, walls, and other housekeeping surfaces.

Glutaraldehydes

Glutaraldehydes are EPA registered as a "sterilant/disinfectant" chemical. They have low surface tension, which allows them to penetrate blood and bioburden. (**Low surface tension** means that the liquid has the ability to flow and penetrate surfaces. **Bioburden** is any visible organic debris.)

Glutaraldehydes may be used as a holding solution for soiled instruments and to remove blood and debris from suction hoses. (A **holding solution** is a disinfecting solution used to cover soiled instruments while they are awaiting processing.)

Because they are slow-acting, glutaraldehydes are *not suitable* for disinfecting surfaces.

Glutaraldehydes are available as *neutral*, *alkaline*, or *acidic* solutions. Each type of glutaraldehyde solution has different properties, and the manufacturer's instructions for mixing and use should be followed exactly.

Some of these glutaraldehyde products must be activated before use by adding an appropriate buffer. These activated solutions have an active life of 14 to

30 days, depending on the preparation. (**Active life** describes how long a reusable solution will remain effective after it has been put into use.)

The active life of the solution can be altered by incorrect mixing, by dilution from water left on instruments, or by heavy debris and contamination from instruments placed in the solution.

A special color-monitor dipstick may be used to test the strength of the solution. A solution that is not of the appropriate strength must be replaced immediately.

Glutaraldehydes produce fumes that are very toxic to lung tissue. Therefore, these chemicals must be used with caution by following the manufacturer's guidelines.

Glutaraldehydes also discolor the skin. Do not put your hand in the solution! Place and remove instruments only while wearing utility gloves.

Iodophors

Iodophors are intermediate-level disinfectants registered with the EPA as *hospital disinfectants with tuberculocidal action.*

Iodophors are recommended for disinfecting surfaces that have been soiled with potentially infectious patient material. When used properly, according to the manufacturer's instructions, they are effective usually within 5 to 10 minutes.

Iodophors are available as antiseptics and hard-surface disinfectants. These two types are *not* used interchangeably.

Antiseptic iodophors are minimally irritating to tissue and do not stain the skin.

Hard-surface iodophor disinfectant solutions have a built-in color indicator that changes from amber to light yellow or clear when the iodophor molecules are exhausted. A fresh solution should be prepared when the amber disappears.

Because iodophors are inactivated by hard water, they must be mixed with soft or distilled water. Iodophors may corrode or discolor certain metals and may temporarily stain clothing and other surfaces.

Synthetic Phenol Compounds

Synthetic phenol compounds are EPA-registered hospital (intermediate-level) disinfectants with broad-spectrum disinfecting action. (**Broad-spectrum** means it is capable of killing a wide range of microbes.) When diluted properly, phenols are used for surface disinfection (provided that the surface has been thoroughly cleaned first).

Because phenols are effective in the presence of detergents, they can be used on metal, glass, rubber, or plastic. They may also be used as a holding solution for instruments; however, phenols leave a residual film on treated surfaces.

Guidelines for Sodium Hypochlorite Dilutions

- Sodium hypochlorite solution is not stable; it must be mixed fresh each day.
- To make a 1:10 dilution, mix 2½ cups of bleach with one gallon of water. (This is an intermediate-level disinfectant and can be used on smooth, hard surfaces such as countertops, walls, and floors.)
- To make a 1:100 dilution, mix ¼ cup of bleach with one gallon of water. (This strength is suitable for general purpose disinfection for which sodium hypochlorite is indicated.)

Synthetic phenol compound is prepared daily. The manufacturer's instructions must be followed for work with phenolic solutions.

Sodium Hypochlorite

The advantages of sodium hypochlorite (common household bleach) are that it is fast-acting, economical, and a broad-spectrum, intermediate-level disinfectant.

It can disinfect surfaces in 3 to 30 minutes. The exact time depends upon the surface to be disinfected and the concentration of the solution.

The disadvantages of sodium hypochlorite are that it has a strong odor and is corrosive to some metals. It is also destructive to fabrics and irritating to the eyes and skin; it may eventually cause plastic chair covers to crack and is not stable.

Treatment Room Cleaning and Disinfection

All treatment room surfaces that were *not covered* with barriers but were touched or exposed to splatter and aerosol spray during the prior procedure are contaminated.

These are referred to as "splash surfaces" and they *must* be cleaned and disinfected between patients. Any surface under a barrier that was torn or dislodged also must be cleaned and disinfected.

PROCEDURE: **Performing the Spray-Wipe-Spray Technique**

Instrumentation

PPE, including utility gloves, goggles, and a mask
Liquid cleaner
Brush, special sponge, or paper towels
Surface disinfectant

Immediately After the Patient Visit

1. While still gloved from the patient visit, discard disposable needles, scalpels, and other sharp items into a puncture-resistant sharps disposal container. (See Chapter 12 for information on proper waste disposal.)
2. Place instruments and other waste, such as used cotton rolls and gauze sponges, on the tray and take it to the contaminated area of the sterilization center.
3. Return to the treatment room and remove the protective barriers used during the visit. Discard these with nonhazardous waste materials.
4. Remove gloves, wash hands, and return the patient's records to the business office.
5. Return to the treatment room to clean and prepare it for the next patient.

Treatment Room Cleaning and Disinfection

1. Wash hands and put on utility gloves.
2. Spray *cleaning solution* on contaminated surfaces (Fig. 13–6).
   □ *RATIONALE:* This is step 1 of "spray-wipe-spray."
3. Vigorously wipe these surfaces clean (Fig. 13–7).
   □ *RATIONALE:* This is step 2 of "spray-wipe-spray."
4. Spray *disinfectant solution* on the clean surfaces.
   □ *RATIONALE:* This is step 3 of "spray-wipe-spray."
5. Do not dry these surfaces.
   □ *RATIONALE:* The disinfectant is left in place to continue working.
6. Wash the exterior of the utility gloves and spray disinfectant on them. Then remove the gloves and wash hands.

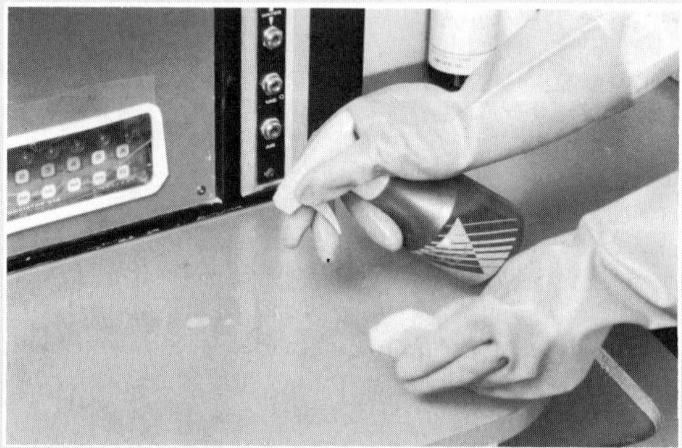

FIGURE 13–6

The surface is sprayed with an EPA-registered cleaner/disinfectant.

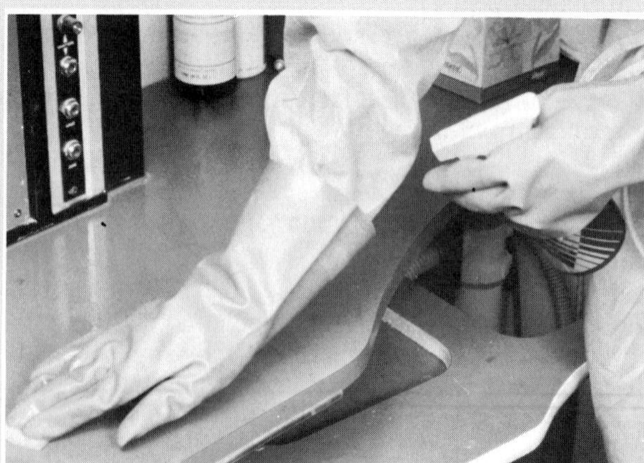

FIGURE 13–7

In the next step, the surface is wiped thoroughly clean. After the surface has been cleaned, it is sprayed with an EPA-registered disinfectant and left wet.

Preparation for the Next Patient

1. Place clean barriers in the treatment room (Fig. 13–8).
2. Place sterile instrument tray ready for the next patient. Do not open the packages yet.
   □ *RATIONALE:* This keeps the instrument sterile as long as possible.
3. Prepare the patient's chart, laboratory work, and radiographs.
4. Seat and drape the patient. (This is discussed in Chapter 14.)
5. Open the instrument package, taking care not to touch the instruments.
   □ *RATIONALE:* Doing this after the patient is seated lets the patient know that sterile instruments are being used.
6. Put on other PPE, then wash hands thoroughly and put on clean gloves and other PPE before assisting in patient care.

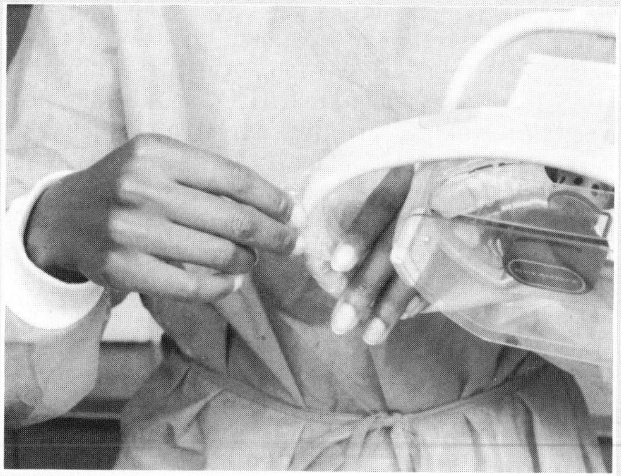

FIGURE 13–8

Clean barriers are placed. Shown here, the assistant places clear wrap barriers on the handles of the operating light.

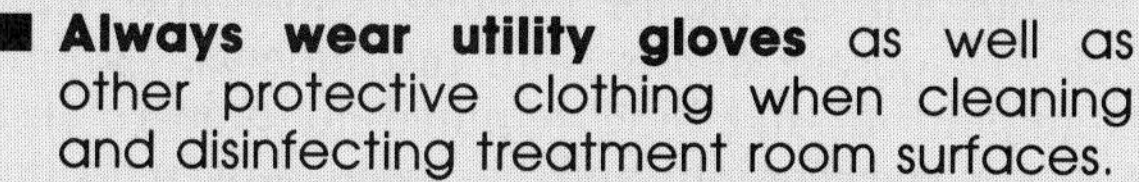

Guidelines for Treatment Room Care

- **Always wear utility gloves** as well as other protective clothing when cleaning and disinfecting treatment room surfaces.
- **Use appropriate solutions** when cleaning and disinfecting treatment room splash surfaces.
- **Carefully follow the manufacturer's directions** when preparing disinfectant solutions.
- **Do not mix materials** that might cause a chemical reaction or toxic fumes.
- **Properly ventilate and wear a mask** while using materials that give off toxic fumes or performing procedures that may create splatter and aerosol spray.
- **Pay special attention to the manufacturer's precautions** such as warnings about surfaces that the solution may stain, crack, or corrode.
- **Clean and disinfect all surfaces** that may have been contaminated during the previous visit. (Other treatment room surfaces are cleaned and disinfected at the end of the day.)

Treatment Room Preparation Procedures

Care of treatment room surfaces is a three-step process known as the "*spray-wipe-spray*" technique. This procedure involves thoroughly cleaning and disinfecting all affected surfaces—and it must be carried out carefully after each patient visit.

Spray. Thoroughly *clean* the surfaces to remove all debris and bioburden. This is done by spraying the surface with a combination *cleaning-disinfecting solution.*

Wipe. Use a special sponge, brush, gauze sponges, or paper towels to *vigorously wipe* the surfaces clean. The area must be completely clean because if any debris or bioburden remains, the disinfectant will not be effective. If gauze sponges are used, they should be at least a 4 × 4 inch size. (The 2 × 2 inch size is too small to be effective.)

Spray. Spray the surface again with the *cleaning-disinfecting solution.* This time, keep it moist for the manufacturer's recommended exposure time.

Instrument Recirculation

Instrument recirculation involves the cleaning, wrapping, and sterilizing of instruments in preparation for use in treating another patient. These procedures take place in the sterilization center.

When handling contaminated materials and instruments, the assistant *must* wear nitrile utility gloves and protective eyewear.

The Sterilization Center

The sterilization center is centrally located to provide easy access from the treatment rooms and other office areas. It must be separate from the laboratory area and from the staff lounge. CDC guidelines prohibit eating, drinking, smoking, applying cosmetics or lip balm, and handling contact lenses in this area.

The sterilization center must be kept clean, neat, and well stocked at all times. The sterilization center is divided into two sections: the contaminated area and the clean area.

THE CONTAMINATED AREA

Soiled instruments and trays are brought *only* into the contaminated zone to be prepared for sterilization (Fig. 13–9).

The contaminated area contains protective eyewear, utility gloves, counter space, a sink, a waste disposal container, holding solution, ultrasonic cleaner, and supplies for wrapping instruments before sterilization.

There may also be cabinets to store trays that are waiting to be sterilized; however, *soiled and clean instruments are never stored in the same cabinet!*

Instrument Holding Solution

The covered container of holding solution is located in the contaminated area of the sterilization center. The purposes of the holding solution are to

- Prevent debris from drying or crusting on the instruments
- Minimize the handling of soiled instruments
- Prevent airborne transmission of dried microorganisms
- Begin microbial kill on the soiled instruments

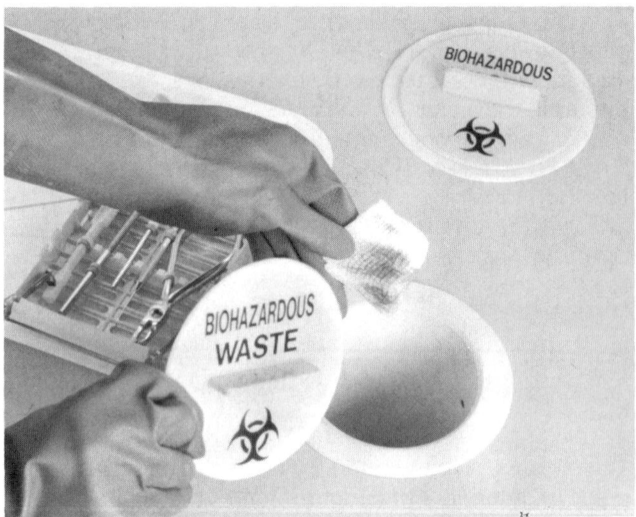

FIGURE 13–9

The contaminated area includes appropriately labeled waste disposal containers.

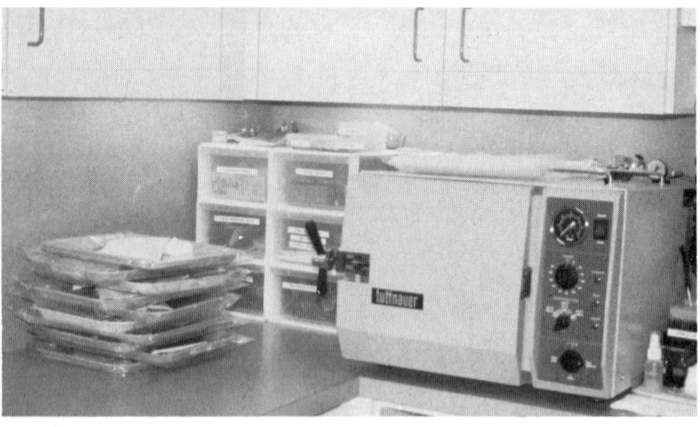

FIGURE 13–10

The clean area includes the sterilizer and space to store prepared trays.

Synthetic phenols, iodophors, household detergent with water, and glutaraldehyde are recommended for use as instrument holding solutions.

If soiled instruments cannot be processed immediately, they are submerged in the holding solution as soon as the soiled tray is brought from the treatment room. The cover is immediately replaced on the holding solution container.

The instruments are kept in the holding solution until they are processed for sterilization. However, the use of the holding solution does *not* replace any of the cleaning or sterilization steps outlined here.

The Ultrasonic Cleaner

Scrubbing contaminated instruments by hand is hazardous and should be avoided. Ultrasonic cleaning effectively loosens debris from instruments, minimizes the amount of handling required to prepare instruments for sterilization, and has been proven to be 16 times more effective than hand scrubbing.

The ultrasonic cleaner works by sound waves, which are beyond the range of human hearing. These sound waves, which can travel through metal and glass containers, cause cavitation. (**Cavitation** is the formation of bubbles in liquid.)

These bubbles, which are too small to be seen, burst by implosion. (**Implosion** means bursting inward, an action that is the opposite of an explosion.)

It is the mechanical action of the bursting bubbles, combined with the chemical action of the cleaning solution, that produces the cleaning effect used to remove the debris from the soiled instruments.

To avoid airborne contamination, the lid is always in place on the ultrasonic unit while it is in operation.

Special Solutions. Specially formulated solutions are used in the ultrasonic cleaner for specific difficult tasks such as removing cements, tartar, stains, plaster, and alginate. These solutions may be placed in the main tank; however, more commonly they are used in small glass beakers with covers. A special cover holds the beakers securely in place in the main tank of solution.

Care of the Ultrasonic Cleaner. The ultrasonic cleaning solution is discarded at the end of the day.

Then the inside of the pan and lid are wiped with a cleaning and disinfecting agent. The next morning the pan is filled with fresh cleaning solution.

Testing the Ultrasonic Cleaner. To determine that the ultrasonic cleaner is working properly, place a 5 × 5 inch sheet of lightweight aluminum foil vertically (like a curtain) half submerged in the solution for 20 seconds while operating the machine. At the end of 20 seconds, hold the foil up toward a light. An effective machine will leave no ½ square inch without visible holes.

THE CLEAN AREA

The sterilizer is located between the contaminated and clean sections of the sterilization center. The clean area has counter space and storage space for sterilized instruments, fresh disposable supplies, and prepared trays or cassettes (Fig. 13–10). *Soiled trays or instruments are never placed in the clean area!*

Preparation of Preset Instrument Trays

The instrument preparation steps shown here include the use of a **plastic instrument carrier**, such as those shown in Figure 13–12. These carriers, which are also known as *mini-cassettes* or *instrument transfer baskets*, are also available in metal.

The use of a carrier is important because it minimizes the handling of soiled instruments and reduces the possibility of injury to the assistant.

PROCEDURE: **Preparing a Preset Instrument Tray**

Instrumentation

PPE, including utility gloves and goggles
Holding solution in container
Scrub brush
Plastic instrument carriers
Sterilizer (autoclave, chemical vapor, *or* dry heat)
Sink with running water
Hazardous and nonhazardous waste receptacles
Paper towels
Ultrasonic cleaner and appropriate solutions
Instrument packs, pouches, or wraps
Clean examination gloves

Cleaning Instruments

1. Wash hands and put on personal protective equipment.
   ☐ *RATIONALE:* PPE *must* be worn when soiled instruments are handled.
2. Discard waste appropriately. The waste shown in Figure 13–11 is nonhazardous.

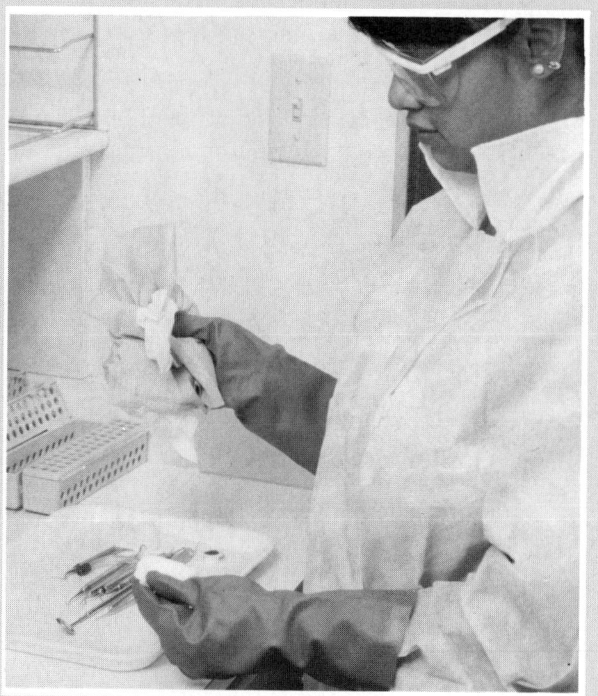

FIGURE 13–11

Waste items are discarded properly.

(continued on following page)

PROCEDURE: **Preparing a Preset Instrument Tray** *(continued)*

3. Place instruments into the carrier (Fig. 13–12). If they are not to be processed immediately, place the carrier in the holding solution.
4. Remove carrier from holding solution and rinse under a steady stream of running warm water for 30 seconds (Fig. 13–13).
   □ *RATIONALE:* This removes holding solution and loose debris.
5. Submerge carrier under the solution of the ultrasonic unit and replace the cover.
   □ *RATIONALE:* The cover prevents airborne contamination while the unit is running.
6. Set the timer for manufacturer's recommended period and run the unit (Fig. 13–14).
   □ *RATIONALE:* This aids in removing visible bioburden, which, if left on, impedes sterilization.
7. Remove instrument carrier and rinse thoroughly under cool running water.
   □ *RATIONALE:* This removes the ultrasonic cleaning solution and loosened bioburden.
8. If visible debris remains, very carefully scrub with an instrument scrubbing brush. Rinse again.
   □ *IMPORTANT:* Hand scrubbing of instruments should be avoided whenever possible because of the splash and splatter created and the hazard of injury from a contaminated instrument.
9. Roll the instruments onto a paper towel on the countertop (Fig. 13–15). Do not touch instruments unless absolutely necessary.
   □ *RATIONALE:* This prevents splashing, as well as inadvertent puncture injuries from sharp instruments.

Wrapping and Sterilizing Instruments

1. Using a second paper towel, pat the instruments dry. Discard paper towels after use in designated waste receptacle.
   □ *RATIONALE:* Drying instruments before placing into some types of sterilizers prevents rusting.
2. Wrap instruments according to type of sterilization (Fig. 13–16).
3. A saliva ejector and cotton supplies for use during treatment (cotton rolls, cotton pellets, and gauze sponges) may be added to the pack just before sterilization.

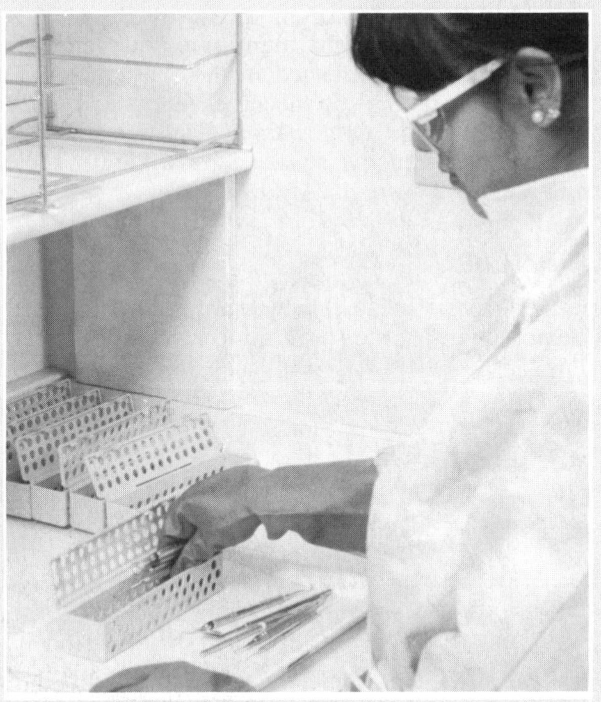

FIGURE 13–12

The soiled instruments are placed in a carrier for cleaning.

Guidelines for PPE During Instrument Preparation

- Nitrile utility gloves and protective eyewear *must* be worn when soiled instruments are handled.
- A mask *must be worn* if the cleaning method generates splash, splatter and/or aerosols (examples are hand scrubbing of instruments and running the ultrasonic cleaner without the cover in place; neither of these is a recommended procedure).
- PPE is not required when preset trays of wrapped sterile instruments are reassembled.

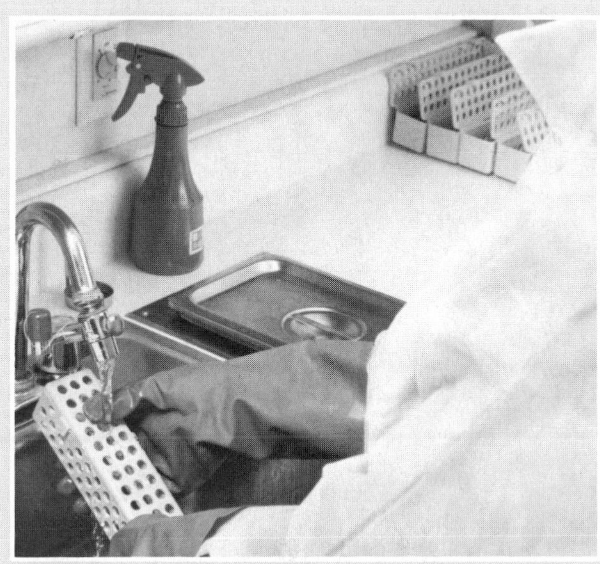

FIGURE 13–13

The carrier is removed from the holding solution and rinsed thoroughly under running water.

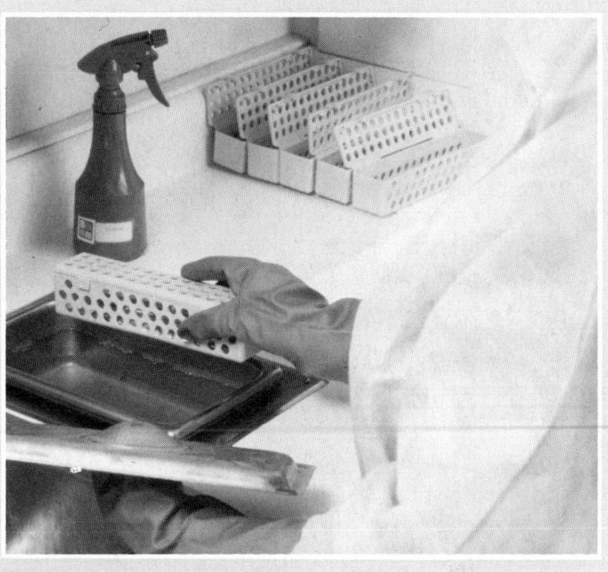

FIGURE 13–14

The carrier is placed in the ultrasonic cleaner, the cover is replaced, and the unit is run. The instruments in the carrier are removed from the ultrasonic cleaner and rinsed thoroughly under running water.

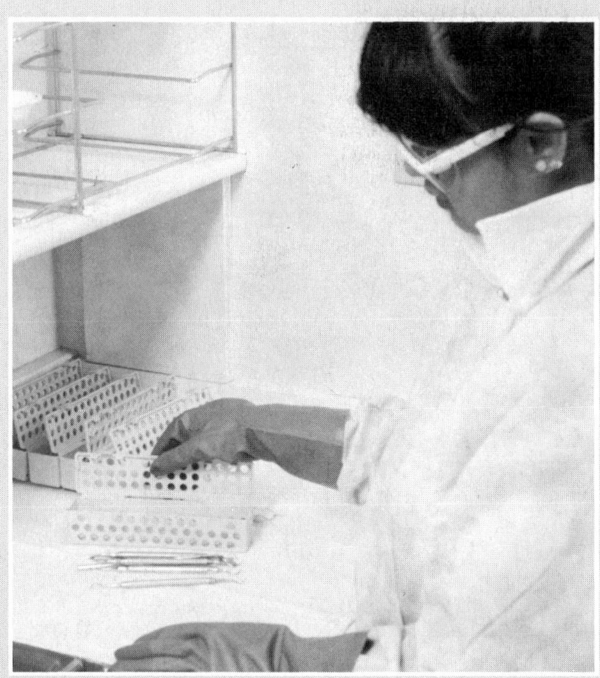

FIGURE 13–15

The cleaned instruments are removed from the carrier and placed on a towel to be dried.

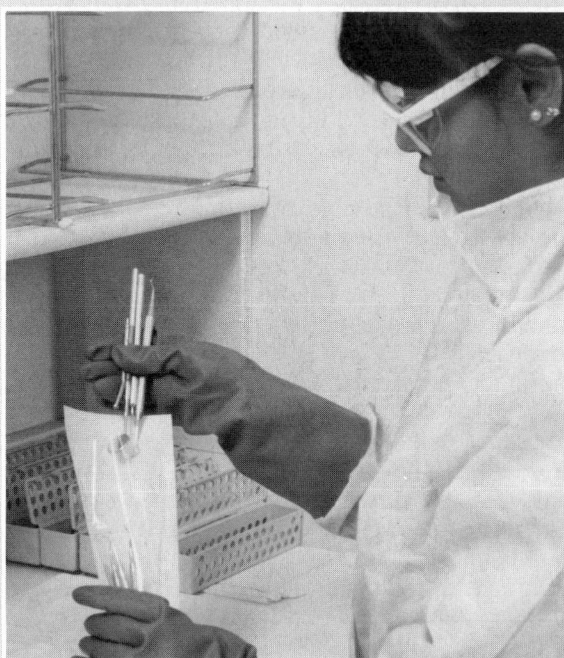

FIGURE 13–16

The dry instruments are bagged for sterilization. Shown here is a biofilm/paper bag.

(continued on following page)

PROCEDURE: Preparing a Preset Instrument Tray *(continued)*

4. *Alternative:* These supplies may be wrapped, sealed, and sterilized in single-use portions. A packet of these supplies is added to the tray before use. (A **single-use portion** contains just enough of a supply for one patient/visit. Any excess is discarded.)
5. Label the pack as to the type of procedure and date of processing.
6. Place the prepared instruments in the pack and seal it. Then sterilize according to manufacturer's directions (Fig. 13–17).

Care of the Tray

1. Working in the contaminated area, use the spray-wipe-spray technique to clean and disinfect the tray with an intermediate-level disinfectant. This may be done while you wait for the instruments to be sterilized.
   □ *RATIONALE:* The tray is a noncritical item.
2. After the tray has been cleaned and disinfected, store it in the clean area, ready to be reused.
3. When finished preparing the instruments and tray, remove utility gloves and wash hands.

Reassembling and Storing Preset Trays

1. Work only in the clean area of the sterilization center and wear clean examination gloves while handling sterile packets and reassembling trays.
2. Remove sealed packets from the sterilizer and place them in the clean area.
3. Reassemble the tray, taking care to include all of the supplies necessary to perform the procedure (Fig. 13–18).
4. *Optional:* A disposable cover may be placed on the tray before placing the instrument packs.
5. *Optional:* In some practices, the necessary gloves and masks are added to the tray at this time. In other practices, these are stored in the treatment room.
6. Store the prepared tray in the clean area until needed.
7. Bagged sterile instruments may be stored in drawers in the clean area of the sterilization center. A few may be stored, in their sealed bags, in the treatment room for emergency use.
8. Just before use, take the appropriate tray to the treatment room. Open the packaging in full view of the patient.
   □ *RATIONALE:* This way, the patient knows that sterile instruments are being used, and the possibility of cross-contamination is reduced.

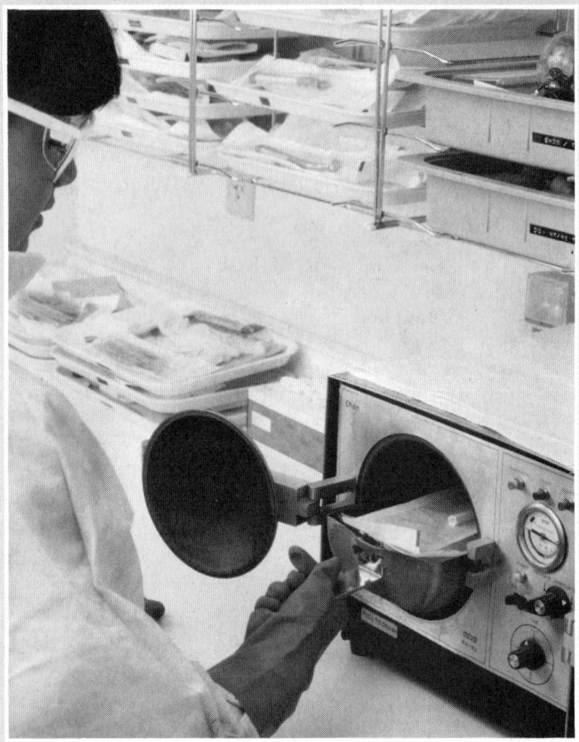

FIGURE 13–17

The prepared instruments are placed into the autoclave to be sterilized.

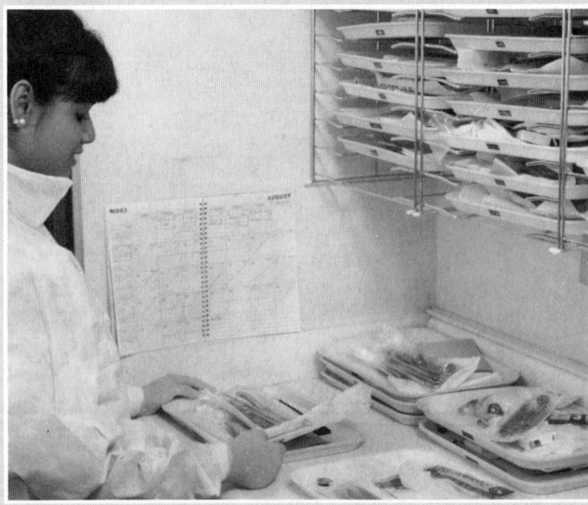

FIGURE 13–18

In the clean area, the preset trays are reassembled and stored ready for use.

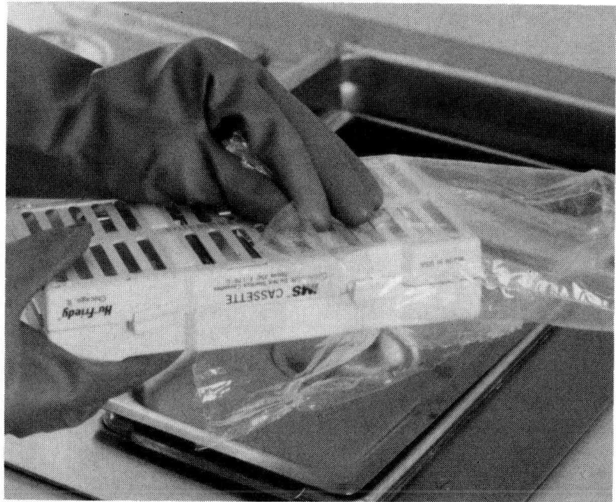

FIGURE 13–19

Instruments can be cleaned, wrapped, and sterilized without being removed from the cassette. Shown here, the prepared cassette is being placed in an autoclave bag that will be labeled and sealed before sterilization.

Preparation of Instrument Cassettes

Resin cassettes, such as the one shown in Figure 13-19, are used to transport and protect instruments through use and sterilization cycle. These cassettes have openings on the bottom and sides that make it possible to clean and sterilize the instruments in the cassette.

When this type of cassette is used, it is necessary to have an ultrasonic cleaner and sterilizing equipment that are large enough to accommodate the cassettes.

RETURN FROM THE TREATMENT ROOM

After use, the soiled instruments are returned to the cassette. The cassette does not have a solid bottom or sides to prevent contaminants from leaking out during transportation. For this reason, it is necessary to place the cassette in a pan or wrap it in a moisture-proof barrier while it is being moved.

CLEANING, WRAPPING, STERILIZATION, AND STORAGE

In the contaminated area, the disposables are discarded. If the instruments are not to be processed immediately, the entire cassette may be placed in a holding solution.

During cleaning and preparation, the instruments are rinsed and cleaned without being removed from the cassette. The time in the ultrasonic cleaner is determined by the manufacturer's specifications.

After cleaning, disposables such as cotton supplies and an air-water syringe tip are added. The entire cassette is then wrapped, labeled, and sterilized.

After sterilization, the wrapped cassette is stored in the clean area until needed in the treatment room.

Special Considerations

Care of the Patient's Chart and Radiographs

The patient's chart and radiographs will be contaminated if touched with gloved hands during or after treatment. Many different methods are used to prevent contamination. The following is a description of one system.

1. Place the patient's mounted radiographs on the view box *before* seating the patient and before gloving.
   ☐ **Rationale:** The hands are clean to this point.
2. Do not touch the chart or radiographs once treatment begins.
   ☐ **Rationale:** Any touching with a gloved hand will contaminate them.
3. To make a chart entry, place an overglove over the examination glove. Touch the chart and pen or pencil *only* with the overgloved hand (Fig. 13–20).
4. After the entry is complete, remove and discard the overglove. Do not touch the chart or the pen again while gloved.
5. When finished performing tasks involving the examination gloves, and before putting on utility

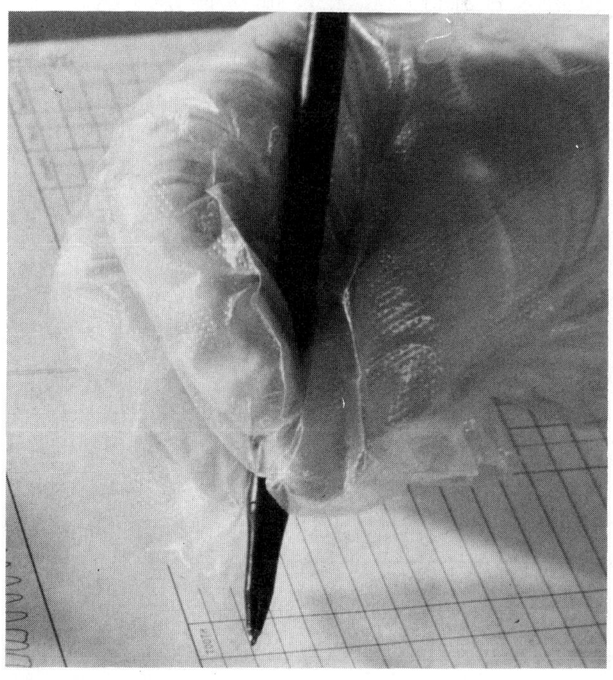

FIGURE 13–20

To prevent contamination, an overglove is worn while a charting entry is made.

gloves, return the radiographs and chart to the business office.

Heat-Sensitive Semicritical Instruments

According to the CDC guidelines, if heat-sensitive semicritical instruments are not disposable and *must* be reused, they should be cared for in the following manner:

1. The instruments are thoroughly cleaned and dried and then placed in an EPA-registered hospital grade disinfectant for up to 10 hours of exposure.
2. After the appropriate time, the instruments are rinsed by an aseptic technique with sterile water. If not to be used immediately, they should be placed in a sterile container after drying.

Curing Light

The handle of the curing light, which is described in Chapter 14, should be covered with a clear plastic protective barrier. If a barrier is not used or if the barrier is damaged, the curing light must be disinfected during treatment room cleanup.

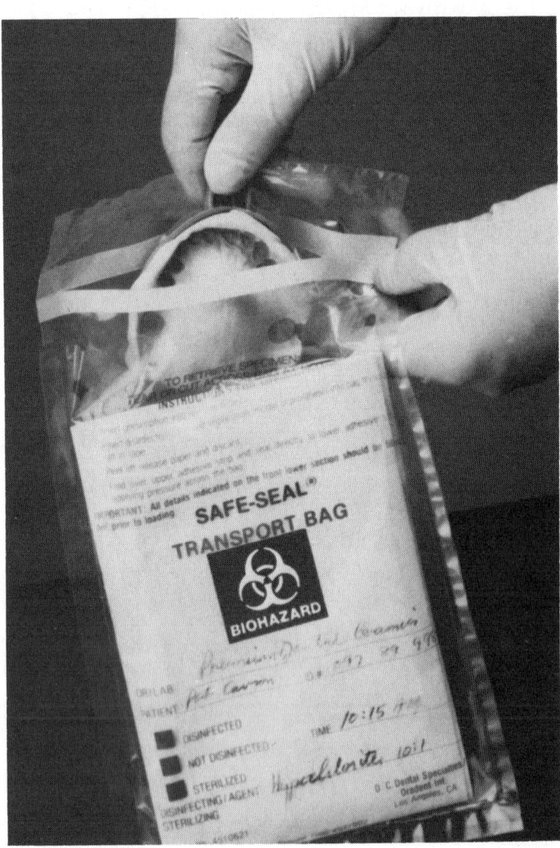

FIGURE 13–21

Impressions are placed in a leakproof bag for transportation to the dental laboratory. The biohazard label is required if the impressions have not been completely disinfected. (Photo courtesy DC Specialties, Los Angeles, CA.)

Handpiece, Prophy Angle, and Bur Sterilization

High-speed handpieces, low-speed handpiece components, reusable prophy angles, and burs *must* be sterilized before reuse. Also, a broken handpiece must be sterilized before it is sent to the manufacturer for repair. (The care and sterilization of this equipment is discussed in Chapter 15.)

Ultrasonic Scalers

Before use, the ultrasonic scaler handpiece should be covered with a plastic barrier, and then a sterile tip is inserted into the handpiece.

At the end of the patient visit, the scaler is run for 30 seconds to flush the water through the lines. The tip is removed and taken to the sterilization center to be autoclaved.

If the barrier on the ultrasonic scaler handpiece was damaged, it is necessary to disinfect with the spray-wipe-spray method. Afterward, it is placed on the bracket table or tray and sprayed with disinfectant to keep it thoroughly wet for at least 10 minutes. It is then wiped clean with gauze sponges or paper towels.

Radiography Precautions

Special precautions are necessary while exposing and processing radiographs. These precautions are discussed in Chapter 17.

Disinfection of Impressions

After the impression is removed from the patient's mouth, the impression is rinsed thoroughly, sprayed with a disinfecting solution, and placed in a sealed plastic bag. If the impression has not been disinfected, the bag must be labeled with a biohazard emblem (Fig. 13–21).

This isolates the impression and maintains the appropriate humidity for transport to the dental laboratory. Gloves are always worn when impressions are handled.

Depending upon the type of impression material, a damp paper towel may be included to increase the humidity. However, each type of impression material is handled and disinfected according to the manufacturer's directions. The following sections describe general recommendations.

POLYSULFIDE AND SILICONE IMPRESSIONS

Polysulfide and silicone impressions can be disinfected by immersion with any accepted disinfectant product. The length of the immersion is determined by the manufacturer's recommendations.

POLYETHER IMPRESSIONS

Some polyether impressions are adversely affected if disinfected by immersion. With other polyether formulas, after a 30-minute wait, the impression can safely be immersed in glutaraldehyde disinfectant. Always follow the manufacturer's directions for the material being used.

ALGINATE IMPRESSIONS

Alginate impressions should be disinfected by spraying rather than by immersion because soaking may distort the impression. After spraying with the disinfectant, the impression should be left in a sealed plastic bag for the recommended disinfection time.

Disinfection of Laboratory Cases

BEFORE THE CASE IS SENT TO THE LABORATORY

Blood and saliva should be thoroughly and carefully cleaned from impressions and from laboratory materials that have been used in the mouth. This includes anything tried in the mouth. These materials must be disinfected before being handled, adjusted, or sent to a dental laboratory.

An acrylic prosthodontic or orthodontic appliance may be disinfected by soaking it for 10 to 30 minutes in a diluted sodium hypochlorite solution. To determine the best method of disinfection, follow the manufacturer's instructions for the material being used.

WHEN THE CASE IS RETURNED FROM THE LABORATORY

Many dental laboratories routinely disinfect all cases (castings and appliances) before returning them to the dentist. Good communication between the laboratory and the dental practice is important to clarify these procedures.

If the laboratory *does* disinfect, gloves are not required. The case is unwrapped and rinsed before use.

If the laboratory has *not* disinfected the case, gloves are worn while it is unwrapped. All packing materials are discarded, and the case is disinfected and rinsed thoroughly before it is inserted in the patient's mouth.

REMOVABLE PROSTHODONTIC AND ORTHODONTIC APPLIANCES

When an appliance is removed from the patient's mouth, it should be placed directly into a disposable plastic cup and covered with a disinfectant.

Laboratory Disinfection Techniques

Because laboratory cases, as well as highly flammable and caustic materials, are potential sources of contamination, staff members may not eat, drink, smoke, apply cosmetics or lip balm, or handle contact lenses in the laboratory. (This is an OSHA regulation.)

Working surfaces should be covered with a barrier, such as a large sheet of paper, which is discarded after each case use. Laboratory work surfaces should be cleaned regularly with the same "spray-wipe-spray" technique used to clean treatment room surfaces.

Gloves, masks, and protective eyewear must always be worn when working on laboratory cases—especially when grinding or polishing equipment is used. Extreme caution is necessary during work in gloves because they could get caught in equipment such as a grinding wheel or rotary bur.

A separate set of laboratory instruments, attachments, and materials is used for each case that has already been in the mouth. These instruments are disinfected or discarded after use.

When polishing appliances, a clean rag wheel and fresh pumice or other polishing materials should be used for each case. Rag wheels are washed and then sterilized in an autoclave. As an alternative, a disposable buffing wheel may be used instead of the rag wheel.

Pumice should be mixed with dilute sodium hypochlorite (5 parts of sodium hypochlorite to 100 parts of distilled water). Adding 3 parts green soap in the disinfectant solution will keep the pumice suspended. If the pumice is used on a case that has been in the mouth, it should be discarded after use.

Chapter 14

Dental Treatment Areas

Introduction

The treatment area, also known as the *clinical area*, is that part of the dental facility directly involved in providing patient care. This includes the treatment rooms, central sterilization and storage, and the dental laboratory.

The treatment areas, as well as other areas of the office, must be kept neat and clean at all times. Attention to this detail is very important, because if the office appears sloppy or if the patient sees debris, he may assume that the staff is careless and the entire office is unclean.

Design of Treatment Rooms

Dental treatment rooms, also known as *operatories*, are the heart of the clinical area of the practice. It is here that patients receive treatment. Most practices have two or more treatment rooms per dentist. To promote efficiency as the dentist moves from one room to another to deliver care, it is desirable that these rooms be designed and furnished in a similar manner.

In addition, there are usually treatment rooms equipped primarily for use by the dental hygienist. In some practices, these rooms also serve as an extra operatory for emergencies or brief procedures such as post-surgical checkups.

The design and configuration of the treatment room depend on the space available and the dentist's preferences (Figs. 14–1 and 14–2).

The goal is to achieve the flexibility of equipment placement to enhance the application of four- and six-handed dentistry. This allows the seated team to provide quality patient care with maximal efficiency and minimal strain while observing exposure (infection) control protocols. (Four- and six-handed dentistry is explained further in Chapter 1.)

CLASSIFICATIONS OF MOTIONS

The motions of the dental team are classified in five categories, listed from the simplest to the most complex:

- **Class I motions** involve fingers-only movement.
- **Class II motions** involve movements of the fingers and wrist.
- **Class III motions** involve movements of the fingers, wrist, and elbow.
- **Class IV motions** involve movements of the entire arm from the shoulder.
- **Class V motions** involve movements of the arm and twisting the body.

The goal is to reduce fatigue by arranging equipment and supplies in the treatment room so that the dentist and assistant use primarily Classes I, II, and III motions that involve a minimum of twisting, turning, or reaching movements.

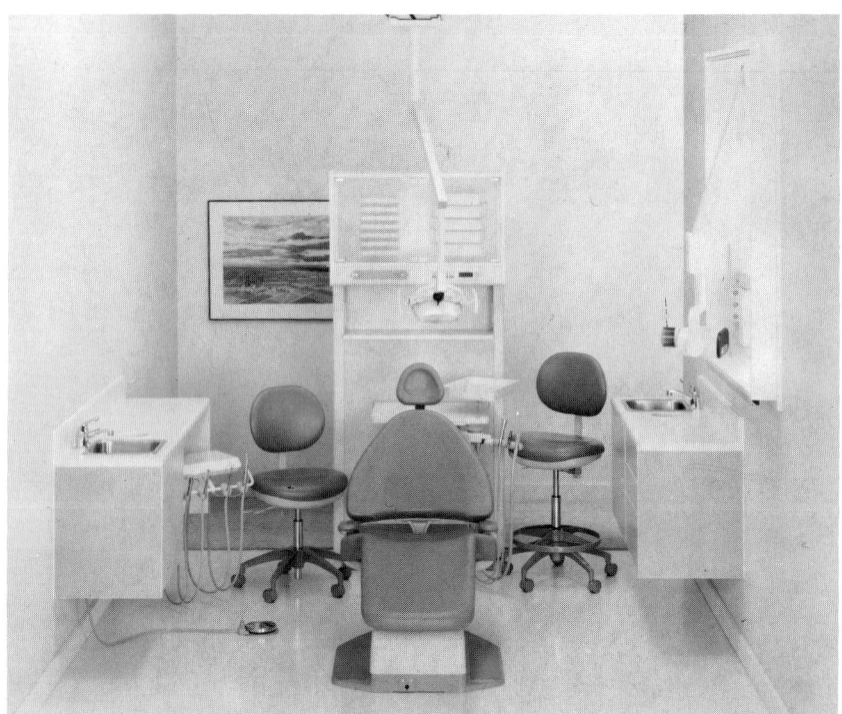

FIGURE 14–1

Dental treatment room equipped for side delivery. To the left of the dental chair are the operator's instrumentation, stool, and sink. The rheostat is on the floor near the operator's stool. To the right are the assistant's cart, stool, and sink. The operating light is suspended from the ceiling, and the x-ray unit is wall-mounted at the far right. (Courtesy of A-DEC, Inc., Newberg, OR.)

EQUIPMENT PLACEMENT

The placement of major pieces of equipment is described in terms of the location of the dental unit in relation to the operator. The three commonly used unit positions are front, side, and rear delivery. These are discussed in the section on dental units.

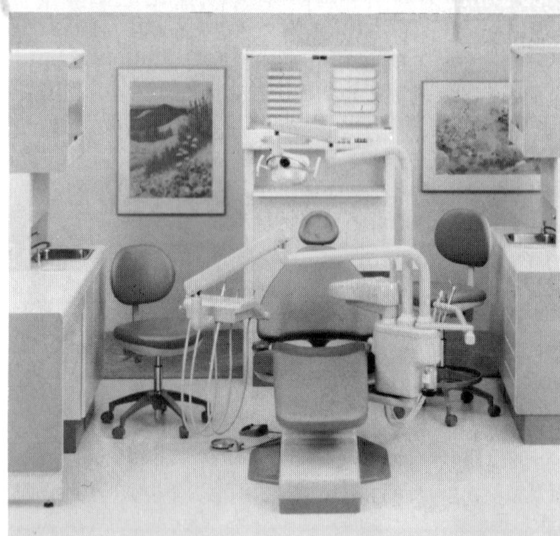

FIGURE 14–2

Dental treatment room equipped with chair-mounted units. The operating light and instrumentation for the operator and assistant are mounted on the dental chair. To the left of the chair are the operator's stool and sink. The rheostat and foot control for adjusting the dental chair are on the floor near the operator's stool. To the right are the assistant's stool and sink. (Courtesy of A-DEC, Inc., Newberg, OR.)

Dental Treatment Room Equipment

The basic equipment in each treatment room includes a lounge-type dental chair, stools for the operator and assistant, one or more dental units or mobile carts, an operating light, fixed and movable cabinets, a wall-mounted x-ray unit, and an x-ray view box (Fig. 14–3).

Care of Dental Equipment

Dental equipment is expensive, complex, and delicate. It must be used carefully and maintained properly in accordance with the manufacturer's instructions.

Responsibility for the routine care of these areas is usually shared by the dental assistants working in the clinical area. However, one staff member may be assigned the responsibility of seeing that preventive equipment care steps are carried out on a routine basis. Larger practices may contract to have maintenance personnel provide this service.

Any equipment contaminated during patient care is cleaned and disinfected according to the infection control protocols discussed in Chapter 13.

Dental Chair

The lounge-type dental chair accommodates a wide range of body sizes, for both children and adults, and

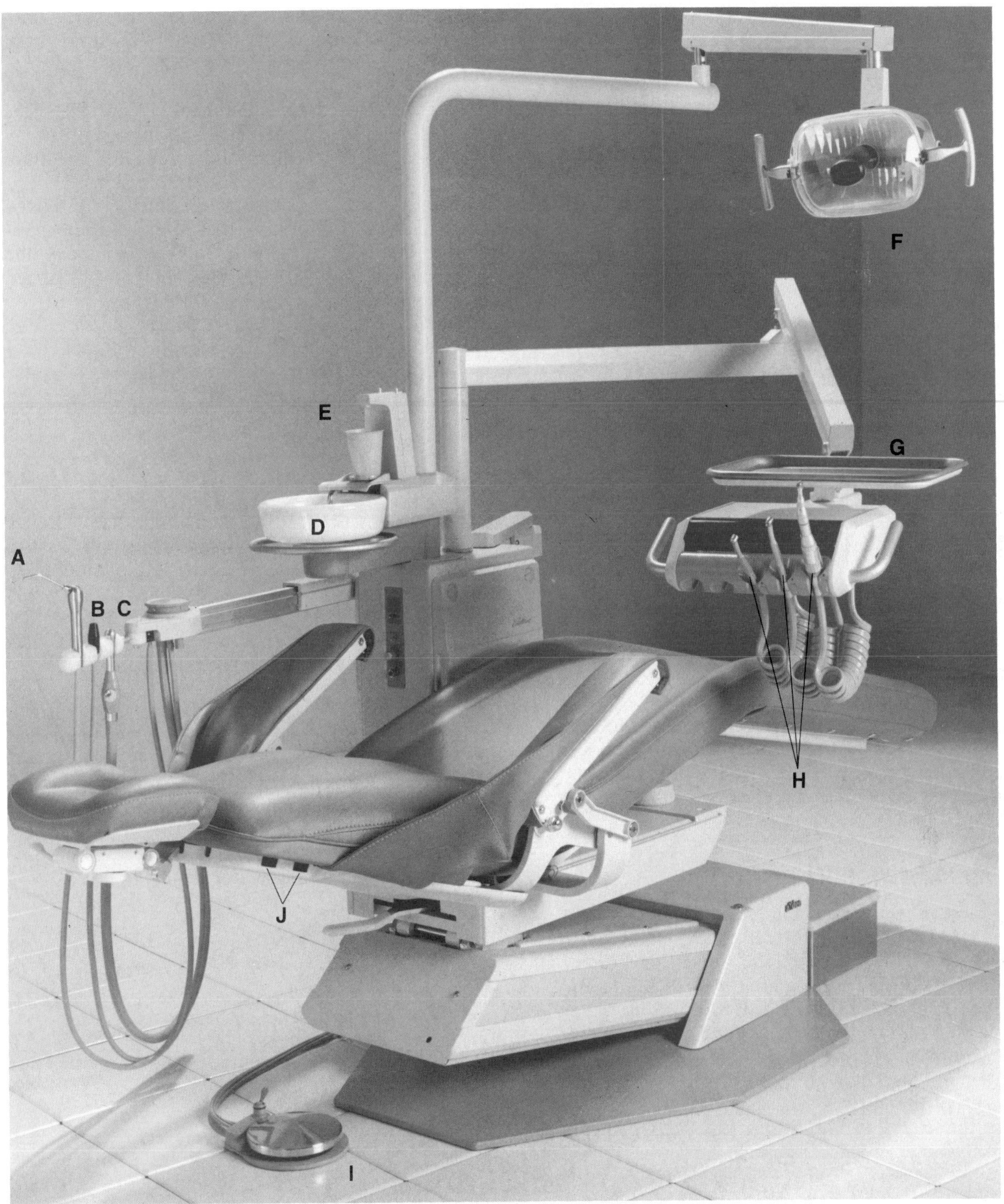

FIGURE 14–3

Dental chair and fixed unit. *A*, Air-water syringe; *B*, saliva ejector housing; *C*, HVE receptacle; *D*, cuspidor; *E*, cup filler, *F*, operating light; *G*, bracket tray, *H*, handpieces; *I*, rheostat; *J*, chair adjustment switches. (Courtesy of A-dec, Inc., Newberg, OR.)

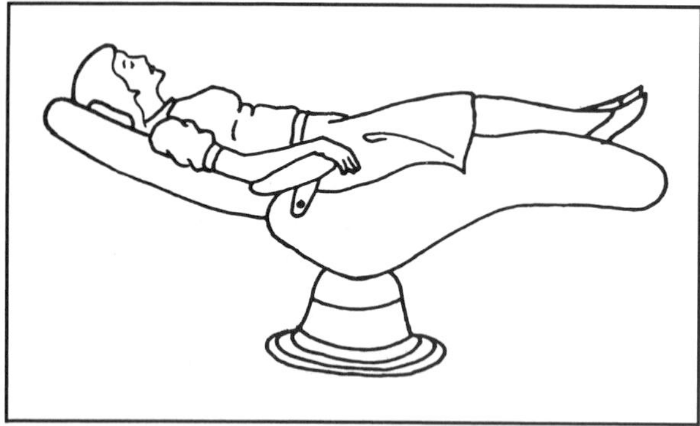

FIGURE 14–4

Patient in a supine position for dental treatment. Notice that the nose and knees are on the same plane.

provides flexibility in positioning the patient during treatment.

Although the type of headrest on the chair varies, all are easily adjusted to hold the patient's head securely and comfortably in the position required for the treatment being provided.

The arms of the chair support the patient's arms and elbows without strain. To facilitate patient seating and dismissal, the arms are made either to be raised or to slide back out of the way.

The chair back and leg rest can be adjusted to seat the patient comfortably with full support in the shoulders, lumbar region of the back, buttocks, and legs. (The **lumbar** region is located below the rib cage and above the pelvis.)

DENTAL CHAIR CONTROLS

Controls on the dental chair make it possible to adjust the back support and footrest, to raise and lower the chair, and to swivel it slightly to the left or right.

Foot controls, which are programmed to automatically move the patient into the desired position, make it possible to position the chair without touching the controls with gloved hands.

Older dental chairs have the controls located on the back or side of the chair. Because it may be necessary to adjust the chair during treatment, these controls should be protected with a disposable barrier.

ADJUSTMENT OF THE DENTAL CHAIR

The position of the chair and patient are determined by the procedure to be performed. Ideally, all chair adjustments (height, back, footrest, and headrest) are completed after the patient is seated and *before* clean examination gloves are put on for patient care.

Whenever the chair is repositioned, the patient must be warned first. Adjustments are made slowly, and patient comfort is taken into consideration. The patient is always returned to an upright position slowly and then is encouraged to sit quietly for a few moments to be certain that he does not feel dizzy from the change of position.

Upright Position. In the upright position, the foot of the chair is lowered and the back is upright. This position is used for patient entry and dismissal. It may also be used when exposing radiographs and for other procedures such as taking alginate impressions.

Supine Position. Most dental treatment is provided with the patient comfortably placed in a supine position with the nose and knees on approximately the same plane (Fig. 14–4). (**Supine** means positioned lying on the back.)

Subsupine Position. In the subsupine position, the patient is lying on the back, face up, with the head *lower* than the feet. This position may be necessary for a procedure such as the extraction of a maxillary third molar.

Operator's Stool

It is important that the assistant understand proper use and positioning of the operator's stool because there may be times when the assistant, functioning as an extended-functions dental assistant (EFDA), is seated in the operator's position. The operator's stool must provide stability, mobility, and comfort and should include the following features (Fig. 14–5):

- Castors to allow the operator to move about easily
- A broad base to prevent tilt when the operator's weight is shifted during use
- A padded seat sized to adequately support the operator's buttocks and thighs without cutting off circulation to the legs and feet
- Adjustable height, from floor to the seat, to accommodate differences in operator height

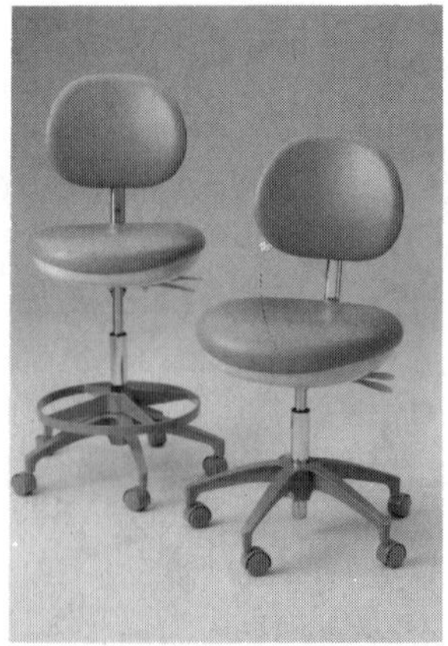

FIGURE 14–5

Assistant and operator stools. The assistant's stool, on the left, has a ring near the base to support the assistant's feet. The operator's stool is on the right. (Courtesy of A-DEC, Inc., Newberg, OR.)

- A back support that is adjustable to the lumbar area of the operator's back

CRITERIA FOR PROPER POSITIONING OF SEATED OPERATOR

1. The operator is seated in an unstrained position with the back straight, feet flat on the floor, and thighs angled so that the knees are slightly above hip level.
2. The rheostat is positioned on the floor near the operator's right or left foot. (A **rheostat** is a foot control that operates the dental handpieces.)
3. The operator's elbows are close to the sides, with shoulders and forearms parallel to the floor.
4. The field of operation, which is the area of the patient's oral cavity being treated, is positioned at the operator's elbow height. This is accomplished with the headrest and patient's head comfortably positioned over the operator's lap.
5. The seated operator, with head erect and eyes focused downward, has a clear line of vision with an optimal focal distance of at least 14 inches. (**Optimal focal distance** means the best, least stressful, distance from the operator's eyes to the patient's mouth.) If it is necessary to lessen the focal distance, the operator's head should be tilted slightly downward but not angled at more than 15 degrees.

OPERATOR POSITION IN RELATION TO THE DENTAL CHAIR

Where the operator's stool is positioned in relation to the dental chair is dependent on the position of the equipment and the treatment to be provided.

These relative positions are described in terms of the clock concept, which is explained in Chapter 16.

Assistant's Stool

The assistant's stool must also provide stability, mobility, and comfort and should include the following features (see Fig. 14–5):

- Castors on a broad base to provide mobility and stability
- A seat of adjustable height to provide support of the assistant's buttocks and upper legs
- A broad platform or ring near the base where the assistant places his or her feet
- An adjustable back support that can be positioned to support the lumbar region of the assistant's back

An optional feature is a curved, padded bar extension from the back of the stool that is adjustable in height and curvature. This support, which swings in front of the seated assistant, provides support at the abdominal level (just below the rib cage) when the assistant leans forward against it toward the operating field.

CRITERIA FOR PROPER POSITIONING OF SEATED ASSISTANT

1. The assistant is seated, with her back straight, in an unstrained position 4 to 5 inches higher than the operator.
   □ *RATIONALE:* This added height is important so that the assistant is able to see into the oral cavity and function efficiently while remaining out of the operator's line of vision.
2. The assistant is positioned well back on the seat with the stool back adjusted to provide lumbar support.
   □ *ALTERNATIVE:* The extension bar is swung forward so that it supports the assistant as he or she leans forward.
3. The assistant's feet are placed firmly on the platform near the base of the stool.
   □ *RATIONALE:* This is very important because the stool is too high for the assistant's feet to reach the floor. Placing the feet on this platform provides the support needed for proper circulation to the legs and feet.
   □ *CAUTION:* Hanging one's heels on the edge of this platform is *not* recommended because it reduces circulation.
4. Once the patient is reclined in the dental chair, the seated assistant is positioned so that his or her hips and thighs are level with the floor and parallel with the patient's shoulders.
   □ *RATIONALE:* From this position, the assistant should be able to easily reach nearby supplies and working areas by pivoting the chair seat only slightly to the right or left.

Treatment Room Cabinets

The treatment room is equipped with wall-mounted cabinets, mobile cabinets, or a combination of both. These provide working surfaces and limited storage space for commonly used disposable supplies. Although some items, such as the sharps container, must be kept on the counter top, other small pieces of equipment should be stored out of the way.

Because of exposure control concerns, the emphasis is on storing supplies away from the treatment room as much as possible. (Anything stored here is in danger of contamination.) Instead, all equipment and supplies needed for the patient's visit are brought into the treatment room through a "tub and tray" system, such as the one described in Chapter 15.

MOBILE CABINETS

A **mobile cabinet**, which is mounted on castors, usually has four drawers and a top that slides either from side to side or from front to back. This top serves as a work surface for the assistant, and the cabinet is moved into position when needed.

The recessed area under the movable top is usually a deep space that is used to store larger items such as the amalgamator. The items stored in the drawers depend on the dentist's preference.

Any instruments and items, such as extra cotton rolls and gauze sponges, that are stored in this cabinet *must* be packaged to maintain sterility. Examples of additional items that might be stored here include

- Topical and local anesthetic supplies
- Dental dam equipment and supplies
- A first aid kit and sterile resuscitation masks
- Sterile dental radiography stabilizing accessories
- Mixing bowls and spatulas
- Sterile impression trays

Treatment Room Sinks

Both the operator and the assistant must wash their hands before gloving and again after the gloves are removed. To ensure easy access for this critical procedure, the operatory is equipped with two sinks: one on the operator's side and the other on the assistant's side (see Figs. 14–1 and 14–2).

So that it is *not* necessary to touch a faucet handle, operatory sinks should be equipped with shoulder, knee, foot, or electronic water controls and a foot-operated liquid soap dispenser. (Bar soap transmits contamination.)

Each sink also is equipped with a supply of paper towels and hypoallergenic hand lotion. (Cloth towels that are reused transmit contamination.)

The sinks, faucets, and surrounding area must be kept clean and free of splatter at all times. During treatment room preparation, a paper towel may be used to wipe and dry this area. At least once daily, these entire areas, including the chrome trim, should be thoroughly cleaned and dried to remove any remaining spots or debris.

Dental Units

The basic function of a dental unit is to provide the necessary attachments and controls for the handpieces, air-water syringe, and high-volume oral evacuation (HVE) systems.

A unit that accommodates handpieces includes a gauge or liquid crystal display (LCD) that is used to monitor the compressed air pressure needed to operate these handpieces.

Dental units are supplied in a range of styles and equipment combinations. The type of unit selected depends upon (1) the space available, (2) the operator's preferred mode of delivery, (3) whether the operator is left- or right-handed, and (4) whether the operator works primarily with or without a chairside assistant. (Positioning for the left- or right-handed operator is discussed in Chapter 16.)

MODES OF DELIVERY

- With **front delivery,** the unit is positioned so that the equipment comes over the patient's chest toward the mouth (see Fig. 14–2).
- In **side delivery,** separate units for the operator and assistant are placed at either side of the chair (see Fig. 14–1).
- With **rear delivery,** equipment is positioned behind the chair near the back of the patient's head (Fig. 14–6).

It is also possible to have a combination of these delivery systems: for example, a fixed unit providing front delivery for the operator while the assistant works from a mobile cart that provides side delivery.

DENTAL UNIT INSTRUMENTATION

The dental units supply the basic instrumentation for the operator and assistant.

- **Operator instrumentation** includes attachments for the high- and low-speed handpieces and an air-water syringe.
- **Assistant instrumentation** includes attachments for the saliva ejector, the HVE system, and the air-water syringe.
- **Solo instrumentation** includes all of the equipment needed by an operator or a hygienist working alone.

TYPES OF DENTAL UNITS

Fixed Units

A fixed unit is mounted on the floor, the wall, or the side of the dental chair pedestal. Floor-mounted units stand on a base or pedestal.

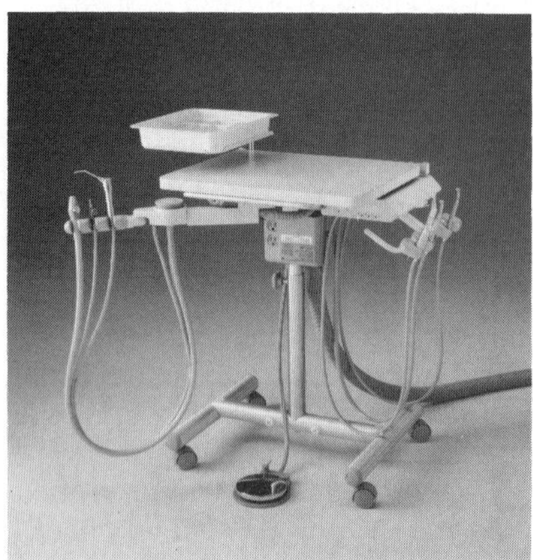

FIGURE 14–6

Mobile dental unit for rear delivery with accessories and controls for the operator and the assistant. (Courtesy of A-DEC, Inc., Newberg, OR.)

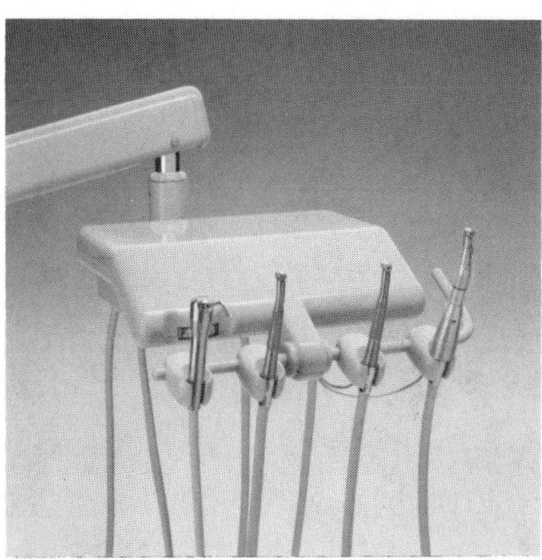

FIGURE 14–7

Moveable arm on a fixed dental unit to allow flexibility in positioning the operator's instrumentation. (Courtesy of A-DEC, Inc., Newberg, OR.)

The console, which is on a movable arm, is easily positioned over the seated patient for front delivery. This arm usually includes space for a tray and attachments for use by the operator (Fig. 14–7).

The attachments used by the assistant are commonly placed on the left side of the unit (Fig. 14–8). An alternative is to have this equipment on a mobile cart.

The fixed unit may include a cup filler, an attachment for the operating light, a filter to catch solid waste from the oral evacuation system, and possibly a cuspidor. These are attached to the pedestal, which is to the left of the chair, as shown in Figure 14–2.

The **cup filler** is used to fill a fresh cup for each patient. At the end of the visit, the cup is emptied and discarded. (Rinsing with an antiseptic mouth rinse by the patient just before treatment greatly reduces the bacteria in spray created by the handpiece.)

The unit may include a **cuspidor** located near the cup filler. Although it is equipped with an automatic rinse function, the cuspidor is unsanitary, and its use is discouraged. (Alternative ways of rinsing the patient's mouth are discussed in Chapter 16.)

Because the fixed unit does not provide necessary work space for the assistant, a mobile cabinet or cart is positioned for his or her use.

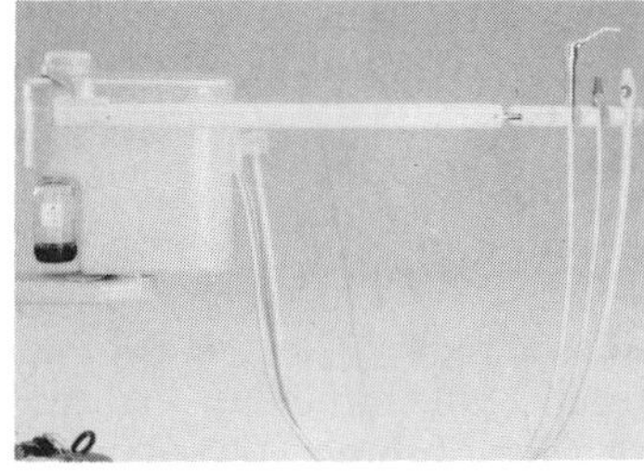

FIGURE 14–8

Assistant's instrumentation on fixed dental unit. The telescoping arm allows flexibility in positioning. Shown to the left is a solids collector for the oral evacuation system. (Courtesy of A-DEC, Inc., Newberg, OR.)

Mobile Carts

Mobile carts have a work surface top with equipment attachments hanging from the sides. Air, water, and electric connections for these carts are through a hoselike cord. This makes it possible to move the units about (within the limits of this cord), and they are used most frequently for side or rear delivery.

The **operator's cart** has attachments for three handpieces and an air-water syringe. This cart is positioned so that the operator can easily reach the equipment.

The **assistant's cart** has an air-water syringe and attachments for a saliva ejector and the HVE system (Fig. 14–9). The assistant's cart is moved into position on the assistant's side of the dental chair with the instrument tray over the assistant's knees.

A **dual cart**, such as the one shown in Figure 14–6, contains all of the equipment found on the other carts. This type of cart is frequently used in rear delivery and is positioned within reach of both the operator and the assistant.

Air-Water Syringe

The air-water syringe is used in three ways. It delivers (1) a stream of water, (2) a stream of air, or (3) a combined spray of air and water.

During tooth preparation, extremely hot or cold air or water can shock or injure the dentin of the tooth. A control on the dental unit is adjusted to maintain the temperature of the water at approximately 130°F.

The tip of the air-water syringe, which is classified as semicritical equipment, is removed during treatment room preparation. Metal tips are sterilized by autoclave before reuse. Plastic tips are discarded after a single use. The handle and tubing are covered with a plastic barrier.

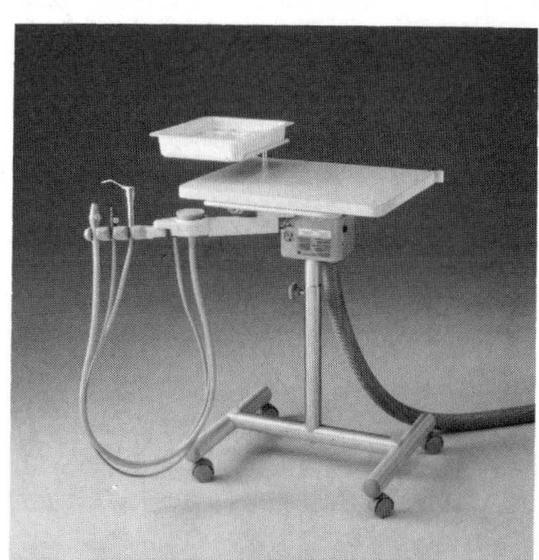

FIGURE 14–9

Assistant's mobile unit with air-water syringe, saliva ejector, and HVE. (Courtesy of A-DEC, Inc., Newberg, OR.)

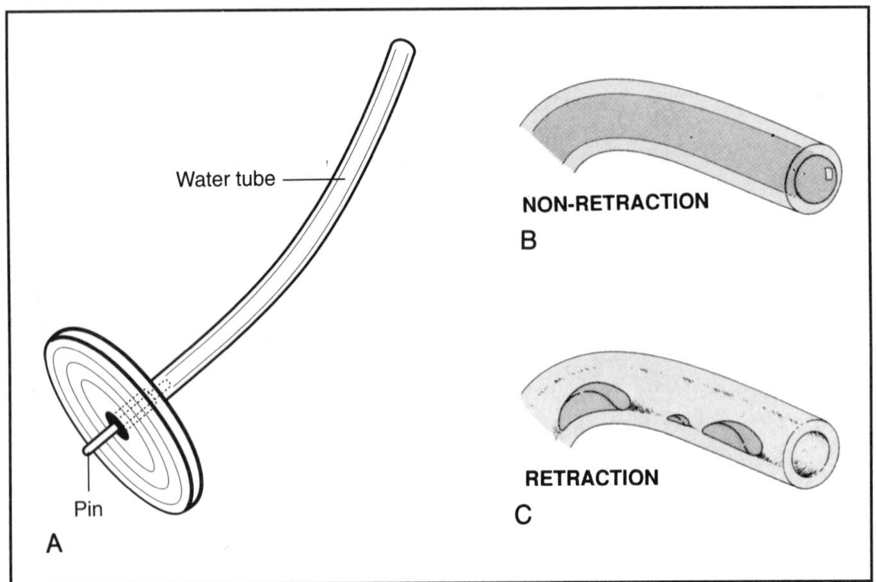

FIGURE 14–10

Schematic representation of a retraction tester. *A*, When the dental unit is turned on, the pin portion is inserted into the coolant hole of the handpiece connection. *B*, If the system is working properly, the water tube remains filled with water. *C*, If the system is not working properly, water will be sucked back out of the tube.

Water Lines to the Handpieces and Air-Water Syringe

The unit supplies the water needed for the air-water syringe and the high-speed handpiece used in the washed field technique. (**Washed field technique** is the use of a water spray from the dental handpiece as a coolant to protect the tooth from injury due to overheating.)

Since this equipment sprays water directly into the patient's mouth, there are two areas of concern regarding the safety of the water supply for this purpose. One concern is the danger of contamination through the retraction of fluids into the lines. (**Retraction** means to draw back in.) The other concern is the danger of contamination of water in the lines coming into the treatment area.

TESTING FOR WATER RETRACTION

The retraction of fluids into the water lines is commonly referred to as *suckback*. Suckback into the handpiece could occur immediately after use when the water is no longer flowing. The retraction of contaminated fluids is a serious exposure control hazard.

To prevent this contamination, these water lines should be equipped with *nonretracting valves* that do not permit suckback after the water is turned off. New units come equipped with these valves, and older units may be fitted with them.

To determine whether water retraction is occurring in the handpiece lines, a water retraction tester is used in accordance with the manufacturer's directions (Fig. 14–10).

SELF-CONTAINED WATER SYSTEM

To ensure that the water supply to the handpieces and air-water syringe is free of sediment and contamination, a self-contained water system may be attached to the unit.

A glass or plastic container, fastened to the post of the unit, is readily checked and refilled when the water supply level becomes low. If the local water is "hard" (contains minerals that cause a build-up in the lines) or contaminated (must be boiled before drinking), distilled or bottled water may be used in these containers.

This controlled water supply is recommended for use during surgery procedures that require a coolant on the dental bur. For this purpose, the unit is filled with sterile water.

CARE OF HANDPIECE AND AIR-WATER SYRINGE TUBING

Because microbial material can build up in the handpiece and air-water syringe tubing, these tubes should be purged (rinsed) by running the water for *3 minutes* at the beginning and end of the day and at least *1 minute* between patients.

For more thorough cleansing of the tubing, it is necessary to remove all of the components (tubing, valves, and filter) from the unit.

The assembly is taken to an operatory sink and flushed thoroughly with warm running water. Before reassembly, the tubing is cleaned and deodorized with a disinfecting solution.

Operating Light

The operating light is on a flexible arm and may be track-mounted from the ceiling or attached to the wall, dental chair, or fixed unit (Fig. 14–11). The light is used to illuminate the operating field for the dentist.

To provide a cool, bright illumination, halogen bulbs are used in most operating lights. The light is very bright, and care is taken to avoid shining it into the patient's eyes.

POSITIONING THE OPERATING LIGHT

The only parts of the light the assistant touches while gloved for patient care are the light handles, which are protected with removable barriers.

After the patient is seated, and before gloves are donned, the assistant positions the light to shine on the patient's chest approximately 25 to 30 inches below the patient's chin. The light is turned on and is then slowly adjusted upward to illuminate the oral cavity.

When properly positioned, the light illuminates the area to be treated without projecting shadows of the operator's or assistant's hands onto the oral cavity.

CARE OF THE OPERATING LIGHT

The light becomes hot during use. Other than changing the removable barrier on the handle, the light is cleaned only when it has cooled.

When the lens is cool, a mild detergent and a soft cloth are used to wipe it free of smudges and debris. (Touching a warm lens with a damp cloth can cause the lens to break.)

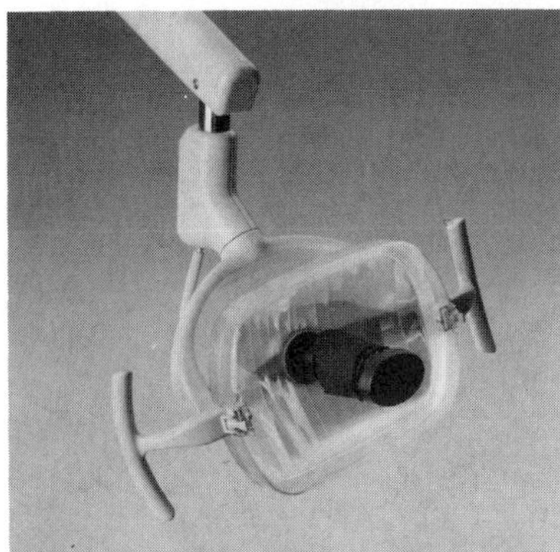

FIGURE 14–11

Ceiling-mounted operating light. (Courtesy of A-DEC, Inc., Newberg, OR.)

When the bulb of the operating light must be replaced, turn the light off and allow the old bulb to cool before removing it.

If using a halogen bulb, follow the manufacturer's instructions. (These bulbs will break if touched with a bare hand.) Extra bulbs should be stored in inventory to ensure immediate replacement as necessary.

Associated Equipment

Oral Evacuation System

The saliva ejector and HVE system make up the oral evacuation system. Their *use* is discussed in Chapter 16.

A disposable **saliva ejector** is used during some procedures to remove excess fluids from the patient's mouth. At the end of the patient visit, it is discarded. During treatment, the receptacle and housing for the saliva ejector are protected with a disposable plastic barrier.

The **HVE system** is used by the assistant to remove debris and excess fluids from the patient's mouth. A sterile HVE tip is provided for each patient. During use, the HVE handle and hose are covered with a protective plastic barrier.

The following are procedures for the *care* of these systems. When cleaning these systems, the assistant should wear appropriate personal protective equipment (PPE), including goggles and utility gloves. After use, this PPE is rinsed well and disinfected.

CARE OF TRAPS

There is a small trap near the top of the saliva ejector holder and HVE handle that catches debris drawn from the mouth. These traps are disposable and should be changed weekly. Utility gloves are worn, and cotton pliers or utility tongs should be used when handling these highly contaminated screens (Fig. 14–12).

CENTRAL VACUUM COMPRESSOR

A central vacuum compressor provides the suction needed for the oral evacuation systems. This equipment actually consists of two parts: the compressor, which creates the flow of air, and the vacuum tank, which is a container that screens the flow of air to create a suction.

This central vacuum compressor should be serviced regularly, in keeping with the manufacturer's directions.

Central Air Compressor

A central air compressor is used to provide compressed air for the air-water syringe and for the air-

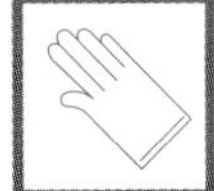
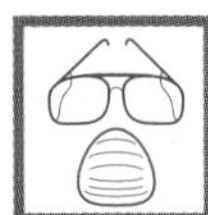

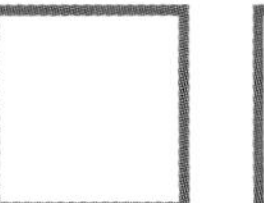
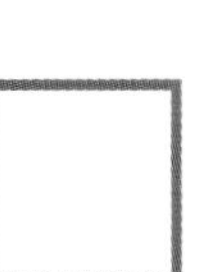

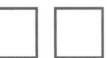

PROCEDURE: **Cleaning Oral Evacuation Hoses**

1. Put on appropriate PPE.
2. Aspirate through the system a solution of 1 quart of hot tap water mixed with 1 tablespoon of automatic dishwasher cleanser.
3. Aspirate through the system 2 quarts of chlorine bleach solution (7 ounces of bleach to 2 quarts of water).
   □ *CAUTION:* Be careful not to spill or splash the bleach solution.
4. Wait 10 to 20 minutes.
   □ *RATIONALE:* This allows the solution time to work within the system.
5. Aspirate another 1 to 2 quarts of hot tap water through the system. Do this by dipping the nozzle in and out of the water several times.
   □ *RATIONALE:* This chugging effect helps to loosen debris and flush it through.

driven handpieces (Fig. 14–13). The capacity of the compressor depends upon the number of treatment rooms and handpieces used in the practice.

Because of the noise level, and for safety reasons, the compressor system is placed outside the treatment area and, frequently, outside the office building.

The air compressor must receive routine service according to the manufacturer's instructions. This includes changing filters and occasionally checking for condensation in the lines. This service is usually handled by trained maintenance personnel.

Condensation in the air lines could cause the presence of moisture, sediment, or algae. (**Condensation** is the process by which a liquid is removed from vapor.) These contaminants can ruin handpieces and can cause debris to be ejected into the patient's mouth. If there is any indication of a condensation problem, the equipment should be serviced immediately.

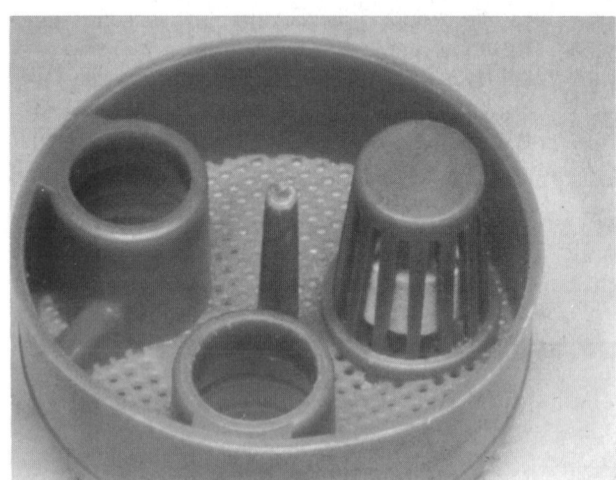

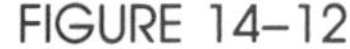

FIGURE 14–12

Disposable trap for evacuation systems. A deodorizing pellet is placed in the "tower" shown at right of photo. (Courtesy of Sultan Dental Products, Inc., Englewood, NJ.)

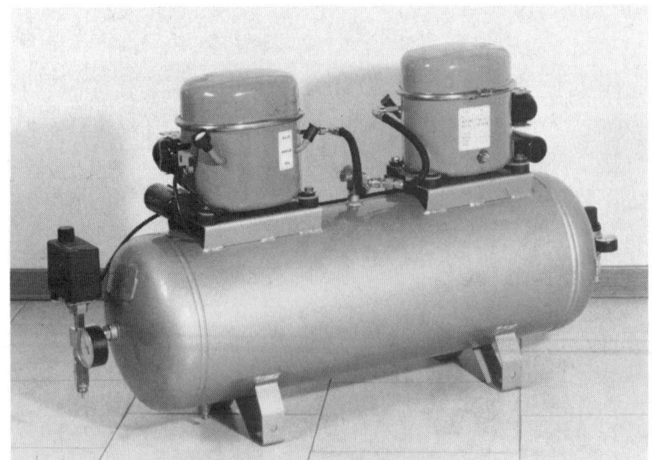

FIGURE 14–13

Central air compressor. (Courtesy of Silent Aire Compressors, Dentalaire Products International, Santa Ana, CA.)

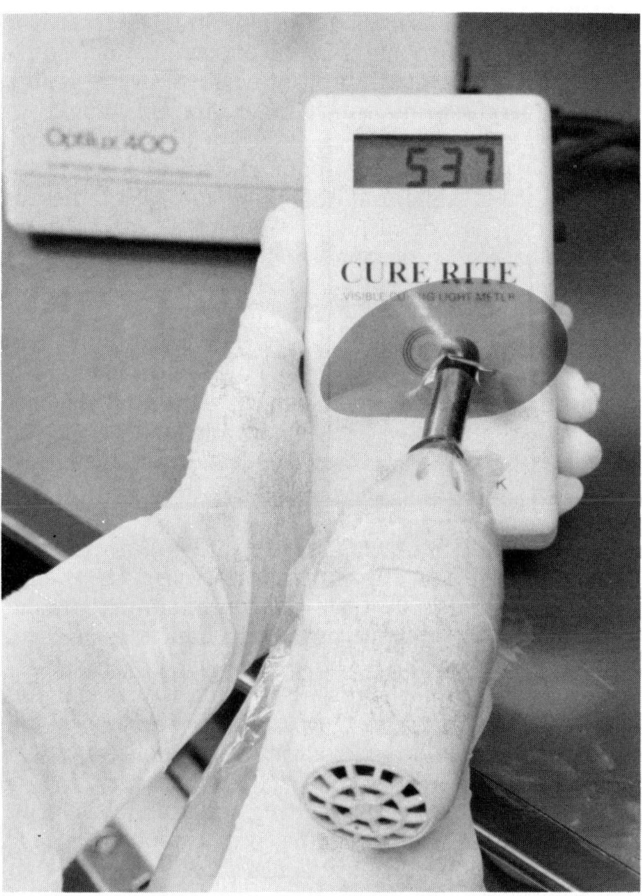

FIGURE 14–14

The curing light is tested periodically to determine that it is working properly.

Dental X-Ray Unit

Most treatment rooms include a dental x-ray unit. The structure and use of the dental x-ray unit are discussed in Chapter 17. The required infection control measures are discussed in Chapter 13.

The master switch of the x-ray unit may safely be turned on at the beginning of the day and left on throughout the day. (Radiation is emitted only while the exposure timer switch is depressed.) Should the x-ray unit require maintenance, it must be disconnected from its electrical source first.

View Box for Radiographs

A view box, used to read and diagnose radiographs, is placed in the cabinetry or flush in the wall of the operatory. It consists of a bright, white light source with a frosted glass or plastic cover.

The glass surface of the view box must be kept free of smudges by wiping it with a soft cloth. If touched during treatment, it must be cleaned and disinfected during treatment room preparation.

Curing Light

The curing light consists of a lighted wand, a protective shield, a handle, and a trigger switch to turn it on and off. This light is used to "cure" light-cured composites, sealants, and bonding agents. The action of the curing light brings about the chemical reaction that causes the material to harden. If the curing light is not working at full strength or is not used correctly, the material will not harden properly, and the results will be unsatisfactory.

TESTING AND MAINTENANCE

As shown in Figure 14–14, the curing light is tested periodically to determine that the light is working at full strength. Should it not reach the desired reading on the testing device, it is necessary to change the light bulb before use.

Most curing lights use a halogen bulb. When it is necessary to replace it, do so according to the manufacturer's instructions and do *not* touch the bulb with your hands. Test the new bulb before operation.

Because the curing light is such an important part of productivity in the operatory, extra bulbs should always be available for replacement as needed.

During use, the curing light is protected with a plastic barrier. If additional cleaning and disinfecting are necessary during treatment room preparation, the light should be cool before it is wiped with the solutions. (A sudden change in temperature might damage the bulb.)

Amalgamator

An amalgamator is used to triturate amalgam and some dental cements by vigorously shaking the ingredients. (**Triturate** means to mix together.)

The amalgamator may be mounted under a countertop or the edge of a mobile cart or stored in the top drawer of a mobile cabinet (Fig. 14–15). To reduce the

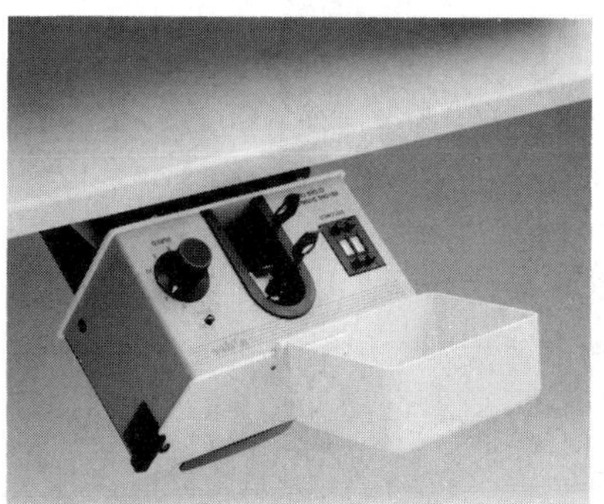

FIGURE 14–15

Amalgamator mounted under a cabinet. The cover must be closed during use. (Courtesy of A-DEC, Inc., Newberg, OR.)

hazard of mercury contamination in the air, the cover must be closed during trituration.

Other Clinical Areas

Sterilization and Supply Center

The sterilization and supply center is centrally located to provide easy access from the treatment rooms and other areas of the office. This center is discussed in Chapter 13.

Reminder: Each assistant is responsible for knowing where the contaminated area is within the sterilization center. Soiled instrument trays are returned only to the contaminated area; they are never placed in the "clean" area.

Dental Laboratory

The dental laboratory is the room where laboratory procedures such as pouring impressions, preparing diagnostic casts, and creating custom impression trays are performed (Fig. 14–16). These tasks are usually performed by the dental assistants. More complex procedures are sent to a commercial dental laboratory.

If the dentist provides extensive reconstructive services such as crowns and bridges and dentures, a larger laboratory is maintained, and a dental technician may be employed on the premises.

It is important to remember that materials coming into the laboratory have been in the patient's mouth, and exposure control is just as important here as it is in the treatment rooms. For this reason, eating, drinking, smoking, the application of cosmetics or lip balm, and the handling of contact lenses are *not* allowed in the laboratory.

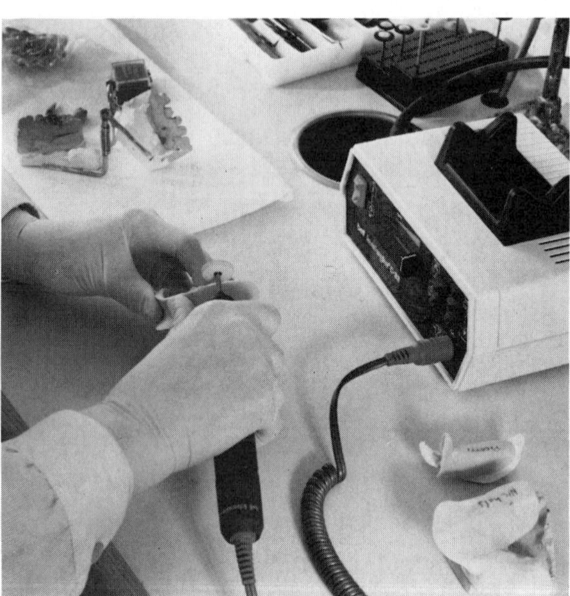

FIGURE 14–16

The dental laboratory includes work benches and equipment used to perform basic laboratory procedures.

When working in the laboratory, safety is always a concern. It is important to follow the safety precautions, which are discussed in Chapter 12, and the infection control procedures, which are discussed in Chapter 13.

LABORATORY STORAGE AND WORK AREAS

The dental laboratory is organized around benches and wall cabinets that provide an adequate work area and safe storage for the supplies and equipment used here. It is important that this entire area be kept neat and clean at all times.

Wall-mounted bins are used to store bulk supplies of plaster, stone, and investment materials. These bins protect the materials from moisture contamination and make it easy to remove gypsum products as needed. After use, the bin should be re-covered immediately.

Work pans are open plastic containers with identification labels that are used to hold the laboratory work in progress for the individual patient (Fig. 14–17).

Pans may be color-coded to indicate the type of procedure: for example, requiring construction of temporary coverage. If a written prescription from the dentist is required, this is attached to the pan.

LIGHTING AND VENTILATION

The dental laboratory must be adequately lighted and ventilated to provide a safe working environment.

Laboratory work requires close attention to detail. Good general lighting and specific work area lighting are important for this reason and for helping ensure safe working conditions.

Adequate ventilation is necessary to remove fumes and particles of debris from the air. An exhaust fan is installed for general laboratory ventilation. Also, protective hoods and vacuum systems on grinding equipment are used when materials such as acrylic trays, diagnostic casts, and metal prostheses are trimmed and polished.

The laboratory personnel must wear protective eyewear and masks to protect themselves from the dust and debris generated as these materials are ground and polished.

BASIC LABORATORY EQUIPMENT

The dental laboratory is generally equipped with a laboratory handpiece, a vibrator, a model trimmer, a vacuum former, and a dental lathe. Each piece of laboratory equipment should receive regular preventive care and maintenance as recommended by the manufacturer.

Laboratory Handpieces. A low-speed laboratory handpiece is used for many tasks such as trimming

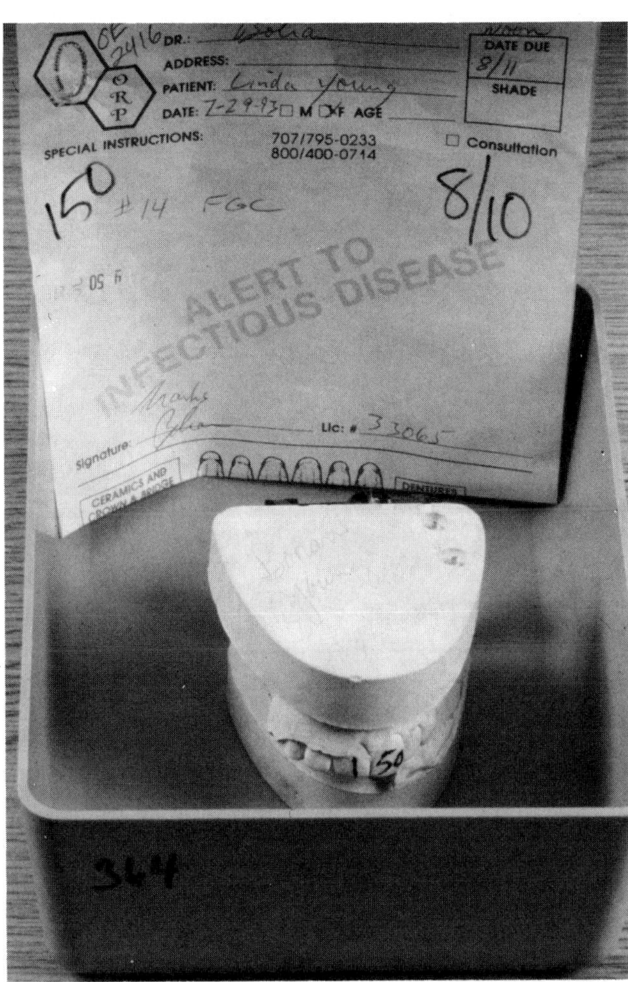

FIGURE 14–17

Laboratory cases are stored in work pans. The dentist's written laboratory prescription is posted on the work pan.

custom impression trays, adjusting dentures, and polishing cast restorations. (This handpiece is discussed further in Chapter 15.)

Vibrator. A vibrator has a flat working surface that vibrates (shakes). It is used to remove air bubbles and to aid in the flow of the plaster or stone mix into an impression when diagnostic casts are poured. To help keep the vibrator clean, a disposable cover is placed on the vibrator work surface before it is used. After use, this cover is discarded.

Model Trimmer. The model trimmer has an abrasive grinding wheel that is used to remove excess plaster or stone when the shape of the diagnostic casts is finalized. The wheel works most effectively if the models are slightly damp.

Casts are placed on the angled work table and held in place with a holding device so that they may be trimmed safely without endangering the fingers.

To control the dust level from the cast and to facilitate cutting, a gentle stream of water is run on the wheel when it is in use. Also, using the wheel without an adequate supply of water will destroy it.

The used water drains directly into a sink that is equipped with a plaster trap that catches the grindings and prevents them from clogging the drain.

The steps in the use of the model trimmer are discussed in Chapter 19.

Vacuum Former. A vacuum former is a small electric appliance that is used to construct plastic (acrylic) appliances such as temporary coverage, bleaching trays, mouth guards, and custom trays. (Construction of these is discussed in Chapter 24.)

The upper part is a heating element that warms and softens a sheet of plastic material (Fig. 14–18). The work surface has holes in it that allow the vacuum to pull and shape the warmed plastic around the cast.

The moist prepared model is placed on the work surface, and a sheet of plastic is placed in the holder

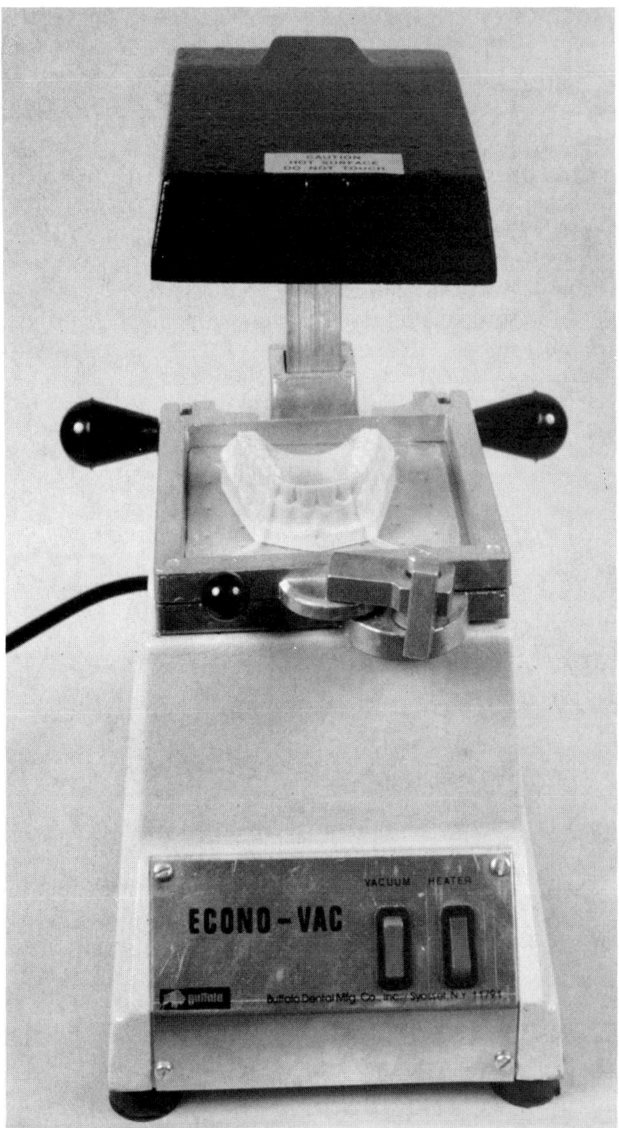

FIGURE 14–18

A vacuum former is used to make custom trays, mouth guards, and bleaching trays.

TABLE 14–1

Treatment Room Preparation Checklist

OK	PREPARATION STEP
	The between-patient routine has been completed, and the treatment room is clean and ready for the next patient.
	The patient's chart, radiographs, laboratory case, appropriate sterile preset tray, and other supplies are in place and ready for use.
	The dental chair has been lowered, the back is upright, and the chair arm (on the entry side) has been raised out of the way.
	Equipment, wires, and hoses have been moved out of the path of entry of the patient and dental team.

on the heating element. The plastic is heated until soft and lowered onto the model. Vacuum from below (through the holes in the base) forms the plastic close about the model.

Dental Lathe. The dental lathe is used to trim custom trays and to polish temporary coverage, dentures, and precious metal castings. To protect the operator, the lathe must have a shield and should also have a vacuum system. Also, the operator must always wear appropriate PPE when using the lathe.

The lathe has a revolving, threaded extension from each end of the motor. Attachments such as abrasive grinding rings and polishing brushes or rag wheels are placed on these extensions.

Pumice and other polishing agents are used during polishing. A protective pan behind and under the wheel is used to hold the pumice and catch the spatter.

Heat Sources. A heat source is often required in the laboratory to heat wax or other materials. A propane or butane torch is used for this purpose. Because of the danger of fire, the laboratory must be equipped with a fire extinguisher. It is the responsibility of anyone working in the laboratory to know where it is and how to use it.

The Patient Visit

Attention to detail and staff attitudes in receiving and dismissing patients are very important in creating a positive experience for the patient.

Table 14–1 is a treatment room preparation checklist that should be completed before the patient is seated. The exposure control steps in treatment room preparation are discussed in Chapter 13.

PROCEDURE: **Admitting the Patient**

1. Go to the reception area, pleasantly greet the patient by name, and request that he follow you to the treatment room.
2. Place the patient's personal items, such as eyeglasses or earrings, in a safe place out of the way of the dental team.
   □ *RATIONALE:* Under exposure control protocols, the patient's coat should not be brought into the treatment room.
3. Make pleasant conversation; however, if the patient obviously does not want to talk, remain busy and quiet.
   □ *RATIONALE:* Chatting about things, other than treatment, may help the patient feel more comfortable and relaxed.
4. Answer any questions about impending treatment honestly. If you do not know the answer, say so and offer to get the information.
   □ *RATIONALE:* Patients frequently ask the assistant questions about treatment that they are reluctant to bring up with the dentist. Willingness to answer these questions helps reassure the patient.

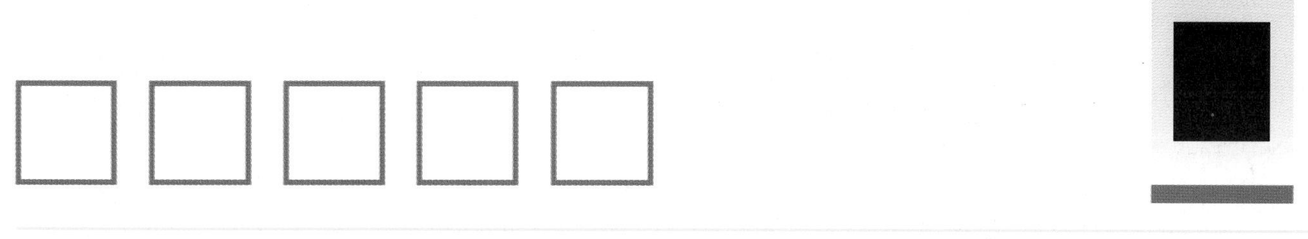

PROCEDURE: **Seating the Patient**

1. Ask the patient to sit on the side of the dental chair and then to swing his legs into position.
   □ *RATIONALE:* The patient should be positioned so that buttocks and shoulder blades are flush against the back of the chair.
2. Lower or slide the chair arm into position.
3. Drape the patient with a disposable patient towel (Fig. 14–19). Depending on the procedure, a plastic drape may also be necessary.
4. Inform the patient before adjusting the chair. Make the adjustments slowly until the patient and chair are in the proper position for the planned dental treatment.
5. Turn on the operating light and check that all treatment room preparations are complete.
6. Wash hands and put on gloves in preparation for assisting in patient care.
7. Touch only the protective barrier on the operating light handle, and slowly adjust the light slowly upward to illuminate the patient's oral cavity.

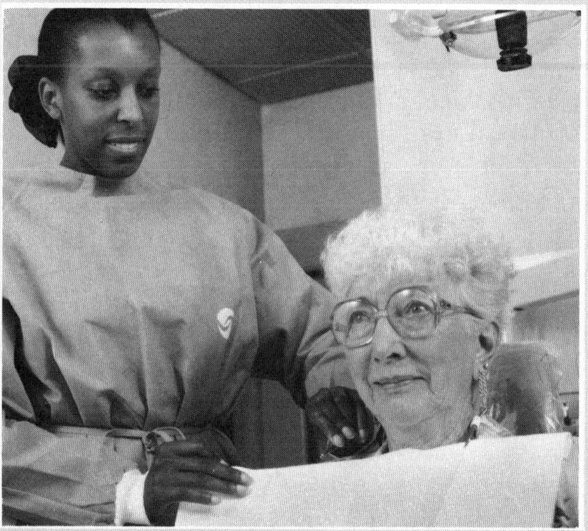

FIGURE 14–19

The assistant seats and drapes the patient.

PROCEDURE: **Dismissing the Patient**

1. While still gloved from patient care, slowly return the chair to the upright position. If necessary, give the patient postoperative instructions.
2. Check the patient's face for smudges or debris. If present, these should be removed gently with a moist tissue.
3. Remove the patient towel and drape, and raise the chair arm. If there is debris on clothing, this should be removed carefully.
4. Remove gloves and wash hands.
5. Return any personal belongings while the patient is still seated (Fig. 14–20).
6. Assist the patient from the chair, if necessary.
7. Direct or escort the patient to the business office.

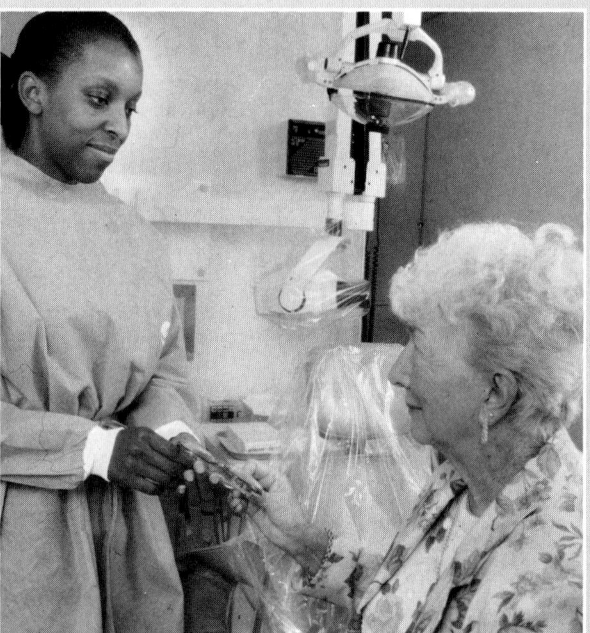

FIGURE 14–20

Dismissing the patient. The back of the chair is raised slowly, the towel and drape are removed, and the patient's belongings are returned.

Evening and Morning Routines for Dental Assistants

In most practices, several assistants are employed in the treatment area, and the important responsibilities of evening and morning care of these areas are divided among them.

Careful completion of all these steps helps ensure the smooth flow of patient care throughout the day. The goal in the evening is to leave the office ready for patient care first thing in the morning.

Failure to complete these steps could cause the loss of productive time for the dentist, inconvenience or discomfort for the patient, and unnecessary stress for everyone.

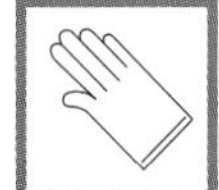
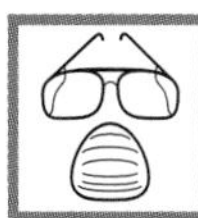

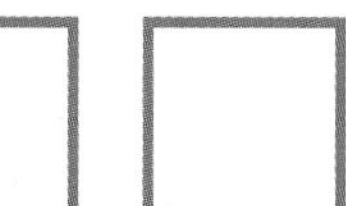

PROCEDURE: **Evening Routine (After the Last Patient)**

1. Complete the treatment room exposure control cleanup and preparation protocols.
2. Wear appropriate PPE while emptying waste receptacles and placing fresh plastic liners.
   ☐ *RATIONALE:* Waste must be disposed of safely, and this is discussed in Chapter 12.
3. Turn off all equipment.
4. Determine that treatment rooms are adequately stocked for the next day.
5. Post appointment schedules for the next work day in treatment rooms.
6. Check the appointment schedule to see that preset trays, patient records, and laboratory work are ready for the next day.
7. Determine that all contaminated instruments have been processed and that the sterilization center has been cleaned.
8. Determine that the treatment rooms are ready for use.
9. Change out of protective clothing and into street clothes. Place soiled protective clothing in the appropriate container.
   ☐ *RATIONALE:* Proper handling of contaminated protective attire is an important part of exposure control.

PROCEDURE: **Morning Routine (Opening the Office)**

1. Arrive 30 minutes before the first scheduled patient of the day.
   ☐ *RATIONALE:* This allows time to complete duties so that the day can start smoothly and on time.
2. Change into fresh protective clothing at the office.
   ☐ *RATIONALE:* Because of the possible danger of spreading contamination, protective clothing is *never* worn outside the office.
3. Turn on the master switches for the central air compressor and vacuum units. Turn on the master switches for the dental and x-ray units.
4. Determine that the treatment rooms are ready for use.
5. Recheck the appointment schedule of patients for the day to be certain that preset trays, patient records, radiographs, and laboratory cases are all available as needed for the planned treatments.
6. Set up treatment rooms for the first patients.

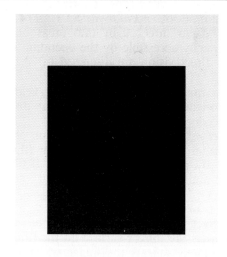

Chapter 15

Dental Instruments and Accessories

Introduction

This chapter discusses the types of instruments most commonly used in restorative dentistry. Dental specialty instruments are discussed in the chapter for each specialty.

There is a wide variety of instruments used in dentistry. The instruments discussed here are the basic designs. Manufacturers make many variations of these basic designs to accommodate the personal preferences of dentists.

Each type of dental instrument has a specific purpose, and these instruments are commonly used in a specific sequence. The terms **order of use** and **sequence of use** describe the order in which the dentist needs these instruments.

There are two broad categories of dental instruments: **hand instruments**, which are held and manipulated by the operator's hand, and **rotary instruments,** which are commonly referred to as the dental handpiece.

Hand Instruments

Hand Instrument Design

Hand instruments are designed with three specific parts: the handle, shank, and working end (Fig. 15–1).

HANDLE

The handle is the portion where the operator grasps or holds the instrument. Handles are manufactured in various shapes and sizes. Some handles are round; others are hexagonal. They can be smooth in texture or have a grooved pattern to prevent them from slipping when grasped with a gloved hand.

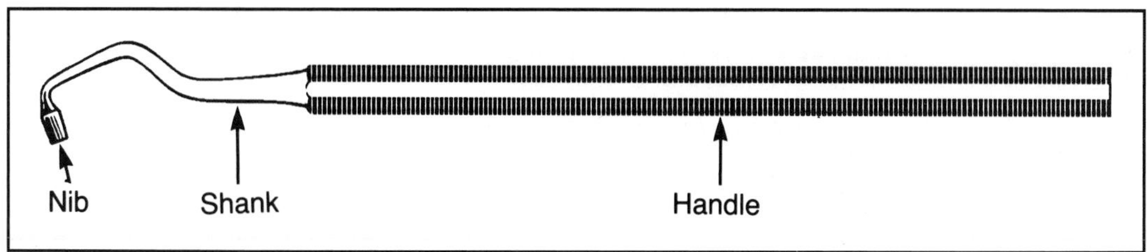

FIGURE 15–1

Basic parts of a dental hand instrument.

SHANK

Shank refers to that part of the instrument that attaches the working end to the handle. The angles in the shank allow the instrument to reach various areas of the oral cavity.

For example, instruments that are used in the posterior areas of the mouth have more angles in the shank, and those instruments used in the anterior regions have fewer angles.

The thickness and strength of the shank dictate the amount of pressure that can be applied to the instrument without breakage.

WORKING END

Working end refers to the end of the instrument used to perform the procedure on the tooth. The working end can have a point, a blade, or a nib. A nib is a blunt tip that may be smooth or serrated. (**Serrated** means notched or toothlike on the edge.)

Hand instruments are single-ended or double-ended. A double-ended instrument has a shank and working end at both ends of the handle.

Often double-ended instruments are mirror images (reverse angles) of each other to allow adaptation to all surfaces of the tooth. These are referred to as being left and right instruments.

The Basic Setup

The term **basic setup** describes the three instruments used for almost every patient visit. These are a mouth mirror, an explorer, and cotton pliers (Fig. 15–2).

MOUTH MIRRORS

Mouth mirrors are used for a variety of purposes, including

- **Indirect vision,** which allows the operator to see into areas of the mouth not visible by direct vision
- **Light reflection,** to direct light into areas of the mouth not directly accessible by the operating light (direct and indirect vision are discussed in Chapter 16)
- **Retraction,** to maintain a clear operating field by keeping the tongue or cheek out of the way during operative procedures
- **Tissue protection,** to guard the tongue or cheek against accidental injury from a dental bur (this is accomplished by placing the mirror head between the handpiece and the tissues)

Types and Sizes of Mouth Mirrors

The **front surface mirror**, which is the one most commonly used, has the mirror surface on the front of the glass. It accurately reflects the image without enlarging it.

The **concave mirror** magnifies the image. Many operators prefer this magnification for better vision. The **flat surface mirror**, also known as a *plane surface mirror,* is the least expensive but can distort the image so that structures viewed indirectly look different from those viewed directly.

Mouth mirrors are available in a variety of sizes, ranging from ¾ inch to 1⅝ inches. The sizes are identified by number, numbers 4 and 5 being the most commonly used.

EXPLORERS

Explorers are multifunctional instruments and are included in the basic setup for every operative procedure. There are many types of explorers available, and each has a thin, flexible, wirelike working end with a sharp point at the tip (Fig. 15–3).

This thin tip enables the operator to use tactile sensitivity to distinguish areas of decay and discrepancies

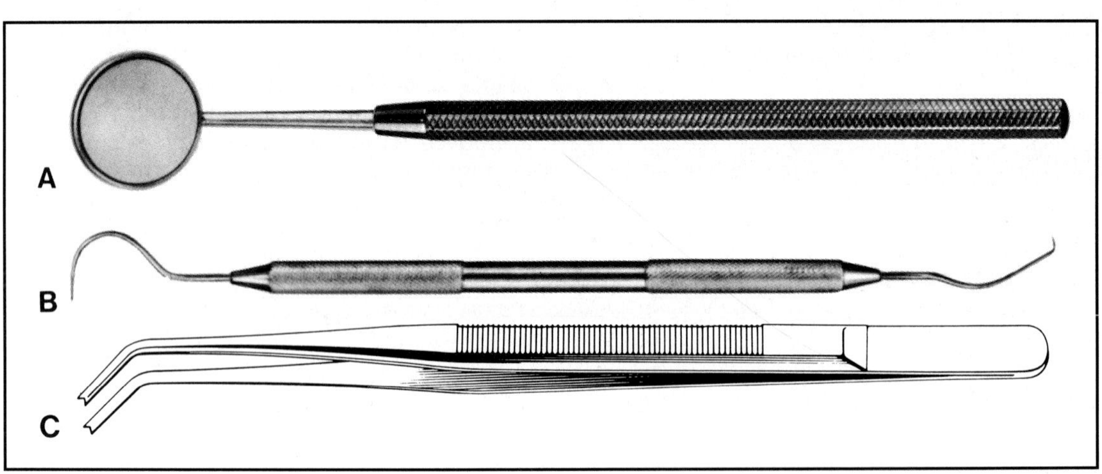

FIGURE 15–2

The basic setup. *A*, Mouth mirror. *B*, Double-ended explorer. *C*, Cotton pliers. (Courtesy of Hu-Friedy, Chicago, IL.)

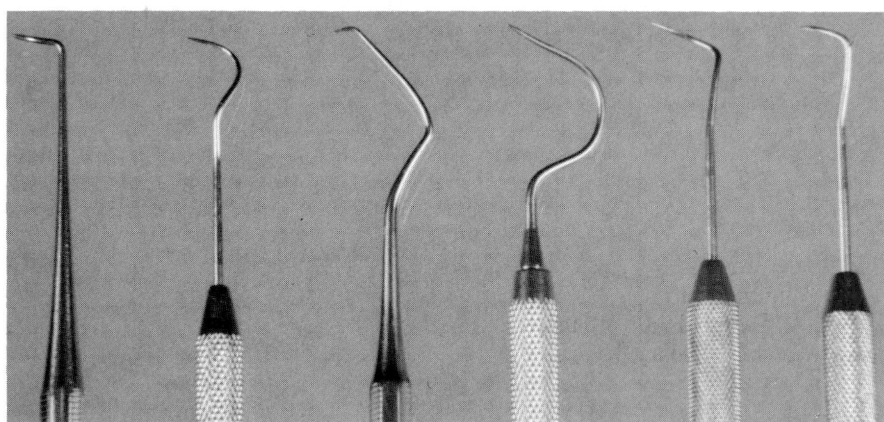

FIGURE 15–3

Basic styles of dental explorers.

on the surface of the teeth. (**Tactile** refers to the sense of touch.)

COTTON PLIERS

Cotton pliers are used to place and retrieve small objects in the mouth, such as cotton pellets, gingival retraction cord, matrix bands, and wedges.

Cotton pliers are available with plain or serrated points, which are also known as *beaks*.

The handles of cotton pliers may be of a locking or nonlocking style. To hold something, such as a cotton pellet, in the beaks of nonlocking pliers, the handles must be held closed with the fingers. With locking pliers, the handles can be locked in a closed position, and the beaks do not open until the lock is released.

PERIODONTAL PROBES

The basic setup for a dental examination and for periodontal treatment includes a fourth instrument. This is a periodontal probe, which is used to measure periodontal attachment.

The periodontal probe is a tapered, rod-shaped instrument calibrated in millimeters. It has a blunt tip and is available in many designs, including color-coded calibrations (see Fig. 18–19).

Hand-Cutting Instrumentation for Restorative Procedures

Hand-cutting instruments are used primarily to remove soft, carious dentin, to plane (smooth) the walls and floor of the cavity, and to refine the cavity preparation. These steps are discussed in Chapter 25.

The six classes of hand-cutting instruments are excavators, hatchets, gingival margin trimmers, chisels, and hoes. The instruments within each class are available in a variety of sizes and designs (Fig. 15–4).

Most dentists use only one or two of these instruments during a cavity preparation. The instruments selected depend upon the dentist's preference.

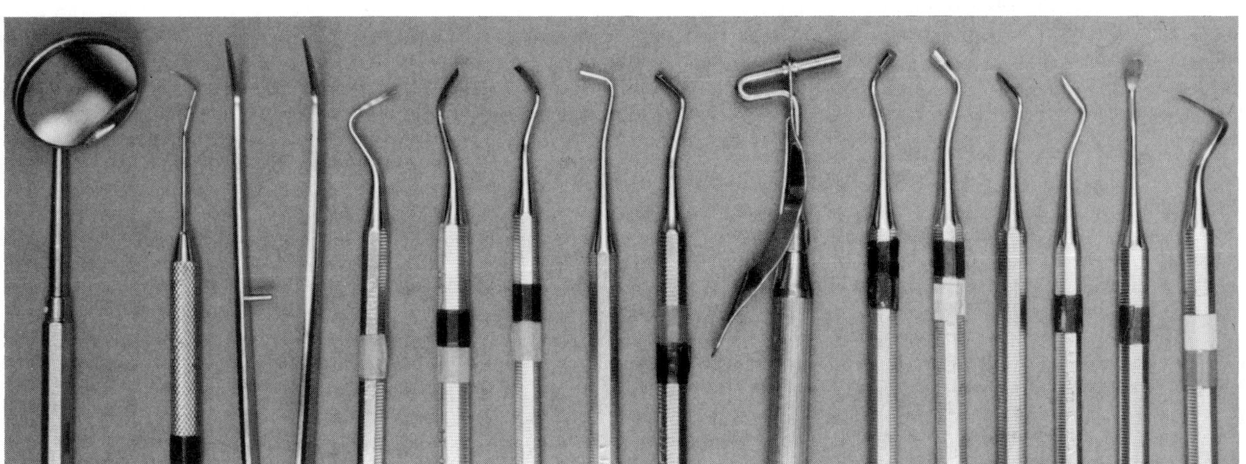

FIGURE 15–4

Working ends of dental hand instruments. *Left to right*, Mirror, explorer, cotton pliers, small spoon excavator, large spoon excavator, binangle chisel, plastic instrument (plugger end), burnisher (acorn), amalgam carrier, small condenser, large condenser, two Hollenback carvers, discoid carver, interproximal knife.

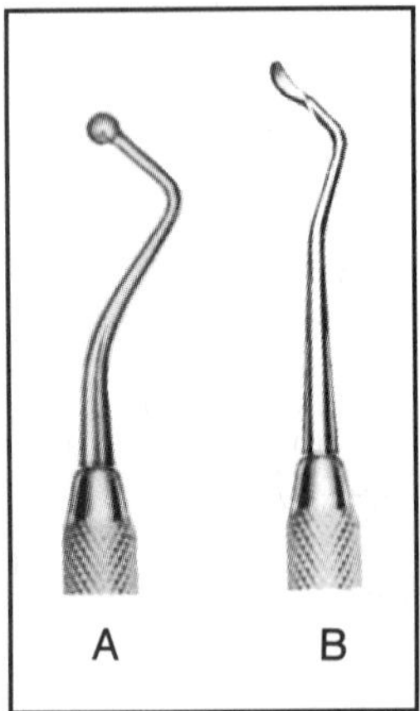

FIGURE 15-5

Spoon excavators. *A*, Round. *B*, Oval. (Courtesy of Hu-Friedy, Chicago, IL.)

EXCAVATORS

An excavator has a spoon-shaped working end with a sharp edge designed primarily for the removal of soft dentin, debris, and caries from the tooth by the dentist (Fig. 15-5).

In states where these functions are legal, the assistant frequently uses a spoon excavator

- To clean temporary cement from cast restorations before final cementation
- To assist in placing the matrix band in a difficult cervical area of a preparation
- To place and shape cavity liners and cement bases
- To remove temporary restorations

A **cleoid-discoid** is a double-ended variety of excavator (Fig. 15-6). The cleoid end is in the form of a claw and sharpened to a point. The discoid end is disc-shaped with sharp edges. This instrument is also commonly used as a carver.

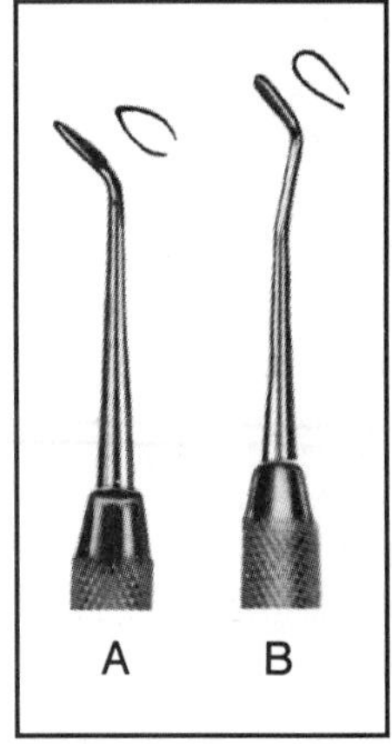

FIGURE 15-6

Cleoid-discoid excavator. *A*, Cleoid. *B*, Discoid. (Courtesy of Hu-Friedy, Chicago, IL.)

HATCHETS

Hatchets are similar in appearance to wood hatchets. The cutting edge is in the same plane as the handle of the instrument, and the instrument contains at least one bend in the shank. Hatchets are used during cavity preparation to smooth the cavity walls and floors and to remove undermined (unsupported) enamel (Figs. 15-7*A* and 15-8*B*).

GINGIVAL MARGIN TRIMMERS

A gingival margin trimmer is a variety of hatchet that has been modified so that the blade is curved slightly (Fig. 15-9*B*). This is a double-ended instrument: one end curves to the right, and the other curves to the left. Both ends of one instrument can be used for either the mesial or distal surfaces.

Gingival margin trimmers are used to place a bevel along the gingival margin of the cavity preparation for amalgam restorations, inlays, or onlays. This instrument can also be used to plane all enamel margins.

CHISELS

A chisel is a straight instrument with a single-beveled cutting edge. Chisels are used to plane (smooth) the enamel margins of the cavity preparation (see Figs. 15-7*B* and 15-8*A*). (A **bevel** is the slanting edge of the instrument. In a cavity preparation, the **margin** is the outside limit of the preparation.)

A **straight chisel** has no angles in the shank; a **bin-angle chisel** has two angles in the shank; and a **Wedelstaedt chisel** has a slight curve in the shank.

An **angle former** is variety of chisel with the cutting edge at an angle, other than a right angle, to the blade (see Fig. 15-9*A*). The *sides* of the blade are sharp to form cutting edges. These instruments are used to form sharp line and point angles of cavity preparations.

HOES

The hoe is similar in appearance to the garden tool. The blade is nearly perpendicular to the handle of the instrument. The hoe is used to plane (smooth) cavity walls and floors.

Instruments for Amalgam and Composite Restorations

Amalgam restorations are discussed in Chapter 25.

AMALGAM CARRIERS

The dental assistant uses the amalgam carrier to pick up an increment of amalgam, carry it to the oral cavity, and place it into the cavity preparation, where it is condensed in place by the dentist (Fig. 15-10).

Most amalgam carriers are double-ended to hold a large increment of amalgam in one end and a small increment in the opposite end.

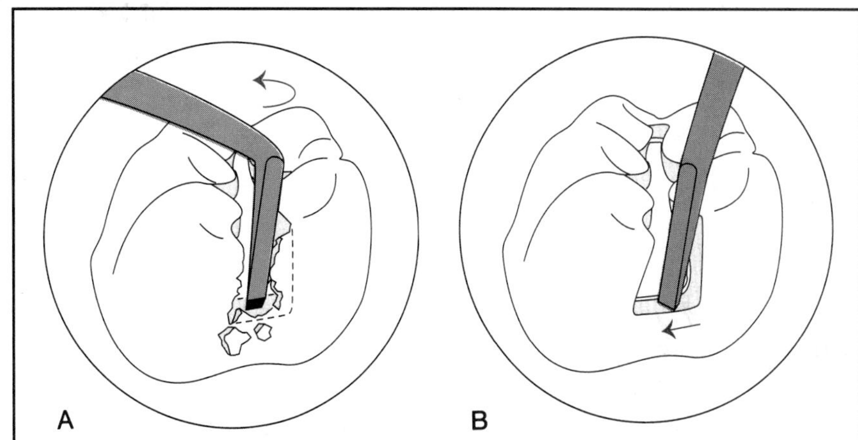

FIGURE 15–7

Dental hand-cutting instruments in use. *A*, Hatchet used to fracture away undermined enamel. *B*, Chisel used to refine the cavity preparation. (Courtesy of Hu-Friedy, Chicago, IL.)

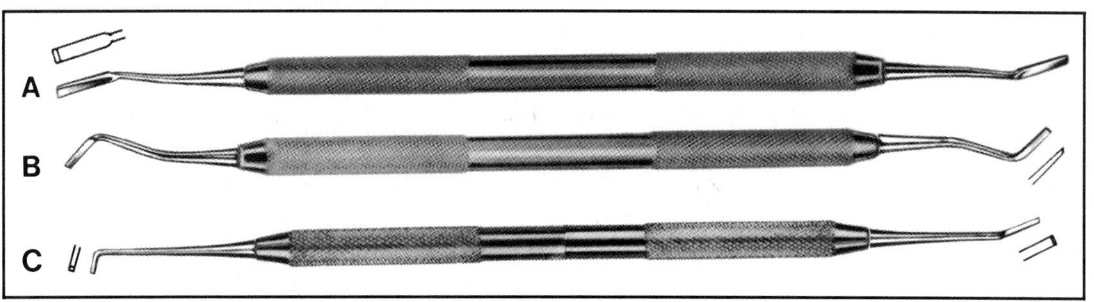

FIGURE 15–8

Dental hand-cutting instruments. *A*, Binangle chisel. *B*, Hatchet. *C*, Hoe. (Courtesy of Hu-Friedy, Chicago, IL.)

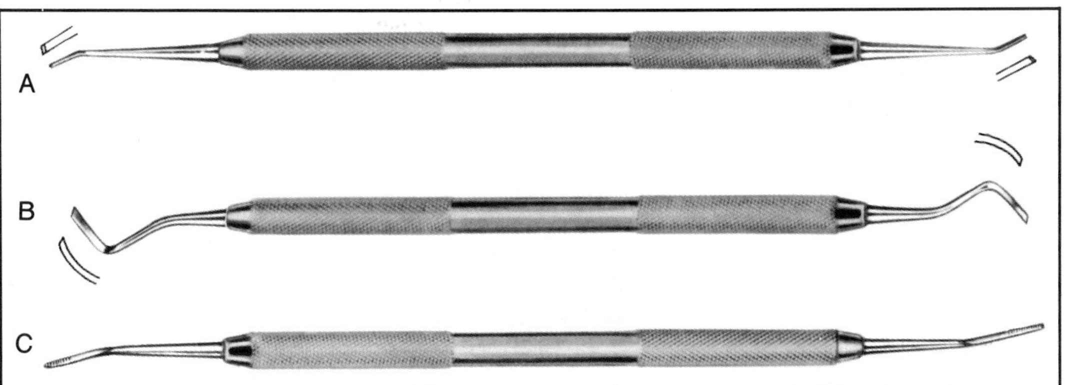

FIGURE 15–9

Dental hand-cutting instruments. *A*, Angle former. *B*, Gingival margin trimmer. *C*, Wedelstaedt interproximal amalgam file. (Courtesy of Hu-Friedy, Chicago, IL.)

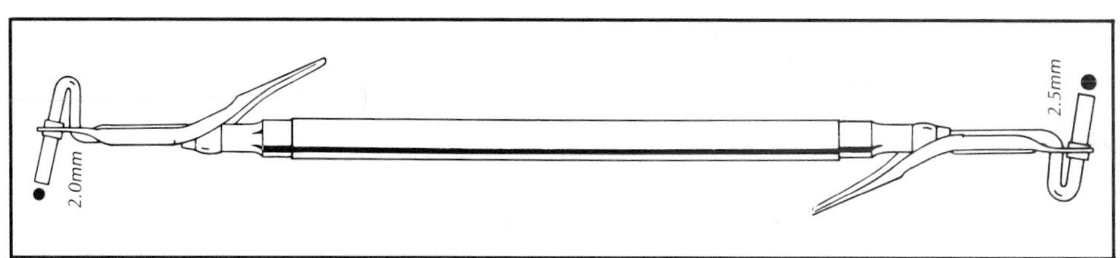

FIGURE 15–10

Double-ended amalgam carrier. (Courtesy of Hu-Friedy, Chicago, IL.)

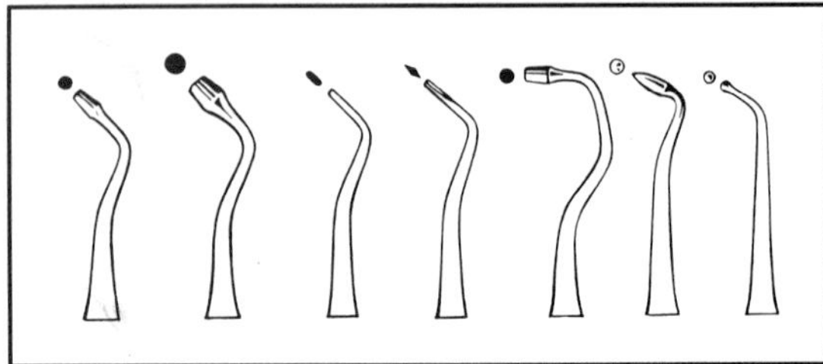

FIGURE 15–11

Amalgam condensers. (Courtesy of Hu-Friedy, Chicago, IL.)

AMALGAM CONDENSERS

The amalgam condenser, also known as a *plugger*, is used to condense (pack down) the freshly placed amalgam into the cavity preparation (Fig. 15–11).

The working end is flat and can be either smooth or serrated. To enable the operator to reach all areas of the cavity preparation, the shank of the instrument is angled.

AMALGAM CARVERS

Carvers are used to carve anatomy in the amalgam restoration before the amalgam hardens. There is a variety of styles of carvers available (Fig. 15–12).

Some are especially useful for occlusal surfaces, some are very thin in order to reach the proximal surfaces, and others can be used on all surfaces. Every dentist has individual preferences for carvers.

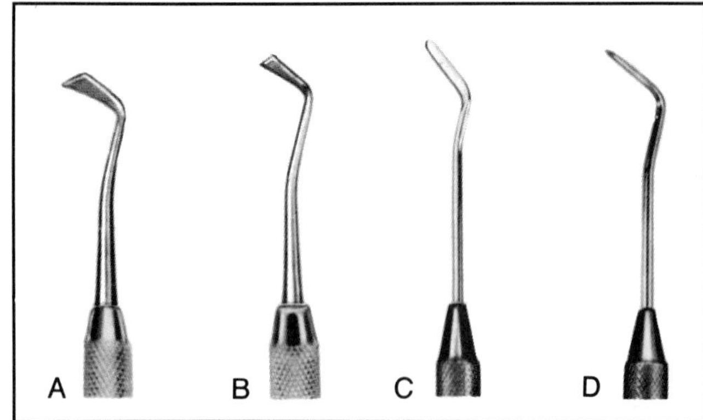

FIGURE 15–12

Assorted amalgam carvers. *A* and *B*, Hollenback carvers. *C* and *D*, Interproximal carvers. (Courtesy of Hu-Friedy, Chicago, IL.)

KNIVES AND FILES

In restorative dentistry, **interproximal knives** and **finishing files** are used to trim away excess restorative material or to smooth off overhanging margins of metal restorations (see Fig. 15–9*C*).

COMPOSITE PLACEMENT INSTRUMENTS

These instruments are designed specifically for placement of composite restorative materials. (A **composite** is a tooth-colored resin material used for dental restorations. These are discussed in Chapter 25.)

Composite placement instruments are made from a special plastic material that prevents the composite from sticking to the instruments during placement. Also, these instruments do not discolor the composite material, as do metal instruments.

Accessories for Restorative Dentistry

BURNISHERS

Commonly used shapes of burnishers include round ball, football or egg, and beavertail (Fig. 15–13). Burnishers are versatile instruments with many uses. (**Burnish** means to smooth the edge of a surface by rubbing against it.)

- A football-shaped burnisher may be used to shape matrix bands.
- A beavertail burnisher may be used to aid the process of inverting the dental dam around the teeth.
- A burnisher may be used to smooth the surface of the freshly placed amalgam restoration.

PLASTIC INSTRUMENTS

The term *plastic* describes the state of a dental material while it is still soft and can be easily placed and

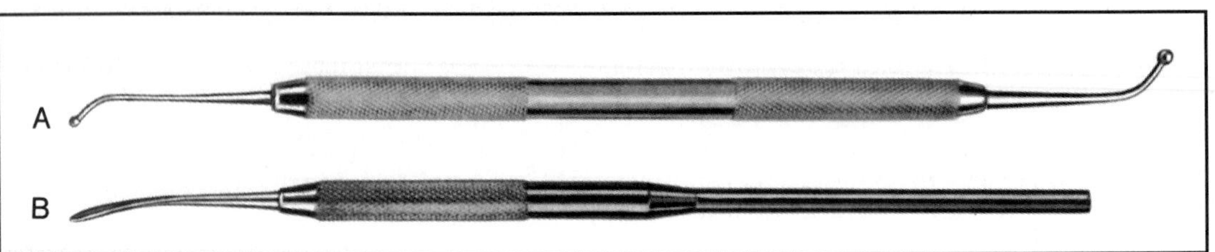

FIGURE 15–13

Burnishers. *A*, Ball burnisher. *B*, Beavertail burnisher. (Courtesy of Hu-Friedy, Chicago, IL.)

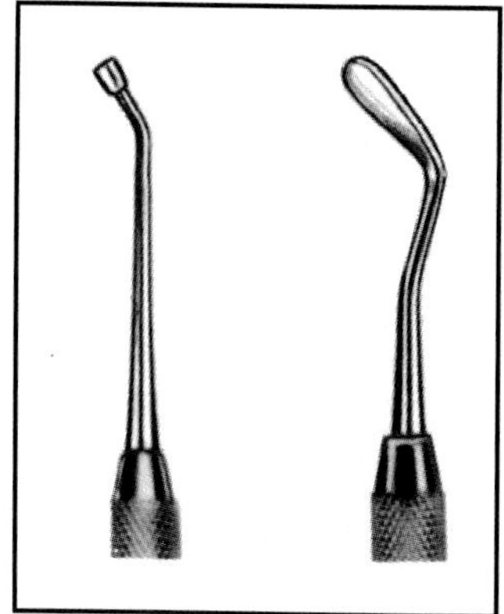

FIGURE 15–14

Woodson plastic instrument. *Left,* Nib end. *Right,* Blade end. (Courtesy of Hu-Friedy, Chicago, IL.)

shaped. Plastic instruments, which are actually made of metal, are used for this purpose. One end of these double-ended instruments is usually a smooth, flat blade, whereas the other end is a rounded nib (Fig. 15–14).

SPATULAS

A variety of spatulas are used to mix dental materials (Fig. 15–15). The selection of the spatula depends on the properties of the material to be mixed. Metal spatulas are used to mix

- Impression materials (see Chapters 19 and 24)
- Dental cements (see Chapter 23)
- Gypsum for diagnostic casts (see Chapter 19)

A metal spatula is *not* used to mix composite restorative materials. For those composites that require mixing, the manufacturer supplies disposable plastic mixing sticks.

SCISSORS

The scissors most commonly associated with restorative dental procedures are the **crown and bridge scissors** (Fig. 15–16). These scissors are available with either curved or straight blades. They are useful for many tasks, including trimming temporary crowns, cutting retraction cord, and shaping matrix bands.

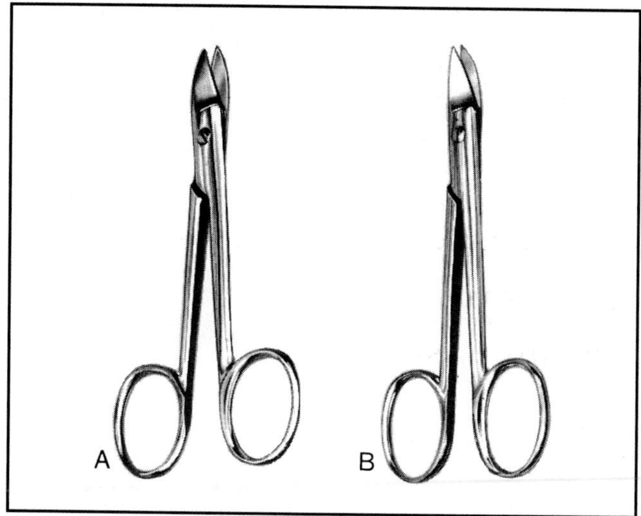

FIGURE 15–16

Crown and bridge scissors. *A,* Straight. *B,* Curved. (Courtesy of Hu-Friedy, Chicago, IL.)

ARTICULATING PAPER HOLDER

Articulating paper, held in place by a metal articulating paper holder, is used to identify high spots in the process of adjusting the occlusion on a newly placed restoration.

The holder and blue articulating paper are shown in the lower left corner of the instrument tray in Figure 15–17. When placed in the mouth, it is positioned so that the handle of the metal holder is next to the cheek.

Preset Trays, Cassettes, and Tubs

The hand instruments and related accessories for a given procedure (such as a composite restoration) are prepared, stored, and transported together as a **preset tray** or **cassette.**

A practice will have enough trays or cassettes for each of the commonly performed procedures to allow

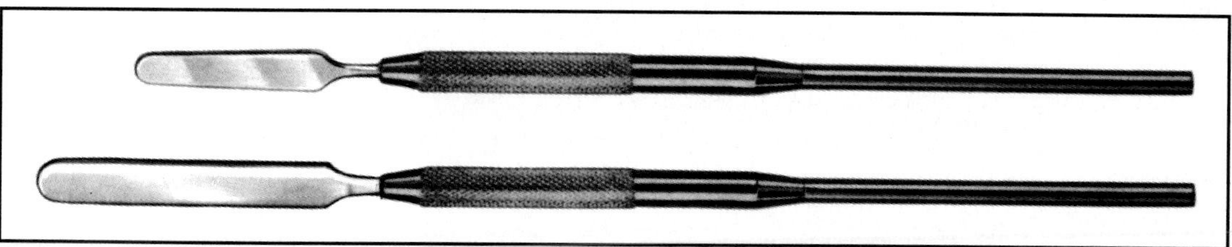

FIGURE 15–15

Cement spatulas. (Courtesy of Hu-Friedy, Chicago, IL.)

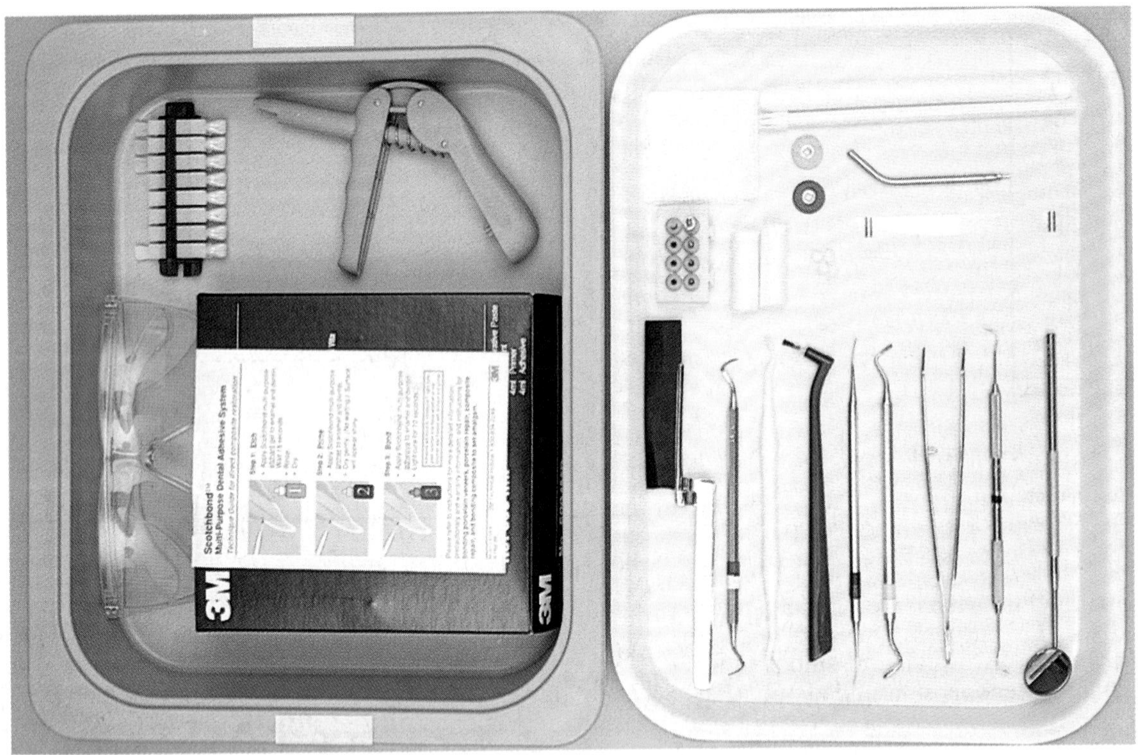

FIGURE 15–17

Tub and tray for composite restorations. *Left*, The tub contains the restorative material and related supplies. *Right*, The tray contains the instruments for this procedure.

adequate sterilization and preparation time before the tray is needed again. (This is discussed in Chapter 13.)

The sterile tray or cassette is taken to the treatment area during preparation for the patient visit. The sterile instruments are unwrapped just before use.

Supplies for a specific procedure, such as a composite restoration, are stored and transported to and from the treatment room in a covered plastic tub. The combination is known as the **tub and tray** system (see Fig. 15–17.)

Color-Coding Systems

Color-coding is one of the most convenient and efficient ways to organize instruments, trays, and supply

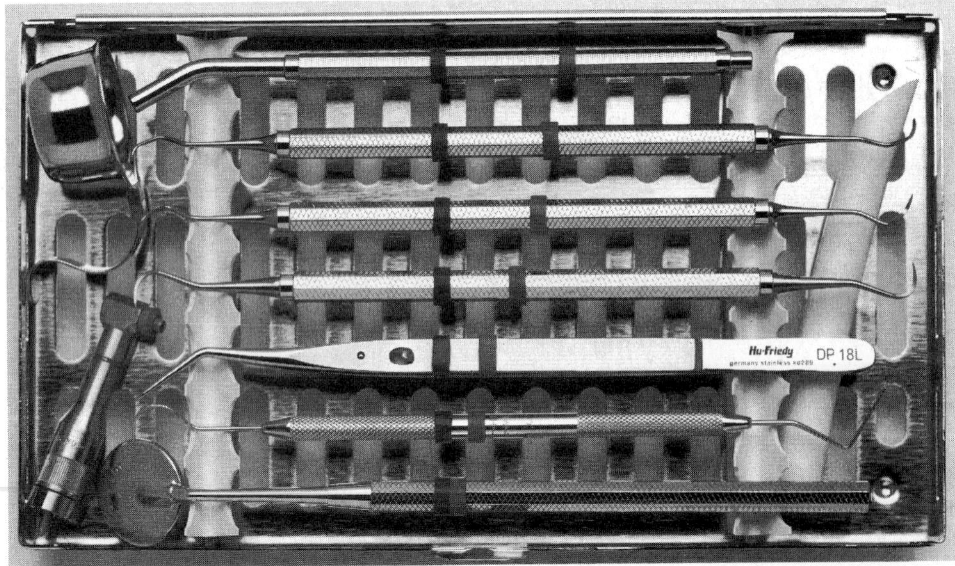

FIGURE 15–18

Color-coded instruments. Color-coded pedodontic prophy and sealant placement instrumentation in a metal instrument cassette. (Courtesy of Hu-Friedy, Chicago, IL.)

tubs for specific procedures (Fig. 15–18). The ways in which color-coding can be used are limited only by the creativity of the user.

COLOR-CODING INSTRUMENTS

Colored identification tape or rubber rings are placed on the handles of instruments. Some dentists prefer to use two or even three colors on the instruments. For example:

- One color is used to designate the procedure.
- The second color may designate the operatory in which it will be used.
- The third color may indicate the operator who prefers a specific tray setup. (This technique is especially helpful in group practices or offices that employ more than one dental hygienist.)

Instruments can be set up on the tray very quickly and in the correct order of use by positioning the color code bands on the instrument in a descending order (see Fig. 15–18).

COLOR-CODING TRAYS AND TUBS

The instrument tray and the tub of related materials are usually also color-coded to indicate the procedure. Thus if blue is the color chosen to indicate composite restorations, each of the instruments has a blue band, the tray has a blue label, and a blue tub is used to transport the related materials.

ROTARY INSTRUMENTS

Rotary instruments refer to the use of the dental handpiece and a bur. This combination is like the industrial power tool in which a drill and bit are used to make holes in wood and metal. Many patients immediately associate "the drill" with dentistry.

Rotary instruments have many uses in restorative dentistry, including

- Cutting the cavity preparation (see Chapter 25)
- Preparing teeth for crowns and other cast restorations (see Chapter 31)
- Removing old amalgam or cast restorations
- Finishing and polishing restorations

Dental Burs

There are many types of dental burs available, and these are designed for very specific uses; however, all burs have three basic parts: the shank, neck, and head (Fig. 15–19).

The **shank** of the bur fits into the handpiece. Shank length varies according to the specific function of the bur. For example, short shank burs are used in areas of the oral cavity with very limited access, such as the maxillary molar area.

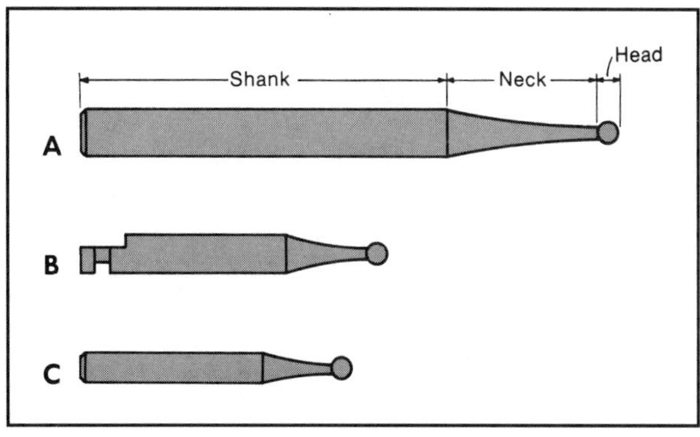

FIGURE 15–19

Bur parts and basic design. *A*, Long-shank friction bur. *B*, Latch-type bur. *C*, Regular friction-grip bur.

The **neck** is the narrow portion of the bur that connects the shank and the head.

The **head** of the bur is the cutting or polishing portion. Heads are manufactured in a large variety of sizes, shapes, and materials.

When burs are ordered, it is necessary to specify the shank type (indicated by letters) and the head shape and size (indicated by a number).

SHANK TYPES

Dental burs are manufactured in three basic styles of shanks. The type of shank on the bur determines in which type of handpiece it may be used. The three styles of shanks are as follows:

Straight. These burs have a long, straight shank and are used in the straight handpiece. They are designated with the letter **HP** (for handpiece).

Latch Type. The latch-type contra-angle handpiece holds this bur in place by mechanically grasping the small groove at the end of the shank. These burs are designated with the letter **RA** (for right angle).

Friction-Grip. The shank is short and smooth and has no retention grooves in the end. It is held in the friction-grip handpiece by a friction chuck (sleeve) that grasps the entire shank. These burs are designated with the letters **FG** (for friction-grip).

Many friction-grip burs are available with shorter-than-normal shanks. These are useful in limited-access areas of the oral cavity. They are designed with the letters **SS** (for short shank).

SHAPES OF CARBIDE BURS

Burs used in restorative dentistry are made from carbide steel and work well when used with light pressure. A carbide bur may be reused up to five times before its cutting edges are dulled and it must be discarded. All burs *must* be sterilized before reuse.

Carbide burs are manufactured in six basic shapes, and each shape is available in a variety of sizes (Fig. 15–20). The size and shape of the head of burs are designated by a number.

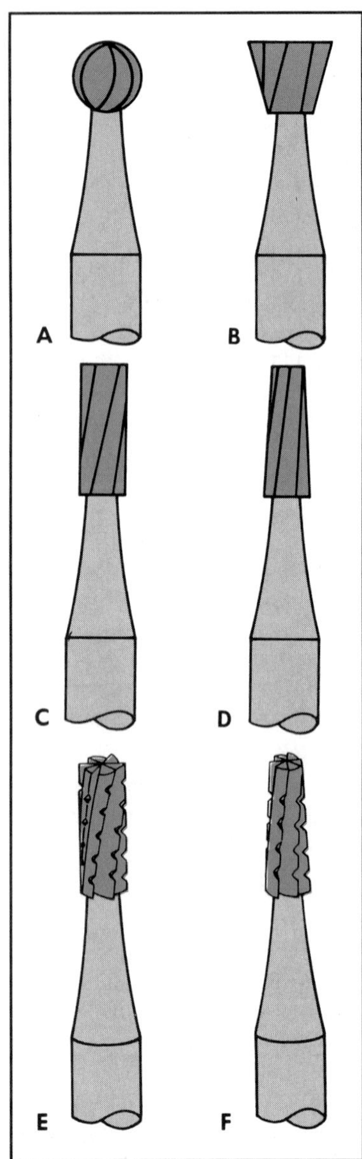

FIGURE 15–20

Basic bur shapes. *A*, Round. *B*, Inverted cone. *C*, Straight fissure, plain. *D*, Tapered fissure, plain. *E*, Straight fissure, cross-cut. *F*, Tapered fissure, cross-cut.

Round. Round burs are used to remove carious tooth structure during cavity preparation. Round burs are also used to open the pulp chamber of a tooth in preparation for endodontic treatment. The commonly used sizes of round burs range from numbers ¼ to 8.

Inverted Cone. This bur is used for removal of caries and to place retention grooves during cavity preparation (see Chapter 25). The commonly used sizes for inverted cones range from numbers 33½ to 37.

Fissure Burs. The term **fissure** means groove, and the burs in this group are characterized by long grooves in the working end. These burs are used to modify axial walls of cavity preparations, place axial retention grooves, and reach inaccessible areas of the preparation near the shoulder of the preparation.

Straight fissure burs have parallel sides, and the commonly used sizes range from numbers 56 to 58. The letter **L** or **S** following the number indicates an extra long or extra short shank length: for example, 58L (long) or 56S (short).

Tapered fissure burs have sides that taper and converge near the tip. (**Converge** means to come together.) The commonly used sizes range from numbers 169 to 171L (long).

Cross-cut straight fissure burs have straight sides and horizontal grooves. The cross-cuts provide additional cutting ability. The most commonly used sizes range from number 556 558L (long).

Cross-cut tapered fissure burs have tapering sides and horizontal grooves for additional cutting ability. The most commonly used sizes range from numbers 669 to 701L (long).

End-cutting burs are similar in design to the straight fissure bur except that the cutting portion is on the *end* of the bur only. Commonly used sizes for end cutting burs are numbers 957 and 958.

Trimming and finishing burs are described by shape and by the number of blades. The more blades on the head, the finer the finish (Fig. 15–21).

DIAMOND INSTRUMENTS

Diamond instruments, also called *diamond burs* or *diamond stones,* have bits of industrial diamonds impregnated into the working surfaces. Many dentists use these diamond rotary instruments as an important part of restorative dentistry because of their cutting ability. However, with multiple use and sterilization, debonding of the diamond particles occurs. This reduces the number of diamond particles on the bur and decreases the cutting efficiency.

Disposable diamonds, designed for a single use, are available prepackaged and sterile. This ensures that the diamond is always working at its maximum cutting rate. This shortens preparation time and increases pro-

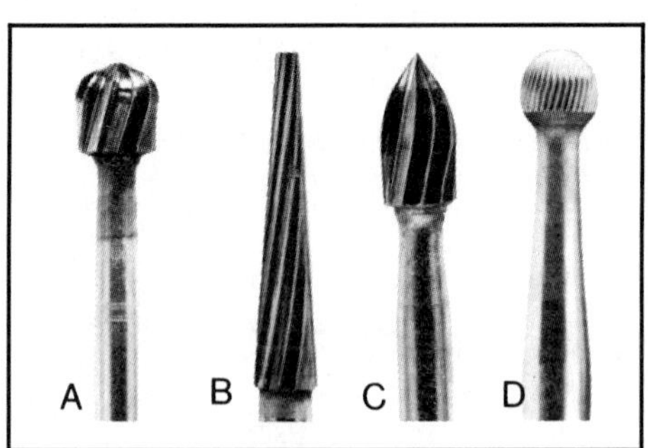

FIGURE 15–21

Assorted trimming and finishing burs. *A*, 12-bladed round. *B*, 12-bladed flame. *C*, 12-bladed flame. *D*, 30-bladed ball fine-finishing bur. (Courtesy of Midwest Dental Products Corp., Des Plaines, IL.)

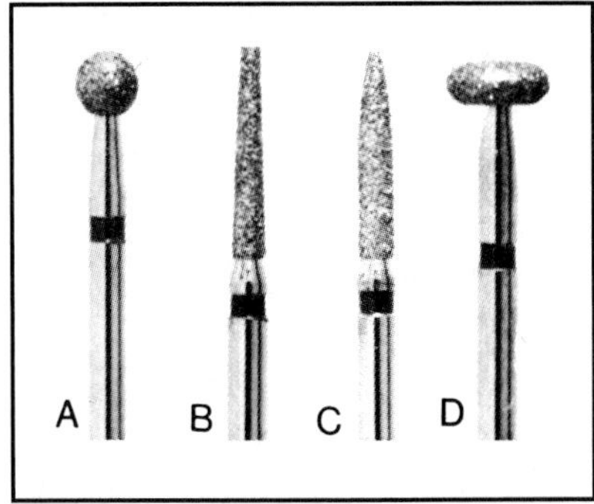

FIGURE 15–22

Sample shapes of diamond burs. *A*, Round. *B*, Flat end taper. *C*, Flame. *D*, Wheel. Notice the identifying band on the shank. (Courtesy of Midwest Dental Products Corp., Des Plaines, IL.)

ductivity. Because these diamonds are discarded after a single use, the time and cost involved in cleaning and sterilizing are eliminated.

Diamond Grit or Cutting Rate. Diamond burs are manufactured in a range of grit (coarseness) classifications to allow selection of the proper grit and cutting rate for each phase of restorative dentistry.

To identify the various grits, some manufacturers use a letter designation at the end of the bur number to indicate the grit or cutting rate; other manufacturers use a color-coded band on the bur. Common letter codes for the cutting classification of diamond burs are

- **P (pre-stressed)**: Fastest cutting rate, used for bulk removal and the rapid cutting of tooth structure
- **M (micro-grain)**: Medium fast cutting rate, used for controlled cutting and contouring
- **F (finisher)**: Fine-grained for removal of striations, used to refine and smooth marginal areas, remove all line angles, and finish subgingivally
- **XF (super-finisher)**: Finest-grained, used for contouring and finishing composite restorative materials

Indications for Using Diamond Burs. The shapes of diamond burs are very similar to those of the carbide steel burs, and burs of most shapes are available in each diamond bur classification (Fig. 15–22).

The indications for each shape are as follows:

Round end taper burs are used to prepare teeth for crowns and to make mechanical retention grooves in amalgam preparations.

Flat end taper burs are used for crown preparations when a square shoulder on the preparation is desired. They are also used to remove the incisal edge in crown preparations of anterior teeth.

Cylinder burs are used to smooth and finish walls in amalgam preparations or in any procedure in which parallel sides and flat floors are desired. They can also be used to extend small fissures for Class I amalgam restorations (see Chapter 25).

Flame-shaped burs are used to make subgingival finish lines (bevels) in crown preparations. (A **finish line** is the point at which the cavity preparation meets the external surface of the tooth.)

Ball, or **round,** burs are used to provide access to the pulp chamber for endodontic treatment or for the preparation of single surface restorations. They are also used to adjust and shape occlusal surfaces.

Wheel-shaped diamond burs are used reduce the lingual surface for anterior crown preparations and to make gross reductions of incisal edges. They can also be used to adjust and shape occlusal surfaces.

Equilibrating burs are available in several designs. Each design creates a concave shape in the tooth being prepared. They are used to reduce the lingual surface during anterior crown preparations. They can also be used to contour and adjust occlusal surfaces.

Composite trimming and finishing burs are available only in the XF (super finisher) designation. These burs are used for interproximal trimming and finishing of composite restorations.

Other Rotary Instruments

MANDRELS

Mandrels are used to attach various finishing (smoothing margins) and polishing devices to dental handpieces (Fig. 15–23). Some of the devices commonly attached to mandrels are polishing discs, points, and stones.

STONES

Stones are used when maximum abrasion is needed during a finishing and polishing procedure such as ad-

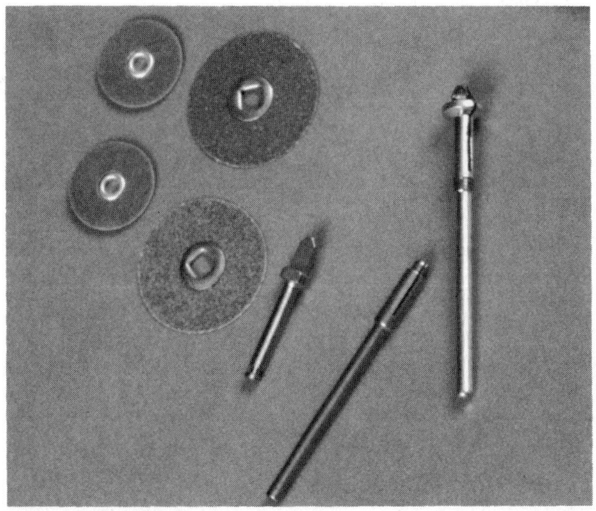

FIGURE 15–23

Assorted mandrels and sandpaper discs.

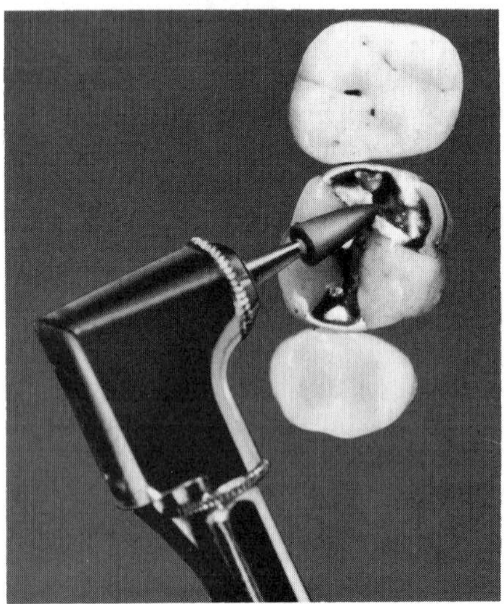

FIGURE 15–24

Mounted stone, in latch-type low-speed handpiece, used for polishing an amalgam restoration. (Courtesy of Shofu Dental Corp., Menlo Park, CA.)

justing the occlusion on an amalgam restoration or a gold crown (Fig. 15–24).

Red stones, gray stones, and black stones are used to finish and polish metallic restorations. White stones are used on tooth-colored restorations.

POLISHING DISCS

A polishing disc is rotary instrument made of various abrasive materials, commonly with a metal or paper backing. A mandrel is used to hold it securely in the handpiece (see Fig. 15–23).

Polishing discs are available in four basic grits: coarse, medium, fine, and super-fine. The coarser discs are used to remove excess filling material from the margins of a restoration. The finer discs are used to smooth and polish the restoration.

RUBBER POINTS

Rubber points impregnated with a polishing agent are used to polish metallic restorations. The tip of the point is handy for polishing the grooves in the anatomy of the restoration.

Dental Handpieces

Dental handpieces are the most frequently used instruments in dentistry. They have applications in every specialty. This chapter discusses uses in restorative dentistry (Fig. 15–25). Use of the handpiece in specialties is discussed in each specialty chapter.

Handpieces Used in Restorative Dentistry

Two types of air-driven handpieces are used in restorative dentistry:

- **Low-speed handpieces,** which operate at speeds up to 25,000 rpm
- **High-speed handpieces,** which operate at speeds up to 450,000 rpm (some of these handpieces are equipped with a fiber optic light system)

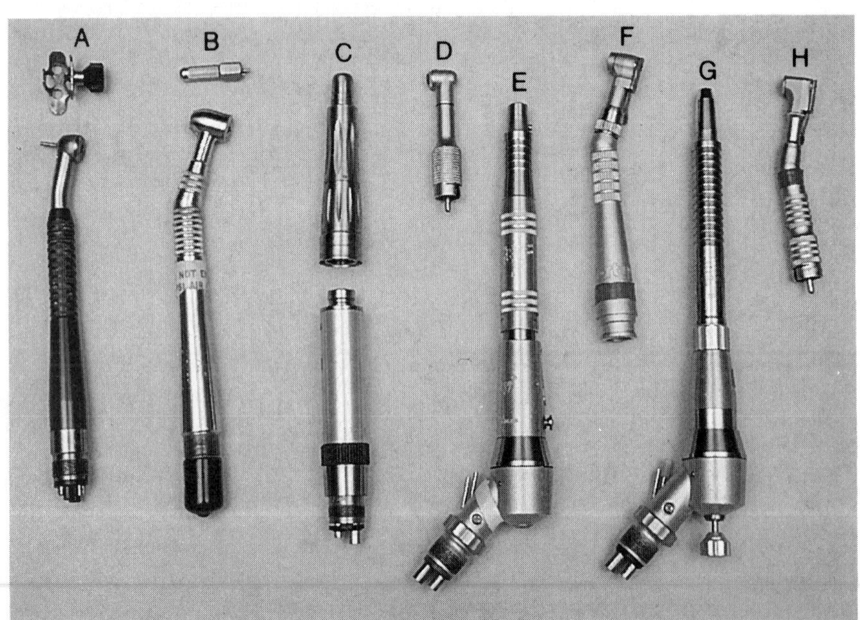

FIGURE 15–25

Assorted dental handpieces. *A*, High-speed handpiece with bur changer above. *B*, High-speed handpiece with bur changer above. *C*, Straight handpiece attachment with motor base below. *D*, Prophy angle attachment. *E*, Straight handpiece. *F*, Latch-type contra-angle attachment. *G*, Straight handpiece. *H*, Latch-type contra-angle attachment.

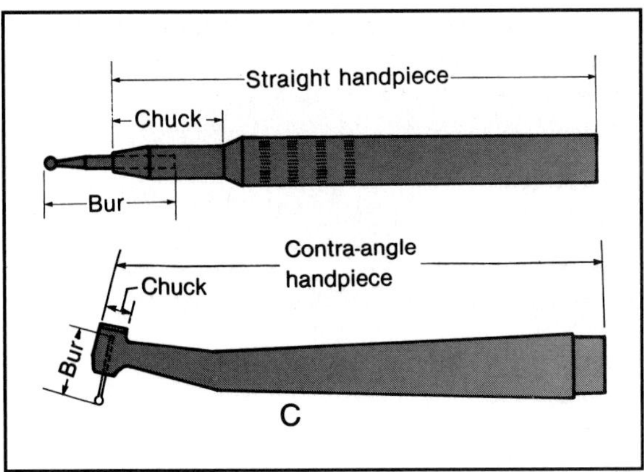

FIGURE 15–26

Straight and contra-angle handpieces.

LOW-SPEED HANDPIECES

The low-speed handpiece is often referred to as the *straight handpiece* because of its straight-line design (Fig. 15–26). This handpiece is used in finishing, polishing, and contouring procedures. On occasion, the low-speed handpiece is used for caries removal and fine finishing of the cavity preparation.

The straight-line design of this handpiece is ideal for use on the maxillary anterior teeth and for procedures done outside the mouth, such as denture adjustments and preparation of temporary crowns. To gain access to the maxillary posterior teeth and all mandibular teeth, a variety of angled attachments (sleeves) must be used.

Two of the most common attachments for the low-speed handpiece are the contra-angle and the prophylaxis angle.

Contra-Angles. Contra-angles are available in both **latch-type** and **friction-grip** varieties. The difference between the types is the method in which the burs are held in the contra-angle handpiece.

The latch-type bur is held in place mechanically by grasping a small notch on the end of the shaft of the bur. The friction-grip angle holds the bur in place by grasping the entire shaft of the bur with a friction chuck in the head of the contra-angle.

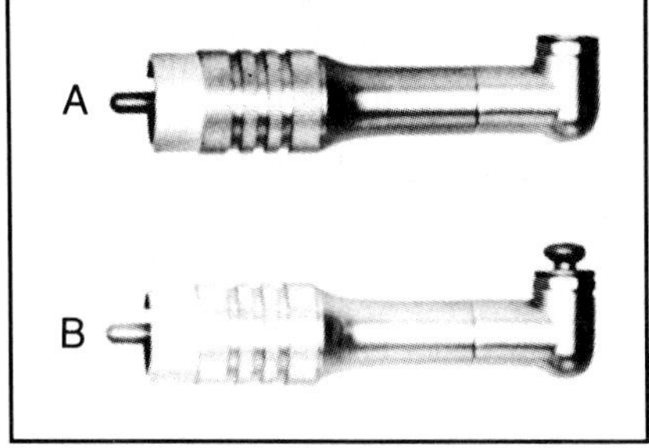

FIGURE 15–27

Two styles of prophy angles. *A*, Screw-type attachment for cup or brush. *B*, Snap-on attachment for cup or brush. (Courtesy of Unitek Corp., Monrovia, CA.)

Prophylaxis Angles. Prophylaxis angles, commonly referred to as *prophy angles,* are used to hold polishing cups and brushes (Fig. 15–27). There are two types of prophy angles available.

The **screw type** holds the cup or brush in place by a threaded shaft. The **snap-on** type holds the polishing device in place by snapping over a smooth button.

Plastic **disposable prophy angles** are discarded after a single use. They are available with either rubber cup attachments or bristle brushes already in place. If the operator wishes to use both a cup and a brush, two angles must be used.

HIGH-SPEED HANDPIECES

The high-speed handpiece operates on air pressure and reaches speeds of 450,000 rpm (see Figs. 15–25*A* and 15–25*B*). During operative procedures, the bulk of tooth structure is removed by using the high-speed handpiece. Refinement of the preparation and removal of caries is accomplished with both the low-speed handpiece and hand-cutting instruments.

The extremely high speed of the bur or stone against tooth structure generates enough frictional heat to cause pulpal damage. To protect against this, high-speed handpieces are equipped with water-spray devices. The tooth and bur are constantly sprayed with cool water during use. The water spray also helps remove debris from the cavity preparation.

FIBER OPTIC LIGHT HANDPIECES

High-speed handpieces are available with fiber optic lights that are mounted in the head of the handpiece. Light ports near the bur deliver the proper amount of light directly onto the operating site (Fig. 15–28).

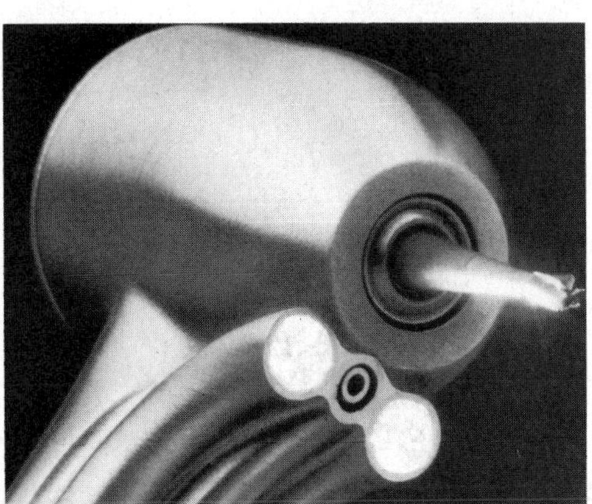

FIGURE 15–28

High-speed handpiece fiber optic lights. (Courtesy of Midwest Dental Products Corp, Des Plaines, IL.)

The tungsten halogen lamp produces a bright, pure white light that is virtually identical to that produced by the overhead lights in the treatment room. This significantly reduces operator eyestrain and improves visibility.

CHANGING BURS

There are a variety of designs of high-speed handpieces on the market, and the method of inserting and removing burs from the handpiece varies according to the manufacturer's design.

Some handpieces require the use of a bur-changing tool (see Figs. 15–25*A* and 15–25*B*). Others have a release built into the head of the handpiece, and a bur-changing tool is not required. Regardless of the manufacturer, all high-speed handpieces use friction-grip burs, diamond stones, and polishing devices.

BUR CARE

Some burs are discarded after a single use. Those burs that are not discarded *must* be sterilized before reuse.

To minimize handling used burs, they should be placed in a bur block before cleaning (Fig. 15–29). This also prevents damage to the blades from rubbing or vibrating against each other or any hard surface during cleaning.

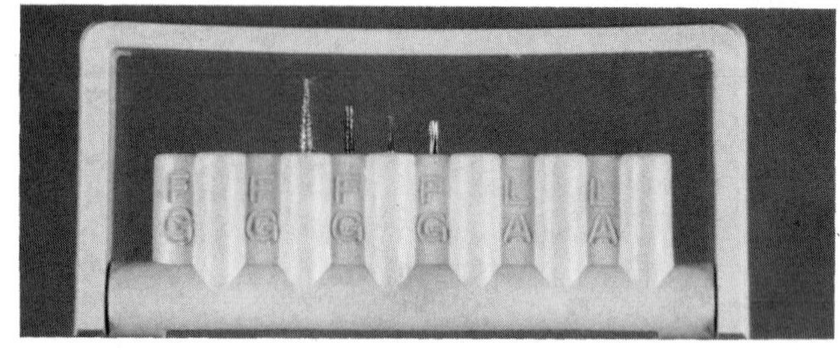

FIGURE 15–29

A bur block holds and protects the burs during processing and sterilization.

These burs may be presoaked *briefly* to prevent debris from drying on them. Burs are cleaned in the ultrasonic cleaner and then packaged with the other instruments before sterilization by autoclaving.

LASER HANDPIECES

The laser light beam is conducted through a fiber optic cable that extends from the console (where the laser energy is generated) to the laser handpiece. The use of laser technology and therapy is discussed in Chapter 26.

The laser handpiece has a removable cannula at the working end. (A **cannula** is a hollow tube.) This is to

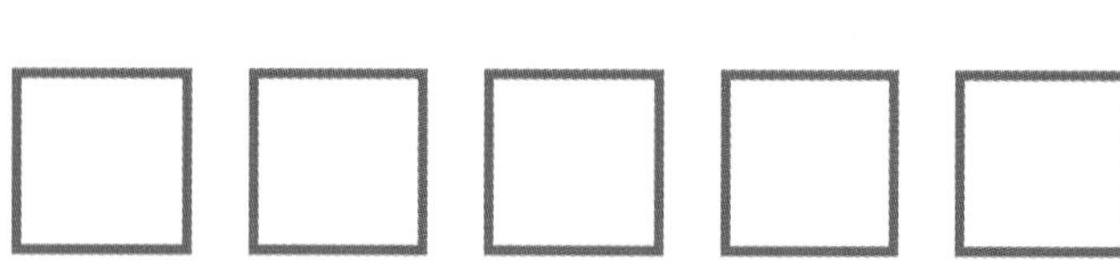

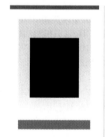

PROCEDURE: Cleaning and Sterilization of Laser Handpieces

1. Turn off the laser controls.
2. Disconnect the fiber from the laser console, and take the fiber to the sterilization center.
3. Wash hands and put on appropriate personal protective equipment (PPE) (utility gloves and protective eyewear).
4. Remove organic debris from the handpiece, cannula, and fiber tip with warm, soapy water. Rinse well with tap water.
5. Place these items loosely in a 7 × 12 inch autoclave bag.

   □ *RATIONALE:* The assembly must not be coiled more tightly than a 5-inch diameter loop. Coiling it more tightly will damage the fiber assembly.
6. Steam autoclave at the following settings: temperature, 121° C; pressure, 15 psi; time, 30 minutes.

   □ *NOTICE:* This is longer than the usual autoclave cycle. Autoclaving is discussed in Chapter 13.
7. Allow the fiber assembly to cool 30 minutes before handling.

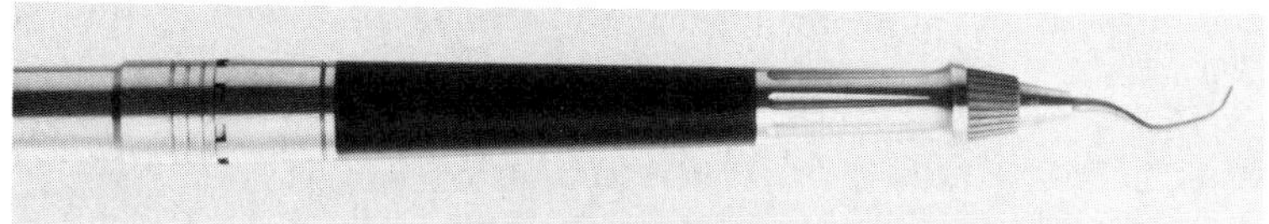

FIGURE 15–30

Sonic scaler (Titan-S-Sonic) with mounted tip. (Courtesy of Syntex Dental Products, Inc., Valley Forge, PA.)

ensure that the fiber tip can be accurately positioned at the intended surgical site. A foot switch is used to operate the laser handpiece.

Care and Handling of Laser Handpieces. Follow these precautions to avoid damage to the fiber optic cables and laser handpiece:

- Do not sharply bend or twist the optical fiber cable, or else it may break and burn during use. (This could result in injury to the user or to the patient.)
- Do not touch the exposed optical fiber cable. (Dirt and fingerprints will damage the fiber optic.)
- Do not touch the end of the fiber optic cable connector. (It contains a small optical fiber that may degrade if contaminated.)
- Do keep the connecting parts clean. (Dirt is damaging to them.)

Laboratory Handpieces

These handpieces are designed to be used in the dental laboratory, not in the mouth. The laboratory handpiece operates at speeds up to 20,000 rpm and uses laboratory burs of various shapes and sizes.

The laboratory handpiece provides greater torque than intraoral handpieces. (**Torque** is the turning power of the instrument when pressure is applied during the cutting procedure). The increased torque is better suited to the heavier pressure required during laboratory grinding and polishing procedures.

Ultrasonic and Sonic Handpieces

Ultrasonic and sonic handpieces are adjuncts to, but not substitutes for, manual scaling and instrumentation. They use vibrations, similar to sound waves, set at various power levels to create energy at the tip of the instrument. (**Sonic** means referring to sound.)

Ultrasonic handpieces work by converting high-frequency electrical current into mechanical vibrations. Vibrations at the tip of the ultrasonic scaler range from 29,000 to 40,000 cycles per second. Water is needed to cool the friction between the tip and the tooth surface. (The ultrasonic handpiece is a separate piece of equipment and is *not* connected to the dental unit.)

Use of the ultrasonic scaler may interfere with the function of a patient's cardiac pacemaker or other electronic life-support device. A consultation with the patient's cardiologist is indicated before an ultrasonic scaler is used.

Sonic handpieces use air pressure to create mechanical vibrations and are attached to the unit in the same manner as conventional air-driven handpieces. (Fig. 15–30).

The vibrations at the tip of the sonic handpiece range from 2,000 to 6,000 cycles per second. Heat is not generated from the sonic handpiece, but water is indicated for debridement. (**Debridement** means the removal of debris.)

Because sonic scalers use air pressure rather than electrical power, they are safe for use on patients with

Indications for Use of Ultrasonic and Sonic Handpieces

- Gross removal of heavy deposits of calculus
- Removal of heavy stain from the tooth surfaces
- Removal of excess cement after cementation of orthodontic bands
- Debridement and enlargement of root canals
- Initial debridement for a patient with necrotizing ulcerative gingivitis

Contraindications to Use of Ultrasonic and Sonic Handpieces

- Patients with a known communicable disease that can be transmitted by aerosols
- Patients with a history of chronic pulmonary disease, including asthma, emphysema, or cystic fibrosis
- Patients with a swallowing or severe gagging problem
- Patients with sensitive areas (sonic and ultrasonic instrumentation can aggravate existing sensitivity)

cardiac pacemakers or other electronic life-support devices.

SPECIAL EXPOSURE CONTROL CONCERNS

The fluid spray that is generated by ultrasonic and sonic handpieces creates an aerosol of water and microorganisms that come into contact with the operator and assistant and settle onto operatory surfaces. It is recommended that the following precautions be taken:

- Operator and assistant should wear a plastic face shield in addition to a mask and eyewear.
- The patient should also be provided protective eyewear and a plastic drape.
- The dental unit should be covered with plastic if possible, and the entire area should be disinfected thoroughly after each use.
- The high-volume oral evacuator (HVE) should be placed immediately adjacent to the instrument tip.
- The patient should rinse with chlorhexidine. This will significantly reduce the bacterial count in the patient's saliva.

Handpiece Maintenance

Problems with dental handpieces most often result from improper cleaning and lubrication. Inadequate cleaning of the handpiece before sterilization can result in collection of debris in the internal parts of the handpiece.

This creates wear similar to sludge within an automobile engine. Excessive lubrication is as damaging as inadequate lubrication. Handpieces are also available with ceramic bearings or heads that require no lubrication at all.

If inappropriate cleaning solutions or techniques are used, the working life of the handpiece is significantly shortened. It is imperative to follow the *manufacturer's directions* for the maintenance of each handpiece. Failure to do so can result in voiding of the handpiece warranty.

Some types of handpieces require lubrication *before* sterilization, some require lubrication *after* sterilization, and others require lubrication both *before and after* sterilization. You must carefully follow the manufacturer's instructions for the handpiece being sterilized.

Handpiece Sterilization

The dental handpiece is a critical instrument (one that comes in contact with blood, saliva, and tissue) that *must* be sterilized before reuse.

Dental handpieces require special considerations for sterilization because blood and saliva may be sucked back into the internal portions of the handpiece. The special valves to prevent this are discussed in Chapter 14.

Before the high-speed handpiece is removed from the dental unit, it should be run into the HVE for a minimum of 20–30 seconds to discharge water and air. This aids in physically flushing out bioburden that may have entered the turbine and air or water lines. Take care not to spread spray, spatter, and aerosols during this process.

GENERAL CONSIDERATIONS FOR HANDPIECE STERILIZATION

Important variations exist between manufacturers' instructions regarding specific details for handpiece sterilization.

The following are general considerations for sterilizing dental handpieces:

1. Wear personal protective equipment (PPE) and follow the Universal Precautions (see Chapter 13).
   ☐ **Rationale**: The used handpiece is contaminated and must be handled with appropriate care.
2. Use mild soap and water, or water alone, to clean debris from the external surfaces of the handpiece.
   ☐ **Rationale**: Disinfectants are neither necessary nor cost effective because the handpiece will be sterilized. Also, disinfectants could cause potential damage to the handpiece.
3. Clean the internal components of the handpiece according to the manufacturer's instructions.

Handpiece	Model	Precleaning	Lubrication	Packaging	Sterilizer
Star	430K	Ultrasonic	3 drops Titan Oil before and after sterilization	No	Steam or dry heat
Midwest		Lifecycle	After sterilization	Yes	Autoclave Chemclave

FIGURE 15–31

Sample handpiece sterilization procedure sheet. Information is listed for each type of handpiece used in the practice.

□ **Rationale:** Some manufacturers recommend ultrasonic cleaning; others do not.

4. Handpieces must be dry before being packaged.
   □ **Rationale**: This is important to avoid corrosion when an autoclave is used.
5. Wrap the handpiece for sterilization according to the type of sterilization and according to the manufacturer's care instructions.
6. Sterilize the handpiece according to the manufacturer's instructions.
   □ **Rationale:** Most manufacturers recommend autoclaving or chemical vapor sterilization.
7. After sterilization, wipe the light port on fiber optic handpieces with an alcohol swab to remove any excess lubricant.
   □ **Rationale**: The light will be dimmed if any lubricant remains.
8. Before attaching the sterile handpiece, flush the air and water lines on the handpiece hose for 30 to 60 seconds.
   □ **Rationale**: This reduces any bioburden that may be sprayed into the patient's oral cavity.

STERILIZATION PROCEDURE SHEETS

It is not uncommon for one dental office to have handpieces made by several different manufacturers. This occurs over time as handpieces are replaced or when new models become available. Sterilization instructions vary not only between manufacturers but also between different models made by the *same* manufacturer.

The use of a "Sterilization Procedure Sheet," such as the one shown in Figure 15–31, is one way to avoid errors in handpiece sterilization. This is particularly helpful if several team members are involved in the process.

"Sterilization Procedure Sheets" can be created for the practice by using the information found in each manufacturer's instruction book.

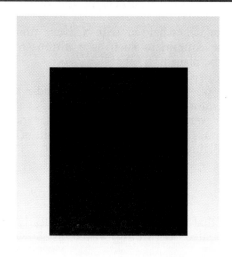

Chapter 16

Oral Evacuation and Instrument Transfer

Introduction

The smooth and efficient team interaction between the dentist and chairside assistant (a) increases patient comfort and aids in providing quality care; (b) reduces the chair time needed for most treatment; and (c) minimizes the stress and fatigue caused by performing complicated dental procedures (Fig. 16–1).

During this treatment, the assistant is responsible for performing the following tasks skillfully and efficiently:

- Use of the high-volume oral evacuator (HVE) to remove saliva, blood, water, and debris from the mouth of the patient in the supine position
- Maintenance of a clear operating field through retraction and by keeping the mouth mirror clear for the operator
- Smooth transfer of instruments and materials as necessary

The Clock Concept of Operating Zones

As shown in Chapter 14, dental offices vary considerably in design, type, and location of equipment. However, the basic concepts required for practicing efficient and comfortable four-handed and six-handed dentistry can be applied to any dental environment.

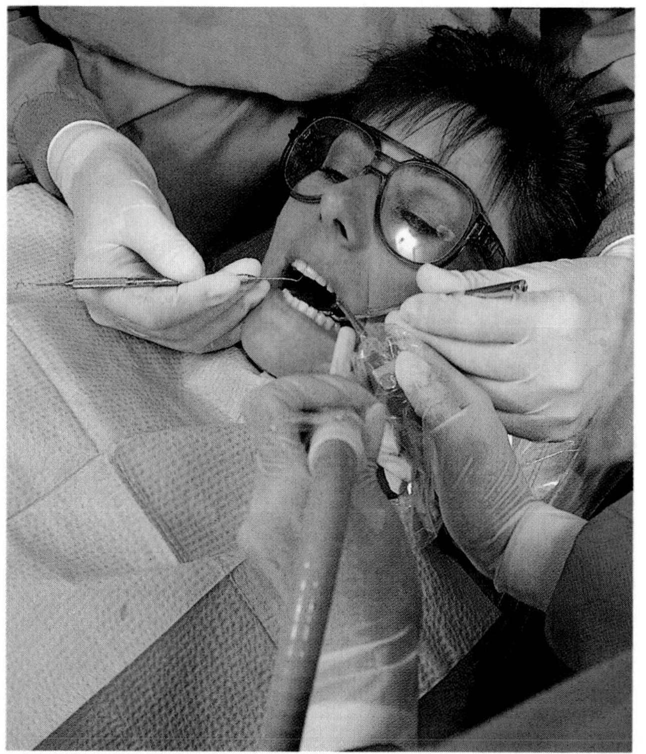

FIGURE 16–1

An efficient team provides quality care with a minimum of stress.

The use of operating zones, based on the "clock concept," is the best way to identify the working positions of the equipment and dental team.

Visualize a circle placed over the dental chair with the patient's face in the center of the circle and the top of the patient's head at the 12 o'clock position. The face of the clock is divided into four zones:

- The **operator's zone** is the area where the dentist is seated. (The dentist moves about in this zone according to the area of the mouth being treated.)
- The **transfer zone** is the area where instruments and dental materials are exchanged. (In front delivery, the dental unit is located in this area so that it is within easy reach of the dentist and/or assistant.)
- The **assistant's zone** allows room for the mobile work surface. (The dental assistant remains seated in the same position regardless of the operator's position.)
- The **static zone** is where a rear delivery unit or other portable equipment such as a nitrous oxide machine can be placed.

The location of the zones varies, depending on whether the operator is right- or left-handed. The operator's position varies within that zone, depending upon the treatment to be delivered. These positions are summarized in Figures 16–2 and 16–3.

Direct and Indirect Vision

It is essential that the dentist be able to clearly see the area being treated. With **direct vision**, as shown in

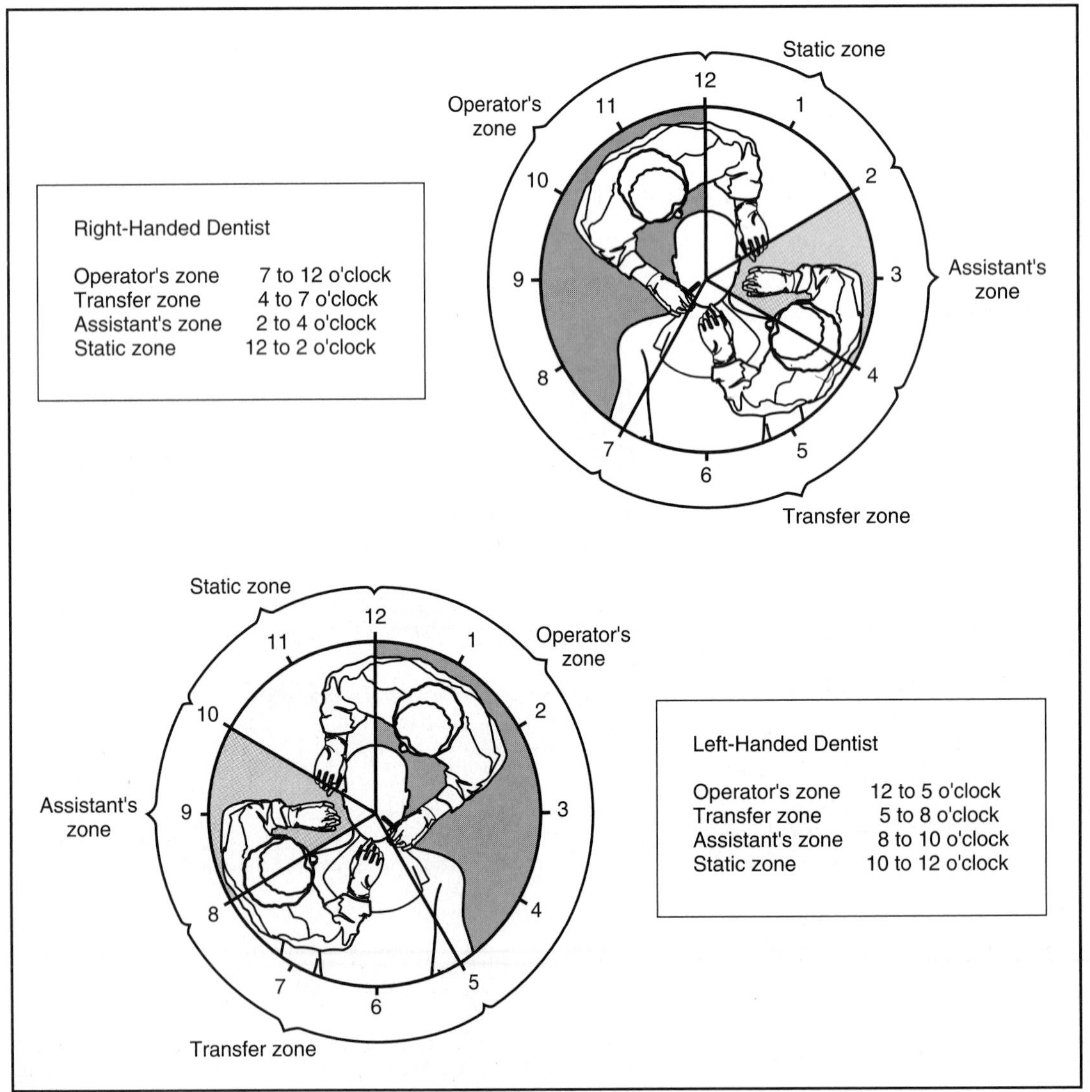

FIGURE 16–2

The clock concept. *Left,* Zones for a right-handed operator. *Right,* Zones for a left-handed operator.

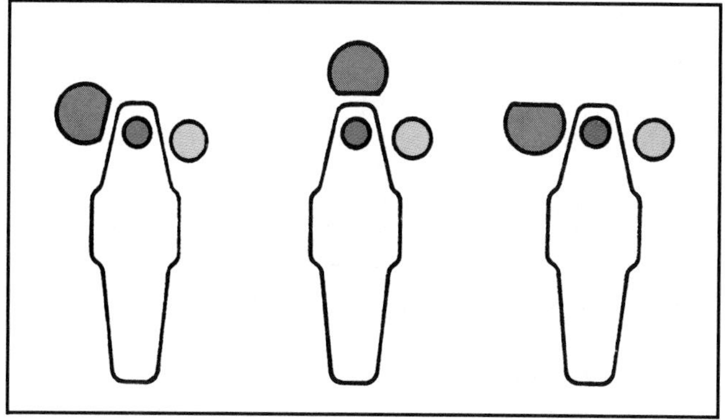

FIGURE 16–3

Diagram illustrating positioning of the dental team and patient when working with a right-handed dentist. The operator's stool is in gray, the assistant's stool is in pink, and the red circle represents the patient's head. Notice that the assistant's position remains the same even as the operator's changes.

Figure 16–1, the dentist is able to look directly at the area being treated.

When working in some areas of the mouth, the dentist must depend upon indirect vision. When using **indirect vision**, the dentist is often seated at the 12 o'clock position and views the treatment area in a mirror (Fig. 16–4).

Retraction and Maintaining a Clear Mirror

As necessary, the assistant retracts the patient's lips or controls the patient's tongue to ensure that the operator can readily see and reach the area being treated.

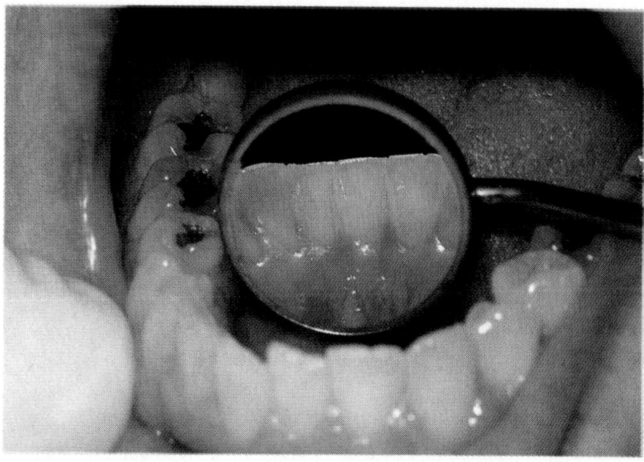

FIGURE 16–4

With indirect vision, the dentist views the area being treated in a mirror. It is essential that the surface of the mirror be kept clean and dry.

Retraction, which means to draw back, is accomplished during most operative procedures by the assistant, using his or her fingers or a mouth mirror. When retracting, it is essential that the assistant position her fingers or instrument so that they do not block the operator's vision or access to the area.

Having a clear mirror is particularly important when the operator is working with indirect vision. To remove debris and prevent fogging of the mirror, the assistant may use the air-water syringe to blow a gentle stream of air across the face of the mouth mirror. As necessary, water may also be used to remove debris.

High-Volume Oral Evacuation

The high-volume oral evacuator (HVE) is used to remove saliva, blood, water, and debris from the mouth of the patient in the supine position.

The HVE system, which is also known as the *oral evacuator*, works on a vacuum principle similar to that of a household vacuum cleaner. It is capable of picking up water and debris when the tip is placed near, but not actually touching, the water or debris. This is possible because high volumes of air are moved into the vacuum hose at a low pressure to create suction.

The HVE tip is used to

- Keep the back of the mouth free from saliva, blood, water, and debris
- Retract the tongue and cheek away from the field of operation
- Reduce the bacterial aerosol caused by the high-speed handpiece

Oral Evacuation Caution

Improper or careless use of the HVE can cause the soft tissues to be accidentally "sucked" into the tip and tissue trauma could result. Keeping the tip at an angle to the soft tissue helps prevent this from happening.

If the soft tissues are accidentally get "sucked" into the tip, rotate the angle of the tip to break the suction or quickly turn the vacuum control off to release the tissue.

Oral Evacuation Tips

A variety of HVE tips made of stainless steel or plastic are available. Stainless steel tips are sterilized before reuse. Depending upon the type of plastic, these tips are sterilized before reuse or are discarded after a single use (Fig. 16–5).

There are advantages and disadvantages to each. For example, some patients complain about the coldness of

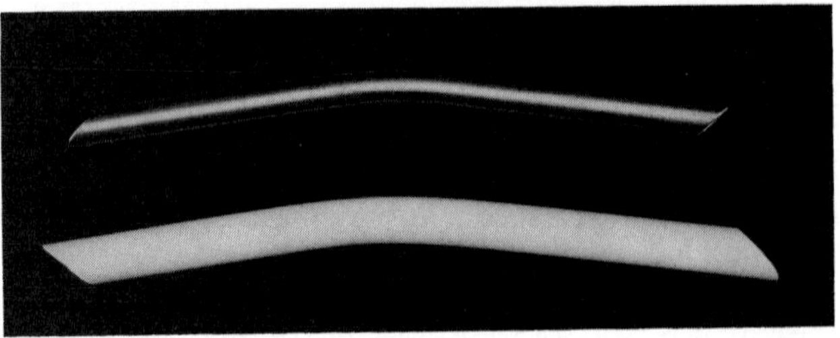

FIGURE 16–5

Two types of HVE tips. A metal tip is shown at the top, and a plastic tip is shown below. Notice the slight angle in the middle of the tips to increase access to all areas of the mouth. The anterior end has a downward slant. The posterior end mouth has an upward slant.

the metal tip. This is caused by air constantly running through the tip. Plastic tips do not get cold, but some are not stiff enough to be used as a retractor for the soft tissues.

The most commonly used HVE tip is slightly angled in the middle and has two beveled working ends. (**Beveled** means slanted.) The bevel for use in the **anterior** portion of the mouth is slanted downward. The bevel for use in the **posterior** portion of the mouth is slanted upward.

When the tip is placed into the handle, the end of the tip *not* being used during the procedure is pushed into place through the plastic protective barrier covering the HVE handle.

Holding the Oral Evacuator

The oral evacuator may be held in either the thumb-to-nose grasp or the modified pen grasp (Fig. 16–6). Either method provides the dental assistant with control of the tip, which is necessary for patient comfort and safety. Many assistants alternate between positions, depending on the resistance of the tissue to retraction and the area being treated.

When assisting a right-handed dentist, the assistant holds the evacuator in the right hand. When assisting a left-handed dentist, the assistant holds the evacuator in the left hand.

The hand not holding the HVE is free to operate the air-water syringe or transfer instruments to the dentist as needed. (HVE positioning and the instrument transfers described in this chapter are for working with a right-handed dentist.)

Positioning the HVE Tip

Usually the most efficient technique is for the assistant to position the HVE tip in the mouth first, and then the dentist can position the handpiece and mouth mirror.

When teeth on the dentist's side of the mouth are being treated, the HVE tip is placed on the lingual aspect of the tooth being prepared. When teeth on the assistant's side of the mouth are being treated, the HVE tip is placed on the buccal aspect of the tooth. (**Aspect**, as used here, means surface.)

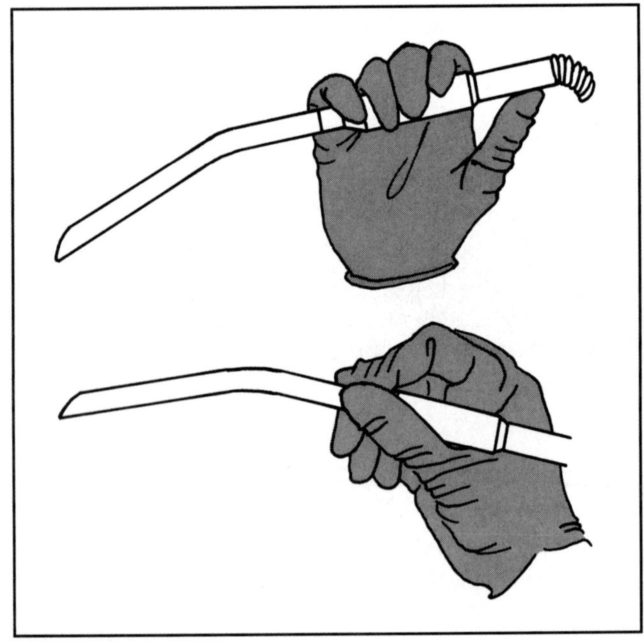

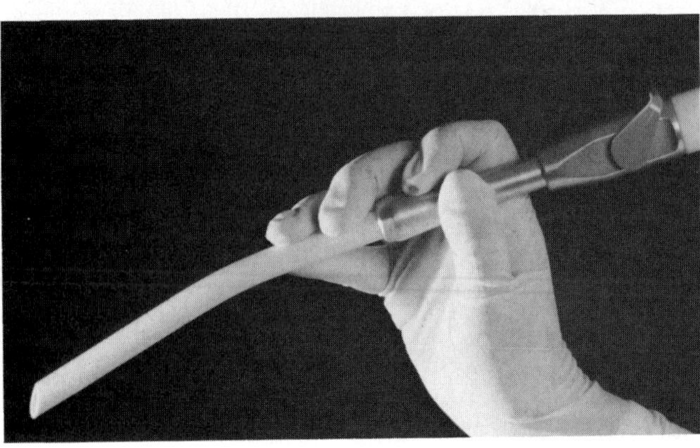

FIGURE 16–6

Methods of holding the oral evacuator tip and hose. *Top left,* The thumb-to-nose method. When this method is used, tubing is tucked under the arm close to the body. *Lower left,* The more commonly used modified pen grasp. *Right,* A photograph of this grasp in use.

 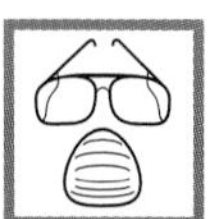 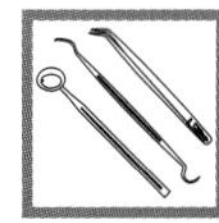 

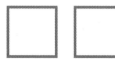

PROCEDURE: **Positioning the HVE Tip**

Posterior HVE Placement

1. Place the HVE tip in the holder by pushing the anterior end of the tip into the holder through the plastic barrier.
   □ *RATIONALE:* This leaves the posterior end exposed and ready for use.
2. When a mandibular tooth is being treated, place a cotton roll under the tip.
   □ *RATIONALE:* This increases patient comfort, aids in stabilizing tip placement, and prevents injury to the tissues.
3. Place the tip as close as possible, and slightly distal to, the tooth being prepared (Figs. 16–7 and 16–8).
   □ *RATIONALE:* This will draw the water into the tip immediately after it leaves the tooth being prepared.
4. Position the bevel on the evacuator tip parallel to the buccal or lingual surface of the tooth being prepared.
5. Place the upper edge of the tip to extend slightly beyond the occlusal surfaces.
   □ *RATIONALE:* This will catch the water spray from the handpiece as it leaves the tooth being prepared.

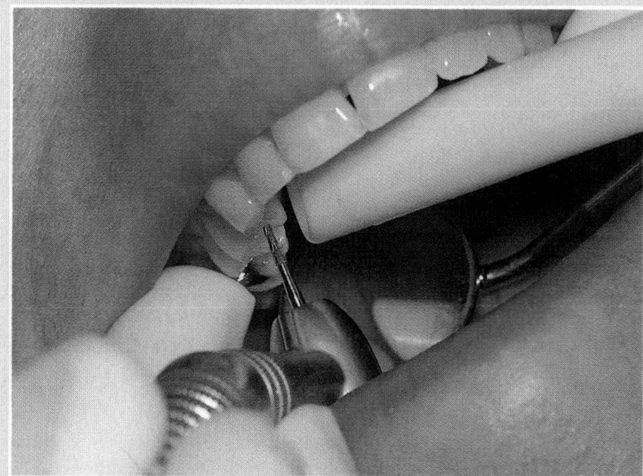

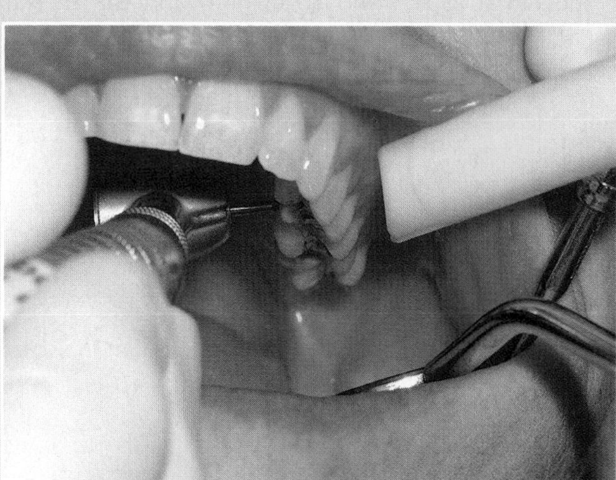

FIGURE 16–7

Posterior maxillary HVE tip placement. Notice that the tip is parallel and slightly distal to the tooth being treated. It does not block the dentist's vision or access. *Left,* Lingual placement of the HVE tip. *Right,* Buccal placement of the HVE tip.

(continued on following page)

PROCEDURE: **Positioning the HVE Tip** *(continued)*

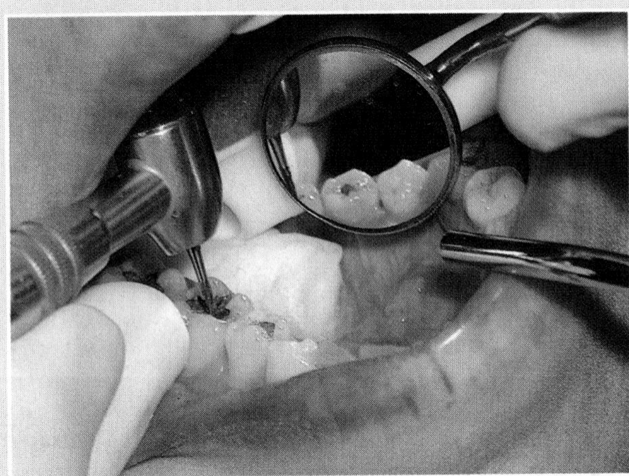

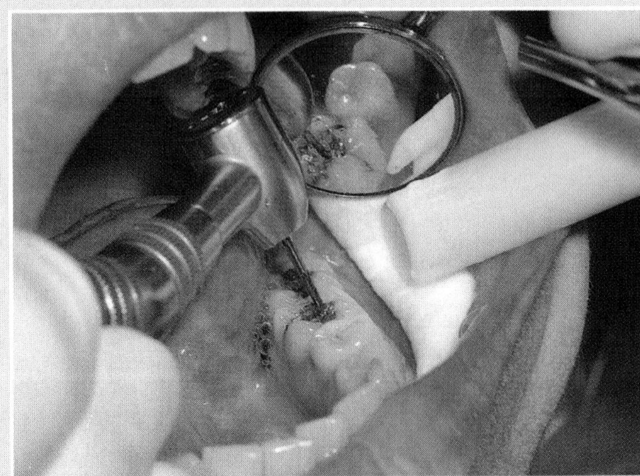

FIGURE 16–8

Posterior mandibular HVE tip placement. Notice the cotton rolls placed under the end of the HVE tip. The assistant is using air (from the air-water syringe) to clear the mirror, which the dentist is holding. *Left,* Lingual placement of the HVE tip. *Right,* Buccal placement of the HVE tip.

Anterior HVE Placement

1. Place the HVE tip in the holder by pushing the "posterior end" of the tip into the holder through the plastic barrier.
   □ *RATIONALE:* This leaves the anterior end exposed and ready for use.
2. When the dentist is preparing a tooth from the lingual aspect, place the beveled tip parallel to the labial aspect and slightly beyond the incisal edge (Fig. 16–9).

   Because the lingual surfaces of the mandibular teeth are difficult to access, it is sometimes necessary for the assistant to retract the tongue and evacuate intermittently as fluid accumulates.
3. When the dentist is preparing the tooth from the facial aspect, hold the beveled tip parallel with the lingual surface and slightly beyond the incisal edge (Fig. 16–10).

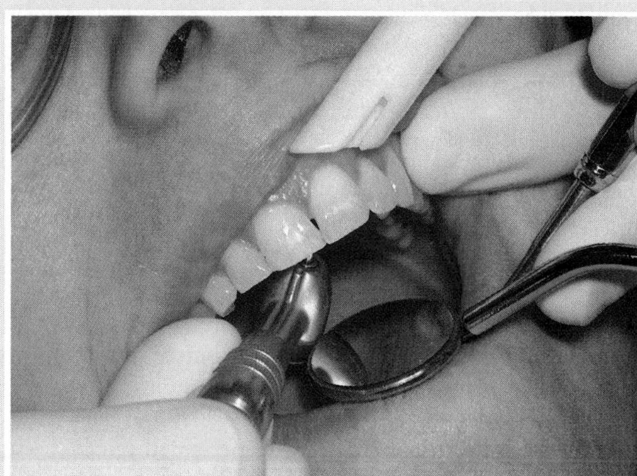

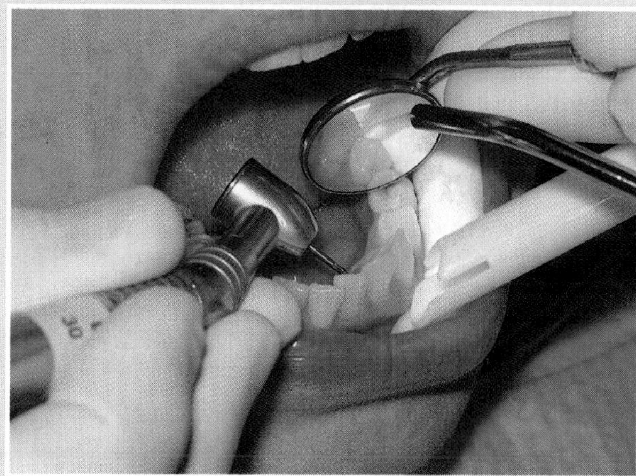

FIGURE 16–9

Anterior HVE placement for a lingual approach. The dentist is using the mirror for indirect vision, and the assistant is using air (from the air-water syringe) to clear the mirror that the dentist is holding. *Left,* Facial placement of the HVE tip for a maxillary preparation. *Right,* Facial placement of the HVE tip for a mandibular preparation.

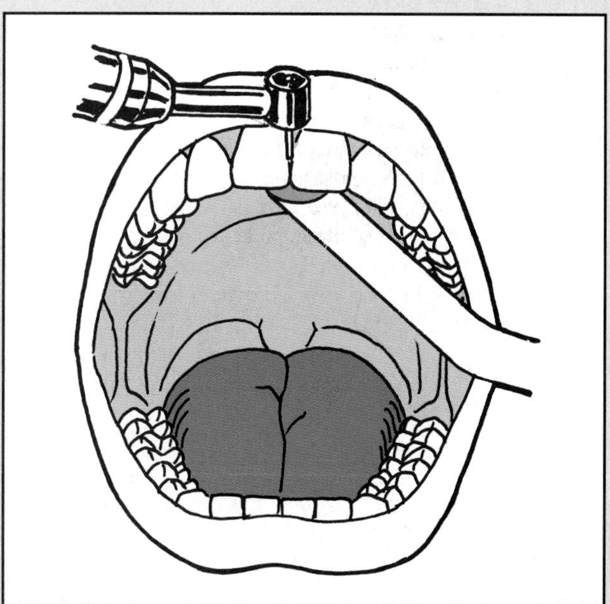

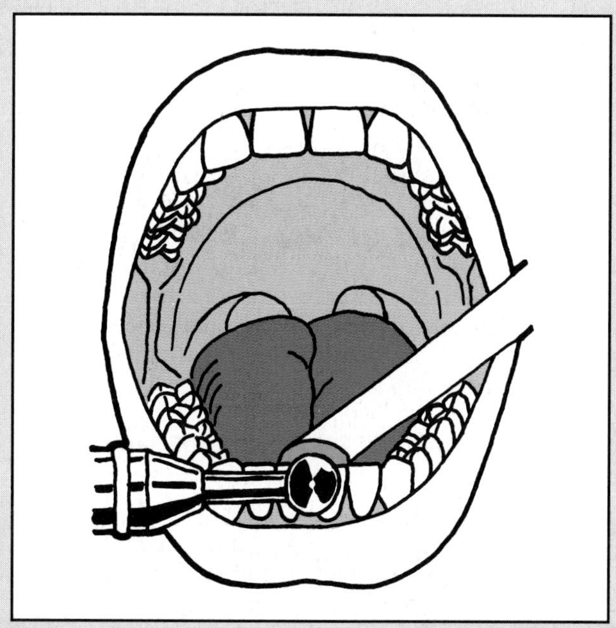

FIGURE 16–10

Anterior HVE placement for a facial approach. Care must be taken to keep the HVE tip out of the dentist's line of vision. *Left,* Lingual placement of the HVE tip for a maxillary preparation. *Right,* Lingual placement of the HVE tip for a mandibular preparation.

Rinsing the Oral Cavity

Frequent rinsing of the oral cavity maintains a clear operating field for the dentist and keeps the patient comfortable. It is also used to remove any debris from the patient's mouth before dismissal.

The two basic types of rinsing procedures used in dentistry are limited-area rinsing and complete mouth rinsing.

Limited-area rinsing is performed frequently as debris accumulates during tooth preparation. This must be accomplished quickly and efficiently without causing any delay in the procedure. Most commonly this is done when the dentist pauses for cavity inspection.

The **complete mouth rinse** is used when it is desirable to freshen the patient's entire mouth. This may be during long restorative procedures, dental prophylaxis, and periodontal treatment. Also, before the patient is dismissed after any dental procedure, a complete mouth rinse is *always* used to leave the patient with a comfortable and fresh feeling.

The saliva ejector can be used as an alternative to the HVE in the complete mouth rinse procedure when the assistant performs this alone.

Instrument Transfer

The smooth, efficient transfer of instruments and materials is a team effort that requires coordination, communication, and practice between the dentist and the dental assistant.

Both the patient and the dental team benefit from a standardized operating sequence. The patient enjoys a

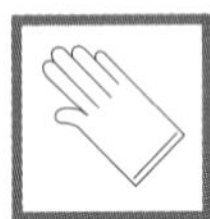
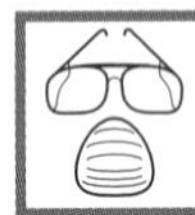
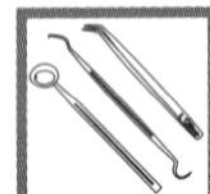

PROCEDURE: **Rinsing the Patient's Mouth**

Limited-Area Rinsing

1. The assistant operates the air-water syringe with the left hand and the oral evacuator with the right hand. Water is sprayed on the area and is removed with the HVE tip.
2. The dentist retracts the cheek or lips as necessary to give the assistant access to the area.
3. If drying is indicated, the assistant uses the air-water syringe to gently blow puffs of air on the tooth and tissues.

Complete Mouth Rinsing, Using the Team Approach

1. The dentist operates the air-water syringe with the right hand and retracts the lips and cheeks with the mouth mirror held in the left hand.
   □ *RATIONALE:* The vigorous spraying of water and air will dislodge debris.
2. The assistant operates the HVE with the right hand and retracts the patient's cheeks and lips with the left hand.
3. The dentist rinses the mouth by quadrants, starting at the maxillary midline. Each side should be finished before the dentist proceeds to the opposite side.
   □ *RATIONALE:* This pattern of rinsing pushes the debris to the posterior of the mouth, since this is the lowest part of the mouth and the easiest area for the assistant to evacuate.
4. The assistant uses the HVE to remove the accumulation from the posterior region of the patient's mouth.
5. The patient is reassured that his mouth is now clean and that he may swallow if he wishes.

Mouth Rinsing, Using a Saliva Ejector

1. Be certain that the saliva ejector is in place and turned on, and explain the procedure to the patient.
2. Use the air-water syringe to place water in the patient's mouth, and instruct the patient to swish the water around vigorously.
3. Place the saliva ejector tip into the patient's mouth, and instruct the patient to close his lips gently around the tip.
4. Repeat as necessary for patient comfort.

reduction in the amount of time required in the dental chair, and the dental team experiences increased productivity with less fatigue and stress.

The techniques discussed in this chapter are based on assisting a right-handed dentist.

Instrument Grasps

The manner in which an instrument is held in the dentist's hand depends upon the type of instrument, how it is used, and which arch is being treated (Fig. 16–11). An understanding of these instrument grasps is essential to smooth instrument exchange. The three basic grasps are

- The **pen grasp,** in which the instrument is held in the same manner as a pen
- The **palm grasp,** in which the instrument is held securely in the palm of the hand
- The **palm-thumb grasp,** in which the instrument is held in the palm of the hand and the thumb is used to stabilize and guide the instrument

Basic Principles of Instrument Transfer

Instrument transfer, which is also referred to as *instrument exchange,* takes place in the transfer zone. The following principles are used to produce the most efficient instrument transfer method:

- The assistant must understand the sequence of the treatment procedure and anticipate when an instrument transfer will be required.
- The transfer of instruments should be accomplished with a minimum of motion involving only the fingers, wrist, and elbow.
- Instruments are passed in the position of use so that the dentist does not need to shift the instrument in his or her hand before using it. (**Position of use** means that the working end of the instrument is pointing downward for mandibular areas and upward for maxillary areas.)
- Pen grasp or modified pen grasp instruments are passed so that the dentist can receive them without moving his or her hand from the finger rest. (A **finger rest**, also known as a *fulcrum*, is used to stabilize the wrist and arm of the operator during use of an instrument.)
- The instrument being transferred must be positioned so that the dentist can receive it without moving his or her eyes from the field of operation.
- The assistant generally uses only the left hand to transfer instruments.

Use of the Assistant's Left Hand

The assistant's right hand is usually occupied with operating the HVE tip. The left hand is used for the following tasks required during a dental procedure:

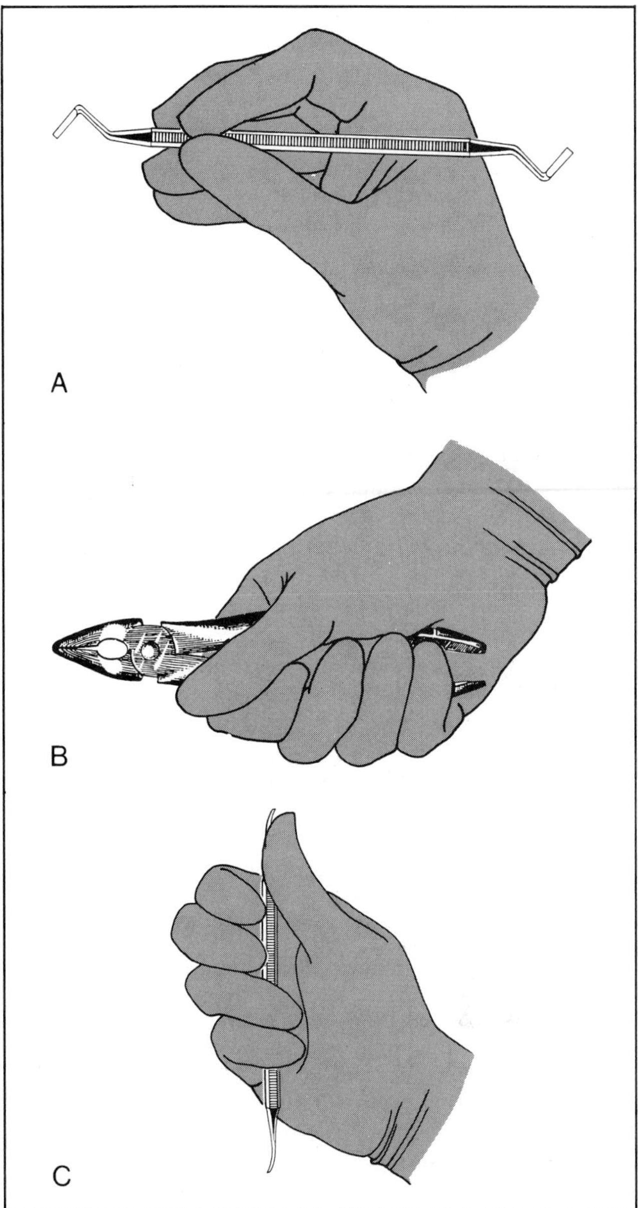

FIGURE 16–11

Basic instruments grasp. *Top,* The operator is holding the instrument in a pen grasp. *Middle,* The operator is holding the instrument in a palm grasp. *Bottom,* The operator is holding the instrument in a modified palm thumb grasp. (Courtesy of Colwell Systems, Champaign, IL.)

- Retraction of the tongue and soft tissue with a mouth mirror or the index finger
- Transfer of dental instruments and handpieces
- Operation of the air-water syringe
- Wiping the working end of instruments as they are withdrawn from the patient's mouth (this is especially helpful with instruments such as the cavity liner applicator where debris may dry on the instru-

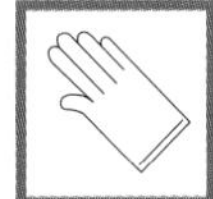 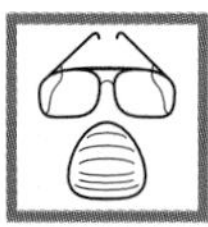 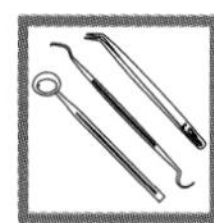  

PROCEDURE: **Transferring Instruments, Using the Single-Handed Technique**

1. The assistant uses the pick-up fingers to take the instrument to be delivered from the instrument tray. This instrument is grasped at the end *opposite* the working end that the dentist will use (Fig. 16–12).
   □ *RATIONALE:* This makes it possible to have the working end in the proper position of use when it is delivered.
2. The assistant holds the instrument in the transfer zone 8 to 10 inches away from the dentist until the signal is given to begin the transfer.
   □ *RATIONALE:* Holding the instrument closer until the dentist is ready for it may crowd the dentist.
3. The dentist signals for the transfer by maintaining the finger rest in the oral cavity and rolling the hand back slightly.
   □ *RATIONALE:* The dentist should not have to reach for the instrument. The instrument should be delivered into the dentist's hand while the finger rest is maintained.
4. The assistant positions the new instrument parallel to the instrument in the dentist's hand (Figs. 16–13 and 16–14).
   □ *RATIONALE:* Keeping the shanks of both instruments parallel avoids tangling them during the exchange.
5. The assistant extends the pick-up fingers and grasps the instrument being held in the dentist's hand near the end opposite to the working end.
6. The assistant folds the pick-up fingers into the palm of the hand and lifts the hand slightly above the dentist's hand.
   □ *RATIONALE:* This removes the unwanted instrument from the dentist's hand and tucks it carefully against the assistant's palm.
7. The assistant delivers the new instrument by lowering it into the dentist's hand (Figs. 16–15 and 16–16).

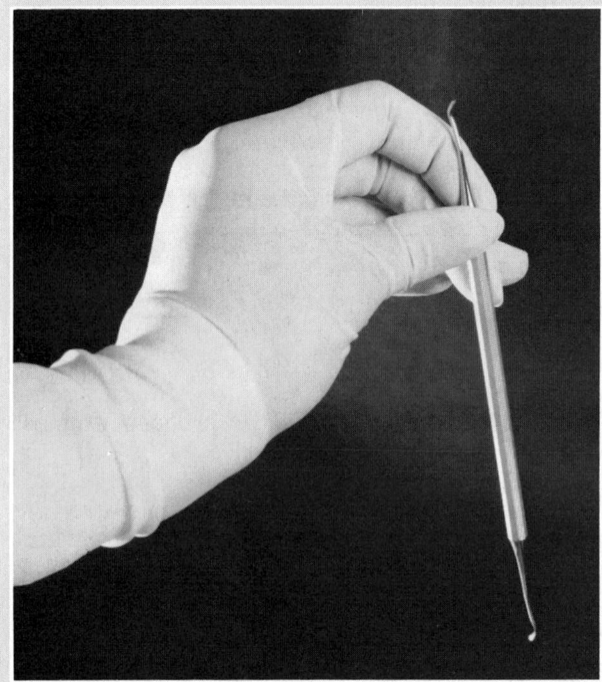

FIGURE 16–12

Demonstration of the assistant grasping the instrument to be transferred away from the working end.

8. If the same two instruments are to be exchanged again, the assistant immediately rolls the retrieved instrument upward between the thumb and pick-up fingers and shifts it to the delivery fingers.
   □ *RATIONALE:* This positions the instrument so that it is ready to be passed to the dentist again when needed.

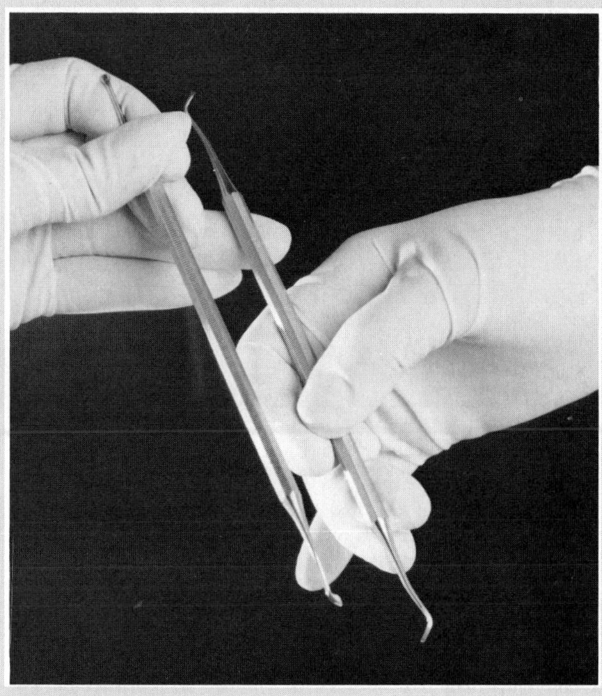

FIGURE 16–13

Demonstration of the instruments being held parallel before the transfer. The assistant's pick-up fingers (hand on the left) are moving into position to take the used instruments. The operator's hand (on the right) is ready for the instrument exchange.

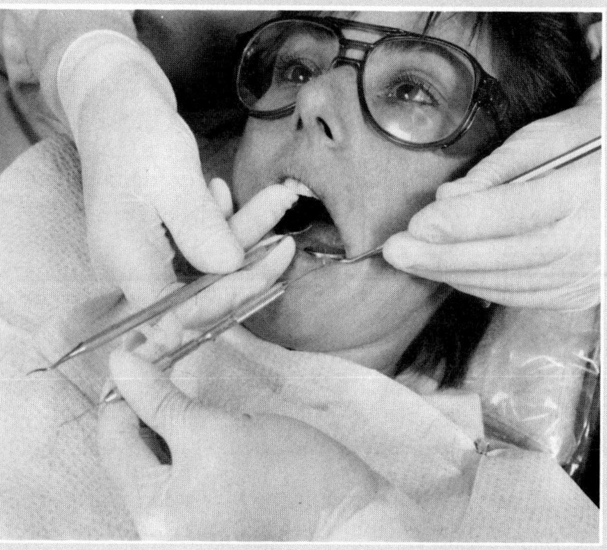

FIGURE 16–14

Actual instrument transfer with the instruments held parallel. Notice that the dentist's right hand has not moved from the fulcrum or position in the mouth. The dentist is holding a mirror in the left hand.

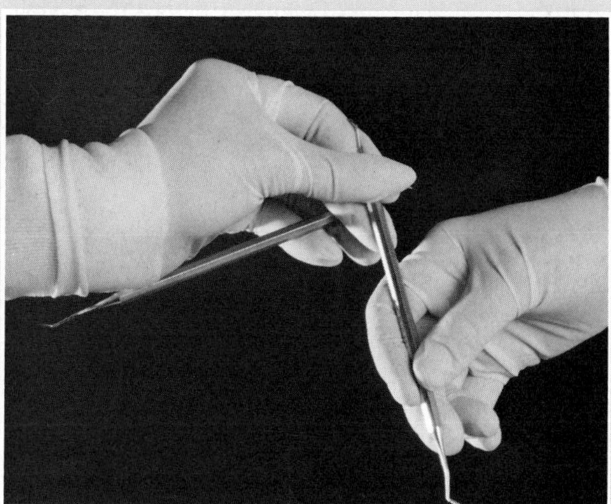

FIGURE 16–15

Demonstration of taking the used instrument and placing the next instrument. The assistant's hand (on the left) is already holding the used instrument in the pick-up fingers as the new instrument is placed into the dentist's hand in the position of use.

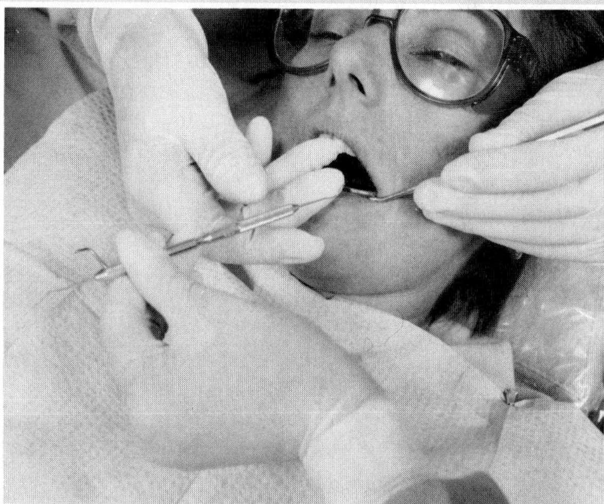

FIGURE 16–16

Actual instrument transfer. The dentist's hand position remains unchanged. The assistant has already taken the used instrument and gotten it out of the way as the new instrument is placed in the dentist's hand, ready for use.

ment; a gauze sponge is held in the assistant's hand for this purpose)

- Transfer of dental materials

Single-Handed Instrument Transfer

The single-handed transfer technique is the method of instrument transfer most commonly used because it is smooth and efficient. When the dentist is finished using an instrument and wants to exchange it for another, in a smooth motion using only the left hand, the assistant picks up the used instrument and "delivers" the new instrument. (Hence the name *single-handed transfer.*)

- The last two fingers (ring and little fingers) are **pick-up fingers** and are used to receive the used instrument.
- The thumb, index, and middle fingers work together as the **delivery fingers** to place the new instrument in the dentist's hand.

The single-handed transfer technique applies to hand instruments, handpieces, and air-water syringes. Forceps and scissors exchanges, which are described later, are made with only slight modifications.

Two-Handed Instrument Transfer

As the name implies, both of the assistant's hands are used in this transfer technique. Depending on the type of treatment or the phase of the procedure, the two-handed transfer is useful and convenient.

Instruments held in the palm, such as surgical forceps, dental dam forceps, and elevators, are easier to transfer by the two-handed method. So too are heavier instruments such as the handpiece and the air-water syringe.

PALM GRASP TRANSFER

The assistant uses the left hand to pick up the new instrument. It is held so that it can be delivered in the position of use.

The assistant uses the right hand to take the used instrument from the dentist. Then the assistant uses the left hand to deliver the new instrument to the dentist. This instrument is oriented with the working end in the appropriate position (Figs. 16–17 and 16–18).

The assistant returns the used instrument to its proper position on the preset tray, where it can be located quickly if needed later in the procedure.

HANDPIECE TRANSFER

The handpiece can be exchanged for an instrument by use of the same technique as when two hand instruments are exchanged as described earlier (Fig. 16–19). When exchanging two handpieces, take care to avoid tangling the hoses during the exchange.

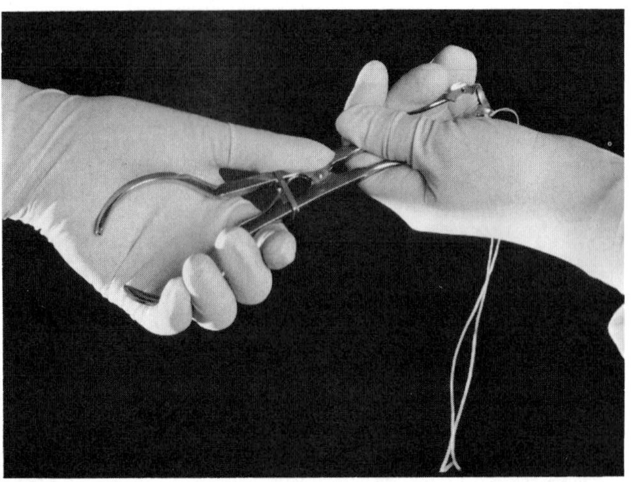

FIGURE 16–17

Demonstration of the transfer of a palm grasp instrument. The assistant, whose hand is on the right, passes a dental dam forceps and clamp to the dentist. Notice the assistant has positioned the jaws of the forceps upward for placement on a maxillary tooth.

AIR-WATER SYRINGE TRANSFER

To transfer the air-water syringe, the assistant holds the nozzle of the syringe in the delivery fingers (Fig. 16–20). The assistant delivers the syringe by bending the wrist slightly as the dentist prepares to receive it.

If the dentist is already holding an instrument, it is removed with the pick-up fingers before the syringe is delivered.

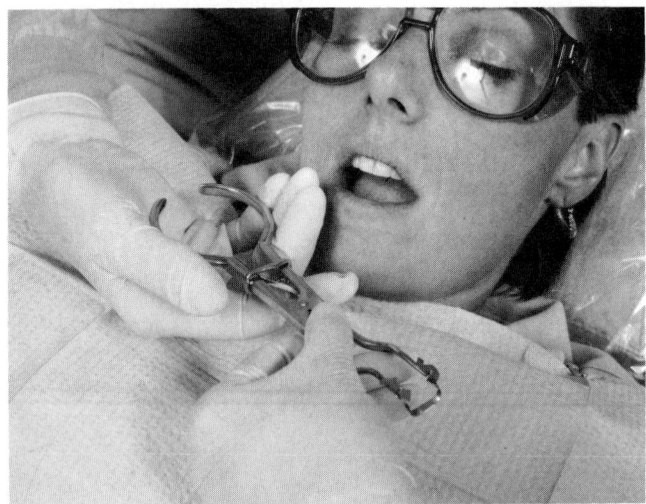

FIGURE 16–18

Simulation of an actual palm grasp instrument transfer. Notice how the instrument is placed into the palm of the dentist's hand. (In an actual transfer, there would be a ligature on the dental dam clamp.)

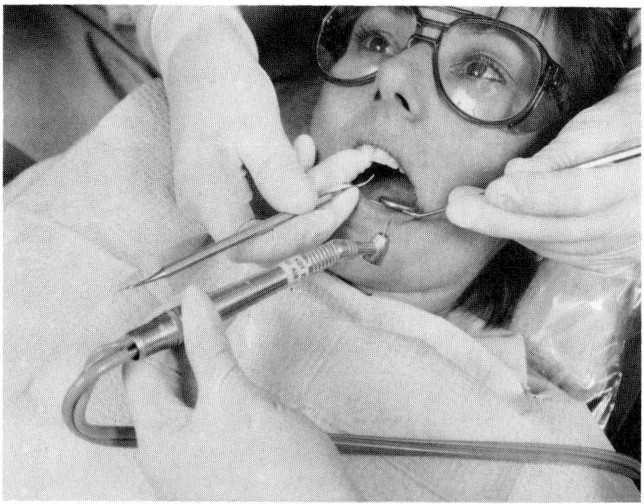

FIGURE 16–19

Handpiece transfer. Notice that the handpiece is positioned parallel to the instrument to be picked up. Also, the bur is oriented upward for use on the maxillary arch.

COTTON PLIERS TRANSFER

When nonlocking cotton pliers are used to transfer small items to and from the oral cavity, a modification in the single-handed transfer technique must be made.

1. The assistant delivers the pliers to the dentist while pinching the beaks together to avoid dropping the item held in the pliers.
2. The pliers are delivered so that the dentist can grasp and hold the beaks together before the assistant releases them.
3. Pick-up of the same pliers must be made by placing the pick-up fingers closer than normal to the working end of the pliers.
   □ **Rationale**: This will prevent the contents of the forceps from slipping out.

SCISSORS TRANSFER

1. The assistant picks up the scissors and grasps them near the working end with the beaks slightly open (Fig. 16–21).
   □ **Rationale**: This will make it easier to position the handles over the dentist's fingers.
2. Before the scissors are delivered, the dentist moves his or her hand away from the oral cavity.
3. The assistant positions handles of the scissors over the dentist's fingers.
4. When the assistant retrieves the scissors after use, the beaks of the scissors should be in the closed position.
   □ **Rationale**: This helps protect the assistant from an accidental cut or injury while handling the used scissors.

MIRROR AND EXPLORER TRANSFER

When beginning a procedure, the dentist frequently needs the mouth mirror and explorer to inspect the area to be treated. The dental assistant can deliver both the mirror and explorer simultaneously, using a two-handed exchange.

The dentist signals the assistant by placing one hand on each side of the patient's mouth in a position ready to receive the instruments.

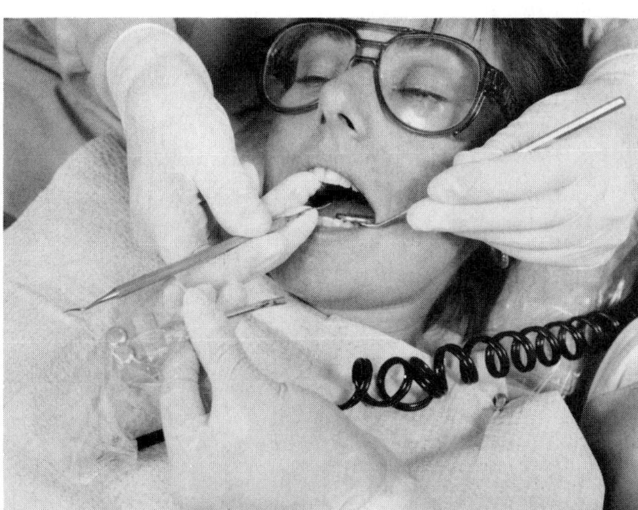

FIGURE 16–20

Air-water syringe transfer. The air-water syringe is positioned parallel to the instrument to be picked up. The assistant is holding the syringe so that the dentist will be able to grasp it by the handle in the position of use.

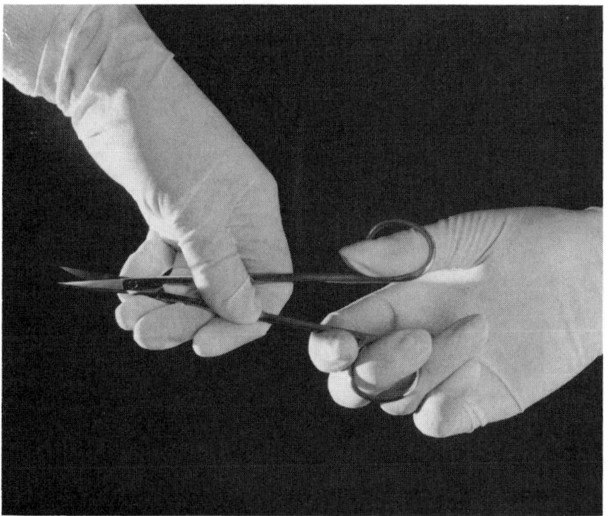

FIGURE 16–21

Scissors transfer. The assistant's hand is on the left, and the scissors are being transferred with the beaks slightly open. When the assistant receives the used scissors, the beaks will be closed.

Solutions to Common Problems

Smooth instrument transfer requires practice to develop the necessary skills. Listed as follows are solutions to some of the more common problems encountered during instrument transfer:

Presenting Past Midline. When the dentist is treating posterior teeth on the patient's right side, it is helpful for the dentist to present the instrument toward the assistant. (As used here, **present** means to tilt the instrument toward the midline.)

The dentist should never present an instrument beyond the patient's midline. Placing the handle at a 45-degree angle to the midline is the most desirable.

Crowding. Crowding occurs when the assistant, in anticipation of the signal to transfer, is holding an instrument too close to the instrument that the dentist is still using.

This is very distracting to the dentist and often leads to a false start in the exchange. Until the transfer is signaled by the dentist, the assistant should continue to hold the instrument ready at a distance of 8 to 10 inches from the dentist's hand.

Shorting. This occurs when the assistant does not grasp the instrument to be delivered far enough from the working end. The result is not enough room left on the handle for the dentist to grasp the instrument.

Tangling of Instruments During Transfer. Such tangling occurs when the handles of the instruments are not parallel to each other before the exchange.

Disorientation. This occurs when the instrument is delivered without having been oriented to the arch being treated. In the position of use, the working ends should be directed upward for the maxillary arch and downward for the mandibular arch.

Delivery of Dental Materials

Dental materials are generally delivered to the dentist in the transfer zone near the patient's chin.

Cements and liners, along with the applicator instrument, are delivered on the mixing slab or pad. The assistant holds the mixing pad in the right hand and a 2 × 2 gauze sponge in the left hand. The dentist can access the material, and the assistant is able to wipe the tip of the insertion instrument with the gauze as necessary (Fig. 16–22).

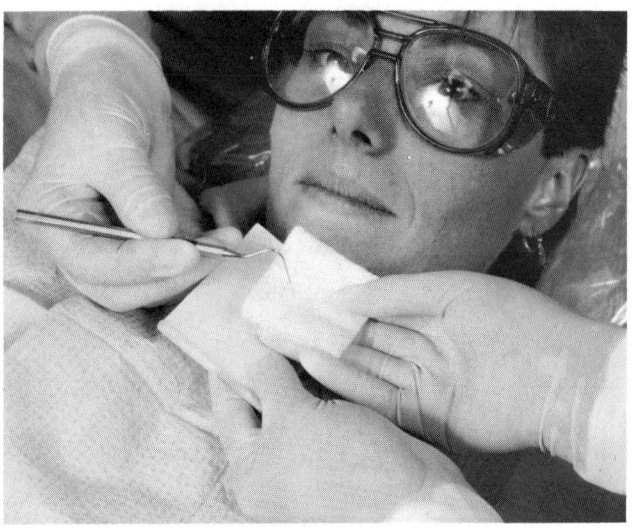

FIGURE 16–22

Delivering cements and liners. Notice that the assistant is using both hands here.

Material in syringes, such as impression material or composite material, can be delivered directly to the dentist. The syringe is passed so that the dentist can grasp the syringe in the position of use with the tip turned upward for maxillary use and the tip turned downward for mandibular use.

Amalgam can be delivered to the dentist for insertion into the preparation or can be placed into the preparation by the assistant.

This is often a matter of the dentist's preference or simply one of convenience. The team member who can conveniently see and reach the cavity preparation should place the material directly into the cavity, thus eliminating unnecessary instrument exchanges.

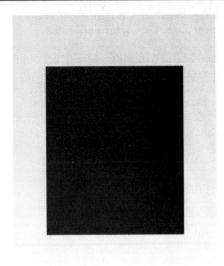

Chapter 17

Dental Radiography

Introduction

Dental radiographs, commonly known as x-rays, are among the most valuable diagnostic tools available to the dentist. Radiographs are used to detect

- Dental caries in the early stages
- Changes in the supporting structures
- Abnormalities in the surrounding hard and soft tissues

Dental radiographs are part of the patient's record and are legal documents. Therefore, it is important that all radiographs be of diagnostic quality. (A **diagnostic quality** radiograph clearly shows the tissues to be examined in a manner that the dentist is able to use it for diagnostic purposes. See Criteria for Diagnostic Quality Radiographs on page 294.)

Diagnostic quality radiographs do not happen by chance. They are taken only by operators who are thoroughly trained in dental radiography and who routinely practice the principles of radiation protection.

Radiation, which is used to produce dental radiographs, has the potential to damage all living tissue. Any exposure to radiation, no matter how insignificant, can cause harm to the operator and the patient. Therefore, radiographs are taken only as necessary and are always produced in the safest manner possible.

Both intraoral and extraoral radiographs are used in dentistry. An **intraoral film** is placed inside the patient's mouth. An **extraoral film** is placed near, but not inside, the mouth.

Responsibilities of the Dentist

1. To prescribe only those radiographs that are necessary for diagnostic purposes
2. To have all radiographic equipment properly installed and maintained in a safe working condition (most states regulate x-ray equipment and have radiation health codes that pertain to the use of radiation)
3. To install appropriate shielding to protect staff and patients from the effects of radiation (depending on the state regulations, dental offices, clinics, and dental schools are inspected every 1 to 3 years to check the safety of x-ray machines and barrier protection)
4. To allow radiographs to be exposed only by personnel who are properly trained, credentialed, and appropriately supervised in keeping with the state regulations regarding individuals who expose dental radiographs

Responsibilities of the Dental Assistant

1. To be knowledgeable about the radiographic licensing requirements, rules, and regulations of the state in which he or she practices (each state deals with

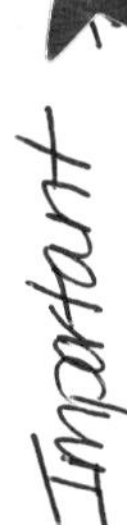

Criteria for Diagnostic-Quality Radiographs

The radiograph should include:

- Adequate contrast and definition to define clearly the detail and structure of the teeth and surrounding area being radiographed.
- An accurate reproduction of the long axis of the tooth or teeth. The overall measurement on the radiograph must be the same as that of the natural tooth.
- At least $\frac{1}{4}$ inch of alveolar bone beyond the apex of the tooth. A periapical radiograph should also include a margin of $\frac{1}{8}$ to $\frac{1}{4}$ inch between the crown of the tooth and the edge of the radiograph.
- On the posterior radiographs, the occlusal plane presented as straight or slightly curved upward toward the distal area.
- The adjacent teeth and their contacts shown without overlapping.
- A clear image of the periodontal space including the alveolus, tissue adjacent to the tooth, and the trabeculae of the bone.
- An accurate representation of anatomic landmarks within the area of the teeth being radiographed.
- Accurate location of pathologic conditions when situated in proximity to the teeth being radiographed.
- Accurate location of an impacted tooth and its position relative to other structures in the dental arch.

From Ehrlich, A., and Torres, H.O.; Essentials of Dental Assisting. Philadelphia, W.B. Saunders Co., 1992, p 252.

dental radiography differently, and one cannot assume that regulations for all states are the same)

2. To meet the radiographic licensing requirements of the state in which he or she practices (being licensed in one state does not mean that the license is recognized in another state)
3. To participate in obtaining **informed consent** (this includes explaining the purpose of taking radiographs to the patient and helping the patient to understand the benefit of dental radiographs; an example would be informing the patient of the diseases that might go undetected without radiographs and what the consequences might be; if the patient is a minor, the parent or guardian must give the consent)
4. To review the health questionnaire (the assistant should call the dentist's attention to any information that might contraindicate or change the number and type of radiographs to be taken)
5. To use *only* those techniques that will produce diagnostic quality radiographs with minimal exposure of radiation to the patient

Radiation Physics

The efficient and safe production of dental radiographs depends upon understanding of the basic principles of radiation physics that are involved in the process.

Atomic Structure

Understanding basic atomic structure is important because it relates directly to the ways in which x-rays are produced, emitted (given off) from the machine, and absorbed by patients and operators.

All matter is made of atoms. Atoms are extremely minute and are composed of (1) an inner core, or **nucleus,** that possesses a positive electric charge and (2) a number of negatively charged particles called **electrons** that orbit around the nucleus. The nucleus of an atom is composed of positively charged subatomic particles called **protons** and subatomic particles called **neutrons** that have no charge.

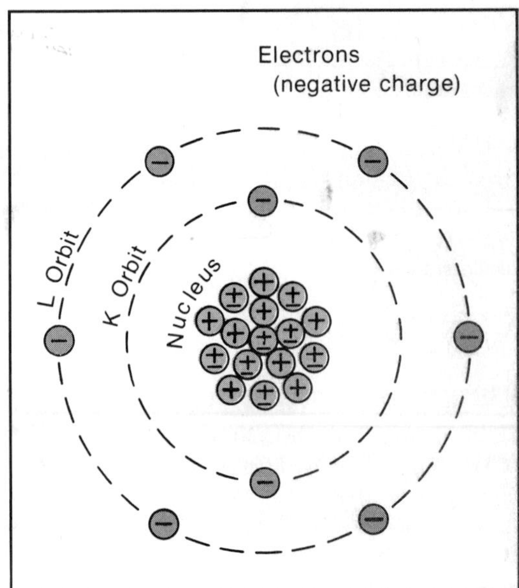

FIGURE 17–1

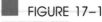

Diagrammatic representation of an oxygen atom.

The arrangement within the atom is similar to that of the solar system. The atom has a nucleus as its center or sun, and the electrons revolve around it like planets (Fig. 17–1). The electrons remain stable in their orbit unless disturbed or removed.

In the neutral or stable atom, the number of orbiting electrons (−) equals the number of protons (+) in the nucleus; hence the atom is electrically neutral.

Atoms in turn join to form molecules. A molecule is the smallest particle of substance that retains the property of the substance.

IONIZATION

Ionization is the process whereby electrons are removed from electrically stable atoms by collisions with x-ray photons. (A **photon** is a minute bundle of pure energy that has no weight or mass.) The atoms that lose electrons become positive ions. As such, they are unstable structures capable of interacting with (and damaging) other atoms, tissues, or chemicals.

It is the harmful ionizing effect of x-rays in humans that can result in a disruption of cellular metabolism and cause permanent damage to living cells and tissues.

Methods of protecting both the patient and operator from exposure to ionizing radiation are discussed later in this chapter.

Properties of X-Rays

X-rays are a form of energy that can penetrate matter. Like visible light, radar, radio, and television waves, they belong to a group called **electromagnetic radiation** (Fig. 17–2).

Electromagnetic radiations are made of **photons,** which travel through space at the speed of light in a straight line with a wavelike motion.

The *longer* the wavelength, the *weaker* its ability to penetrate matter. These longer waves are of limited usefulness in dental radiography.

The *shorter* the wavelength, the *greater* the energy of a photon. Because of the high energy of short wavelengths, they are able to penetrate matter more easily than longer wavelengths. X-rays have unique properties that make them especially useful in dentistry. These properties include the abilities to

- Travel at the speed of light
- Travel in straight lines
- Penetrate matter
- Produce a latent image (a **latent image** is an image on the film that is not visible until the film has been processed)
- Produce fluorescence (glowing) in certain materials (this is important in extraoral radiography)
- Produce ionization

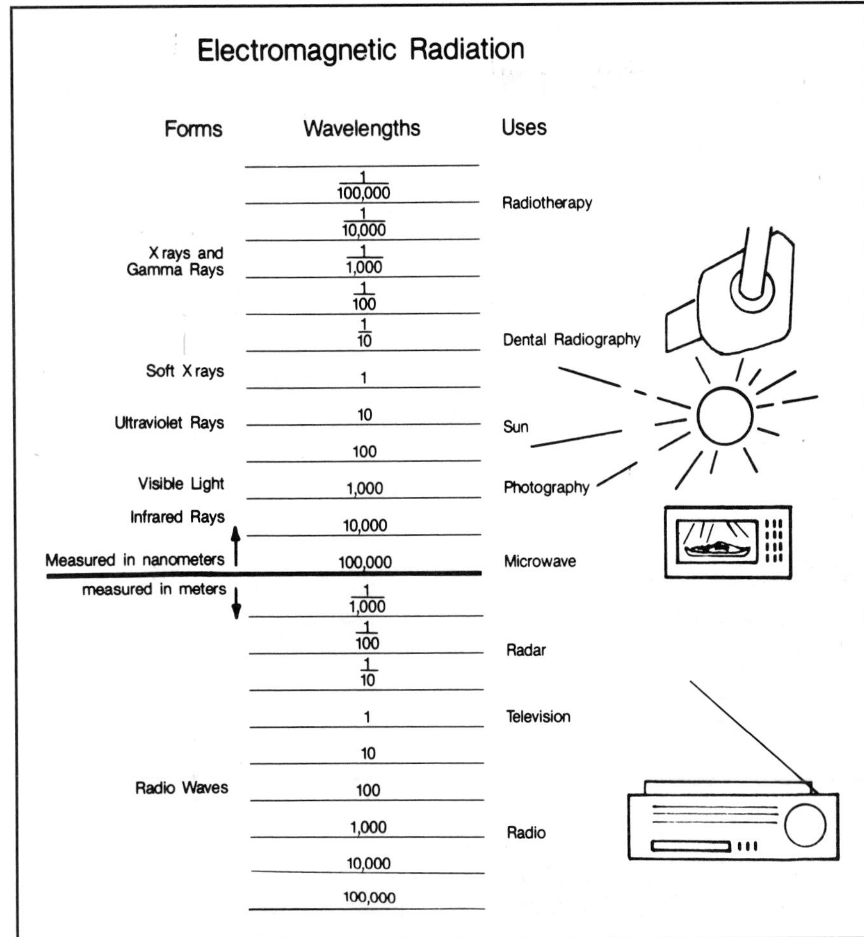

FIGURE 17–2

Electromagnetic spectrum, showing the various wavelengths of commonly used radiations. The upper part of the scale is measured in nanometers. A nanometer is one-billionth of a meter. (From Miles, D.A., VanDis, M.L., Jensen, C.W., and Ferretti, A.: Radiographic Imaging for Dental Auxiliaries, 2nd ed. Philadelphia, W.B. Saunders Co., 1994, p 78.)

TYPES OF X-RADIATION

Primary radiation, also known as the *central ray* or *primary beam*, is the stream of radiation as it is emitted from the x-ray unit tubehead through the open end of the lead-lined position indicator device (PID).

The primary beam travels in a straight line and contains powerful short waves. It is the short waves in the central ray that produce the diagnostically useful radiograph.

Secondary radiation is given off by matter exposed to radiation. This form of radiation is created the moment the primary beam comes into contact with matter. For example, during the exposure of a dental radiograph, adjacent tissues of the face and head become irradiated. (**Irradiated** means exposed to radiation.) This irradiation may continue to expose the film and harm the adjacent tissues.

Scatter radiation is radiation that has been deflected from its path during the impact with matter. (**Deflected** means turned aside.) The terms *secondary* and *scatter radiation* are often used interchangeably.

Scatter radiation travels in all directions and is impossible to confine. As the patient is exposed to radiation, the radiation changes direction on impact. Without adequate protective barriers, the operator and others nearby may be affected by exposure to scatter radiation.

Units of Radiation Measurement

There are two sets of terminology currently used to define the way radiation is measured. In 1985, an international system (SI) of measurement was adopted worldwide. However, the traditional terminology is also still in use. Both systems are presented here, and the units are compared in Table 17–1.

RADIATION EXPOSURE

The amount of radiation a person is exposed to is measured in SI units as **coulombs per kilogram** (C/kg). This is a measure of electric charge in a certain mass of air. The traditional term is the **roentgen** (R). One coulomb per kilogram (C/kg) equals 1 roentgen (R).

TABLE 17–1

Comparative Units of Radiation Measurement

MEASUREMENT	SI AND TRADITIONAL COMPARED
Radiation exposure	1 coulomb per kilogram (C/kg) = 1 roentgen (R)
Absorbed dose	1 gray (Gy) = 100 radiation absorbed doses (rads)
Dose equivalence	1 sievert (Sv) = 100 roentgen equivalent man (rem)

ABSORBED DOSE

The amount of radiation energy actually absorbed by the tissues is the absorbed dose. The SI unit of absorbed dose is called a **gray** (Gy). A gray is defined as the transfer of 1 joule (a unit of energy and work) per gram of tissue.

The traditional system used the term **radiation absorbed dose** (rad) as the unit of measurement. One rad is equivalent to the transfer of 100 ergs (another unit of energy and work) per gram of tissue. One gray (Gy) equals 100 radiation absorbed doses (rads).

DOSE EQUIVALENCE

Dose equivalence is defined as the absorbed dose of any form of radiation that produces the same biological effect in a human as does 1 rad of x-radiation.

The SI unit of dose equivalence is the **sievert** (Sv). The traditional unit is a **roentgen equivalent man** (rem). One sievert (Sv) equals 100 rems. Technically, there are some differences between the units of radiation measurement; however in dental radiology, the units are virtually interchangeable.

Maximum Permissible Dose

The maximum permissible dose (MPD) represents the exposure limits for those who are occupationally exposed to radiation. This amount of radiation to the whole body produces very little chance of injury.

The MPD for whole body exposure for occupationally exposed personnel is 0.05 Sv (5 rems). These personnel include dental healthcare workers who expose radiographs.

An age-based formula has been developed as a guideline for any accumulated dose: $(N - 18) \times 0.05$ Sv per year = MPD. In this formula, N equals age in years.

Occupationally exposed women who are pregnant are allowed an MPD of only 0.005 Sv per year. This is the same dose limit that applies to the general population.

Dental personnel should strive for an occupational dose of zero by adhering to strict radiation protection practices.

RADIATION MONITORING

A film badge (pocket dosimeter) is used to measure the amount of occupational exposure. The badge contains a film packet, similar to dental film, embossed with the wearer's name and identification number.

Employees wear the badge at all times while at work, and at the end of the reporting period (usually every 3 to 4 weeks), the badge is returned to the monitoring service company. The company processes the badge and prepares a report that is returned to the dental office.

The report contains the radiation exposure results for the reporting period and the accumulated quarterly, yearly, and lifetime exposure of the individual. These reports should be retained by the dentist with other important employee records.

Film badges should *not* be worn outside the office, especially in bright sunlight. Film badges must be removed when the person being monitored is having medical or dental x-rays, because it is intended to measure only occupational exposure.

Radiation Health and Safety

We are exposed to radiation every day of our lives. **Background radiation** comes from natural sources such as radioactive materials in the ground and cosmic radiation from space.

Exposure from medical or dental sources is an additional radiation risk. Because of their concern, patients frequently say, "I've heard x-rays are bad for me. Do you really need to take them?" The dental assistant must anticipate this patient reaction and be able to explain to the patient the risks and diagnostic benefits of dental radiation.

The benefits of the use of x-rays in dentistry certainly outweigh the risks when proper safety procedures are followed.

Biological Effects of Radiation

X-rays in sufficient doses may produce harmful effects in human beings. X-rays can bring about changes in body chemicals, cells, tissues, and organs. The effects of the radiation may not become evident for a great number of years after the time the x-rays were absorbed. This time lag is called the **latent period.**

CUMULATIVE EFFECTS

Exposure to radiation has a cumulative effect over a lifetime. When tissues are exposed to x-rays, some damage occurs. Tissues have the capacity to repair some of the damage; however, the tissues do not return to their original state.

This can be compared to the wrinkles and skin damage that can occur from repeated exposure over the years to the sun. The cumulative effects of repeated exposure to radiation are summarized in Table 17–2.

ACUTE AND CHRONIC RADIATION EXPOSURE

Acute radiation exposure occurs when a large dose of radiation is absorbed in a short time, such as in a nuclear accident.

Chronic radiation exposure occurs when small amounts of radiation are absorbed repeatedly over a long time. It may be years after the original exposure that the effects of chronic x-ray exposure are observed.

TABLE 17–2

Cumulative Effects of Repeated Radiation Exposure

CRITICAL ORGAN	RESULTING DISORDER
Lens of eye	Cataracts
Bone marrow	Leukemia
Salivary gland	Cancer
Thyroid gland	Cancer
Skin	Cancer
Gonads	Genetic abnormalities

From Miles, D.A., VanDis, M.L., Jensen, C.W., and Ferretti, A.: Radiographic Imaging for Dental Auxiliaries, 2nd ed. Philadelphia, W.B. Saunders Co., 1994, p 276.

SOMATIC AND GENETIC EFFECTS

Table 17–3 compares the relative radiation sensitivity of cells and tissues. Note that the skin, eye, and oral mucosa, all of which might be affected by dental radiographs, are high on the list.

X-rays affect both genetic and somatic cells. **Genetic** cells are the reproductive cells (sperm and ova). Damage to genetic cells *is* passed on to succeeding generations. These changes are referred to as **genetic mutations.**

TABLE 17–3

Relative Radiation Sensitivity of Cells and Tissues

SENSITIVITY TO RADIATION	CELL TYPE OR TISSUE
High	Small lymphocyte
	Bone marrow
	Reproductive cells
	Intestinal mucosa
Fairly high	Skin
	Lens of the eye
	Oral mucosa
Medium	Connective tissue
	Small blood vessels
	Growing bone and cartilage
Fairly low	Mature bone and cartilage
	Salivary gland
	Thyroid gland
	Kidney
	Liver
Low	Muscle
	Nerve

From Miles, D.A., VanDis, M.L., Jensen, C.W., and Ferretti, A.: Radiographic Imaging for Dental Auxiliaries, 2nd ed. Philadelphia, W.B. Saunders Co., 1994, p 275.

Somatic Effects. All other cells in the body belong to the group of somatic tissue. (**Somatic** means referring to the body.) Somatic tissue can be damaged by x-rays, but the damage is *not* passed on to future generations.

Minimizing Genetic Effects. The dose to reproductive cells from dental radiography is very small. A lead apron *must* be worn on by every patient during radiographic procedures, and this reduces the exposure to the reproductive cells to virtually zero (0.0001–0.0003 mGy). (A milligray, or mGy, is one-thousandth of a gray.)

Because of any possible risk of radiation during pregnancy, women of childbearing age are asked to let the dental personnel know if they are pregnant. The exact amount of x-radiation that may produce damage to a developing human embryo or fetus is unknown. It is believed that doses below 100 mGy entail little risk.

Nevertheless, it is advisable to postpone routine radiographs until after pregnancy. In case of a dental emergency, a minimal number of films can be taken. As with all patients, the lead apron must cover *all* of the patient's abdomen.

The levels of radiation involved in dental radiography are only about 1/25 to 1/1,000 of the levels that are associated with possible somatic injury. The benefits of detecting disease in a patient, disease that might not otherwise be detected, far outweighs the risks from receiving small doses of radiation.

The key is to follow all safety procedures and to minimize the number of retakes by using skillful exposure techniques. (A **retake** means that the radiograph must be taken again because the first film is not of diagnostic quality. This is time consuming and exposes the patient to excess radiation.)

Protection of the Patient

The amount of radiation exposure to the dental patient can be reduced to a very small amount by adhering to the ALARA concept. (**ALARA** stands for "as low as reasonably achievable.") This goal can be achieved by always using

- Well-calibrated, properly installed, and properly maintained x-ray equipment
- The fastest speed of dental film
- Position indicator devices (PID) and film-holding instruments to reduce exposure to radiation
- Good film exposure techniques
- Lead aprons and thyroid collars for all patients during all radiographic procedures

PROPER FILM EXPOSURE TECHNIQUE

Retakes are the leading source of unnecessary exposure to radiation in the dental office. Every retake of a film as a result of poor operator technique or processing error doubles the radiation exposure to the patient for that film.

FILM-HOLDING INSTRUMENTS

The use of a film-holding instruments keeps the patient's hands from being exposed to radiation. Film-holders also hold the film in a stable position and aid the operator in properly positioning the film and the PID.

To avoid cone cuts, film-holders are absolutely necessary when a rectangular PID is used. (A **cone cut** is a clear area of the film that was not exposed to radiation.)

LEAD APRONS AND THYROID COLLARS

A lead apron and a thyroid collar must be used on *all* patients for *all* exposures (Fig. 17–3). This rule applies to all patients regardless of the patient's age, sex, or the number of films being exposed. The lead apron should cover the patient from the thyroid and extend over the gonadal area.

Thyroid collars, also known as *cervical collars*, can be separate shields or can be part of the lead apron. The collar covers the thyroid gland during exposure and reduces radiation exposure of the gland. Thyroid disease has *not* been shown to be caused by the low exposure from dental x-rays, but the use of collars further minimizes patient exposure to x-radiation.

Lead aprons and thyroid collars are *not* folded when

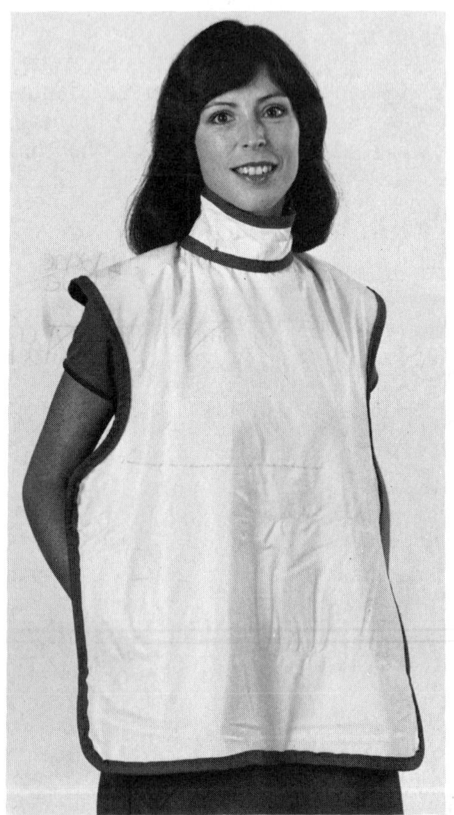

FIGURE 17–3

Combination lead apron and thyroid collar.

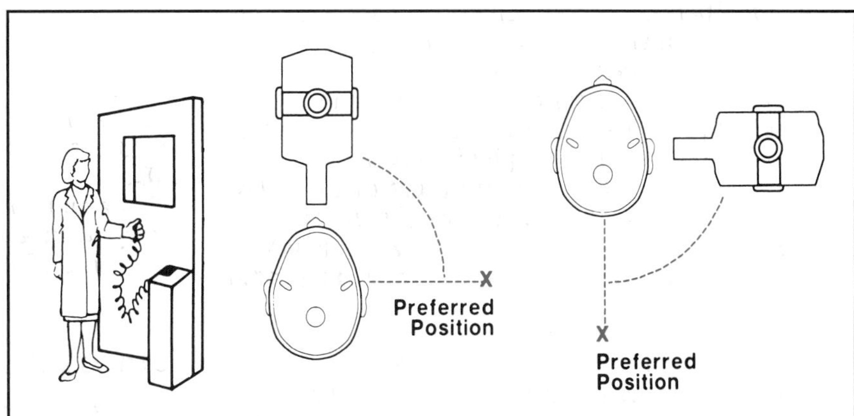

FIGURE 17–4

Preferred positions for operator. *A*, Behind a protective lead barrier. *B* and *C*, **X** represents the safest operator positions if no lead barrier is available. (Modified from Miles, D.A., VanDis, M.L., Jensen, C.W., and Ferretti, A.: Radiographic Imaging for Dental Auxiliaries, 2nd ed. Philadelphia, W.B. Saunders Co., 1994, pp 3 and 4.)

not in use. (Folding eventually cracks the lead and allows leakage.) Instead, they should be hung up, preferably over a rounded bar.

Protection of the Operator

An assistant who fails to follow the rules of radiation protection may suffer the results of chronic exposure. By following these rules, dental personnel can keep their radiation exposure to zero (Fig. 17–4 and Rules of Radiation Protection).

If the Patient Cannot Hold the Film

If the patient is a child who is unable to cooperate, the child is seated on the parent's lap in the dental chair. Both parent and child are covered with the lead apron, and the parent holds the film. (Having the parent hold the film is acceptable because this is a single exposure for the parent. If the assistant were to hold films in this manner, he or she would have repeated exposure and would suffer the cumulative effects of this radiation.)

Infection Control in Dental Radiography

Dental radiographic procedures present special infection control challenges, primarily because the operator contacts the patient's saliva and then moves about and must touch many things while exposing and processing the films (see Sources of Disease Transmission During Radiography).

Rules of Radiation Protection

- *Never* stand in the direct line of the primary beam.
- *Always* stand behind a lead barrier if one is available. (If a lead barrier is not available, stand at right angles to the beam.)
- *Never* stand closer than 6 feet to the x-ray unit during an exposure (unless you are behind a lead barrier).
- *Never* use x-ray equipment that is faulty. (Use the unit again only after it has been repaired.)
- *Never* hold a film in the patient's mouth. (There are no exceptions to this rule.)

Sources of Disease Transmission During Radiography

- X-ray machine arm, head, and position indicator device (PID)
- Film packets or cassettes and film positioning instruments
- Control panel and exposure button
- Dental chair headrest and chair adjustment controls
- Operating light handle
- Counter tops and film transfer cup
- Doorknobs, door frames, light switches, and walls
- Processors and darkroom equipment
- Patient records
- Any object the operator touches after placing the film packet in the patient's mouth

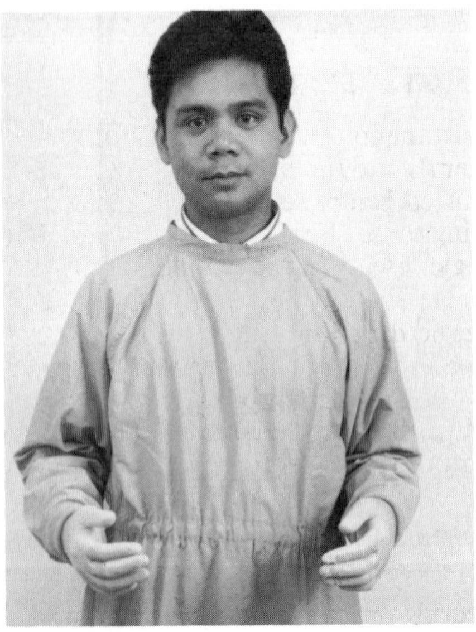

FIGURE 17–5

Operator wearing personal protective equipment before exposing radiographs. (From Ehrlich, A., and Torres, H.O.: Essentials of Dental Assisting. Philadelphia, W.B. Saunders Co., 1992, p 258.)

Protective Equipment

PERSONAL PROTECTIVE EQUIPMENT

Gloves must be worn whenever contaminated films are handled; however, because radiographic procedures do not involve the aerosol spray produced by the dental handpiece, a mask and glasses are not required while radiographic films are exposed (Fig. 17–5). The exception is if either the patient or operator has a cough or a cold; then the operator should wear a mask.

PROTECTIVE BARRIERS

Any object that the operator touches while producing radiographs *must* be covered with a removable barrier or disinfected after the patient is dismissed. Household plastic wrap and plastic bags are most commonly used as these barriers.

Barriers must be placed over the **dental chair headrest**, the **countertops**, the **extension arm**, **tubehead** and **PID** of the x-ray machine, **control panel**, and **exposure button** (Figs. 17–6 and 17–7).

Any object without a barrier that was touched *must* be disinfected. This situation is not desirable for two reasons: (1) disinfecting solutions may not reach irregular surfaces, and (2) disinfecting solutions may be damaging to the electrical connections of the equipment.

BARRIER ENVELOPES

To minimize contamination by saliva, a clear plastic barrier envelope may be placed over the film packet. Films are available already enclosed in a clear plastic barrier packet (Fig. 17–8). Another option is the use of barrier envelopes that are placed on each new film by the operator *before* the radiographic procedure begins.

The film packet in the barrier envelope is exposed and brought to the processing area. With gloved hands and taking care not to touch the film packet, the assistant opens the barrier envelope and allows the film packet to drop onto a clean surface (Fig. 17–9). The contaminated barrier packets are discarded, and the films are processed.

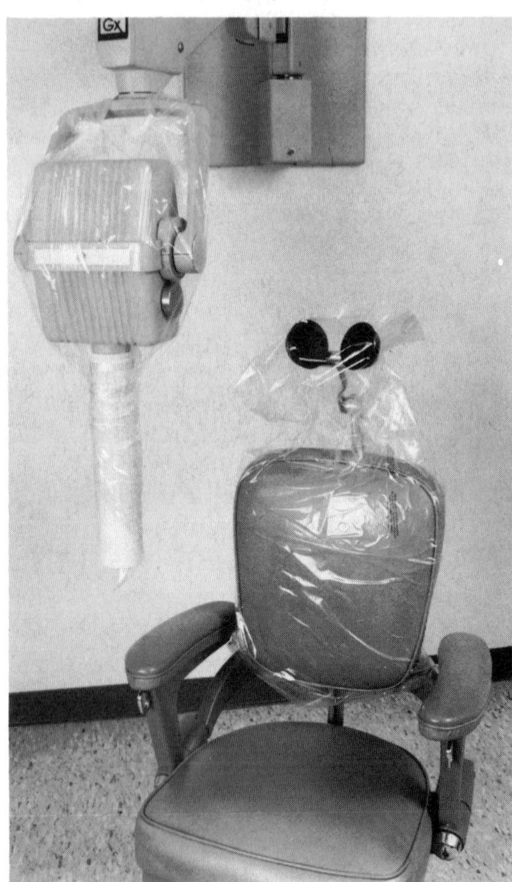

FIGURE 17–6

Protective barriers placed over the x-ray machine and head of the dental chair. (From Ehrlich, A., and Torres, H.O.: Essentials of Dental Assisting. Philadelphia, W.B. Saunders Co., 1992, p 258.)

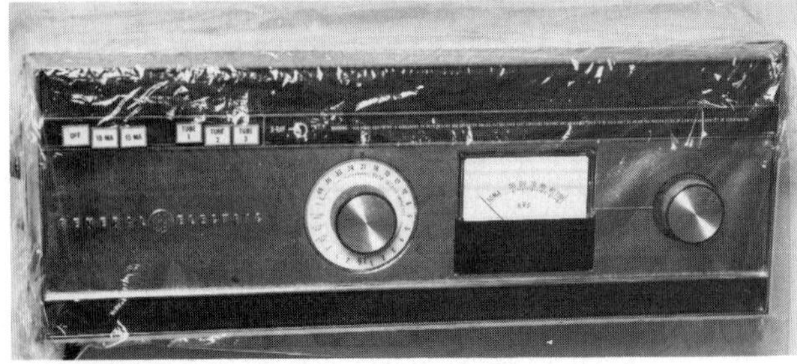

FIGURE 17–7

Protective barrier placed over the control panel. (From Ehrlich, A., and Torres, H.O.: Essentials of Dental Assisting. Philadelphia, W.B. Saunders Co., 1992, p 258.)

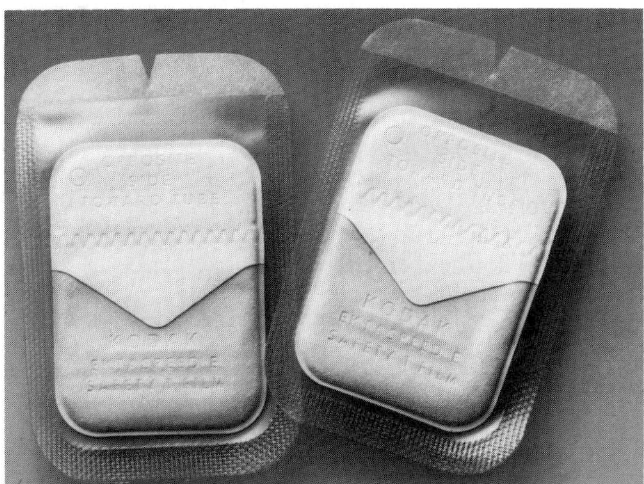

FIGURE 17–8

Protective barrier on x-ray film. (Courtesy of Eastman Kodak Co., Dental Products, Rochester, NY.)

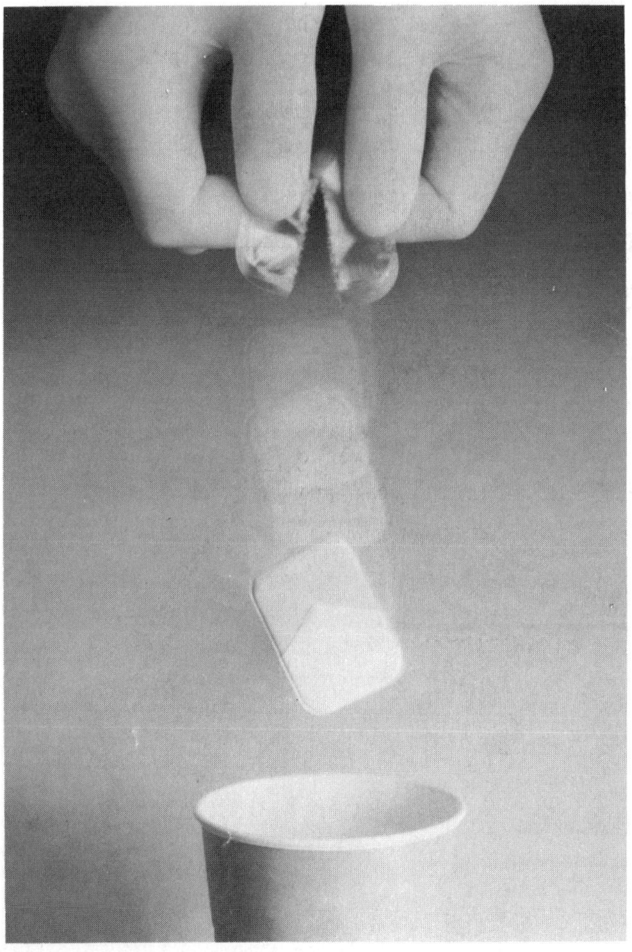

FIGURE 17–9

While the assistant is still gloved, the exposed film is removed from the barrier packet. (Courtesy of Eastman Kodak Co., Dental Products, Rochester, NY.)

Care of Films and Equipment

CARE OF FILM-HOLDING INSTRUMENTS

Film-holding instruments and bite-blocks that are placed in the patient's mouth are critical items and must either be sterilized before reuse or disposable and discarded after a single use. Foam bite-blocks are discarded after a single use. Most film-holding instruments are autoclavable and are clearly labeled as such.

Some plastic film-holding instruments may be damaged by heat. In accordance with the manufacturer's recommendations, these must be sterilized in an EPA-registered sterilant/disinfectant chemical solution in the appropriate concentration and for the recommended length of time. (See Chapter 13.)

CARE OF FILM PACKETS

The contaminated film packet is the major source of cross-containation during radiographic procedures. When the packet is removed from the patient's mouth, it is contaminated with saliva (or on occasion with blood). For this reason, the operator *must* always wear gloves while handling contaminated films.

Decontamination of Film Packets. Wipe saliva from the film packet, using a dry 2 × 2 inch gauze sponge or a paper towel. Do *not* sterilize the film packet. Heat sterilizing will destroy the image.

Some manufacturers permit lightly spraying the film packets with a disinfectant spray; however, immersing the packet in a disinfecting solution is not recommended because this can result in the solution's seeping into the emulsion and damaging the image.

Components of the Dental X-Ray Machine

Dental x-ray machines may vary slightly in size and appearance, but all have three primary components: the tubehead, an extension arm, and the control panel.

The Tubehead

The primary function of the tubehead is to house the dental x-ray tube. The tubehead is made of metal and has a protective lead lining to prevent any radiation from escaping. (Lead is used because it is very effective at blocking radiation.)

The tubehead is filled with oil to help absorb the heat created by the dental x-ray tube during the production of x-rays.

COMPONENTS OF THE DENTAL X-RAY TUBE

The dental x-ray tube is made of glass and is about 6 inches long and 1½ inches in diameter (Fig. 17–10). The air has been removed from the tube to create a vacuum. This vacuum environment allows the elec-

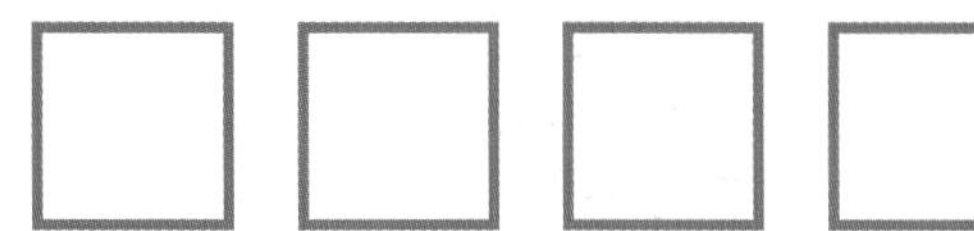

PROCEDURE: **Infection Control Steps During Film Exposure**

1. Before starting to expose the radiographs, place the appropriate barriers. Include a barrier on a work surface where films will be stored just after they have been exposed. Place a paper towel and a transfer cup on this barrier. (The transfer cup is a small paper cup labeled with patient identification information.)
   □ *RATIONALE:* The towel is used to wipe excess saliva from the film packets. The transfer cup is used to carry the films from the treatment room to the processing center.
2. Always wear gloves when exposing radiographs and handling exposed radiographs.
3. After taking each radiograph, place the packet on the paper towel to remove excess saliva. Then put the exposed film in the paper cup. Do not touch the exterior of the cup.
4. When finished exposing films and while still gloved, discard the paper towel.
5. Remove gloves and wash hands before leaving the treatment room.
6. Take the transfer cup of exposed radiographs to the processing area.
7. Before processing films, wash hands and put on fresh gloves.
   □ *RATIONALE:* Exposed films are contaminated with the patient's saliva. Film processing is discussed later in this chapter.

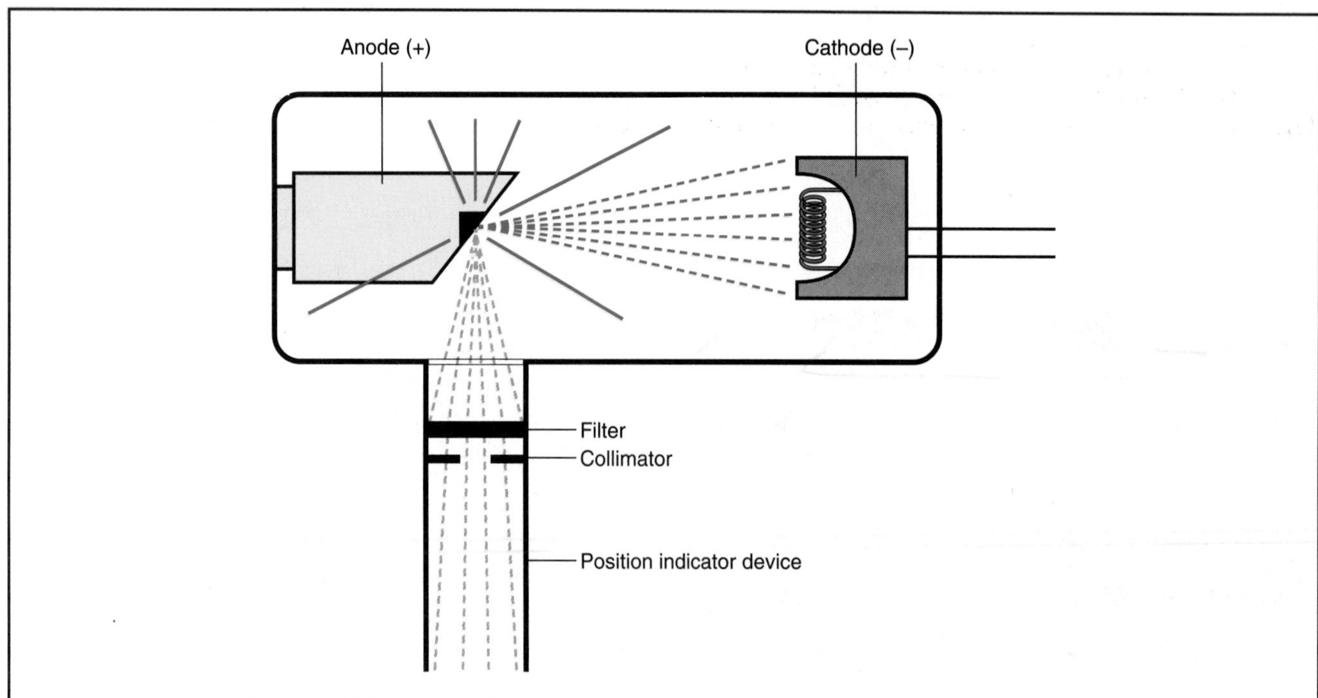

FIGURE 17–10

Schematic drawing of a dental x-ray tube. (Modified from Miles, D.A., VanDis, M.L., Jensen, C.W., and Ferretti, A.: Radiographic Imaging for Dental Auxiliaries, 2nd ed. Philadelphia, W.B. Saunders Co., 1994, p 85.)

trons to flow with minimum resistance between the electrodes (cathode and anode).

Cathode. The cathode (−) is a tungsten filament. Electrons are generated in the x-ray tube at the cathode. The hotter the filament becomes, the more electrons are produced. (Tungsten is a metal capable of withstanding the intense heat given off during the generation of x-rays.)

Focusing Cup. The focusing cup, also part of the cathode, keeps the electrons suspended in a cloud at the cathode. When the exposure button is pressed, the circuit within the tubehead is completed, and the electrons very rapidly cross from the cathode (−) to the anode (+).

Anode. The anode (+) acts as the target for the electrons. It is composed of a **tungsten target** (a small block of tungsten) that is embedded in the larger copper stem. The copper around the target conducts the heat away from the target, thus reducing the wear and tear on the target.

About 99 percent of the x-rays generated by this process are absorbed by the oil, and this energy is given off as heat. The remaining 1 percent exit the tubehead through the port (opening) as a divergent beam toward the patient. The x-rays at the center of this beam are known as the central ray.

FILTER

The filter is an aluminum disc located at the port of the tubehead where the PID is connected. The filter removes low-energy, long-wavelength x-rays, which may be absorbed by the patient but are not necessary for producing the radiograph.

By law, dental x-ray machines operating below 70 kilovolts (kV) must have 1.5 mm. of added aluminum filtration. Those with a kilovoltage of 70 or above must have 2.5 mm. of aluminum filtration. (A **kilovolt** is a unit of electrical force that equals 1000 volts.)

The additional filtration required for the higher kilovoltage machines is necessary because of the higher energy of the x-rays produced in these machines.

COLLIMATOR

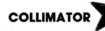

The collimator, like the filter, is a metal disc, usually lead, that has a small round opening in the center to control the size and shape of the x-ray beam as it leaves the tubehead.

The collimator limits the size of the x-ray beam to a circular 2¾ inches. When the size and shape of the beam are changed to a rectangle that is *just* slightly larger than the film, the amount of tissue exposed could be reduced by more than half.

The result of this collimation is a reduction in the amount of radiation to the patient, and the American Dental Association and the American Academy of Maxillofacial Radiology strongly recommend the use of rectangular collimation.

POSITION INDICATOR DEVICE

The PID, which is lead-lined, is used to aim the x-ray beam at the film in the patient's mouth, thereby minimizing the amount of radiation exposure to the patient.

The open end of the PID is placed against the patient's face during film exposure. The PID may be cylindrical or rectangular in shape. The rectangular PID limits the beam size to that of a number 2 size (periapical) dental film (Fig. 17–11).

PIDs used in dentistry are usually 8, 12, or 16 inches in length. The length selected is determined by the radiography technique being used.

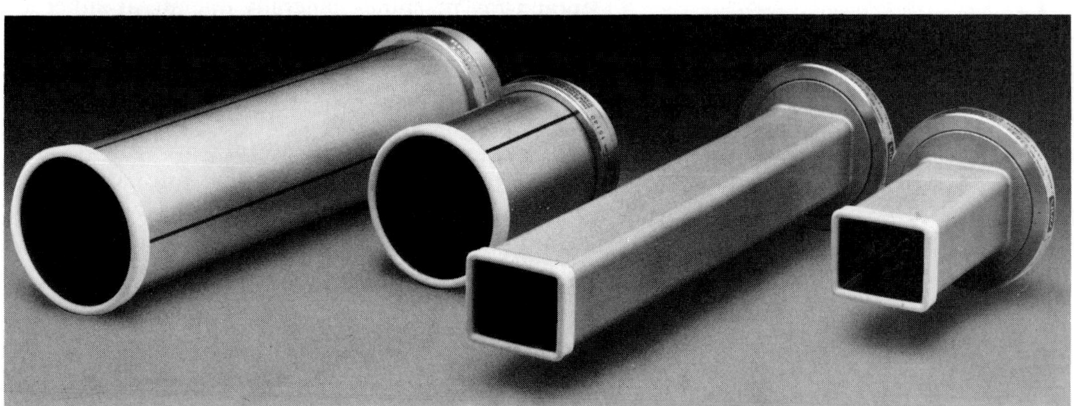

FIGURE 17–11

Lead-lined position indicator devices. These are available in round and rectangular shapes and in 8-, 12-, and 16-inch lengths. (Courtesy of Rinn Corporation, Elgin, IL.)

However, a long (12- to 16-inch) PID is more effective in reducing exposure to the patient than a short (8-inch) PID because there is less divergence of the beam.

The Extension Arm

The extension arm, which is hollow, encloses the wires between the tubehead to the control panel. It also has an important function in positioning the tubehead.

The tubehead is attached to the extension arm by means of a yoke that can be turned 360 degrees horizontally. (**Horizontally** means to move in a side-to-side motion.) In addition, the tubehead can be rotated vertically within the yoke. (**Vertically** means to move in an up-and-down motion.) This design permits maximum flexibility in positioning the tubehead.

The extension arm folds up and can be swiveled from side to side. If the extension arm is left in an extended position when the machine is not in use, the weight of the tubehead can cause it to become loose, and the tubehead will drift (slip out of position) after it is positioned for an exposure. This movement can cause a cone cut (central ray positioned off the film).

If the tubehead drifts, the arm should be repaired immediately. The patient or the auxiliary must *never* hold the tubehead in place during exposure.

The Control Panel

The control panel of an x-ray unit contains: the master switch and two indicator lights, exposure timer, milliamperage (mA) selector, and kilovoltage (kV) selector (Fig. 17–12). A single centrally located control panel may be used to operate several tubeheads located in separate treatment rooms.

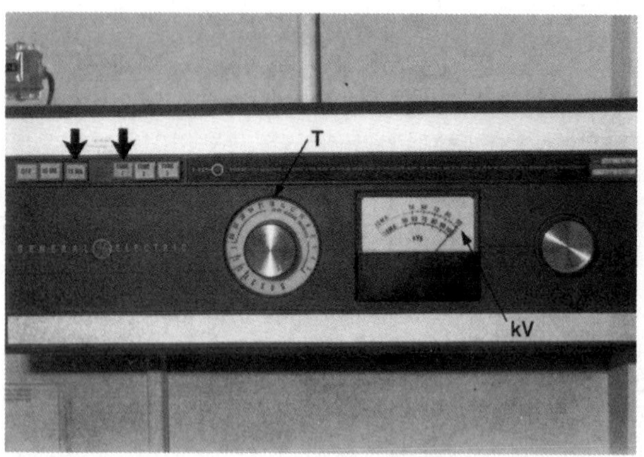

FIGURE 17–12

The control panel. The left arrow shows the button to set milliamps. The arrow next to it indicates the tubehead in use. T indicates the dial to set impulses for time. (From Miles, D.A., VanDis, M.L., Jensen, C.W., and Ferretti, A.: Radiographic Imaging for Dental Auxiliaries, 2nd ed. Philadelphia, W.B. Saunders Co., 1994, p 79.)

MASTER SWITCH AND INDICATOR LIGHTS

The **master switch** turns the machine on and off. An **indicator light** (orange) shows when the machine is on. The x-ray machine may be safely left on all day because is does not produce radiation unless the electronic timer is being pushed.

The red emission indicator light comes on *only* when the electronic timer is being pushed and radiation is being emitted.

EXPOSURE TIMER

The exposure timer controls the flow of electricity to generate the x-rays. The timer is electronically controlled to provide precise exposure time, and x-rays are generated *only* while the exposure timer is pressed.

The exposure time is measured in fractions of a second called **impulses**. Thirty impulses equal one-half second.

MILLIAMPERAGE SELECTOR

The **milliamperage (mA)** of a dental x-ray machine is a measure of the electric current that passes through a tungsten filament.

The **milliamperage selector** controls the number of electrons that are produced. Increasing the milliamperage increases the *quantity* of electrons available for the production of x-rays. The combination of milliamperage and the time of exposure in seconds is described as **milliamperage seconds** (mAs.) To calculate the mAs, the milliamperage used is multiplied by exposure time in seconds (mA × exposure time = mAs).

KILOVOLTAGE SELECTOR

The **kilovoltage** selector is used to control the penetrating power, or the *quality*, of the x-ray.

Dental x-ray machines generally operate at either 70 kV or 90 kV. The kV setting determines the contrast of the resulting film. (**Contrast** refers to the shades of gray on the x-ray film.)

- A 90-kV setting requires less exposure time and produces a radiograph that has low contrast.
- The 70-kV setting requires a slightly longer exposure time and produces a radiograph with high contrast.

Intraoral Dental X-Ray Film

Composition

Intraoral dental film consists of a semi-flexible plastic film base coated on both sides with an emulsion containing x-ray–sensitive crystals of silver bromide, silver halide, and silver iodide embedded in gelatin.

The image on the film is produced when radiation interacts with the chemicals in the film emulsion. (Before the film has been processed, this image, which is not visible, is known as the **latent image**.)

Film Packets

Because the emulsion is sensitive to light as well as to radiation, the film is enclosed in an opaque light-tight packet. The packet is also water resistant to prevent the patient's saliva from penetrating the packet and destroying the image.

The front of the packet has a small embossed dot, or a raised "bump." This side is always placed *toward* the PID. The back, which has the tab used for opening the packet before processing, is always placed *away* from the PID.

Within the packet, the film is protected on either side by a sheet of black paper (Fig. 17–13). In back, behind the black paper, there is a thin sheet of lead that absorbs most of the x-rays that pass through the film (thus protecting the patient) and also prevents film fog (a slight increase in darkness).

This lead sheet is embossed with a herringbone pattern. This pattern appears on the finished radiograph *only* if the film was positioned with its back toward the PID (see Fig. 17–37).

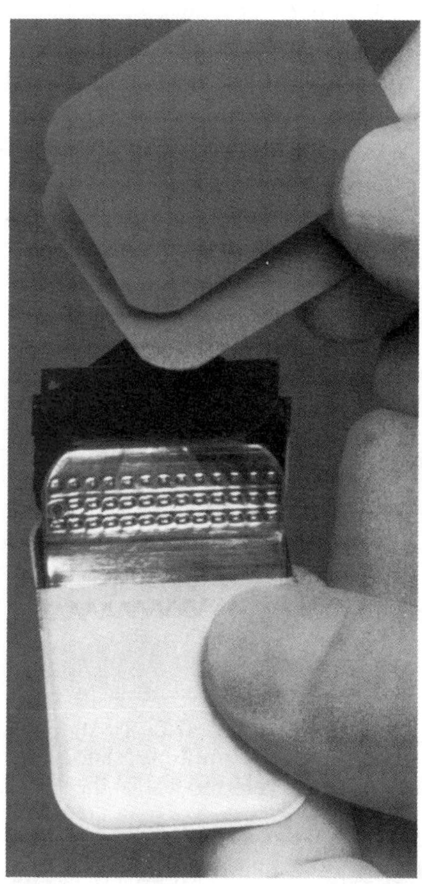

FIGURE 17–13

Contents of film packet: lead foil, x-ray film, and black paper. (From Miles, D.A., VanDis, M.L., Jensen, C.W., and Ferretti, A.: Radiographic Imaging for Dental Auxiliaries, 2nd ed. Philadelphia, W.B. Saunders Co., 1994, p 52.)

DOUBLE FILM PACKETS

Double film packets contain two pieces of film between the black paper lining. This makes it possible to produce an exact duplicate set of the films without exposing the patient to additional radiation.

Double film packets are useful when radiographs are requested by the insurance company or when a patient is referred to a specialist.

Film Speed

The film speed reflects the film's sensitivity to radiation and determines the amount of x-radiation needed to produce a diagnostic quality radiograph. The *faster* the film speed, the *less* radiation needed for each exposure.

Fast film speed is a major factor in reducing patient exposure to radiation, and dental film speed is rated in a range from A to E, A being slowest and E being the fastest. (These speeds are rated according to standards adapted by the American National Standards Institute [ANSI].)

In comparison with D speed, film speed E reduces the patient's radiation exposure by 50 percent. In dentistry, film slower than D should never be used, and the faster E film should be used whenever possible.

Film Sizes

Intraoral film packets come in five basic sizes (Fig. 17–14). These are numbered from 0 to 4, 0 being the smallest.

- Full mouth radiographic surveys for adults normally involve film sizes No. 1 and No. 2.
- Adult bite-wing surveys normally involve No. 2 film.
- For children younger than 3, film size No. 0 may be used.
- For occlusal radiographs, film size No. 4 is used.

Care of Dental Films

FILM STORAGE

All dental films should be stored according to the manufacturer's instructions. This includes storing them so that they are protected from light, heat, moisture, chemicals, and scatter radiation.

To avoid exposure from stray radiation, film kept in

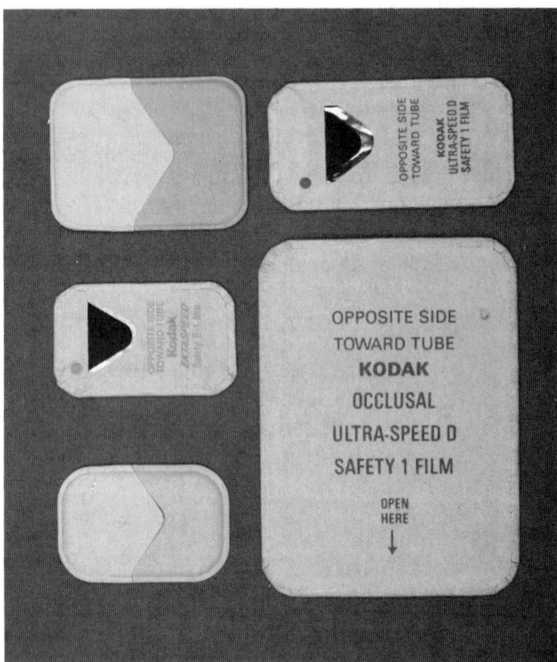

FIGURE 17–14

Commonly used sizes of dental x-ray film. Shown here is the back of the packet. This side is positioned *away from* the position indicator device (PID).

the treatment room or near the x-ray unit should be stored in a lead container.

The box of radiographic film is marked with an expiration date. The film should be used before that date. If it is not, the radiographs produced may be fogged and not of diagnostic quality. This effect is known as **age fog.**

FILM CARE DURING EXPOSURE

Never leave either exposed or unexposed films in the room where other radiographs are being exposed. This could result in the exposure of the films to scatter radiation and can cause film fog, which reduces the diagnostic value.

Films to be exposed are dispensed before the radiographic procedure begins. They are placed on a clean towel or cup just outside the room where the radiographs are to be exposed.

A paper cup labeled with the patient's name and the date is used to store the films as they are exposed. This cup is placed just outside the room where the radiographs are to be exposed. When film exposure has been completed, the films are transported in this cup to the processing area.

Image Characteristics

Two very important terms are used in discussing the characteristics of a radiographic image: **radiolucent** and **radiopaque** (Fig. 17–15).

Radiolucent means that the substance allows radiant energy to pass through it. A radiolucent substance appears to be *black* on the radiograph. Air, soft tissues of the body, and the dental pulp are radiolucent. They appear as black or dark gray areas.

Radiopaque means that the substance does *not* allow radiant energy to pass through it. A radiopaque substance appears to be *white* on the radiograph. Metal, enamel, and dense areas of bone are radiopaque. They appear as white or light gray areas.

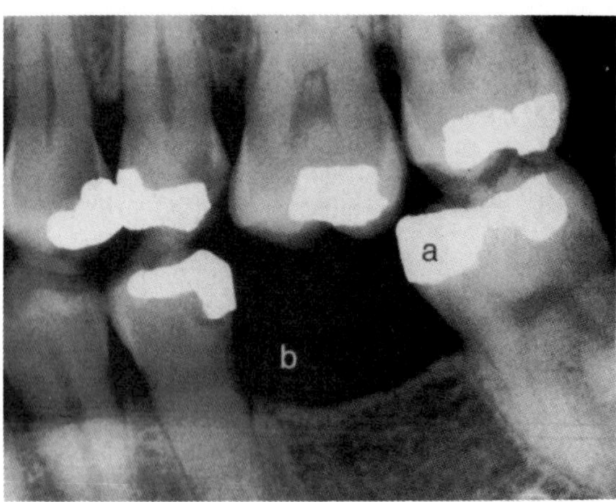

FIGURE 17–15

Radiolucent and radiopaque objects in a bite-wing radiograph. The white (radiopaque) area marked *a* is an amalgam restoration. The black (radiolucent) area marked *b* is air and soft tissue of the cheek. (From Miles, D.A., VanDis, M.L., Jensen, C.W., and Ferretti, A.: Radiographic Imaging for Dental Auxiliaries, 2nd ed. Philadelphia, W.B. Saunders Co., 1994, p 94.)

Radiographic Quality

The factors that influence how much diagnostic information the dentist is able to gain for the amount of radiation expended are contrast, density, image detail, and image distortion.

CONTRAST

The image on a radiograph appears in a range of shades from black to white with multiple shades of gray in between. This range is referred to as the **gray scale** (Fig. 17–16).

The differences between the shades of gray is called the **contrast**. The ideal contrast of a film clearly shows the white of a radiopaque metal restoration, the radiolucent black of air, and the many shades of gray between.

The amount of contrast in a film must also reflect the dentist's preferences. Some dentists prefer radiographs with more contrast, whereas others prefer low

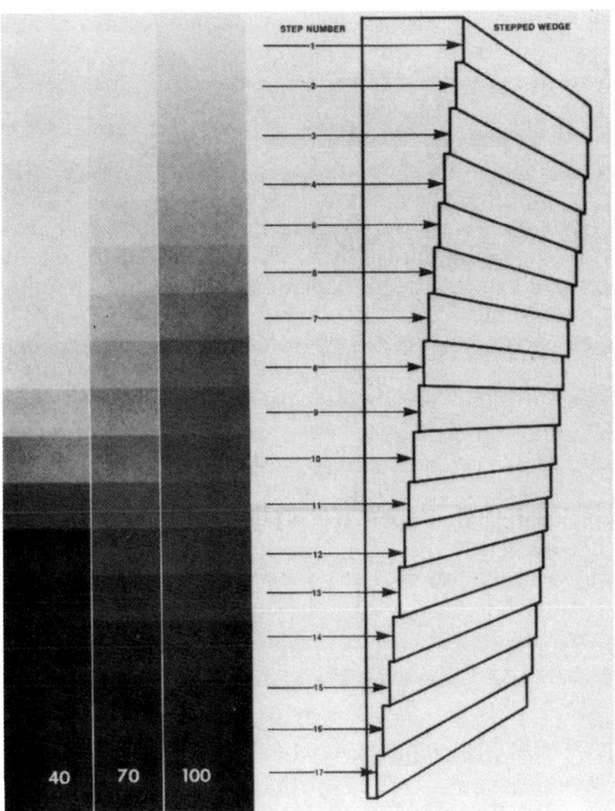

FIGURE 17–16

Contrast is affected by kilovolts. X-rays taken at 40 kV are mostly black and white (a short scale of contrast). They have high contrast. Those taken at 100 kV show many shades of gray (a long gray scale.) Shown at the right is a stepped wedge, which is a device used to measure contrast in radiographs. (From Miles, D.A., VanDis, M.L., Jensen, C.W., and Ferretti, A.: Radiographic Imaging for Dental Auxiliaries, 2nd ed. Philadelphia, W.B. Saunders Co., 1994, p 99.)

contrast. The two basic factors affecting the contrast of a film are

1. The kVp during the exposure: higher kilovoltages produce more penetrating x-rays and lower radiographic contrast.
2. The temperature of the developer solution: higher film-developing temperature produces higher contrast.

DENSITY

Density is the degree of overall darkness of a film. The degree of density is determined by the following factors (Table 17–4):

- The amount of radiation reaching the film
- The distance from the x-ray tube to the patient
- The processing times and temperatures
- The patient thickness

The term *patient thickness* refers to the patient's body size. For example, a small child or a thin elderly person would require less radiation than a husky, heavy boned individual.

IMAGE DETAIL

An x-ray image is said to have good image detail, also referred to as *sharpness*, if small objects can be easily identified in the film without distortion. (**Distortion** is a change in shape or dimension.)

In general, intraoral films have greater detail than extraoral films. The quality of image detail is determined by focal spot size, contrast, and the factors that influence film distortion.

Focal Spot Size. The smaller the focal spot size at the anode, the better the image detail. The dentist has no control over the focal spot size, except when purchasing an x-ray machine. Newer dental x-ray machines are equipped with the smallest focal spot possible.

IMAGE DISTORTION

Image distortion is influenced by object-film distance, source-film distance, and movement. (As used here, **distortion** means not accurately showing position, length or width.)

Object-Film Distance. The term **object-film distance** (OFD) describes the distance between the object (teeth) being radiographed and the radiographic film.

Casting an image of teeth onto a dental radiograph is like the game of "shadow casting" with your hands. If you move your hand nearer to the screen and away from the light source, the shadow is close to the actual size. If you move your hand away from the screen and nearer to the light source, the image is magnified (larger) but distorted.

In dental radiography, placing the film near the teeth reduces the OFD. Having the film close to the object reduces the distortion or lack of sharpness that results when the film is at a greater distance from the object.

Source-Film Distance. Source-film distance (SFD) refers to how far the source of radiation (tubehead) is

TABLE 17–4

Factors Affecting the Density of a Radiograph

FACTOR	DENSITY EFFECT
Kilovoltage	Density increases with kVp
Milliamperage	Density increases with mA
Exposure time	Density increases with time
Film	Density increases with film speed
Developing time	Density increases with time
Developing temperature	Density increases with temperature
Fixing time	Density decreases with overfixing
Patient size	Density decreases with thickness
Source-film distance (SFD)	Density decreases with SFD

from the film. Increasing the SFD reduces distortion due to magnification.

If a film cannot be placed close to the teeth, the image can be made sharper by increasing the SFD and then placing the object and film parallel to each other and positioning the central ray perpendicular to them.

Movement. Movement of the patient, film, or tubehead can result in an image that is blurred (not sharp). Therefore, it is very important that the patient remain still and not disturb the film during the exposure. When properly maintained, the tubehead and arm do not vibrate or drift out of position. If they do move during use, they should be serviced immediately to correct this problem.

Basic Principles of Intraoral Radiography

Types of Intraoral Radiographs

There are three types of intraoral radiographs: periapical, bite-wing, and occlusal.

PERIAPICAL RADIOGRAPHS

Periapical radiographs record images of the entire length of the teeth plus 3 to 4 mm. of supporting tissues beyond the apex. Periapical films are used to interpret normal anatomy and pathology in the crown, root area, and surrounding bony structures.

BITE-WING RADIOGRAPHS

Bite-wing radiographs show images of the crowns and interproximal regions of the maxillary and mandibular teeth on the same film. Root structure is not visible on these films. (A bite-wing radiograph is shown in Figure 17–15.)

This type of radiograph is used to reveal interproximal or recurrent carious lesions, overhanging restorations, calculus, crestal bone levels, internal pulpal pathology, and occlusal relationships.

A **bite-wing survey (BWX)** normally consists of two or four posterior films. In a two-film survey, one film is centered on the premolar and molar region on both left and right sides of the patient. In a four-film survey, a film is centered on the premolar region and another on the molar region on both left and right sides of the patient.

OCCLUSAL RADIOGRAPHS

Occlusal radiographs record images of one entire arch on a single film (Fig. 17–17). This type of radiograph is useful for locating supernumerary, unerupted, and impacted teeth. Occlusal films are used in some pediatric dental offices when periapical radiographs are difficult to take.

Intraoral Radiography Techniques

The two most frequently used intraoral dental radiography techniques are the bisecting angle technique and the paralleling technique (Fig. 17–18).

PRINCIPLES OF THE BISECTING ANGLE TECHNIQUE

The bisecting angle technique is based on a geometric principle of bisecting a triangle. (**Bisecting** means dividing into two equal parts.)

In this technique, the film is placed directly against

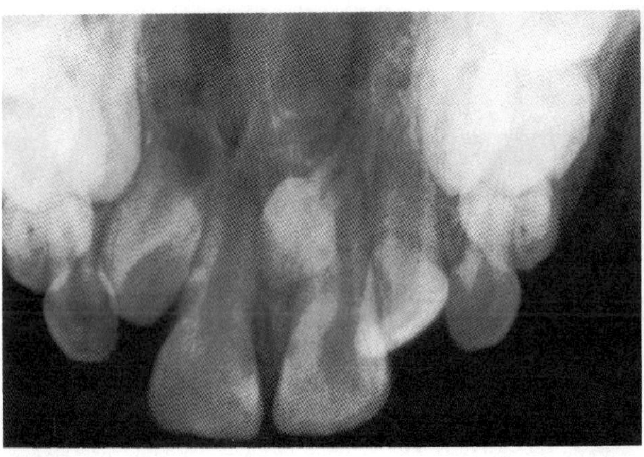

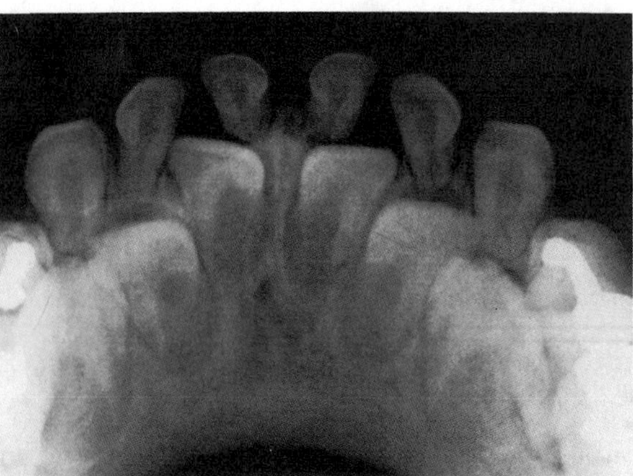

FIGURE 17–17

Occlusal radiographs of 4-year-old child. On the left is the maxillary view. On the right is the mandibular view. (From Miles, D.A., VanDis, M.L., Jensen, C.W., and Ferretti, A.: Radiographic Imaging for Dental Auxiliaries, 2nd ed. Philadelphia, W.B. Saunders Co., 1994, p 8.)

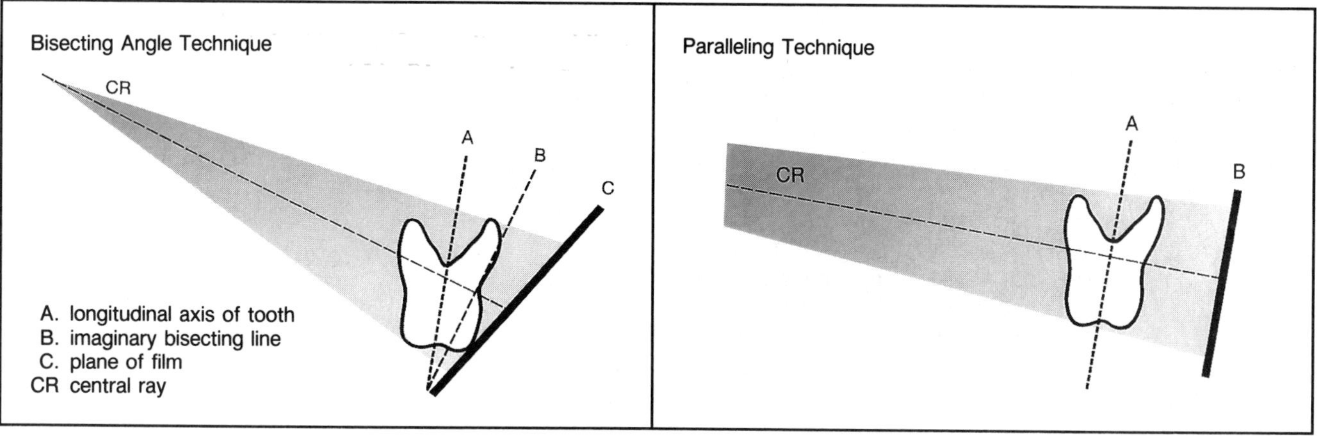

FIGURE 17–18

Intraoral radiographic techniques compared. *A* is the long axis of the tooth; *B* is the imaginary bisecting line; *C* is the plane of the film; and *CR* is the central ray. (Courtesy of Rinn Corporation, Elgin, IL.)

the teeth to be radiographed. The angle that is formed by the long axes of the teeth and the film is bisected, and the x-ray beam is directed perpendicular to the bisecting line. (**Perpendicular** means at a right angle.)

The bisecting angle technique uses a short SFD. This is a PID length of only 7 or 8 inches, and for this reason, this is also referred to as the *short cone technique.*

The bisecting angle technique produces dimensional distortion and increased radiation to the patient. This is because the shorter SFD results in greater magnification of the image and causes the x-ray beam to cover a greater area of the head, thus adding to the patient's absorbed dose.

The distortion is an inherent characteristic of the technique and cannot be totally avoided even when the bisecting angle principle is used by the most skillful operators.

Elongation and Foreshortening

Two very common errors that occur in the bisecting technique are elongation and foreshortening (see Fig. 17–37). The cause of these two errors can be compared to the position of the sun in the sky.

Elongation (lengthening of the image on the film) can be caused by inadequate vertical angulation or improper patient position. When the sun is low in the sky, your shadow is long (elongated).

Foreshortening (shortening of the image on the film) is usually caused by excessive vertical angulation. When the sun is high in the sky, your shadow is short (foreshortened).

Applications of the Bisecting Angle Technique

Bisecting angle technique is not recommended as a standard technique, but it does have a place in dental radiography in some circumstances. For example, difficult or unusual anatomy, small children, and some endodontic films may require the use of this technique.

PRINCIPLES OF THE PARALLELING TECHNIQUE

The paralleling technique is used in dental radiography to minimize image distortion and to reduce x-radiation dose to the patient's head and neck.

The geometric principle of this technique is to place the film parallel to the long axes of the teeth to be radiographed while aiming the central x-ray beam at right angles to both the film and the teeth. In this text, the paralleling technique is considered to be the method of choice.

Application of the Paralleling Technique

Important factors to be considered in exposing periapical radiographs include the dental chair position; film position and placement; point of entry of the x-ray beam; vertical and horizontal angulation; and the use of film-holding instruments.

Dental Chair Position. The dental chair is positioned so the midsagittal plane of the patient's head is perpendicular to the floor (Fig. 17–19*A*). For most exposures, this means that the patient is seated in an upright position.

This position is adjusted so that the occlusal plane of the jaw being radiographed is parallel to the floor when the film packet is in position (Fig. 17–19*B*).

In the maxilla, this plane corresponds to the ala-tragus line on the face (Fig. 17–19*C*). In the mandible, this is the occlusal plane of the teeth with the jaw open.

Film Position and Placement. The film packet is placed in a vertical position for anterior projections and in a horizontal position for posterior periapical projections. The film is held in position by the patient closing on a bite-block or other film-holding device.

The film is placed so that the raised dot is toward the occlusal surface and facing the PID. This places the front of the packet toward the PID, prevents the dots from being superimposed over the apex of a tooth, and later aids in mounting the processed film.

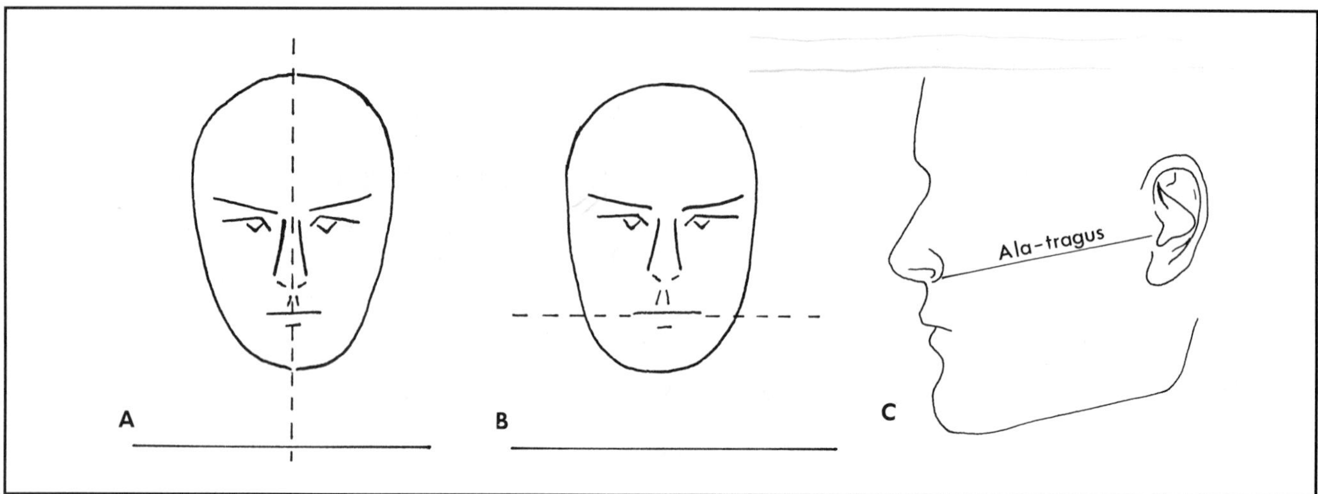

FIGURE 17–19

Planes used for guidance in positioning the patient's head. *A*, Midsagittal plane. *B*, Occlusal plane. *C*, Ala-tragus plane. (Courtesy of Drs. Stephen Taylor and C.R. Parks, University of California School of Dentistry, San Francisco, CA.)

The film position must be parallel to the *whole tooth*, not just parallel to the crown. This is an important concept to understand. Although the crowns of the teeth appear to tilt one way, the entire structure actually tilts another.

For example, the apices of the most of the maxillary teeth tilt inward toward the palate. The mandibular premolars are more nearly vertical, and the mandibular molars tilt inward slightly.

Point of Entry. The point of entry is the position on the patient's face at which the central x-ray beam is aimed. The goal is to completely cover only the film with the beam of radiation.

Vertical Angulation. The vertical angulation is the movement of the tubehead in an up-and-down direction, similar to shaking your head "yes." In the paralleling technique, the vertical angulation must be perpendicular to the film *and* to the long axes of the teeth.

Horizontal Angulation. The horizontal angulation is the movement of the tubehead in a side-to-side direction, similar to shaking your head "no." In the paralleling technique, the horizontal angulation of the x-ray beam must be directed through the contacts of the teeth and be as perpendicular to the horizontal plane of the film as possible.

Film-Holding Instruments

The paralleling technique requires the use of film-holding instruments to place and keep the film packet in its proper position in relation to the tooth. One of the most commonly used types is the Rinn XCP (extension cone paralleling) instrument (Fig. 17–20).

In addition to film positioning, these instruments include a **localizing ring**, also known as an *aiming*

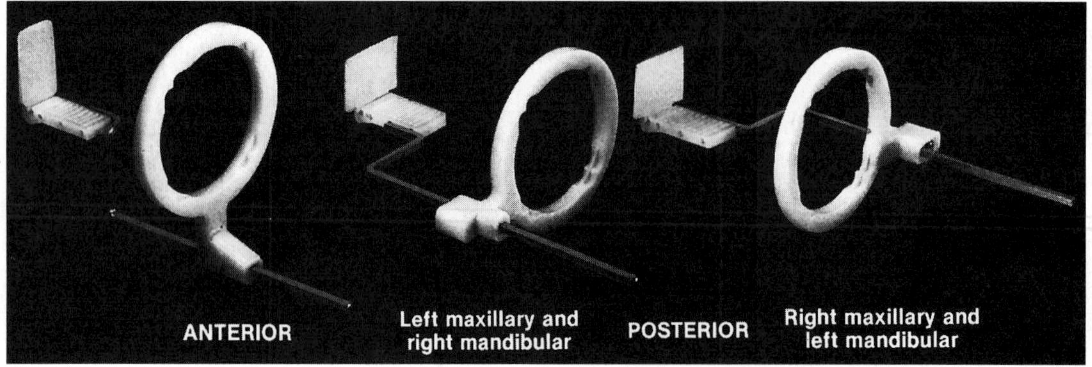

FIGURE 17–20

XCP holding instruments for paralleling technique. (Courtesy of Rinn Corporation, Elgin, IL.)

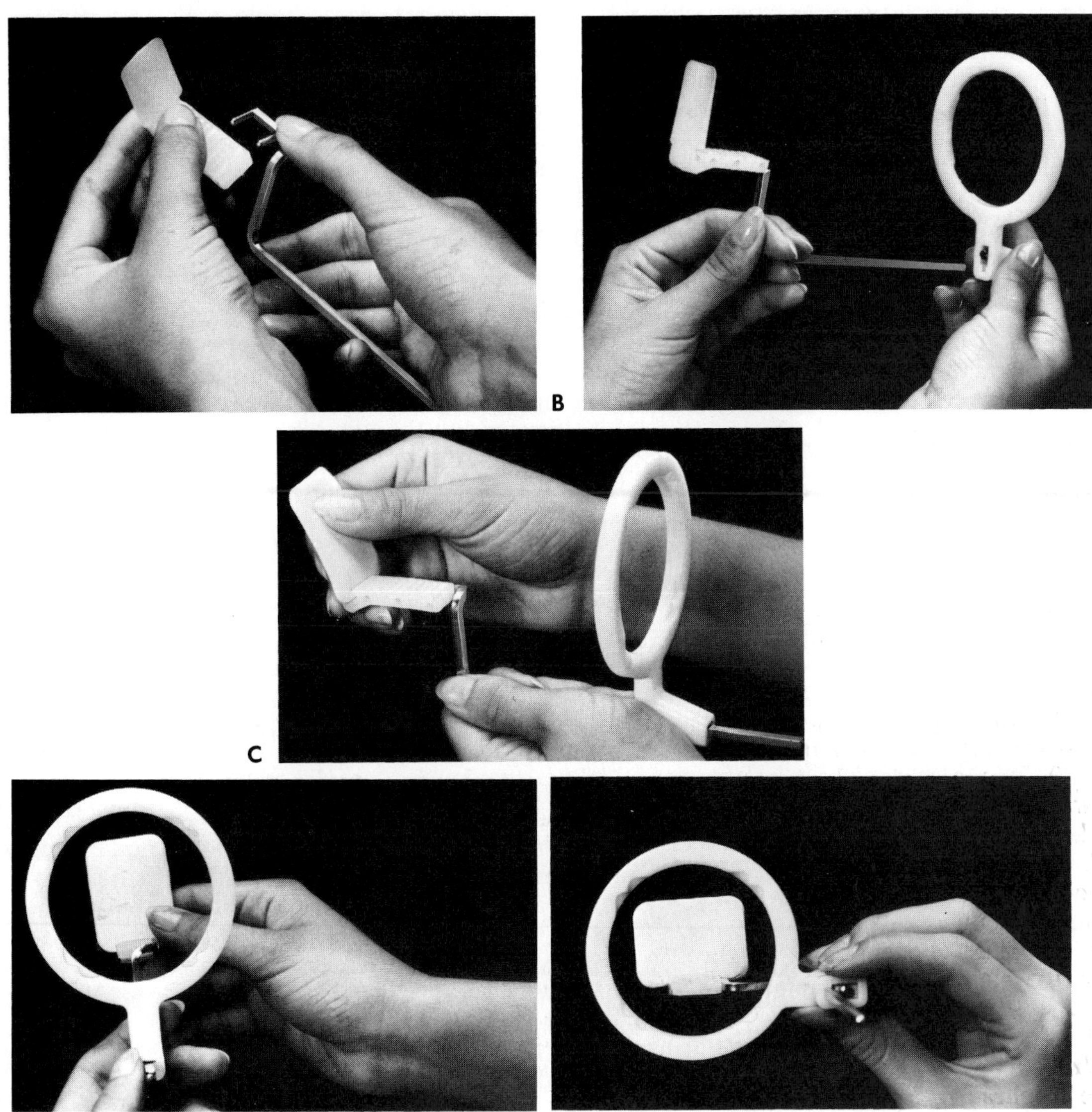

FIGURE 17–21

Demonstrating assembling XCP instruments for paralleling technique. *A*, Insert the two prongs of the indicator rod into the bite block. On three-hole blocks, use the forward holes (away from the backing plate). Use the third opening when the bite block is shortened for use with children. *B*, Insert indicator rod into the aiming ring slot. *C*, Flex the backing plate of the bite block to open the film slot for easy insertion of the film packet. *D*, Assembly is correct when film can be seen through aiming ring on "target." (Courtesy of Rinn Corporation, Elgin, IL.)

ring, which facilitates aligning the PID with the film in both the horizontal and vertical planes. This increases accuracy and reduces the need for retakes.

The procedures that follow include the use of the XCP holding instruments; however, the basic principles of placement and paralleling are similar regardless of the film-holding instrument that is used.

Guidelines for Use of Film-Holding Instruments

The steps in assembling this equipment are demonstrated in Figure 17–21. (If this were an actual treatment situation, the assistant would be gloved.) As shown here, the arrangement of the holder and film depends upon the teeth being radiographed; however, the following principles apply to all views.

1. Assemble the instrument appropriately for the area to be radiographed.
2. Place the side of the film that does *not* have the raised dot toward the backing plate. (This is the side with the tab for opening of the packet.)
3. Use the *entire* horizontal length of the bite-block to position the film as far away from the teeth as possible.
4. Place the bite-block on the incisal or occlusal surfaces of the teeth being radiographed.

5. Instruct the patient to close slowly but firmly to retain position of the film packet.
6. To increase patient comfort, a cotton roll may be placed between the bite-block and the teeth of the opposite arch.
7. When the film is in place, slide the localizer ring down the indicator rod to the skin surface. Align the PID so that it is centered and in close approximation to the aiming ring.
8. Expose the radiograph and remove the film from the patient's mouth.

Guidelines for Patient Comfort During Dental Radiography

1. Set the timer and exposure controls before the film is placed.
   □ **Rationale**: The patient should not have to wait with film in his mouth while the operator makes these adjustments.
2. Position the film in the patient's mouth for as short a time as possible.
   □ **Rationale**: This increases patient comfort and decreases the likelihood of gagging and patient movement.
3. Start with anterior films, which normally do not trigger the gag reflex.
   □ **Rationale**: This lets the patient become accustomed to the procedure without danger of gagging.
4. If necessary, gently curve or "roll" the film to allow the film to follow the contours of the patient's anatomy.
   □ **Caution**: Do not actually bend the film. This will cause distortion of the film.
5. Observe the patient from behind a barrier during exposure.
   □ **Rationale:** If the patient moves, the film will be blurred and a retake will be necessary.
6. After the exposure has been made, remove the film from the patient's mouth and place the exposed film in the paper cup labeled with the patient's name and date.

MANAGEMENT OF THE PATIENT WHO GAGS

Skillful placement of the film helps to reduce patient gagging; however, for those patients in whom this is still a problem, the following steps may help:

- Have the patient take several deep breaths and then breathe out through his nose while the film is being placed.
- Distract the patient by asking him to concentrate on something other than the procedure at hand.
- A liquid topical anesthetic to numb the gag reflex may be used just before the films are exposed.

Producing a Full Mouth Radiographic Survey

A full mouth radiographic survey (FMX), also referred to as an *intraoral complete series*, is composed of a number of periapical and bite-wing radiographs.

Each of the following landmarks or structures must appear *at least once*, somewhere on the survey:

- Every crown
- Every apex
- Every contact (interproximal) area
- 3 to 4 mm. of supporting structure periapically
- Edentulous areas

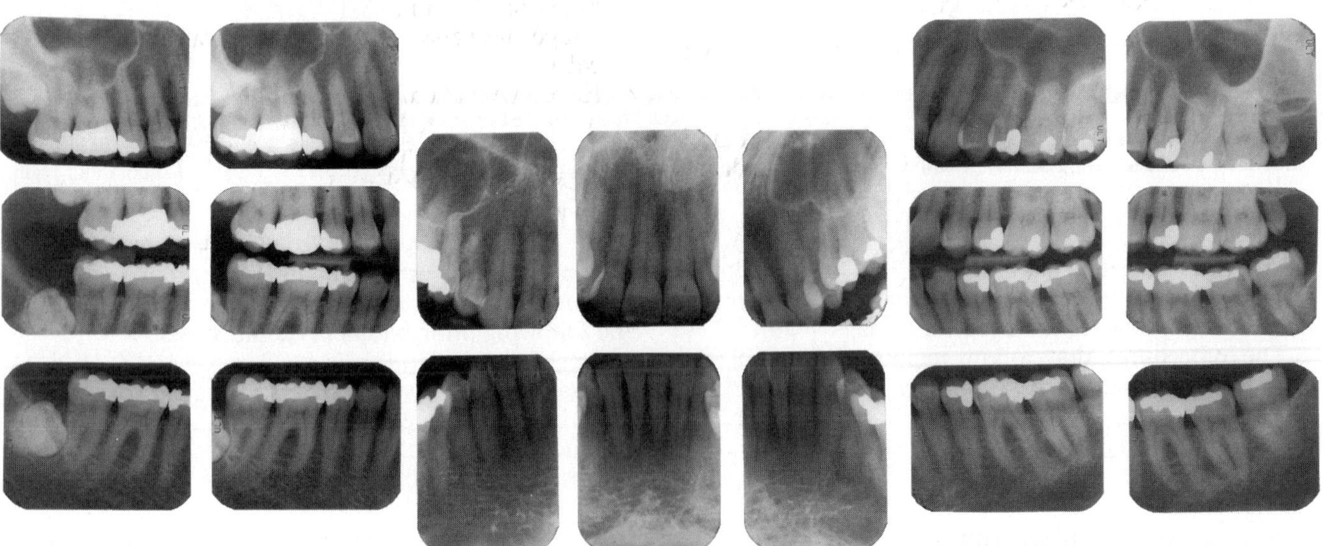

FIGURE 17–22

Complete radiographic survey with bite-wings.

The number and size of the film to be used depends upon the dentist's instructions, which take into consideration

- Number of teeth present
- Size of the oral cavity
- Anatomic structures within the mouth
- Age of the patient
- Level of patient cooperation

To complete the full mouth survey, an operator may expose as few as 10 or as many as 18 periapical films, plus whatever bite-wing films are indicated.

In exposing a full mouth series of radiographs, always follow a definite order. Skipping from one area to another without a pattern will result in an omitted film. Also, take care not to mix unexposed film with those that have been exposed. This could result in a double exposure.

The procedure described here includes positioning and steps for each exposure in one half of the maxillary arch and one half of the mandibular arch with the use of the paralleling technique, XCP film instrument, and a round PID.

When the opposite side of each arch is radiographed, the same procedures are followed. The completed radiographic survey is shown in Figure 17–22.

(text continued on page 319)

PROCEDURE: **Producing a Full Mouth Radiographic Survey**

Instrumentation

Appropriate number and size of radiographic films
Paper cup
Lead apron and thyroid collar
Sterile XCP instruments
Cotton rolls
Patient chart

Preparation Before Seating the Patient

1. Turn on the x-ray machine and check the basic settings (mA, kV, and exposure time).
2. Place all necessary barriers.
   □ *RATIONALE:* Anything that is touched and was not covered with a barrier must be disinfected after the patient is dismissed.
3. Assemble the sterile film-holding instruments.
4. Determine the number and type of films to be taken. This is accomplished by reviewing the patient's chart and/or is based on directions from the dentist.
5. Dispense the desired number of films and store them outside of the room where the x-ray machine is being used.
   □ *RATIONALE:* This prevents fogging caused by scatter radiation.
6. Label a paper cup with the patient's name and the date, and place this outside of the room where the x-ray machine is to be used.
   □ *RATIONALE:* This is the transfer cup for storing and moving exposed films.

Positioning the Patient

1. Seat the patient comfortably in the dental chair, with the back in an upright position and the head supported.
2. Ask the patient to remove any eyeglasses or bulky earrings.
   □ *RATIONALE:* Failure to do this can result in radiopaque images of these items being superimposed on the film.
3. Drape the patient with a lead apron and thyroid collar.
4. Have the patient remove any removable prosthetic appliances from his mouth.
5. Position the occlusal plane of the jaw being radiographed parallel to the floor when it is in the open position.
6. When preparations are complete, wash your hands and put on clean examination gloves before exposing the radiographs.

Maxillary Central/Lateral Incisor Region

1. Insert the No. 1 film packet vertically into the anterior block. (An alternative technique is to use No. 2 film and center the two central incisors on the film.)
2. Center the film packet between the central and lateral incisors, and position the film as posteriorly as possible.
3. With the instrument and film in place, instruct the patient to close slowly but firmly.

PROCEDURE: **Producing a Full Mouth Radiographic Survey** *(continued)*

4. Position the localizing ring and PID, and then expose the radiograph (Fig. 17–23).

Maxillary Cuspid Region

1. Insert the No. 1 film packet vertically into the anterior bite-block. (If No. 2 film is used, slightly roll the upper anterior corner of the film packet to facilitate positioning.)
2. Position the film packet with the cuspid and first premolar centered. Position film as far posteriorly as possible.
3. With the instrument and film in place, instruct the patient to close slowly but firmly.
4. Position the localizing ring and PID, and then expose the radiograph (Fig. 17–24).
   □ *NOTE:* The image of the lingual cusp of the first premolar is often superimposed on the distal surface of the cuspid. This is because of the curvature of the maxillary arch. This contact area must be "opened" on the view of the premolar region.

Maxillary Premolar Region

1. Insert the film packet horizontally into the posterior bite-block, pushing the film packet all the way into the slot.
2. Center the film packet on the second premolar. Position film in the midpalatal area.
3. With the instrument and film in place, instruct the patient to close slowly but firmly.
4. Position the localizing ring and PID, and then expose the radiograph (Fig. 17–25).

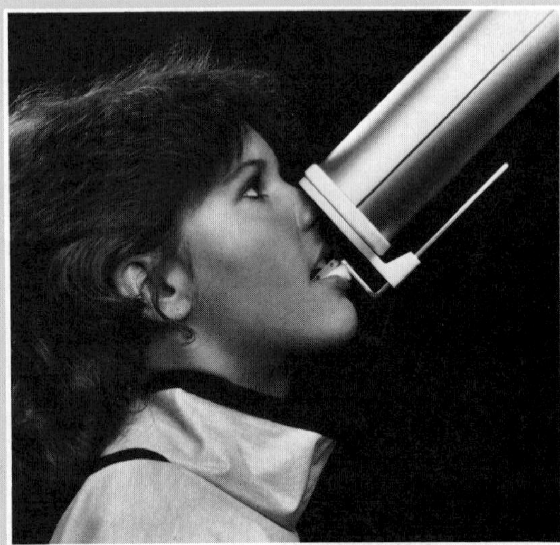

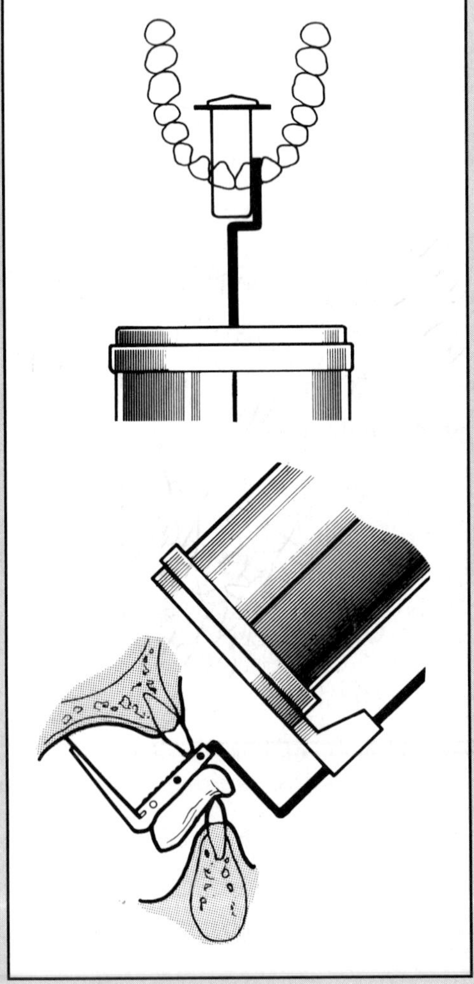

FIGURE 17–23

Maxillary central incisor region. (Courtesy of Rinn Corporation, Elgin, IL.)

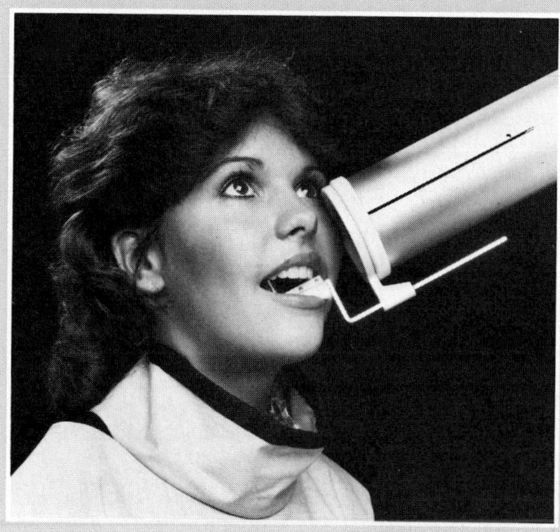

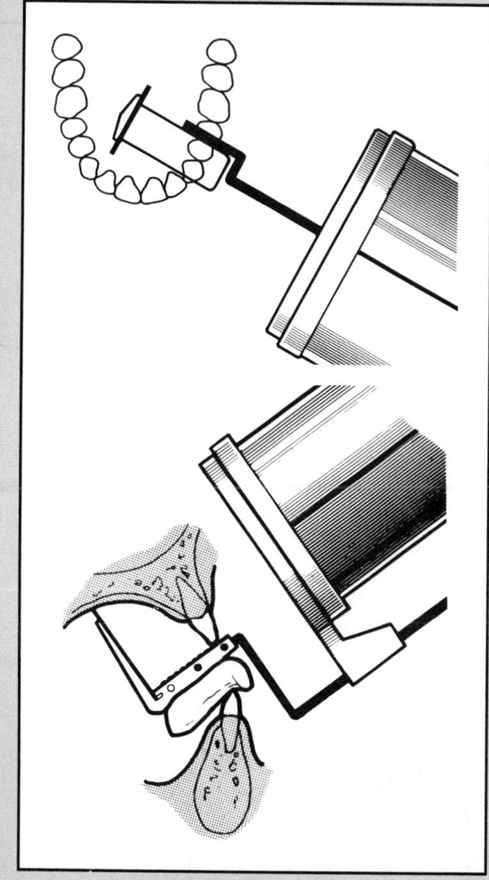

FIGURE 17–24

Maxillary cuspid region. (Courtesy of Rinn Corporation, Elgin, IL.)

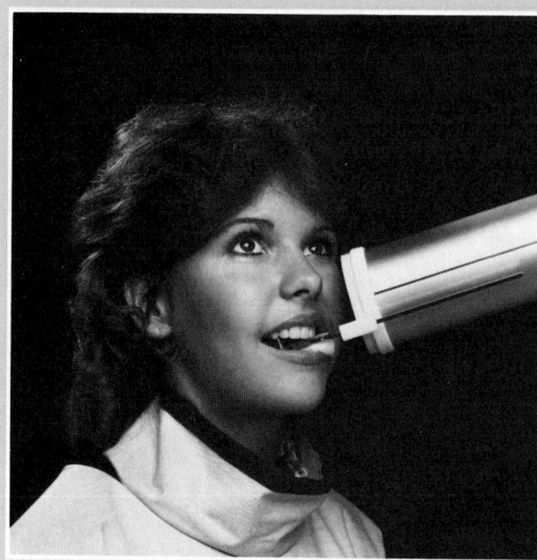

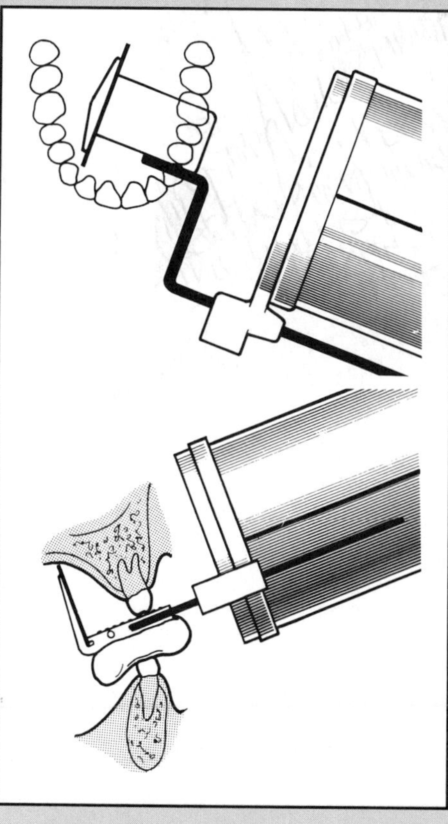

FIGURE 17–25

Maxillary premolar region. (Courtesy of Rinn Corporation, Elgin, IL.)

(continued on following page)

PROCEDURE: Producing a Full Mouth Radiographic Survey *(continued)*

Maxillary Molar Region

1. Insert the film packet horizontally into the posterior bite-block.
2. Center the film packet on the second molar. Position the film in the midpalatal area.
3. With the instrument and film in place, instruct the patient to close slowly but firmly.
4. Position the localizing ring and PID, then expose the radiograph (Fig. 17–26).

Mandibular Central/Lateral Incisor Region

1. Insert the No. 1 film packet vertically into the anterior bite-block. (When using No. 2 film, slightly roll the lower anterior corners to facilitate positioning.)
2. Center the film packet between the central incisors. Position the film as far in the lingual direction as the patient's anatomy will allow.
3. With the instrument and film in place, instruct the patient to close slowly but firmly.
4. Slide the localizing ring down the indicator rod to the patient's skin surface.
5. Position the localizing ring and PID, and then expose the radiograph (Fig. 17–27).

Mandibular Cuspid Region

1. Insert the No. 1 film packet vertically into the anterior bite-block. (When using No. 2 film, slightly roll the lower anterior corners to facilitate positioning.)
2. Center the film on the cuspid. Position the film as far in the lingual direction as the patient's anatomy will allow.
3. A cotton roll may be placed between the maxillary teeth and bite-block to prevent rocking of the bite-block on the cuspid tip and to increase patient comfort.
4. With the instrument and film in place, instruct the patient to close slowly but firmly.
5. Slide the localizing ring down the indicator rod to the patient's skin surface.
6. Position the localizing ring and PID, and then expose the radiograph (Fig. 17–28).

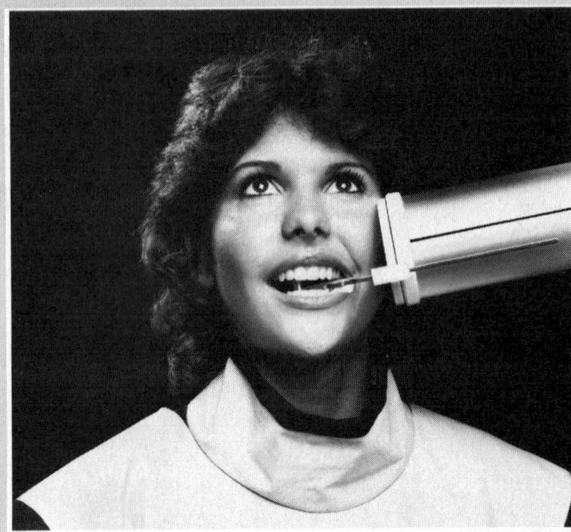

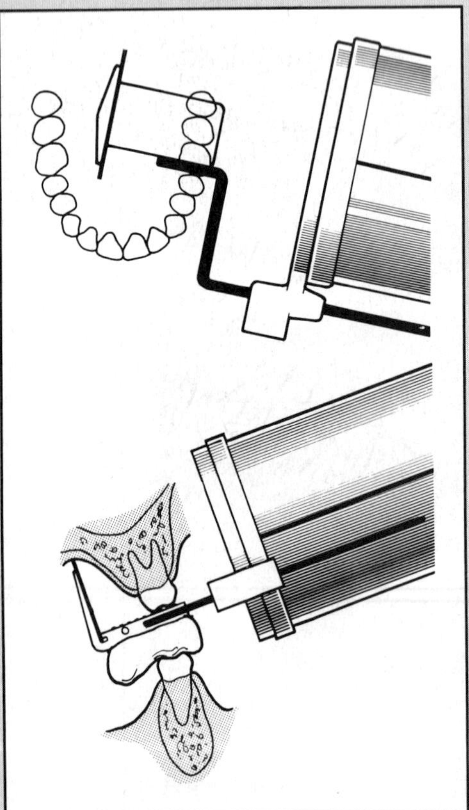

FIGURE 17–26

Maxillary molar region. (Courtesy of Rinn Corporation, Elgin, IL.)

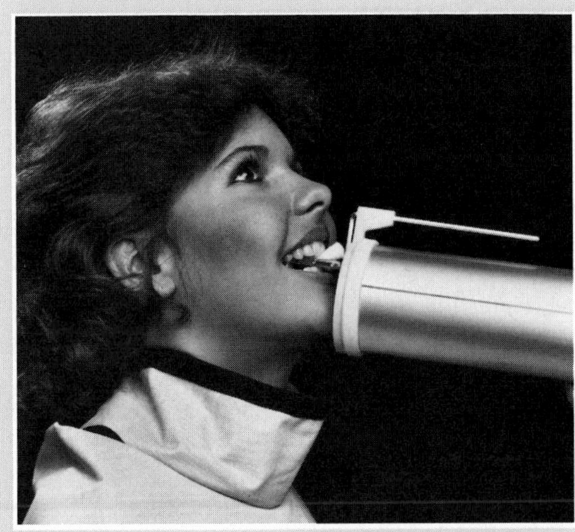

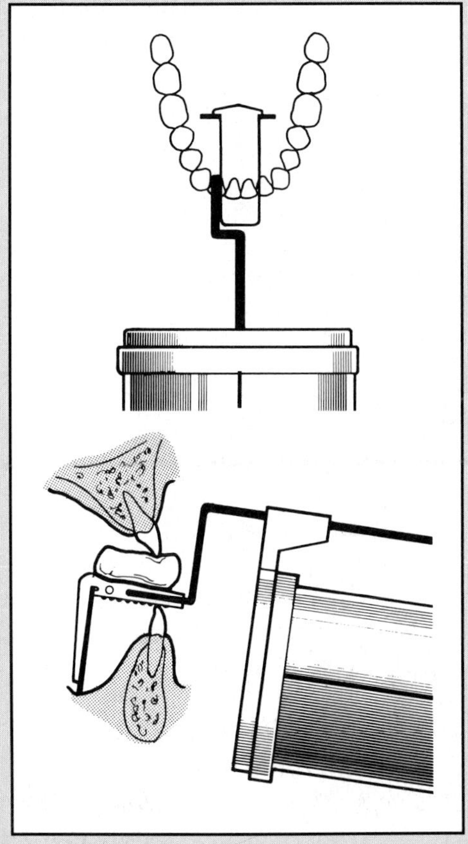

FIGURE 17–27

Mandibular incisor region. (Courtesy of Rinn Corporation, Elgin, IL.)

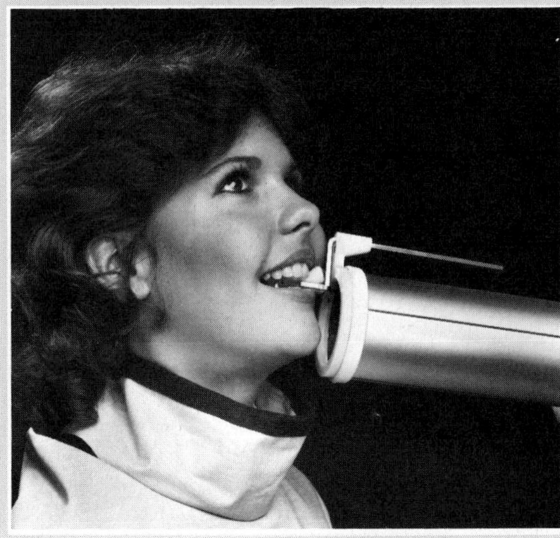

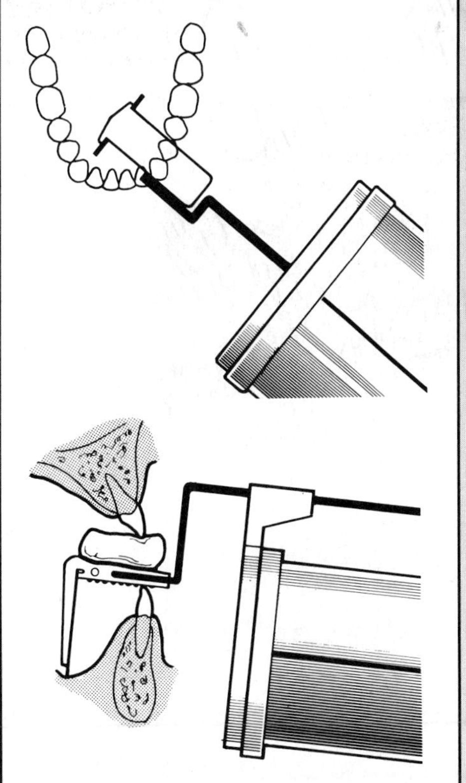

FIGURE 17–28

Mandibular cuspid region. (Courtesy of Rinn Corporation, Elgin, IL.)

(continued on following page)

PROCEDURE: **Producing a Full Mouth Radiographic Survey** *(continued)*

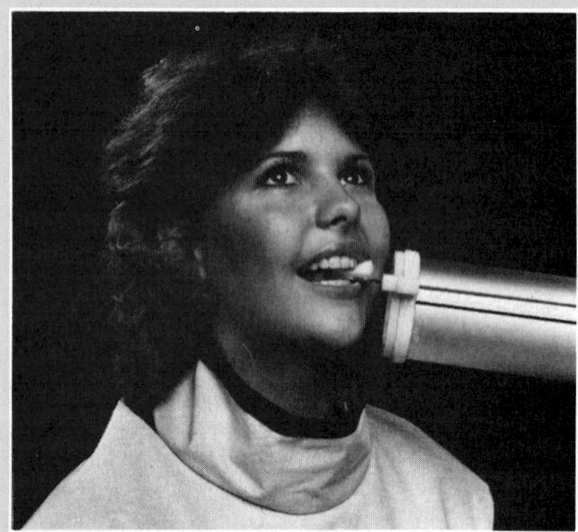

FIGURE 17–29

Mandibular premolar region. (Courtesy of Rinn Corporation, Elgin, IL.)

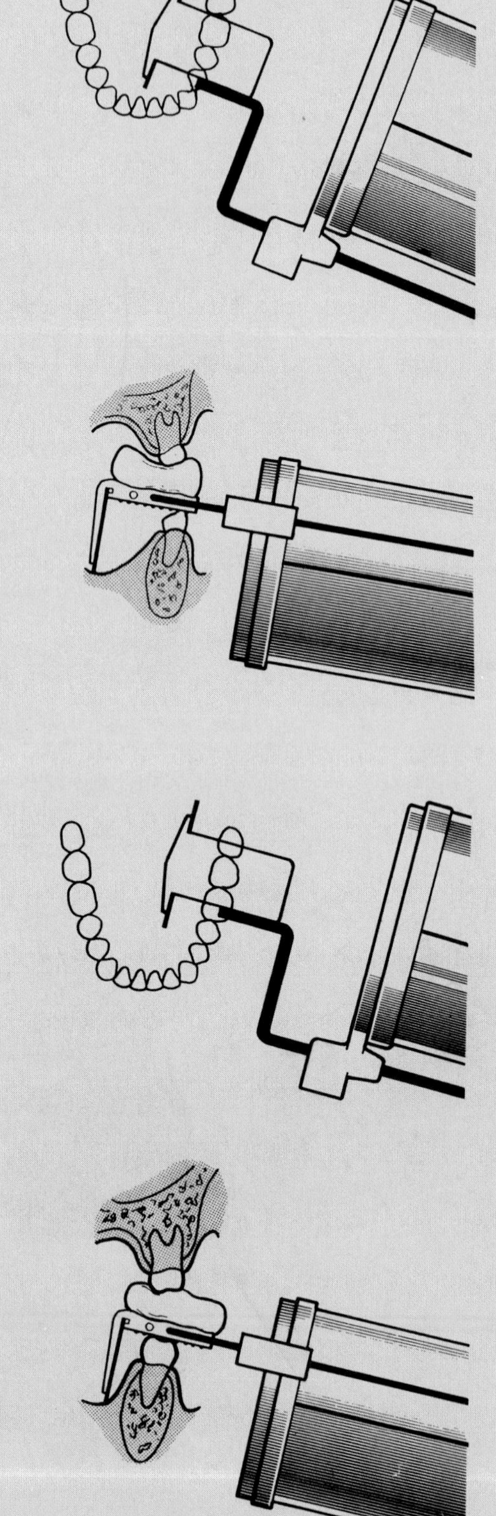

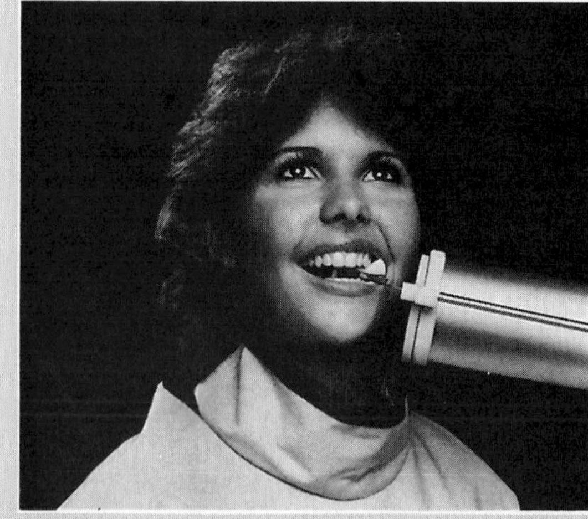

FIGURE 17–30

Mandibular molar region. (Courtesy of Rinn Corporation, Elgin, IL.)

Mandibular Premolar Region

1. Insert the No. 2 film horizontally into the posterior bite-block.
2. Center the film on the contact point between the second premolar and first molar. Position the film as far lingually as the patient's anatomy will allow.
3. With the instrument and film in place, instruct the patient to close slowly but firmly.
4. Slide the localizing ring down the indicator rod to the patient's skin surface.
5. Position the localizing ring and PID, and then expose the radiograph (Fig. 17–29).

Mandibular Molar Region

1. Insert the No. 2 film horizontally into the posterior bite-block.
2. Center the film on the second molar. Position the film as far lingually as the tongue will allow. This position will be closer to the teeth than that for the premolar and anterior views.
3. With the instrument and film in place, instruct the patient to close slowly but firmly.
4. Slide the localizing ring down the indicator rod to the patient's skin surface.
5. Position the localizing ring and PID, and then expose the radiograph (Fig. 17–30).

Producing Bite-Wing Radiographs

The procedure for bite-wing radiographs is the same in the paralleling and bisecting techniques. Bite-wing films are always parallel films regardless of the technique used for the periapical films (Fig. 17–31).

The film is positioned (either by a bite tab or by a film-holding device) parallel to the crowns of both upper and lower teeth, and the central ray is directed perpendicular to the film.

Correct horizontal angulation is crucial to the diagnostic value of the bite-wing radiograph. Even a slight amount of overlapping of the proximal (contact) surfaces on the film may lead to a misdiagnosis.

Producing Occlusal Radiographs

The occlusal technique is a supplementary technique to periapical and bite-wing radiography because it shows teeth and pathological conditions in the *bucco-lingual* dimension.

For example, a periapical film of an impacted mandibular molar (which shows the tooth from the side) shows the mesiodistal location and the vertical distance from the crest of the alveolar ridge. But the periapical film does not show the location of the molar in a buccolingual dimension.

An occlusal radiograph, which shows the tooth from above, is taken to determine whether the impacted

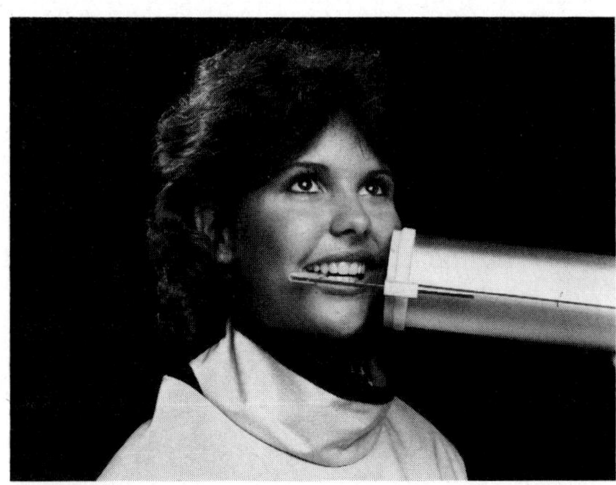

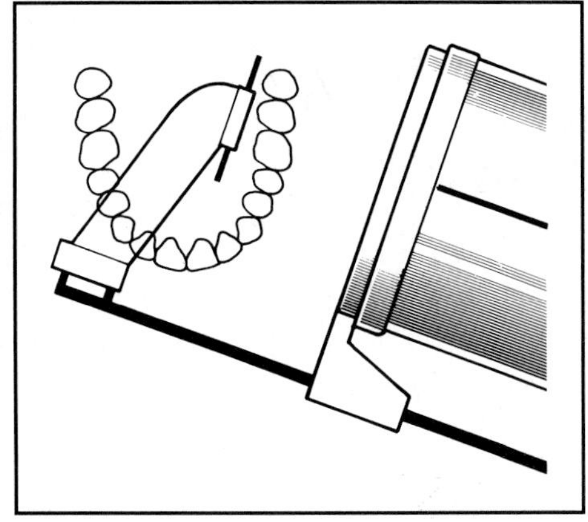

FIGURE 17–31

Instrumentation and placement for a molar bite-wing exposure. (Courtesy of Rinn Corporation, Elgin, IL.)

PROCEDURE: **Producing Occlusal Radiographs**

Maxillary Occlusal Technique

1. Position the patient's head so the film plane is parallel to the floor.
2. Place the film packet in the patient's mouth on the occlusal surfaces of the maxillary teeth with the front of the packet toward the teeth.
3. Place the film as far posterior as possible.
4. Position the PID so that the central ray is directed at a 65-degree angle through the bridge of the nose, perpendicular to the center of the film packet.
5. Press the x-ray machine activating button and take the exposure.

Mandibular Occlusal Technique

1. Tilt the patient's head back to a comfortable position. The midsagittal plane should be vertical.
2. Place the film packet in the patient's mouth on the occlusal surfaces of the mandibular teeth with the front of the packet toward the teeth.
3. Position the film as far posterior on the mandible as possible.
4. Position the PID so that the central ray is directed at 90 degree to center of the film packet.
5. Press the x-ray machine activating button and take the exposure.

mandibular molar lies toward the buccal or lingual side of the alveolar ridge.

A larger film (No. 4) is used and therefore shows a larger area of the jaw. The angulation of the occlusal projection may vary from 45 to 75 degrees, depending on the anatomic area.

Specialized Intraoral Radiographic Techniques

Pedodontic Radiography

The type and number of films for a pedodontic full-mouth survey vary, depending on the child's age, the size of the mouth, and the willingness of the child to cooperate.

PEDODONTIC EXPOSURE FACTORS

Exposure factors are generally reduced for children. Less exposure time and sometimes less milliamperage can be used because a child's tissues are not thick and therefore require less radiation than do those of an adult.

The exact exposure settings depend upon the size of the child, the type of film used, and the recommendations of the x-ray machine manufacturer.

FILM SIZE

In children up to the age of 5, it is often necessary to use the pedodontic-size film No. 0 for anterior, posterior, and bite-wing projections. Oversize film will cause discomfort, and you will lose the child's cooperation. Size No. 1 film may be used for a child with mixed dentition; sizes No. 1 and No. 2 are used for preadolescent and adolescent dentitions.

PEDODONTIC BITE-WINGS

Normally, until the second molars have erupted, only two bite-wing radiographs are necessary (one on each side). All erupted posterior teeth usually fit on one film (Fig. 17–32).

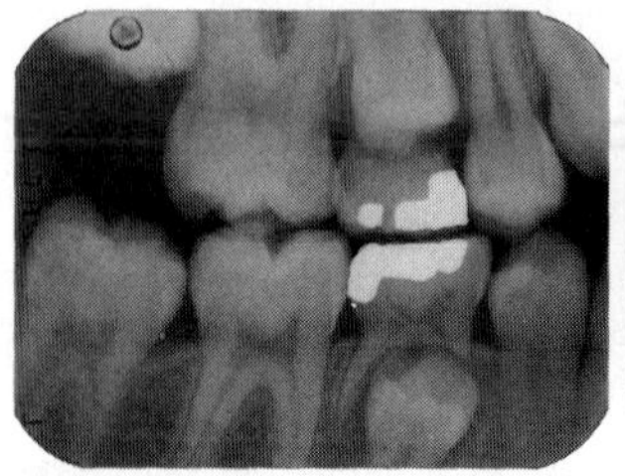

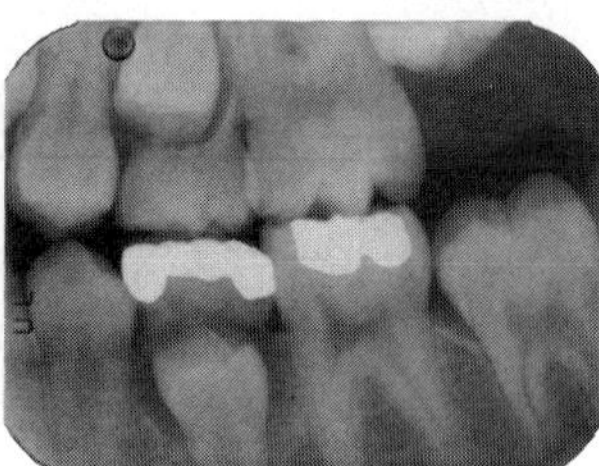

FIGURE 17–32

Pedodontic bite-wing radiographs.

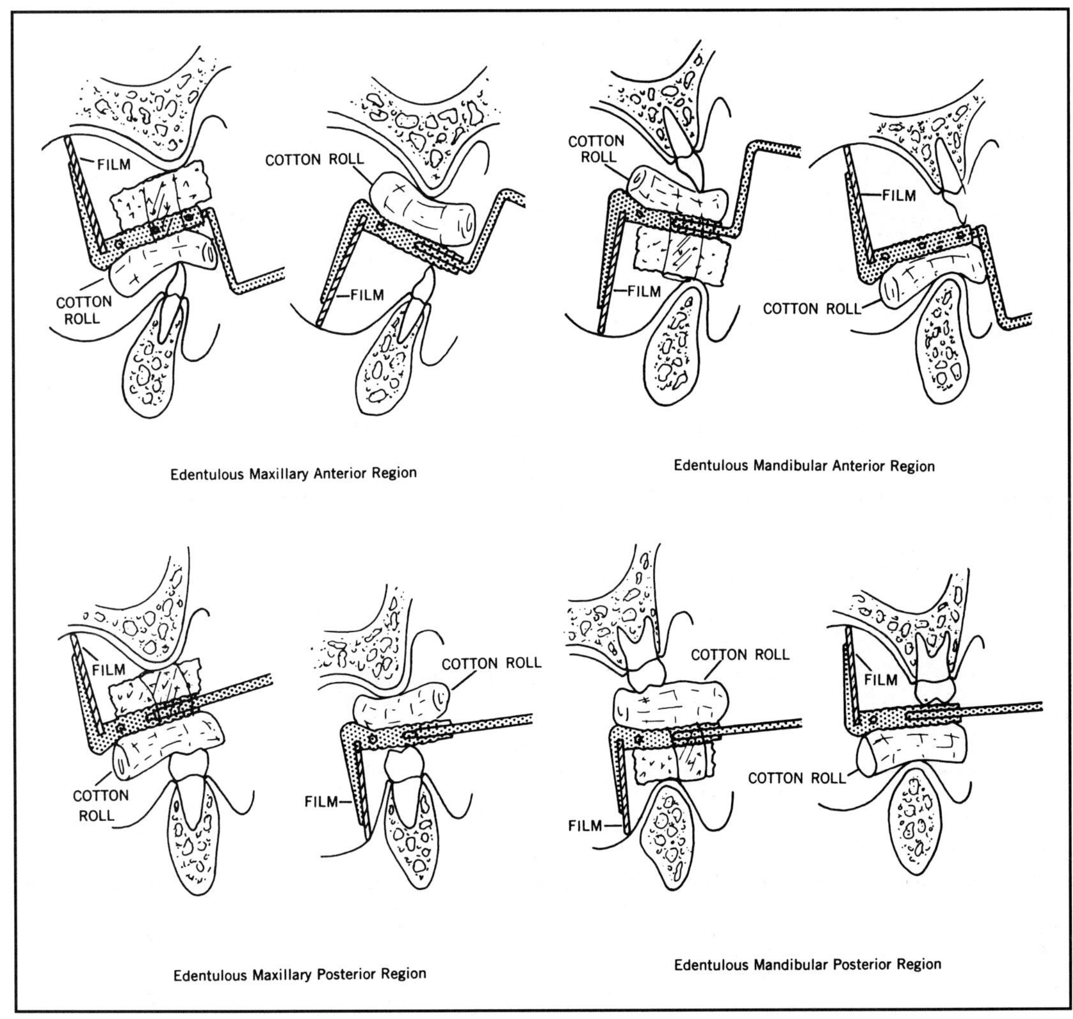

FIGURE 17–33

Partially edentulous survey technique. Cotton rolls and foam blocks are used to help stabilize the film. (Courtesy of Rinn Corporation, Elgin, IL.)

Edentulous Radiography

Full mouth radiographic surveys are often recommended for edentulous patients. Just because there are no teeth present does not mean that there are no retained roots, impacted teeth, cysts, or other pathological conditions in the bone.

EDENTULOUS EXPOSURE FACTORS

The exposure time for each edentulous region should be reduced by approximately one-fourth the normal exposure time, to avoid overexposure (dark films). This is because there are no teeth present and the bone may be thinner.

NUMBER OF FILMS

The edentulous survey may contain as many as 14 films (six anterior and eight posterior), or as few as 10 (two anterior and eight posterior). Bite-wings radiographs are *not* required because there are no teeth present.

Acceptable alternatives for a full mouth survey on an edentulous patient may be occlusal films with posterior periapical films or a panoramic radiograph.

EDENTULOUS EXPOSURE TECHNIQUE

For **partially edentulous** patients, film-holding instruments can be used by substituting a cotton roll for the space normally occupied by the crowns of the missing teeth and then following the standard exposure procedures (Fig. 17–33).

For **edentulous** patients, either the bisecting angle or the paralleling technique may be used. Because no teeth are present, the distortion inherent in the bisecting angle technique does not interfere with the diagnosis of intrabony conditions (Fig. 17–34).

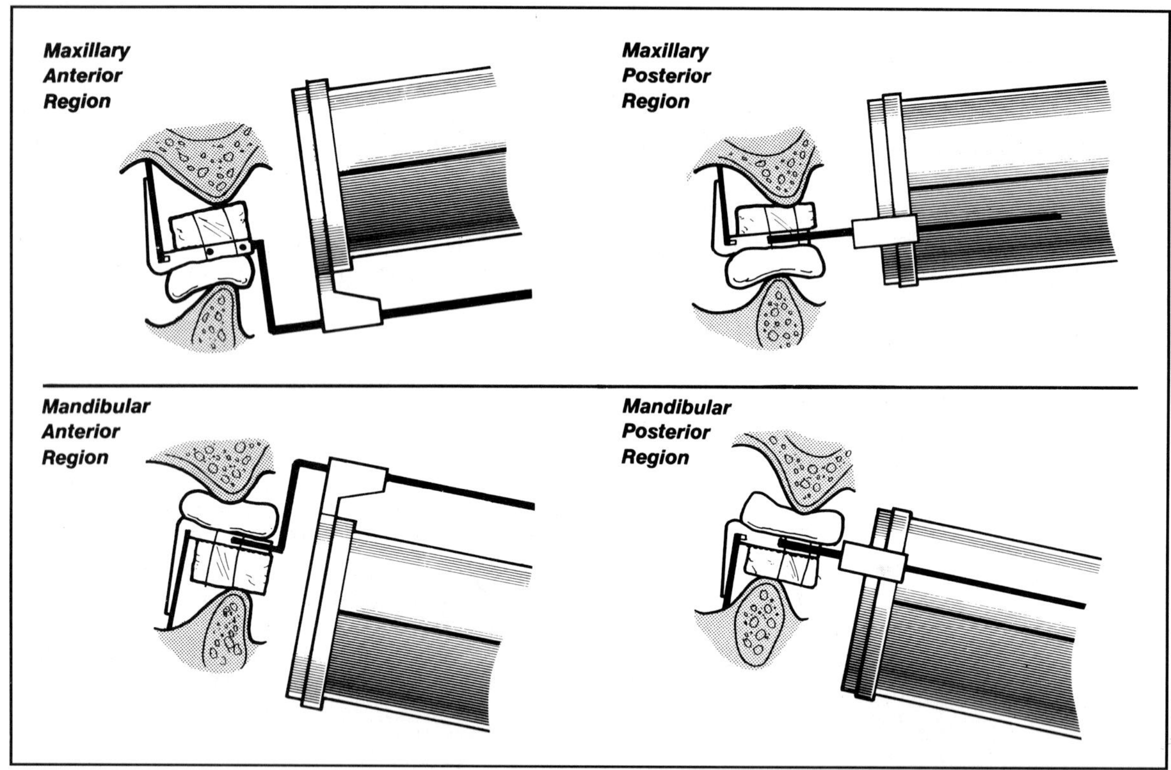

FIGURE 17–34

Modified paralleling technique for the completely edentulous mouth. Foam blocks are used to position the film parallel to the ridge being examined. (Courtesy of Rinn Corporation, Elgin, IL.)

Endodontic Radiography

It is often difficult to obtain accurate radiographs during endodontic treatment. This is because of the rubber dam clamp, endodontic instruments, or filling material extending from the tooth.

It is sometimes necessary to use a "modified bisecting angle" technique during this phase of treatment. A diagnostic quality endodontic film requires that

- The tooth is centered on the film.
- At least 5 mm. of bone beyond the apex of the tooth is visible.
- The image is as anatomically correct as possible.

The preoperative diagnostic film and the postoperative follow-up film should be taken with the standard paralleling technique. The bisecting angle technique is *not* recommended for these films because of the inherent dimensional distortion.

Processing Radiographs

Before the exposed radiographs can be used, they must be **processed.** This is also known as **developing.**

Many dental radiographic films are of poor quality because of improper film processing. Because films damaged in processing also necessitate retakes, proper processing is as important as the exposure technique in producing good diagnostic quality radiographs.

If a film is *overexposed* or *overdeveloped,* it will be *dark.* If a film is *underexposed, underdeveloped,* or *overfixed,* it will be *light.*

Radiographic film is sensitive to daylight until it has been processed. For this reason, it is necessary to use the appropriate precautions to safeguard against daylight during processing.

It is also necessary to always handle contaminated films with gloved hands. Fresh examination gloves are worn while this procedure is performed.

Processing Solutions

In most practices, intraoral films are processed in an automatic processor. However, in some situations, it is necessary to know how to process the film manually.

No matter which system is used, the use of developer and fixer solutions is required. These photographic processing solutions are considered hazardous substances and are discussed further in Chapter 12.

DEVELOPER SOLUTION

The processing of exposed film begins with the developer solution. When the film is placed in the developer solution, the gelatin softens and swells, and the developer solution permeates the gelatin to react with *all* of the silver halide crystals.

Those crystals struck by the x-rays readily react with the developer chemicals. This reaction causes the silver halide to separate into bromide (or iodine) and metallic silver, which is black. The black metallic silver is deposited on the film to form the black (radiolucent) areas.

The silver halide crystals that were not struck by radiation do not react with the developer chemicals and will be rinsed away. When processing is complete, these are the white or light gray radiopaque areas indicating where the film did not receive exposure to radiation.

FIXER SOLUTION

"Fixing" is the step in film processing that removes the undeveloped crystals from the emulsion. The fixer solution penetrates the gelatin and comes in contact with all the crystals. The dark crystals that were "developed" have completed their chemical reaction and do not react further. In this process, the developed crystals are fixed and preserved on the film.

The fixer solution removes from the gelatin those crystals that were not developed. These are expelled with the fixer solution and thereby leave the radiopaque areas white.

After the films have been fixed, they are rinsed to remove all of the chemicals. Then they are dried to allow the gelatin to harden again.

Manual Processing

Manual processing depends upon a combination of temperature (of the solutions) and time (how long the film remains in each solution). Both are critical for successfully processing the films.

THE DARKROOM

Manual film processing requires that the darkroom have adequate working space, that it be kept clean at all times, and that it be equipped with the following:

- A light-tight room with no cracks around doors or corners that would allow light leaks
- Separate processing tanks for developer, rinse water, and fixer solution
- A hot and cold running water supply with mixing valves to adjust the temperature
- A safelight and a source of white (normal) light (a **safelight** is a device that provides enough illumination in the darkroom to work by without the danger of fogging the films)
- A timer accurate in minutes and seconds
- An accurate thermometer that floats in the tanks to monitor the temperature of the solutions
- Safe storage space for chemicals
- Film hangers
- A film-drying rack and a film dryer

Processing Tanks

In most darkrooms, the developer solution is in the left tank, the water bath (rinse) in the center tank, and the fixer solution in the right tank. *Always* check before processing.

The fixer can be identified by its odor and feel. It has an odor similar to that of vinegar and feels slippery to the touch.

The tanks are kept covered except when films are placed and removed. Leaving the tanks uncovered allows the solutions to evaporate, and this lowers the solution level so that it may not cover the films.

Solution levels are raised by adding the appropriate replenisher. Because it dilutes the solution, water is never added to raise the solution level.

To equalize the temperature and evenly mix the chemicals, the solutions should be stirred before use. To avoid contamination, use a separate stirring paddle for each solution.

Automatic Film Processing

An automatic film processor is composed of a series of rollers that transport the films through the steps and solutions necessary for complete processing (Figs. 17–35 and 17–36).

The temperatures of the developer in automatic processors range from 85 to 105°F. This significantly reduces the developing and overall processing time.

Units with daylight loading capability do not require a darkroom as they have light-tight baffles into which

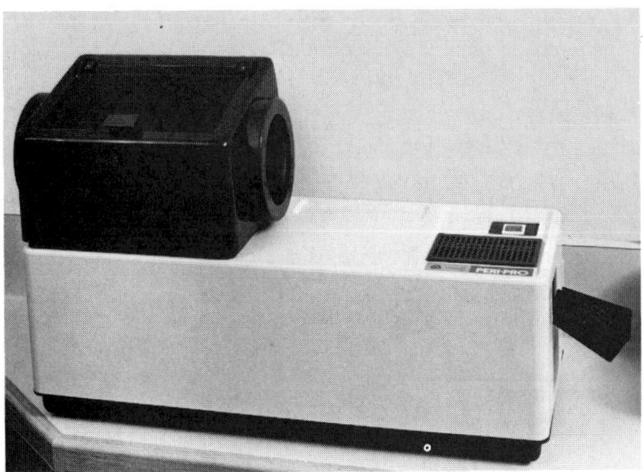

FIGURE 17–35

A daylight loading automatic film processor.

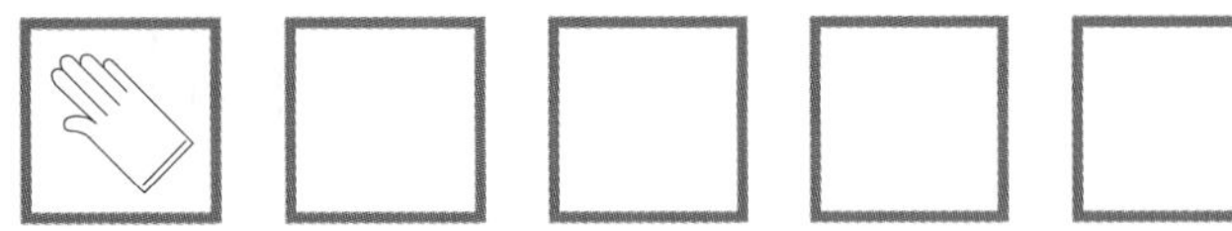

PROCEDURE: **Processing Films Manually**

Preparations

1. Cover the work area with a barrier, and place a clean paper towel on the barrier.
2. Stir the solutions, and check solution levels and temperature. The temperature should be between 65 and 70°F.
   □ *RATIONALE:* Manual processing is based on a combination of time and temperature as specified by the solution manufacturer.
3. Label the film rack with the patient's name and the date of exposure.
4. Wash hands and put on gloves.
5. Turn on the safelight; then turn off the white light.
6. Open the film packets and allow the films to drop on the clean paper towel. Take care not to touch the films.
   □ *RATIONALE:* Untouched films are not contaminated. Films that have been touched are contaminated, and the image may be damaged.
7. Discard the transfer cup and film packets.
8. Remove contaminated gloves and carefully wash and dry hands.
   □ *RATIONALE:* Water on the hands or powder from gloves may cause artifacts on the films. (An **artifact** is a structure or appearance that is produced by artificial means and is not normally present in the radiograph.)

Processing

1. Attach each film to the film rack so that films are parallel and not touching each other.
2. As you immerse the film rack in the developer, agitate the rack slightly to prevent air bubbles from adhering to the film.
   □ *RATIONALE:* Air bubbles prevent the solution from coming into contact with the film.
3. Start the timer. The timer is set according to the manufacturer's instructions on the basis of the temperature of the solutions.
4. When the timer goes off, remove the rack of films and rinse it in the running water in the center tank.
5. Immerse the rack of films in the fixer tank. Set the timer for 10 minutes. If the films must be viewed, they can be removed from the fixer after 3 minutes. However, they *must* be returned to the fixer for a total of 10 minutes.
6. Return the rack of films to the center tank with circulating water for 20 to 30 minutes.
   □ *RATIONALE:* Failure to do this will result in an incomplete wash, and the films will eventually turn brown.
7. Remove the rack of films from the water and hand it to dry.
8. When the films are completely dry, remove them from the rack and mount them in an appropriately labeled mount.

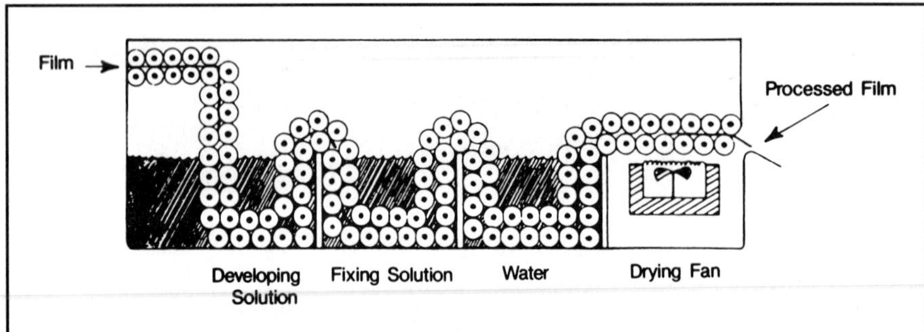

FIGURE 17–36

Schematic of the interior of an automatic film processor. (From Miles, D.A., VanDis, M.L., Jensen, C.W., and Ferretti, A.: Radiographic Imaging for Dental Auxiliaries, 2nd ed. Philadelphia, W.B. Saunders Co., 1994, p 64.)

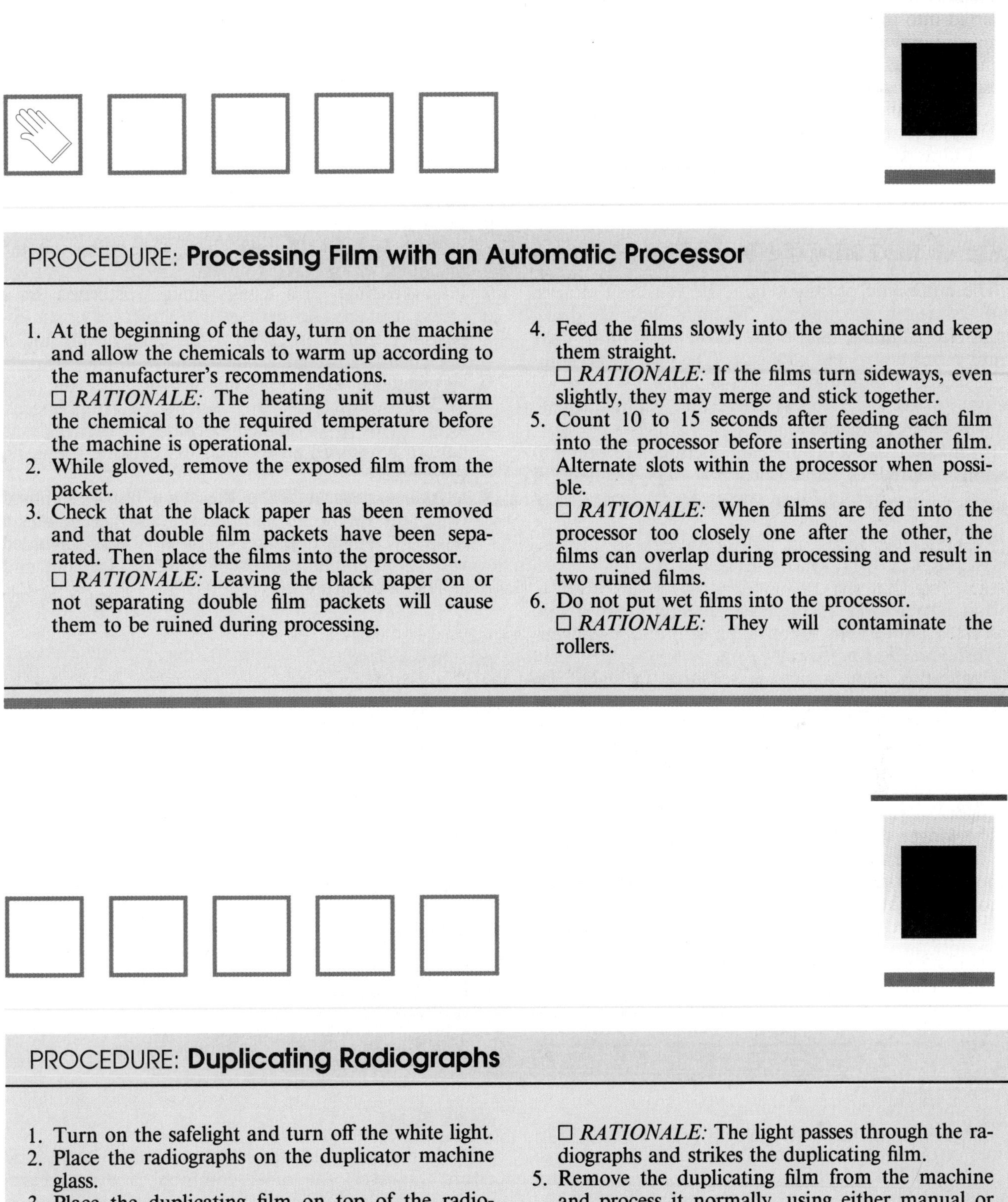

PROCEDURE: **Processing Film with an Automatic Processor**

1. At the beginning of the day, turn on the machine and allow the chemicals to warm up according to the manufacturer's recommendations.
   □ *RATIONALE:* The heating unit must warm the chemical to the required temperature before the machine is operational.
2. While gloved, remove the exposed film from the packet.
3. Check that the black paper has been removed and that double film packets have been separated. Then place the films into the processor.
   □ *RATIONALE:* Leaving the black paper on or not separating double film packets will cause them to be ruined during processing.
4. Feed the films slowly into the machine and keep them straight.
   □ *RATIONALE:* If the films turn sideways, even slightly, they may merge and stick together.
5. Count 10 to 15 seconds after feeding each film into the processor before inserting another film. Alternate slots within the processor when possible.
   □ *RATIONALE:* When films are fed into the processor too closely one after the other, the films can overlap during processing and result in two ruined films.
6. Do not put wet films into the processor.
   □ *RATIONALE:* They will contaminate the rollers.

PROCEDURE: **Duplicating Radiographs**

1. Turn on the safelight and turn off the white light.
2. Place the radiographs on the duplicator machine glass.
3. Place the duplicating film on top of the radiographs with the emulsion side against the radiographs.
4. Turn on the light in the duplicating machine for the manufacturer's recommended time.
   □ *RATIONALE:* The light passes through the radiographs and strikes the duplicating film.
5. Remove the duplicating film from the machine and process it normally, using either manual or automatic processing techniques.

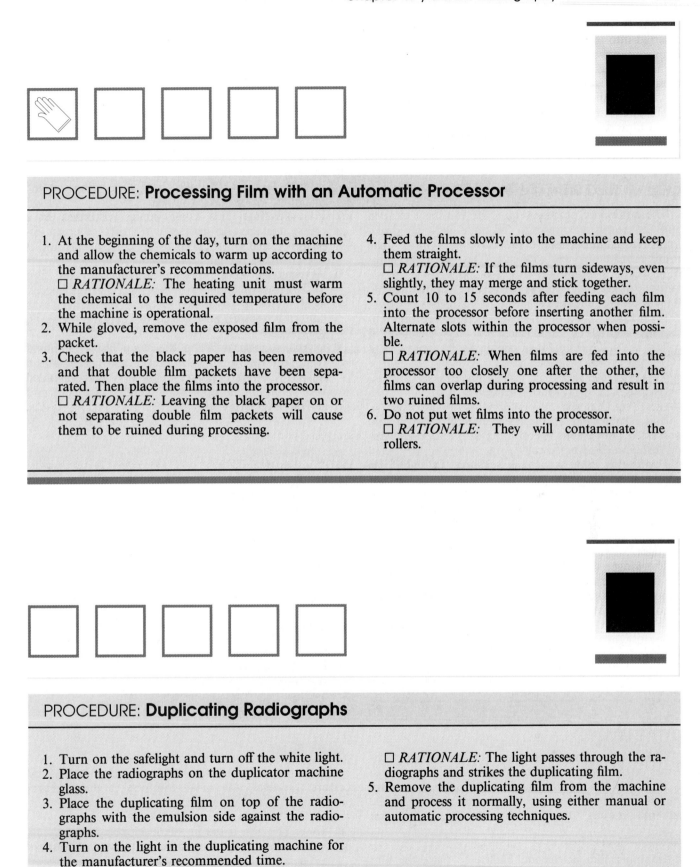

the hands are placed while the films are opened and inserted into the rollers. In a daylight loading unit, the films are unwrapped and processed within the machine. (Gloves are worn while films are handled in these machines.)

An automatic processor without daylight loading capability requires the use of a darkroom while the exposed films are unwrapped and placed into the processor. (Gloving protocols are the same here as for manual processing.)

CARE OF THE AUTOMATIC PROCESSOR

The automatic processor must be routinely cleaned and disinfected according to the manufacturer's directions. In addition, automatic processors *must* have routine preventive maintenance. The two most common causes of automatic processor breakdown are (1) failure to keep the rollers clean and (2) inadequate replenishing of chemicals.

A schedule, based on the manufacturer's recommendations, should be established for daily cleaning of rollers and replenishment of chemicals.

Film Duplicating Techniques

If it is necessary to duplicate already exposed and processed radiographs, duplicating film and a film duplicating machine are used.

Duplicating film, which is sensitive to light, has emulsion on one side only. The emulsion side is normally gray or lavender.

The **duplicating machine** uses white light to expose the film. Because the film is light sensitive, the duplication process is performed in the darkroom with the safelight.

The longer the duplicating film is exposed to light, the lighter the duplicate films will become. This is the opposite of x-ray films, which become darker when exposed to light.

Troubleshooting Technique and Processing Errors

Exposure Errors

The most common error in the paralleling technique, even with the use of film-holding instruments, is improper film placement (Fig. 17–37). If the film packet and film-holder are not placed correctly in the patient's mouth, the paralleling technique will not work.

- **Improper film placement:** Failure to place the film packet deep enough in the floor of the mouth or high enough in the palate results in cutting off the apices of the teeth.
- **Overlapping:** Improper selection of the horizontal angulation results in overlapping of interproximal contact areas. (This is especially critical in bite-wing radiography.)
- **Cone cutting:** Unexposed areas on the radiograph result when the x-ray beam is not centered on the film packet.
- **Light films:** Those films that do not have enough density result from *underexposure* or *underdevelopment.*
- **Dark films:** These films result from *overexposure* or *overdevelopment.* (Always check the settings on the machine before making an exposure.)
- **Film bending:** This causes image distortion or a crease artifact. (An **artifact** is a structure or an appearance that is produced by artificial means and is not normally present in the radiograph.)
- **Herringbone effect:** Placing the *back* of the film packet toward the PID causes the "herringbone effect." (This is so named because the herringbone pattern embossed on the lead foil backing shows on the film.)
- **Double exposure:** When the same film is exposed twice, the resulting film is useless and necessitates a retake. (Double exposure of films is easily avoided with a systematic approach to film placement and storage after exposure.)

Processing Errors

STAINED FILMS

Stained films can result when any fluid drops on a dental x-ray film (Fig. 17–38).

- **Water:** dissolves or dilutes the film emulsion, and the result may be a dark stain or a clear spot
- **Developer solution:** if dropped or splashed onto a film, causes a black stain
- **Fixer:** when dropped on an unprocessed film, causes a white spot
- **Fixer:** left on a processed film, results in yellow or brown stains (this is caused by not properly rinsing the film after it has been fixed)
- **Fluoride:** on the gloved fingers of the operator handling the film, can result in black stains

DARK FILMS

Dark films can be the result of many processing errors; however, the most common is overdevelopment. Dark films are most commonly caused by

- **Time:** The film is left in the developer too long.
- **Solution strength:** The developer concentration is too strong.
- **Temperature:** The developer solution is too warm.
- **Light leaks:** The film is exposed to light before processing.

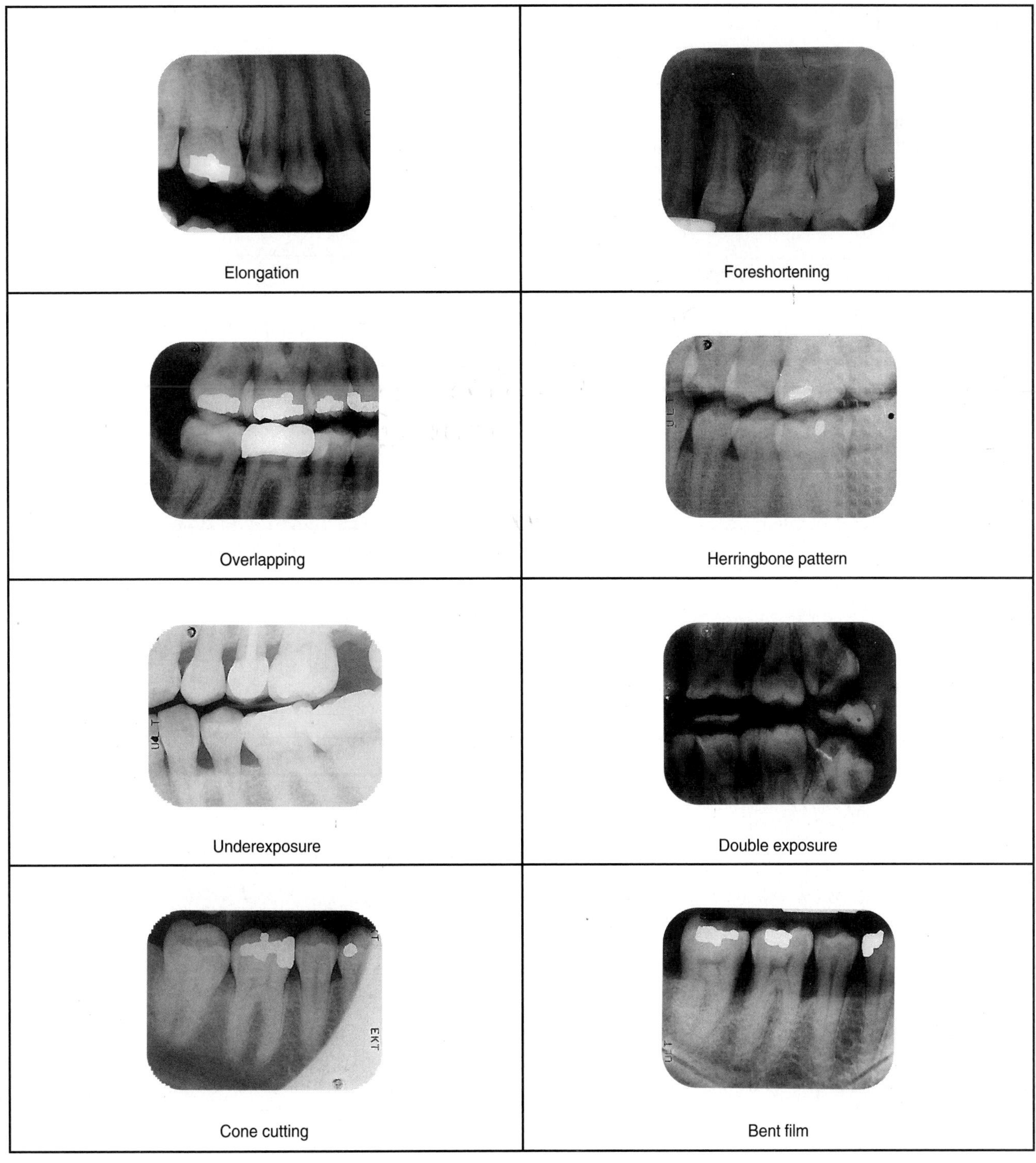

FIGURE 17–37

Exposure errors.

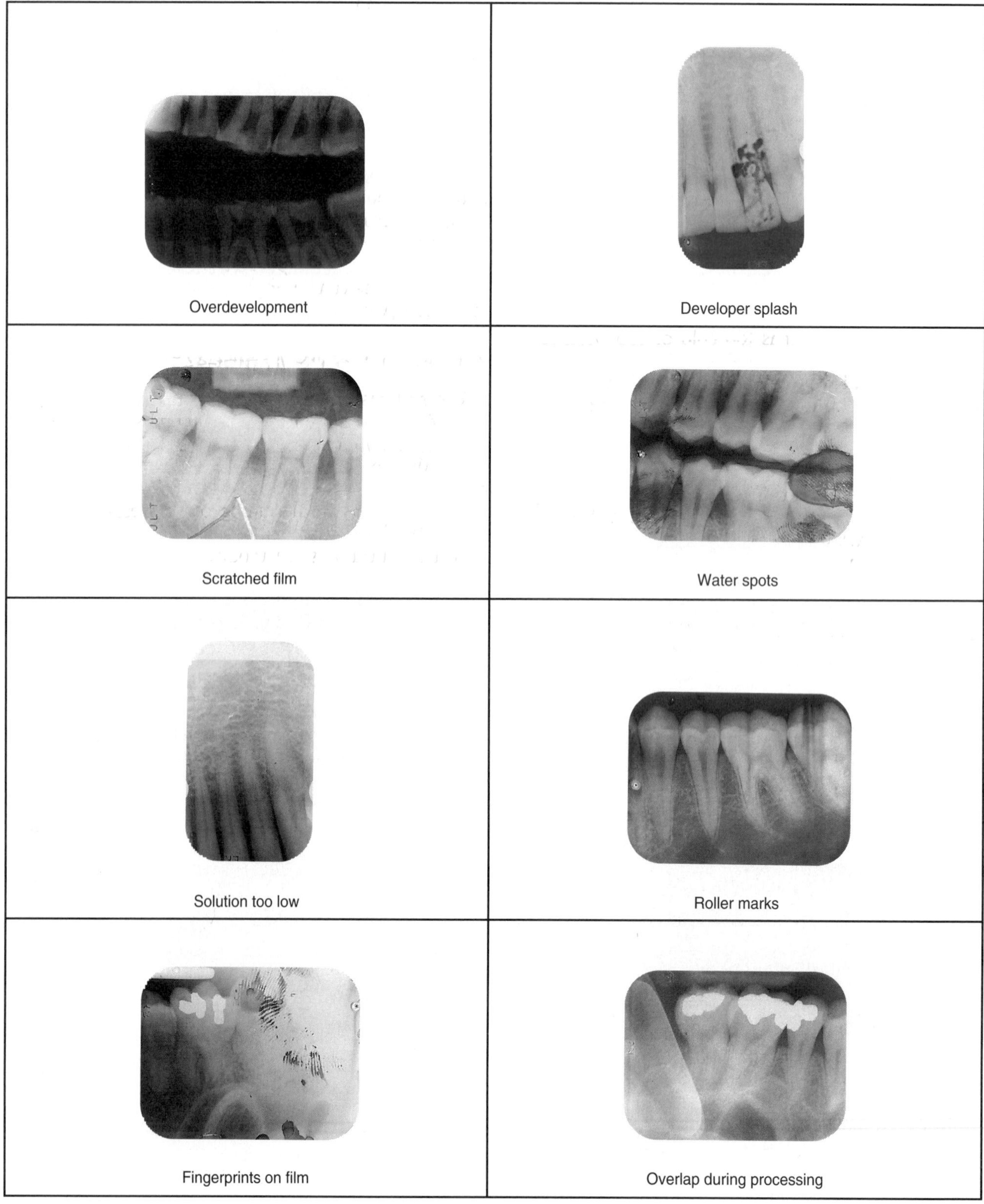

FIGURE 17–38

Processing errors.

- **Improper fixation:** The film is not left in the fixer for a long enough time or at the proper temperature.
- **Paper left on film:** Failure to remove the paper backing prevents the solutions from reaching the film.

LIGHT FILMS

Films that are too light have insufficient contrast or detail for diagnostic interpretation. This lack of diagnostic quality means that a retake is required. Light films result when

- The **developing time** is too short
- The **developer solution** is too cold or too weak (exhausted)
- The **fixer solution** is contaminated with developer, or films are left in the fixer solution too long

FOGGED FILMS

Fogged films usually appear almost uniformly gray. There is reduced contrast, and it may be difficult to diagnosis early carious lesions in the enamel. Fog may be caused by improper safelighting in the darkroom (light leaks or cracks in the safety light filter), storage in a warm to hot environment, or expired (out-of-date) film.

Mounting Radiographs

Processed radiographs are arranged in anatomic order in holders, called **mounts**, to make it easier for the dentist to study and review them. The mount is always labeled with the patient's name and the date that the radiographs were exposed. The dentist's name and address should also be on the mount.

Selecting the Mount

The mounts most commonly used for radiographic surveys are available in black, gray, and clear plastic. Mounts also come in many sizes, with different numbers and sizes of windows (openings) to accommodate the number and sizes of exposures in the patient's radiographic survey.

All the radiographs of a single series should be in the same mount, and the size of the mount selected is determined by the number and size of windows needed.

If there are more windows in the mount than there are radiographs in the series, the extra windows should be blocked with a black piece of paper or a cardboard blank. This is done to keep the light from shining through the opening into the dentist's eyes when he or she is studying the radiographic series on a lighted x-ray view box.

Left-Right Orientation of Mounted Films

Before mounting radiographs, it is necessary to know the dentist's preferred method of mounting, because it determines where the left and right sides of the oral cavity as represented in the radiograph mount.

This is extremely important, for mistakes in mounting radiographs can result in errors in the treatment of the dental patient.

THE RAISED DOT ON RADIOGRAPHS

The systems of mounting are based on the orientation of the raised dot on the radiographs.

If the bump of the raised dot is placed *outward* (convexly), toward the person mounting or reading the radiographs, it represents the facial surface of the teeth, and the left side of the radiograph corresponds to the right side of the patient's oral cavity.

When radiographs are mounted this way, the upper left of the mount represents the upper right molar area (Fig. 17–39). That is, when you look at the mounted radiographs, it is as though you are looking at the patient, the patient's right side is on your left, and the patient's left side is on your right side. This method of mounting radiographs complies with the Universal Tooth Numbering System.

If the dot faces *inward* (concavely), away from the person mounting or reading the radiographs, it represents the lingual surface of the teeth. The left side of the radiograph corresponds to the left of the patient's oral cavity.

When radiographs are mounted this way, the upper left of the mount represents the upper left molar area. It can be compared to being inside the mouth looking out: your right is the patient's right also.

The Radiographic Appearance of Anatomic Structure

Before radiographs are mounted, it is necessary to recognize the radiographic appearance of normal anatomic structures, for these are helpful in properly placing the films in the mount (see Fig. 17–39). It is also helpful to be able to recognize the radiographic appearance of dental restorations and some dental materials (Fig. 17–40).

THE TEETH AND SURROUNDING STRUCTURES

Enamel, which is the hardest tooth structure, appears almost white on a radiograph. **Dentin**, which is not as hard, appears to be slightly darker gray.

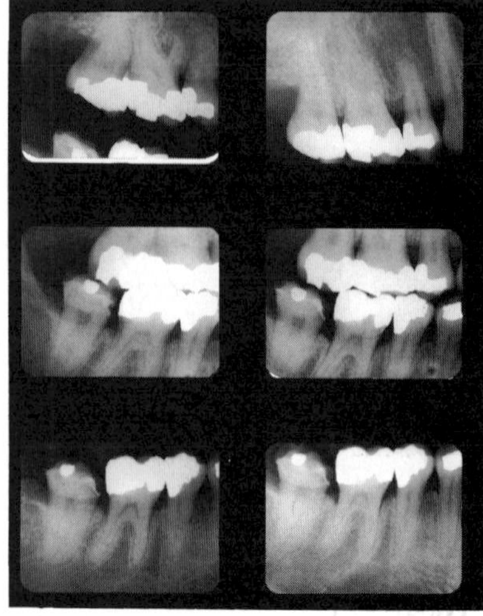
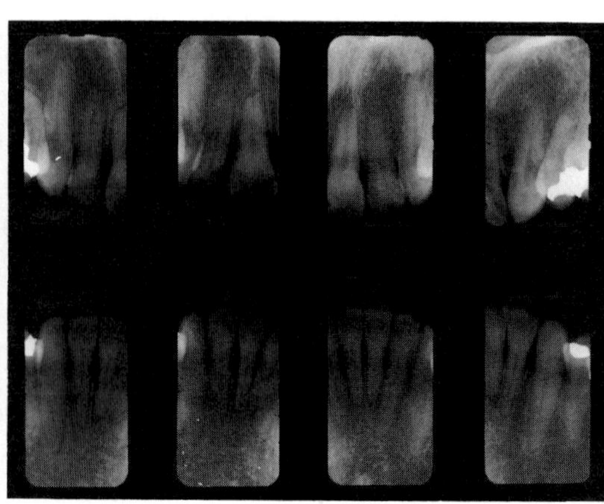
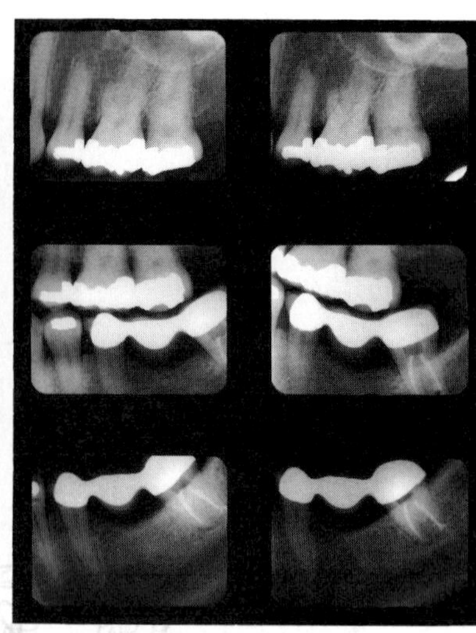

FIGURE 17–39

Radiographic survey mounted with the raised dot outward. These films are mounted with the raised dot outward. Therefore, the upper left of the mount represents the upper right molar area.

Dentin and **cementum** are similar in hardness. On a radiograph showing the root of the tooth, the junction between the dentin and the cementum covering the root is not visible.

Because the **pulp** is soft tissue, it appears as a dark area within the tooth.

The periodontal ligament is soft tissue and therefore not visible on the radiograph; however, the **periodontal ligament space** is visible as a continuous dark line around the root of the tooth.

The **lamina dura**, which lines the tooth socket, is dense, like cortical bone, and it appears as a white line around the roots of the teeth.

On radiographs, **cancellous bone** appears as irregularly shaped random patterns called *trabecular patterns*. The trabecular pattern of bone is extremely variable between patients.

Cortical bone is denser than cancellous bone and therefore appears lighter. Cortical bone forms the exterior surface of the mandible and forms the crests of the alveolar processes.

LANDMARKS OF THE MAXILLARY ARCH

The maxillary molars have *three* roots, and the maxillary first premolar has *two* roots.

The **maxillary sinus** is evident in the cuspid and premolar views of the teeth and, in some instances, in views of the central and lateral incisors.

The **zygomatic process** may be visible on the apices of the maxillary molars.

The **trabeculae** of the bone are more loosely structured in the maxillary arch than in the mandibular arch.

The **tuberosity** and the **hamulus** of the sphenoid bone are evident in radiographs of the third maxillary molar.

The **maxillary midsagittal suture,** the **nasal cavity,** and frequently the **incisive foramen** are evident in the central incisor area.

LANDMARKS OF THE MANDIBULAR ARCH

The mandibular molars have two roots. The mandibular premolars have single roots.

The cortical bone surrounding the mandible is visible in views showing the edge of the bone.

The **mental foramen** is visible near the apex of the first premolar, and the **mandibular canal** may be seen parallel to the apices of the molars.

In radiographs of the premolars and molars, the **mylohyoid ridge** may appear to be superimposed over the roots of these teeth. The **retromolar area** and the **ramus** of the mandible are evident posterior to the second or third molar area.

Storage of Radiographic Records

The mounted radiographs are stored with the patient's dental treatment record.

On instructions from the dentist, inactive radiographs may be removed from their mount and placed in a small envelope. The envelope must be clearly identified with the patient's name and the date that the films were taken. This is permanently filed with the patient's treatment record.

If the patient-identifying information was in pencil, this may be removed from the mount, and the mount may be reused for another patient.

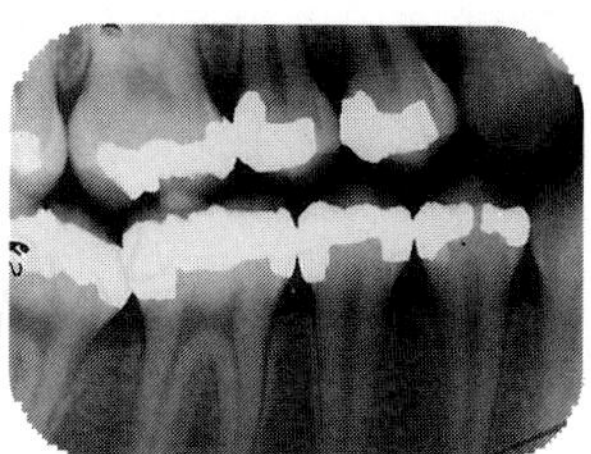

Lamina dura, alveolar crest, and periodontal ligament space

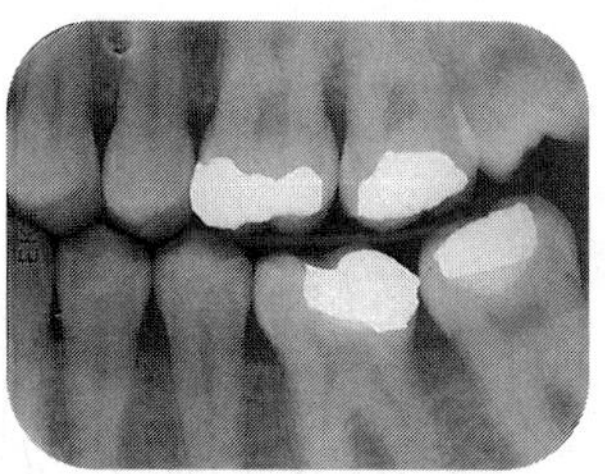

Bone loss due to periodontal disease

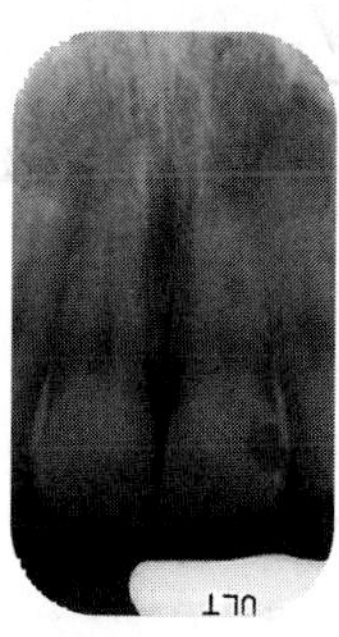

Maxillary incisive canal

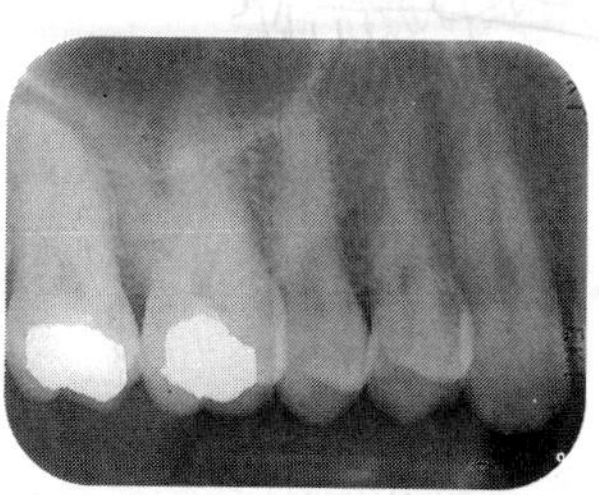

Floor of maxillary sinus

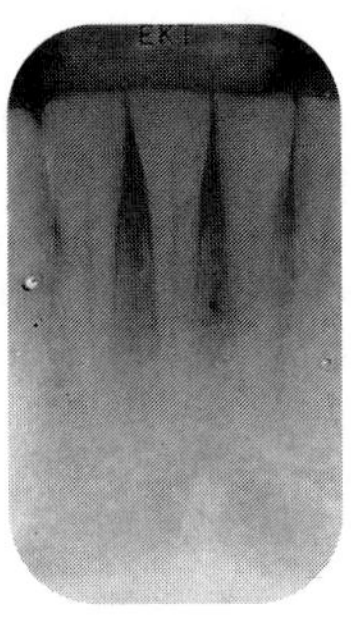

Mandibular incisive canal

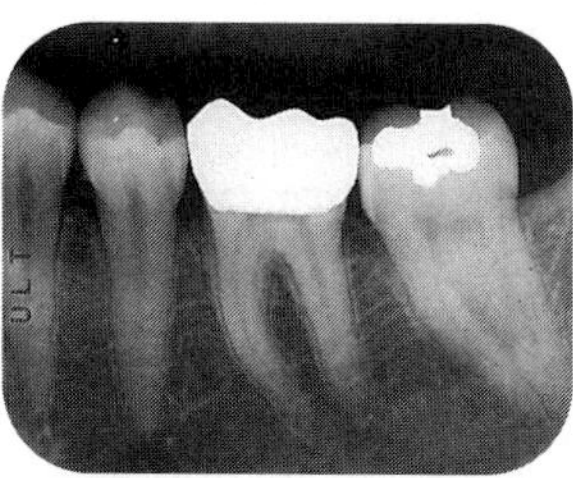

Mental foramen, gold crown, and amalgam restoration

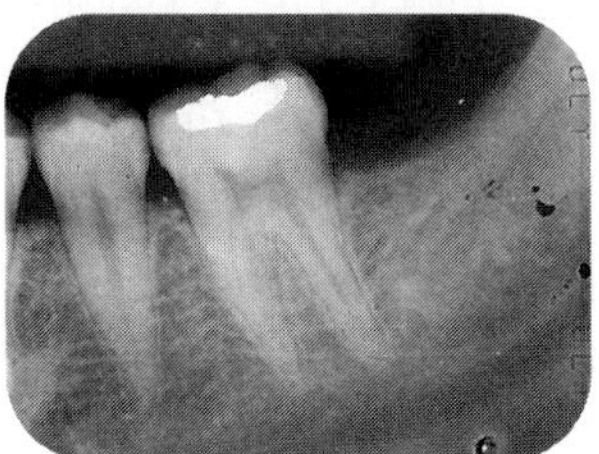

Mandibular canal and trabecular bone pattern

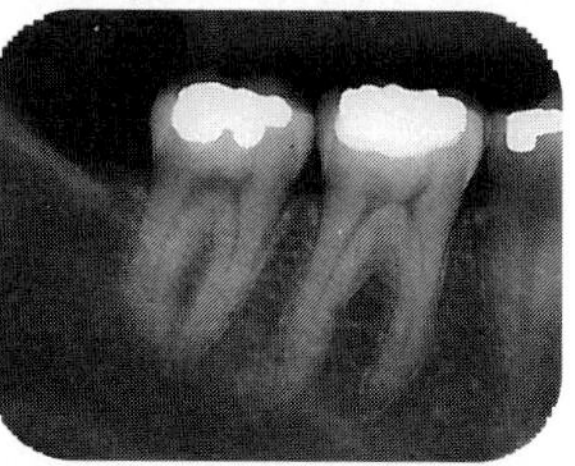

External oblique line and amalgam restorations

FIGURE 17–40

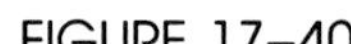

Anatomic landmarks.

PROCEDURE: **Mounting Radiographs**

1. Hands should always be clean and dry when radiographs are handled. Films are grasped only at the edges, never on the front or back.
   □ *RATIONALE*: Dirt or smudges may spoil the diagnostic quality of the film.
2. Select the appropriate size mount, and label it with the patient's name and the date that the radiographs were exposed.
3. Arrange the dry radiographs in anatomic order on a piece of clean white paper or on a flat view box. (A **viewbox**, which has a light behind a frosted surface, aids in mounting and viewing radiographs.)
4. Once the films are arranged properly, place them neatly in the mount. In many practices, the next step is to place the mounted radiographs and the patient's chart on the dentist's desk to be reviewed.

Extraoral Radiography

Extraoral radiographs (outside the mouth) are taken when large areas of the skull or jaw need to be examined or when patients are unable to open their mouths for film placement. Extraoral films are available in 5 × 7, 8 × 10, and 10 × 12 inch sizes. These radiographs do not show details as well as do intraoral films. They are useful for evaluating large areas but are not recommended for detection of subtle changes such as dental decay or early periodontal changes.

There are many different types of extraoral radiographs. Some types are used to view the entire skull, whereas other types focus on the maxilla and mandible.

Extraoral Radiographic Equipment

Extraoral films are contained in a holder called a **cassette.** These cassettes can be rigid or flexible and come in a variety of sizes corresponding to the size of film being used. The cassette must be light-tight and yet allow x-rays to pass through.

Because there is no embossed dot on extraoral film to tell the patient's left from the right as on intraoral films, the cassettes are marked with lead letters "L" or "R." After exposure, the letter will be superimposed on the radiograph.

INTENSIFYING SCREENS

Intensifying screens are built into film cassettes. The purpose of intensifying screens is to reduce the amount of radiation to the patient. This happens because the screens are coated with a substance called phosphor. A phosphor has the property of fluorescence and emits either a blue or green light when struck by x-radiation.

The type of film used in extraoral radiography is the **screen-type**. This means that the film is more sensitive to the light emitted by the phosphor in the intensifying screen than it is to radiation.

Intensifying screens vary in their speed or exposure requirements. (This is the same concept as the D or E speed of intraoral film.) The speed of the screen depends on the type of phosphor and the size of the crystal. The larger the crystal, the faster the screen but the poorer the definition. One type of screen uses a common type of phosphor called **calcium tungstate,** which produces a blue light.

The other type of phosphors are called the **rare earth elements,** which produce a green light. The rare earth element screens are four times more efficient in converting x-ray energy into light than are calcium tungstate screens and therefore are faster and require less exposure time. It is important to use the appropriate film for the intensifying screen.

The two types of film used in extraoral radiography are

- **Green-sensitive:** This type of film is used with cassettes that have rare earth–intensifying screens.

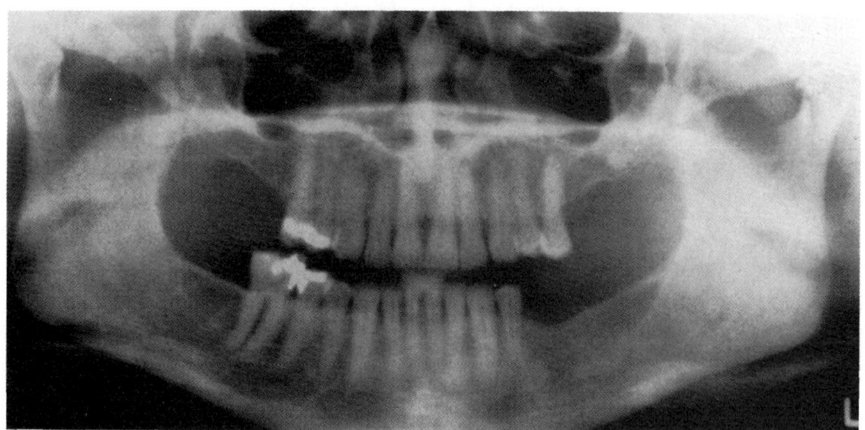

FIGURE 17–41

A typical panoramic radiograph. Notice the absence of posterior teeth. (From Miles, D.A., VanDis, M.L., Jensen, C.W., and Ferretti, A.: Radiographic Imaging for Dental Auxiliaries, 2nd ed. Philadelphia, W.B. Saunders Co., 1994, p 163.)

- **Blue-sensitive:** This type of film is used with cassettes that have calcium tungstate–intensifying screens.

When cassettes are loaded or unloaded in the darkroom, care must be taken not to scratch the intensifying screen. If an intensifying screen is badly scratched and the phosphor removed, a white streak will appear on any films taken with this cassette.

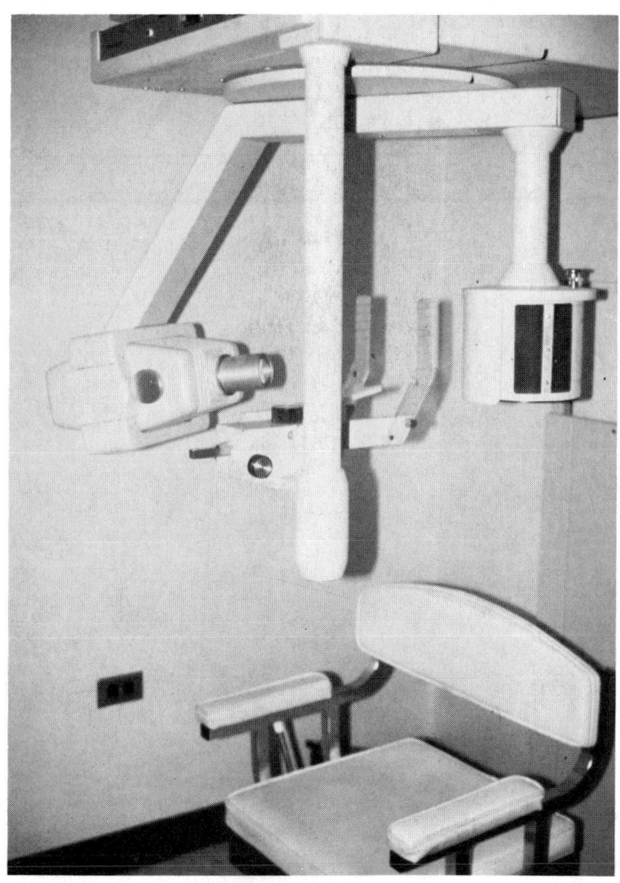

FIGURE 17–42

Extraoral panographic dental x-ray unit.

Panoramic Radiography

Panoramic radiography provides a view of the entire maxilla and mandible on a single film that is 5 × 12 or 6 × 12 inches (Fig. 17–41).

There are many types of panoramic x-ray machines made by different manufacturers; however, the basic operating principles are the same for most machines (Fig. 17–42).

The x-ray tube and the cassette holder are connected to each other across the top of the unit. These components rotate simultaneously around the patient, with the x-ray beam always aimed at the film. With any of the panoramic units, positioning the patient and maintaining that position during the movement of the tubehead are critical. If these are not done, the area to be radiographed may appear blurred on the radiograph. The manufacturer's instructions for patient positioning and film exposure should be followed carefully.

A lead apron should be always be used, but a thyroid collar can interfere with a portion of the image and is not used on all types of panoramic unit.

Cephalometric Projections

The cephalometric projection is an 8 × 10 inch lateral view of the entire skull. The right and left sides of the skull are superimposed on each other.

Most orthodontists use a cephalometric radiograph to assess a patient's profile and to assist in predicting growth patterns. Because the film is used for measuring changes, it must be taken with the patient fixed in a position that can be repeated in the future (Fig. 17–43).

Temporomandibular Joint Projections

There are many ways to obtain a radiographic image of the temporomandibular joint (TMJ) for use in the diagnosis of TMJ disorders.

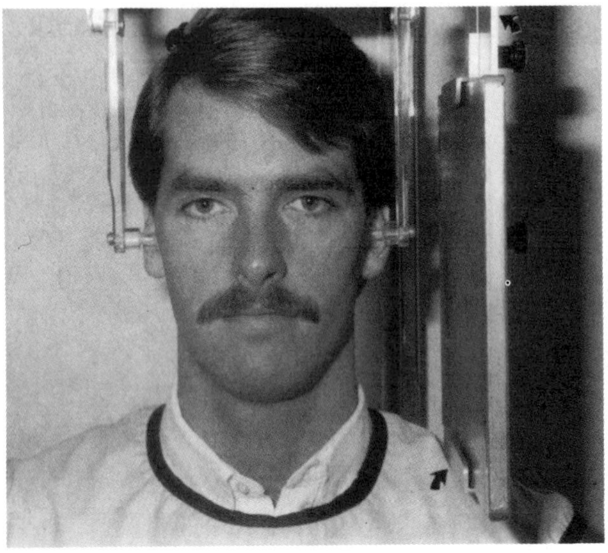

FIGURE 17–43

Patient positioned in a cephalometric unit. (From Miles, D.A., VanDis, M.L., Jensen, C.W., and Ferretti, A.: Radiographic Imaging for Dental Auxiliaries, 2nd ed. Philadelphia, W.B. Saunders Co., 1994, p 161.)

Panoramic units in which variations in patient position and exposure permit better views of the TMJ are available.

Arthrography is a technique for imaging the soft tissues of the TMJ in which a special radiopaque dye is injected into the joint space. The joint space, which is filled with dye, appears as a white area on the radiographs. The condyle and glenoid fossa are also visible.

Tomographs show the dentist a "slice" of the joint in focus, while the surrounding structures are "blurred out." Adjustments to the machine allow specific areas of the joint to be in focus at one time. A special tomographic unit is required for this radiograph.

Transcranial (meaning through the skull or cranium) is the most commonly used TMJ radiographic technique (Fig. 17–44). This technique provides a view down the long axis of the condyle and also shows the glenoid fossa and its relationship to the condyle.

The cassette is positioned against the ear and cheekbone of the side being radiographed. There are several commercial devices for correctly positioning the patient when this technique is used.

Other Imaging Systems

Digital Imaging

Digital imaging systems use x-rays to record images of the teeth and surrounding structures and transmit those images to a computer monitor screen. The ability of the computer to zoom in and magnify any area of the image, such as the apex of a tooth, makes this a valuable diagnostic and teaching tool.

Digital radiography eliminates the need for processing films, and it gives the dentist the advantage of being able to adjust the contrast and density of the image on the monitor without exposing the patient to additional radiation during a retake.

Digital radiography does *not* substitute for the basic principles of intraoral radiography. A digital image receptor (which looks like a hard plastic x-ray film with a cord attached to it) is positioned in the mount, just as a traditional film would be. The PID is aligned with the digital image receptor, and the exposure is made.

This means that any errors in film positioning or in PID placement that result with traditional techniques will also result with digital radiography.

Xeroradiography

Xeroradiography is an imaging system used in medical radiology. The system uses the xerographic copying process to record images produced by x-rays from a standard dental x-ray machine.

The system replaces conventional x-ray film as the image receptor; however, it does not replace the con-

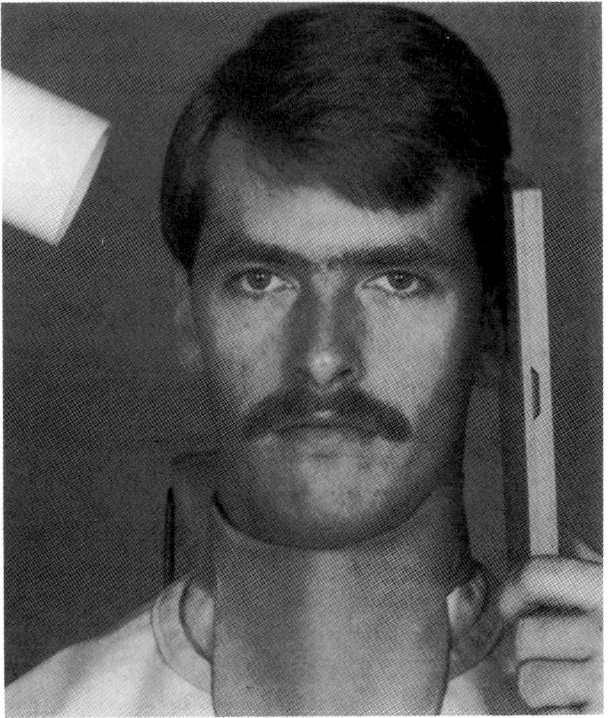

FIGURE 17–44

Patient positioned for a transcranial radiograph of the temporomandibular joint. (From Miles, D.A., VanDis, M.L., Jensen, C.W., and Ferretti, A.: Radiographic Imaging for Dental Auxiliaries, 2nd ed. Philadelphia, W.B. Saunders Co., 1994, p 188.)

ventional x-ray unit. A photoreceptor plate is used to record the image. The exposed photoreceptor plate is placed into a processing machine, and the image is recorded on opaque paper.

The quality of xeroradiographs is superior to that of traditional radiographs. The radiation exposure to the patient is about the same as that with the use of E speed film.

The major disadvantages with this system are its limitations to only No. 0 and No. 2 (pediatric and adult size) film and the use of rigid intraoral cassettes. The rigid cassettes are difficult to place in some mouths.

Computed Tomography

Computed tomography, also known as *CT scanning*, is an imaging method by which a computer reconstructs two-dimensional cross-section images of the body as a three-dimensional image. In this process, the patient is placed in the CT unit, and the x-ray source and image detector rotate around the patient.

Although CT scanners are not found in dental offices, the dentists may refer a patient to a hospital with CT scanning equipment. The dentist then uses the CT report in the diagnosis of pathologic conditions and in the planning of implant placement in the jaws.

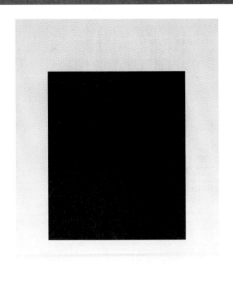

Chapter 18

Diagnosis and Treatment Planning

Introduction

Diagnosis and treatment planning for each patient involves three major steps: data gathering, examining the patient, and preparing and presenting treatment plans to the patient.

The assistant has several important roles in each of these steps, including

- Aiding patients in completing information forms
- Generating diagnostic aids such as radiographs, diagnostic casts, and photographs
- Recording the dentist's findings during the examination
- Making financial arrangements with a patient who has accepted a treatment plan

Diagnosis and Treatment of the Emergency Patient

A patient's first contact with the practice may be an emergency call for the relief of pain. When this happens, the patient should be seen as quickly as possible. At the beginning of the emergency visit, basic information (medical history and personal data) must be gathered, and radiographs may be required.

Once the patient's **chief complaint** (reason for seeking dental treatment at this time) has been determined, the dentist will strive to relieve the discomfort as quickly as possible.

If the emergency patient has a regular dentist, he is referred back to that dentist for continuing treatment. If the patient does not have a regular dentist, he may be rescheduled for a complete diagnosis and treatment plan.

Exposure Control for the Dental Staff

In all contacts with all patients, staff members must follow the exposure (infection) control protocols described in Chapter 13.

Recording the Dental Examination

During the examination, the dentist's findings must be recorded completely and accurately. This information is organized and stored in the patient's **clinical record,** which is commonly referred to as the *patient chart.* This record is discussed further in Chapter 2.

In a **manual charting system,** the dentist dictates examination findings, and the assistant records the data on the patient chart (Fig. 18–1). On the tooth diagram portion of the chart, color-coded pencils may be used to indicate conditions of the teeth. Although these entries are made in pencil, all treatment entries must be in ink.

In a **computerized charting system,** examination findings are stored as a computerized record. With a voice-activated system, the dentist wears a microphone and dictates information directly into the computer.

LAST NAME	FIRST NAME	RESIDENCE TEL	RESIDENCE ADDRESS	CITY	STATE
Peterson	David	370-5140	2916 Harvest Drive	Anywhere	U.S.A.

GUARDIAN

BUSINESS TEL	BUSINESS ADDRESS	CITY	STATE
894-0101	1900 Park Avenue	Anywhere	U.S.A.

SS # 168-20-5841 | OCCUPATION computer sales | NAME OF PHYSICIAN Mary Devlin, MD | RECOMMENDED BY Simon Klein | DATE OF EXAM 8/15/xx

REFERRED TO OR BY DR. | ADDRESS OR TELEPHONE 894-7201 | ADDRESS | DATE OF ESTIMATE 9/10/xx | NO. OF PATIENT

1 2 3 4 5 6 7 8 9 10 11 12 13 14 15 16

RIGHT — LEFT

32 31 30 29 28 27 26 25 24 23 22 21 20 19 18 17

A B C D E F G H I J

R L

T S R Q P O N M L K

X-RAYS - F M ✓ B-W AREA

STUDY MODELS ✓ AGE

PHOTOGRAPHS - BEFORE

AFTER

ORAL FINDINGS

HYGIENE 1 (2) 3 4

DEPOSITS 1 (2) 3 4

PERIODONT 1 (2) 3 4

OCCLUSION

ABNORMALITIES

CONDITION OF TEETH

PRESENT FINDINGS
1 missing
2
3 missing*
4-A
5-B
6-C
7-D
8-E composite veneer
9-F composite veneer
10-G
11-H
12-I
13-J DO amalgam
14 MOD amalgam
15
16 missing
17 missing
18 abutment crown
19 pontic
20-K abutment crown
21-L
22-M
23-N
24-O
25-P
26-Q
27-R
28-S
29-T
30 gold crown
31
32 missing
OTHER–

DATE	TOOTH	SERVICE PLANNED	EST 1	EST 2	EST 3

CHIEF COMPLAINT

WHEN WAS LAST DENTAL VISIT 2 years ago

PROPHYLAXIS RESTORATIONS EXTRACTIONS

OTHER TREATMENT

GENERAL PHYSICAL CONDITION?

UNDER PHYSICIAN'S CARE NOW?

WHOM

NATURE OF TREATMENT

PREVIOUS HISTORY OF BLEEDING

REACTION TO ANESTHETIC

ALLERGIES INFECTIOUS HEPATITIS

CHRONIC AILMENTS? HEART DIABETES

RHEUMATIC FEVER ANEMIA

NERVOUSNESS BLOOD PRESSURE-

DENTURES: UPPER TYPE HOW LONG

LOWER TYPE HOW LONG

PARTIALS: TYPE HOW LONG

TYPE HOW LONG

REMARKS
Patient wants to discuss implant to replace tooth #3. Wants amalgams replaced

WORK SCHEDULE

TOOTH	MOULD		SHADE	
	UPPER	LOWER	UPPER	LOWER
CENT.				
LAT.				
CUSP.				
POST				

Form 9420 Colwell Co., Champaign, Illinois

An alternative is for the assistant to enter the data into the system.

A computerized charting system generates a color-coded printout of the examination findings. A copy is kept in the patient's chart, and a second copy may be given to the patient. This examination information is used in treatment planning and in conjunction with the accounts receivable system.

Data Gathering

The goal of data gathering is to bring together all of the information needed by the dentist to make an accurate diagnosis of the patient's condition. The following information must be gathered on each patient:

- Personal information
- Medical history
- Dental history
- Clinical observations
- Clinical examination
- Intraoral imaging and photographs (if necessary)
- Radiographs (see Chapter 17)
- Diagnostic casts (see Chapter 19)

Personal Information

Personal information, which is gathered on a **patient registration form** such as the one shown in Figure 34–4, includes the patient's full name, address, telephone numbers, and employment and dental insurance information and the referral source.

This information is used primarily by the administrative assistant in making financial arrangements and in collecting the fees owed to the dentist. Because this is financial information, not clinical information, it is *not* included in the patient's clinical chart.

Medical History

It is essential that the dentist have a current medical history on every patient. New patients are requested to complete a medical history form before initial treatment. Returning patients are asked to update their medical history information at each recall visit.

The medical history may be recorded on a written form, such as the one shown in Figure 18–2, or stored as a computerized data file.

This record includes questions concerning the patient's past medical history, present physical condition, chronic conditions, allergies, and medications. This information helps the dentist evaluate the patient's physical condition and identify any special treatment needs.

The dentist may also wish to consult the patient's physician regarding health problems, particularly if the patient is medically compromised. (**Medically compromised** means that the patient has an illness or physical condition that may influence the proposed dental treatment.)

A **release of information form** must be signed by the patient giving his consent before this consultation between the dentist and physician can take place.

MEDICATION HISTORY

A confidential medication history is a record of *all* the drugs the patient is currently taking. This includes prescription, over-the-counter, and any other drugs.

The dentist needs to know about these medications because either the medication or the condition for which it was prescribed may modify the selection of drugs and procedures in providing dental treatment.

A complete medication history is particularly important in older patients, many of whom have chronic conditions and are taking several prescribed medications.

ALLERGIES

If the patient has any known allergies or suspected allergies, it is extremely important that the dentist be aware of these. Of particular concern are allergies to antibiotics, latex products, and local anesthetic solutions.

MEDICAL ALERT

If the patient has a medical condition (such as a heart condition) that could impact decisions regarding dental treatment, this information is highlighted in the chart. A sticker may also be placed on the outside of the chart to alert the staff to this condition.

MEDICAL TESTS

On the basis of data from the medical history, clinical examination, and consultation with the patient's physician, the dentist may order medical laboratory tests such as blood tests or a biopsy. When required, a blood work-up is performed by a clinical medical laboratory. Biopsies are discussed in Chapter 30.

FIGURE 18–1

A dental chart used to record the dental examination. Treatment is recorded on the reverse side of the chart. (Courtesy of Colwell Systems, Champaign, IL.)

Date ____________

Name *James A. Gridley* Date of Birth *04/05/55*

Address *670 Northridge Terrace, Champaign Ill.* Telephone *351-4498*

Business Address ____________ Business Phone *322-0987*

Soc. Sec. No. ____________

Patient Name ____________

PATIENT MEDICAL HISTORY

Physician *Dr. Grace Hardy* Office Phone *322-0643* Home Phone ____________

Approximate date of last physical examination *one year*

		Yes	No
1.	Are you under any medical treatment now?	☑	☐
2.	Have you had any major operations? If so what?	☐	☑
3.	Have you ever had a serious accident involving head injuries?	☐	☑
4.	Have you had any adverse response to any drugs including penicillin?	☐	☑
5.	Has a physician ever informed you that you had: A Heart Ailment?	☐	☑
6.	High Blood Pressure?	☑	☐
7.	Respiratory Disease?	☐	☑
8.	Diabetes?	☐	☑
9.	Rheumatic Fever?	☐	☑
10.	Rheumatism or Arthritis?	☐	☑
11.	Tumors or Growths	☐	☑
12.	Any Blood Disease?	☐	☑
13.	Any Liver Disease?	☐	☑
14.	Any Kidney Disease?	☐	☑
15.	Any Stomach or Intestinal Disease?	☐	☑
16.	Any Venereal Disease?	☐	☑
17.	AIDS?	☐	☑
18.	Yellow Jaundice or Hepatitis?	☐	☑
19.	Do you have night sweats accompanied by weight loss or cough?	☐	☑
20.	Are you on a diet at this time?	☑	☐
21.	Are you now taking drugs or medications?	☑	☐
22.	Are you allergic to any known materials resulting in hives, asthma, eczema, etc.?	☐	☑
23.	Are you in general good health at this time?	☑	☐
24.	Have any wounds healed slowly or presented other complications?	☐	☑
25.	Are you pregnant?	☐	☑
26.	Do you have a history of fainting?	☐	☑
27.	Have you ever had any X-RAY TREATMENTS (other than diagnostic)?	☐	☑

PATIENT DENTAL HISTORY

		Yes	No
28.	Do you have pain in or near your ears?	☐	☑
29.	Do you have any unhealed injuries or inflamed areas in or around your mouth?	☐	☑
30.	Have you experienced any growth or sore spots in your mouth?	☐	☑
31.	Does any part of your mouth hurt when clenched?	☐	☑
32.	Have you ever had Novocaine anesthetic?	☑	☐
33.	Any reactions or allergic symptoms to Novocaine?	☐	☑
34.	Any difficult extractions in the past?	☐	☑
35.	Prolonged bleeding following extractions in the past?	☐	☑
36.	Trench Mouth?	☐	☑
37.	Do your gums bleed?	☐	☑
38.	Have you ever had instruction on the correct method of brushing your teeth?	☑	☐
39.	Have you ever had instructions on the care of your gums?	☑	☐
40.	Do you chew on only one side of your mouth? If so why?	☐	☑
41.	Do you at the present time have any dental complaints?	☐	☑
42.	Do you habitually clench your teeth during the night or day?	☐	☑
43.	When was your last full mouth X-RAY taken? *6 months ago* Where? ____________		
44.	Any part of your mouth sore to pressures or irritants (cold, sweets, etc.) If so locate ____________	☐	☑

Signature *James A. Gridley*

FORM 9879 COLWELL SYSTEMS, INC., CHAMPAIGN, IL 61820

FIGURE 18–2

Medical history form. (From Ehrlich, A., and Torres, H.O.: Essentials of Dental Assisting. Philadelphia, W.B. Saunders Co., 1992, p 225.)

Dental History

The patient's dental history offers important clues concerning previous dental care, how recently the patient has received dental treatment, the frequency of dental visits, the patient's home care program, and the patient's attitude concerning the importance of dental care.

Clinical Observations

Vital signs, which are important clinical observations, include the patient's pulse and respiration rates, blood pressure, and temperature. These are discussed in Chapter 9.

The patient's appearance also offers important clues as to his general health and mental well-being. These too are discussed in Chapter 9.

Examination Techniques and Equipment

The purpose of the clinical examination is to provide a record of the patient's current dental health and to detect disease or abnormal conditions that may be present in the soft and hard tissues of the face, neck, and oral cavity.

If a suspicious lesion is discovered, a biopsy may be required. **Lesion** is a broad term describing tissue damage caused by either injury or disease. A lesion is described by its

- Exact location
- Size (in millimeters)
- Color
- Form
- Other characteristics

Terms used to describe the form include **indurated** (hard or firm), **bulbous** (round), and **pedunculated** (extended or hanging from a cordlike length of tissue).

Other characteristics include whether the lesion is fixed or movable, whether it is smooth or rough, and what its relationship is to the surface of the tissue. It may be elevated (above the surface), flat (even with the surface), or ulcerated (below the surface).

Part of the examination is performed visually and by palpation. (**Palpation** is an examination technique in which the examiner's hands are used to feel the texture, size, and consistency of certain body parts.)

A **digital** examination is a form of palpation in which the examiner uses the fingers and thumb of one hand. A **bimanual** examination is a form of palpation in which both hands are used simultaneously.

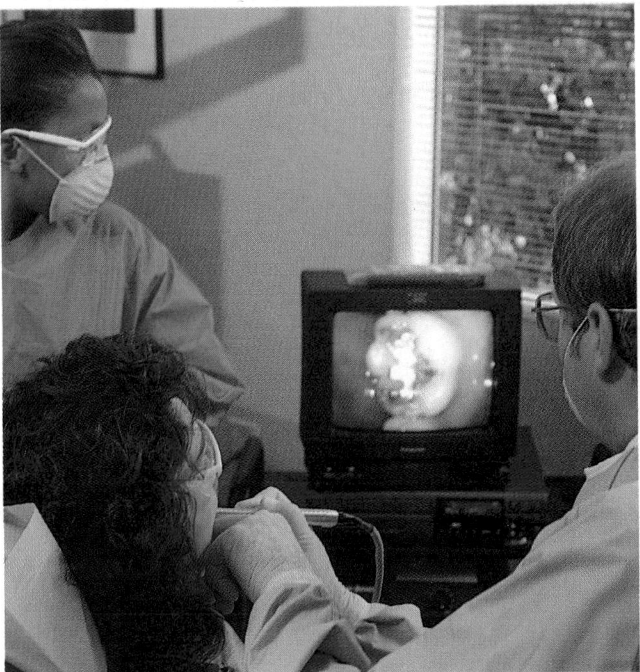

FIGURE 18–3

An intraoral imaging system is a powerful diagnostic and patient education tool.

Intraoral Imaging

An intraoral imaging system, which is similar to a miniature video camera, may be used as a diagnostic aid and a patient education tool. An intraoral imaging system consists of

- A **handpiece** to capture the images
- A **computer** to process and store the images
- A **color monitor** to project the images
- A **color printer** to create "prints" of selected images

The handpiece may be used extraorally at low magnification to record a full face or smile view before and/or after treatment. In addition, the system may digitize (capture) radiographs so that they too can be viewed on the monitor and stored in the system.

The handpiece is used intraorally at high magnifications primarily as a diagnostic aid to view all areas of the mouth. Because it is used in the patient's mouth, the handpiece must be sterilized after each use.

These images are displayed on the color monitor for both the dentist and the patient to see (Fig. 18–3). Because of the magnification and access into hard-to-see areas, this is a very powerful diagnostic and patient education tool.

Color prints of selected images may be used during the case presentation to the patient, to document treatment, and for submission with insurance claims.

(text continued on page 348)

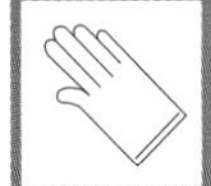
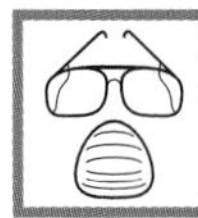
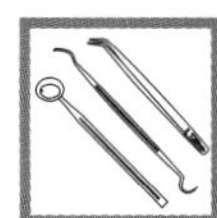

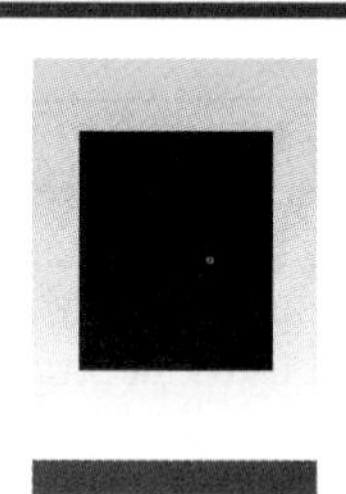

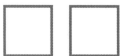

PROCEDURE: **Assisting During the Clinical Examination**

Instrumentation (Fig. 18–4)

Periodontal probe
Gauze sponges (2 × 2 or 4 × 4 inch)
Dental floss
Tongue depressor (optional)
Patient chart
Pencils: black, blue, red, green

Patient Preparation

1. The assistant observes the patient's general appearance, speech, and behavior as he enters the operatory.
   □ *RATIONALE:* Unusual occurrences are immediately noted or called to the dentist's attention.
2. The assistant seats and drapes the patient in an upright position.
3. The operator explains the procedure, and the need for it, to the patient before the examination.
   □ *RATIONALE:* The patient who knows what to expect will be more comfortable. He will also be able to give informed consent for this treatment.

Examination of the Face

1. The operator examines the face, neck, and ears, looking for asymmetry or abnormal swelling (Fig. 18–5).
   □ *RATIONALE:* Normally both sides of the face are symmetric. (**Symmetric** means divided into halves that are mirror images of each other. When the halves are not the same, this is referred to as **asymmetry.**)
2. The operator looks for abnormal tissue changes, skin abrasions, and discolorations.
   □ *RATIONALE:* Unusual bruising, scratches, or cuts may indicate that the patient has been abused.
3. The operator notes the texture, color, and continuity of the vermilion border; the commissures of the lips; the philtrum; and the smile line (Fig.

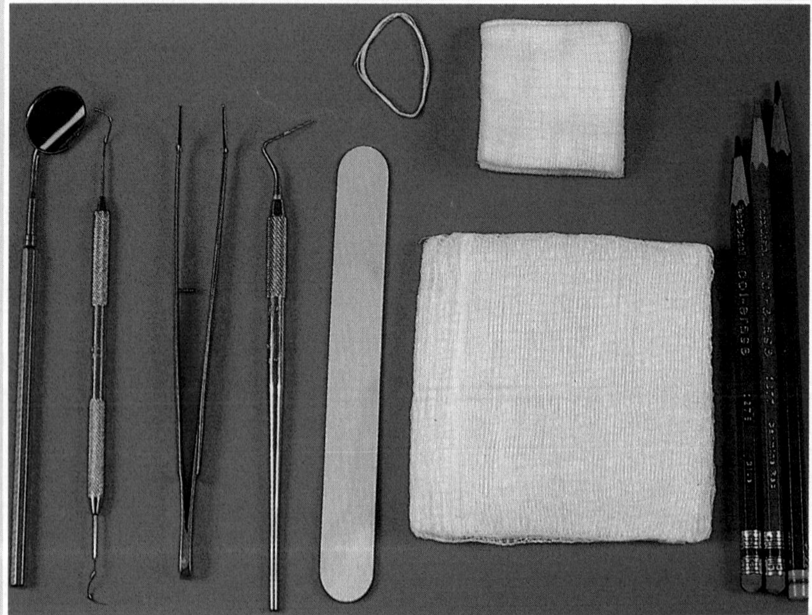

FIGURE 18–4

Instrumentation for a dental examination. *Left to right:* mouth mirror, explorer, cotton pliers, periodontal probe, tongue blade (optional), dental floss, gauze sponges, and colored pencils (optional).

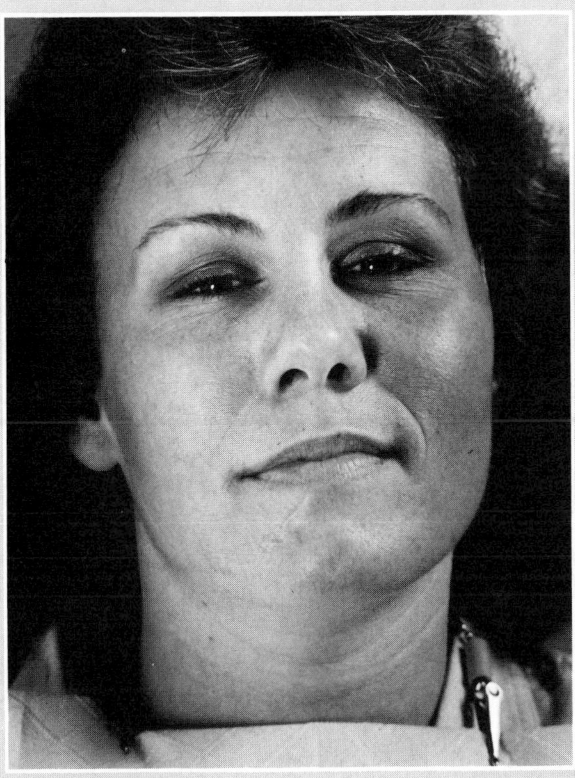

FIGURE 18–5

The patient's face is examined for symmetry.

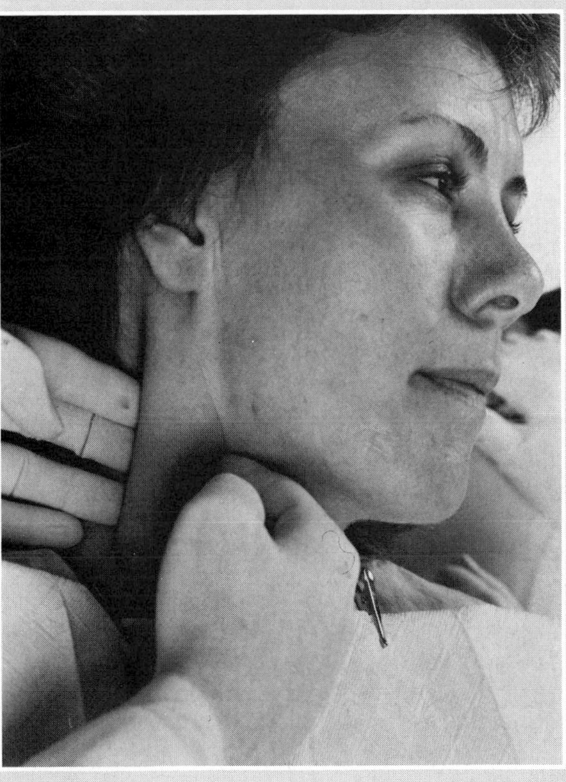

FIGURE 18–7

Palpating the right cervical chain of lymph nodes. This procedure is repeated on the left.

18–6). (The **smile line** is the level at which the lip covers the teeth when the patient smiles.)
□ *RATIONALE:* Indurations, lump formation, dryness, and cracking of the tissues are all deviations from normal.

Examination of the Cervical Lymph Nodes

1. The operator is positioned in front and to the side of the patient.
2. To examine the right side of the neck, the operator's right hand steadies the patient's head. The fingers and thumb of the operator's left hand gently follow the chain of lymph nodes downward, starting in front of the right ear and continuing to the collarbone (Fig. 18–7).
□ *RATIONALE:* The operator is looking for swelling, abnormal formation, and/or tenderness of the area.
3. To examine the left side of the neck, the operator's left hand steadies the patient's head. The fingers and thumb of the operator's right hand gently follow the chain of lymph nodes downward, starting in front of the left ear and continuing to the clavicle (collarbone).

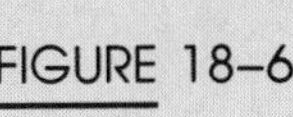

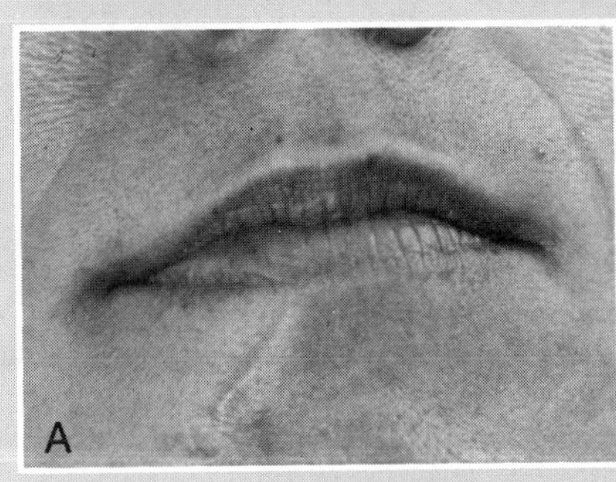

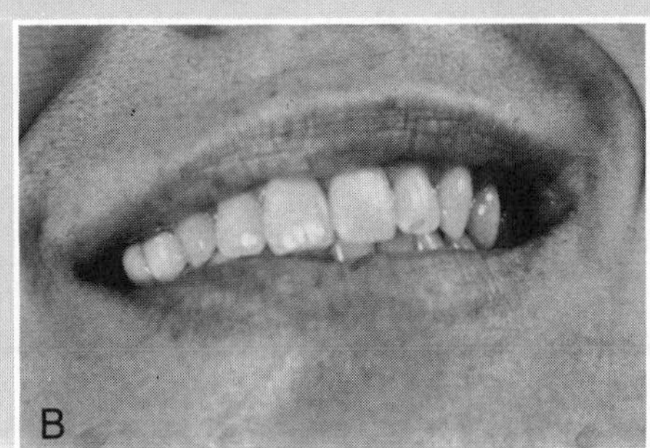

FIGURE 18–6

External examination of the lips. *A*, Checking the vermilion border and commissures. *B*, Checking the smile line.

(continued on following page)

PROCEDURE: **Assisting During the Clinical Examination** *(continued)*

Examination of the Temporomandibular Joint (TMJ)

1. To determine whether tenderness of the TMJ is present, the operator gently places fingers of each hand just anterior to the tragus of each ear (Fig. 18–8*A*).
2. To evaluate TMJ movements in centric, lateral, protrusive, and retrusive movements, the operator asks the patient to open and close his mouth normally and then to move his jaw from side to side (Fig. 18–8*B*).
3. To further evaluate the movement of the TMJ, the operator gently places fingers in the external opening of the ear. The patient is asked to open and close his mouth normally (Fig. 18–9).
4. To determine whether there is noise in the TMJ during movement, the dentist listens as the patient opens and closes his mouth. A stethoscope, placed on the joint, may be used for this purpose.
5. Any abnormalities or patient comments regarding pain, tenderness, or other problems relating to opening and closing the mouth are noted on the patient's chart.

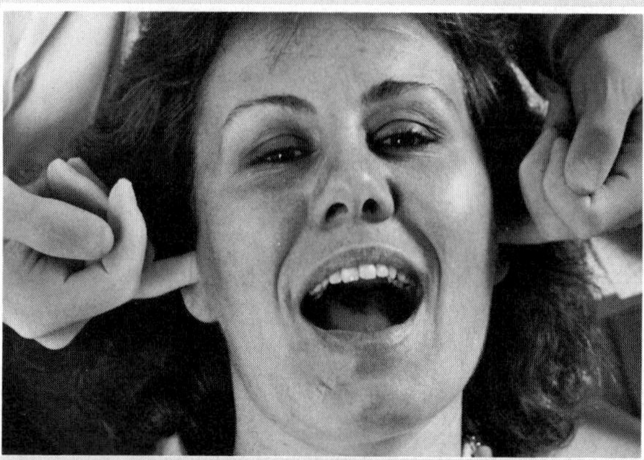

FIGURE 18–9

Palpating the temporomandibular joint during motion by placing the fingers gently into the external opening of the ear.

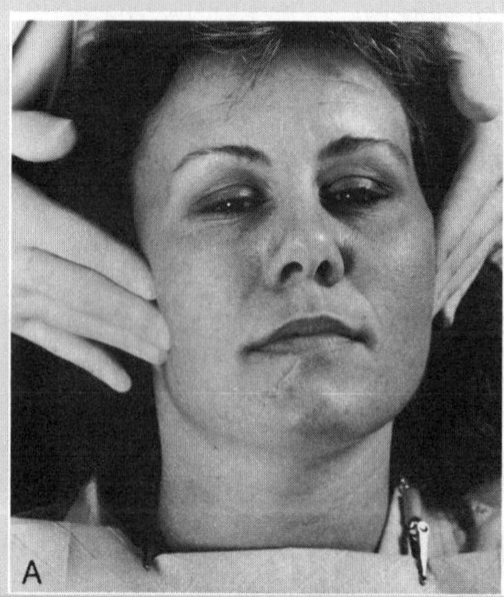

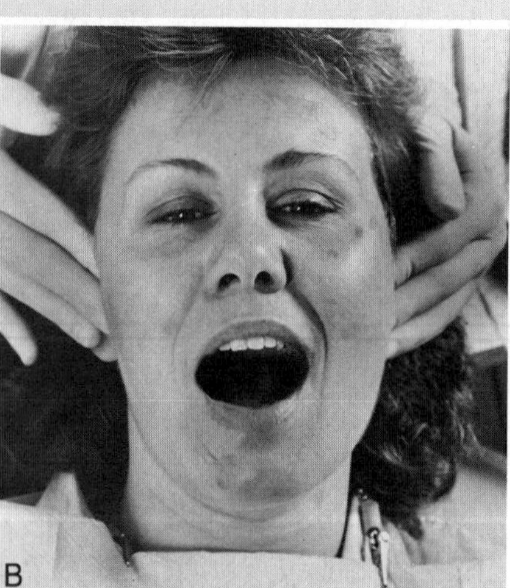

FIGURE 18–8

Palpating the function of the temporomandibular joint. *A*, With the mouth closed. *B*, With the mouth open.

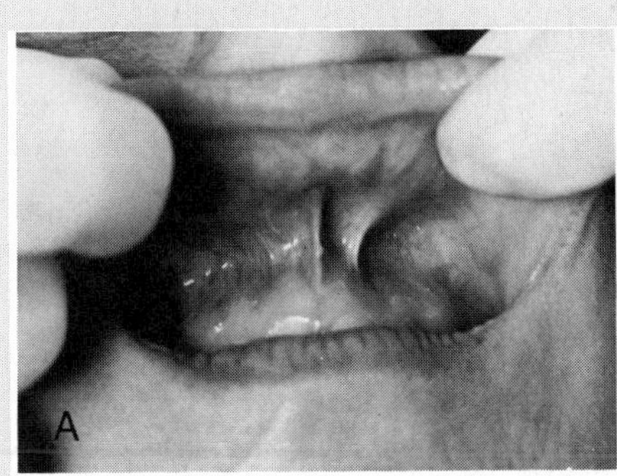

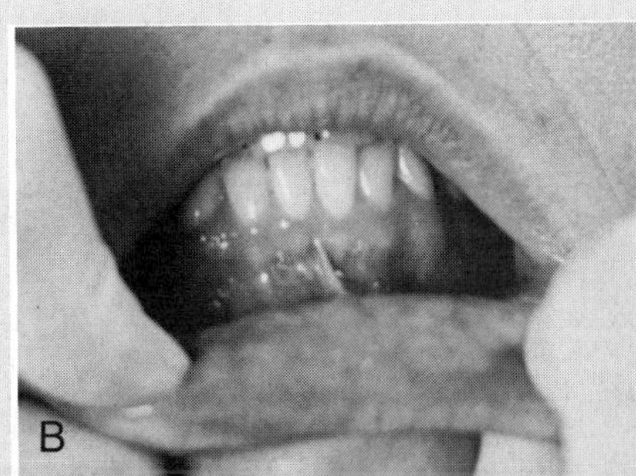

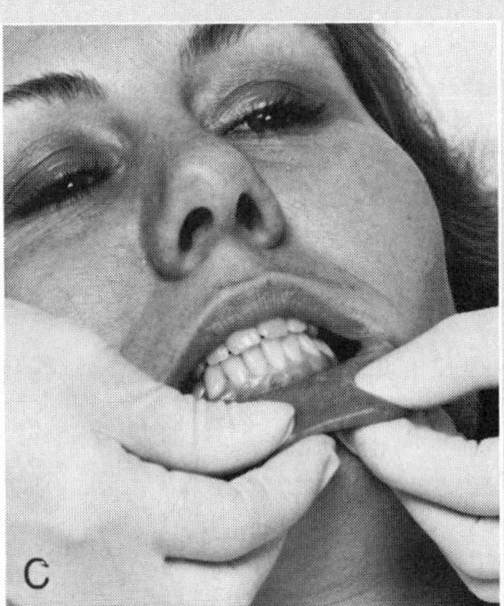

FIGURE 18–10

Examining the mucosa and frenum of the upper and lower lips. *A*, Visually examining the maxillary tissues. *B*, Visually examining the mandibular tissues. *C*, Gently palpating the tissues.

Examination for Indications of Oral Habits

1. The dentist looks for indications of oral habits such as thumb sucking, tongue-thrust swallow, and mouth breathing.
   □ *RATIONALE:* The habits may impact the occlusion or cause irritation around the lips.
2. The dentist looks for signs of oral habits such as bruxism, grinding, and clenching. These indications include abnormal wear on the teeth and problems in the TMJ.

Examination of the Interior of the Lips

1. The patient is asked to open his mouth slightly.
2. The mucosa and labial frenum of the upper lip are examined by gently retracting the lip with the thumbs and index fingers (Fig. 18–10*A*).
3. The mucosa and labial frenum of the lower lip are examined by gently retracting the lip with the thumbs and index fingers (Fig. 18–10*B*).
4. These tissues are gently palpated to detect lumps or similar abnormalities (Fig. 18–10*C*).

Examination of the Oral Mucosa and Stensen's Duct

1. The tissues of the buccal mucosa are gently palpated by placing the thumb of one hand inside the mouth and the index and third fingers of the other hand on the exterior of the cheek (Fig. 18–11).
2. The tissue covering the hard palate is palpated very gently with an index finger (Fig. 18–12).
3. The buccal mucosa and the opening of Stensen's duct are examined visually (Fig. 18–13). A warm mouth mirror may also be used to note the flow of saliva from the duct.
   □ *RATIONALE:* The mouth mirror is warmed to prevent fogging.

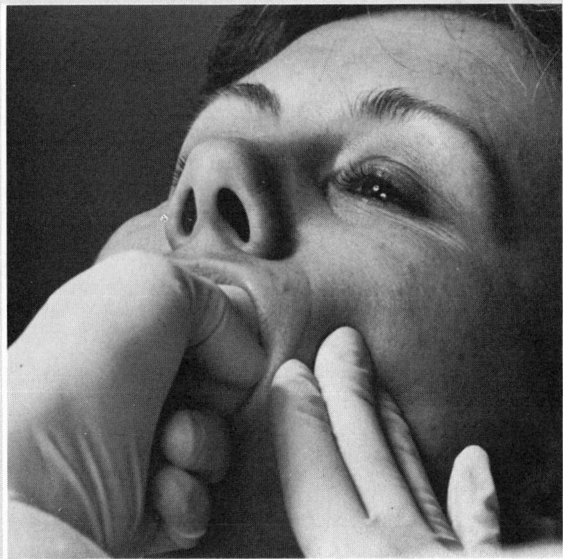

FIGURE 18–11

Bimanually palpating of the left buccal mucosa. The procedure is repeated on the right.

(continued on following page)

PROCEDURE: **Assisting During the Clinical Examination** *(continued)*

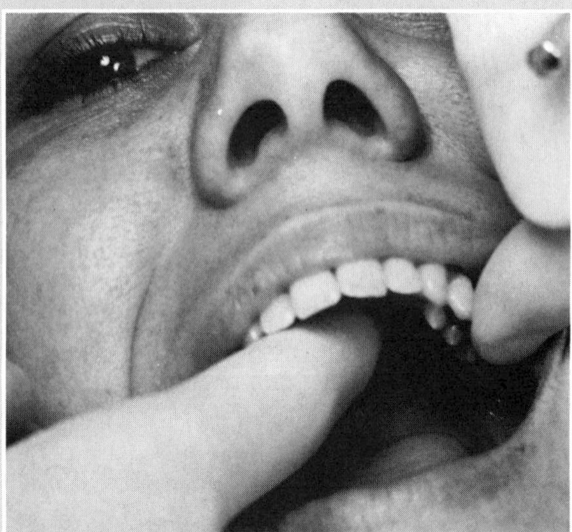

FIGURE 18–12

Palpating the anterior portion of the hard palate.

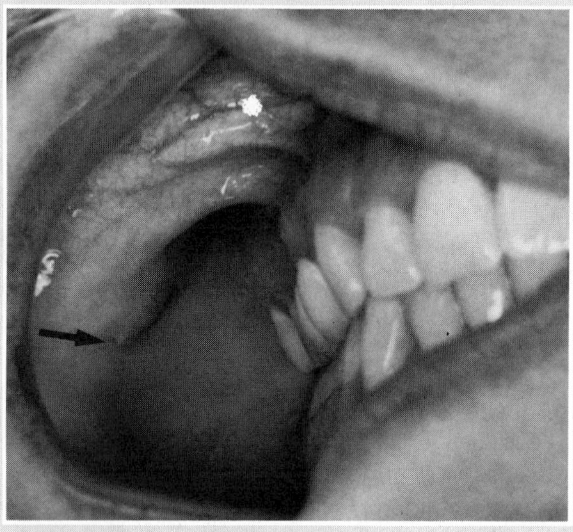

FIGURE 18–13

Visual examination of the buccal mucosa. The arrow indicates the opening of Stensen's duct.

Examination of the Tongue and Throat

1. The patient is asked to extend his tongue and to relax it. Using a sterile gauze sponge, the operator gently grasps the tip of the tongue and gently pulls it forward (Fig. 18–14*A*).
2. The operator observes the dorsum (top) of the tongue for color, papillae, presence or lack of a coating, and abnormalities.
3. The operator gently moves the tongue from side to side to examine the lateral (side) and ventral (under) surfaces.
4. A warm mouth mirror is used to observe the posterior area of the palate and oropharynx (Fig. 18–14*B*).

   □ *CAUTION:* To avoid triggering the gag reflex, this mirror is placed very carefully and moved very little.
5. The uvula, the base of the tongue, and the posterior area of the mouth are examined by placing a mouth mirror firmly at the base of the tongue (Fig. 18–15).

   □ *RATIONALE:* Firm but gentle placement reduces the possibility of triggering the gag reflex.
6. With the mouth mirror firmly depressing the base of the tongue, the patient is asked to say "eh-eh."

   □ *RATIONALE:* This action causes the oropharynx to expand, so the operator can view the upper portion of the throat.

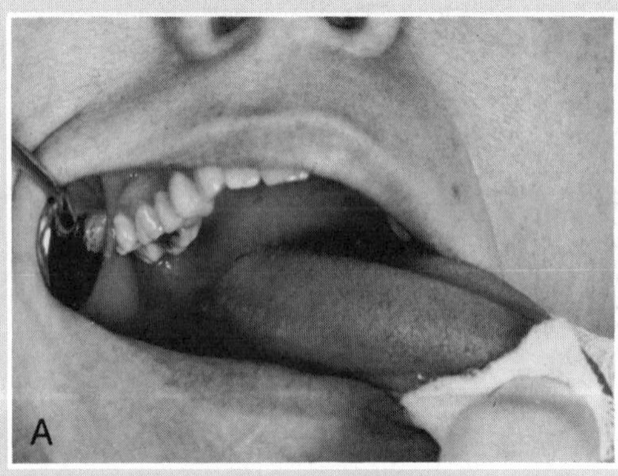

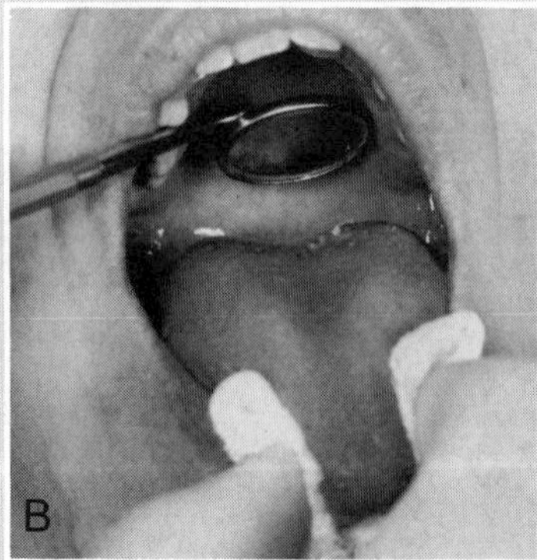

FIGURE 18–14

Examining the tongue and posterior of the mouth. *A*, The tongue is grasped with a gauze sponge and gently pulled forward. *B*, A mouth mirror is used to examine the base of the tongue.

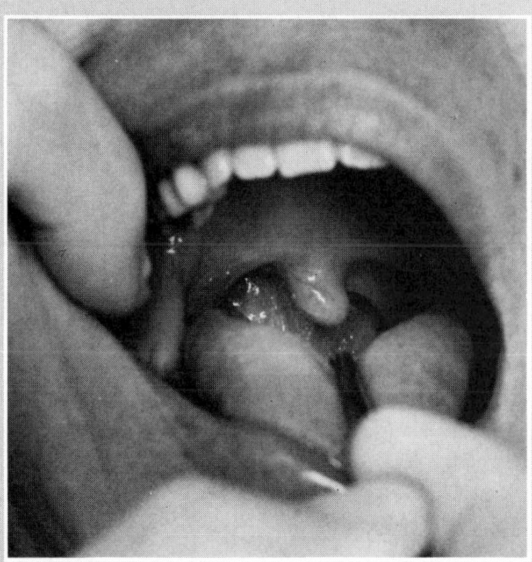

FIGURE 18–15

Examining the uvula and the tissues of the oropharynx.

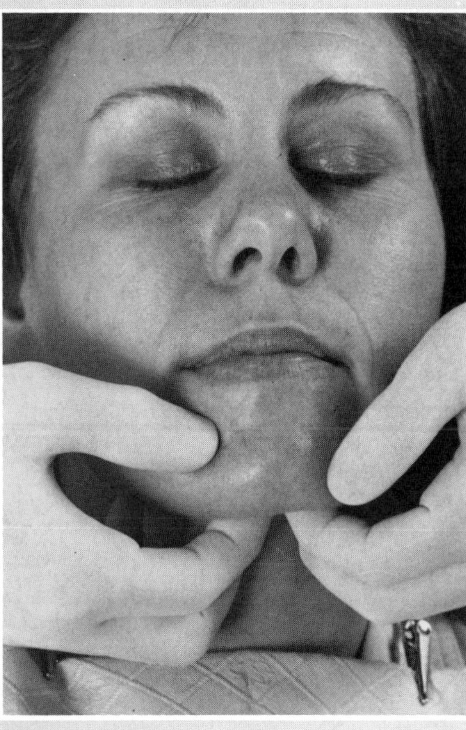

FIGURE 18–16

Gently palpating the external tissues of the mandible and floor of the mouth.

Examination of the Floor of the Mouth

1. With the patient's mouth closed, the operator gently palpates the soft tissues of the face above and below the mandible (Fig. 18–16).
   □ *RATIONALE:* The operator is looking for the presence of tori and other abnormalities.
2. The interior of the floor of the mouth is gently palpated by placing the index finger of one hand on the floor of the mouth and placing the fingers of the other hand on the outer surface under the chin (Fig. 18–17*A*).
3. The patient is instructed to touch the tongue to the hard palate. This allows the operator to visually examine the floor of the mouth, the lingual frenum, and the salivary ducts (Fig. 18–17*B*).
4. The quantity and consistency of the flow of saliva are observed. Depending on the patient's general health or diet, the saliva may vary in consistency from watery to thick and ropey.

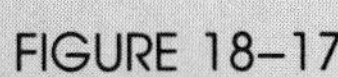

FIGURE 18–17

Internal examination of the tissues of the mandible and floor of the mouth. *A*, Bimanually palpating the floor of the mouth. *B*, Visually examining the ventral side of the tongue and the floor of the mouth.

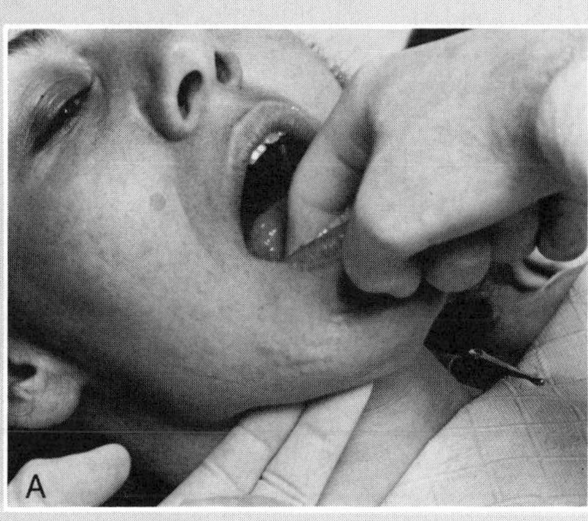

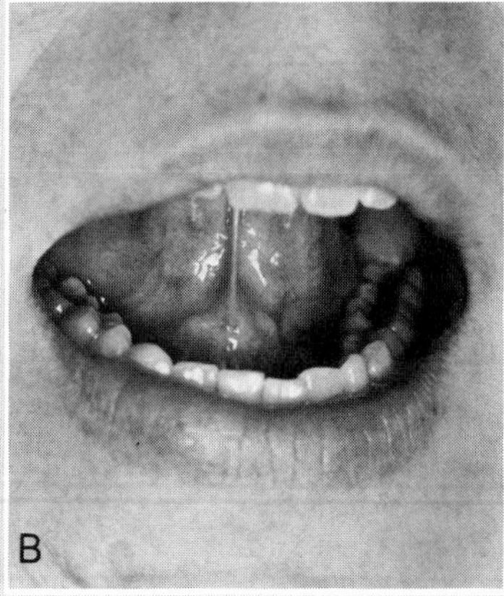

Intraoral Photography

A flash camera and color film are frequently used to document conditions of the tongue or soft tissues of the oral cavity and as "before" and "after" records before orthodontic treatment, major restorative treatment, or the placement of esthetic restorations.

Depending upon the use, these photographs may include full face and profile views. For intraoral views, sterile clear plastic retractors are used to hold back the cheeks.

Periodontal Screening and Recording

The American Dental Association and the American Academy of Periodontology recommend that periodontal screening and recording (PSR) be part of *all* adult periodic oral examinations.

PSR is a system for the early detection of periodontal disease. Its purpose is to permit the dentist to very quickly determine whether the patient needs a more thorough periodontal examination. (This is discussed in Chapter 26.)

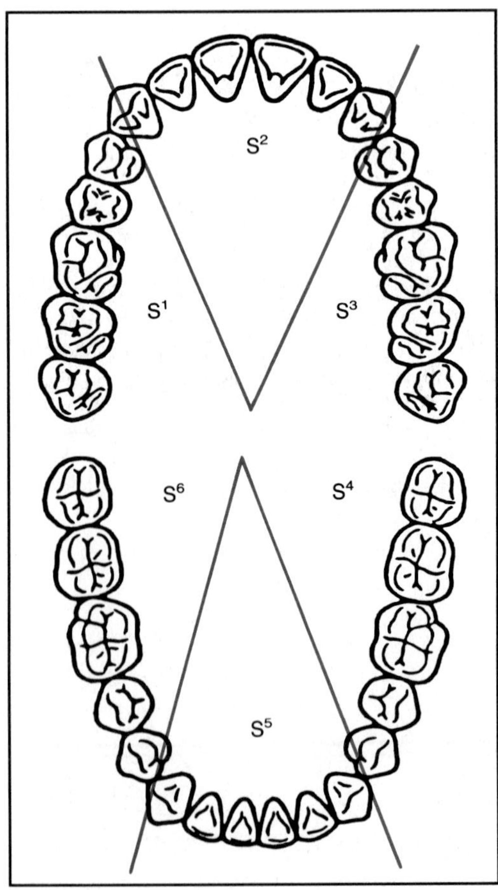

FIGURE 18–18

For recording purposes during the PSR examination, the arch is divided into sextants.

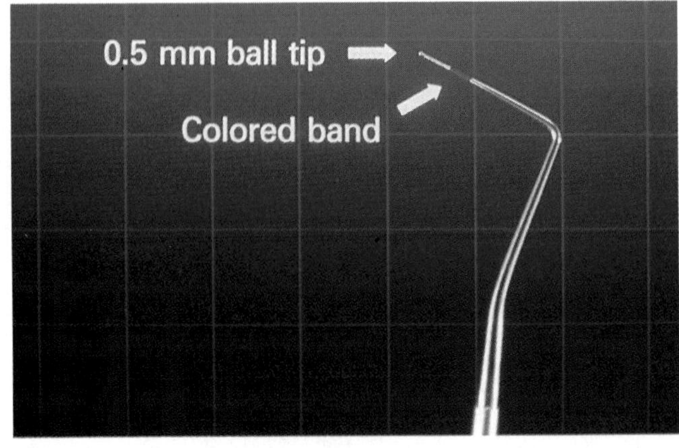

FIGURE 18–19

A special color-coded periodontal probe is used during the PSR examination. (Courtesy of American Academy of Periodontology, Chicago, IL.)

LIMITATIONS OF THE PSR

- The PSR is not intended to replace a periodontal examination.
- The PSR is designed to be used on adults and is *not* recommended for patients under the age of 18.
- The PSR should not be used for those patients who have already been treated for periodontal diseases and are now in a maintenance phase. These patients need a comprehensive periodontal examination.

PERIODONTAL SCREENING AND RECORDING

For ease in examination and charting, the dentition is divided into sextants (Fig. 18–18). Using gentle pressure, the dentist inserts the color-coded periodontal probe into the gingival sulcus until resistance is met (Fig. 18–19). The depth of insertion is read by noting the position of the color coding in the sulcus.

The dentist may choose to probe only one or two teeth in each sextant or to probe every tooth in the sextant. Six surfaces on the selected teeth are probed:

- Mesiofacial
- Buccal
- Distofacial
- Mesiolingual
- Lingual
- Distolingual

The system for scoring these readings is outlined in Table 18–1. The highest score in each sextant is recorded in a simple box chart (Fig. 18–20).

In addition to these scores, an asterisk (*) is written next to the sextant scores if any of the following clinical abnormalities are present:

- Furcation involvement
- Mobility

TABLE 18–1

Periodontal Screening and Recording Scores

SCORE	DESCRIPTION
0	The colored area of the probe remains *completely visible* in the deepest sulcus in the sextant; no calculus or defective margins are detected
1	The colored area of the probe remains *completely visible* in the deepest probing in the sextant; no calculus or defective margins are detected; there is bleeding after gentle probing
2	The colored area of the probe remains *completely visible* in the deepest probing in the sextant; supra- or subgingival calculus and/or defective margins are detected
3	The colored area of the probe remains *partly visible* in the deepest probing depth in the sextant
4	The colored area of the probe *completely disappears*, indicating probing depth of greater than 5.5 mm

- Mucogingival problems
- Recession extending to the colored area of the probe (3.5 mm or greater)

If two or more quadrants have teeth with scores of 3 or 4, a comprehensive full-mouth periodontal examination and charting is indicated.

Clinical Examination of the Teeth

A clinical examination of the teeth includes detailed scrutiny of each tooth from the incisal edge or occlusal surface of the crown to the free gingival margin. The natural pits and grooves of each tooth are explored carefully as the operator looks for

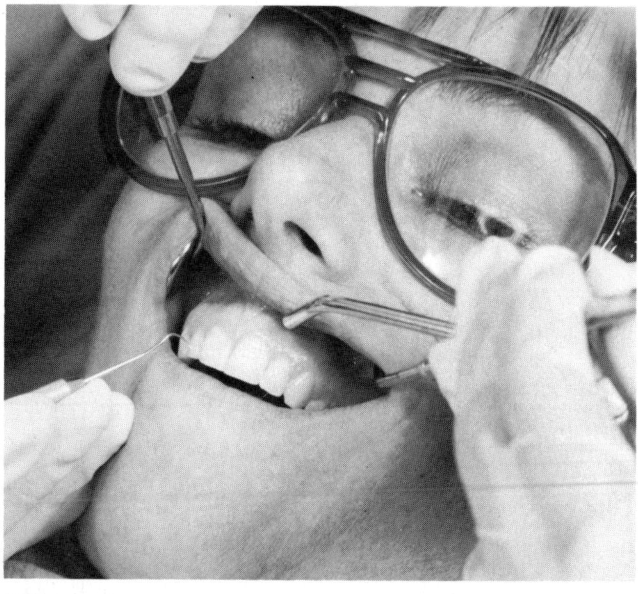

FIGURE 18–21

The assistant may be asked to dry the tooth surface with air from the air-water syringe.

- Malpositioned or missing teeth
- Structural defects, staining, or fractures of the teeth
- Decalcified areas and minute breaks in the enamel
- Carious lesions and indications of recurrent decay
- Rough interproximal surfaces and an overhang of the margins of amalgam or cast restorations
- Poorly adapted cast restorations and poorly fitting prostheses
- Abnormal wear patterns on the teeth

To improve the operator's view of the tooth surfaces, the assistant may be asked to use the air syringe to dry the teeth (Fig. 18–21).

Using an explorer and mouth mirror, the operator examines each surface of the tooth. Unwaxed dental floss is passed through the contacts of adjacent teeth to examine for interproximal caries and overhanging restorations. (These conditions will cause the floss to catch or fray.)

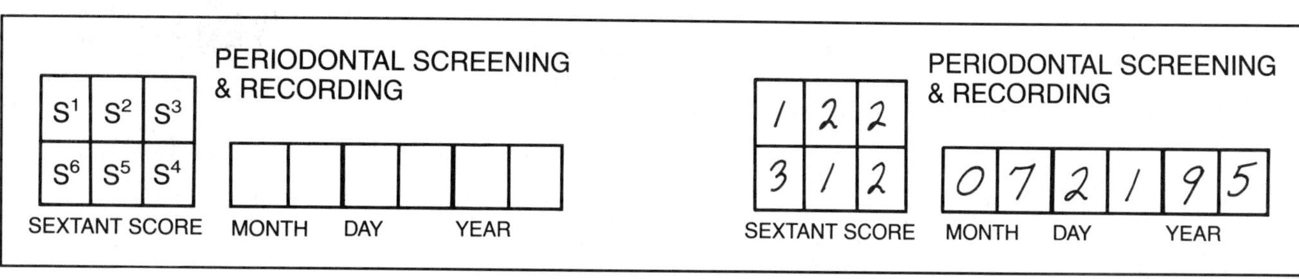

FIGURE 18–20

A box chart is used to record the scores for each sextant. *Left*, Chart showing where each sextant score is recorded. *Right*, Chart showing sample entries.

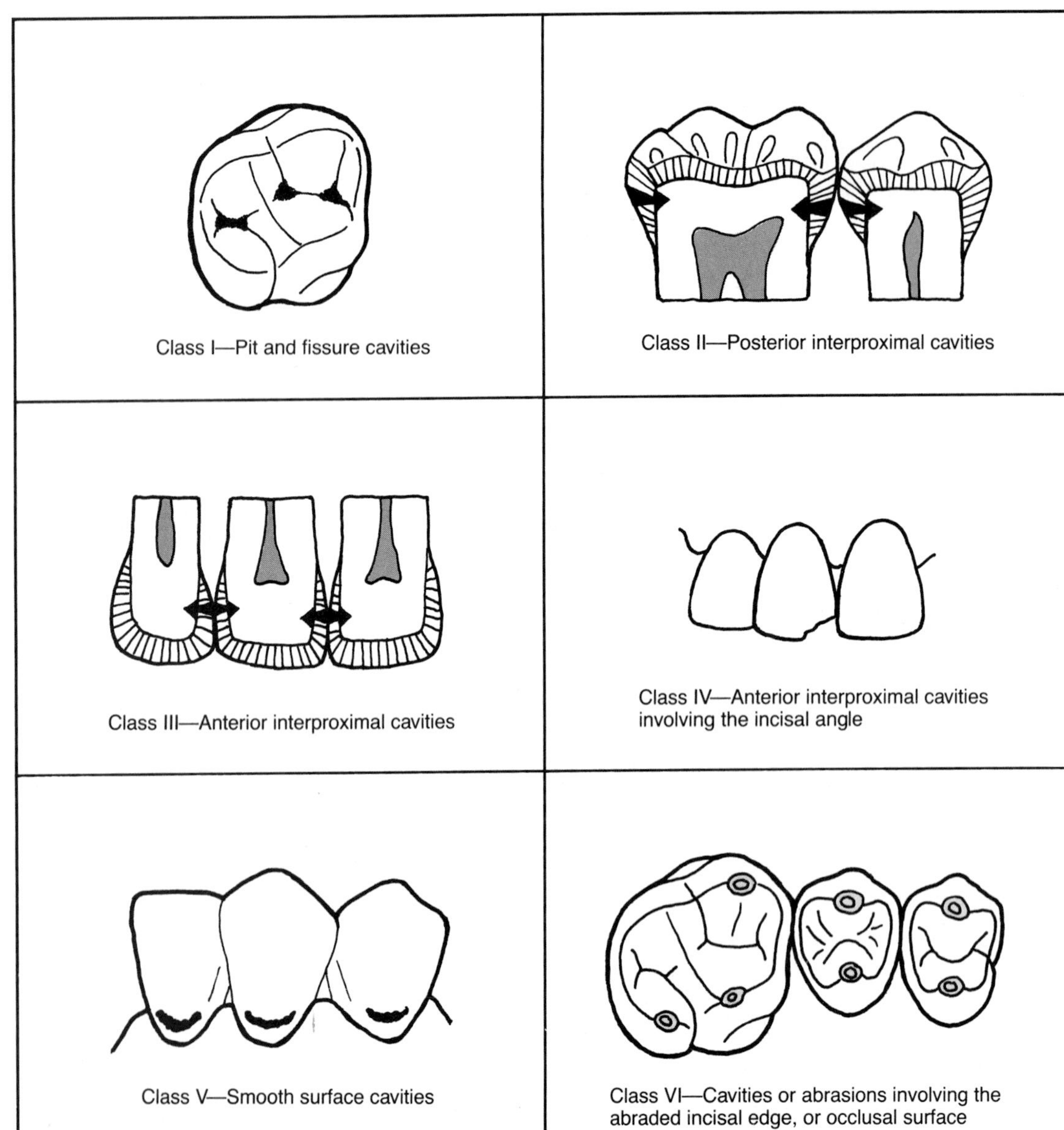

FIGURE 18–22

Black's classification of cavities. (From Ehrlich, A., and Torres, H.O.: Essentials of Dental Assisting. Philadelphia, W.B. Saunders Co., 1992, p 232.)

Charting Conditions of the Teeth

During the clinical examination, the dentist usually dictates findings to the assistant, who records them on the patient's chart. Whether charting findings are recorded manually or by computer, it is essential that all entries be accurate.

A tooth diagram on the chart is used to graphically record examination findings. When dictating, the dentist uses the Universal Numbering System to identify the teeth. The tooth diagram is labeled according to the same system: the permanent teeth are numbered from 1 to 32, and the primary teeth are lettered from A to T.

BLACK'S CLASSIFICATION OF CAVITIES

When cavities or restorations are present, they are described and classified according to the system developed by G. V. Black in about 1900. The original classes were I to V. Class VI was added at a later date (Fig. 18–22).

Class I cavities (pit and fissure) occur in the following sites:

- Occlusal surfaces of premolars and molars
- Occlusal two-thirds of the facial surfaces of mandibular molars
- Occlusal one-third of the lingual surfaces of the maxillary molars
- Lingual surfaces of maxillary incisors most frequently in the pit near the cingulum

Class II cavities (posterior interproximal) occur in the proximal surfaces of premolars and molars and involve the occlusal surfaces of the teeth.

Class III cavities (anterior interproximal) occur in the proximal surfaces of incisors and cuspids.

Class IV cavities (anterior interproximal cavities involving the incisal angle) occur in the proximal surfaces of incisors and cuspids and involve the incisal angle.

Class V cavities (smooth surface) occur in the gingival third of the facial (or lingual) surfaces of any tooth. They may also occur on the root of the tooth near the cementoenamel junction (CEJ).

Class VI cavities or abrasions involve the abraded incisal edge of anterior teeth or occlusal surfaces of posterior teeth. (**Abraded** means worn away.)

NUMBER OF SURFACES INVOLVED

In addition to the classification just described, the following terms are used to describe the number of tooth surfaces involved:

- **Simple:** involving only one tooth surface
- **Compound:** involving two surfaces of a tooth
- **Complex:** involving more than two surfaces of a tooth

Color Coding Charting

Color coding systems may be used in both manual and computerized systems to indicate restorations and defects that are present. The following are the color codes most commonly used in manual systems:

- Carious lesions are outlined on the tooth surface in black pencil.
- After the tooth has been restored, the outlined area is filled in with the appropriate color.
- Amalgam restorations are colored in blue.
- Composite restorations may be *shaded* in green to distinguish the difference in restorative material.
- Gold restorations are colored in red (an alternative is to outline the area and fill it with cross-hatching).
- If a previously restored tooth needs a new restoration, the involved area is *outlined* in the color corresponding to the color of the intended restoration.

Charting Symbols

Charting symbols are used on the tooth diagram to represent various conditions and restorations (Figs. 18–23 and 18–24). There are many systems of charting symbols, and the ones used depend upon the operator's preference. It is important that the assistant quickly learn to use the dentist's preferred system. As examples:

- In some systems, an **X** is used to indicate a missing tooth. (In other systems, a single slash [/] is used for this purpose.)

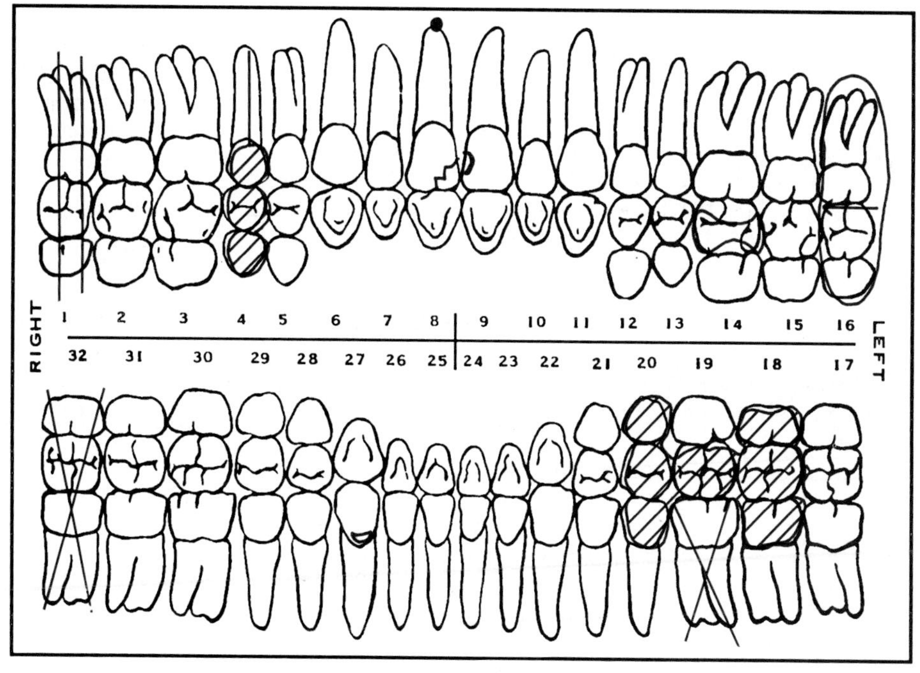

FIGURE 18–23

Tooth diagram portion of a dental chart showing conditions and restorations present. (This was recorded in one color.) 1: To be extracted. 4: Completed endodontic treatment, restored with a full crown. 8: MI fracture, periapical abscess. 9: M composite restoration. 14: MOD amalgam restoration. 16: Impacted, mesial drift. 19: Missing, replaced with a three-unit bridge. 18 and 20 are abutments and have full crowns. 27: Class V caries. 32: Missing. (Courtesy of Colwell Systems, Champaign, IL.)

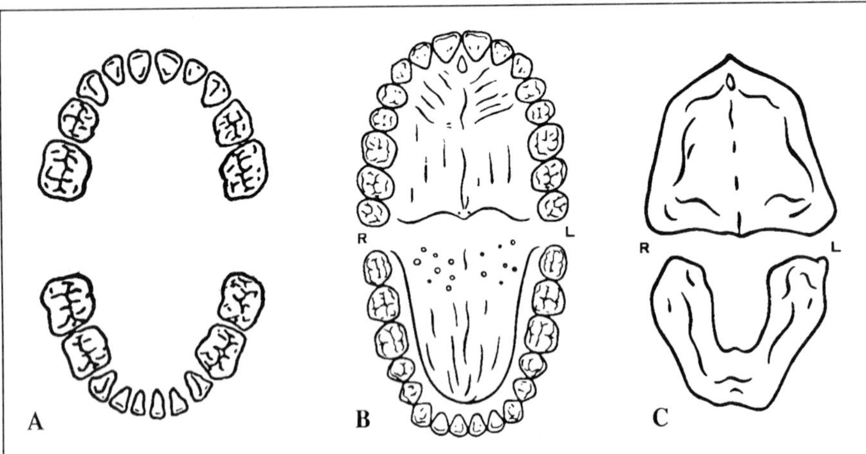

FIGURE 18–24

Specialized dental diagrams. *A*, Occlusal view of the primary dentition. *B*, Occlusal view of the permanent dentition with space to indicate findings on the palate and tongue. *C*, Occlusal view of the edentulous arches. (Courtesy of Colwell Systems, Champaign, IL.)

- In some systems, a tooth to be extracted is indicated with two parallel lines. (In other systems, a tooth to be extracted may be marked with an **X**.)

Charting Abbreviations

Abbreviations are used to indicate a single surface or a combination of tooth surfaces. Single surface abbreviations are summarized in Table 18–2.

When two or more tooth surfaces restored as a single restoration are described, a new term is formed. This is done by (a) dropping the last letter of the first word of the combination and (b) changing the word ending to "o." As shown in Table 18–3, sometimes the word parts are connected directly. Other times, they are joined by a hyphen.

To simplify things when dictating these findings, the dentist simply gives the letters involved: for example, "MI fracture" instead of "mesioincisal fracture."

Recording Treatment

The treatment record contains all details concerning the patient's treatment. This record is a log of the date, condition treated, materials used, and all other details pertinent to the patient's visit. Guidelines for making these entries are discussed in Chapter 2.

TABLE 18–2

Single Surface Abbreviations

ABBREVIATION	SURFACE NAME
B	buccal
D	distal
F	facial
I	incisal
L	lingual
M	mesial
O	occlusal

Often abbreviations are used when recording the treatment, and each dentist has his or her personal preferences. Some of the more commonly used abbreviations are summarized in Table 18–4.

However, accuracy and completeness of these records is essential. If there is any doubt about the meaning of an abbreviation, it is better to spell out what has taken place.

If the assistant records the treatment, the entry should be initialed by the operator providing that treatment.

Treatment Planning

After the dentist has gathered sufficient information and studied it carefully, he or she will diagnose the patient's dental conditions. On the basis of this diagnosis, the dentist may prepare one or more treatment plans for presentation to the patient.

A written treatment plan demonstrates that the dentist has made a thorough study of the patient's condition and is prepared to offer the patient options to help him manage his dental treatment according to his needs, priorities, and financial resources.

TABLE 18–3

Combination Abbreviations

ABBREVIATION	SURFACE NAME
BO	bucco-occlusal
DI	distoincisal
DL	distolingual
DO	disto-occlusal
LO	linguo-occlusal
MI	mesioincisal
MO	mesio-occlusal
MOD	mesio-occlusodistal
MODBL	mesio-occlusodistobuccolingual

TABLE 18–4

Treatment Abbreviations

ABBREVIATION	TREATMENT
am or amal	amalgam
anes	local anesthetic
Br	bridge
C&B	crown and bridge
com or comp	composite
CR	crown
GR	gold restoration
MandFD or LFD	mandibular (or lower) full denture
MandPD or LPD	mandibular (or lower) partial denture
MFD or UFD	maxillary (or upper) full denture
MPD or UPD	maxillary (or upper) partial denture
PFM	porcelain fused to metal
prophy	prophylaxis

Types of Treatment Plans

Each treatment plan includes a description of the proposed treatment and an estimate of the fee involved. Many dentists prepare three treatment plans for the patient's consideration. These plans represent the following levels of care:

Level I—Emergency: Relieves distressful conditions and provides comfort to the patient.

Level II—Standard: Restores the dental components to normal function. As needed, this includes restoring teeth with composite or amalgam restorations, saving teeth with endodontic treatment, conservative treatment of periodontal problems, and the replacement of missing teeth with removable prostheses.

Level III—Optimum: Restores the dental components to maximum function and esthetics. When appropriate, this includes restoring teeth with cast restorations (crowns, inlays, or onlays); treatment of periodontal, orthodontic, or endodontic problems; and the replacement of missing teeth with fixed prostheses (fixed bridges) or with dental implants.

Presenting Treatment Plans to the Patient

At least a 15- to 20-minute appointment is scheduled for the uninterrupted presentation of the treatment plans to the patient.

Rather than seating the patient in a treatment room, the dentist conducts the case presentation in a private, well-ventilated, and lighted room containing an x-ray view box, a table or a desk, and at least two chairs.

The dentist has ready the patient's chart, radiographs, diagnostic casts, treatment plans, and other visual aids. These might include

- "Before" and "after" photographs or diagnostic casts of similar cases
- Models of proposed appliances such as full or partial dentures, dental implants, or fixed crowns and bridges
- Anatomic models to demonstrate conditions

The dentist tries to make the patient comfortable and relaxed in this setting and takes care to present all information in terms that the patient can understand. Then the dentist explains his or her findings regarding the patient's diagnosis and prognosis.

After this, the treatment plans are presented with the supporting rationale and fee estimates for each option. The patient is cautioned that it may be necessary to modify the treatment plan because of conditions encountered during treatment.

The patient is encouraged to ask questions and to discuss the advantages and disadvantages of each plan. When the patient makes a decision and accepts a treatment plan, he is giving informed consent for treatment. (Informed consent is discussed in Chapter 2.)

At this time, the administrative assistant explains the payment plans offered through the practice and makes the necessary financial arrangements with the patient. (Making financial arrangements is discussed in Chapter 34.) When all of these arrangements have been completed, the patient is scheduled for treatment. (This is discussed in Chapter 33.)

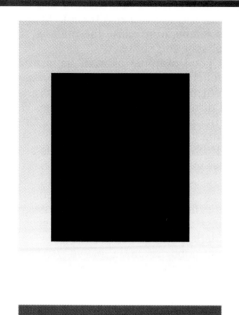

Chapter 19

Alginate Impressions and Diagnostic Casts

Introduction

Diagnostic casts, also called *study casts* or *primary casts*, are accurate three-dimensional reproductions of the teeth and surrounding soft tissues of the patient's maxillary and mandibular arches.

Diagnostic casts are created from alginate impressions. These impressions are a negative reproduction of the structures of the arches and surrounding tissues. These impressions are poured in a gypsum product to create the completed diagnostic cast (Fig. 19–1).

Because these casts show a three-dimensional view of conditions existing in the mouth before, during, and after treatment, they are a particularly valuable diagnostic tool. Also, using diagnostic casts allows the dentist to study the patient's mouth from angles impossible during the clinical examination. These casts are used during diagnosis and treatment planning for the following:

Fixed Bridges or Partial Dentures. The casts provide information about the size, shape, and position of the teeth that is used when planning fixed and removable prostheses.

Orthodontic Treatment. The casts record conditions before, during, and after treatment and become part of the patient's permanent record.

Periodontal Treatment. The casts record the size, shape, and position of the gingivae and papilla.

Full Mouth Dental Reconstruction. The dentist can

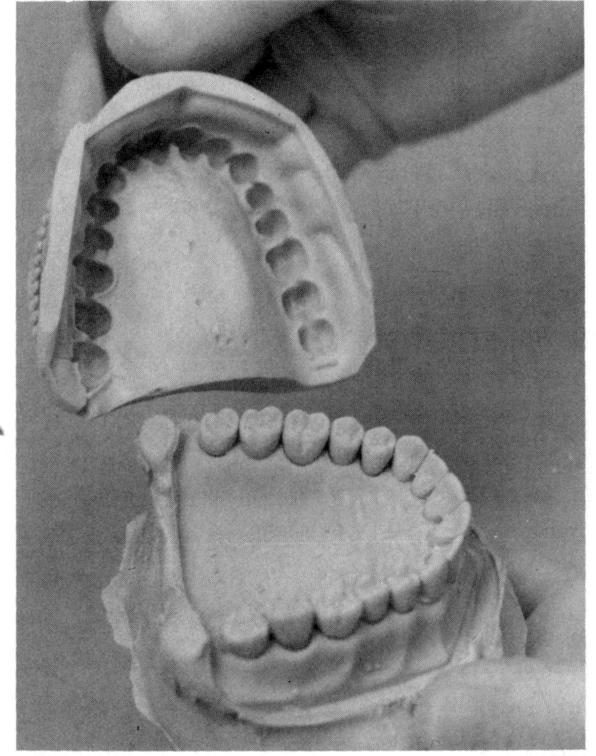

FIGURE 19–1

An alginate impression is poured in gypsum to create the completed diagnostic cast.

evaluate jaw movements when designing appliances, restorations, and implant placement.

Visual Aid. During the case presentation, the dentist can use the casts to illustrate problems and possible solutions.

Fabrication of Custom Trays and Temporary Appliances. Diagnostic casts are also used in the fabrication of the following:

- Custom trays for elastomeric impressions (see Chapter 24)
- Bleaching trays (see Chapters 24 and 25)
- Athletic mouth guards (see Chapter 27)
- Orthodontic appliances (see Chapter 28)
- Temporary coverage (see Chapter 31)

Hydrocolloid Impression Materials

Alginate is a member of the family of impression materials known as hydrocolloids. (The prefix *hydro-* means water, and a **hydrocolloid** is a solution in which water is used as the mixing agent.)

Physical Characteristics of Hydrocolloid Impression Materials

ELASTOMERIC PROPERTIES

Hydrocolloids, also referred to as *aqueous elastomeric impression materials*, are so called because they are somewhat elastic. This allows the completed impression to be stretched as it is being removed from the mouth. Then, like elastic, the impression springs back into its previous shape.

The elastomeric properties of alginate are not as great as those created in the elastomeric impression materials discussed in Chapter 24.

PHYSICAL PHASES

Hydrocolloid impression materials have two physical phases. The first phase is known as a **sol** (as in solution). In the sol phase, the material is in a liquid or semi-liquid form. The second phase is known as a **gel.** In the gel phase, the material is semi-solid, similar to a gelatin dessert.

The **gel strength** of hydrocolloid gels are not as great as that of other elastomeric impression materials. The hydrocolloids have difficulty withstanding tensile fracture (tearing) and elastic strain (stretching).

REVERSIBLE AND IRREVERSIBLE HYDROCOLLOIDS

Depending on the type of hydrocolloid, the physical change from sol (solution) to gel (solid) is either reversible (changed by thermal factors) or irreversible (changed by chemical factors).

Reversible Hydrocolloids. Hydrocolloid impression materials that change physical states (from a sol to a gel, then back to a sol) are called reversible hydrocolloids. Changes in temperature cause the material to go from one physical state to another.

Ice cream is a good example of what happens to a reversible hydrocolloid. When ice cream is frozen, it is in the gel state. When left at room temperature, the ice cream melts and turns into a sol (solution) state. When returned to the freezer, the ice cream once again becomes a gel (solid).

Reversible hydrocolloid impression materials are no longer widely used in dentistry.

Irreversible Hydrocolloids. Hydrocolloid impression materials that cannot return to the sol state after they become a gel are called irreversible hydrocolloids. The change in the physical state results from a chemical change in the material.

Cake mix is a good example of an irreversible change. When water is added to the powder in a cake mix, a chemical reaction occurs. It is impossible to remove the water and return the mixture to powder.

Alginate impression material is an irreversible hydrocolloid. Once it has solidified, it cannot be returned to the solution state.

Alginate Impression Materials

Alginate is not as accurate as the other impression materials used in dentistry. For this reason, it is not recommended for impressions for which accuracy and very fine detail are important; however, it is an ideal impression material for diagnostic casts because it

- Is easy to mix and use
- Requires little equipment
- Is much less expensive than other impression materials
- Is sufficiently accurate for diagnostic casts

Properties of Alginate Impression Materials

COMPOSITION AND CHEMISTRY

The chief ingredient is **potassium alginate**, from which the material gets its name. This material, which comes from sea kelp, is also used in other foods (such as ice cream) as a thickening agent.

Calcium sulfate reacts with the potassium alginate to form the gel. Because the rate of gelation must be controlled to allow adequate working time, **trisodium phosphate** is added as a retarder. (**Gelation** is the change from the solution to the solid state.)

Diatomaceous earth and sometimes **zinc oxide** are added as fillers to add bulk to the material.

Alginate impression ingredients interfere with the setting and surface strength of gypsum products used to pour the cast. To minimize this problem, **potassium titanium fluoride** is added to the alginate impression material.

PACKAGING AND STORAGE

Alginate impression material can be purchased in a variety of ways. **Containers**, which are about the size of a coffee can, are the most commonly used form of packaging.

Premeasured Packages. These are more expensive than other types of packaging but do save chair time by eliminating the need for measurement of the powder. They also limit the assistant's exposure to alginate dust.

Alginate impression material deteriorates very quickly (1) at elevated temperatures, (2) in the presence of moisture, or (3) under both conditions. This deterioration results either in the material's failure to set or in setting much too rapidly.

Only as much material as can be used in 1 year should be purchased at a time. When a new supply is purchased, it is stored behind the current supply so that the older material is used first.

WORKING AND SETTING TIMES

The **gelation time** is the total time required from the beginning of the mix until gelation occurs and the impression is complete. This is divided into two parts:

- **Working time,** which is the time allowed for mixing the alginate, loading the tray, and positioning the tray in the patient's mouth
- **Setting time,** which is the time required for the chemical action to be completed and after which the impression is ready to be removed from the mouth

Altering the Setting Times. Room-temperature water (21°C or 70°F) should be used when mixing alginate. Warmer water increases the setting time. Cooler water decreases the setting time.

STRENGTH OF THE IMPRESSION MATERIAL

It is important for alginate to be strong enough to resist tearing when the impression is being removed from the patient's mouth. Within limits, the strength of alginate can be increased by using a slightly thicker mix. However, if the mix is too thick, the material will not have enough flow to obtain a good impression. (**Flow** is the ability of the material to adapt to the surfaces it encounters.)

The strength of the material continues to increase even after it appears to be set. Therefore, leaving the impression in the mouth for the full length of time recommended by the manufacturer is also important in achieving maximum strength.

DIMENSIONAL STABILITY

The most serious problem associated with alginate impressions is the loss of accuracy when the impression is stored before pouring. This loss is due to the water content in these materials.

- If the impression is stored in water, or in a very wet paper towel, the alginate absorbs additional water and expands. (This absorption of water is called **imbibition.**)
- If the impression is stored in air, the water evaporates from the alginate, and the impression shrinks.
- The least amount of distortion occurs when the impression is stored in 100% humidity.

Storing the disinfected impression in a sealed plastic bag, or other sealed container, along with a moistened piece of gauze provides an atmosphere of 100% relative humidity.

Alginate impressions can be stored this way for about 1 hour without serious dimensional changes. (See Chapter 13 for disinfection techniques.)

Working with Alginate Impression Materials

TYPES OF ALGINATES

Alginate is available in two types: normal set and fast set. The types refer to the **working time** and **setting time** of the alginate.

- **Normal set alginate** has a working time of 2 minutes and a setting time up to 4½ minutes after mixing
- **Fast set alginate** has a working time of 1¼ minutes and a setting time of 1 to 2 minutes.

There is no difference in the completed impression between the two setting types of alginates. The decision as to which type to use is based on time-related factors, including

- Difficulties in seating the tray (normal set allows more time for insertion and placement of the tray)
- The operator working alone (normal set will give the operator more time to mix the alginate and load the impression tray)
- Children and patients with a severe gag reflex (fast set allows the tray to be removed from the mouth much sooner)

ALGINATE POWDER AND WATER RATIO

It is important to accurately measure the alginate powder and the water it is to be mixed with. To help ensure accuracy, the manufacturer supplies a plastic scoop for dispensing the bulk powder and a plastic cylinder for measuring the water (Fig. 19–2).

The water-to-powder ratio for mixing alginate is clearly marked on these measures. The ratio is one scoop of powder to one "measure" of water.

- A **mandibular impression** requires two scoops of powder and two measures of water.
- A **maxillary impression** generally requires three scoops of powder to three measures of water.

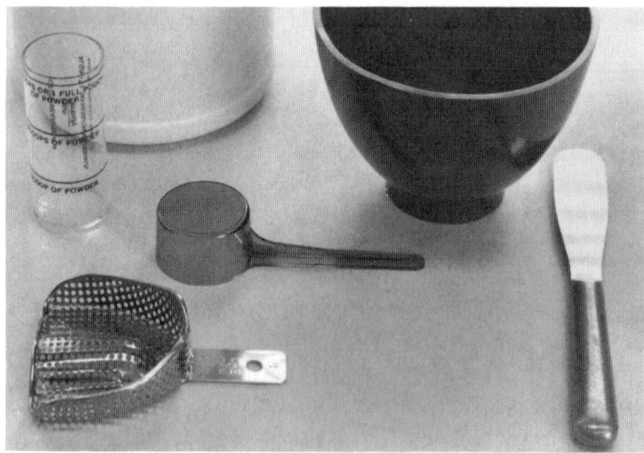

FIGURE 19–2

Plastic measuring device and scoop. Also shown are the mixing bowl, spatula, and maxillary impression tray. (From Ehrlich, A., and Torres, H.O.: Essentials of Dental Assisting. Philadelphia, W.B. Saunders Co., 1992, p 284.)

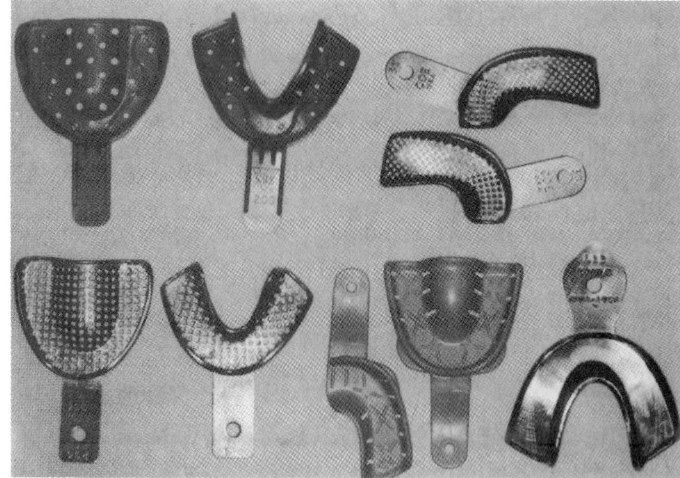

FIGURE 19–3

Metal and disposable plastic impression trays used with alginate impression materials. (From Phillips, R.W., and Moore, K.B.: Elements of Dental Materials for Dental Hygienists and Dental Assistants, 5th ed. Philadelphia, W.B. Saunders Co., 1994, p 72.)

ALGINATE IMPRESSION TRAYS

Impression trays for use with alginate impression materials are perforated (have holes in them) to allow the alginate to ooze through the holes in the tray as it sets. This forms a "lock" and keeps the alginate from pulling out of the tray when it is removed from the patient's mouth.

These trays are available in two types (plastic and metal) and a range of sizes (Fig. 19–3). **Plastic impression trays** are discarded after a single use. **Metal impression trays** are sterilized after each use.

Selecting Impression Trays. Impression trays are selected for size by trying the tray in the patient's mouth. Trays that have been tried in the mouth and not selected for use must be sterilized before they are returned to storage. The correct tray will

- Be comfortable to the patient
- Extend slightly beyond the facial surfaces of the teeth
- Extend approximately 2 to 3 mm. beyond the third molar, retromolar, or tuberosity area of the arch
- Be deep enough to allow 2 to 3 mm. of alginate between the tray and the incisal or occlusal edges of the teeth

Adapting Impression Trays. If necessary, the depth or length of the tray can be extended by adding utility wax to the border of the tray. This might be necessary if the tray does not completely cover the third molars.

For a patient with an unusually high palate, softened utility wax can be added to the palate area of the impression tray (Fig. 19–4).

Taking Alginate Impressions

Some states allow the qualified dental assistant to take alginate impressions for diagnostic casts. In other states the assistant may mix the alginate, load the trays, and help keep the patient comfortable while the dentist actually takes the impression.

The procedures described here describe the roles of both the assistant and the dentist. The assistant who is taking the impressions alone fills both roles.

EXPLAINING THE PROCEDURE TO THE PATIENT

Before taking the impressions, the procedure should be explained to the patient to ensure his comfort. The patient needs to know the following:

- A plastic drape is used to protect his clothing against any spilled material.
- The material will feel cold, there is no unpleasant taste, and the material will set quickly.

(text continued on page 363)

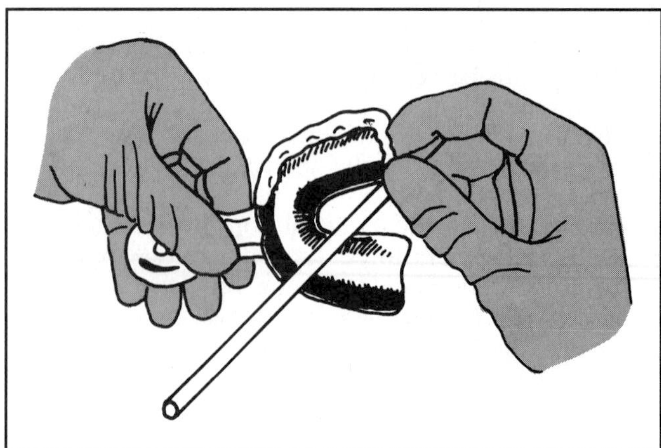

FIGURE 19–4

Placing wax beading on the impression tray.

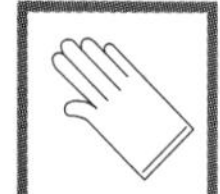 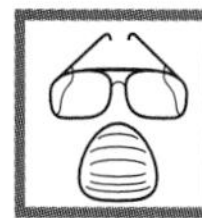 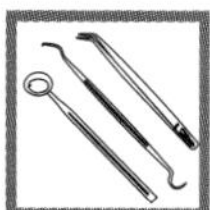 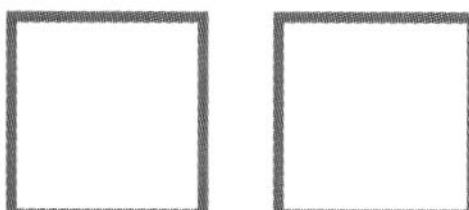

PROCEDURE: **Preparing to Take Alginate Impressions**

Instrumentation

Fast-setting alginate powder
Alginate measure (scoop provided by manufacturer)
Water measure (provided by the manufacturer)
Room-temperature water (21°C or 70°F)
Rubber bowl (flexible, medium size)
Wide-blade mixing spatula (beaver-tail shape)
Sterile impression trays
Utility wax
Facial tissues

Preparing the Patient

1. Seat the patient and place the plastic drape.
2. Explain the procedure to the patient.
3. Ask the patient to rinse his mouth before the impression to remove any food debris from the teeth. If the patient has very thick and ropy saliva, a mouth rinse is used instead of water to thin and remove the excess saliva.
4. Ask the patient to take out any removable full or partial denture and to rinse his mouth. The denture must be stored in a safe place in water or mouth rinse. After the impression has been taken, the denture is rinsed and returned to the patient.
5. Adjust the dental chair in the upright position.
   □ *RATIONALE:* This increases patient comfort and prevents the material from running down the patient's throat. In some circumstances, the supine position may be used.

Measuring Alginate Powder and Water

1. Use room-temperature water.
   □ *RATIONALE:* Cold water lengthens the setting time, and hot water shortens the setting time.
2. Read the water level by holding it at eye level. The amount of water should come to the "line" of the measure.
3. Before taking alginate from a container, shake the can to "fluff" the material.
   □ *RATIONALE:* The material tends to pack down in the can and the measure will not be accurate. (When premeasured packages are used, "fluffing" is not necessary.)
4. After fluffing the material, lift the lid very carefully to avoid having the very fine particles fly into the air.
5. Slightly overfill the powder scoop and then tap the side of the scoop with the spatula.
   □ *RATIONALE:* This fills any voids in the measure and ensures an accurate measurement.
6. Use the blade of the spatula to scrape the excess powder from the top of the scoop and back into the can. While doing this, take care not to compact the powder into the scoop.

Mixing Alginate for the Mandibular Impression

1. Place two measures of room-temperature water into the rubber bowl.
2. "Fluff" the contents of the alginate can, carefully lift the lid, and measure two scoops of powder.
3. Add the powder to the water and mix with a stirring action until the powder has been moistened.
4. Use the broad side of the spatula blade to mix the alginate with a spreading stroke that squeezes the alginate between the spatula and the side of the rubber bowl.
5. Mix for 30 to 45 seconds. The mixture should be smooth and creamy.
   □ *RATIONALE:* Inadequate mixing of alginates results in mixes that are grainy and in poor detail in the impression.
6. Wipe the alginate mix into one mass on the inside edge of the bowl.

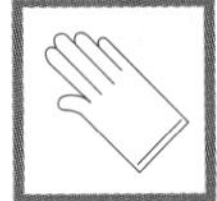
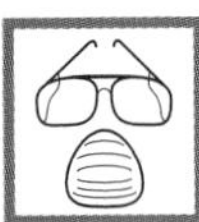
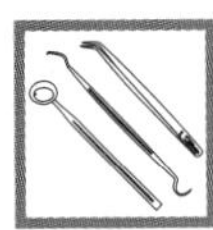

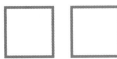

PROCEDURE: **Taking a Mandibular Impression**

Loading the Mandibular Impression Tray

1. Load the tray quickly, using two increments. The tray must be ready and placed in the mouth before it sets (in 1 to 2 minutes).
2. Gather about half of the alginate onto the spatula. Wipe the alginate from the spatula into the tray from the lingual edge.
3. Quickly press the material down to the base of the tray.
   □ *RATIONALE:* This will remove any air bubbles trapped in the tray.
4. Gather the remaining half of alginate in the bowl onto the spatula and load the other side of the tray in the same way.
5. Smooth the surface of the alginate by wiping a moistened finger along the surface (Fig. 19–5).
6. Pass the loaded tray facing downward, and with the handle first, to the operator's right hand.
7. *Optional:* Some operators wipe a small amount of alginate on the occlusal surfaces before placement of the tray (Fig. 19–6).
   □ *RATIONALE:* This minimizes the formation of air bubbles on these surfaces.

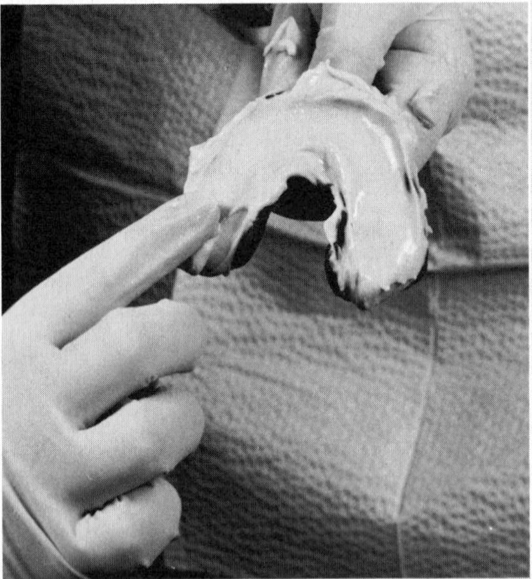

FIGURE 19–5

Smoothing alginate impression material in mandibular tray.

Making the Mandibular Impression

1. Retract the right cheek with your left finger.
2. Turn the tray slightly to the left and ease it into the mouth in a slightly sideways position.
3. Center the tray over the teeth.
4. Press the posterior border of the tray down first.
   □ *RATIONALE:* This will form a seal.
5. Push the anterior portion of the tray down and ask the patient to lift his tongue and then relax it.
   □ *RATIONALE:* This will allow the alginate to make an impression of the lingual aspect of the alveolar process.
6. Instruct the patient to breathe normally while the tray is in place.
7. Use the fingers to hold the tray firmly in position while the alginate sets (Fig. 19–7).
8. Check the excess alginate around the edges of the

tray to determine when the set has occurred. The material should not register a dent when pressed with the finger.

Removing the Mandibular Impression

1. Place the fingers of the left hand on top of the impression tray.
   □ *RATIONALE:* This protects the maxillary teeth from damage during removal of the mandibular tray.
2. Move the inside of the cheeks or lips gently with your finger.
   □ *RATIONALE:* This breaks the seal between the impression and the peripheral tissues.
3. Place the thumb and index finger of the right hand on the handle and exert a firm lifting motion.
4. Snap the tray and impression upward, off the dentition, and out of the patient's mouth.
5. Instruct the patient to rinse with water to remove any excess alginate impression material.
6. Check the impression for accuracy. (See "Criteria for Alginate Impressions" in this chapter.)
7. Set the impression aside for completion.

Completing the Mandibular Impression

Before the mandibular impression can be poured, the tongue space in the center of the tray must be filled in to create a smooth "floor of the mouth" on the cast.

This space may be filled with utility wax or a piece of moist paper towel. However, the following technique is commonly used in creating a smooth floor that is important in the appearance of the cast.

This technique requires a fresh mix of a single scoop of alginate. Some assistants complete this step while the operator is taking the maxillary impression. Others do this just before pouring the impression.

1. Use a clean bowl and spatula to mix one scoop of alginate and a single measure of water.
2. Scoop the mix of alginate onto the spatula.
3. Place the thumb of one hand into the tongue space of the mandibular impression tray.
4. Wipe the mass of alginate over the thumb. The new alginate should be placed about 2 mm. below the lingual periphery of the impression.
   □ *RATIONALE:* This ensures an accurate reproduction of the alveolar ridge.
5. Moisten the fingers of the other hand, and blend the two masses of alginate together.
6. When the alginate is set, remove the thumb. The mandibular impression is now ready to pour.

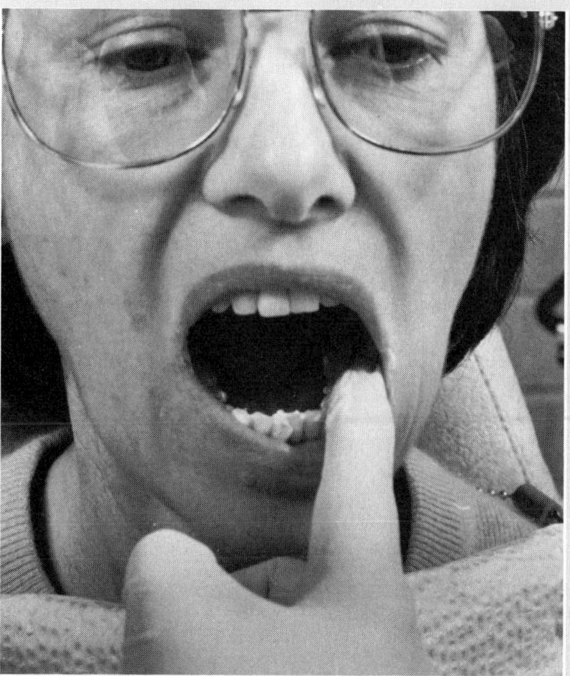

FIGURE 19–6

Spreading alginate impression material on the occlusal surfaces before placement of the tray.

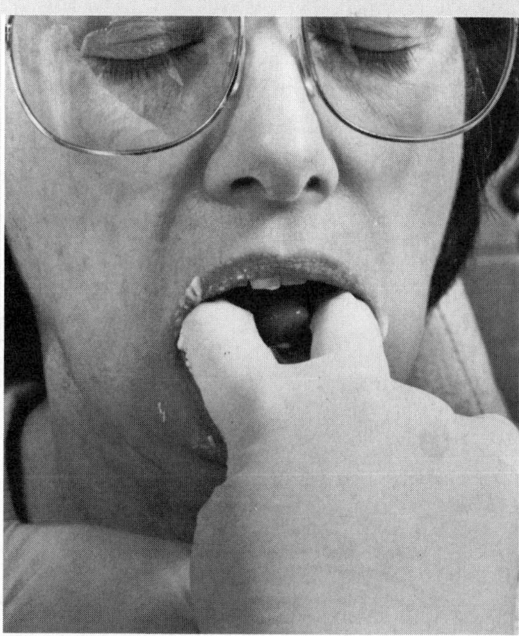

FIGURE 19–7

Lower impression tray held firmly in place with two fingers. Note the tongue is up out of the floor of the mouth.

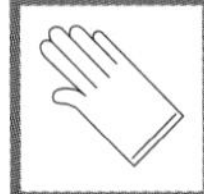
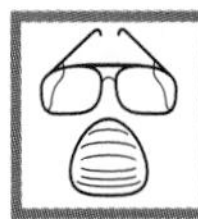
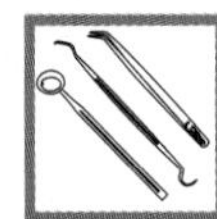

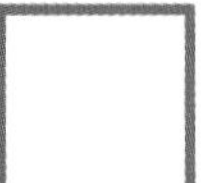

PROCEDURE: **Taking a Maxillary Impression**

Mixing Alginate for the Maxillary Impression

1. A maxillary impression usually requires three scoops of powder and three measures of water.
2. If the same bowl and spatula are being reused, they must be clean *and* dry before the next mix is begun.
3. Mix the alginate in the same manner as for the mandibular impression.

Loading the Maxillary Impression Tray

1. The maxillary tray is loaded in one large increment.
2. Use a wiping motion to fill the tray from the posterior end.
   □ *RATIONALE:* This prevents the formation of air bubbles between the tray and the material.
3. Place the bulk of the material toward the anterior and palatal area of the tray.
   □ *RATIONALE:* This helps prevent impression material from flowing into the patient's throat during tray placement.
4. Moisten fingertips with tap water and smooth the surface of the alginate.
5. Use the moistened fingers to make a slight trough, or indentation, in the alginate in the area of the alveolar ridge (Fig. 19–8).
   □ *RATIONALE:* This helps prevent air bubbles on the occlusal surfaces and to ensure recording the mucobuccal areas.
6. Pass the loaded tray facing upward with the handle first to the operator.

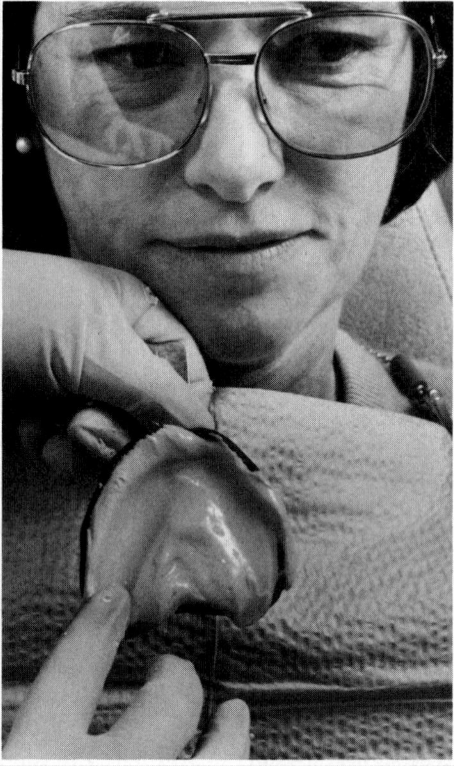

FIGURE 19–8

Smoothing impression material before insertion of the maxillary tray.

Making the Maxillary Impression

1. Use the left index finger to retract the patient's right cheek (Fig. 19–9).
2. Turn the tray slightly to the left, and insert the tray in a slightly sideways position.
3. Center the tray over the teeth.

4. Gently press the posterior border (back) of the tray up against the posterior border of the hard palate to form a seal.
   □ *RATIONALE:* The patient may experience a gag reflex when the material touches the soft palate.
5. Rotate the anterior portion of the tray upward over the teeth.
6. Use your left hand to lift the patient's lips and cheeks out of the way as the tray is seated.
   □ *RATIONALE:* This retraction allows the material to flow into the vestibular areas.
7. Pull the upper lip over the anterior portion of the tray to shape the anterior border of the seated tray.
8. Check the posterior border of the tray to make sure no material has oozed into the patient's throat. (If necessary, excess material can be wiped away with a mouth mirror or finger.)
9. Instruct the patient to tip his head downward and breathe through his nose.
10. Place a saliva ejector in the floor of the patient's mouth to control any excessive flow of saliva.
11. Hold the tray firmly in place while the alginate sets.

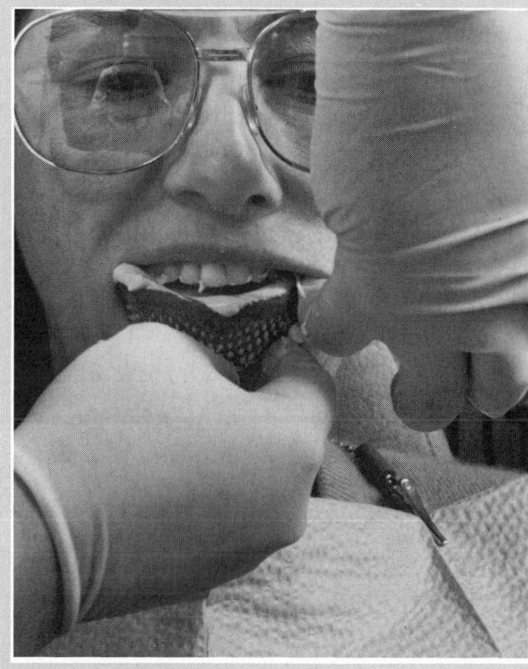

FIGURE 19–9

Retraction of the cheek as the tray is placed.

Removing the Maxillary Impression

1. Keep a finger between the mandibular teeth and the impression tray.
   □ *RATIONALE:* This protects the mandibular teeth from injury while the maxillary impression tray is removed.
2. Place a finger from the other hand along the lateral borders of the tray, and push down to break the seal.
3. Use a straight, downward snapping motion to remove the tray from the teeth and the mouth.
4. Instruct the patient to rinse with water to remove any excess alginate impression material.
5. Check the impression for accuracy.

- His mouth will feel full with the tray in place, and he will be more comfortable if he breathes deeply through his nose throughout the procedure.
- He must use agreed-upon hand signals to indicate discomfort.

If impressions are being taken of both arches, the mandibular impression is usually obtained first. This is because the mandibular impression is generally more comfortable for the patient than the maxillary. It also allows the patient to become familiar with the material and process.

Evaluating Alginate Impressions

An acceptable alginate impression meets the following criteria:

- The impression tray was centered over the central and lateral incisors.
- There is a complete "peripheral roll," which included all of the vestibular areas.
- The tray was not "overseated" (pushed down too far), which would have resulted in exposure of areas of the impression tray.

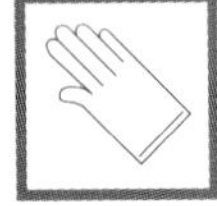
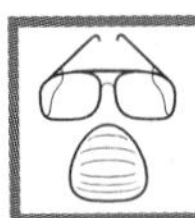
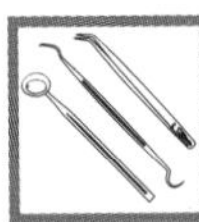
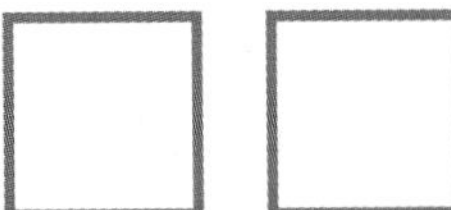

PROCEDURE: **Before Dismissing the Patient**

1. Use an explorer and dental floss to remove any remaining fragments of alginate from interproximal areas.
2. Provide the patient with a mouth rinse to rinse again.
3. Use a moist facial tissue to remove any alginate from the patient's face and lips.
4. If applicable, rinse and return the patient's denture.

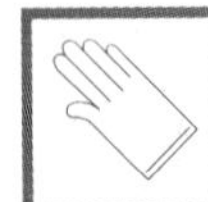
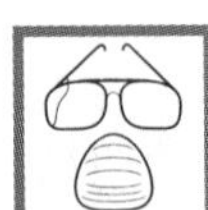

PROCEDURE: **Caring for Alginate Impressions**

1. Gently rinse the impression under tap water to remove any blood or saliva.
   □ *RATIONALE:* These materials will interfere with the setting of the gypsum products.
2. Spray the impression with an approved surface disinfectant (Fig. 19–10) (see Chapter 13).
3. If the impression must be stored before pouring, wrap it in a damp paper towel and store it in a covered container or plastic bag labeled with the patient's name.

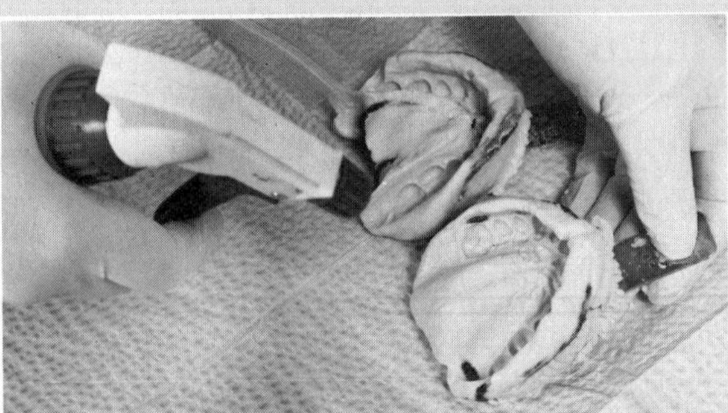

FIGURE 19–10

Completed impressions are sprayed with a surface disinfectant before placement in a plastic bag for storage.

- The impression is free from tears or voids (holes).
- There is sharp anatomic detail of all teeth and soft tissues.
- The retromolar area, lingual frenum, tongue space, and mylohyoid ridge are reproduced in the mandibular impression.
- The hard palate and tuberosities are recorded in the maxillary impression.

Wax-Bite Registration

A wax-bite registration is used to show the occlusal relationship of the maxillary and mandibular teeth. It is particularly useful when the diagnostic casts are trimmed.

The most common technique is to use a softened horseshoe-shaped wafer of wax. Some brands have a piece of foil between the layers of wax to add strength (Fig. 19–11).

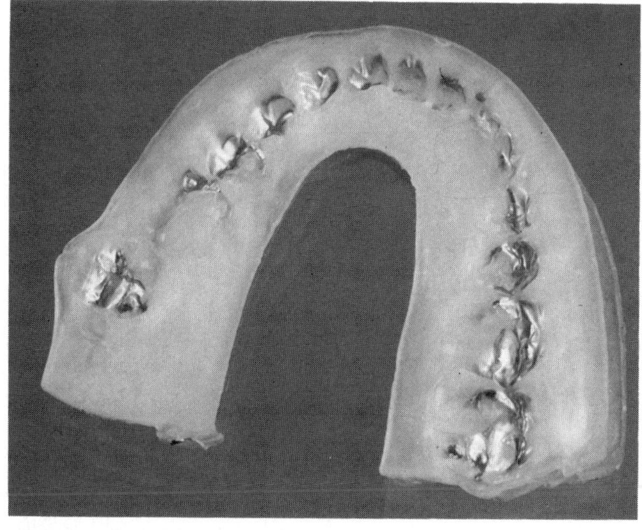

FIGURE 19–11

Commercially prepared wax-bite registration wafer after patient has bitten into it.

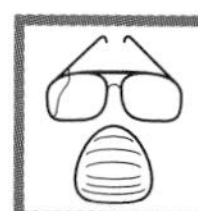

PROCEDURE: Taking the Wax-Bite Registration

Instrumentation

Bite registration wax
Laboratory knife
Heat source (warm water, Bunsen burner, or torch)

Taking the Wax-Bite Registration

1. Explain the procedure to the patient. Reassure him that the wax will be warm, not hot, in his mouth.
2. Have the patient practice opening and closing normally.
   □ *RATIONALE:* When the wax is in place, the patient may close his front teeth together instead of biting directly into the wax. This will result in an inaccurate bite registration. This is to be sure that the correct position will be recorded in the wax.
3. Place the wax over the biting surfaces of the teeth and check the length. If the wax extends so far beyond the last tooth that the patient is uncomfortable, remove the wax from the patient's mouth. Use the laboratory knife to shorten the length of the wax.
4. Use heat source to soften the wax.
5. Place the softened wax against the biting surfaces of the mandibular teeth.
6. Instruct the patient to bite gently and naturally into the wax.
7. Allow the wax to cool. (It will cool quickly and may be removed from the mouth in 1 to 2 minutes.)
8. Remove the wax-bite registration very carefully to avoid distortion.
9. Write the patient's name on a piece of paper and keep it with the wax-bite registration.
10. Store the wax-bite registration with the impressions or casts until it is needed during the trimming of the casts.

Gypsum Products

Gypsum products are used extensively in dentistry to make diagnostic casts and dies (extremely accurate reproductions of a single tooth).

Characteristics and Properties of Gypsum Products

CHEMICAL PROPERTIES

Gypsum is a mineral that is mined from the earth. In the raw state, gypsum is the dihydrate form of calcium sulfate. (**Dihydrate** means that there are two parts of water to every one part of calcium sulfate.)

Heating during the manufacturing process removes water, and the gypsum is converted into a powdered **hemihydrate**. This means that there is now only one-half part of water to one part of calcium sulfate.

SETTING REACTIONS

When the gypsum powder is mixed with water, the hemihydrate crystals dissolve in water and begin to form clusters known as the **nuclei of crystallization.**

These nuclei are so close together that as the gypsum crystals grow during the setting process, they intermesh and become entangled with each other. The more intermeshing of crystals, the greater the strength, rigidity, and hardness of the final product.

PHYSICAL FORMS

Three forms of gypsum products are commonly used:

- Model plaster
- Dental stone
- High-strength stone

Model plaster, dental stone, and high-strength stone are made up of hemihydrate crystals whose size, shape and porosity differ for each material. It is these differences in the hemihydrate crystals that determine the characteristics and water-to-powder ratios for each type of gypsum product.

Model plaster, also commonly called *plaster of Paris*, is used primarily for pouring primary impressions and making diagnostic casts. The crystals in plaster are irregular in shape and very porous, similar in appearance to a sponge. Because of the porous and irregular crystals, model plaster requires the most water for mixing and produces a weaker cast.

Dental stone is used when a more durable diagnostic cast is required or for use as a working model in the fabrication of dentures.

The crystals in dental stone are uniform in shape and less porous than those in plaster. The resulting cast is much stronger and denser than one made from plaster.

High-strength stone is also known as *Densite* or *improved dental stone.* Its strength, hardness and dimensional accuracy make it ideal to create the dies used in the production of crowns, bridges, and cast restorations. (See Chapter 31.)

The crystals in high-strength stone are smooth and very dense and require the least amount of water for mixing.

WATER-TO-POWDER RATIOS

The water-to-powder ratio has a dramatic effect on the setting time and strength of any gypsum product. Recommended ratios are shown in Table 19–1. The exact water-to-powder ratio depends, in part, on the intended use of the finished product.

Each type has an optimal water-to-powder ratio, which has been specified by the manufacturer. These ratios should be carefully observed because deviations will change both the consistency of the material and the properties of the set cast.

When too little water is used, the mix will be difficult to manipulate and have a shorter working time. If additional water is added to try to thin it out, the crystallization (setting) process is disturbed, and the cast will not have the desired strength.

When too much water is used, the mix will be thin and runny and will take longer to set, and the cast will be considerably weaker. If additional powder is added after the stirring begins, the continued stirring will break up the crystals that have begun to form. The result is a cast that is weak and brittle.

Measuring the Water and Powder. Measurements for the water and powder in each mix must be exact. The water is measured by volume with a measuring device such as a large syringe or milliliter graduated cylinder (Fig. 19–12)

The powder is measured by weight with the use of a dietetic scale (Fig. 19–13). A paper towel is placed on the scale to receive the powder. The scale is adjusted for this weight *before* the powder is weighed. If a scale is not available, the powder may be measured by volume.

TABLE 19–1

Recommended Water-to-Powder Ratios for Gypsum Products

GYPSUM PRODUCT	MIXING WATER
Model plaster (100 gm.)	45–50 ml.
Dental stone (100 gm.)	30–32 ml.
High-strength dental stone (100 gm.)	19–24 ml.

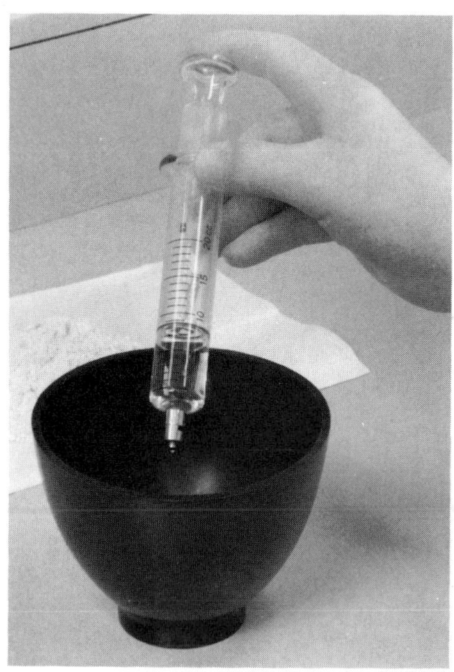

FIGURE 19–12

A large glass syringe is used to measure the water accurately. (From Ehrlich, A., and Torres, H.O.: Essentials of Dental Assisting. Philadelphia, W.B. Saunders Co., 1992, p 295.)

INFLUENCES ON SETTING TIME

Setting time is the length of time it takes for the mixture of gypsum to turn into a rigid solid. It is important to have enough working time to mix the material and pour it into the impression.

The setting time of gypsum products is influenced by several factors:

- **Type of gypsum:** model plaster sets faster than dental stone.
- **Water-to-powder ratio:** the less water used, the faster the set.
- **Mixing:** the longer and faster the mixing, the faster the set.
- **Water temperature:** the warmer the water that is used, the faster the set.
- **Humidity:** on a very humid day, the gypsum can absorb moisture from the atmosphere and take longer to set.

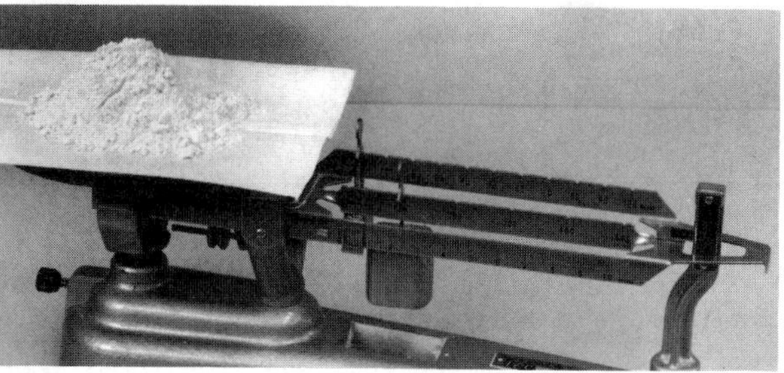

FIGURE 19–13

A dietetic scale is used to measure the powder accurately. (From Ehrlich, A., and Torres, H.O.: Essentials of Dental Assisting. Philadelphia, W.B. Saunders Co., 1992, p 295.)

Diagnostic Casts

A cast consists of two parts: the **anatomic portion,** which is created from the alginate impression, and the **art portion,** which forms the base of the cast.

There are three different pouring methods used to create the art portion. In the **double-pour** method, the anatomic portion of the cast is poured first. Then a second mix of plaster is used to prepare the art portion.

In the double-pour method, a free-form base may be created. An alternative is the use of commercial rubber molds for making bases. These molds provide symmetry to the casts and reduce the need for trimming.

In the **box-and-pour** method and **inverted-pour** methods, the anatomic portion of the cast is *not* poured first. Instead, one large mix of plaster is used to pour both portions of the cast in a single step.

In this method, the impression is surrounded with a "box" made of wax before it is poured. The completed "box" should extend at least ½ inch above the palatal area of the maxillary impression and ½ inch above the tongue area of the mandibular impression.

(text continued on page 372)

PROCEDURE: **Mixing Model Plaster**

Instrumentation

Flexible rubber mixing bowl (clean and dry)
Metal spatula (stiff blade with a rounded end)
Dietetic scale
Paper towel (for use on the scale)
Plaster (100 gm.)
Water-measuring device
Room-temperature water (70°F)
Vibrator with a disposable cover on the vibrator platform

Mixing Plaster

1. Measure 45 ml. of room-temperature water into a clean rubber mixing bowl.
2. Place the paper towel on the scale and make necessary adjustments.
3. Weigh out 100 gm. of model plaster.
4. Add the powder to the water in steady increments. Allow the powder to settle into the water for about 30 seconds.
   □ *RATIONALE:* This prevents trapping of air bubbles.
5. Use the spatula to slowly incorporate the powder into the water. A smooth and creamy mix should be achieved in about 20 seconds.
   □ *RATIONALE:* This is to avoid spilling the powder.
6. Turn the vibrator to low or medium speed, and place the bowl of plaster mix on the vibrator platform.
7. Lightly press and rotate the bowl on the vibrator (Fig. 19–14.). Air bubbles will rise to the surface.
8. Complete mixing and vibration of the plaster in *no more* than 2 minutes.

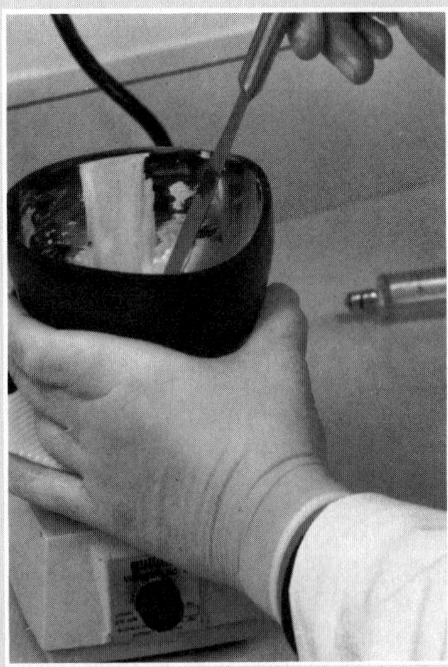

FIGURE 19–14

The vibrator is used to complete mixing and to eliminate air bubbles from the mix. (From Ehrlich, A., and Torres, H.O.: Essentials of Dental Assisting. Philadelphia, W.B. Saunders Co., 1992, p 296.)

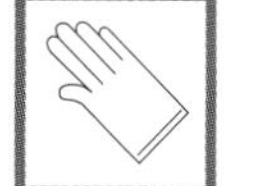

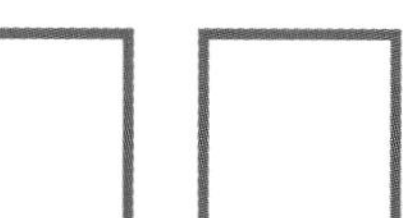
 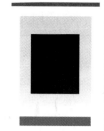

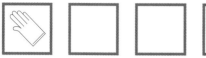

PROCEDURE: **Pouring Diagnostic Casts**

Instrumentation

Maxillary and/or mandibular impressions
100 gm. of freshly mixed model plaster
Glass slabs or tiles
Beading wax (square or rope type)
Boxing wax
Laboratory spatula
Laboratory knife (to trim alginate impression)
Heat source

Impression Preparation

1. Use a gentle stream of compressed air to remove excess moisture from the impression. Be careful not to dehydrate the impression and cause distortion.
2. Use the laboratory knife to carefully remove excess impression material that will interfere with pouring the cast (Fig. 19–15).

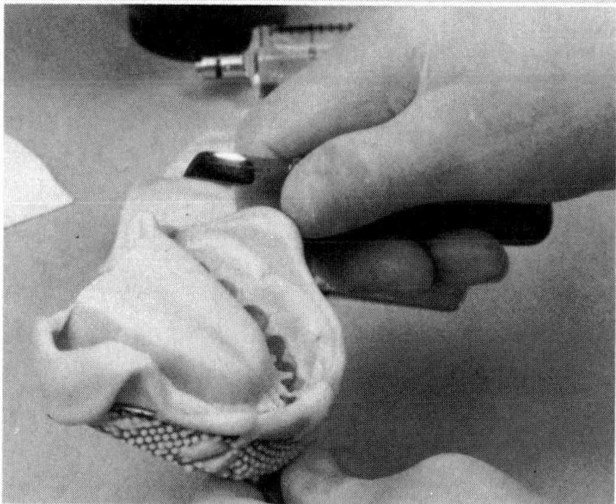

FIGURE 19–15

Before the model can be poured, any excess alginate must be carefully trimmed away. (From Ehrlich, A., and Torres, H.O.: Essentials of Dental Assisting. Philadelphia, W.B. Saunders Co., 1992, p 292.)

Pouring the Anatomic Portion

1. Set the vibrator at low to medium speed.
2. Hold the impression tray by the handle, and place the edge of the handle base on the vibrator (Fig. 19–16).
3. Dip the spatula into the plaster mix to pick up a small increment (about 1 tsp.).
4. Place that small increment at the palatal area of the impression near the most posterior tooth.
5. Guide the material as it flows down from the palatal area (for maxillary impressions) or above the retromolar pad area (for mandibular impressions) into the impression of the most posterior tooth.
   □ *RATIONALE:* The flowing action pushes out the air ahead of it and eliminates air bubbles.
6. Continue to place small increments in the *same area* as the first increment, and allow the plaster to flow toward the anterior teeth.
7. Rotate the tray on its side to provide the continuous flow of material into each tooth impression.
8. Once all of the teeth in the impression are covered with plaster, begin to add larger increments on the palatal area until the entire impression is filled.

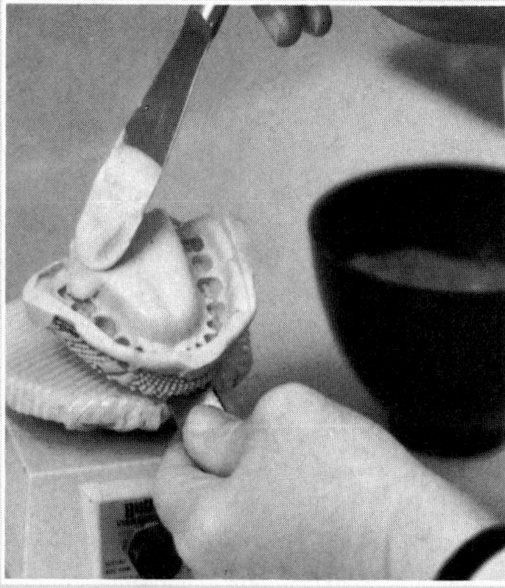

FIGURE 19–16

The base of the handle of the tray is placed on the vibrator, and the mix is flowed into the posterior portion of the maxillary impression. (From Ehrlich, A., and Torres, H.O.: Essentials of Dental Assisting. Philadelphia, W.B. Saunders Co., 1992, p 297.)

(continued on following page)

PROCEDURE: **Pouring Diagnostic Casts** *(continued)*

Pouring the Art Portion, Using the Double-Pour Method

1. Pour the art portion of the cast and allow it to set for approximately 5 to 10 minutes.
2. Use a clean bowl and spatula to create a second mix of plaster. Use the formula of 50 gm. of powder to 20 ml. of water.
   □ *RATIONALE:* This will produce a slightly thicker mix, which is desirable for a base.
3. Place the mix on a glass slab (or tile), and shape the base to approximately 2 × 2 inches, ¾ to 1 inch thick (Fig. 19–17).
4. Invert the impression onto the new mix (Fig. 19–18). Do not push the impression into the base.
   □ *RATIONALE:* When the poured impression is inverted onto the new mix, the fresh material will tend to flow excessively. This can result in a base that is too large and too thin.
5. Hold the tray steady and parallel with the glass slab. Use a spatula to smooth the plaster base mix up onto the margins of the initial pour (Fig. 19–19). Be careful not to cover the impression tray with plaster.
   □ *RATIONALE:* If plaster covers part of the impression tray, you will have difficulty in removing the cast from the impression.
6. Place the impression tray on the base so that the handle and occlusal plane of the teeth on the cast are parallel with the surface of the glass slab (or tile).
   □ *RATIONALE:* This will help form a base with uniform thickness.

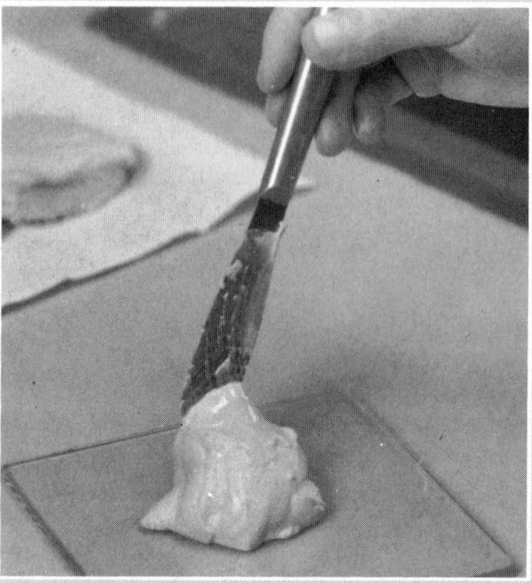

FIGURE 19–17

A mass of fresh plaster is placed on a glass slab to form the base of the completed cast. (From Ehrlich, A., and Torres, H.O.: Essentials of Dental Assisting. Philadelphia, W.B. Saunders Co., 1992, p 299.)

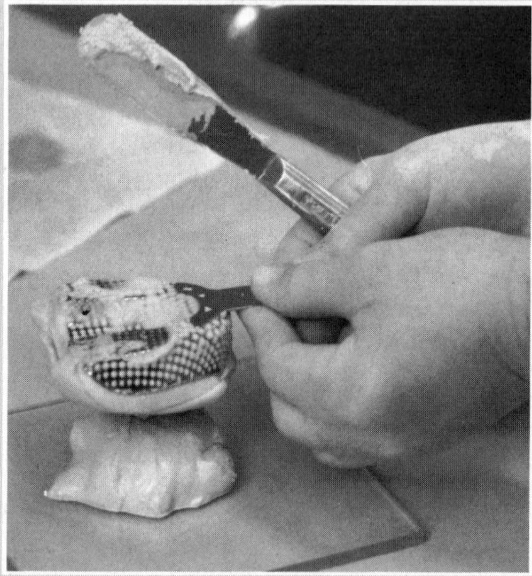

FIGURE 19–18

The poured base is inverted and carefully placed on the base. (From Ehrlich, A., and Torres, H.O.: Essentials of Dental Assisting. Philadelphia, W.B. Saunders Co., 1992, p 299.)

Pouring the Anatomic and Art Portions Using the Inverted-Pour Method

1. Mix the plaster, using the formula of 150 gm. powder to 90 ml. water.
   □ *RATIONALE:* This produces the larger mix needed for both portions of the cast.
2. Pour the plaster mix into the anatomic portion, using the method previously described.
3. Place the remaining plaster on the glass slab (or tile) to create a mass approximately 2 × 2 inches, ¾ to 1 inch thick.
4. Wait 2 to 3 minutes for the initial set, and then invert the impression onto the base.
5. Do *not* push the impression into the base material.
6. Use the same method as in the double-pour method to smooth the base material up and over the plaster in the impression. Be careful not to cover the impression tray.

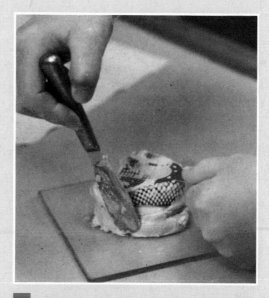

FIGURE 19–19

The base material is carefully dragged up over the edges of the cast without covering any of the impression tray. (From Ehrlich, A., and Torres, H.O.: Essentials of Dental Assisting. Philadelphia, W.B. Saunders Co., 1992, p 299.)

Pouring the Anatomic and Art Portions, Using the Box-and-Pour Method

1. Use the laboratory knife to trim the alginate impression. Remove any alginate that extends beyond the post dam area or over the posterior part of the impression tray.
   □ *RATIONALE:* Just enough of the alginate is removed to allow you to wrap the boxing wax around the impression. (Be careful not to remove any of the essential anatomic landmarks.)
2. Place a strip of beading wax around the tray approximately 3 mm. below the peripheral roll of the impression.
3. Warm the spatula over the flame of the heat source. Use the warm, not hot, spatula to attach the wax to the tray.
4. Wrap the strip of boxing wax around the impression and attach it to the beading wax, using a warm spatula.
5. Pour the anatomic portion, using the method described until all of the landmarks are covered.
6. Scrape the remaining plaster from the bowl onto the spatula. With the impression still on the vibrator, wipe the spatula and plaster over the edge of the boxing wax to fill the base.

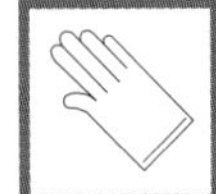

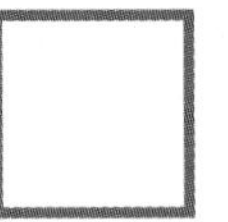

PROCEDURE: **Separating the Cast from the Impression**

1. Wait 40 to 60 minutes after the base has been poured before separating the impression from the cast.
2. Use the laboratory knife to gently separate the margins of the tray (Fig. 19–20).
3. Apply firm, straight, upward pressure on the handle of the tray to remove the impression.
4. If the tray does not separate easily, check to see where the tray is still attached to the impression. Again, use the laboratory knife to free the tray from the plaster.
5. Again pull the tray handle straight up from the cast. *Never* wiggle the impression tray from side to side while it is on the cast (Fig. 19–21).
   ☐ *RATIONALE:* This can cause the teeth on the cast to fracture.

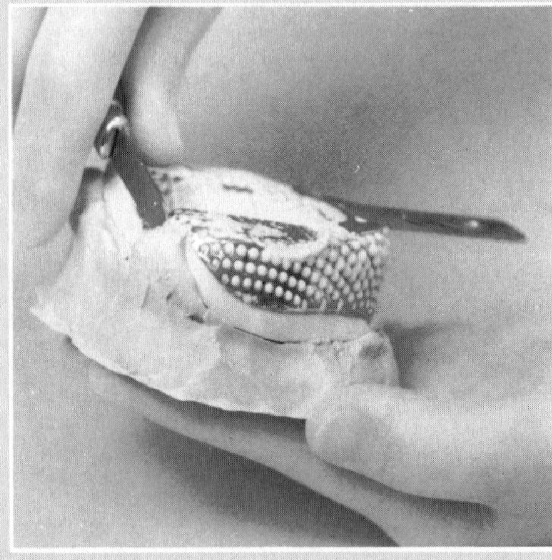

FIGURE 19–20

A laboratory knife is used to trim away excess carefully before the impression and cast are separated. (From Ehrlich, A., and Torres, H.O.: Essentials of Dental Assisting. Philadelphia, W.B. Saunders Co., 1992, p 300.)

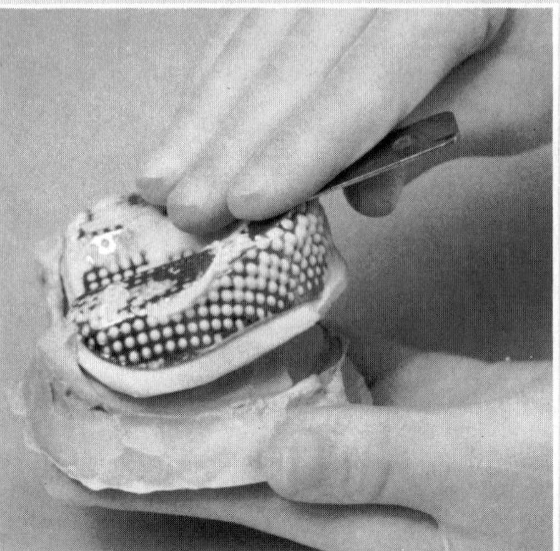

FIGURE 19–21

The impression and tray are lifted off with a straight-up motion. (From Ehrlich, A., and Torres, H.O.: Essentials of Dental Assisting. Philadelphia, W.B. Saunders Co., 1992, p 300.)

Finishing Diagnostic Casts

When diagnostic casts are to be used for a case presentation or as part of the patient's permanent record, they must have an attractive appearance. This is accomplished by trimming the casts to a geometric standard. The wax-bite registration is used to articulate the casts during the trimming process.

Appearance of the Anatomic and Art Portions

The **anatomic portion**, which includes the teeth, oral mucosa, and muscle attachments, should make up

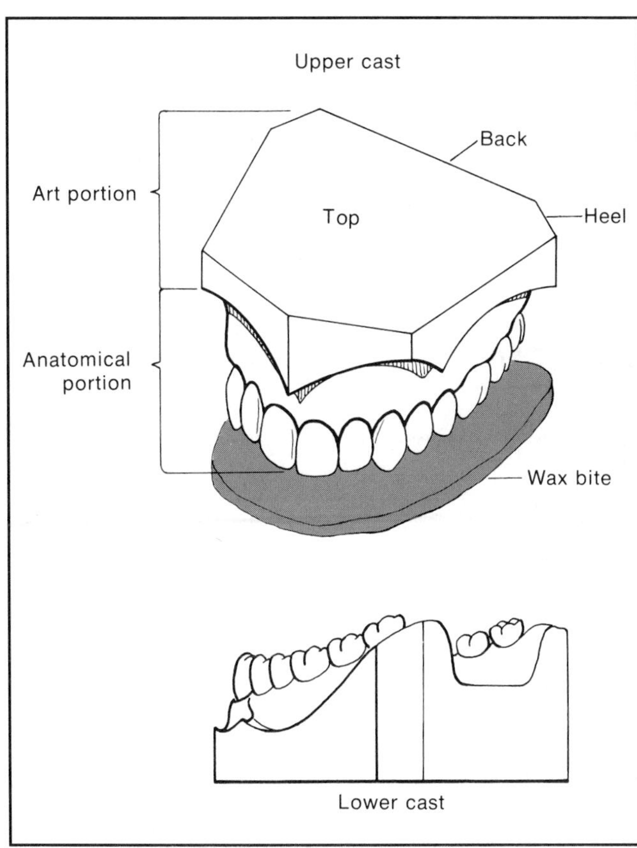

FIGURE 19–22

Landmarks of diagnostic casts.

two-thirds of the overall trimmed cast (Figs. 19–22 and 19–23).

The **art portion**, which forms the base, should make up one-third of the overall trimmed cast. However, the art portion should be no more than ½ inch thick.

The angles for trimming the art portion are shown in Table 19–2 and Figure 19–24.

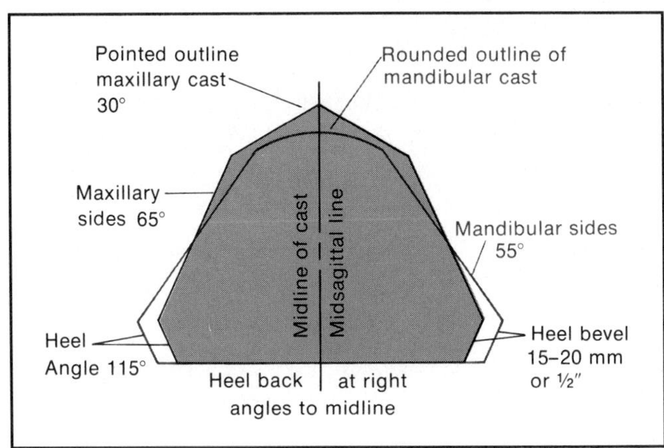

FIGURE 19–23

Outline of the maxillary cast (shaded) superimposed over the outline of the mandibular cast.

TABLE 19–2

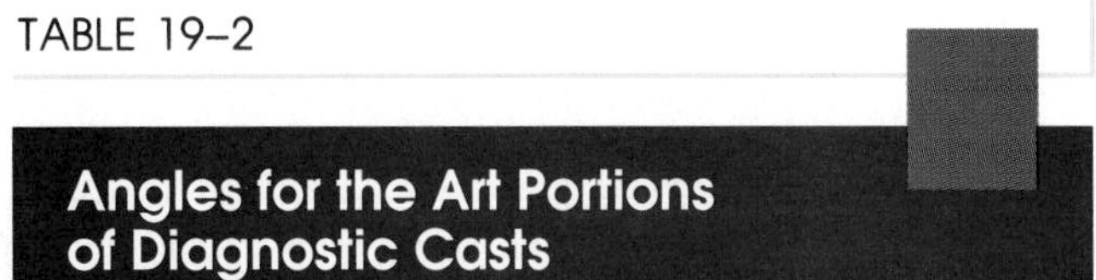

Angles for the Art Portions of Diagnostic Casts

ART PORTION OF MAXILLARY CAST	ART PORTION OF MANDIBULAR CAST
Cast comes to a point at the midline. This point results from a 30° angle from the cuspid to the midline.	The midline is rounded from cuspid to cuspid.
Sides are angled at a 65° angle.	Sides are angled at a 55° angle.
Heels are angled at a 115° angle.	Heels are angled at a 115° angle.

Trimming Diagnostic Casts

The wheel of the model trimmer works best when the casts are damp. Therefore, the casts should be soaked in cool water for 5 minutes before trimming. If the casts have been recently poured and are still damp, additional soaking is not necessary.

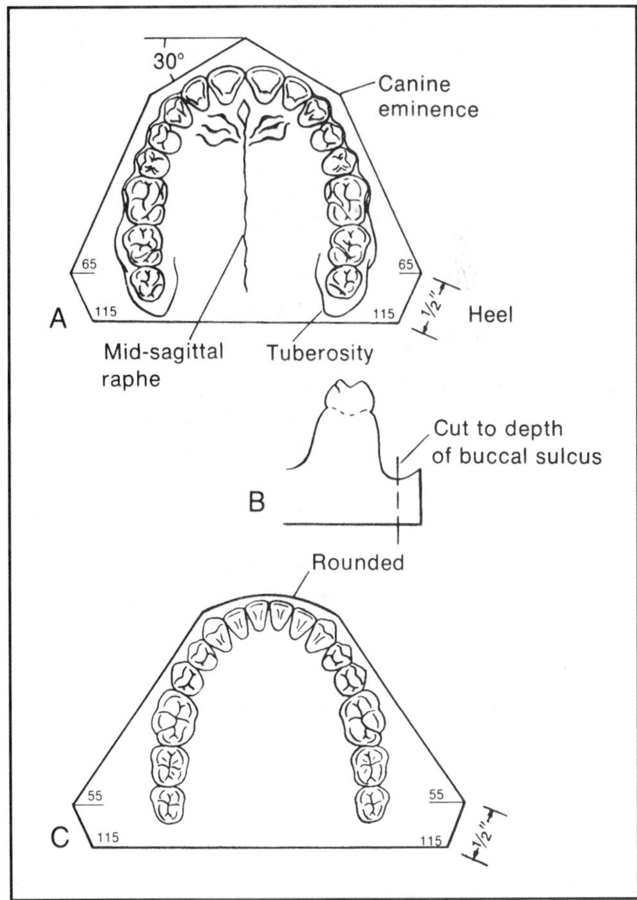

FIGURE 19–24

Landmarks, angles, and cuts on art portion of casts. *A*, Maxillary cast. *B*, Cut to depth of buccal sulcus. *C*, Mandibular cast.

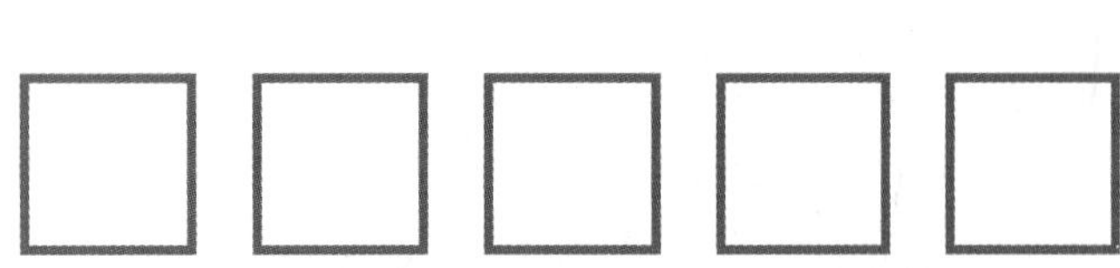

PROCEDURE: Trimming Diagnostic Casts

Instrumentation

Damp maxillary cast
Damp mandibular cast
Wax-bite registration
Ruler
Pencil
Laboratory knife
Measuring device
Model trimmer
Safety goggles

Preliminary Trimming

1. Measure the overall height of each cast.
   □ *RATIONALE:* The art portion should not be greater than one-third of the overall height of the cast.
2. Use the pencil to mark areas to be trimmed.
   □ *RATIONALE:* Excessive amounts must be removed.
3. Articulate the casts into the wax-bite registration.
4. Put on safety goggles, and turn on the power and water to the model trimmer.
5. Place the base of the mandibular cast flat on the trimmer table (Fig. 19–25).
6. Use the holding device on the trimmer to hold the model firmly against the trimming wheel.
7. Push the base of the cast against the wheel to reduce the excess. Check frequently to avoid reducing the base too much.
8. Repeat these steps for the maxillary cast.
9. Check to see that the cast sits flat when placed on a flat surface.

Refining Trimming

1. Use a laboratory knife to remove any bulky or rough edges from both casts.
   □ *RATIONALE:* These could interfere with obtaining accurate measurements.
2. Select the larger of the two casts. Draw a straight line with a pencil across the posterior of the cast.
   If the mandibular cast is larger, the line should be 3 mm. (¼ inch) in back of the retromolar pad.

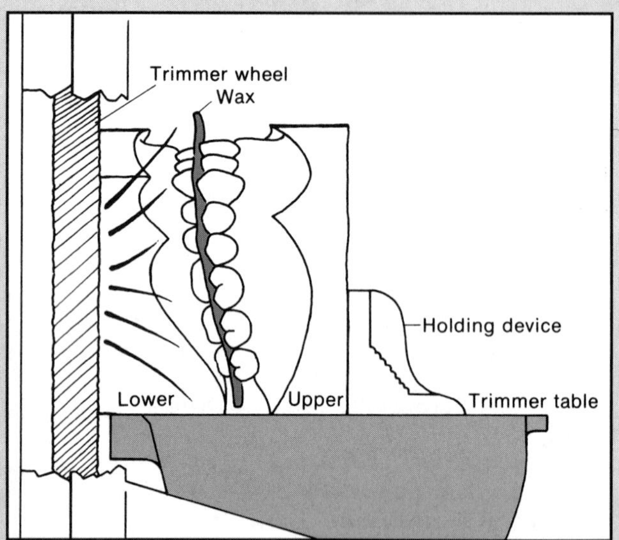

FIGURE 19–25

Trimming the back of the mandibular cast on the model trimmer.

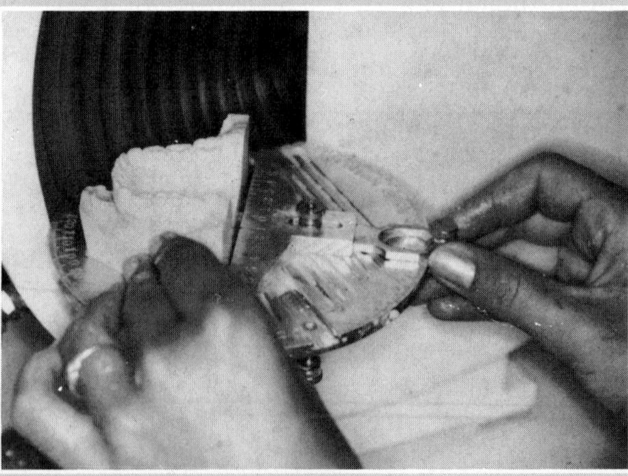

FIGURE 19–26

Trimming the rough edges of the cast on the model trimmer. (Courtesy of Harry W. Humphreys, DDS, MS, San Rafael, CA.)

If the maxillary cast is larger, the line should be 3 mm. (¼ inch) in back of the tuberosity.
3. Place the cast on the model trimmer and trim straight to the line. There should be 2 to 3 mm. of plaster remaining in back of the landmark *after* the cast is trimmed.

Creating Angles on the Mandibular Cast

1. Set the angulator of the model trimmer at 55 degrees (Fig. 19–26).
2. Place the heel of one side of the mandibular cast against the angulator and the base on the trimmer table.
3. Trim the side of the mandibular cast. Do not trim into the mucobuccal fold or remove the buccal frenum.
4. Repeat this process on the opposite side of the mandibular cast.
5. Trim the anterior portion of the mandibular cast, following the curve of the arch. Be careful not to remove the vestibular area or the labial frenum (Fig. 19–27).
6. Set the angulator at 115 degrees. Place the base of the mandibular cast on the trimmer table. Now cut the heels on each side of the cast.
   □ *RATIONALE:* This cut will align the heel line and the sides of the cast.

Creating Angles on the Maxillary Cast

1. Articulate the maxillary and mandibular casts on the wax-bite.
2. Place the mandibular cast on the trimmer table. Trim the heels of the maxillary cast to match the heel trim on the mandibular cast.
3. Place the articulated casts on their heels and trim the base of the maxillary cast parallel to the base of the mandibular cast (Fig. 19–28).
4. Separate the casts. Set the angulator at 65 degrees.
5. Place the base of the maxillary cast on the trimming table. Make the side cuts to the lowest portion of the mucobuccal fold. Be careful not to remove the buccal frenum attachment.
6. Place the maxillary cast base on the trimmer table with the anterior portion against the wheel.
7. Make a 25-degree angle cut from the cuspid to the central (midline). Repeat for the opposite side. (Be careful not to remove the labial frenum attachment.)
   □ *RATIONALE:* These cuts are important because they provide the point at the anterior portion of the cast.

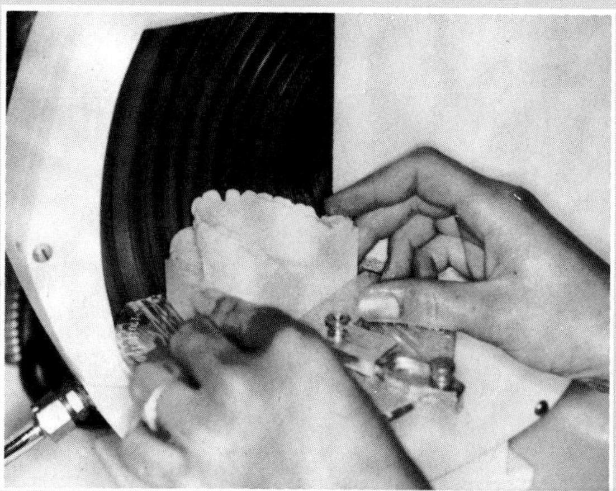

FIGURE 19–27

Trimming the anterior portion of the maxillary cast. (Courtesy of Harry W. Humphreys, DDS, MS, San Rafael, CA.)

Finishing the Casts

1. Remove any beads of plaster from the occlusal surfaces of the teeth on both casts.
2. *Optional:* Use a thick mix of plaster to fill up voids or bubbles in the moist base or body portion of the casts.
3. Place a typed label on the posterior of the casts. This label should include the patient's name, age, and date.
4. Store the casts in containers to prevent breakage.

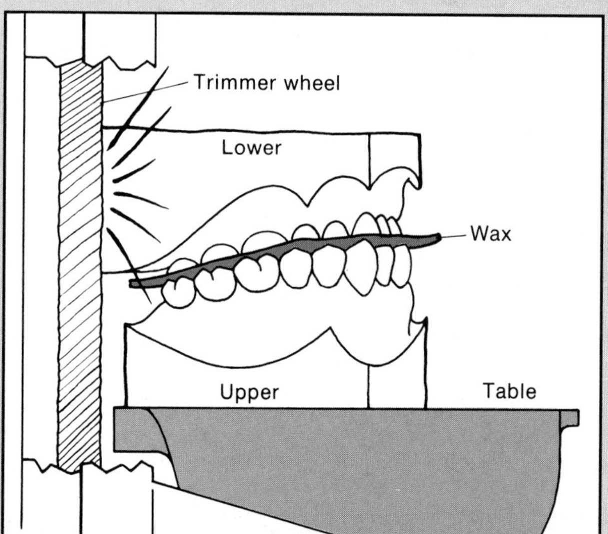

FIGURE 19–28

Trimming the back of the maxillary cast on the model trimmer.

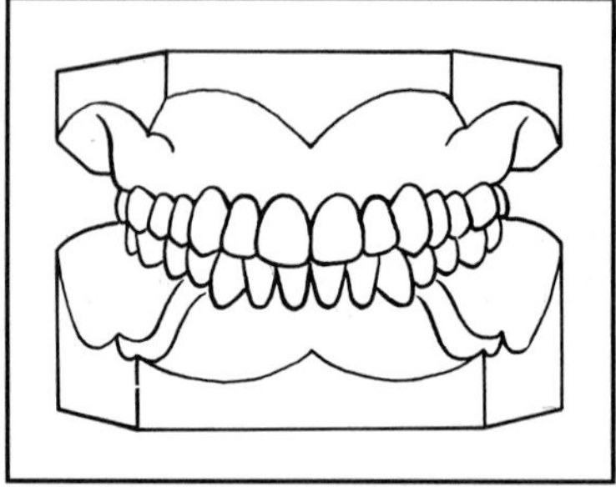

FIGURE 19–29

The completed diagnostic casts.

Polishing Diagnostic Casts

Many dental offices display casts to demonstrate "before and after" treatment results, and polishing provides these casts with a professional quality appearance (Fig. 19–29).

A commercial model gloss spray may be used for this purpose. An alternative is to soak the casts for 24 hours in a soap-and-water solution.

After the casts are dry, a soft dry cloth is used to gently buff the surfaces until there is a high gloss.

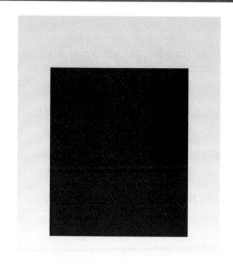

Chapter 20

Pharmacology and Pain Control

Introduction

Pharmacology is the study of drugs, especially as they relate to medicinal uses. It also deals with reactions and properties of drugs. Drugs, or medicines, are substances administered to help the body overcome disease and the effects of disease by aiding one or more of the body's physiological and reparative functions.

Under no circumstances may a dental assistant prescribe medication! He or she may dispense medicine only according to the explicit instructions and under the direct supervision of the dentist.

Effective **pain control** in dentistry is very important, and the means of achieving this are discussed in this chapter. The difficulties of patients with excessive fear of pain that they associate with dental treatment are discussed in Chapter 8.

Different types of anesthetic agents are used in dentistry. **Anesthesia** means the absence of pain. An **anesthetic** is the agent (drug) used to create this pain-free state.

Pharmacology

Drug Names

Drug names are divided into two broad classes: brand names and generic names. **Brand names** are those names controlled by business firms and that are registered trademarks. Brand names are always capitalized.

Generic names are those names that any business firm may use. Common names that are *not* registered trademarks fall into this second group. Generic names are not capitalized. For example, Valium is the brand name of a drug used to treat anxiety. The generic name for this same drug is diazepam.

Drugs are also classified legally on the basis of their availability to the public. Those in containers that bear the legend "Federal law prohibits dispensing without prescription" are called **prescription** items.

Those in containers not bearing such a legend are referred to as **over-the-counter** (OTC) items, and they may be purchased without restriction.

Controlled Substances Act

The drugs and drug products covered under the Federal Comprehensive Drug Abuse Prevention and Control Act are divided into five schedules. These schedules depend largely on the drug's potential for abuse, its medical usefulness, and the degree to which it may lead to physical and psychological dependence.

Many states also have controlled substances acts patterned after the federal law. Some state laws are more restrictive, but none are less restrictive, than the federal law.

The dentist must comply with the provisions of the federal laws and those of the state in which he or she practices.

Under these laws, a professional who is authorized to prescribe these medications is issued a Federal Drug Enforcement Agency (DEA) identification number.

(This DEA number is *not* printed on prescription blanks.)

SCHEDULE I

Schedule I drugs have no current accepted medical usefulness and have a high potential for abuse. Normally, Schedule I drugs cannot be prescribed. This schedule includes opium derivatives (such as heroin), hallucinogenic substances (including lysergic acid diethylamide [LSD] and marijuana), depressants (including methaqualone), and certain stimulants. (A hallucinogenic substance causes hallucinations. A **hallucination** is a sense perception such as sight, touch, sound, smell, or taste that has no basis in reality.)

SCHEDULE II

Schedule II drugs have a high potential for abuse and have accepted medical usefulness. Prescriptions for Schedule II drugs must be in writing and cannot be renewed.

This schedule includes morphine, hydromorphone (Dilaudid), methadone, meperidine (pethidine) (Demerol), oxycodone (Percodan), codeine, cocaine, short-acting barbiturates, and stimulants such as amphetamine and methylphenidate (speed).

SCHEDULE III

Schedule III drugs have less abuse potential than the drugs in Schedule I and II and have accepted medical usefulness. Prescriptions for Schedule III and Schedule IV drugs may be written or oral. If authorized, these prescriptions may be refilled up to five times within 6 months after the date of issue.

This schedule includes some stimulants and depressants that are not included in other schedules and preparations that contain a limited quantity of codeine (such as acetaminophen [Tylenol] with codeine).

SCHEDULE IV

Schedule IV drugs have a low abuse potential and have accepted medical usefulness. The prescribing information is the same as for Schedule III drugs. This schedule includes phenobarbital, diazepam (Valium), and propoxyphene (Darvon).

SCHEDULE V

Schedule V drugs have a low abuse potential and have accepted medical usefulness. Under federal law, Schedule V drugs are not required to be prescribed; however, they are available only under controlled circumstances. Some states do require that these drugs be dispensed only on prescription.

This schedule includes a few OTC preparations containing very limited quantities of codeine combined with other medications, such as cough preparations containing a very small quantity of codeine.

Ordering Narcotics for the Office Supply

Most general practitioners do *not* keep a supply of narcotics in the dental office. Specialists who require an office supply of narcotics keep only a minimum quantity, and this is always stored in a locked cabinet. Narcotics for "office use" cannot be ordered through your local pharmacy by prescription.

An official Schedules I and II order form, which is supplied by the Drug Enforcement Administration (DEA), must be used for this purpose. Two copies of each order must be sent to the supplier (a medical wholesale or supply house). A third copy must be filed in the office narcotics record book.

INVENTORY OF DRUG SUPPLIES

When these controlled substances are administered or dispensed from the dental practice, the dentist must comply with the federal recordkeeping requirements. These records must account for all narcotics used in the dental office.

The State Board of Dentistry is responsible for checking suspected abuse of prescription drugs. When abuse is suspected, deputized agents of the board may gain access to all prescription and drug inventory records in the practice.

Prescriptions

A prescription is a written order authorizing the pharmacist to furnish certain drugs to a patient (Fig. 20–1). A prescription may be written only by a professional who is legally authorized to prescribe medications. Table 20–1 shows the English equivalents of Latin abbreviations that are frequently used in writing prescriptions.

WRITING PRESCRIPTIONS

Prescription pads should never be used as note paper or left out where they might be stolen. The format and

TABLE 20–1

Latin Abbreviations Frequently Used for Prescriptions

LATIN ABBREVIATION	ENGLISH EQUIVALENT
bid	Twice daily
prn	When needed
qid	Four times daily
tid	Three times daily

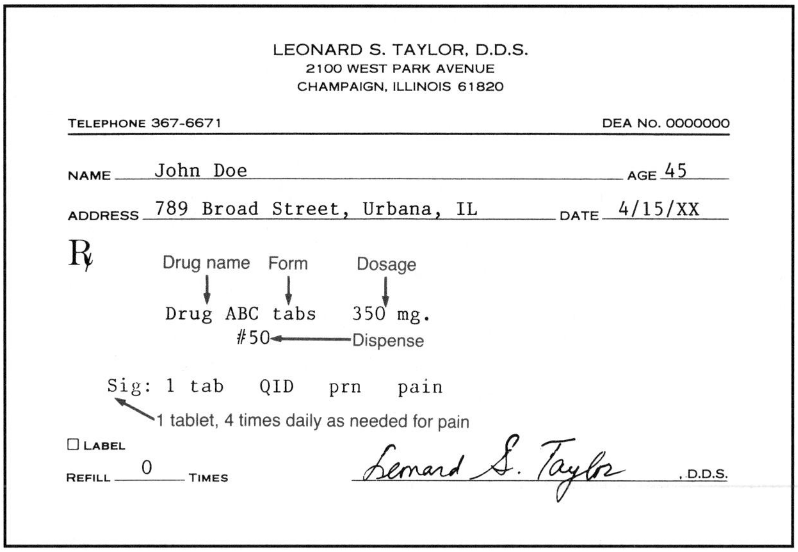

LEONARD S. TAYLOR, D.D.S.
2100 WEST PARK AVENUE
CHAMPAIGN, ILLINOIS 61820

TELEPHONE 367-6671 DEA No. 0000000

NAME John Doe AGE 45

ADDRESS 789 Broad Street, Urbana, IL DATE 4/15/XX

℞ Drug name Form Dosage

Drug ABC tabs 350 mg.
#50 ← Dispense

Sig: 1 tab QID prn pain
1 tablet, 4 times daily as needed for pain

☐ LABEL

REFILL 0 TIMES Leonard S. Taylor, D.D.S.

FIGURE 20–1

Sample prescription blank. (Courtesy of Colwell Systems, Champaign, IL.)

information to be included on the prescription may be regulated by state law. Also, some states require duplicate or triplicate prescription blanks for some or all controlled substances.

In general, a prescription must include the following information:

- The prescriber's name, address, and telephone number
- The name of the patient and the date the prescription was written
- The name, strength, and quantity of the drug to be dispensed
- Directions for use by the patient
- The prescriber's signature
- If the prescription is for a controlled substance, the prescriber's DEA number must be included

State laws may require additional information such as

- The patient's address and age
- Whether or not the pharmacist may substitute a generic brand of this medication
- Whether or not the prescription may be refilled (if refills are permitted, the number of refills must be specified)

RECORDING PRESCRIPTIONS

A record must be kept of each drug prescribed for or administered to a patient. The doctor may elect to write the prescription in duplicate so that a copy is retained in the patient's records.

An alternative is to make a notation in the patient's chart giving complete information about the prescription.

PRESCRIPTIONS AND THE TELEPHONE

The following are guidelines for the assistant regarding telephone procedures related to drugs:

1. Narcotics cannot be ordered without a written prescription.
2. It is against the law for an assistant to "call in" any prescription.
3. When a pharmacist calls, notify the dentist immediately. Do not try to relay information in a call from the pharmacist.
4. If the dentist is unable to come to the phone, take the pharmacist's name and phone number so that the call may be returned.
5. Never try to evaluate a patient's reaction to a drug (whether over the phone or in person). Only the dentist is qualified to do this!

The Terminology of Drug Effects

A **drug interaction** is a response resulting from two or more drugs or other therapeutic measures acting simultaneously. For example, aspirin taken with an anticoagulant increases the possibility of the patient's having a bleeding problem.

Potentiation, also known as *synergism*, is the action of drugs together so that the combined effect is greater than the effect of either drug taken alone. For example, Tylenol and codeine taken together are more effective than either drug taken separately.

Antagonism, which is the opposite of potentiation, occurs when the action of the drugs together creates an undesirable effect.

Drug tolerance is usually acquired through the repeated use of a drug. The result is that the patient requires larger and larger amounts of the drug to produce the same effect.

Intolerance is a reaction greater than the expected effect of a drug produced by an unusually small dose: for example, marked sedation from a small dose of a barbiturate.

Hypersensitivity, commonly known as an *allergic reaction*, is a response resulting from the altered reactivity of an individual. For example, a patient may have a severe, life-threatening allergic reaction to penicillin.

A **side effect** is an unavoidable effect that results from administration of an average dose of a drug. For example, constipation is a frequent side effect from the use of codeine.

A **secondary effect** is an indirect consequence of the action of a drug: for example, a superinfection that follows prolonged use of broad-spectrum antibiotics.

Idiosyncrasy is an unsuspected, abnormal response to a drug: for example, central nervous system (CNS) stimulation by a barbiturate that would normally be expected to depress the CNS.

An **overdose** is an undesirable effect due to an excessive amount of a drug present in the body. An overdose that causes poisoning is called a **toxic dose**. One that causes death is called a **lethal dose**.

Substance Abuse

Substance abuse is the use of medically prescribed drugs or illegal drugs to escape reality.

Addiction is drug-oriented behavior that includes the compulsive abuse of the drug, an obsession about securing its supply, and great difficulty in discontinuing its use.

Chemical dependence (CD) is the state of psychological and/or physical dependence on a mood-altering substance.

Physical dependence is a state of chronic intoxication with a drug, characterized by tolerance (the need for ever larger quantities to achieve the desired effect) and withdrawal illness.

Withdrawal illness is the experience of physical symptoms associated with stopping the use of a drug of dependence, including convulsions, headaches, trembling, and nervousness.

Psychological dependence is the habitual, compulsive use of a substance, despite the risk of adverse consequences. The degree of dependence ranges from a fairly mild desire for the drug to an uncontrollable craving for it.

Psychological dependence differs from physical dependence in that abstinence does not cause withdrawal illness.

COCAINE

Cocaine is a powerful CNS stimulant and a vasoconstrictor. (A **vasoconstrictor** causes blood vessels to narrow and stimulates the heart.) It may produce extreme restlessness, excitement, tachycardia (rapid heart rate), and talkativeness.

The cocaine abuser may also abuse prescription drugs such as analgesics and/or antianxiety drugs to "come down" gently from the "high" produced by the cocaine.

It is essential that the dentist know whether the patient uses cocaine because cocaine may interact with the epinephrine in local anesthetic solution. This can possibly cause a dangerous increase in heart rate and blood pressure. Also, cocaine-induced alterations in the pulmonary gas exchange can make nitrous oxide administration hazardous.

ALCOHOL

Alcohol is a depressant and a very commonly abused drug. Symptoms of use include impaired judgment, slurred speech, staggering, and drowsiness. It may also cause confusion and aggressive behavior.

NARCOTIC ANALGESICS

Narcotic analgesics may be abused because they produce euphoria. (**Euphoria** is an exaggerated feeling of physical and mental well-being.) These drugs, which are discussed further in the section "Strong Analgesics," depress the CNS and may cause pinpoint pupils, drowsiness, lethargy, or stupor. (**Lethargy** is a condition of drowsiness or indifference. **Stupor** is a state of lethargy in which a person seems unaware of his surroundings.)

BARBITURATES AND ANTIANXIETY AGENTS

Barbiturates, also known as downers, are depressants. They may produce drowsiness, staggering, slurred speech, confusion, and aggressive behavior.

Included in this group are antianxiety agents such as chlordiazepoxide (Librium), ethchlorvynol (Placidyl), diazepam (Valium), and methaqualone (Quaaludes). When combined with alcohol, these drugs can have a deadly effect.

AMPHETAMINES AND HALLUCINOGENS

Amphetamine drugs, also known as uppers, are stimulants. They may produce excitement, increased wakefulness, talkativeness, and hallucinations.

Hallucinogens, such as LSD and phencyclidine (PCP), cause excitement, hallucinations, and rambling speech. They may also produce bizarre behavior, psychotic symptoms, and violent reactions.

DENTAL IMPLICATIONS OF SUBSTANCE ABUSE

Any behavior suggesting that a patient is under the influence of one or more drugs when he comes to the dental office should be called to the dentist's attention immediately (in private).

Also, some individuals go from doctor to doctor collecting prescriptions to control a vague but severe pain that tends to "come and go" and yet defies diagnosis. If you suspect that a patient is doing this, you should alert the dentist (in private).

Some patients with chemical dependencies tend to consume large quantities of refined carbohydrates. This may result in a high caries rate. Poor diet also contributes to deteriorating general health and increased periodontal disease.

Drug-induced xerostomia (dry mouth), which may result from narcotic and stimulant abuse, also may be responsible for rampant dental decay and numerous abscessed teeth.

Some drug use increases bruxism. This may result in an increased incidence of advanced general periodontitis and a high rate of dental attrition.

Routes of Drug Administration

- **Inhalation** administration is by breathing a gaseous substance. Example: nitrous oxide sedation.
- **Topical** administration is by application on the surface of the mucosa or skin. Example: topical anesthetic ointments.
- **Transdermal** administration is also through the skin. Most commonly this is through a patch that continuously releases a controlled quantity of the medication. Example: nicotine patches to aid in smoking cessation.
- **Rectal** administration is by suppositories or enemas. These are used most often with infants and young children who are unable to take drugs by mouth.
- **Oral** administration may be in the form of pills, tablets, capsules, or liquids.
- **Sublingual** administration is placement of the medication under the tongue and absorption through the oral mucosa.
- **Parenteral** administration is by injection through a hypodermic syringe.
- A **subcutaneous** (SC) injection is administered just under the skin.
- An **intramuscular** (IM) injection is administered within the muscle tissue.
- In **intravenous** (IV) administration, the medication is administered directly into a vein.

PREMEDICATION

Premedication is the administration of an anti-anxiety drug, sedative, or hypnotic to an apprehensive patient before dental treatment. The drug of choice and the amount and time of administration are determined by the dentist, on the basis of the needs of the patient.

Premedication is used most frequently with very young children, extremely apprehensive patients, and patients who are scheduled for extensive surgical or restorative procedures. Administration may begin the night before the appointment, several hours before the appointment, or just before treatment.

Antibiotics

Antibiotics are chemical substances that inhibit the growth of, or destroy, bacteria and other microorganisms. The use of any antibiotic is based on four major considerations:

1. A clearly established need for antibiotic therapy (antibiotics are not effective against viral infections)
2. Knowledge that the microorganism is susceptible to this particular antibiotic (the antibiotics specific in their action against certain bacteria; for best results, the dentist must determine the cause of the infection and then select an antibiotic known to be most effective against that bacteria)
3. A thorough medical history to determine that the patient has not experienced any previous allergic or adverse reactions to this agent (allergic reactions to antibiotics can be very serious)
4. Awareness of the potential side effects of this antibiotic (the doctor must weigh any possible adverse effects against the anticipated therapeutic effects)

PROPHYLACTIC ANTIBIOTIC ADMINISTRATION

For high-risk patients, prophylactic antibiotic administration is recommended in conjunction with all dental procedures that are likely to cause bleeding. Included in this list of high-risk patients are those with various forms of heart disease, a history of rheumatic fever, open heart surgery, pacemakers, an artificial joint, or a dental implant.

As a preventive measure, the antibiotic may be administered before treatment and then continued for several days after treatment.

This prophylactic administration of antibiotics is controversial. Some experts believe that it is essential. Others state that it unnecessarily exposes the patient to the possibility of adverse drug reactions.

The dentist, who may consult the patient's physician, must decide whether or not this treatment is advisable for his or her high-risk patients.

SUPERINFECTIONS

All antibiotics, to a greater or lesser degree, disrupt the normal microbial balance of the skin, mucous membranes, and intestinal tract. This may allow drug-resistant bacteria or fungi to proliferate.

This may produce a new infection at the original site or elsewhere in the body. Such an infection is known as a superinfection. For example, after antibiotic therapy, there may be an overgrowth of the fungus *Candida albicans* in the mouth.

PENICILLINS

Penicillin is a generic term for a group of antibiotics similar in chemical structure and adverse drug reactions but differing in antibacterial spectrum and oral absorption rate. Penicillins may be administered orally or parenterally.

There are many types of penicillins, and they are referred to by either their generic or trade names. (They are described here by generic name.)

Penicillin V. Penicillin V is the antibiotic of choice against most orofacial infections. Penicillin V is most useful in dentistry to combat infections caused by gram-positive bacteria such as streptococci. However, it is not effective in the treatment of infections caused by many gram-negative microorganisms and by viruses or fungi.

Extended-Spectrum Penicillins. Amoxicillin and **ampicillin** are extended-spectrum penicillins with a greater gram-negative spectrum than penicillin V. They are used to treat staphylococci infections and some infections that are resistant to other forms of penicillin.

CEPHALOSPORINS

The cephalosporin group of antibiotics are chemically related to the penicillins. They are broad-spectrum antibiotics that are active against both gram-positive and gram-negative organisms.

In general, their dental use is limited to the treatment of infections with sensitive organisms when other agents are ineffective or cannot be used. However, they may be the drugs of choice for patients who are allergic to penicillins.

ERYTHROMYCIN

Erythromycin closely resembles penicillin in its spectrum of antibacterial activity and may be used with penicillin-sensitive patients or when organisms have become penicillin-resistant.

Erythromycin is usually administered orally and is most effective when taken on an empty stomach; however, the most common adverse effect of erythromycin is gastrointestinal distress.

TETRACYCLINES

The tetracyclines are broad-spectrum antibiotics affecting a wide range of microorganisms. They are *not* generally considered the drugs of choice for the majority of oral infections; however, they are of concern to dentistry because of tetracycline staining of the teeth.

Tetracycline Staining. The administration of tetracycline antibiotics from the second trimester of pregnancy to approximately 8 years of age may produce permanent discoloration of the teeth. These stains cannot be removed by polishing; however, in less severe cases, bleaching may be helpful.

The variation in severity, extent, coloration, depth, and location of the stains depends on the dosage time, the duration of drug use, and the type of tetracycline received. Tetracycline stains can be classified as slight, moderate, or severe.

Slight tetracycline staining appears as a light-yellow or light-gray discoloration of the entire dentition. It is small in extent, uniformly distributed throughout the crown, and exhibits no banding or localized concentrations.

Moderate tetracycline staining is observed as a darker, deeper hue of uniform yellow or gray discoloration without banding.

Severe tetracycline staining is characterized by dark-gray or blue to purple discoloration and often exhibits banding with a concentration of stain in the cervical regions (Fig. 20–2.)

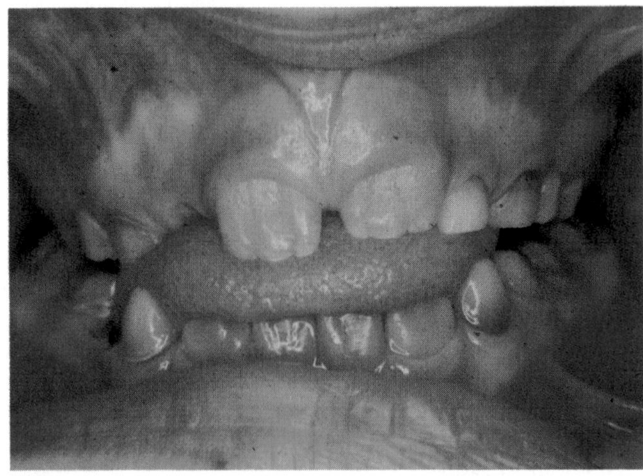

FIGURE 20–2

Tetracycline staining in mixed dentition. Notice the stains on the cervical region of the primary molars.

Antifungal Agents

Nystatin is an antifungal agent effective against *Candida albicans.* It is administered orally as a suspension that should be held in the mouth for some time before it is swallowed. To prevent a relapse, medication should be continued for at least 48 hours after the disappearance of clinical signs.

Epinephrine

Epinephrine, which is sometimes referred to as *adrenaline,* acts as both a vasoconstrictor and a vasodilator depending upon the amount used. (A **vasoconstrictor** narrows the blood vessels and stimulates the heart. A **vasodilator** causes the blood vessels to expand, thereby increasing circulation and potentially bleeding.)

Although epinephrine must be used with caution, it has many applications in dentistry.

USE IN LOCAL ANESTHETIC

Epinephrine is added in small quantities to local anesthetic solutions as a vasoconstrictor. This use is discussed later in this chapter.

USE IN GINGIVAL RETRACTION

Vasoconstrictors are frequently used to aid in the temporary retraction of gingival tissue from the margins of the cavity preparation. (Gingival retraction is discussed in Chapter 31.)

USE IN CONTROLLING DIFFUSE BLEEDING

Epinephrine may be used to control diffuse bleeding such as that immediately following periodontal surgery, in which the surgical area is not covered by sutured tissue.

Immediately after periodontal surgery, a gauze strip saturated with 1:1000 epinephrine may be placed over the surgical site to control the bleeding. It is left in place for several minutes while surgical dressings are prepared.

USE IN TREATING SEVERE ALLERGIC REACTIONS

In the event of a severe anaphylactic allergic reaction such as anaphylactic shock, epinephrine may be injected subcutaneously or intramuscularly to relieve swelling and as a cardiac stimulant. (This is discussed in Chapter 9.)

Atropine Sulfate

Atropine sulfate controls the secretion of saliva and mucus so that the mouth and throat become dry. This control of salivary flow is particularly important during a dental procedure performed when the patient is under general anesthesia.

Corticosteroids

Corticosteroids, such as hydrocortisone (cortisol), are used to reduce inflammation. In dental practice, corticosteroids may be applied topically for symptoms related to inflammation and for treatment of oral ulcers.

Their effectiveness in reducing swelling also makes corticosteroids useful as adjuncts to epinephrine in emergency situations such as anaphylaxis.

Agents for the Control of Anxiety

Anxiety is defined as a generalized feeling of fear and apprehension. Drugs employed to control anxiety are classified as antianxiety agents, sedatives, and hypnotics.

ANTIANXIETY AGENTS

Antianxiety agents are most commonly used in dentistry as either premedication or sedation to reduce patient fears, tension, and anxiety. The most frequently used antianxiety agents in dentistry include diazepam (Valium), chlordiazepoxide (Librium), and lorazepam (Ativan).

These drugs are CNS depressants and may cause drowsiness. They should *not* be administered in combination with other depressants such as alcohol.

SEDATIVE AND HYPNOTIC AGENTS

Hypnotics produce sleep. **Sedatives** reduce excitability, create calmness, and allow sleep to occur as a secondary effect. The same drugs, which produce varying degrees of CNS depression, are effective as either sedatives or hypnotics depending upon the dose given.

Sedatives and hypnotics may be administered as premedication shortly before a dental procedure to relieve apprehension. In some cases, a hypnotic drug may be prescribed for the night before an operation in order to promote sleep.

Premedication with a sedative before general anesthesia may also minimize the occurrence of undesirable side effects. These drugs are also used to supplement the action of analgesics and are used in combination with some of them to induce sleep in the presence of pain.

Barbiturate Sedative–Hypnotics. The uses of the barbiturates are determined by their duration of action: **Ultra-short-acting** barbiturates, such as methohexital sodium (Brevital) and thiopental sodium (Pentothal), are used intravenously for the induction of general anesthesia.

Short-acting barbiturates, such as pentobarbital sodium (Nembutal) and secobarbital sodium (Seconal), can be used orally for their hypnotic or calming effect. These agents may be given preoperatively to allay anxiety.

Intermediate-acting barbiturates, such as butalbital (Fiorinal), may also be used to relieve anxiety before a dental appointment.

Long-acting barbiturates, such as phenobarbital, are used primarily for sedation.

Nonbarbiturate Sedative–Hypnotics. In general, nonbarbiturate sedative–hypnotics are less effective and are associated with a higher incidence of side effects than barbiturates. Phenergan and chloral hydrate are nonbarbiturate sedative–hypnotics that are used in dentistry.

Pain Control in Dentistry

Analgesics

Analgesics are drugs that dull the perception of pain without producing unconsciousness. Non-narcotic and narcotic analgesics are available individually, in combination with other analgesics, or in combination with other substances such as barbiturates.

Analgesics may be used preoperatively to relieve pain such as toothache, or they may be prescribed to relieve postoperative pain following surgery or other extensive procedures.

MILD ANALGESICS

Mild analgesics are used for the relief of pain of low intensity, such as some headaches and most dental postoperative discomfort. These analgesics, which have minimal side effects, are not addictive and are available without a prescription.

The medications commonly recommended are **ibuprofen** (Motrin, Advil), **aspirin**, and **acetaminophen** (Tylenol).

Of these, ibuprofen, which is classified as a nonsteroidal anti-inflammatory drug (NSAID), is considered to be the most effective for controlling this type of pain. However, patients who are allergic to aspirin are also likely to be allergic to ibuprofen.

All three pain relievers have analgesic, antipyretic, and anti-inflammatory properties. (**Analgesic** means it reduces pain. **Antipyretic** means it reduces fever. **Anti-inflammatory** means it aids in reducing inflammation.)

MODERATE ANALGESICS

To control moderate pain, dentists most commonly prescribe a mild analgesic in combination with codeine. Because of the potentiation effect between these two drugs, more pain relief is achieved with a smaller amount of codeine.

STRONG ANALGESICS

Narcotic drugs used as strong analgesics for the relief of severe pain are capable of producing physical and psychological dependence. Their extended use should be avoided.

Codeine is often used when an analgesic stronger than aspirin is required. Codeine is frequently used in combination with acetaminophen or aspirin. This combination potentiates (increases) the pain-relieving effects of both drugs and permits the use of smaller quantities of both drugs.

Oxycodone hydrochloride (Percodan) is also employed in dentistry for the relief of severe pain. Its analgesic effect appears to be similar to that of codeine but can be of longer duration. Its habit-forming potential is somewhat less than that of morphine but greater than that of codeine.

TABLE 20–2

The Stages of Anesthesia

STAGE 1	Maintained analgesic stage Plane 1: relative analgesia Plane 2: relative analgesia Plane 3: total analgesia
STAGE 2	Delirium (excitement)
STAGE 3	Surgical anesthesia Plane 1 Plane 2 Plane 3 Plane 4
STAGE 4	Respiratory paralysis (death)

Meperidine hydrochloride (Demerol) has both morphine-like and atropine-like properties. It can be used when morphine is indicated for patients who cannot tolerate morphine because of the nausea it produces. Continued use may result in tolerance and addiction.

Morphine has the strongest narcotic, analgesic, and hypnotic effects of all analgesics. It is administered by injection. Its side effects include constipation, nausea, and vomiting. It is highly addictive.

Hydromorphone (Dilaudid) is similar to morphine and it may be administered orally. It too has a high addiction potential.

Sedation

Sedation is used during treatment to ease patient anxiety and to raise the patient's pain threshold. For more complete pain control, a local anesthetic agent is commonly used in conjunction with the sedation.

Sedatives may be administered orally, intravenously, or by inhalation (gasses). Before administering any form of sedation, the dentist is required to have received specialized training covering the choice of agents and the modes of delivery.

THE LEVELS OF SEDATION

Sedation is divided into three levels: conscious sedation (also known as analgesia), deep sedation (a level of analgesia), and general anesthesia. These levels are summarized in Table 20–2.

Conscious Sedation. Conscious sedation is a minimally depressed level of consciousness that retains the patient's ability to independently and continuously maintain an airway and respond appropriately to physical stimulation and verbal commands.

Diazepam (Valium) may be administered intravenously to achieve conscious sedation. However, nitrous oxide sedation is the most commonly used form of conscious sedation. (This consists of the gasses nitrous oxide and oxygen and is described later in this chapter.)

Deep Sedation. Deep sedation is a controlled state of depressed consciousness, accompanied by partial loss of protective reflexes, including inability to respond purposefully to verbal command.

In contrast to general anesthesia, the patient is not totally unconscious. Deep sedation, rather than general anesthesia, may be used when oral surgery is performed in the dental office. (General anesthesia is further explained later in this chapter.)

MODES OF ADMINISTRATION OF SEDATIVES

Oral or Intramuscular Administration. A barbiturate sedative may be given orally or by IM injection about 15 to 20 minutes before surgery. This form of sedation may be indicated for

- Very young children (under age 5) who require extensive treatment

- Moderately to severely mentally retarded children or adults
- Patients in severe pain from an acute infection who require immediate treatment (a local anesthetic cannot be administered into an infected area)
- Patients who are extremely nervous and fearful of dental treatment

With these sedatives, the patient will be drowsy but conscious. The patient should not be allowed to leave alone or drive until the effects of the sedative have worn off.

Intravenous Sedation. IV sedation involves the use of drugs administered directly into the vein to produce conscious or deep sedation. Special training is required for the doctor or anesthetist administering IV sedation.

Diazepam (Valium) or midazolam (Versed) are commonly used for this purpose. In addition to controlling anxiety, these drugs also produce amnesia so that the patient does not remember much of what occurred during treatment.

With IV sedation, the patient remains conscious; however, it may also be used as an induction to general anesthesia. These patients require close monitoring of their vital signs at all times, and the dental team must be prepared to react quickly in the event of an emergency.

Nitrous Oxide Sedation

A combination of nitrous oxide and oxygen gasses is widely used to achieve conscious sedation, which is also known as *nitrous oxide-oxygen analgesia* or *relative analgesia.*

Nitrous oxide sedation acts to relieve apprehension and to relax the patient; however, significant pain control still depends upon the use of effective local anesthesia.

ADVANTAGES

- Administration is relatively simple and easily managed by the operator.
- Although special training is required, the services of an anesthetist or other special personnel are not necessary.
- This type of sedation has an excellent safety record, and the side effects are minimal.
- The patient is awake and able to communicate at all times.
- Recovery is rapid and complete within a matter of minutes.
- Nitrous oxide sedation may be used with patients of all ages.

INDICATIONS FOR USE

- The patient is fearful of the dental experience.
- The patient has a low pain threshold.
- The patient has a sensitive gag reflex.
- The use of local anesthesia is contraindicated, and/or good local anesthesia cannot be obtained.
- The patient has a cardiac condition or high blood pressure. (These patients benefit from the increased concentration of oxygen and from the reduction of stress.)

CONTRAINDICATIONS FOR USE

- The patient has an upper respiratory tract infection or a nasal obstruction that makes breathing through the nose difficult.
- The patient is a very young child, a mentally retarded individual, or any patient with whom communication is not possible.
- The patient has multiple sclerosis or advanced emphysema, both of which impair breathing function.
- The patient is emotionally unstable, such as a drug addict or an individual undergoing psychiatric treatment.

THE PLANES OF ANALGESIA

Table 20–2 illustrates the four stages of general anesthesia. Stage 1, the analgesia stage, is divided into three planes. Of these three planes, only the first two are the desired levels for nitrous oxide sedation.

Analgesia Plane 1. Respiration, blood pressure, pulse, muscle, tone, and eye movements are normal. The patient is able to keep his mouth open without a mouth prop and is capable of following directions.

The patient appears to be fully conscious and relaxed. There may be a tingling in fingers, toes, the lips, or the tongue. There is a marked elevation of the pain reaction threshold and a reduction of fear.

Analgesia Plane 2. Respiration, blood pressure, pulse, and muscle tone are normal. The patient appears to be relaxed and euphoric; however, he is still able to keep his mouth open and to follow directions. The patient has a pleasant feeling of lethargy. He feels safe, is less aware of his immediate surroundings, and is less concerned with activity around him.

He may feel a wave of warmth or a vibratory sensation, somewhat like the soft purring of a motor, throughout his body. At this time, the patient may also describe a feeling of headiness or drowsiness similar to light intoxication.

His voice becomes throaty, losing its natural resonance. The patient's thoughts may wander beyond those of activity in the treatment room.

Analgesia Plane 3. The patient in analgesia plane 3 is moving toward the excitement stage of general anesthesia. Usually the first indication of the shift into this plane is nausea, vomiting, or restlessness.

Additional indications that the patient is in analgesia plane 3 include the following:

- He becomes totally unaware of his surroundings.
- His jaw may become rigid, his mouth tends to close, and his body may stiffen.
- He may appear to stare and have an angry or very sleepy look.

- His respiration, pulse, and blood pressure remain normal; however, the patient may have hallucinatory dreams or experience fear.

Should these indications appear, immediate increased oxygen and decreased nitrous oxide help to quickly return the patient to the desired plane.

SAFETY PRECAUTIONS

Under the Dental Practice Act in some states, the assistant is allowed to aid in monitoring the administration of nitrous oxide *only* under the direct supervision of the dentist. To ensure the patient's safety, it is vital that the auxiliary understand the process and his or her role in its administration.

Nitrous oxide sedation is a pleasant, relaxing experience, but it is not without danger. It is a drug, and it must not be abused. It should never be used for recreational purposes or used regularly to help one relax.

There is also some danger to personnel from escaping waste gasses. (These hazards are discussed further in Chapter 12 in the "Flammable Gasses" section.)

The following steps are necessary to reduce the possibility of gasses' escaping into the treatment room air.

- All equipment must meet current safety standards, including the use of a scavenging system. (**Scavenging equipment** is a vacuum apparatus that attaches to the mask and removes exhaust gasses so they are not released into the air.)
- Equipment must be kept in proper working condition and be monitored regularly for leaks in the hoses.
- The patient's mask must be the correct size and fit snugly.
- The high-volume evacuation (HVE) system should be used during treatment to reduce levels of ambient nitrous oxide released through the patient's mouth.

NITROUS OXIDE–OXYGEN EQUIPMENT

Built-In Installation or Mobile Equipment. The office may be equipped with built-in nitrous oxide–oxygen equipment in the treatment rooms. An alternative is the use of a portable unit that is moved from room to room as needed. Both types of equipment are the same except for the size of the tanks of gas. Regardless of the tank size used, this basic rule applies: In addition to the tank in use, there should always be a reserve tank ready.

In most states, ordering of a new supply of these gasses involves the dentist's signature and license number. It is also necessary to comply with Occupational Safety and Health Administration (OSHA) and state requirements for safe installation and storage of these supplies.

Gas Tanks. The large size "E" tanks are used for a built-in installation. These are stored in an enclosed and locked area outside of the dental office. Maintaining the security of these tanks is important, and this responsibility may be delegated to the company that supplies the tanks.

- **Nitrous oxide** is supplied in *blue* steel tanks.
- **Oxygen** is supplied in *green* steel tanks.

Controls and Gauges. The gasses are dispensed through controls and gauges attached to either a fixed-wall installation or a portable unit. The flowmeter of a fixed unit is shown in Figure 9–8.

The flow of gasses is measured in liters per minute. During the entire procedure, the patient is maintained at a maximum of 6 to 7 total liters of combined gasses.

The equipment also includes a rubber bag, which is lightly inflated during the administration of the gasses.

Masks. The gasses are administered through a scavenging mask that fits snugly over the patient's nose. Masks are available in adult and child sizes to ensure proper fit. The mask may be disposable (discarded after a single use) or must be sterilized before reuse.

A scavenging mask has an inner and an outer mask. The nitrous oxide and oxygen are delivered into the inner mask. The patient's breath, which contains waste gasses, is removed through a tube connecting the outer mask to the central evacuation system.

The mask should fit snugly, and comfortably, on the patient's face to prevent gaps around the edges.

DETERMINING THE PATIENT'S BASELINE

The baseline is the ratio of nitrous oxide to oxygen that is most effective for each patient. At the baseline the patient is conscious and cooperative but pleasantly relaxed. The protective reflexes are intact and active.

The ratio of oxygen to nitrous oxide needed to achieve this baseline varies from patient to patient. In general, however, 50 percent nitrous oxide *or less* is effective.

As an example, for an adult patient with a 7-liter-per-minute flow, the baseline may be 3 liters of nitrous oxide and 4 liters of oxygen. Small children may require a lower percentage of nitrous oxide.

Once the baseline has been determined for a patient, this is recorded on the patient's chart. During future dental treatment, the patient may be started at the level recorded on his chart; however, the patient's reaction may vary from visit to visit. As necessary, adjustments are made to accommodate the patient's needs at each visit.

Nausea. If the patient feels nauseated (as if he is going to vomit) or becomes restless and excited, he is receiving too much nitrous oxide.

Should this happen, turn off the nitrous oxide immediately and administer 100 percent oxygen until the patient is comfortable again. Then the flow of nitrous oxide may be resumed, at a lower baseline, and the dental procedure is continued.

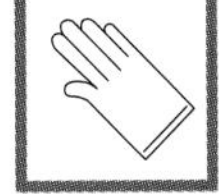 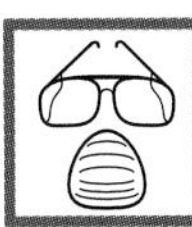  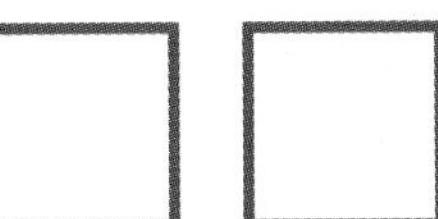 

PROCEDURE: **Assisting the Dentist in Monitoring the Administration of Nitrous Oxide Sedation**

Note: The monitoring of nitrous oxide sedation is accomplished with the dentist in direct supervision of the assistant. (Direct supervision is discussed in Chapter 2.)

Instrumentation

Tanks of nitrous oxide and oxygen gasses (with spares in reserve)
Nitrous oxide equipment (controls and gauges)
Sterile scavenger masks (adult or child size)

Preparation

1. The assistant checks the tanks of nitrous oxide and oxygen to determine that the tanks are full and that the gauges are operating correctly.
   □ *RATIONALE:* Running out of gas during a procedure would be disruptive to both dentist and patient.
2. The assistant places a sterile mask on the tubing connection of the gas unit. The mask must be of an appropriate size to fit the patient.
   □ *RATIONALE:* A mask that does not fit properly allows gasses to leak into the air.
3. The patient is placed in a supine position, and the dentist explains to the patient the effects and sensations of nitrous oxide–oxygen.
4. The patient gives informed consent and is instructed to breathe slowly and deeply throughout the procedure.
5. The assistant begins the flow of oxygen, and the mask is placed over the patient's nose so that it fits comfortably and snugly.
   □ *RATIONALE:* It is more comfortable for the patient to have oxygen flowing when the mask is placed.

Administration

1. The patient is given a flow of 5 to 8 liters of 100 percent oxygen for 1 minute.
   □ *RATIONALE:* This allows the patient to become accustomed to the mask and the flow of gas.
2. The assistant observes the rise and fall of the rubber bag on the gas unit, which indicates the patient's breathing volume.
3. Nitrous oxide is increased at the rate of 1 liter per minute while the oxygen flow is decreased at a similar rate. A 60-second pause is made between each adjustment until the baseline area is achieved.
   □ *RATIONALE:* A sudden increase may startle the patient and can cause nausea.
4. To determine when the patient has reached his baseline, the dentist or assistant quietly asks the patient how he feels.
5. When the patient has reached and is maintained at this optimum level, local anesthetic solution is administered, and the dental procedures are performed.

Recovery

1. When the dental procedure is completed, the nitrous oxide control value is returned to 0, and the oxygen is increased to the original 5- to 8-liter flow per minute.
2. The patient breathes 100 percent oxygen for about 2 minutes or until all signs of sedation are gone.
   □ *RATIONALE:* This allows all of the nitrous oxide gas to be expelled from the patient's system.
3. The patient's mask is removed, and he is slowly seated upright and questioned as to how he feels. Usually the response is a positive one: that the patient feels relaxed and comfortable.
4. Details regarding the administration of the nitrous oxide sedation are recorded on the patient's chart. These include

   a. The levels of gasses administered
   b. The duration of nitrous oxide administration
   c. The duration of oxygenation (oxygen-only administration) at the end of the procedure
   d. The condition of the patient at this time (for example, the patient was alert and relaxed)

5. During treatment room cleanup, a disposable mask is discarded. If the mask is the type that can be sterilized, it is removed from the tubing and sent to the sterilization center.

General Anesthesia

General anesthesia is a controlled state of loss of consciousness produced by chemical induction. Its purpose is to render the patient free of pain and to provide treatment that the patient cannot receive in any other manner.

Although nitrous oxide sedation is superficially similar to general anesthesia, it is important to remember that these are distinctly different techniques and applications. Just administering more nitrous oxide will not achieve the desired effect!

General anesthesia is most safely administered in a hospital setting or another facility with the necessary equipment for administration and the management of any emergencies that might arise.

STAGES OF GENERAL ANESTHESIA

General anesthesia, also known as *surgical anesthesia,* is the third of the anesthesia stages described in Table 20–2. Stage 1 precedes the loss of consciousness.

Stage 2, the excitement stage, is continual from the loss of consciousness to the onset of surgical anesthesia. Because of the retching at this stage, it is highly desirable that the stomach be empty before general anesthesia.

Stage 3, surgical anesthesia, includes the condition from the onset of regular breathing to the occurrence of respiratory failure. Because the patient's protective gag and cough reflexes are suppressed in this stage, it is necessary to place throat packs that will prevent the aspiration of foreign materials. It is also essential to maintain a patent (open) airway for the patient at all times.

In **stage 4,** respiratory paralysis, breathing stops. The patient's blood pressure and pulse are feeble, and the circulatory flow is drastically reduced. Unless this situation is reversed quickly, the patient will die.

AGENTS FOR GENERAL ANESTHESIA

General anesthesia may be achieved by using a combination of gasses and intravenous medications.

Induction may be by intravenous anesthetic agents such as thiopental sodium and methohexital sodium. After induction, anesthesia may be maintained by a gas combination such as nitrous oxide–oxygen and halothane or enflurane mixtures.

GENERAL ANESTHESIA CAUTIONS

- General anesthetics may be administered only by qualified individuals with hospital-based training in anesthesiology.
- An **anesthetist**, a specialist in the administration of anesthetics, may work with the dentist to administer the drugs, monitor the patient's vital signs, and maintain airway patency. (**Patency** means the condition of being wide open.) (Vital signs are discussed in Chapter 9.)
- If general anesthesia is administered in the dental office, it is necessary to have ready the staff and equipment necessary for administration of the anesthetic, for delivering dental treatment to an unconscious patient, and for the management of medical emergencies.
- The dental equipment and seating of the dental team may need to be altered to accommodate the presence of the anesthetist and the anesthesia equipment.
- Properly equipped recovery areas must be available for the postanesthetic patient. (This usually includes suctioning equipment and oxygen that can be delivered with positive pressure.)
- All personnel must be trained to deal with life-threatening emergencies that may arise as adverse reactions to the anesthetic.

PATIENT PREPARATION

The dentist may request that the patient have a preoperative physical examination and/or laboratory tests performed before the administration of the general anesthetic. The patient or his legal guardian must sign a written consent form for the anesthesia and the procedure to be performed.

Preoperative Instructions to the Patient

1. The dentist explains to the patient the procedure to be performed and the risks and probable reactions to the general anesthesia.
2. If the procedure is scheduled for morning, the patient is NPO after midnight the night before. (**NPO** means nothing by mouth, and the patient is instructed not to eat or drink anything after that time.)
3. The patient must have another adult with him to accompany him home from the dental office.

Documentation

At the end of the procedure, the dentist and/or the anesthetist will enter on the patient's permanent record information regarding the preoperative and operative findings, duration of anesthesia, dosage of drugs, and notations of any unusual or untoward reactions.

Recovery from General Anesthesia

After the conclusion of the dental treatment, the patient is monitored closely until his normal reflexes return. The patient should respond to his name and should be capable of moving his limbs, turning his head, and speaking under the direction of the dentist.

The recovering patient should **not** be left alone as he regains consciousness after sedation or general anesthesia. Although fully conscious, the patient should not be allowed to walk alone or to drive an automobile immediately upon leaving the dental office. Therefore, someone *must* accompany him to his home.

Local Anesthetics

Local anesthetic agents are the most frequently used form of pain control in dentistry. These agents provide safe, effective, and dependable anesthesia of suitable duration for virtually all forms of dental treatment. They are compounded to

- Be nonirritating (not harmful) to the tissues in the area of the injection
- Produce minimal toxicity (cause the least possible damage to the body systems)
- Be of rapid onset (take effect quickly)
- Provide profound anesthesia (completely eliminate the sensation of pain during the procedure)
- Be of sufficient duration (remain effective long enough for the procedure to be completed)
- Be completely reversible (leave the tissue in its original state after the patient's recovery from anesthesia)
- Be sterile or capable of being sterilized by heat without deterioration

CHEMISTRY AND COMPOSITION

Local anesthetic solutions for dental use may be broadly classified as **amides** or **esters.**

- Examples of amide solutions include bupivacaine (Marcaine), etidocaine (Duranest), lidocaine (Xylocaine), mepivacaine (Carbocaine), and prilocaine (Citanest).
- Examples of ester solutions include procaine (Novocain), propoxycaine (Ravocaine), and tetracaine (Pontocaine).

Although similar in action, these solutions differ in their chemical compositions. A patient who has an adverse reaction to one type of local anesthetic may tolerate another type well.

MODES OF ACTION

The effect of local anesthetic agents is by temporarily blocking the normal generation and conduction action of the nerve impulses. This is accomplished primarily by producing a conduction block to decrease the permeability of the nerve membrane to sodium ions.

Local anesthesia is obtained by depositing the anesthetic agent near the nerve in the area intended for dental treatment. After the deposition of the local anesthetic in the soft tissue, the anesthetic molecules diffuse into the nerve and block its normal action. (**Diffuse** means to spread from an area of high concentration to one of low concentration.)

To obtain complete anesthesia after an injection, the nerve must be permeated by a concentration of the anesthetic base sufficient to inhibit conduction in all fibers.

The action of a local anesthetic is reversed as the blood stream carries the solution away. Local anesthetic solutions are metabolized primarily in the liver and excreted through the kidneys.

DURATION

Induction time is the length of time from the deposition of the anesthetic solution to complete and effective conduction blockage. **Duration** is the length of time from induction until the reversal process is complete.

Depending upon the procedure to be performed, the dentist may select the local anesthetic on the basis of its duration.

- A **short-acting** local anesthetic lasts less than 30 minutes. (An example is 4 percent prilocaine by infiltration. This might be used for a brief procedure, particularly on a child.)
- An **intermediate-acting** local anesthetic lasts about 60 minutes. (An example is 2 percent lidocaine plus epinephrine. The majority of local anesthetics are in this group and are used for most dental procedures.)
- A **long-acting** local anesthetic lasts more than 90 minutes. (An example is 1.5 percent etidocaine plus epinephrine by nerve block. This is used for surgical procedures to aid in pain control during and after treatment.)

EPINEPHRINE IN LOCAL ANESTHETICS

A very small quantity of epinephrine is added to the local anesthetic solution, usually in the ratio of 1:50,000, 1:100,000, or 1:200,000 parts of epinephrine to anesthetic solution.

In these ratios, the lower the second number, the higher the percentage of epinephrine there is in the solution.

In most situations, it is desirable to use as low a ratio as possible. Local anesthetic solutions are also available without epinephrine. The vasoconstrictor action of the epinephrine

- Prolongs the duration effect of the anesthetic by decreasing the blood flow in the immediate area of the injection
- Causes the tissue to turn white as the anesthetic solution is being injected
- Decreases bleeding in the injected area during surgical procedures

Contraindications for Use of Epinephrine. Because the vasoconstrictor action may cause strain on the heart as the local anesthetic solution is absorbed into the body, the use of an anesthetic solution *without epinephrine* is recommended for patients with a history of heart conditions such as unstable angina (heart-related chest pain), recent myocardial infarction (heart attack), recent coronary artery bypass surgery, untreated or uncontrolled severe hypertension (high blood pressure), and untreated or uncontrolled congestive heart failure.

The vasoconstrictor action may also interact with other drugs that the patient is taking. This is one of the reasons why it is important that the dentist be aware of the medications that the patient is taking and always check the patient's medical history.

When in doubt: before preparing a syringe, always double-check with the dentist as to the type of local anesthetic solution and the desired epinephrine ratio.

LOCAL ANESTHETIC CAUTIONS

Administration into a Blood Vessel. Local anesthetic solution administered directly into the blood stream can alter the function of vital organs, notably the heart. To be certain that the solution is not being injected directly into the blood stream, the dentist always aspirates before depositing any local anesthetic solution. (To **aspirate** means to draw back or inward.)

To do this, an aspirating-type syringe is used. The dentist inserts the needle into the mucosa and advances it to the desired depth. When the tip of the needle reaches the target area, the dentist slowly pulls back on the thumb ring of the syringe. This creates a negative pressure within the anesthetic cartridge.

If the needle has entered a blood vessel, a thin line of red blood cells will be drawn into the anesthetic cartridge. Should this happen, the dentist repositions the needle before depositing the solution.

The injection is also performed slowly to avoid shock to the heart caused by a sudden surge of anesthetic solution in the system. There is also the danger during injection of causing extensive bruising due to damage to a blood vessel.

Infected Areas. Local anesthetics are not effective when injected into an infected area. Also, with injection into an infected area, there is always the danger of spreading the infection.

Localized Toxic Reactions. Local anesthetic solutions are, as a rule, exceptionally well tolerated by the tissues. However, they may produce a variety of local tissue changes. In some sensitive individuals, even slight contact with solutions containing local anesthetic agents may cause **contact dermatitis,** which is an inflammation of the tissues due to an allergic reaction to the anesthetic solution.

Anyone with a history of hypersensitivity should avoid unnecessary contact with all local anesthetics. If a patient is thought to be allergic to a particular anesthetic, another chemical formulation may be substituted by the dentist.

Systemic Toxic Reactions. Although local anesthetic solutions are remarkably safe in therapeutic usage, the importance of their systemic toxicity cannot be ignored. Manifestations of these toxic actions are variable and depend upon

- Individual differences in patients
- The local anesthetic solution used
- The rate of injection
- The rate of absorption
- The quantity of material injected
- Other drugs that may already be present in the patient's system

Temporary Numbness. Because local anesthesia effectively blocks all pain sensation, the patient must be cautioned against biting himself while his tongue, cheek, or lip is numb. This temporary numbness disappears as the effect of the anesthetic wears off.

Because normal nerve sensations are not being received by the brain, the numb area may feel swollen when it is not. For this reason the patient may complain that his lip feels "fat."

Paresthesia. Paresthesia is a condition in which numbness lasts after the effects of the local anesthetic solutions should have worn off.

This complication of local anesthesia may be caused by

- The use of contaminated anesthetic solution: most often this is contamination with alcohol or sterilizing solution used to disinfect the anesthetic cartridge before use
- Trauma (injury) to the nerve sheath during the injection or surgery
- Hemorrhage (bleeding) into or around the nerve sheath

Paresthesia may be temporary or permanent. Most paresthesias resolve in approximately 8 weeks without treatment. The paresthesia is permanent only if the damage to the nerve is severe.

When paresthesia occurs, the patient may call the dental office several hours after receiving local anesthesia and complain of continued numbness. If this happens, the assistant should *not* try to reassure the patient. Instead, the patient should be allowed to speak to the dentist as soon as possible.

MINIMIZING UNFAVORABLE REACTIONS

Unfavorable reactions to local anesthetic solutions can be minimized by taking the following precautions:

- Having a complete and current medical history on the patient
- Using an aspirating syringe to detect blood before making the injection
- Using a sharp needle and injecting the solution very slowly
- Using the smallest quantity and lowest concentration of the least toxic anesthetic that will produce satisfactory anesthesia

Patient Observation. The patient must be kept under observation after the injection. If unusual reactions develop, the dental team should be prepared to start resuscitative or supportive measures immediately. (See Chapter 10.)

Topical Anesthetics

Topical anesthetic agents temporarily numb the sensory nerve endings of the surface of the oral mucosa. This numbing effect makes it possible to inject a local anesthetic agent with minimal discomfort to the patient.

Topical agents, which are similar in action to local anesthetic agents, are selected for their ability to penetrate the oral mucosa and diffuse to reach their site of action.

To facilitate diffusion, the concentration of topical anesthetic solution used for surface application is 2 to 5 percent. This percentage is much higher than that of injectable preparations. As a consequence, the potential toxicity of these preparations is proportionately much greater.

The **rate of onset** of topical anesthesia is slower than that of anesthesia by injection, and 1 to 5 minutes are required for optimum effectiveness. The **duration** of topical anesthesia also is shorter than that of injection anesthesia.

LIQUID TOPICAL ANESTHETICS

Liquid topical anesthetics are in the form of a viscous (thick) liquid that contains a flavoring agent. They are applied by having the patient swish a small amount of the liquid around in his mouth. The excess is removed with the saliva ejector or HVE tip.

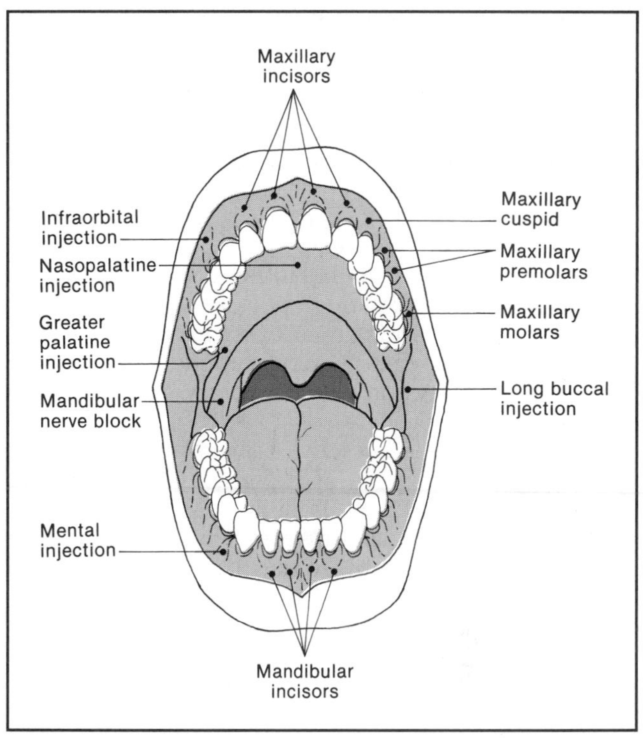

FIGURE 20–3

Sites for application of topical anesthetic in preparation for injection of local anesthetic.

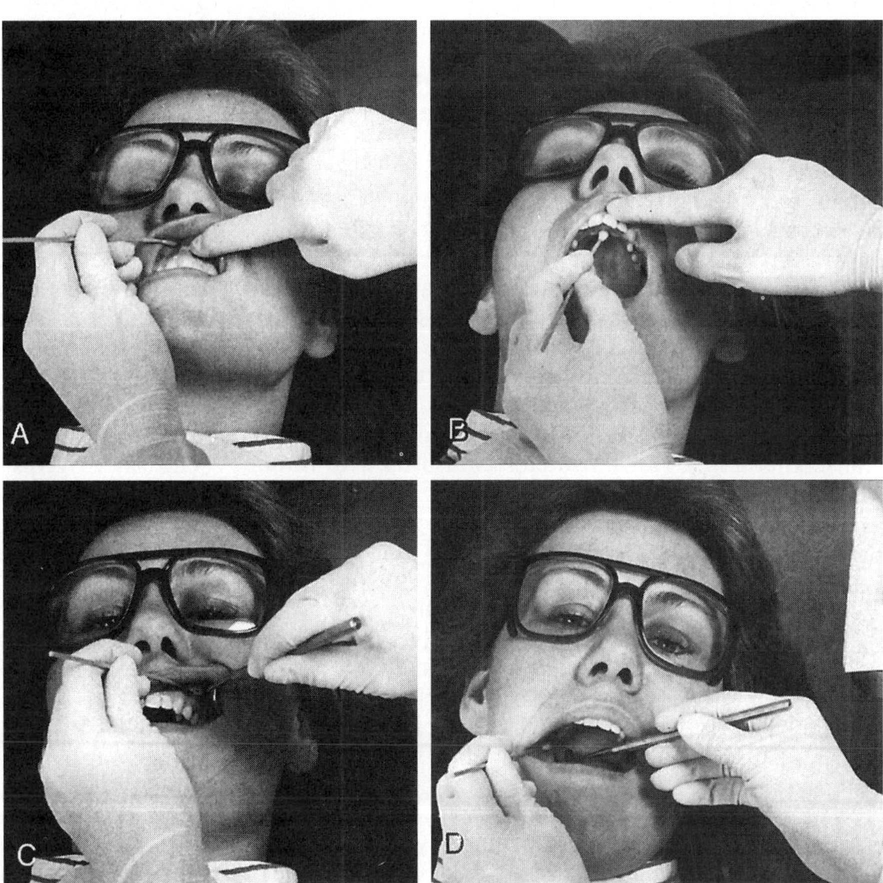

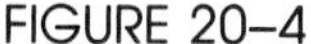

FIGURE 20–4

Topical anesthetic placement. *A,* Maxillary central incisor. *B,* Nasopalatine injection. *C,* Maxillary premolar. *D,* Inferior alveolar block.

These liquids are used to numb the surfaces of the oral tissues just before impressions are taken or intraoral radiographs are exposed in patients who have an excessive gag reflex. They may also be used to provide temporary relief of the pain of ulcers, wounds, and other injured areas in the mouth.

OINTMENT TOPICAL ANESTHETICS

The primary use of these ointment topical anesthetics is before the injection of a local anesthetic (Figs. 20–3 and 20–4). They are also used to provide temporary numbness during deep periodontal curettage and may be used to provide temporary relief from the pain of oral injuries.

This ointment is usually applied with a sterile cotton-tipped applicator. To prevent contamination when ointment is taken from a container, a sterile applicator is used each time. An applicator is never dipped into the container more than once. Also, the cover is replaced on the container immediately.

Injection Techniques

The location and innervation of the tooth or teeth to be anesthetized determines the topical anesthetic placement and the type of injection to be used. These factors are explained in Tables 20–3 and 20–4.

Figures 20–5 and 20–6 show the maxillary and mandibular injection sites.

INFILTRATION ANESTHESIA

Infiltration anesthesia, which is the technique is most frequently used to anesthetize the maxillary teeth, is achieved by depositing the material directly into the tissue and alveolus at the site of the dental procedure.

Infiltration anesthesia is possible for the maxillary teeth because the porous nature of the alveolus cancellous bone allows the solution to diffuse through the bone and reach the apices of the teeth. It may also be used as a secondary injection to block gingival tissues surrounding the mandibular teeth.

Infiltration administration of a local anesthetic solution containing a vasoconstrictor is also used to minimize localized bleeding.

BLOCK ANESTHESIA

Infiltration anesthesia is not possible for general use in the mandible. Because the extremely dense, compact nature of the mandibular bone does not permit the solution to diffuse through it, block anesthesia is required for most mandibular teeth. In block anesthesia, the solution is deposited near the nerve, and the entire area served by that nerve is numbed.

Inferior Alveolar Nerve Block. An inferior alveolar nerve block (IANB), which is commonly referred to as a *mandibular block,* is obtained by injecting the anesthetic solution near, but not in, the branch of the inferior alveolar nerve close to the mandibular foramen. The nerve and blood supply are very close here, and the dentist must be very careful not to make the injection directly into a blood vessel.

This injection permits the nerve tissue and its vascular supply to take up the anesthetic and carry it along the nerve within the mandibular canal. Desensitizing the teeth occurs through the apices and pulp.

The patient experiences numbness of half of the lower jaw including the teeth, tongue, and lip.

Incisive Nerve Block. The inferior alveolar nerve branches at the mental foramen. One branch, the mental nerve, emerges here toward the cheek. The incisive branch continues on, within the mandibular canal, to the apices of the anterior teeth.

If anesthesia is needed only for the mandibular anterior teeth or premolars, solution is deposited at the site of the mental foramen.

PERIODONTAL LIGAMENT INJECTION

An alternative infiltration anesthesia method is a technique whereby the anesthetic solution is injected, under pressure, directly into the periodontal ligament and surrounding tissues.

The periodontal ligament injection technique is generally used as an adjunct to conventional injection techniques. This may be done by using either a conventional syringe or a special periodontal ligament injection syringe.

INTRAOSSEOUS ANESTHESIA

Intraosseous anesthesia involves injecting the local anesthetic solution through the gingiva and cortical plate, directly into the spongy portion of the bone.

This technique has the advantage that it provides anesthesia in cases in which other techniques do not work. It also makes it possible to anesthetize only one tooth and to eliminate the "fat lip" sensation and numbness that some patients find objectionable.

Intraosseous anesthesia involves the use of a special needle that fits on a standard dental syringe. The needle is stabilized with a sliding sleeve that retracts into the needle body as the needle penetrates the tissues. The sleeve gives the needle the necessary stability to penetrate the bone without bending or breaking during injection.

Topical anesthetic is applied first to numb the tissues; however, bone in this area is not sensitive because it does not contain nerve endings. The injection site is always slightly anterior to the tooth to be anesthetized.

The Anesthetic Syringe

Figure 20–7*A* is a diagram of the kind of syringe used in the administration of local anesthesia. It is made up of the following parts:

(text continued on page 397)

TABLE 20–3

Maxillary Local Anesthesia

NAME OF INJECTION AND/OR AREA ANESTHETIZED	NAME OF NERVE	INJECTION TYPE (NEEDLE LENGTH)	TOPICAL ANESTHESIA PLACEMENT SITE
Maxillary central incisor	Anterior superior alveolar nerve	Infiltration (short)	Mucogingival junction above the root
Maxillary lateral incisor	Anterior superior alveolar nerve	Infiltration (short)	Mucogingival junction above the root
Maxillary cuspid	Anterior superior alveolar nerve	Infiltration (short)	Mucogingival junction at a point midway between the roots of the cuspid and the lateral incisor
Maxillary first premolar	Middle superior alveolar nerve	Infiltration (short)	Mucogingival junction above the roots
Maxillary second premolar	Middle superior alveolar nerve	Infiltration (short)	Mucogingival junction above the roots
Maxillary first molar	Middle superior alveolar nerve (mesiobuccal root)	Infiltration (short)	Mucogingival junction at the roots of second premolar
	Posterior superior alveolar (distobuccal and lingual roots)	Infiltration (short)	Mucogingival junction above second molar
Maxillary second and third molars	Posterior superior alveolar nerve	Infiltration (short)	Mucogingival junction over the maxillary second molar
Nasopalatine injection (soft tissues, anterior third of the palate; used primarily for surgery)	Nasopalatine nerve	Block (short)	Surface of the palate beside the incisive papilla (in the midline just posterior to the central incisor teeth)
Greater palatine injection (soft tissues of the hard palate from the tuberosity to the cuspid region and from the midline to the gingival crest on the side injected; used primarily for surgery)	Anterior palatine nerve	Block (short)	Bisect an imaginary line drawn from the gingival border of the maxillary second molar along its palatal root to the midline
Infraorbital injection (maxillary second and first premolars, cuspids, lateral and central incisors)	Infraorbital nerve	Block (long)	Opposite second maxillary premolar about 5 mm. outward from the buccal surface

TABLE 20–4

Mandibular Local Anesthesia

NAME OF INJECTION AND/OR AREA ANESTHETIZED	NAME OF NERVE	INJECTION TYPE (NEEDLE LENGTH)	TOPICAL ANESTHESIA PLACEMENT SITE
Mandibular nerve block (a complete block of the inferior alveolar nerve)	Inferior alveolar nerve	Block (long)	With patient's mouth wide open, deep depression of mandibular retromolar area
Long buccal injection (buccal soft tissues in the mandibular molar region; used primarily for surgery)	Buccal nerve	Block (long)	Mucogingival junction at a point just distal to the region to be treated or distal to the third molar
Lingual injection (soft tissues on the lingual surface of the mandible; used primarily for surgery)	Lingual nerve	Block (long)	Lingual gingiva halfway down the root of the tooth to be anesthetized
Mental injection (mandibular premolar and cuspid teeth for restorative procedures)	Mental nerve (subdivision of the inferior alveolar nerve)	Block (long)	Mucous membrane between the premolar teeth about 1 cm. laterally from the buccal plate of the mandible
Mandibular incisors	Incisive nerve (subdivision of the inferior alveolar nerve)	Infiltration (short)	Mucogingival junction opposite the apex of the root of the tooth

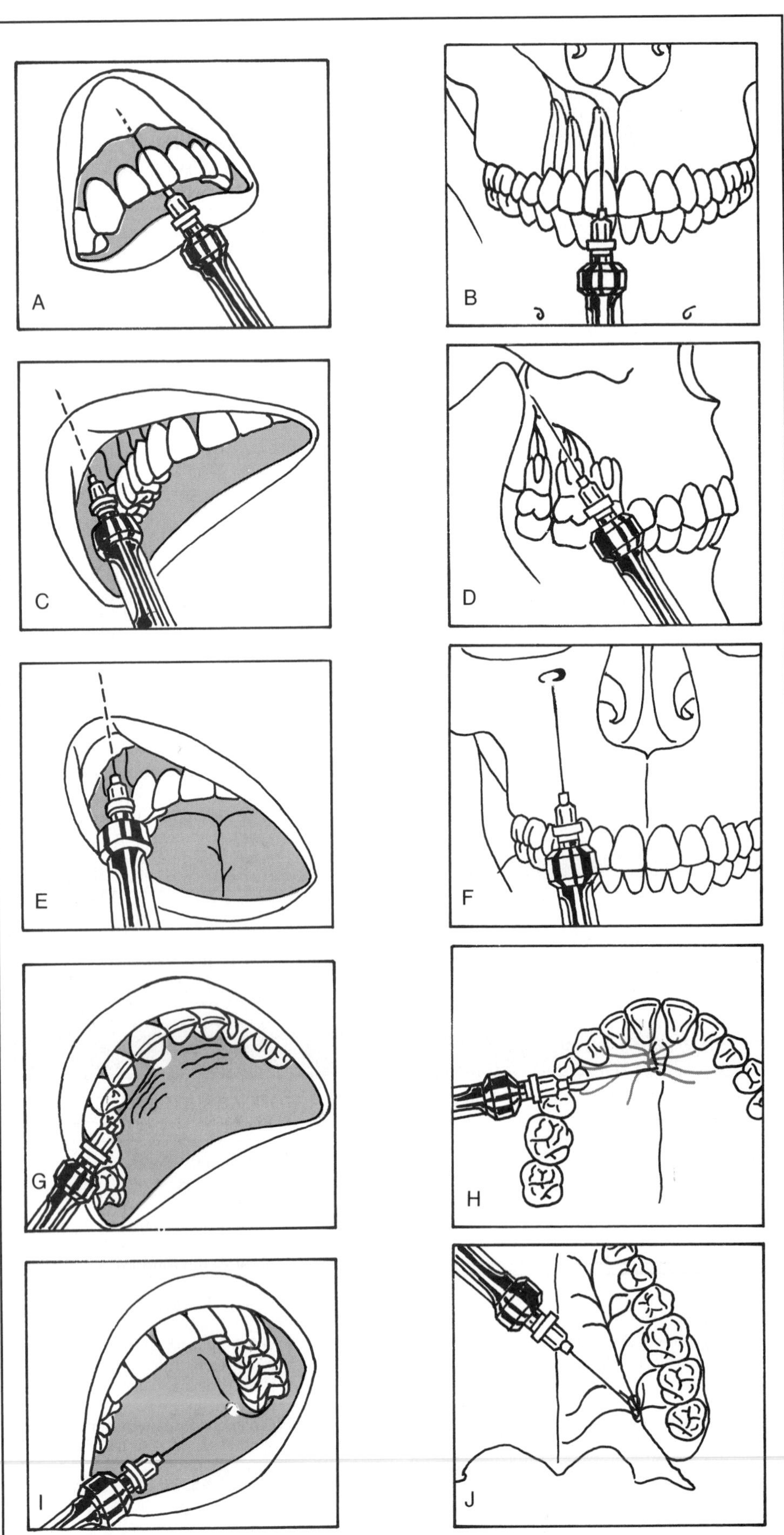

FIGURE 20–5

Sites for maxillary injections. (The left column shows the needle inserted at injection site. The right column shows a cut-away of the same site.) *A* and *B,* Anterior superior infiltration site. *C* and *D,* Posterior superior alveolar infiltration injection site. *E* and *F,* Infraorbital nerve block injection sites. *G* and *H,* Nasopalatine nerve block injection site. *I* and *J,* Anterior palatine nerve block injection site.

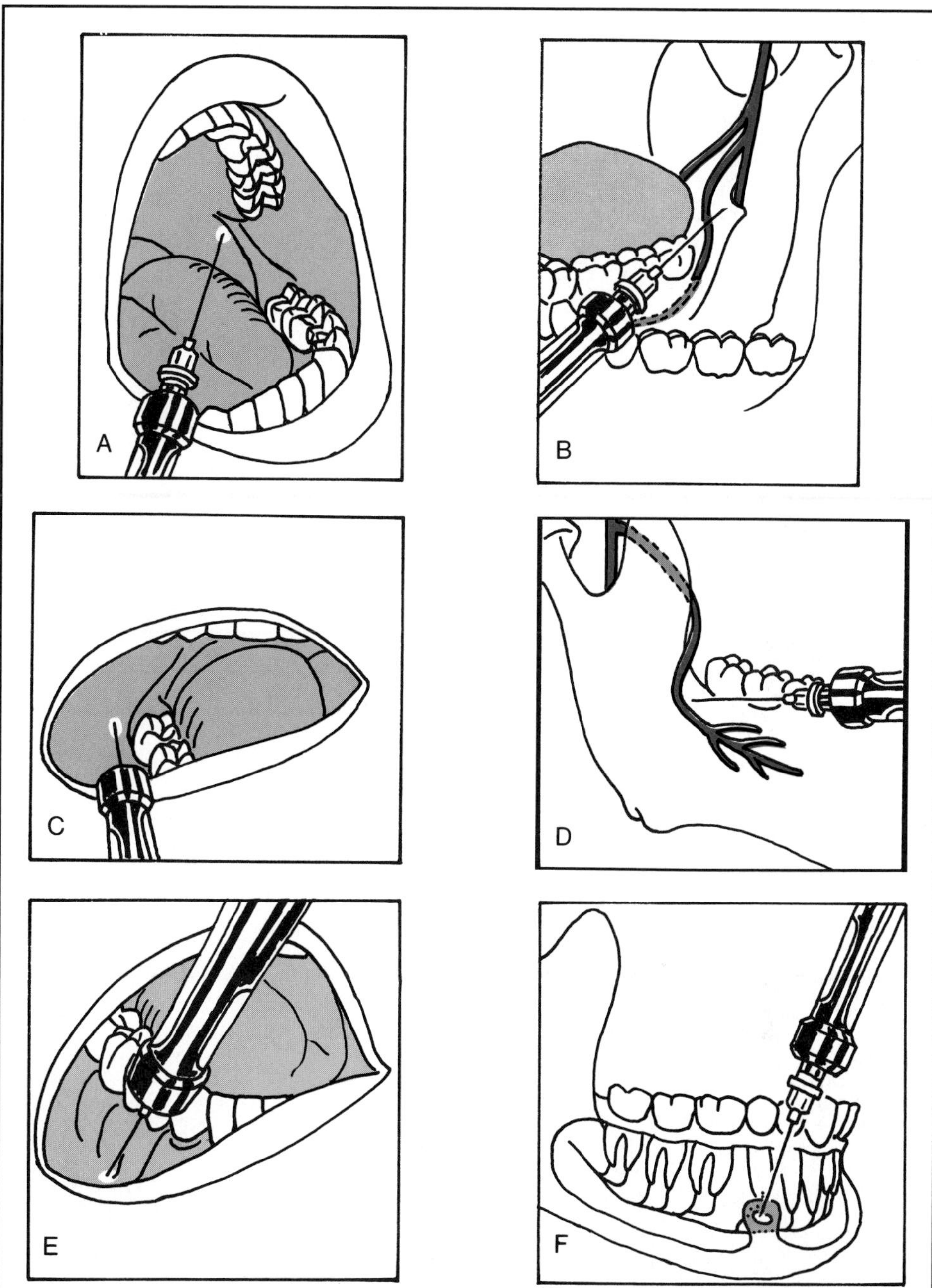

FIGURE 20–6

Sites for mandibular injections. (The left column shows the needle inserted at injection site. The right column shows a cut-away of the same site.) *A* and *B*, Inferior alveolar nerve block injection site. *C* and *D*, Buccal nerve block injection site. *E* and *F*, Mental nerve block injection site.

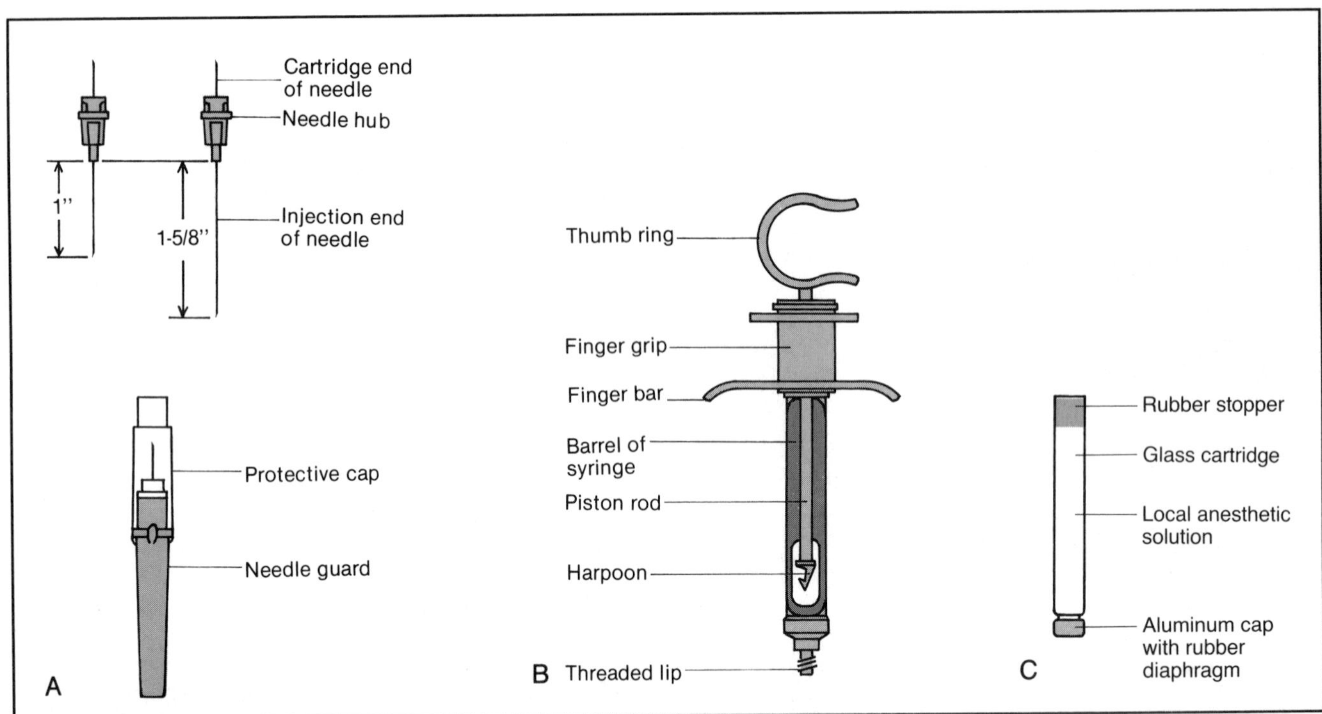

FIGURE 20–7

Equipment for local anesthetic administration. *A,* Disposable needle. *B,* Aspirating syringe. *C,* Local anesthetic cartridge.

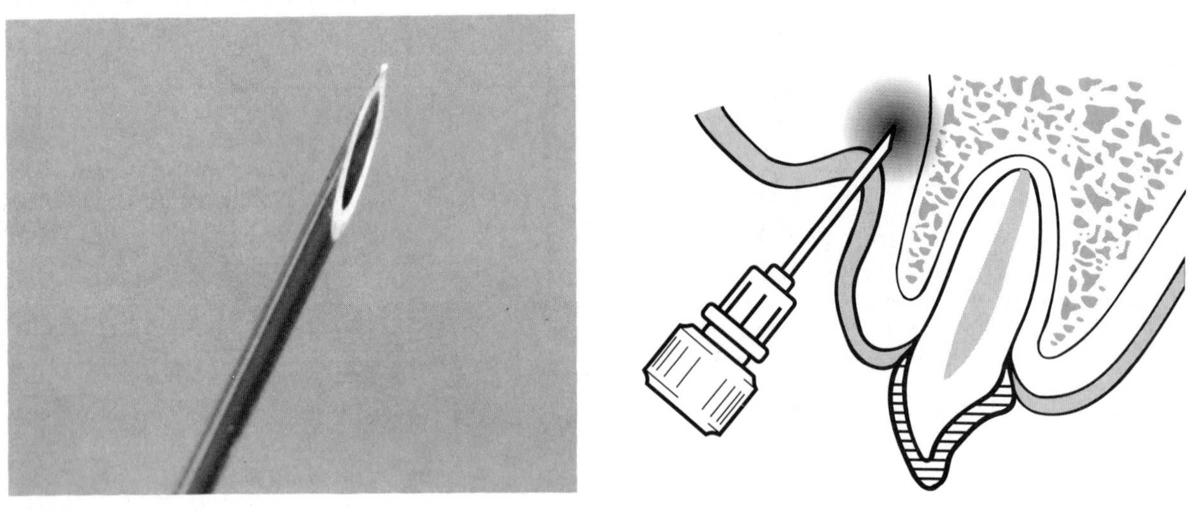

FIGURE 20–8

The bevel of the needle is positioned toward the bone. *Left,* A photo of the bevel. *Right,* A diagram showing the bevel oriented toward the bone.

Thumb Ring, Finger Grip, and Finger Bar. These are the parts that make it possible for the dentist to control the syringe firmly and to aspirate effectively, using one hand.

Harpoon. The harpoon is hooked into the rubber stopper of the anesthetic cartridge so that the stopper can be retracted by pulling back on the piston rod. It is this action that makes aspiration possible.

Piston Rod. This rod pushes down the rubber stopper of the anesthetic cartridge and forces the anesthetic solution out through the needle.

Barrel of the Syringe. The barrel firmly holds the anesthetic cartridge in place. One side of the barrel is open, and the cartridge is loaded through this area. The other side has a window so that the dentist can watch for blood cells during aspiration.

Threaded Tip. The hub of the needle is attached to the syringe on the threaded tip. The cartridge end of the needle passes through the small opening in the center of the threaded tip. This enables it to puncture the rubber diaphragm of the anesthetic cartridge.

The Disposable Needle

The sterile needle to be used for the injection is protected by a two-part plastic covering. The two parts are sealed together to ensure sterility. The needle should not be used if this seal is broken (see Fig. 20–7*B*).

The **cartridge end of the needle** is the shorter end of the needle. It fits through the threaded tip of the syringe and punctures the rubber diaphragm of the anesthetic cartridge. The protective plastic cap covers the cartridge end of the needle.

The **needle hub**, which may be either self-threading plastic or a prethreaded metal, is used to attach the needle to the threaded tip of the syringe.

The **injection end of the needle**, which is protected by the needle guard, may be either 1 inch or 1⅝ inch. Most commonly, the 1-inch "short" needle is used for infiltration anesthesia and the 1⅝-inch "long" needle is used for block anesthesia.

The tip of the needle is **beveled** (angled). Before the injection, the needle is turned so that the bevel angle is toward the bone. This enables the dentist to deposit the solution next to the bone without actually contacting the bone (Fig. 20–8).

The **lumen** is the hollow center of the needle through which the anesthetic solution flows. The **needle gauge** refers to the thickness of the needle. Gauges are numbered so that

- The larger the gauge number, the thinner the needle.
- The lower the gauge number, the thicker the needle.

Because a longer needle needs more strength, these needles are generally used in a lower gauge number. The most commonly used gauge numbers are 25, 27, and 30.

Anesthetic Cartridges

Local anesthetic solutions are supplied in glass cartridges with a rubber or silicone stopper at one end and an aluminum cap, with a rubber diaphragm, at the other (see Fig. 20–7*C*).

Color coding indicates the epinephrine ratio of the solution. This may be shown by the color of the stopper or by a colored band around the glass cartridge.

Learn to identify these color codes and always take care to select the ratio specified by the dentist. Also, always take the precaution of double-checking the patient's chart before selecting the anesthetic solution.

PRECAUTIONS

- Cartridges should be stored at room temperature and protected from direct sunlight. (Heat and sun may cause the solution to deteriorate and be less effective.)
- Never use a cartridge that has been frozen. (An extruded rubber stopper and a large air bubble are signs that the solution may have been frozen.)
- Do not use a cartridge if it is cracked, chipped, or damaged in any way. (The glass may shatter under the pressure of the injection.)
- Never use a solution that is discolored, is cloudy, or has passed the expiration date shown on the package. (The solution may no longer be effective.)
- Do not leave the syringe preloaded with the needle attached for an extended period of time. (This allows metal ions from the needle to be released into the solution. This may cause swelling edema after use of the solution.)
- Once the needle and syringe have been assembled, the cartridge must either be used or be discarded. (Once the cartridge has been punctured, there is always danger of contamination.)
- Never save a cartridge for reuse. (The cartridge started for a patient is discarded during cleanup—even if there is solution left.)

DISINFECTING CARTRIDGES

Cartridges are supplied with the contents already sterilized. If packaged in a "blister pack" so that the cartridge is in a sealed environment, the cartridge is ready for use.

If the cartridge is not in a sealed wrapper, just before use the ends may be disinfected by wiping them with a gauze sponge moistened with either 70 percent ethyl alcohol or undiluted isopropyl alcohol.

IN THE EVENT OF A NEEDLESTICK INJURY

Any such injury must be reported to the dentist or supervisor immediately. In addition to receiving appropriate treatment, it is necessary to complete a written report of the incident.

The care of a needlestick injury and the necessary reports are discussed in Chapter 12.

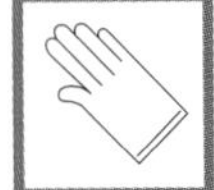

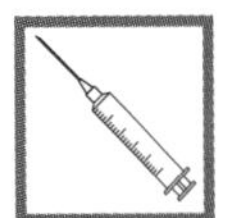

PROCEDURE: Assembling the Local Anesthetic Syringe

Instrumentation

Sterile syringe
Sealed disposable needle(s)
Sterile local anesthetic cartridges

Selecting the Supplies

1. The dentist will specify the type of anesthetic solution (brand and epinephrine content) plus the needle length and needle gauge to be used.
   □ *RATIONALE:* These choices depend upon the patient's medical and dental history and the procedure to be performed.
2. The assistant gathers the supplies as specified by the dentist and positions them at chairside out of the patient's view (Fig. 20–9).
   □ *RATIONALE:* Accuracy is essential! An error in anesthetic solution could endanger the patient's life.
3. The assistant washes his or her hands and puts on clean examination gloves before preparing the syringe.

Loading the Anesthetic Cartridge

1. Hold the syringe in one hand, and use the thumb ring to pull back the plunger. With the other hand, load the anesthetic cartridge into the syringe. The stopper end goes in first, toward the plunger (Fig. 20–10).

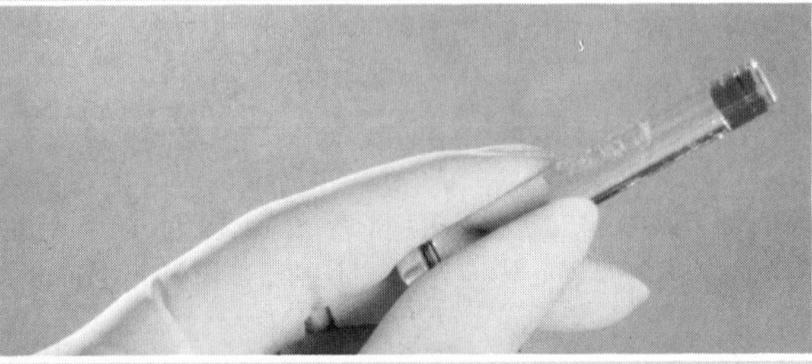

FIGURE 20–9

Double-check that the local anesthetic selected is the one specified by the dentist.

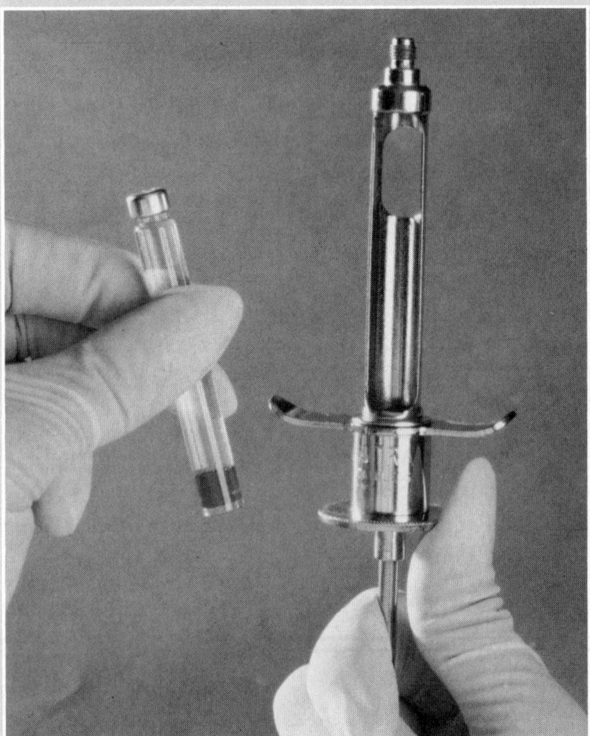

FIGURE 20–10

Pull back on the harpoon before loading the anesthetic cartridge.

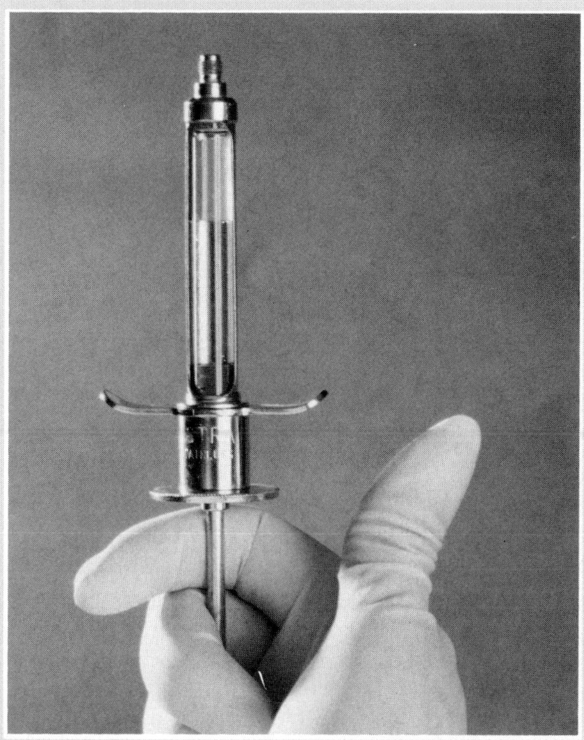

FIGURE 20–11

Release the pressure, and allow the harpoon to seat in the rubber stopper of the anesthetic cartridge.

2. Release the thumb ring and allow the harpoon to engage into the stopper (Fig. 20–11).
3. Use the other hand to apply firm pressure (tapping the plunger handle if needed) until the harpoon is engaged (hooked) into the stopper.
4. To check that the harpoon is securely in place, gently pull back on the plunger.
   □ *RATIONALE:* The harpoon must be securely engaged so that the dentist can aspirate during the injection.

Placing the Needle on the Syringe

1. Break the seal on the needle and remove the protective cap from the needle (Fig. 20–12). Do *not* remove the needle guard.
   □ *RATIONALE:* This protects the sterility of the needle and guards against a puncture injury.
2. Screw the needle into position on the syringe (Fig. 20–13). Take care to position the needle so that it is straight and firmly attached.
   □ *RATIONALE:* If this is not positioned correctly, the anesthetic solution may leak or not flow properly.
3. Place the prepared syringe on the tray ready for use and out of the patient's sight.

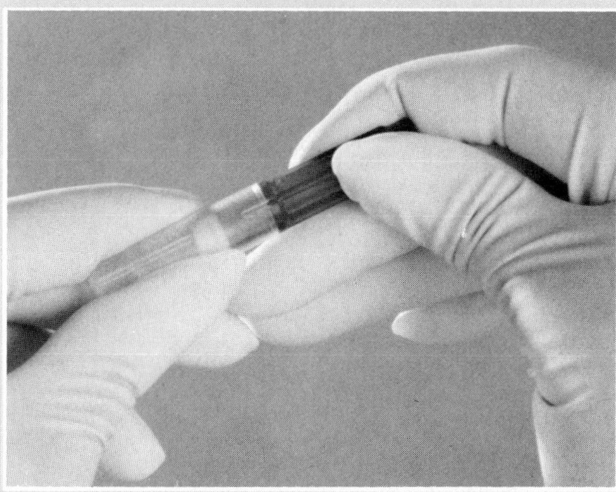

FIGURE 20–12

Break the seal on the sterile needle. The protective guard (clear plastic) is removed at this time. The needle guard is not removed yet.

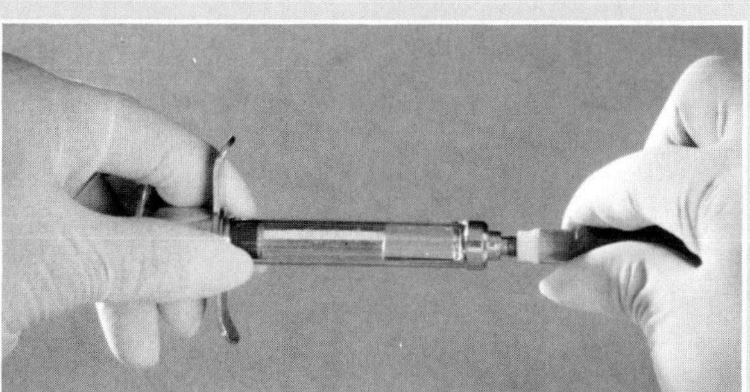

FIGURE 20–13

Carefully screw the end of the needle onto the syringe so that it is straight.

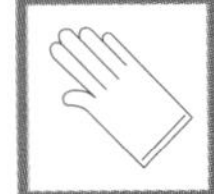
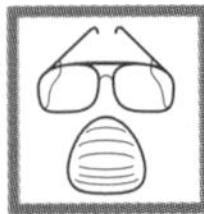
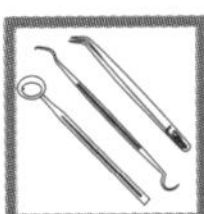
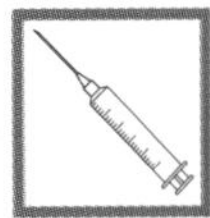

PROCEDURE: **Administering Local Anesthetics**

Instrumentation (Fig. 20–14)

Topical anesthetic ointment
Sterile cotton-tipped applicators
Sterile gauze sponges
Sterile assembled local anesthetic syringe

Applying Topical Anesthetic

1. Place the ointment on a sterile cotton-tipped applicator.
2. Use a sterile gauze sponge to dry the injection site.
   □ *RATIONALE:* Dry tissues absorb the topical anesthetic more quickly and saliva dilutes the topical anesthetic.
3. Remove the gauze sponge, and position the applicator with the ointment directly on the injection site.
4. Repeat these steps if more than one injection is to be given. A new sterile cotton-tipped applicator is used for each site.
5. Leave the applicator in place for the time recommended by the manufacturer. It is removed by the operator just before injection of the local anesthetic solution.
   □ *RATIONALE:* Leaving the topical anesthetic in place too long may cause damage to the tissues.

Passing the Syringe

1. The assistant loosens the needle guard and rotates the needle so that the bevel is toward the bone as the dentist gives the injection. The needle guard is loosely replaced on the needle.
2. The assistant receives the used topical anesthetic applicator with the left hand and passes the syringe to the operator with the right hand (Fig. 20–15). (This exchange is made just below the patient's chin and out of the patient's line of vision.)
   □ *RATIONALE:* The assistant may pass the syringe the first time it is used because the needle is still sterile.
3. In passing the syringe to the operator, the assistant places the thumb ring over the operator's thumb and then the syringe is laid into the operator's open hand (Fig. 20–16).
4. The operator gives the injection (Fig. 20–17).
5. If a second injection may be necessary, the needle is carefully recapped by using a one-handed

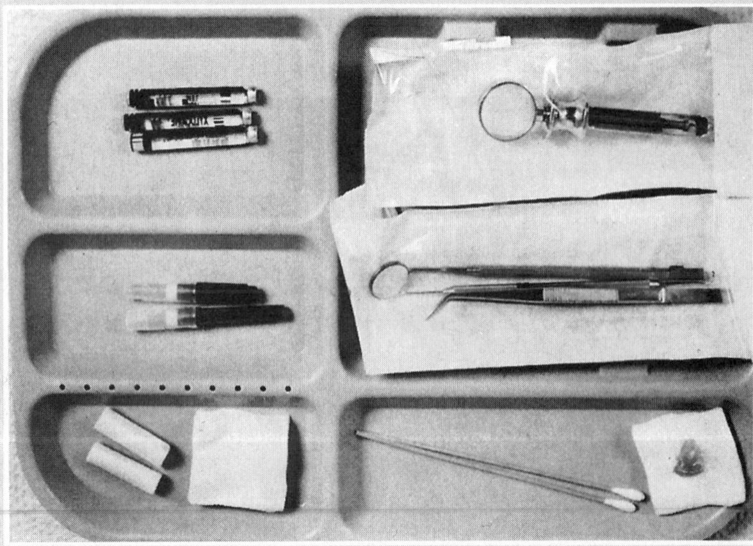

FIGURE 20–14

Tray of local anesthesia supplies. *Top left,* Anesthetic cartridges. *Top right,* A wrapped sterile syringe. *Middle left,* Two sizes of local anesthetic needles. *Middle right,* A sterile basic setup. *Bottom left,* Sterile cotton rolls and gauze sponges. *Bottom right,* Cotton-tipped applicators and topical anesthetic ointment.

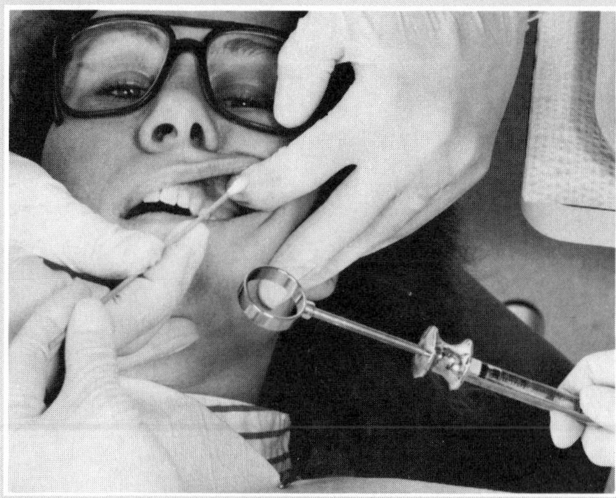

FIGURE 20–15

The assistant receives the used topical anesthetic applicator and passes the syringe to the dentist.

scoop technique or mechanical recapping device. The syringe is placed where the dentist can reach it.

☐ *RATIONALE:* The needle is now contaminated, and passing it again would increase the possibility of a needlestick injury. For this reason, the dentist will pick up the syringe for any additional injections.

Recapping the Used Syringe

1. The dentist or assistant replaces the needle guard on the syringe by using a one-handed scoop technique or a recapping device.
   ☐ *RATIONALE:* This protects against an accidental needlestick injury, and OSHA regulations forbid holding the syringe in one hand while recapping it with the other. Recapping techniques are discussed further in Chapter 12.
2. The person who recaps the needle returns the used syringe to the tray.

After the Injection

1. After the injection, the assistant hands the operator the air-water syringe to rinse the patient's mouth.
2. The HVE is used to remove the excess water and the taste of the anesthetic solution.

Care of the Used Syringe

1. Remove the used needle, with the needle guard still in place, and dispose of it in the sharps container.
2. Remove the anesthetic cartridge and place the syringe on the tray to be returned to the sterilization center.
   ☐ *RATIONALE:* The syringe is sterilized for reuse.
3. Discard the glass anesthetic cartridge appropriately.
   ☐ *RATIONALE:* The criteria for appropriate disposal are discussed in Chapter 12.

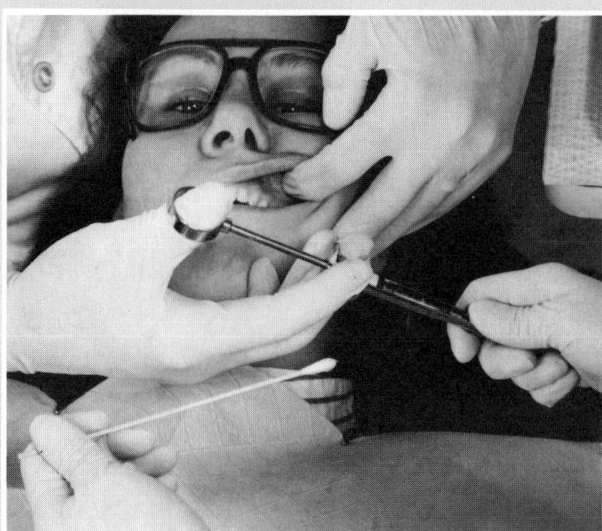

FIGURE 20–16

The assistant secures the thumb ring on the dentist's finger and loosens the needle guard.

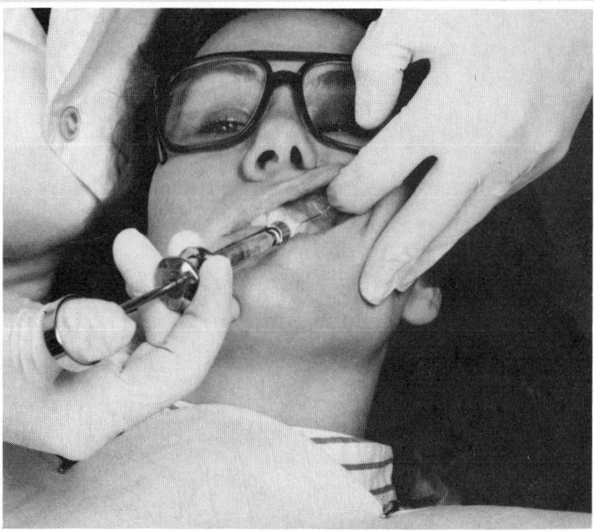

FIGURE 20–17

The dentist administers the injection.

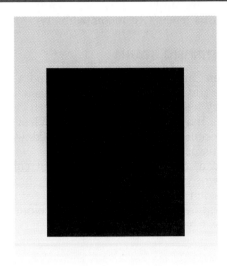

Chapter 21

Coronal Polishing

Introduction

Coronal polishing is a procedure in which plaque and extrinsic stains are removed from the coronal surfaces of the teeth. (Plaque is discussed in Chapter 6.)

In some states, this responsibility is delegated to registered or extended-function dental assistants who are trained in this function; however, it is important to note that coronal polishing is strictly limited to the clinical crowns of the teeth. (The **clinical crown** is that portion of the tooth that is visible in the oral cavity.)

Coronal polishing is not a substitute for a dental prophylaxis. A **prophylaxis,** commonly known as a *prophy,* is the complete removal of calculus, debris, and plaque from the teeth. The dentist and the registered dental hygienist are the only members of the dental team licensed to perform this function.

Indications for Coronal Polishing

Coronal polishing is indicated when plaque and stain, but no calculus, are present on the teeth. (**Calculus** is a hard mineralized deposit attached to the teeth.)

Selective polishing means that only certain teeth or surfaces are polished. Selective polishing is indicated when some but not all surfaces are affected by stain or plaque. It is also indicated before the following procedures:

- Placement of the dental dam
- Placement of temporary crowns
- Cementation of orthodontic bands
- Application of acid etching solution on enamel (if indicated in the manufacturer's recommendations)
- Cementation of crowns and bridges

Contraindications for Coronal Polishing

- Lack of stain and/or debris (because the patient does not need this service)
- Patients at high risk for dental caries (because small amounts of enamel are removed during the polishing procedure)
- Patients at risk for transient bacteremia who require the prophylactic administration of antibiotics as discussed in Chapter 20 (unless these medications have been administered)
- Sensitive teeth (because abrasive agents can increase the areas of sensitivity)
- Newly erupted teeth (because the mineralization of the surfaces may be incomplete)
- The presence of infectious disease such as active hepatitis or tuberculosis (because the aerosols created when a rotary instrument is used may spread the disease).

Stains of the Teeth

Stains, which are pigmented deposits in or on the teeth, vary in type and difficulty to remove. They are primarily esthetic problems (because of their appearance). Stains are caused by foods, chemicals, and chromogenic bacteria (bacteria that give color to the stain).

Before coronal polishing is undertaken to remove stains, it is important to distinguish between extrinsic and intrinsic stains. **Extrinsic stains** occur on the *external* surfaces of the teeth and may be removed by scaling and/or polishing. **Intrinsic stains** are found *within* the enamel and cannot be removed by polishing.

Extrinsic Stains

Black stain occurs as a thin black line on the teeth near the gingival margin. It is a difficult stain to remove and tends to be more common in females, even those with excellent oral hygiene.

Brown stain is most commonly found on the buccal surfaces of the maxillary molars and the lingual surfaces of the lower anterior incisors. It is caused by insufficient brushing or by using a toothpaste with inadequate cleansing action.

Chlorhexidine stain is caused by the use of prescription mouth rinses that contain chlorhexidine. (**Chlorhexidine** is a disinfectant with broad antibacterial action.) The yellowish-brown stain appears on the interproximal and cervical areas of the teeth. It can also appear on restorations, in plaque, and on the surface of the tongue.

Green stain is common in children. It appears as a green or greenish-yellow stain usually occurring on the facial surfaces of the maxillary anterior teeth. It has been considered to be the remnants of the enamel cuticle, but this has not been substantiated.

Orange stain is less common than either brown or green stains. It may occur on both the facial and lingual surfaces of the anterior teeth. It is believed to be caused by bacteria that give the color to the stain.

Tobacco stain is a very tenacious dark brown or black stain. It is caused by the products of coal tar in the tobacco and from the penetration of tobacco juices into pits and fissures, enamel, and dentin of the teeth.

Intrinsic Stains

Intrinsic stains may be **endogenous** (occurring during tooth development), or they may be **exogenous** (acquired after eruption).

ENDOGENOUS INTRINSIC STAINS

Tetracycline antibiotics may stain the teeth light green to dark yellow or a gray-brown. (Tetracycline stains are discussed and illustrated in Chapter 20.)

Dental fluorosis is characterized by varying degrees of discoloration ranging from a few white spots to extensive white areas or distinct brown stains. (Fluorosis is discussed and illustrated in Chapter 11.)

Other systemic conditions can cause tooth discolorations. Examples are prolonged jaundice early in life and erythroblastosis fetalis (Rh incompatibility).

EXOGENOUS INTRINSIC STAINS

Silver amalgam can cause the enamel around a restoration to turn gray or black. **Copper amalgam** used for filling primary teeth can cause a bluish-green color.

Non-vital teeth may or may not discolor. When discoloration does occur, it is caused by the breakdown of blood and pulp tissue within the tooth.

These stains can appear in a wide range of colors: light yellow-brown, gray, reddish brown, dark brown, bluish black, or even black.

Endodontic treatment can also result in discoloration of the tooth. (See Chapter 29.)

Methods of Removing Plaque and Stains

Every stain removal technique has the potential for damage by removing small amounts of enamel from the teeth. There is also the potential for injury to the gingivae. Therefore, these techniques must always be carried out with the utmost caution.

Air-Powder Polishing

The air-powder polishing technique uses a specially designed handpiece that has a nozzle that delivers an air-powder slurry of warm water and sodium bicarbonate. (**Slurry** is a watery mixture of insoluble material.)

This slurry removes stain rapidly and efficiently. It may also be used to prepare teeth for sealant placement and bonded resin restorations.

The flow rate is adjusted to control the rate of abrasion. As with all contaminated aerosols, a health hazard can exist. The air-powder technique is *not* used for patients with

- A restricted sodium diet (this is because of the high sodium content of the slurry)
- A respiratory disease or other conditions that limit swallowing or breathing
- A communicable disease that can be spread by the aerosols produced

Rubber Cup Polishing

The most common technique for removing stains and plaque and polishing the teeth is the use of an abrasive polishing agent in a **rubber polishing cup** that is rotated slowly by a prophy angle attachment to the handpiece. This is the form of coronal polishing that is described in this chapter.

Equipment for Rubber Cup Coronal Polishing

The Prophylaxis Angle and Handpiece

The prophylaxis angle, commonly called a *prophy angle*, attaches to the slow speed handpiece. (See Chapter 15.)

If not properly cleaned and sterilized, the prophy angles can take up and expel the patient's blood and saliva during a coronal polishing procedure, which could result in patient cross-contamination. For this reason, a disposable angle that is discarded after a single use is preferable.

If the prophy angle is not disposable, it must be sterilized and cared for in accordance with the manufacturer's directions. Handpiece maintenance is discussed in Chapter 15.

When attaching the polishing attachment to the prophylaxis angle, take special care to determine that it and the rubber cup or brush are securely fastened. If a rubber cup or brush falls off during the procedure, the patient could swallow or inhale it.

THE HANDPIECE GRASP

The handpiece and prophylaxis angle are held in a pen grasp with the handle resting in the V-shaped area of the hand between the thumb and index finger. (See Chapter 15.)

A proper grasp is important because if the grasp is not secure and comfortable, the weight of the handpiece can cause hand fatigue.

HANDPIECE OPERATION

1. For polishing, a low-speed handpiece that operates to a maximum of 20,000 revolutions per minute (rpm) is recommended.
   ☐ **Rationale:** The low speed minimizes frictional heat and gingival trauma from the rubber cup.
2. The rheostat (foot pedal) controls the speed (rpm) of the handpiece.
3. The toe of the foot is used to activate the rheostat. The sole of the foot remains flat on the floor.
4. To produce a slow, even speed, a steady pressure is applied with the toe.

THE FULCRUM AND FINGER REST

The terms **fulcrum** and **finger rest** are used interchangeably to describe the placement of the third, or ring, finger of the hand that is holding the instrument or handpiece.

The fulcrum provides stability for the operator and must be placed in such a way as to allow for movement of the wrist and forearm.

The fulcrum is repositioned throughout the procedure as necessary. The fulcrum may be either intraoral or extraoral, depending on a variety of circumstances such as

- The presence or absence of teeth
- The area of the mouth being treated
- How wide the patient can open the mouth

Improper movement of the hand and fingers will greatly increase operator fatigue and over time can cause painful inflammation of the ligaments and nerves of the wrist.

Rubber Cups

Soft, webbed rubber cups are used to clean and polish the smooth surfaces of the teeth (Fig. 21–1). The rubber cup attaches to the reusable handpiece by either a snap-on or screw-on attachment.

These cups are made from either natural or synthetic rubber. The natural rubber cups are more resilient and do not stain the teeth. The synthetic rubber cups are stiffer than natural rubber. If synthetic rubber cups are used, white synthetic cups are preferable because black synthetic cups may stain the teeth.

RUBBER CUP POLISHING STROKE

1. Begin with the distal surface of the most posterior tooth in the quadrant and work forward toward the anterior.
2. The stroke should be from the gingival third toward the incisal third of the tooth (see Fig. 21–1).
3. Fill the rubber cup with the polishing agent and spread it over several teeth in the areas to be polished.

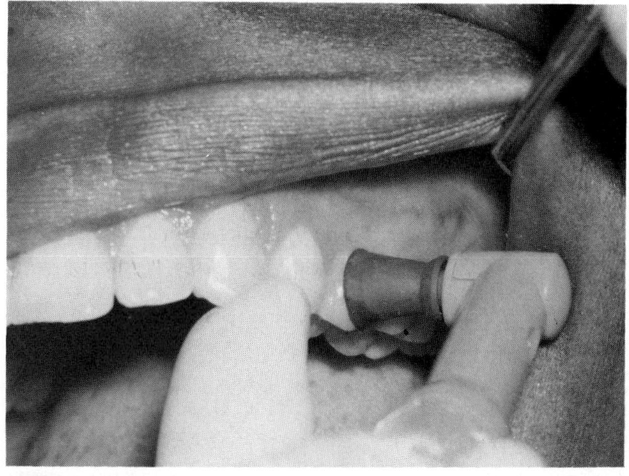

FIGURE 21–1

Stroke from the gingival third to the incisal third with just enough pressure to make the cup flare. (Notice the placement of the fulcrum.)

4. Establish your finger rest, and place the cup almost in contact with the tooth.
5. Use the slowest speed, and then apply the revolving cup lightly to the tooth surface for 1 to 2 seconds.
   ☐ **Rationale:** Higher speeds produce frictional heat that can damage the tooth and burn the gingivae.
6. Use light pressure but enough to make the edges of the rubber cup flare slightly (see Fig. 21–1).
7. Move the cup to another area on the tooth, using a patting, wiping motion.
8. Reapply polishing agent frequently.
9. Turn the handpiece to adapt the rubber cup to fit every area on the tooth.
10. If using two polishing agents with different degrees of coarseness, always use a separate rubber cup for each abrasive. Use the most abrasive first and finish with the finest (least abrasive).

Bristle Brushes

Bristle brushes may be used to remove stains from deep pits and fissures of the enamel surfaces. Bristle brushes can cause severe gingival lacerations and must be used with special care.

These brushes are made from either natural or synthetic materials. Neither type is recommended for use on exposed cementum or dentin because these surfaces are soft and are easily grooved.

BRISTLE BRUSH POLISHING STROKE

1. Soak stiff brushes in hot water to soften them.
2. Apply a mild abrasive polishing agent to the brush and, using a wiping stroke, spread the polishing agent over the occlusal surfaces to be polished.
3. Use your free hand and fingers to both retract and protect the cheek and tongue from the revolving brush.
4. Establish a firm finger rest, and bring the brush almost into contact with the tooth surface before activating the brush.
5. Use the slowest speed, and then apply the revolving brush lightly to the occlusal surfaces. Use care to avoid contacting the gingivae.
6. Use a short-stroke brushing motion from the inclined planes to the cusps of the tooth.
7. Move frequently from tooth to tooth to avoid generating frictional heat.
8. Replenish the supply of polishing agent frequently to minimize frictional heat.

Abrasive Agents

Dental abrasive agents (polishing agents) are used to remove stain and to polish natural teeth, prosthetic appliances, restorations, and castings.

Abrasive agents are available in various grits. (**Grit** refers to the degree of coarseness of that agent.) Examples are extra coarse, coarse, medium, fine, and extra fine. The coarser the agent, the more abrasive the surface.

Even a fine-grit agent removes small amounts of the enamel surface. Therefore, the goal is to always use the abrasive agent that will produce the *least* amount of abrasion to the tooth surface.

The following are additional factors that influence the amount of abrasion that is produced during polishing:

- The amount of abrasive agent that is used (the more agent used, the greater the degree of abrasion)
- The amount of pressure that is applied to the polishing cup (the lighter the pressure, the less abrasion)
- The rotation speed of the polishing cup (the slower the rotation of the cup, the less abrasion)

Abrasive powders are mixed with water or mouthwash to form a slurry used on the polishing cup. The abrasive agents should be as wet as possible (but not runny) to minimize frictional heat. If the mixture is too wet, there will be spatter and difficulty in keeping the material in the cup.

Some of the abrasives most commonly used for polishing the natural teeth are

- **Silex** (silicon carbide), which is fairly abrasive and is used for cleaning more heavily stained tooth surfaces
- **Super-fine silex,** which is used for removal of light stains on tooth enamel
- **Fine pumice,** which is mildly abrasive and is used for more persistent stains such as tobacco stains
- **Zirconium silicate** (sodium and potassium aluminum silicates), which is used for cleaning and polishing tooth surfaces (this material is highly effective and does not abrade tooth enamel)
- **Chalk**, also known as *whiting*, which is precipitated calcium carbonate (it is frequently incorporated into toothpaste and polishing pastes to whiten the teeth)

Commercial preparations contain an abrasive, water, a humectant (to keep the preparation moist), a binder (to prevent separation of the ingredients), flavoring agents, and color.

Some commercial preparations are available in small plastic containers or individual packets that contribute to the cleanliness and sterility of the procedure.

Fluoride prophylaxis pastes replace some of the fluoride that is lost from the surface layer when small amounts of enamel are removed during the polishing process. However, these pastes are not a substitute for topical application of fluoride. Also, their use is contraindicated before acid etching of the enamel.

Rubber Cup Coronal Polishing Steps

Positioning the Patient and Operator

Proper positioning of both the operator and the patient is necessary so that coronal polishing may be performed with maximum comfort and efficiency.

POSITIONING THE PATIENT

- The dental chair is adjusted so that the patient is approximately parallel to the floor with the back of the chair raised slightly.
- The movable headrest is adjusted for patient comfort and operator visibility.
- For access to the *mandibular arch*, position the patient's head with the chin down. (When the mouth is open, the lower jaw should be parallel to the floor.)
- For access to the *maxillary arch*, position the patient's head with the chin up.

POSITIONING THE OPERATOR

The operator positions described in this chapter are in reference to the face of a clock. (This concept is discussed in Chapter 16.)

- The operator should be seated comfortably at the patient's side and must be able to move around the patient to gain access to all areas of the oral cavity.
- The seated operator's feet should be flat on the floor with the thighs parallel to the floor.
- His or her arms should be at waist level and even with the patient's mouth.
- When performing a coronal polish, the right-handed operator generally begins by being seated at the 8 to 9 o'clock position.
- When performing a coronal polish, the left-handed operator generally begins by being seated at the 3 to 4 o'clock position.

The Sequence of Polishing

If full mouth coronal polishing is indicated, it must be done in a predetermined sequence to be certain that no area is missed. The best sequence is based on the operator's preference and the individual needs of the patient.

One very effective sequence is described here. This is the positions and fulcrums for a right-handed operator. The concepts of direct and indirect vision are discussed in Chapter 16.

As necessary to maintain patient comfort throughout the procedure, the patient's mouth is rinsed with water from the air-water syringe. Excess water and debris are removed either with the high-volume evacuation (HVE) tip or by having the patient close his lips around the tip of the saliva ejector.

Flossing After Coronal Polishing

Dental floss and tape have two purposes after coronal polishing. The first is to polish the interproximal tooth surfaces. The second is to remove any abrasive agent or debris that may be lodged in the contact area.

To polish these areas, abrasive is placed on the contact area between the teeth, and the floss or tape is worked through the contact area with a back-and-forth motion. Because both operator's and patient's preferences about floss and tape vary, there are many kinds available. Used properly, floss or tape or both are effective.

After the interproximal surfaces are polished, a fresh piece of dental floss or tape is used to remove any remaining abrasive particles between the teeth.

If necessary, a floss threader can be used to pass the floss under any fixed bridgework to gain access to the abutment teeth. Flossing is discussed further in Chapter 7.

Evaluation of Polishing

When you have completed polishing and flossing, evaluate the effectiveness of your technique by reapplying the disclosing agent. Then use a mouth mirror to determine that the following criteria have been met:

- There is no remaining disclosing agent on any of the tooth surfaces.
- The teeth are glossy and reflect light from the mirror uniformly.
- There is no evidence of trauma to the gingival margins or any other soft tissues in the mouth.

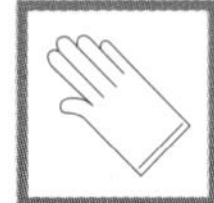
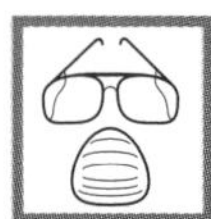
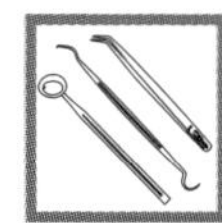

PROCEDURE: **Performing Coronal Polishing**

Instrumentation (Fig. 21–2)

Prophy angle, sterile or disposable
Rubber cup accessory, snap-on or screw type
Bristle brush, snap-on or screw type
Prophy paste or other abrasive in slurry
HVE tip or saliva ejector
Disclosing agent (tablets, gel, or solution)
Cotton-tipped applicator (if disclosing solution is used)
Dental tape
Dental floss
Floss threader
Gauze sponges

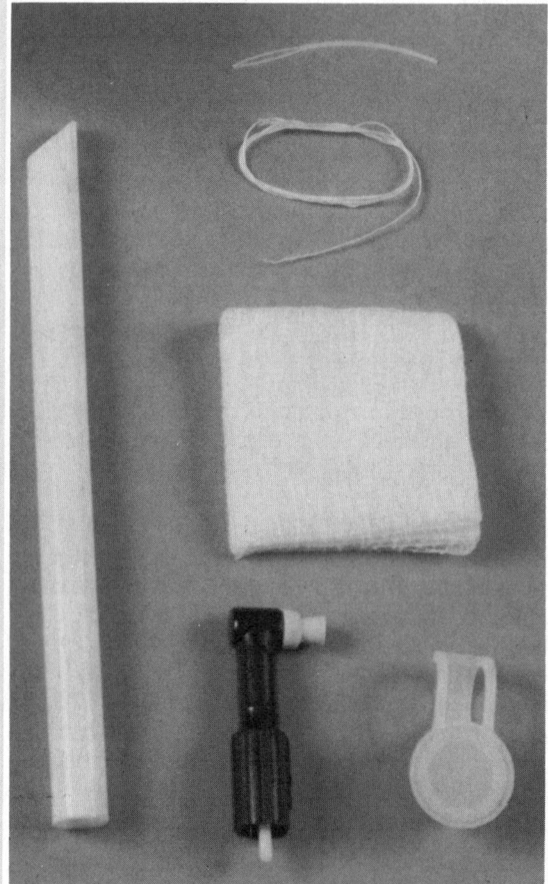

FIGURE 21–2

Instrumentation for coronal polishing. HVE tip, disposable prophy angle with rubber cup, prophy paste, gauze sponges, dental floss, and a bridge threader. The operator will also use a basic setup.

Patient Preparation

1. Check the patient's medical history for any contraindications to the coronal polish procedure.
2. Seat and drape the patient with a waterproof napkin. Provide the patient with protective eyewear.
3. Explain the procedure to the patient and answer any questions.
4. Apply a disclosing agent to identify areas of plaque (Fig. 21–3).

Maxillary Right Posterior Sextant, Buccal Aspect

1. Sit in the 8 to 9 o'clock position.
2. Have the patient tilt his head up and turn slightly away from you (Fig. 21–4).
3. Hold the dental mirror in your left hand. Use it to retract the cheek or for indirect vision of the more posterior teeth.
4. Establish a fulcrum on the maxillary right incisors.

Maxillary Right Posterior Sextant, Lingual Aspect

1. Remain seated in the 8 to 9 o'clock position.
2. Have the patient turn his head up and toward you.
3. Hold the dental mirror in your left hand. Direct vision is good from this position, and the mirror will provide a view of the distal surfaces.
4. Establish a fulcrum on the lower incisors and reach up to polish the lingual surfaces.

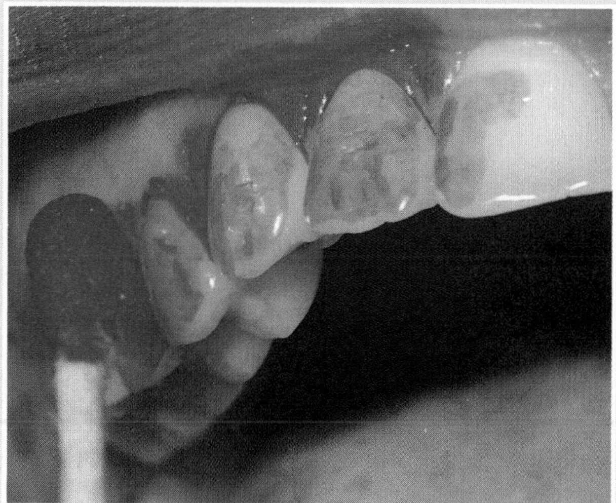

FIGURE 21–3

Application of disclosing solution.

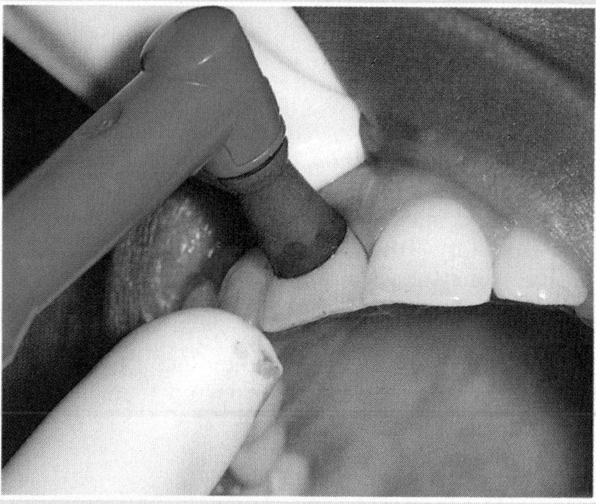

FIGURE 21–5

Polishing the facial surfaces of the maxillary anterior sextant.

Maxillary Anterior Sextant, Facial Aspect

1. Remain in the 8 to 9 o'clock position.
2. Position the patient's head tipped up slightly and facing straight ahead (Fig. 21–5). Make necessary adjustments by turning the patient's head slightly either toward or away from you.
3. Use direct vision in this area.
4. Establish a fulcrum on the incisal edge of the teeth adjacent to the ones being polished.

Maxillary Anterior Sextant, Lingual Aspect

1. Remain in the 8 to 9 o'clock position, or move to the 11 to 12 o'clock position.
2. Position the patient's head so that it is tipped slightly upward (Fig. 21–6).
3. Use the mouth mirror for indirect vision and to reflect light on the area.
4. Establish a fulcrum on the incisal edge of the teeth adjacent to the ones being polished.

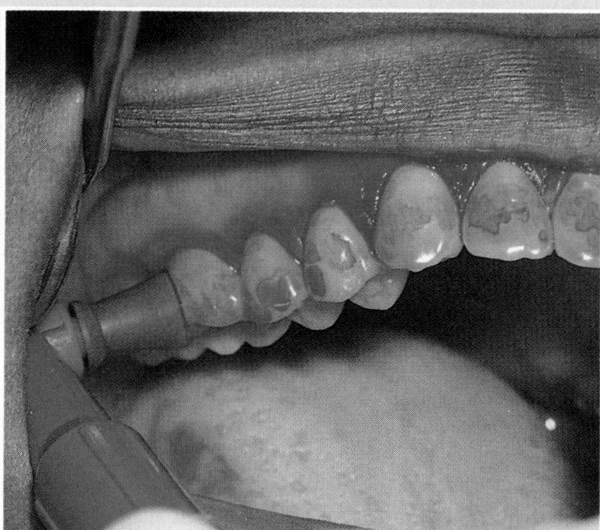

FIGURE 21–4

Polishing the buccal surfaces of the maxillary right sextant.

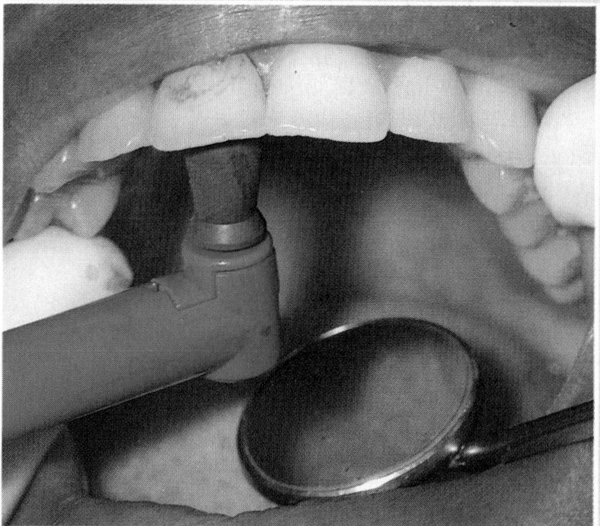

FIGURE 21–6

Polishing the lingual surfaces of the maxillary anterior sextant.

(continued on following page)

PROCEDURE: Performing Coronal Polishing *(continued)*

Maxillary Left Posterior Sextant, Buccal Aspect

1. Sit in the 9 o'clock position.
2. Position the patient's head tipped upward and turned slightly toward you to improve visibility.
3. Use the mirror to retract the cheek and for indirect vision.
4. Rest your fulcrum finger on the buccal occlusal surface of the teeth toward the front of the sextant.

   ☐ *ALTERNATIVE:* Rest your fulcrum finger on the lower premolars and reach up to the maxillary posterior teeth.

Maxillary Left Posterior Sextant, Lingual Aspect

1. Remain in the 8 to 9 o'clock position.
2. Have the patient turn his head away from you.
3. Use direct vision in this position. Hold the mirror in your left hand and use it for a combination of retraction and reflecting light.
4. Establish a fulcrum on the buccal surfaces of the maxillary left posterior teeth or on the occlusal surfaces of the mandibular left teeth.

Mandibular Left Posterior Sextant, Buccal Aspect

1. Sit in the 8 to 9 o'clock position.
2. Have the patient turn his head slightly toward you.
3. Use the mirror to retract the cheek and for indirect vision of distal and buccal surfaces.
4. Establish a fulcrum on the incisal surfaces of the mandibular left anterior teeth and reach back to the posterior teeth.

Mandibular Left Posterior Sextant, Lingual Aspect

1. Remain in the 9 o'clock position.
2. Have the patient turn his head slightly away from you (Fig. 21–7).
3. For direct vision, use the mirror to retract the tongue and reflect more light to the working area.
4. Establish a fulcrum on the mandibular anterior teeth and reach back to the posterior teeth.

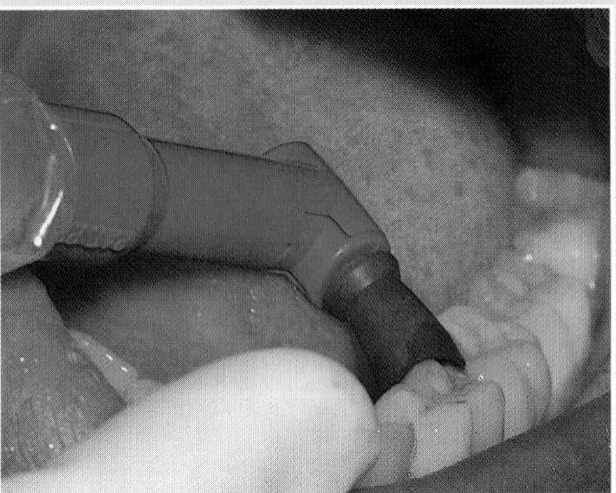

FIGURE 21–7

Polishing the lingual surfaces of the mandibular left sextant.

Mandibular Anterior Sextant, Facial Aspect

1. Sit in either the 8 to 9 o'clock position or the 11 to 12 o'clock position.
2. As necessary, instruct the patient to make adjustments in his head position by turning either toward or away from you or by tilting his head up or down.
3. Use your left index finger to retract the lower lip. Both direct and indirect vision can be used in this area.
4. Establish a fulcrum on the incisal edges of the teeth adjacent to the ones being polished.

Mandibular Anterior Sextant, Lingual Aspect

1. Sit in either the 8 to 9 o'clock position or the 11 to 12 o'clock position.
2. As necessary, instruct the patient to make adjustments in his head position by turning either toward or away from you or by tilting his head up or down (Fig. 21–8).
3. Use the mirror for indirect vision, to retract the tongue, and to reflect light onto the teeth. Direct vision is often used in this area when the operator is seated in the 12 o'clock position, but indirect vision can also be helpful.
4. Establish a fulcrum on the mandibular cuspid incisal area.

Mandibular Right Sextant, Buccal Aspect

1. Sit in the 8 o'clock position.
2. Have the patient turn his head slightly away from you (Fig. 21–9).
3. Use the mirror to retract tissue and reflect light. The mirror may also be used to view the distal surfaces in this area.
4. Establish a fulcrum on the lower incisors.

Mandibular Right Sextant, Lingual Aspect

1. Remain in the 8 o'clock position.
2. Have the patient turn his head slightly toward you.
3. Retract the tongue with the mirror.
4. Establish a fulcrum on the lower incisors.

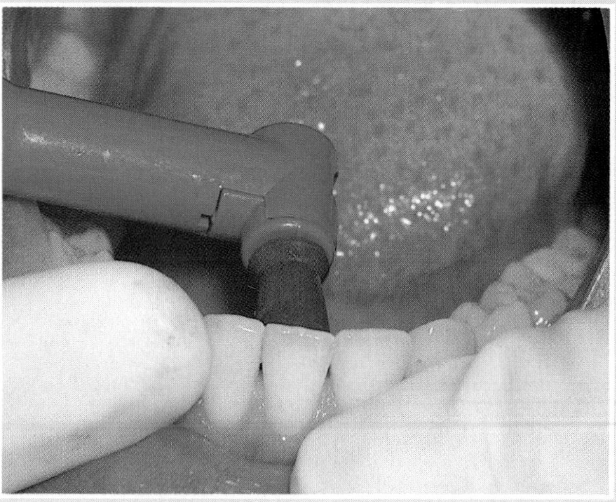

FIGURE 21–8

Polishing the lingual surfaces of the mandibular anterior sextant.

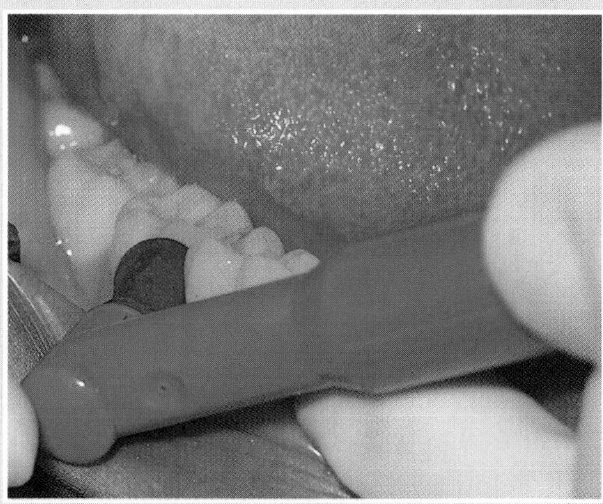

FIGURE 21–9

Polishing the buccal surfaces of the mandibular right sextant.

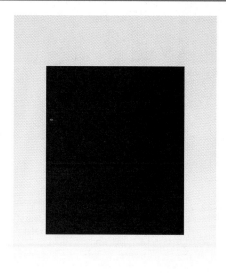

Chapter 22

Dental Dam

Introduction

Dental dam is a thin latex barrier applied to isolate the teeth during treatment. When the dam is in place, only selected teeth are visible through the dam. These teeth are referred to as being **isolated** or **exposed**.

Dental dam is usually applied after the local anesthetic has been administered and while the dentist is waiting for it to take effect. An efficient dental team can place the dam in about 2 minutes. An assistant working alone can accomplish this in about 3 to 5 minutes.

Before the application of the dental dam, the tooth must be clean and free of plaque or debris. If these are not removed, they may be dislodged and pushed into the gingival sulcus, where they may injure the gingival tissues. When indicated, selective coronal polishing is performed before dam placement. (See Chapter 21.)

Also before placement of the dental dam is started, the patient's medical history should be reviewed for any indications of latex sensitivity. If this is a problem, the dentist is consulted before the application is continued.

Indications for the Use of Dental Dam

- It serves as an important infection control protective barrier.
- It safeguards the patient's mouth against contact with debris, acid-etch materials, or other solutions during treatment.
- It protects the patient from accidentally aspirating or swallowing debris such as a small fragments of a tooth or scraps of restorative material. (As used here, **aspirating** means to inhale into the lungs.)
- It protects the tooth from contamination by saliva or debris if pulpal exposure accidentally occurs.
- It protects the remainder of the oral cavity from exposure to infectious material when an infected tooth is opened during endodontic treatment.
- It provides the moisture control that is essential for the placement of restorative materials and for the cementation of cast restorations.
- It improves access during treatment by retracting the lips, tongue, and gingiva from the field of operation.
- It provides better visibility because of the contrast of color of the dam and of the tooth.
- It retracts the interdental papilla, providing better accessibility in the preparation and placement of a restoration in the gingival third of a tooth.
- It increases dental team efficiency, discourages patient conversation, and may reduce time required for some treatment.

Dental Dam Equipment

The specialized equipment used for the rapid and efficient placement of the dental dam is shown in Figure 22–1.

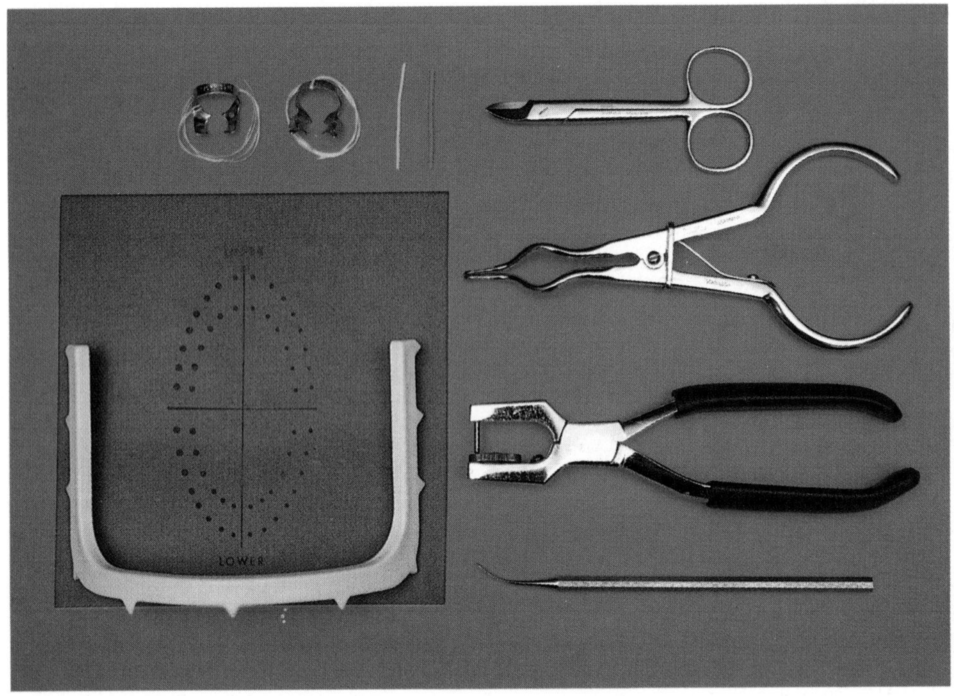

FIGURE 22–1

Basic equipment for dental dam placement and removal. *Lower left,* dental dam and plastic frame. *Upper left,* dental dam clamps with ligatures, dental dam stabilizing cord in two sizes. *Right (top to bottom),* scissors, dental dam clamp forceps, dental dam punch, and burnisher. A basic setup, cotton rolls, and lubricants are also needed.

Dental Dam Material

The dental dam selected for each application is based on the operator's choice of size, color, and thickness (see Fig. 22–1).

Size. Dental dam is available in a continuous roll or in two precut sizes. These are the 6 × 6 inch size, which is used for applications on the posterior teeth in the permanent dentition, and the 5 × 5 inch size, which is used for primary dentition and anterior applications on the permanent dentition.

Color. Dental dam is available in a wide range of colors from light to dark, including green, blue, and pastels. Some colors are also scented or flavored. The brighter colors are widely used and have good patient acceptance; however, some operators prefer dark dam because it provides color contrast and reduces glare.

Thickness. The commonly used dam thicknesses (gauges) are thin (light), medium, and heavy. Thin is most frequently used for endodontic applications. Medium is widely used because of its ease of handling. Heavy may be selected when tissue retraction and extra resistance to tearing are important, such as in placement over crowns, fixed bridges, or teeth with tight contacts.

Dental Dam Frames

A frame or holder is necessary to stabilize and stretch the dam so it fits tightly around the teeth and is out of the operator's way. Plastic and metal frames are available, and both may be sterilized by autoclaving.

The **Young frame** is a stainless steel U-shape holder with sharp projections on its outer margin. This frame is shown later in Figure 22–13.

The Young frame is placed on the *outside* of the dam, and the dam is stretched over the projections of the frame. This increases patient comfort by holding the dam away from the patient's face.

The **plastic U-shaped frame**, shown in Figure 22–1, is placed *under* the dam (next to the face). Because this frame is radiolucent (does not block x-rays), it is not necessary to remove the frame when radiographs are required during treatment.

The **Ostby frame** is a round plastic frame with sharp projections on its outer margin. It too is placed *outside* the dam, and the dam is stretched over the projections of the frame.

Dental Dam Napkins

An option is the use of a disposable dental dam napkin, which is placed between the patient's face and the dam. The primary purpose of the napkin is to increase patient comfort by absorbing moisture. It also protects the patient's face from direct contact with the dam.

Lubricants

When the dam is placed, two types of lubricants are needed. One is placed on the lips to ensure patient comfort. Some operators use zinc oxide ointment for this purpose; others use petroleum jelly.

A second lubricant is also used on the *underside* of the dam to help slide it over the teeth and between the contacts. Some operators use water-soluble lubricant for this purpose. Others use petroleum jelly; however, the disadvantage of this is that it may leave an oily film on the teeth that is difficult to remove.

Dental Dam Punch

The dental dam punch is used to create the holes in the dental dam needed to expose the teeth to be isolated (see Fig. 22–1). The working end of the punch has an adjustable **stylus** (cutting tip) that makes the hole as it strikes an opening in the punch plate.

The **punch plate** is a rotary platform with five or six holes of different sizes cut into the face of the plate. These holes are approximately 1 mm. deep with sharp edges to accommodate the stylus.

The position of the punch plate is rotated to produce holes of different sizes. When the punch plate is turned, a slight click may be heard as the plate falls into the position. This indicates that the stylus is positioned directly over the hole in the punch plate.

The correct position of the stylus is checked by *slowly* lowering the stylus point over the hole in the punch plate. If the stylus is not placed properly, it may be dulled or broken.

Also, the holes may not be punched cleanly. If the holes have ragged edges, they may tear easily as the dam is placed over the crown of the tooth. They may also irritate the gingiva and can allow the leakage of moisture around the tooth.

SIZES OF HOLES ON DENTAL DAM PUNCH PLATE

The holes on the punch plate are graduated in size from very small to approximately 0.75 mm. in diameter. In a five-hole punch, these are numbered 1 to 5, the smallest being hole number 1. The recommended uses for each size are summarized in Table 22–1.

Dental Dam Stamp and Templates

The **dental dam stamp** and an ink pad are used to mark the dental dam with predetermined markings for "average" adult and pediatric arches (Fig. 22–2). The use of a **dental dam template**, which has holes where the teeth should be marked, provides more flexibility when one or more teeth in the arch are out of alignment.

The template is placed on the dental dam, and a pen is used to mark through the template to indicate the location of the punch holes. The use of a specialized template is shown later in Figure 22–17.

Dental Dam Clamp Forceps

Dental dam clamp forceps are used in the placement and removal of the dental dam clamp (see Fig. 22–1).

TABLE 22–1

Dental Dam Punch Hole Sizes

HOLE SIZE	MOST COMMON USE
No. 1	Mandibular incisors
No. 2	Maxillary incisors
No. 3	Premolars and cuspids
No. 4	Molars and bridge abutments
No. 5	Posterior anchor tooth or long-span fixed bridge

The beaks of the forceps fit into holes on the jaws of the clamp.

The handles of the forceps work with a spring action. A sliding bar keeps the handles of the forceps in a fixed position while the clamp is being held. The handles are squeezed to release the clamp.

When the forceps are passed to the operator, they are always passed handles first. The beaks of the forceps are turned toward the arch being treated. This permits the operator to place or remove the clamp without having to rotate the forceps to get them into position.

Dental Dam Clamps

A dental dam clamp, which is made of chrome or nickel-plated steel, is the primary means of anchoring and stabilizing the dental dam (Figs. 22–3 and 22–4).

Most commonly, the clamp is placed on the end of the dam nearest the tooth or teeth to be treated. A second clamp, or an alternative means of stabilization,

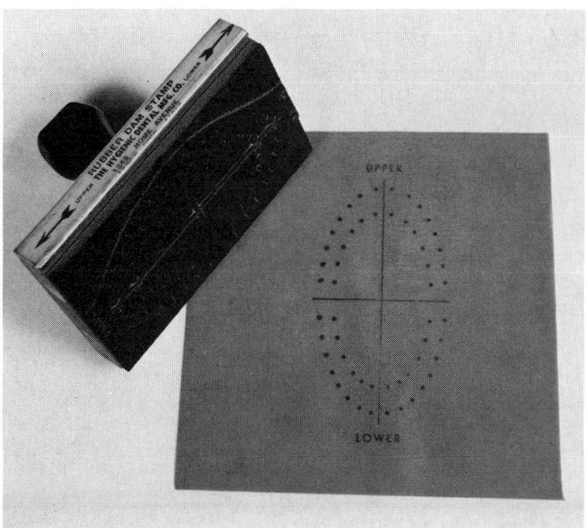

FIGURE 22–2

Dental dam stamp and stamped dam.

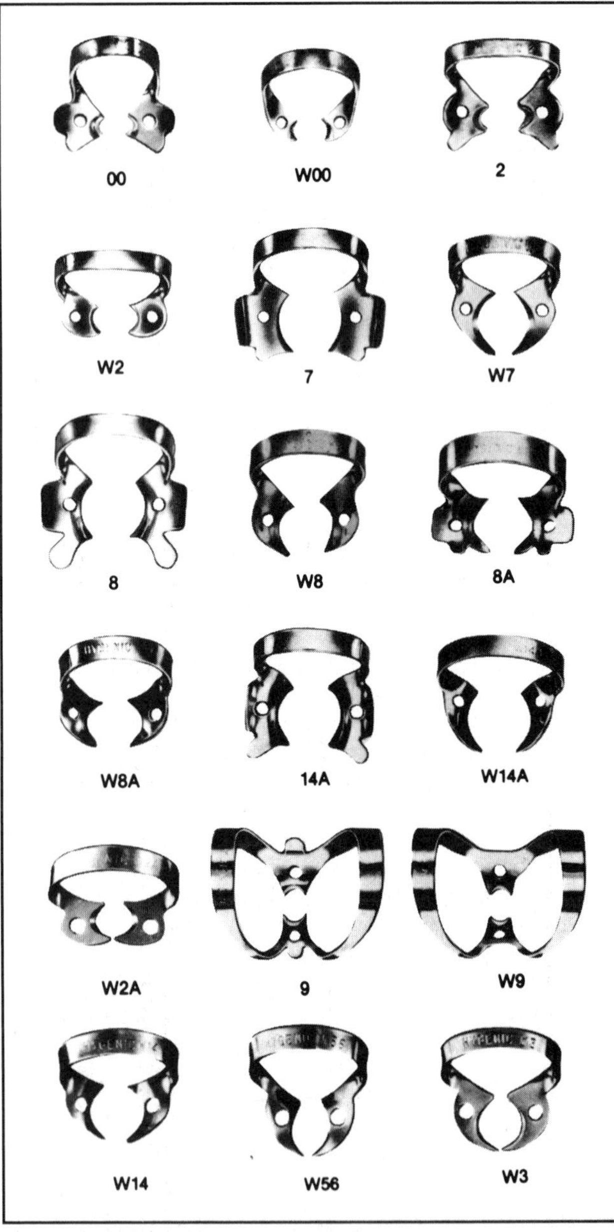

FIGURE 22–3

Basic assortment of dental dam clamps (clamp number and use). 00: Small maxillary or mandibular premolars and incisors (winged). W00: Small maxillary or mandibular premolars and incisors (wingless). 2: Larger mandibular premolars and primary molars (winged). W2: Larger mandibular premolars and primary molars (wingless). 7: General-purpose, flat-jawed, mandibular molar clamp (winged). W7: General-purpose, flat-jawed, mandibular molar clamp (wingless). 8: General-purpose, maxillary molar clamp (winged). W8: General purpose, maxillary molar clamp (wingless). 8A: Partially erupted or irregularly shaped primary molars (winged). W8A: Partially erupted or irregularly shaped primary molars (wingless). 14A: Partially erupted or irregularly shaped larger molars (winged). W14A: Partially erupted or irregularly shaped larger molars (wingless). W2A: Premolars and primary molars (wingless). 9: Double-bowed anterior clamp for cervical Class V restorations (winged). W9: Double-bowed anterior clamp for cervical Class V restorations (wingless). W14: Partially erupted or irregularly shaped molars (wingless). W56: Molar clamp (wingless). W3: Primary molar clamp (wingless). (Courtesy of The Hygienic Corp, Akron, OH.)

is used to secure the other end of the dam application. (See the section "Stabilizing the Dam Application.")

Whenever a clamp has been used or tried in the mouth but not selected, it *must* be sterilized before reuse.

PARTS OF DENTAL DAM CLAMPS

The **bow** is the rounded portion of the clamp that extends through the dental dam (see Fig. 22–4*A*). The clamp is always positioned on the tooth so that the bow is toward the distal. Locating the bow in this manner keeps it out of the operator's way during treatment.

Clamps have **jaws** that are shaped into four prongs. All four prongs must be firmly seated on the tooth in order to create the tension and facial-to-lingual balance necessary to stabilize the clamp.

The jaws of the clamps for use on fully erupted teeth are flat. Those designed for use on partially erupted permanent teeth are tilted inward to provide a firmer grasp (see Fig. 22–4*B*.)

There is a hole in each jaw of the clamp. The tips of the dental dam forceps fit into these holes to allow placement and removal of the clamp.

A **winged** clamp is designed with extra extensions to help retain the dental dam. **Wingless** clamps do *not* have extra projections to engage the dam. In Figure 22–3, wingless clamps have names beginning with a "W."

FITTING THE DENTAL DAM CLAMP

Normally, the clamp fits on the cervical area of the tooth below the height of contour and at, or slightly below, the cementoenamel junction (CEJ). (The **height of contour** is the bulge [widest point] in the facial and lingual contours of the tooth.)

The clamp must be positioned with all four prongs firmly in place on the tooth before the clamp forceps is loosened. If the clamp is not placed properly, it may be displaced (spring off the tooth) and can cause injury to the patient, operator, or assistant.

TYPES OF DENTAL DAM CLAMPS

Dental dam clamps are available in many sizes and styles to accommodate different needs.

Posterior Dental Dam Clamps. When maxillary and mandibular posterior clamps are applied, the term **universal** means that the same clamp may be placed on the same type of tooth in the opposite quadrant. In Figure 22-3, clamps 7 and W7 are universal mandibular molar clamps. Clamps 8 and W8 are universal maxillary molar clamps.

Pediatric Dentistry Dam Clamps. Clamps for pediatric dentistry, such as clamp W3 in Figure 22–3, are designed to accommodate the smaller size and shape of the primary teeth or partially erupted permanent teeth.

Cervical Dental Dam Clamps. Cervical clamps,

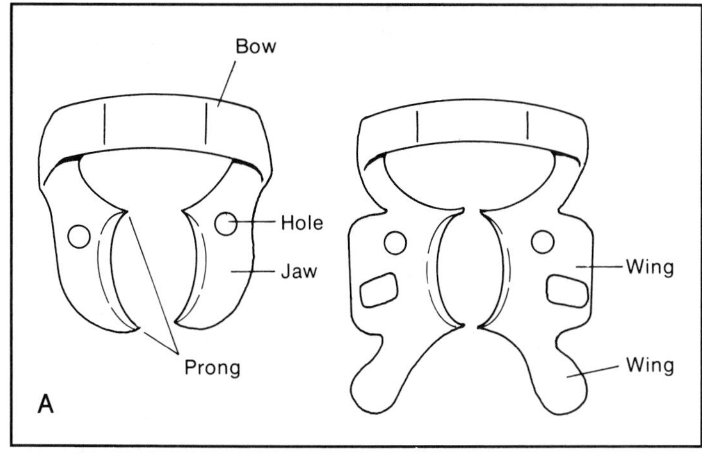

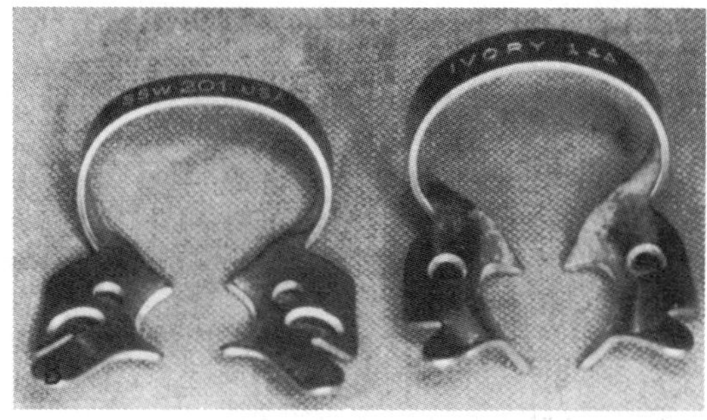

FIGURE 22–4

Clamp designs. *A*, Dental dam clamps with and without wings. *B*, Flat prongs, on the left, are used on fully erupted teeth. Inverted prongs, on the right, are used on partially erupted teeth. (From Baum, L., Phillips, R.W., and Lund, M.R.: Textbook of Operative Dentistry, 2nd ed. Philadelphia, W.B. Saunders Co., 1985, p 177.)

which are also known as *anterior clamps,* such as clamps 9 and W9 in Figure 22–3, are specially designed to

- Retract the gingiva on the facial surface
- Improve visibility for the restoration of cervical Class V cavities
- Permit isolation of an anterior tooth during endodontic treatment
- When stabilized, serve as finger support for the operator during the procedure

CLAMP MODIFICATION

Occasionally a standard clamp must be modified so it can be placed on sound tooth structure even if the tooth is malposed, irregularly shaped, or fractured or has a carious lesion that makes normal placement impossible. For example, the operator may remove the wings from the winged clamps to permit placement of the clamp.

In a modification known as **festooning**, the operator uses a carbide bur, disc, or stone to reshape the jaws or contour of the clamp. (**Festooning** means to trim or shape.) For example:

- If the carious lesion is at the left on the gingival third of the facial surface, the left facial jaw of the clamp might require modification.
- If the right margin of the tooth is carious in this area, the right facial jaw of the clamp might require modification.

LIGATURES ON DENTAL DAM CLAMPS

An 18-inch length of dental floss is *always* attached to the bow of the dental dam clamp as a ligature *before* the clamp is placed in the patient's mouth (Fig. 22–5).

This is an important safety step that must not be omitted. The ligature makes it possible to retrieve a clamp should it accidentally be dislodged, swallowed, or aspirated by the patient. Without this safeguard, such an accident could have extremely serious consequences for the patient.

The ends of this ligature are always kept out of the patient's mouth on the outside of the dental dam material and within easy reach. During treatment, the ligature may be attached to the dam frame to keep it available and yet out of the operator's way.

Stabilizing the Dam Application

The clamp holds the dental dam secure on the end nearest the tooth being treated. The opposite end of

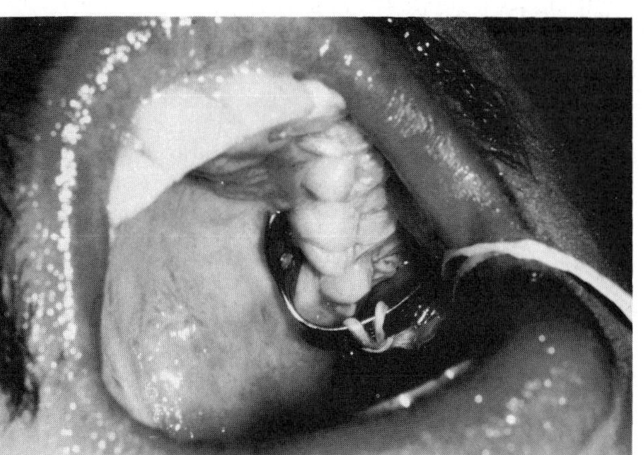

FIGURE 22–5

The clamp with the ligature in place on the tooth and checked for stability. (Courtesy of Steve Eakle, DDS, University of California, San Francisco, School of Dentistry.)

the dental dam application must also be stabilized. Also known as *ligating the dam,* this may be accomplished by using another clamp, a dental dam stabilizing cord, or a ligature.

DENTAL DAM STABILIZING CORD

Dental dam stabilizing cord, which is shown in Figure 22–1, is a disposable latex cord that is available in three sizes: extra-small, small, and large. During insertion, the cord is stretched so that it narrows and slips easily between the teeth. Once placed and released, the cord resumes its original shape and holds tightly.

The size of the cord selected depends upon the amount of contact space available. The length of cord used depends upon the application.

When a single anterior tooth is isolated, a single length of cord is cut. After the dam and frame have been placed, the stretched cord is inserted mesially, wrapped cross the facial surface, and then inserted distally so that both ends of the cord are behind the tooth.

When several teeth are isolated, two lengths of cord are cut. One piece of cord is placed on the distal side of the anchor tooth. The other is placed on the distal side of the last isolated tooth on the opposite side of the arch.

STABILIZING THE "OPPOSITE END" OF THE DAM

A dental dam clamp is commonly used to stabilize the posterior end of the dam application. Several methods are used to stabilize the "opposite end" of the application.

A double loop of dental floss or a small piece of dam material may be used for this purpose. Whichever is selected, the material is wedged between the last two isolated teeth.

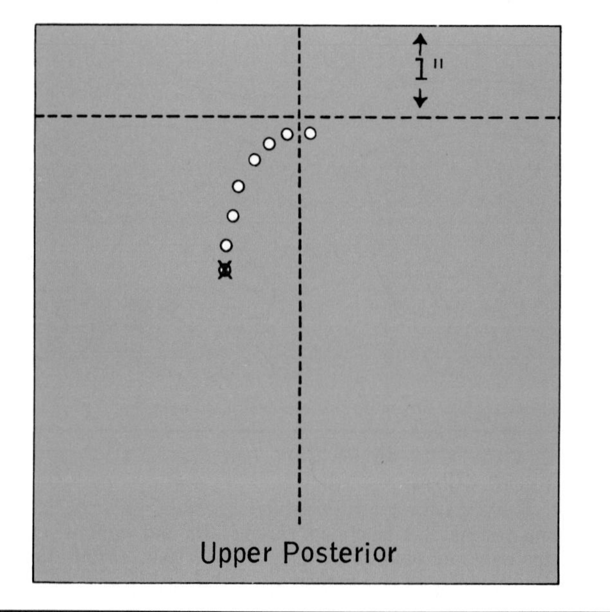

FIGURE 22–6

Punching 6 × 6 inch dental dam for maxillary posterior placement. The dam is divided into imaginary halves, and the holes for the anterior teeth are punched 1 inch from the upper edge of the dam. The key punch hole is on the maxillary second molar.

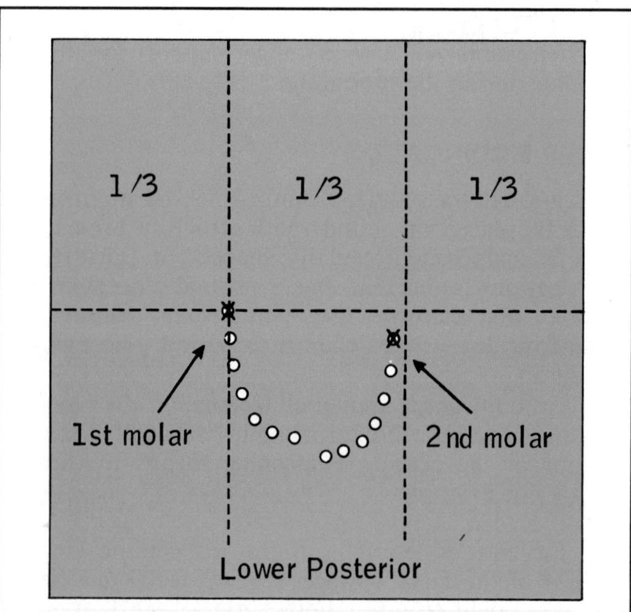

FIGURE 22–7

Punching 6 × 6 inch dental dam for mandibular posterior placement. The dam is divided into half and then into imaginary thirds. *Left,* the key punch hole is placed on the first molar. *Right,* the key punch hole is placed on the second molar. Notice how placement of these holes alters the distance of the anterior holes from the lower edge of the dam.

Dental Dam Application and Removal

Planning the Dental Dam Application

Each application of the dam is preplanned to accommodate operator preferences, the tooth or teeth involved, and the procedure to be performed.

There are several important factors that must be included in planning for the holes to be punched in the dental dam: (1) the arch, its shape, and any irregularities such as missing teeth or a fixed prosthesis; (2) the teeth to be isolated; (3) identification of the anchor tooth and the location of the key punch hole; and (4) the size and spacing of the other holes to be punched. (The **anchor tooth** holds the dental dam clamp, and the **key punch hole** covers the anchor tooth.)

MAXILLARY ARCH APPLICATIONS

In preparation for maxillary application, the dam material is divided vertically into imaginary halves and the holes are punched (Fig. 22–6; see Fig. 22–8).

Because the holes for the maxillary anterior teeth are punched 1 inch down from the upper edge of the dam, it is helpful to place a mark on the extension in back of the punch plate of the dental dam punch to indicate 1 inch. This mark automatically designates the margin of dam for these holes.

If the patient has a mustache or a very thick upper lip, it is necessary to allow extra space here.

MANDIBULAR ARCH APPLICATIONS

In preparation for mandibular application, the dam is divided vertically into imaginary thirds and horizontally into halves, and the holes are punched (Figs. 22–7 and 22–8). Because of the small size of the mandibular anterior teeth, the holes are punched closer together than those for posterior teeth.

CURVE OF THE ARCH

It is necessary to make the adjustments to accommodate an extremely narrow or wide arch. Failure to do this will increase the difficulty with inverting the edges of the dam.

- Punching the curve of the arch too flat or too wide results in bunching and stretching of the dental dam on the lingual aspect.
- Punching the arch too curved or too narrow results in folds and stretching of the dam on the facial aspect.

MALALIGNED TEETH

If a tooth or teeth are malaligned within the dental arch, special consideration of their position is taken *before* the dental dam is punched. (**Malaligned** and **malposed** mean that the individual tooth is not in its normal position within the dental arch.)

- If the tooth is *lingually malposed,* the hole punch size remains the same, but the hole is placed about 1 mm. lingually from the normal arch alignment.
- If the tooth is *facially malposed*, the hole punch size remains the same, but the hole is placed about 1 mm. facially from the normal arch alignment.

THE TEETH TO BE ISOLATED

Single-tooth isolation is used commonly for endodontic treatment and for selected restorative procedures such as Class V restorations. Some operators isolate only the tooth to be treated. Others prefer to have two teeth isolated so that the second tooth acts as an anchor tooth to hold the clamp. During treatment in the posterior area, this provides more stability and better visibility.

For **multiple-tooth isolation**, many operators expose only three or four teeth; however, for optimum stability, it is desirable to have eight to ten teeth isolated.

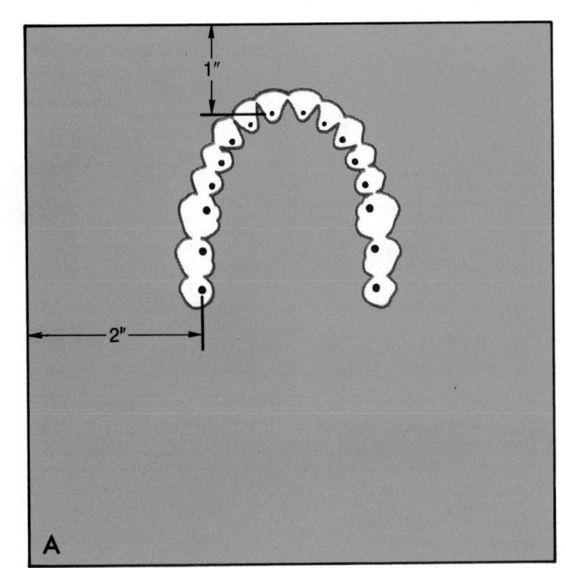

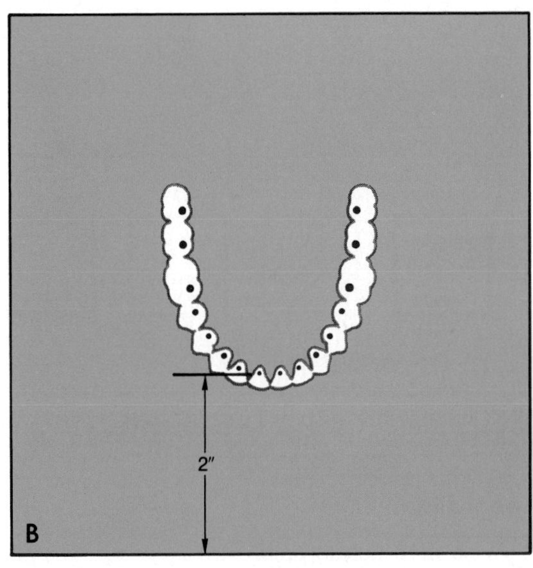

FIGURE 22–8

Diagram for punching dental dam. Dots represent punch holes. *A*, Maxillary arch. *B*, Mandibular arch.

Having this many teeth isolated counteracts the pull on the dam that is created by the curvature of the teeth in the arch.

At a minimum, at least one tooth posterior to the tooth being treated should be isolated. When possible, having two posterior teeth isolated is preferable.

When anterior maxillary teeth are to be treated, maximum stability is achieved by isolating the six anterior teeth (cuspid to cuspid).

KEY PUNCH HOLE

The **anchor tooth** holds the dental dam clamp. The **key punch hole** is punched in the dental dam to cover the anchor tooth. A larger, number 5 size hole, is necessary for the key punch because it must also accommodate the clamp.

The selection of the anchor tooth and the location of the key punch hole are important considerations in the application of the dental dam. For maximum stability and operator ease of access, the key punch hole is placed one to two teeth beyond the tooth to be prepared.

HOLE SIZE AND SPACING

The size of each hole selected on the dental dam punch must be appropriate for the tooth to be isolated (see Table 22–1). A correctly sized hole allows the dam to slip easily over the tooth and fit snugly in the cervical area. This is important to prevent leakage around the dam.

In general, the spacing between the holes is from 3 to 3.5 mm. between the edges, not the centers, of the holes. This allows adequate spacing between the holes to create a septum that can slip between the teeth without tearing or injuring the gingiva.

The **septum** is the dental dam between the holes of the punched dam. During application, this portion of the dam is passed between the contacts. (*Septum* is singular; the plural is *septa.*)

Troubleshooting Hole Size and Spacing

- If the holes are *too large*, the dam will not fit tightly around the tooth. (This may allow saliva to leak through the hole.)
- If the holes are *too small*, the dam will not slip easily over the tooth. (This may cause the dam to stretch or tear and leave gingiva exposed.)
- If the holes are *too close*, the dam may tear or stretch. (The stretched holes may leave the gingiva exposed and may cause leakage.)
- If the holes are *too far* apart, there is excess material between the teeth. (This may block the dentist's vision or catch in instruments.)

Placement and Removal of Dental Dam

There are two commonly used methods of dental dam placement. The difference is in the timing of the placement of the clamp and dam. The other steps are the same.

In the **one-step method**, the dam and clamp are placed at the same time. In the **two-step method,** the clamp is placed first and then the dental dam material is stretched over it.

The description here is of the one-step method on permanent dentition by an operator and assistant using a Young frame.

(text continued on page 425)

 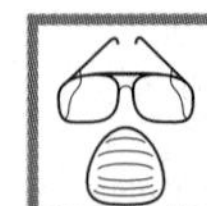 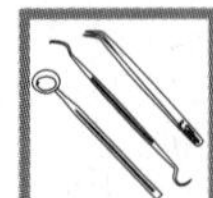 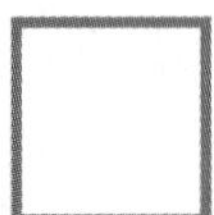 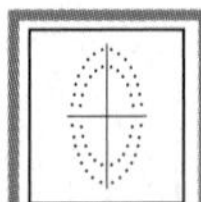

PROCEDURE: Placing and Removing a Dental Dam

Instrumentation

Precut 6 × 6 inch dental dam
Dental dam stamp and ink pad *or* template and pen
Dental dam punch
Dental dam clamp(s) with ligature attached
Dental dam clamp forceps
Young's frame
Dental floss or tape
Cotton rolls
Lubricant for patient's lips
Lubricant for dam
Beavertail burnisher, No. 2 or 34
Scissors

Patient Preparation

1. Check the patient's chart for contraindications and to identify the area to be isolated. Then inform the patient of the need to place a dental dam, and explain the steps involved.
2. The local anesthetic is administered, the operator determines which teeth are to be isolated, and notes whether there are any malposed teeth to be accommodated.
3. *Optional:* The assistant may apply lubricating ointment to the patient's lips with a cotton roll.
   □ *RATIONALE:* The patient's comfort is of concern throughout the placement and removal of dental dam.
4. The assistant passes the mouth mirror and explorer to the operator, who also checks the surfaces for debris or plaque.
   □ *RATIONALE:* If debris or plaque is present, selective coronal polishing is performed on these teeth before the application of the dental dam.
5. The assistant passes a length of floss to the operator, who checks contact areas of teeth to be isolated.
   □ *RATIONALE:* This is to detect contacts that are too snug and may create problems during placement. It also discloses rough contacts that may require smoothing before continuing.

Punching the Dental Dam

1. The assistant uses a template or stamp to mark on the dam the teeth to be isolated. If the assistant is to punch the dam, it is done at this time (Fig. 22–9).
2. If the operator is to punch the dam, the assistant hands the dental dam punch to the operator and holds the dam toward the operator without stretching it.
   If the *anterior teeth* are to be clamped, the superior (upper) border of the dam is held toward the operator.
   If *posterior teeth* are to be clamped, the inferior (lower) border of the dam is held toward the operator.
3. The assistant lightly lubricates the holes on the tooth surface (undersurface) of the dam.
   □ *RATIONALE:* This eases placement of the dam over the contact area of the teeth.

Placing the Clamp and Frame

1. The assistant places the clamp onto the dental dam forceps and slides the bar so that the clamp is held securely on the forceps.
   □ *Important*: A ligature is already attached to the bow of the clamp.
2. The assistant passes the forceps, handles first, positioned so that the operator receives them with the clamp pointed toward the arch for placement on the anchor tooth (Fig. 16–17).
   □ *RATIONALE:* This permits the operator to use the forceps without having to shift their position.
3. The operator checks the clamp for fit (see Fig. 22–5). The clamp is removed, and the forceps and clamp are returned to the assistant.
4. The assistant passes the bow of the clamp through the keyhole of the dam. The ligature is also pulled through the hole.
   □ *RATIONALE:* Throughout the placement procedure, this ligature is kept free of the dam to ensure a quick retrieval if necessary.
5. The assistant returns the forceps, clamp, and dam to the operator, who receives them in the right hand and gathers the excess dental dam edges and ligature in the left hand.
   □ *RATIONALE:* This permits visibility into the mouth for placement of the clamp.
6. The operator places the lingual jaws of the clamp first and then the facial jaws. During placement, the operator keeps the index finger on the clamp to prevent it from coming off before it has been stabilized on the tooth.
   □ *RATIONALE:* This lingual jaw placement serves as a fulcrum for placement of the facial jaws.

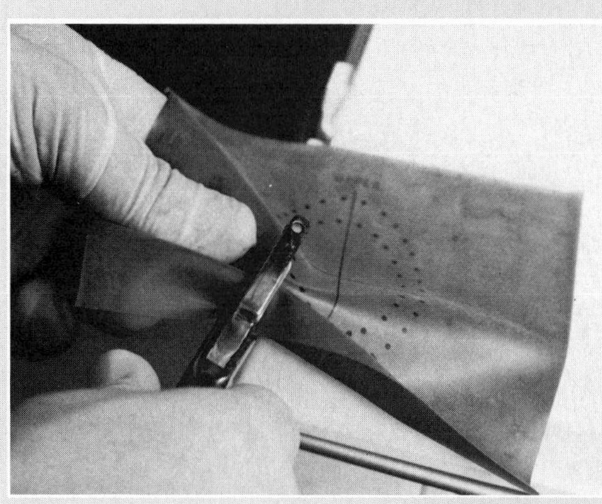

FIGURE 22–9

Punching the dental dam.

(continued on following page)

PROCEDURE: **Placing and Removing a Dental Dam** *(continued)*

7. The operator places the dam over the bow of the clamp and eases the margin of the dam under the clamp to ensure clearance at the cervix of the tooth (Fig. 22–10).
8. The operator holds the edges of the dam, releases the forceps from the clamp, and returns the forceps to the assistant. If a dental dam napkin is to be used, it is placed at this time.
9. The Young frame is placed on the outside of the dam and is hooked onto the projections of the frame.
   □ *RATIONALE:* This will ensure a smooth and stable fit.
10. The operator places the last hole of the dam over the last tooth to be exposed at the opposite end of the arch (Fig. 22–11).
    □ *RATIONALE:* This stabilizes the dam and aids in locating the remaining punch holes for the teeth to be isolated.

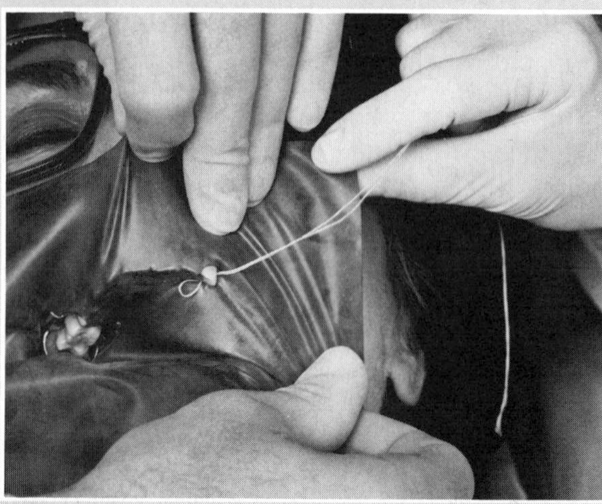

The dam is placed over the last tooth on the opposite end of the arch. Floss is used to ease the dam between the teeth.

Positioning and Ligating the Dam

1. The assistant hands a length of dental floss to the operator, who uses it to pass the dam septum as it is stretched between proximal contacts of each tooth to be isolated (Fig. 22–12).
2. *Optional*: Since the stretched dam septum slips more easily through the contacts when they are dry, the assistant may use the air syringe to dry these surfaces.
3. The assistant may place the index fingers of both hands on lingual and facial surfaces, stretching the dam and aiding the operator in slipping the dam septum through the contact areas.
4. If the contacts are extremely tight, the operator may use floss, a wooden wedge, or the beavertail burnisher wedged into the interproximal area to separate the teeth slightly.
   □ *RATIONALE:* In most cases, this slight action encourages the septum to slip through the tight contacts.

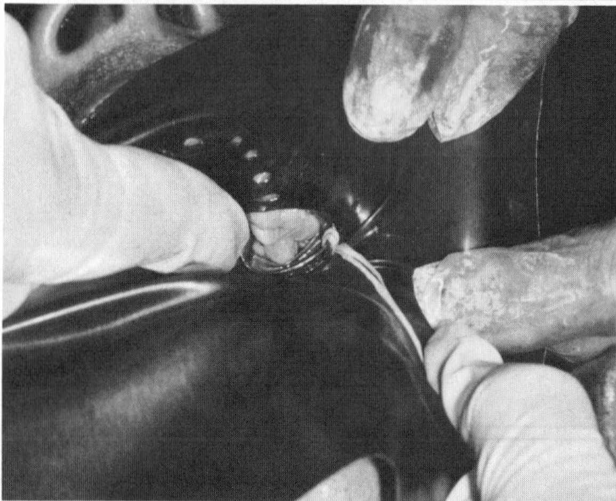

FIGURE 22–10

The dam is placed over the stabilized clamp. (Courtesy of Steve Eakle, DDS, University of California, San Francisco, School of Dentistry.)

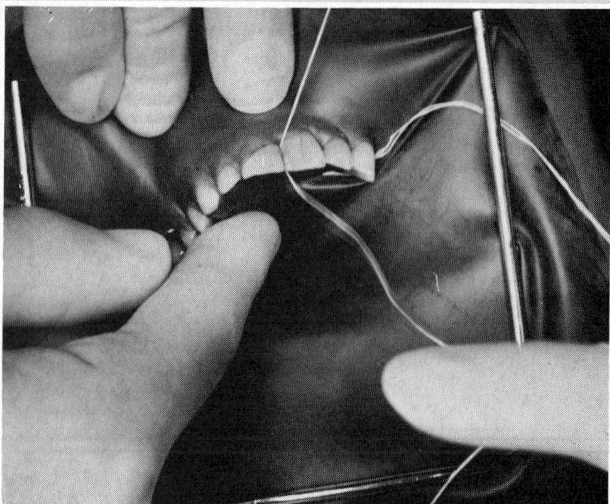

FIGURE 22–12

Dental floss is used to pass the dental dam septum through contacts.

5. A ligature is placed to stabilize the dam between the last two teeth isolated at the *opposite* end of the quadrant.
6. The ligature on the clamp is attached to the frame to keep it out of the way during the dental procedure.

Inverting the Dam

1. The operator inverts the dam by gently stretching it near the cervix of the tooth. (**Invert** means to turn inward or to turn under.)
   □ *RATIONALE:* Inverting the dam creates a seal to prevent the leakage of saliva.
2. Just before inverting the dam, the operator may ask the assistant to dry the tooth with air from the air-water syringe.
   □ *RATIONALE:* When the tooth surface is dry, the margin of the stretched dam usually inverts into the gingival sulcus as the dam is released.
3. *Optional:* The operator may use a beavertail burnisher when inverting the edges of the dam. If so, the assistant will blow air on the tooth as the burnisher is used.
4. *Optional:* The assistant may gently pass a length of dental floss between the teeth to ease the dam material through. The floss is pulled out sideways from the interproximal area.
5. With all rubber margins properly inverted, the field is prepared for the dental procedure (Fig. 22–13).
6. *Optional*: If necessary for patient comfort, a saliva ejector may be placed under the dam. This is positioned on the floor of the patient's mouth on the side *opposite* the area being treated.
7. *Optional*: If the patient complains of being unable to breathe comfortably, the operator may cut a small hole in the palatal area of the dam by pinching up a bit of dam with cotton pliers and cutting a small hole near the palatal area.
8. *Optional:* The assistant passes an applicator of lubricant, and the operator covers any porcelain or composite restorations that may become dehydrated while isolated by the dental dam.
   □ *RATIONALE:* Lengthy drying of these restorations may be harmful to them.

Removing the Dental Dam

1. The dam may be removed while the patient is still in a supine position, or the chair may be moved into an upright position.
2. If the dam is stabilized by a ligature, the operator removes this and passes it to the assistant. If a saliva ejector was used, the assistant removes it.
3. The assistant hands scissors to the operator and then holds the margins of the dam.
4. The operator holds the scissors in one hand and places the index finger and thumb of the other hand under the superior edge of the dam. Working from posterior to anterior, each septum is stretched and cut (Fig. 22–14).
   □ *RATIONALE:* This finger placement guides the operator's use of the scissors and protects the patient's tissues from accidental injury.

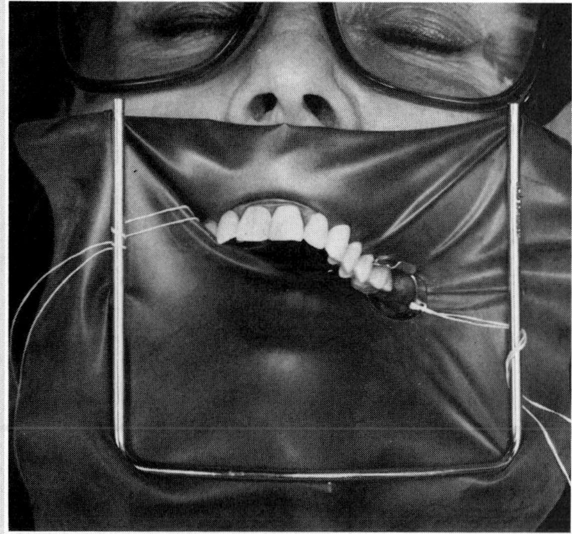

FIGURE 22–13

Completed dental dam application with a Young frame.

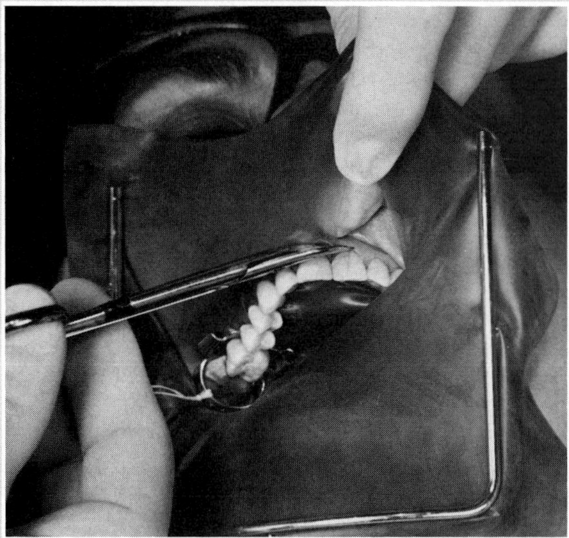

FIGURE 22–14

The dental dam septum is carefully cut before removal of the dam.

(continued on following page)

PROCEDURE: **Placing and Removing a Dental Dam** *(continued)*

5. When all septa are cut, the dam is pulled lingually to free the rubber from the interproximal space. The scissors are returned to the assistant.
6. The assistant passes the dental dam clamp forceps to the operator, who receives the forceps and removes the clamp. The forceps and clamp are then returned to the assistant (Fig. 22–15).
7. The operator removes both dam and frame and returns them to the assistant. A tissue, or the dam napkin, is used to wipe the patient's mouth lips and chin free of moisture.
8. The used dam is placed over a light-colored surface and inspected in order to ensure that the total pattern of the torn septa of the dental dam has been removed (Fig. 22–16).
9. If a fragment of the dental dam is missing, the operator uses dental floss to check the corresponding interproximal area of the oral cavity.
   □ *RATIONALE:* If fragments of dental dam are left under the free gingiva, they can cause gingival irritation.

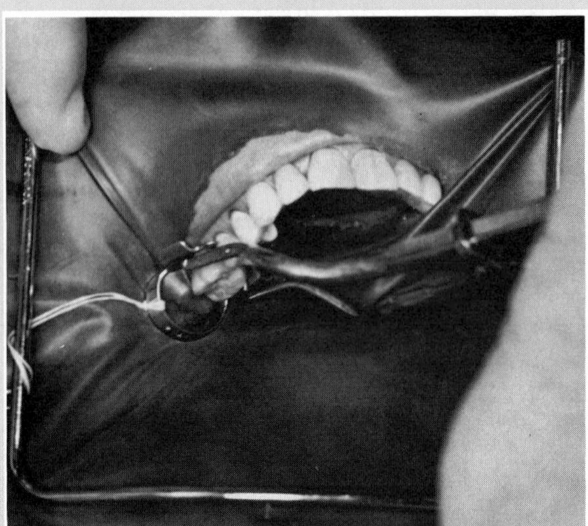

FIGURE 22–15

The clamp is removed.

Checking Hard and Soft Tissue Condition

1. The operator uses an explorer and a mouth mirror to check the condition of the teeth, the mucosa, and interproximal gingiva.
   □ *RATIONALE:* The goal is to determine that the tissues are intact and that no trauma from the dental dam placement or removal has occurred.
2. If indicated, dental floss is gently placed through each contact to be certain that all interproximal areas are free of dental dam or other debris.
3. The operator massages the gingiva of the area covered by the dam to increase circulation, especially the tissues supporting the anchor clamp.
4. *Optional*: The assistant rinses the patient's mouth with warm water and use the high-volume evacuator (HVE) to remove excess water and debris.
5. If a restoration has been placed, the patient's occlusion is checked after removal of the dental dam.

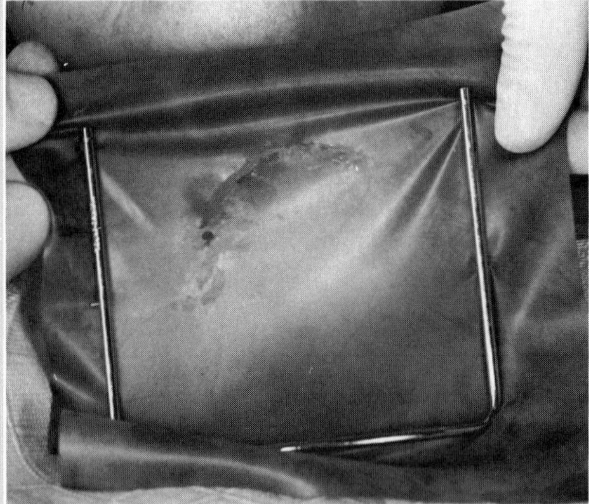

FIGURE 22–16

The used dam is inspected to detect any tears or missing pieces.

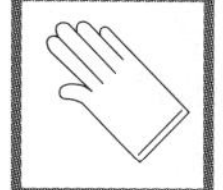
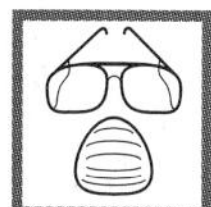
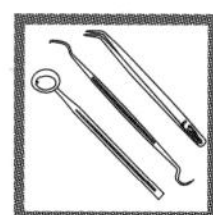

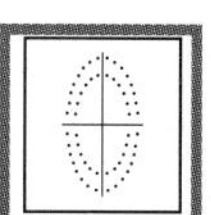

PROCEDURE: **Placing Cervical Ligatures**

1. Cut a length of waxed floss, about 18 inches, for each tooth to be ligated.
   □ *RATIONALE:* Waxed floss is used so that it will not absorb bleaching or etching solutions. This length allows working room in preparing and placing the floss.
2. Loosely tie a slip knot in each piece of floss to form a loop that is slightly larger than the tooth.
3. Slip the preformed loop over the tooth and down to the cervix. Then pull the slip knot firmly to hold the loop in place.
4. Hold the facial portion of the floss in the gingival sulcus. Use a burnisher or plastic instrument to gently tease the lingual portion over the cingulum and into the sulcus.
5. After all of the ligatures have been placed, cut the floss approximately ¼ inch from the knot.

Special Situations

Cervical Ligation of Anterior Teeth

When dental dam is placed before in-office bleaching and placement of some composite restorations on anterior teeth, it is necessary to place a waxed floss ligature around the cervix of each tooth to be treated. This is placed after the dam has been inverted. (Bleaching and composite restorations are discussed in Chapter 25.)

Alternative Style Dental Dam Placement

An alternative to traditional dam placement is a small dental dam and frame combination known as Quickdam. For some applications, it has the advantages of being faster and easier to place.

This dam and frame combination may be placed without additional stabilization. When stabilization is required, stabilizing cord, a dental dam clamp, a floss ligature, or a piece of dental dam may be used for this purpose. (When a clamp is used, follow the steps and precautions as with other dam applications.)

Placing Dental Dam Over a Fixed Bridge

A fixed bridge is a prosthetic device that is cemented in place to replace one or more adjacent missing teeth. A **pontic** is used to replace the missing tooth. The adjacent natural teeth, which are usually covered with full crowns, are used as **abutments**. These units are soldered together so the abutments support the pontic.

Because the units of the bridge are joined together, it is not possible to place the dental dam septum between them. For this reason, placement of a dental dam on fixed bridgework requires a specialized technique.

BASIC TECHNIQUE

The basic technique for this purpose exposes each of the abutment teeth and leaves the pontic covered with dental dam. Because of the added stresses in this application, a heavy or extra-heavy dam may be required.

The dam is punched with large holes for each abutment tooth but *no* hole is punched for the pontic. A clamp is placed on the distal abutment. In some situations, a second clamp is placed on the mesial abut-

(text continues on page 428)

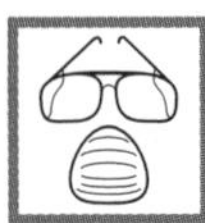
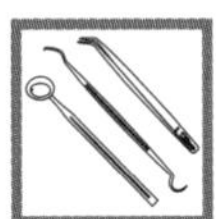

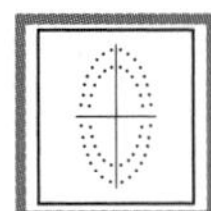

PROCEDURE: **Placing and Removing Quickdam**

Instrumentation

Preformed dental dam and frame
Template for preformed dam
Dental dam punch
Waxed dental floss
Piece of dental dam

Placing and Removing Quickdam

1. Use the template to mark on the dam the teeth to be isolated (Fig. 22–17).
2. Use the punch to make the appropriately sized holes. Hole sizes here are similar to those selected for traditional dam application (Fig. 22–18).
3. Fold the dam double across the width and lightly press the sides together to insert the dam into the patient's mouth (Figs. 22–19 and 22–20).
4. Release the sides of the frame and check to see that the rim is lying in the vestibule of the mouth.
5. Fit the dam over the teeth to be isolated (Fig. 22–21). If necessary, use floss to pass the rubber dam septum through the interproximal contact.
6. If indicated, use a piece of dam to stabilize the application.
7. If indicated, place a ligature around the cervical area of each tooth to be treated (Fig. 22–22).
8. When treatment is finished, remove the stabilization and complete removal as for other types of dam. Check to determine that none of the dam has torn off or been left in the mouth.

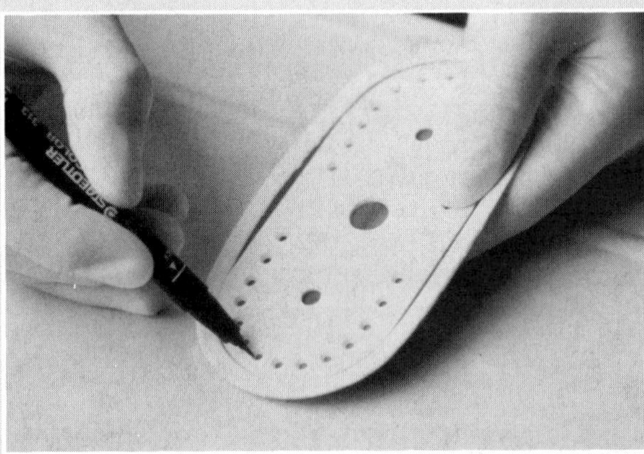

FIGURE 22–17

A specialized template is used to mark each tooth to be isolated. (Courtesy of Ivoclar Vivadent, Amherst, NY.)

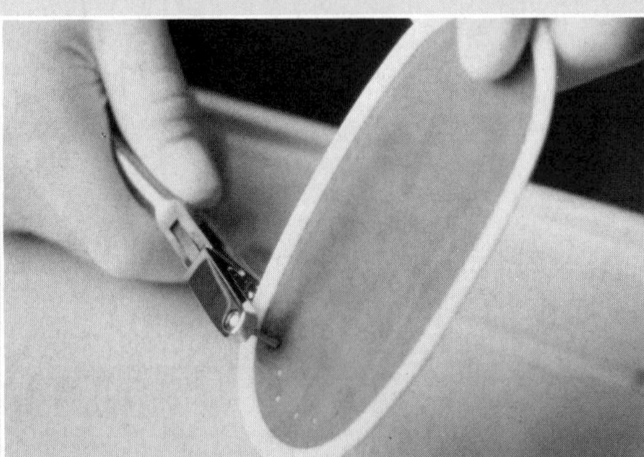

FIGURE 22–18

A dental dam punch is used to create the holes at the positions marked. As with other dental dam applications, each hole must be the appropriate size for the tooth to be exposed. (Courtesy of Ivoclar Vivadent, Amherst, NY.)

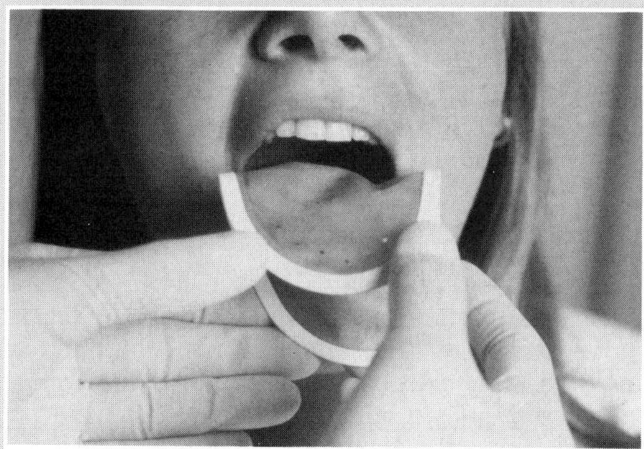

FIGURE 22–19

Before the dam is inserted into the patient's mouth, the dam is folded double. (Courtesy of Ivoclar Vivadent, Amherst, NY.)

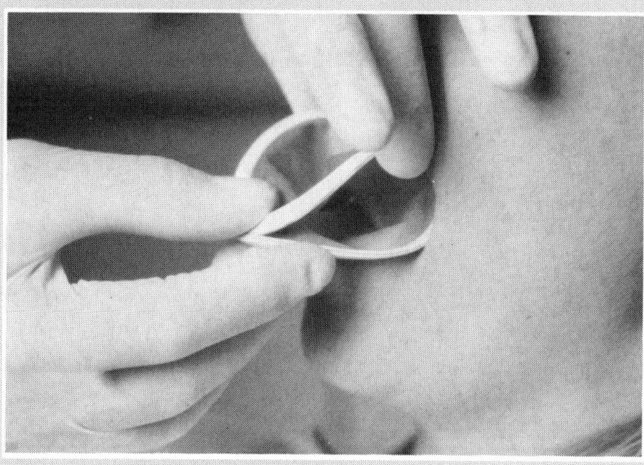

FIGURE 22–20

The sides of the dam are lightly pressed together, and the dam is inserted into the patient's mouth. After the sides are released, the dam should be lying in the vestibule of the mouth. (Courtesy of Ivoclar Vivadent, Amherst, NY.)

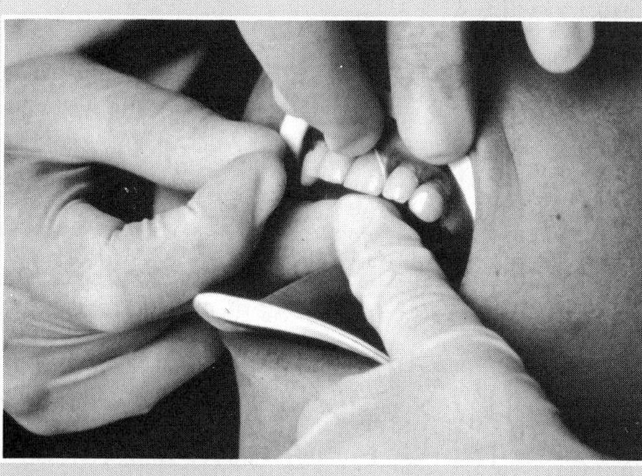

FIGURE 22–21

The dam is fitted over the teeth to be isolated. If necessary, floss is used to slip the dam between the contacts of the teeth. (Courtesy of Ivoclar Vivadent, Amherst, NY.)

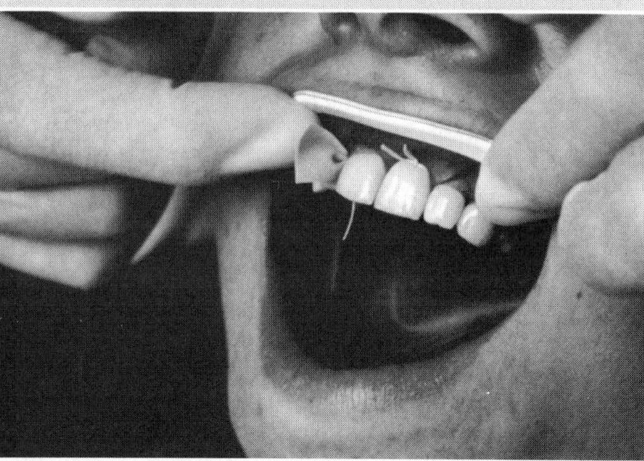

FIGURE 22–22

If necessary, the dam is secured with ligature or clamp. Notice the floss ligature around the cervix of the left central incisor. (Courtesy of Ivoclar Vivadent, Amherst, NY.)

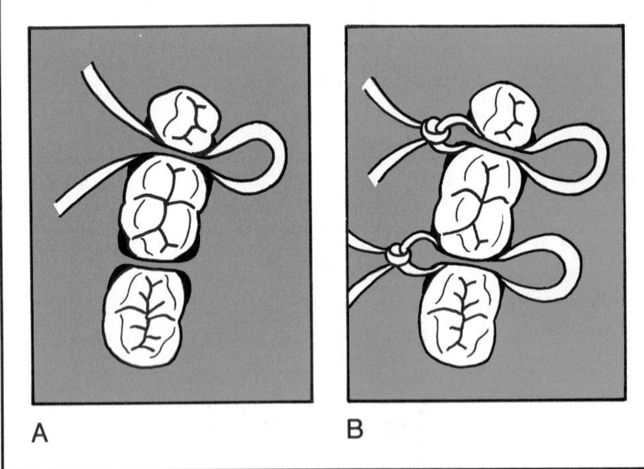

FIGURE 22–23

Placement of a dental dam on a three-unit bridge. *A*, The ligature is placed first between the anterior abutment and the pontic. *B*, The completed application. The ligature has been placed between the posterior abutment and the pontic, and both ligatures have been tied.

ment. (Both clamps are applied so that the bows are toward the distal of the tooth.)

The remainder of the application and removal are as usual.

LIGATURE OF THE PONTIC TECHNIQUE

In some situations, it is necessary to ligate the dam around the pontic. For this technique, in addition to the normal instrumentation, a dulled No. 4 suture needle threaded with dental floss and a needle holder are required. An alternative to the suture needle is a plastic bridge threader.

Holes are punched in a routine manner, including larger sized holes for each bridge unit. Placement is completed except for ligating the septum around the bridge abutments (Fig. 22–23).

Placing Dental Dam for Class V Cervical Restorations

Placement of dental dam for the restoration of Class V cervical caries requires several modifications of the usual technique.

MODIFICATIONS

- A cervical clamp is selected to fit the tooth to be treated.
- Because the caries is low on the gingival third of the tooth surface and may even be below the CEJ, it is necessary to place the jaws of the clamp lower than usual on the tooth surface.
- The jaws are positioned lightly on the cementum of the root just below the carious lesion. (When the clamp is placed, care must be taken *not* to injure the cementum or surrounding tissues.)
- The hole in the dam for the tooth to be restored is punched 1 mm. facially from the normal location.
- Also, 1 mm. of extra rubber should be allowed between the neighboring teeth in the arch.

STABILIZING THE CERVICAL CLAMP

Occasionally, additional stabilization of the cervical clamp is necessary, and softened stick compound may be used for this purpose. This requires the use of a heat source such as a butane torch or Bunsen burner.

1. Soften red or green stick compound by holding it over a flame until the tip bends. Then place the tip in hot water for 5 seconds.
2. Twist off approximately ⅜ inch of the tip and shape it into a cone.
3. Very carefully reheat the cone of compound in the flame, and then place the softened compound under the bow of the clamp (facial surface), away from the area to be treated.
   □ *Caution*: Avoid filling the notch holes of the clamp with compound. The compound would prevent placement of the tips of the dental dam clamp forceps into the notches for removal of the clamp after treatment.
4. Repeat this procedure for the second bow on the opposite side of the clamp (facial surface).
5. Upon completion of treatment, remove the compound before removing the dam and clamp.

Separators

The purpose of a separator is to temporarily create a small interproximal space between teeth that are too tight to allow necessary access (Fig. 22–24). A separator is used only after usual attempts at gaining this space have failed. The use of a separator may be necessary to

- Create space for passage of the dental dam septum or retract the dental dam and interproximal papillae
- Gain and maintain space required for access during restorative procedures
- Detect caries on the proximal surfaces of malaligned teeth that were not evident on radiographs of the area
- Inspect the interproximal papillae and the cervical margin of a tooth

Separators are available in several brands and in sizes to be used according to the teeth involved. Each is used according to the manufacturer's directions.

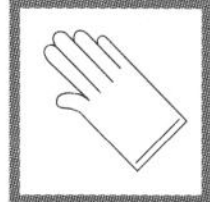
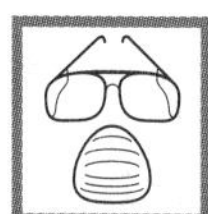
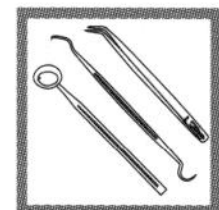

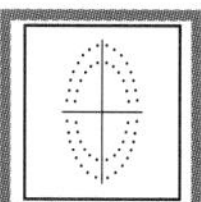

PROCEDURE: **Ligating the Septum Around a Bridge**

1. Pass the needle threaded with floss through the distal portion of the hole covering the anterior abutment in a facial-to-lingual direction. The needle enters on the facial side, goes under the solder joint, and comes out on the lingual side of the same hole.
2. Pass the needle through the mesial portion of the hole covering the pontic in a lingual-to-facial direction. The needle enters on the lingual side, goes under the solder joint, and comes out on the facial side of the same hole.
3. Tie the two ends of the floss and trim the excess.
4. Pass the needle threaded with floss through the mesial portion of the hole covering the posterior abutment in a facial-to-lingual direction. The needle enters on the facial side, goes under the solder joint, and comes out on the lingual side of the same hole.
5. Pass the needle through the distal portion of the hole covering the pontic in a lingual-to-facial direction. The needle enters on the lingual side, goes under the solder joint, and comes out on the facial side of the same hole.
6. Tie the two ends of the floss and trim the excess.
7. When it is time to remove the dam, cut the ligatures on the lingual side. Use the knot on the facial side to pull them out of the dam.

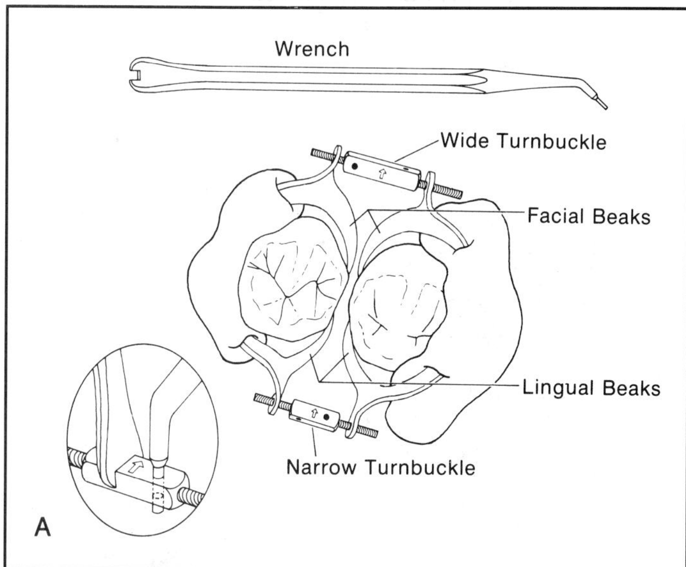

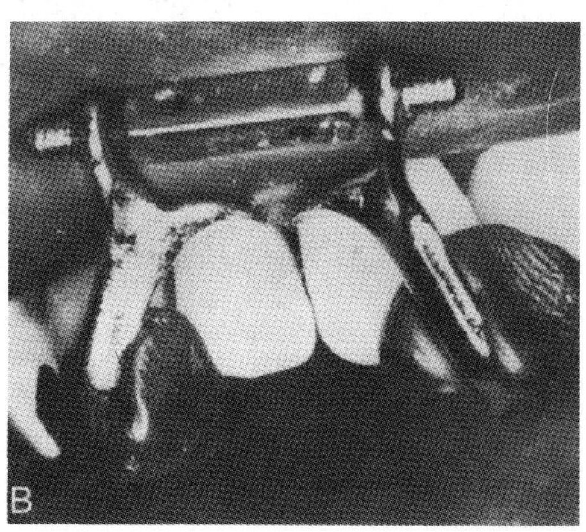

FIGURE 22–24

A Ferrier separator in position and stabilized with compound. *A*, Diagramatic representation. The wrench is used to make the adjustments. *B*, Photograph of separator in position. (Modified from Baum, L., Phillips, R.W., and Lund, M.R.: Textbook of Operative Dentistry, 2nd ed. Philadelphia, W.B. Saunders Co., 1985, p 335.)

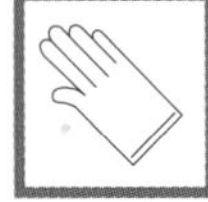 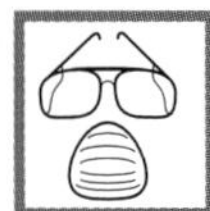 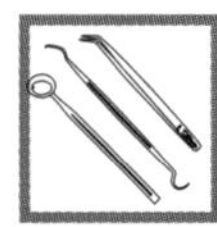 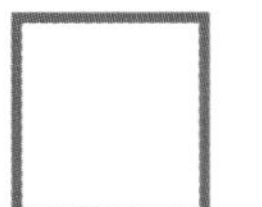 

PROCEDURE: **Placing and Removing a Separator**

1. Before placement, the patient is informed of the need for use of the separator and advised that some discomfort may be felt as the separator applies pressure to the teeth.
2. As the separator is placed and stabilized, care is taken not to impinge on the surrounding tissues or the dental dam.
3. To open the separator, the control screw is turned very slowly for one-quarter turn. A second one-quarter turn may be necessary.
   □ *RATIONALE:* The goal is to obtain the required separation with minimum opening and little patient discomfort.
4. If the separator is being used only to create space for the dam septum to pass through, the pressure of the separator is released immediately.
5. If the tooth is to be prepared for a restoration, stick compound is used to stabilize the separator in the open position.
6. The pressure of the separator is released as quickly as possible.
7. To remove the separator, the operator reverses the turn of the adjustment screw gradually. Brief pauses between the turns reduce the discomfort to the patient.
8. After the separator is removed, the area is inspected to be certain that all compound has been removed. The gingival tissues are gently massaged to restore circulation.

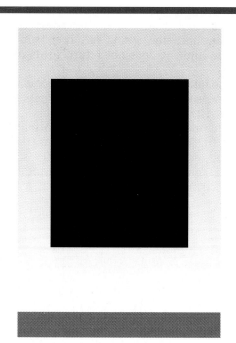

Chapter 23

Restorative Materials

Introduction

Restorative materials play important roles in dentistry. Knowing the characteristics of each and how it must be manipulated is very important; however, in preparation for learning about this, it is necessary to understand the shared characteristics of *all* dental materials. (**Manipulated** means mixed or handled.)

In this chapter, the general discussion of materials is followed by details about dental cements, cavity liners, and restorative materials. The uses and manipulation of these restorative materials are discussed in Chapter 25.

Exposure Control and Dental Materials

Maintaining exposure control protocols while mixing and handling dental materials presents a challenge for the chairside assistant, whose gloves are contaminated from aiding the dentist in the preparation of the tooth.

The chairside assistant must take the appropriate precautions while handling and mixing these materials. One option is to put on overgloves. Another option is to use a tissue, paper towel, or gauze sponge when touching containers of materials.

INSTRUMENT AND EQUIPMENT CARE

With most cements, the slab and spatula must be cleaned before the material has a chance to set on them. This should be done before removing the overgloves and returning to direct patient care.

Although the slab and spatula do not come into direct contact with the patient's mouth, they are often contaminated during use. For example, during crown cementation, the spatula is used to fill the crown. The crown is contaminated because it has been in the patient's mouth.

Because such contamination is so common, the slab and spatula should be sterilized before reuse. Applicators used to place the materials directly into the mouth must be either disposable (and discarded after a single use) or sterilized before reuse.

General Characteristics of Dental Materials

Any material that is used in the mouth is subjected to a warm, moist environment that includes corrosive conditions plus the effects of strong biting forces and rapid thermal changes.

In addition to having the ability to resist these difficult conditions, cements and other materials used in the mouth must meet these five criteria:

1. They must *not* be poisonous or harmful to the body.
2. They must *not* be harmful or irritating to the tissues of the oral cavity.
3. They must help protect the tooth and oral tissues.

4. They must resemble the natural dentition as closely as possible so as to be esthetically pleasing. (**Esthetic**, which is also spelled *aesthetic*, means beautiful or pleasing to the eye.)
5. They must be easily formed and placed in the mouth to restore natural contours and functions despite limited access, wet conditions, and poor visibility.

Factors Affecting Dental Materials

The following factors affect dental materials: biting forces, thermal changes, galvanic action, acidity, curing, solubility, adhesion, and retention.

BITING FORCES

The average biting and chewing force of a person with natural dentition is approximately 170 pounds (77 kg.) in the posterior area of the mouth. This is approximately 28,000 pounds of pressure per square inch (psi) on a single cusp of a molar tooth. Materials used in restoring chewing surfaces must have sufficient strength to withstand these forces.

A **force** is any push or pull upon matter (Fig. 23–1). In response to every force, there is a stress and a strain. **Stress** is the reaction *within* the material to an externally applied force. **Strain** is the *change* produced within the material as the result of stress.

There are three types of force, each with accompanying types of stress and strain:

- **Tensile force** pulls and stretches material. (A tug-of-war is an example of tensile force.)
- **Compression force** pushes material together. (Chewing is an example of compressive force.)
- **Shearing force** tries to slice material apart. (Cutting with scissors is an example of shearing force.)

Elastic Limit is the maximum stress that a structure or material can withstand without being permanently deformed. Once an elastic material has been subjected to stress that is above its elastic limit, it will not return to its original shape.

For example, a spring strained within its elastic limit returns to its original shape when the stress is removed. However, once the spring has been strained beyond its elastic limit, it does not return to its original shape.

The **elastic modulus**, also known as the *modulus of elasticity*, is a measure of the rigidity or stiffness of a material at stresses *below* its elastic limit. This is the resistance of the material to strain or deformation. (**Deformation** means a change in shape or form.)

A rubber band, which changes easily under stress, has a low elastic modulus. An amalgam restoration, which does not change easily under stress, has a high elastic modulus.

It is desirable that dental restorative materials have a high elastic limit and a high elastic modulus rating.

THERMAL CHANGES

When a person drinks hot coffee and eats ice cream, the temperature changes in the mouth can be as great as 100 to 150°F (38 to 66°C) within seconds. These thermal changes are of major concern for two reasons: (1) contraction and expansion and (2) the need to protect the pulp from thermal shock.

Contraction and Expansion. With temperature changes, each type of material contracts (shrinks) or expands (enlarges) at its own rate. It is essential that the tooth structure and the restorative material have, as nearly as possible, the same rate of contraction and expansion.

Significantly different rates of contraction and expansion can cause the restoration to pull away from the tooth, and this produces microleakage. (**Microleakage** is a microscopically small opening between the tooth and restoration that allows fluids and debris to seep downward into the tooth. This can cause recurrent decay and possibly damage to the pulp.)

Protection of the Pulp from Thermal Changes. One of the important functions of dentin is to protect the pulp from sudden thermal changes. The restorative material that is replacing lost dentin must also be able to protect the pulp against these thermal changes.

Metals, such as amalgam or cast metal restorations, are excellent thermal conductors. They transmit heat and cold through the tooth much more rapidly than

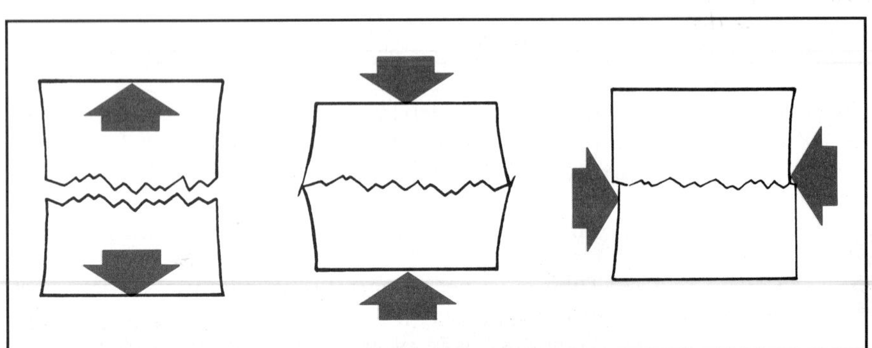

FIGURE 23–1

Types of stress and strain. *A*, **Tensile** pulls and stretches a material. *B*, **Compressive** pushes it together. *C*, **Shearing** tries to slice it apart.

does dentin. When metals are used, it is necessary to place an insulating base *under* the restoration to protect the pulp against these sudden temperature changes.

GALVANIC ACTION

Galvanic action is the term for the small electrical currents created when two different or dissimilar metals are present in the oral cavity.

Because both metals are wet with saliva, a reaction similar to that which occurs in a battery is produced. Thus when the two metals touch, an electrical current in the form of a small shock is created.

A similar effect may occur when a metallic restoration is touched by the edge of a metal fork.

ACIDITY

Acidity (pH) in the mouth varies greatly. (**pH** is a scale of 0 to 14 that expresses the acidity or alkalinity of a solution. A pH of 7 is considered neutral.)

Some foods, such as citrus fruits, and the bacteria in plaque are very acidic. Although saliva helps to neutralize this acidic environment, resistance to acidity is nevertheless an important factor in determining how well restorative materials will function.

A separate concern is the acidic property of dental materials. If applied directly over the sensitive tissues of the tooth, an acidic dental material will irritate the pulp. For this reason, when a very acidic material, such as zinc phosphate cement, is used, it is necessary to place a liner under the cement to protect the pulp.

CURING

Most dental materials are mixed into a paste form for placement in the mouth so that they can be shaped to the tooth. After they are in place, they must be cured (hardened) so they will stay in place and can perform their function.

A **self-curing** material hardens as the result of a chemical interaction of the materials being mixed together. The curing action proceeds from start to finish by itself. For this reason, the material must be mixed and placed within the working and setting times for that material.

A **light-cured** material does not harden until it has been exposed to a curing light. This allows more flexible mixing and working time. (The curing light is discussed in Chapter 14.)

In a **dual-cure** material, some curing takes place as the material is mixed; however, the final cure does not occur until the material has been exposed to the curing light.

When the curing light is used, it is necessary to protect the eyes from exposure to the rays of the curing light. Most lights are equipped with a special shield (see Fig. 14–14). If there is no shield, it is necessary to wear tinted protective glasses such as those shown on the left side of the tub in Figure 15–17.

SOLUBILITY

Solubility is the degree to which a substance will dissolve in a given amount of another substance. For example, sand has low solubility because it does not dissolve easily; sugar has high solubility because it does dissolve easily.

Solubility of a material placed in the mouth is a concern. A material that dissolves easily in the oral environment is of limited usefulness because it will wash away and leave the tooth structure exposed.

ADHESION

Adhesion is the force that causes unlike materials to adhere (stick) to each other. Adhesion between the dental material and the tooth structure is a major concern. Without proper adhesion, microleakage may result and the restoration may be lost. The characteristics of dental materials that affect adhesion are wetting, viscosity, surface characteristics, and film thickness.

Wetting. Wetting is the ability of a liquid to flow over the surface and to come into contact with the small irregularities that may be present. For example, water has high wetting ability because it flows easily.

Wetting is expressed in terms of the **contact angle** (Fig. 23–2). When a liquid has a low contact angle on a solid, it is said to wet the solid well. The ideal adhesive would spread out into such a thin film that the contact angle would be zero.

Viscosity. Viscosity is the property of a liquid that causes it *not* to flow easily. A liquid with high viscosity, such as heavy syrup, does not flow easily and is not effective in wetting a surface.

Surface Characteristics. The type of surface also influences the wetting ability of the material. A liquid flows more easily on a rough surface than on a very

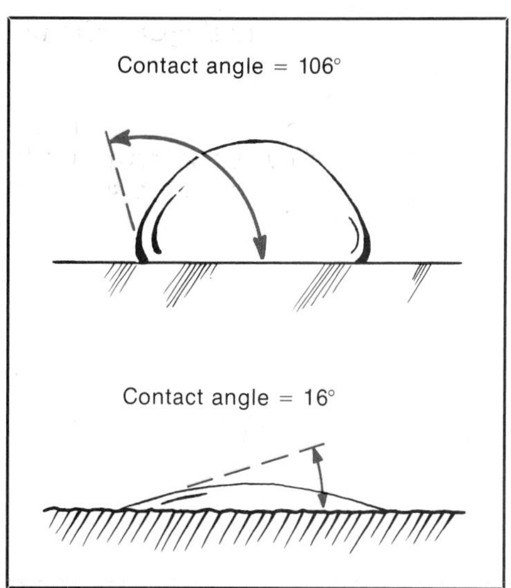

FIGURE 23–2

Contact angle. The lower the contact angle, the better the wetting properties of the liquid.

smooth surface. For example, water usually flows easily on a rough surface; however, on a waxed surface, it beads up and does not flow as readily.

Film Thickness. For adhesion to take place, the materials being joined must be in close contact with each other, and this requires a thin film thickness. (**Film thickness** refers to the thickness of the adhesive film.)

In general, the thinner the film, the stronger the adhesive junction. For example, the ideal film thickness for cementing a permanent restoration is 25 microns or less. (A **micron**, also known as a *micrometer*, is a unit of measure equal in length to one millionth of a meter.)

RETENTION

Retention is the ability to hold two things firmly together when they will *not* adhere (stick) to each other. For example, amalgam and cast metals do not adhere directly to tooth structure.

Retention is an extremely important concept in dentistry because dental restorations, castings, and appliances all must be held in place by using materials and methods that are not harmful to the body.

Since amalgam and tooth structure do not adhere to each other, a traditional cavity preparation includes retention form. (**Retention form** is shaping the sides of the prepared tooth to lock the amalgam in place.) Although this holds the amalgam in place, microleakage may occur between the amalgam and the tooth.

Therefore, retention is accomplished through the use of bonding, cements (as luting agents), and a combination of these methods.

Bonding

Many of the retention problems in dentistry have been solved through bonding, which improves retention by creating micromechanical retention between the tooth structure and the restoration. (**Micromechanical retention** means that the retention bonds created are extremely small.) With these materials, it is possible to bond restorative materials to enamel and dentin.

Enamel Bonding

Examples of enamel bonding include the placement of sealants, bonded orthodontic brackets, resin bonded bridges, and bonded veneers. Most of these are attached directly to the intact enamel surface. For some, such as the veneers, a thin layer of enamel is removed before bonding.

Enamel bonding, commonly referred to as **acid etching**, is a technique in which acid is used to dissolve some of the inter-rod substance between the enamel prisms. This creates a rough surface consisting of **enamel tags** (Fig. 23–3).

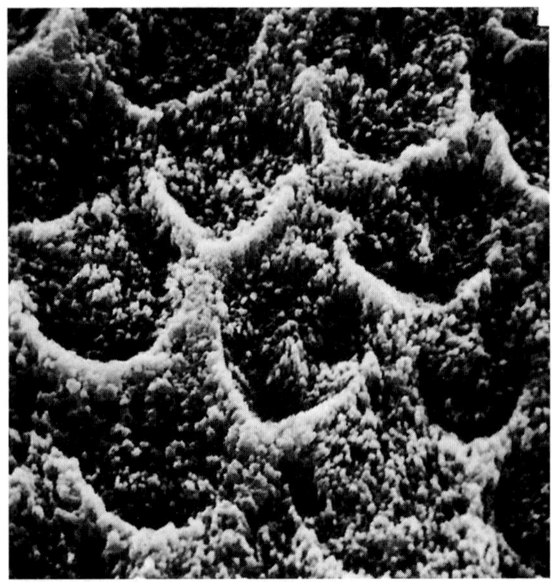

FIGURE 23–3

Etched enamel. Scanning electron micrograph of an enamel surface that has been etched by phosphoric acid (original magnification 5000×). (From Phillips, R.W., and Moore, B.K.: Elements of Dental Materials for Dental Hygienists and Dental Assistants, 5th ed. Philadelphia, W.B. Saunders Co., 1994, p 130.)

When the resin cement or restorative material is placed on the etched surface, it flows in and around the enamel tags. It hardens here to form a strong mechanical bond with the enamel (Fig. 23–4).

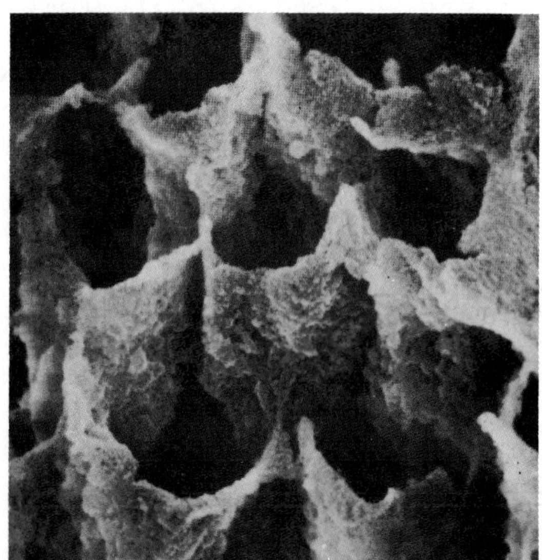

FIGURE 23–4

Resin tags formed by penetration into etched enamel. In this scanning electron micrograph, the enamel was removed to reveal the resin tags (original magnification 5000×). (From Phillips, R.W., and Moore, B.K.: Elements of Dental Materials for Dental Hygienists and Dental Assistants, 5th ed. Philadelphia, W.B. Saunders Co., 1994, p 131.)

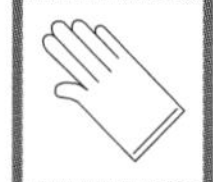 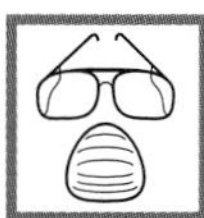 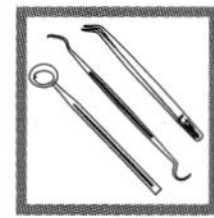  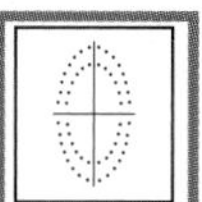

PROCEDURE: **Acid Etching of Enamel Surface**

1. The prepared tooth must be protected from contamination. Dental dam, placed before the etching process begins, provides this protection.
   □ *RATIONALE:* Dental dam placement also protects the patient from possible contact with the acid etchant.
2. The enamel surface must be thoroughly cleaned of all debris, plaque, or calculus before etching. Either pumice and water or a fluoride-free and oil-free polishing paste is used for this purpose.
   □ *RATIONALE:* Debris on the surface may interfere with the etching process. A polishing paste containing fluoride and/or oil also interferes with the etching process.
3. After cleaning, the surface is carefully dried but not desiccated. (**Desiccate** means to make too dry.)
   □ *RATIONALE:* Moisture interferes with the etching process. Excessive drying damages the tooth.
4. An etchant gel of 37 percent phosphoric acid is most commonly used. This gel is provided by the manufacturer of the bonding agent to be used on the etched surface.
   □ *RATIONALE:* The gel allows the etchant to be carefully placed *only* where it is needed. The gel and bonding agent must be from the same manufacturer.
5. The enamel is etched for the time recommended by the manufacturer. This is approximately 15 to 30 seconds.
   □ *RATIONALE:* The exact time depends upon the material and the use. For example, etching time for placing sealants is not the same as the etching time for bonding orthodontic brackets.
6. After etching, the surface is thoroughly rinsed and dried.
7. Etched enamel has a frosty white appearance. If the surface does not have this appearance, or if the surface has been contaminated with water or saliva, it is necessary to repeat the etching process.

Dentin Bonding

Dentin bonding presents special challenges:

- Unlike enamel, dentin consists of a range of organic substances, and this makes bonding more difficult.
- The smear layer, which is described in the next section, must be removed so the material can reach the dentin to bond with it.
- The bonding material must be able to work in an area that always contains some moisture.
- The material used must protect, not irritate, the pulp.

THE SMEAR LAYER

A major factor in the success of bonding to dentin is the removal of the smear layer. The **smear layer** is a very thin layer (5 to 10 microns) of debris composed of fluids and tooth components remaining on the dentin after a cavity preparation.

During the preparation of a tooth for a restoration, thousands of dentinal tubules are cut. The open ends of these tubules can transmit fluids and microorganisms to the pulp of the tooth. This may result in postoperative sensitivity, pain, or even damage to the pulp.

The smear layer, which has been described as "nature's bandage," protects the tooth by obliterating (closing off) the openings of these dentinal tubules. However, before dentin bonding, the smear layer must be removed and these tubules opened. As part of the bonding process, the tubules are sealed again, and this protection is restored to the tooth.

THE DENTIN BONDING PROCESS

There are two basic components of the bonding process: the etchant and the adhesive. The following is a general description of what happens in dentin bonding; however, specifics vary according to brand, and the manufacturer's instructions must always be followed.

The **etchant** removes the smear layer. Then it selectively dissolves away the hydroxyapatite phase of the dentinal structure and opens small defects, or microcracks, on the cut dentinal surface. (As used here, **hydroxyapatite** refers to a form of calcium that makes up part of the dentin structure.)

The **resin component**, which is sometimes referred to as the *adhesive component*, is allowed to flow into these small defects and into the partially opened tubules. This material must be cured to cause it to harden.

After the dentin bonding material is cured, there are numerous hardened resin projections below the surface of the dentin. These projections form strong micromechanical retention with the dentin.

The resulting combination of dentin and resin is called the **hybrid layer**. This hybrid layer is important because it is a very effective barrier against the invasion of microorganisms or any chemical component of the overlying composite resin. It is also the basis of a strong bond with the restorative material.

Amalgam Bonding

With specialized dentin bonding systems, it is possible to create a bond between amalgam and the tooth structure. This reduces the possibility of microleakage and recurrent decay.

Metal Bonding

It is possible to achieve improved retention of cast metal restorations, such as full crowns, by treating the inner surfaces of the crown to permit a bond to be formed between the metal, the cementing agent, and the tooth.

This preparation is usually performed in the dental laboratory with sandblasting or a similar process to roughen the surface of the metal on the interior of the crown.

Working with Bonding Systems

Some dentin bonding systems are self-curing. Others are light-cured or dual-cured. Some systems use two liquids; others use three.

Each bonding system is different, and the materials for one system are *not* interchangeable with those from another. It is essential that the manufacturer's instructions are followed exactly for each product.

Dental Cements

Dental cements are versatile materials that are widely used in dentistry. Each cement has special characteristics and is manipulated in a different way. Cements, their uses, and mixing tips are summarized in Table 23–1.

TABLE 23–1

Uses and Manipulation of Dental Cements

CEMENT USES	MIXING TIPS
Zinc Phosphate Luting agent Protective base Temporary restoration	Mix on a cool thick glass slab. Add powder slowly in small increments. Mix over a wide area to dissipate heat. Clean slab and spatula with baking soda.
Zinc Oxide–Eugenol Temporary luting agent Sedative treatments Insulating bases	Avoid contaminating other materials with eugenol. Clean spatula with alcohol or oil of orange solvent.
Ortho-Ethoxybenzoic (EBA) Luting agent	Incorporate powder all at once. Initial mix (30 seconds) is thick. Continue mixing another 30 seconds, and mix will soften.
Intermediate Restorative Material (IRM) Intermediate restorations	If mixing manually, use paper pad and bring powder into mix quickly. Wipe mix vigorously back and forth on mixing pad. Must be completed in 1 minute.
Polycarboxylate Luting agent Insulating bases Intermediate restorations	Mix all at once within 30 seconds. Mix should have a glossy surface. If liquid is thick, do not use it. If mix has lost gloss and become stringy, do not use it.
Glass Ionomer Restorations Luting agent Bonding agent Core build-up	Follow manufacturer's instructions for each formulation.
Calcium Hydroxide Protective base	Mix equal lengths on small area of mixing pad. Placed next to the pulpal wall, under any insulating base or cavity varnish.

Uses of Dental Cements

The primary uses of cements are as restorations, luting agents, and bases.

CEMENT RESTORATIONS

Cements are used as restorations when strength is *not* the key factor. For example, glass ionomer may be used as a Class V restoration that does not need to withstand the pressures of biting forces. Cement restorations may be

- **Permanent** (expected to last several years)
- **Intermediate** (expected to last about 6 months)
- **Temporary** (expected to last only a few weeks)

Sedative Treatments. Certain cements are used to soothe and promote healing in a traumatized tooth.

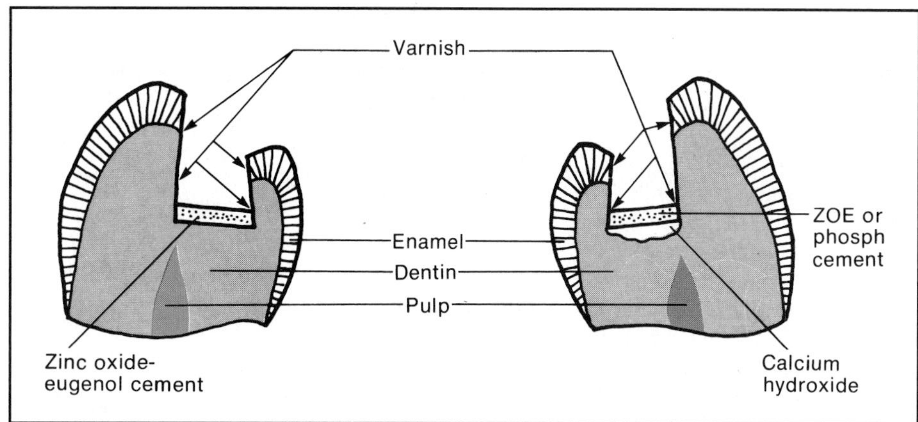

FIGURE 23–5

The use of cements as bases. Varnish, as a cavity liner, is placed over the base and on the walls of the prepared cavity.

(**Traumatized** means injured.) This injury may be caused by deep caries, a fracture of the tooth, or inflammation of the tissues after dental treatment, such as gross reduction of the tooth structure in preparation for placement of a full crown.

These sedative treatments, which are also known as *palliative treatments*, are actually a form of temporary restoration. (**Palliative** mean to ease discomfort.)

LUTING AGENTS

Cements are often used as luting agents. (A **luting** agent is an adhesive in that it holds two things together.)

- Cements are used for the permanent seating of cast crowns, inlays, onlays, and cosmetic laminate veneers. (**Seating**, as used here, describes the final placement of a restoration or prosthesis.)
- Cements are used to hold provisional coverage. (**Provisional coverage** is a temporary crown placed on a tooth that has been prepared for a cast restoration. It protects the tooth until the permanent restoration is ready to be seated.)
- Cements hold orthodontic bands on the teeth.
- Cements secure anchorage of pins and posts in teeth for retention of permanent restorations.

BASES

Different types of cements are used to form specialized types of bases under restorative materials (Fig. 23–5).

Protective Bases. After a tooth has been prepared, it is necessary to protect the pulp before the restoration is placed. Without this protection, there may be postoperative sensitivity and possible damage to the pulp.

Calcium hydroxide is most commonly used for this purpose because it soothes the pulp and promotes the formation of reparative dentin. It is placed directly over the pulpal floor of the preparation. (**Reparative dentin**, also known as *tertiary dentin*, is a protective layer of dentin formed by the tooth over the pulpal area in response to irritation or injury.)

Insulating Bases. When the cavity is deep, it is necessary to place an insulating base under the restoration to protect the tooth from thermal shock. This base is placed *over* the protective base.

The thermal qualities of metal allow it to conduct hot and cold more quickly than does dentin. For this reason, an insulating base is particularly important under a metal restoration.

Sedative Bases. Sometimes a sedative base, of a material such as zinc oxide–eugenol cement, is placed to soothe the pulp. When a sedative base is used, it is placed directly over the pulpal area of the tooth.

Zinc Phosphate Cement

Type I (fine-grain) zinc phosphate cement is frequently used for the cementation of cast restorations such as crowns, inlays, and onlays. It creates the very thin film layer necessary for accurate seating of these precision castings.

Type II (medium-grain) zinc phosphate cement is recommended for all uses *except* the cementing of precision appliances. These uses include use as an insulating base in deep cavity preparations. Because the phosphoric acid of the liquid is irritating to the pulp, it is necessary to place a cavity liner under a zinc phosphate insulating base.

POWDER AND LIQUID

Zinc phosphate is supplied as a powder that is primarily zinc oxide. The liquid is phosphoric acid and water. The water content of the liquid is carefully controlled by the manufacturer and must be maintained without change.

If exposed to air, the water in the liquid may evaporate or the liquid may absorb more water from the air. Either event will alter the setting time and properties of the material. If the liquid has become viscous (very thick) or has turned yellow, it should be discarded.

To avoid these problems, measure the liquid onto the slab just before mixing. Then replace the cap on the bottle immediately.

The powder-to-liquid ratio for a mix is determined by the manufacturer for each intended use. A thick mix for an insulating base has more powder than does the thin mix needed for cementation.

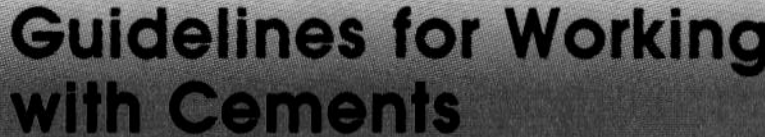

Guidelines for Working with Cements

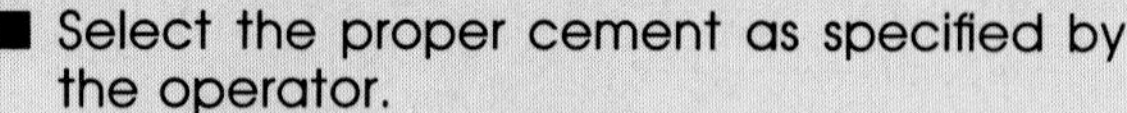

- Select the proper cement as specified by the operator.
  Rationale: The choice depends upon the intended use of the cement and the operator's preferences.
- Always use liquid and powder from the same manufacturer.
  Rationale: Cement formulas vary, and different brands cannot be combined.
- Carefully follow the manufacturer's directions.
  Rationale: The instructions are specific and must be followed exactly.
- Plan the mix to achieve the proper consistency for the intended use.
  Rationale: A thin mix is used for cementation. A thicker mix is necessary for a restoration or base.
- Use the appropriate equipment (glass slab or paper pad) as specified by the manufacturer.
- Use the appropriate spatula. A **narrow, flexible spatula** is used if the cement is thin and must be mixed over a wide area, A spatula with a wider blade is recommended if the cement is thick and heavy.
  Rationale: The equipment used is important for the success of the mix.
- Always measure the powder and liquid carefully.
  Rationale: The powder-to-liquid ratio is critical. Use the measuring devices and instructions provided by the manufacturer.
- When dispensing materials, replace the covers on the containers immediately.
  Rationale: Evaporation of liquids and aging of the product can cause a mix of the wrong consistency or prevent the mix from setting properly.
- Use the appropriate technique to mix the material.
  Rationale: Not all materials are mixed in the same way. Technique is an important part of creating a usable mix.
- Produce a homogeneous mix. (**Homogeneous** means a mix with a uniform quality throughout.)
  Rationale: If the powder and liquid are not evenly distributed throughout the mix, the cement will not set properly or have the appropriate strength.
- Complete the mix within the working time.
  Rationale: Working time is critical, and it is not the same for all cements. If the working time is incorrect, the mix will not be usable.
- If the mix is too thick, discard the mix and start over. Do *not* add more liquid.
  Rationale: Adding more liquid weakens the mix.
- If *placing* the cement, know and follow the manufacturer's instructions for placement.
  Rationale: If conditions are not correct during placement, the mix may not set or have the desired strength. (Placement of cements is discussed further in Chapters 25 and 31.)

These manufacturer's recommendations must be followed. Adding less than the recommended amount of powder increases the working time; however, it also decreases the strength of the material.

TEMPERATURE SENSITIVITY

Zinc phosphate cement is exothermic in action. (**Exothermic** means giving off heat.) To dissipate this heat before placement in the cavity preparation, the cement must be spatulated (mixed) slowly over a wide area of a cool, dry, thick glass slab.

Also, the temperature of the glass slab is an important variable in the mixing time for zinc phosphate cement. The ideal slab temperature is 68°F. This temperature allows a longer working time and permits a maximum amount of powder to be incorporated into the liquid without making the mix too thick. A higher temperature will accelerate (speed) the set of the cement.

Although a cool slab is desirable, the slab should not be cooled below the dew point. (The **dew point** is the temperature at which condensation occurs.) If condensation occurs, the moisture on the slab is incorporated into the mix. This adversely affects the setting time and possibly the strength of the mix.

It is critical that the powder be added to the liquid in very small increments. Each increment is spatulated slowly and thoroughly before the next increment is added. This procedure dissipates the heat of the chemical action and retards the set of the cement.

MIXING AND SETTING TIMES

Depending on the manufacturer's formula, the maximum mixing time for zinc phosphate cement is 1 to 2

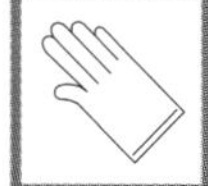
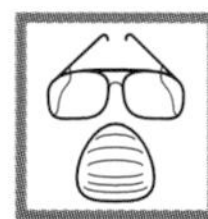
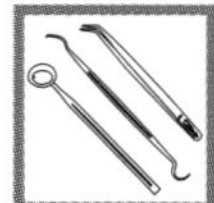
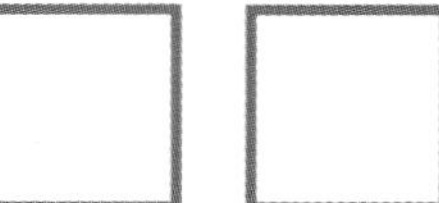

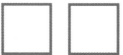

PROCEDURE: **Mixing Zinc Phosphate Cement**

The following are general, not brand-specific, instructions for mixing zinc phosphate cement by a right-handed assistant.

Instrumentation

Glass slab (cool and dry), 1 × 3 × 6 inches
Spatula (flexible stainless steel)
Powder and liquid (from the same manufacturer)
Powder dispenser (from the manufacturer)
Additional placement instruments (determined by the use of the cement and the operator's preferences)

Mixing the Cement

1. Place the measured powder toward one end of the glass slab. Immediately replace the cap on the powder bottle.
   □ *RATIONALE:* Recapping immediately prevents accidentally spilling or contamination of the powder.
2. Use the flat side of the spatula to flatten the powder. Then use the edge of the spatula to divide the powder into sections according to the manufacturer's instructions.
3. Just before mixing, use a circular swirling motion to mix the liquid in its bottle. Use the dropper to dispense the liquid onto the opposite end of the slab. Expel excess liquid from the dropper back into the bottle and recap the bottle immediately.
   □ *RATIONALE:* Contact with the rubber dropper may contaminate the liquid. Leaving the bottle uncapped may alter the water content of the liquid. It could also accidentally spill.
4. Incorporate each increment in the sequence, and for the length of time, specified by the manufacturer (Fig. 23–6).
5. Mix the powder and liquid with the flat side of the spatula over a wide area of the slab (Fig. 23–7).
   □ *RATIONALE:* It is important to spread the material enough to dissipate the heat. It is also important to avoid wasting material.
6. Complete the mix within the allowed mixing time. The mix should be of the appropriate consistency for the intended use.

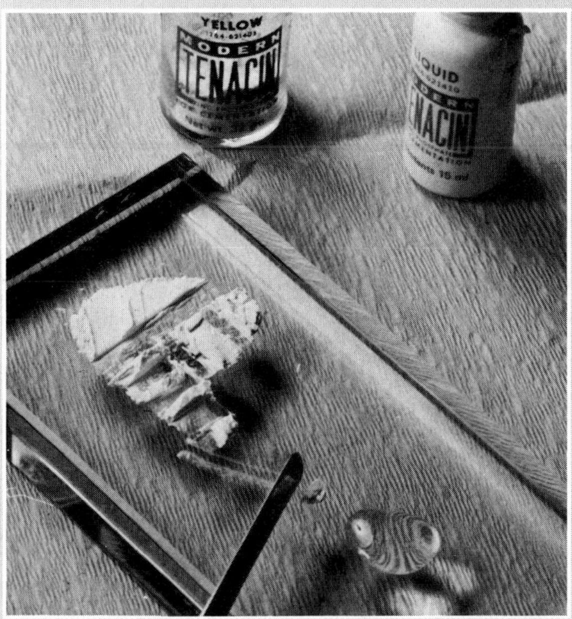

FIGURE 23–6

Starting to mix zinc phosphate cement. The initial increments are very small and made slowly.

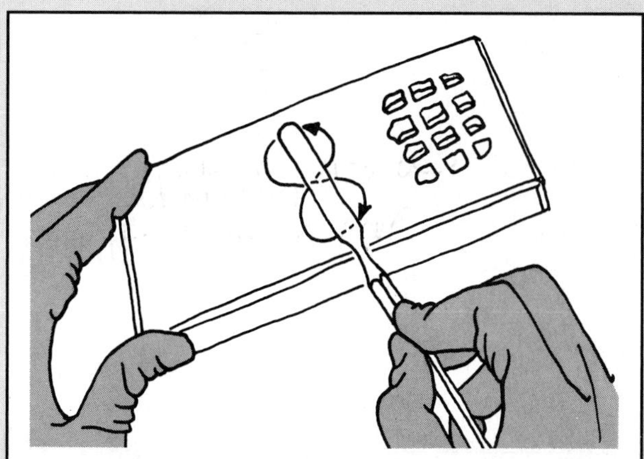

FIGURE 23–7

Mixing zinc phosphate cement, using a figure-eight motion.

minutes. With correct mixing, the setting time in the mouth is 5 to 9 minutes. (The mix does not set as quickly on the slab because the slab is cooler than the mouth.)

Prolonging the setting time allows the operator more working time. This is particularly important during cementation and may be accomplished by

- Using a cool, dry slab
- Decreasing the rate at which the powder increment is incorporated into the liquid at each increment
- Allowing a pause after *initially* incorporating a pinhead amount of powder into the liquid. (The length of the pause varies; check the manufacturer's directions for exact time.)

MANIPULATING ZINC PHOSPHATE CEMENT

All brands of zinc phosphate cement are manipulated in basically the same manner:

- Before mixing, read and carefully follow the manufacturer's directions for the brand being mixed.
- Determine the use and then measure the powder and liquid according to the manufacturer's instructions.
- Place the powder toward one end of the slab and the liquid toward the opposite end. (The space between allows room for mixing.)
- Divide the powder into small sections. (Each manufacturer uses a slightly different system for sectioning the powder.) Some divide it into equal parts; others divide the powder into progressively smaller increments. When increment sizes vary, the smaller increments are used first.)
- Slowly incorporate each powder increment into the liquid, and then mix thoroughly. (Mixing time per increment also varies. The time is approximately 15 to 20 seconds.)
- Mix by using broad strokes or a figure-eight movement over a large area of the slab. (This aids in dissipating the heat generated during mixing.)
- Total mixing time is approximately 1½ minutes. (Here too there are differences from one brand to another.)

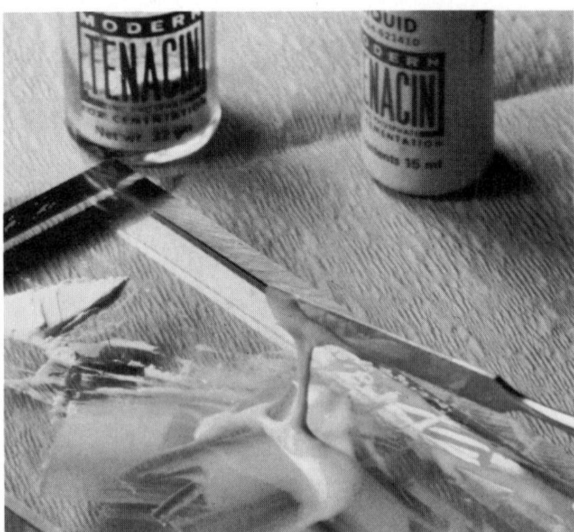

FIGURE 23–8

Testing the mix of zinc phosphate for cementation.

ZINC PHOSPHATE FOR AN INSULATING BASE

A thick, putty-like mix is needed for an insulating base. This is obtained, as specified by the manufacturer, by using a larger portion of powder to the amount of liquid.

The completed mix is formed into a ball on the slab. An explorer, a plastic instrument, or a spoon excavator is used to place the mix in the cavity preparation. The base is gently packed into place with the use of smooth amalgam condensers of graduated sizes.

To prevent the mix from sticking to the instruments, the tips of the condensers are dipped into alcohol or cement powder before use.

ZINC PHOSPHATE FOR CEMENTATION

For cementation, the consistency is correct when the mix adhering to the spatula elongates into a strand when held about 1 inch from the slab (Fig. 23–8).

The cement is distributed so that all *inner* surfaces of the crown are covered, including the margins but not the exterior of the crown.

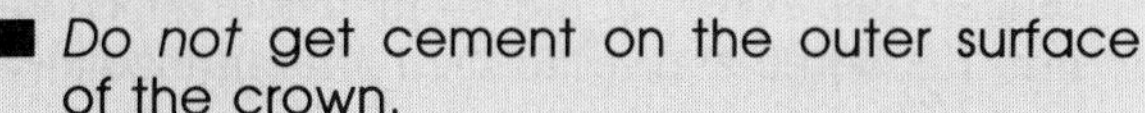

Guidelines for Cementation

- *Do not* get cement on the outer surface of the crown.
  Rationale: This is wasteful and difficult to remove.
- *Do not* trap air bubbles in the cement.
  Rationale: Bubbles will prevent satisfactory seating of the crown.
- *Do not* completely fill the crown with cement.
  Rationale: Excess cement may be forced under the gingiva and injure these tissues. The goal is a thin film thickness over the entire inner surface.
- *Do* complete this quickly.
  Rationale: The crown must be ready to seat before the cement begins to set.

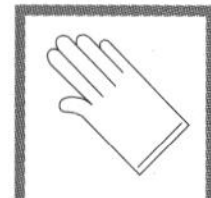 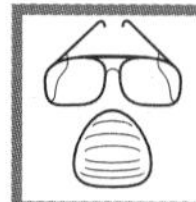 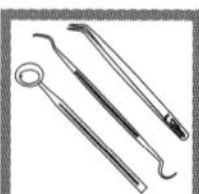 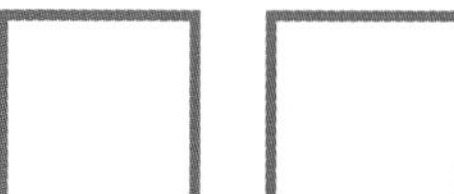

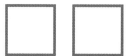

PROCEDURE: **Placing Cement in the Crown**

1. Hold the crown with the inner portion of the crown facing upward.
2. Use the spatula to scoop up the cement. Scrape the edge of the spatula along the crown margin.
   □ *RATIONALE:* This permits the cement to flow from the spatula into the crown.
3. Press the tip of the spatula, or an explorer, into the bulk of the cement in the crown and use a circular motion to break up any air bubbles that might have formed.
   □ *RATIONALE:* Air bubbles in the cement prevent proper seating. This motion also ensures that the inner surfaces are covered.
4. Hold the crown in the proper position for placement. This is with the buccal/lingual and mesial/distal surfaces oriented as they will be when the crown is seated in the patient's mouth.
   □ *RATIONALE:* This enables the operator to seat the crown without having to first shift its position in his or her hand.
5. Pass crown to operator for cementation.
6. Pass cotton roll or wooden bite-stick so the patient can help seat the crown and displace the excess cement.

CARE OF THE SLAB AND INSTRUMENTS

It is important to avoid scratching the glass slab, because any rough areas on the slab will retain particles of the previous mix. If incorporated into a new mix, these particles will cause acceleration (faster set) of the zinc phosphate cement.

Before the cement has hardened, it can be removed from the glass slab and spatula by holding them under running water.

If the mix has hardened, it can be loosened by permitting a solution of bicarbonate of soda and water to stand on the slab and spatula. This solution dissolves the cement.

After the slab and spatula have been cleaned, the appropriate exposure control steps are followed before the slab and spatula can be used again.

Zinc Oxide–Eugenol Cement

Zinc oxide–eugenol (ZOE) cement consists of a liquid (eugenol) that is mixed with a powder that is primarily zinc oxide.

Unlike the phosphoric acid in zinc phosphate cement, the eugenol in ZOE does not irritate the pulp, and ZOE is often used as a sedative treatment for sensitive teeth and in situations in which postoperative sensitivity is a potential problem.

Zinc oxide–eugenol Type I lacks strength and long-term durability. For this reason, it is used for temporary or provisional cementation of cast restorations.

Zinc oxide–eugenol Type II has reinforcing agents added and is used for the permanent luting of cast restorations. (See section on ortho-ethoxybenzoic acid cements.)

Zinc oxide–eugenol is *not* used as an insulating base under amalgam restorations because it lacks the strength to resist the pressure during condensation of the amalgam. This weakness may cause the restoration to crack.

Zinc oxide–eugenol is *not* used under composite, glass ionomer, or other resin restorations because the eugenol in the liquid retards the setting of the resin materials.

EUGENOL PRECAUTIONS

Eugenol has a very strong odor. This is similar to that of cloves. To prevent other materials from being contaminated by this odor, eugenol should be stored away from other materials. When eugenol is dispensed, the bottle is recapped immediately.

Also, avoid getting eugenol into the rubber bulb of the dropper on the liquid bottle. The eugenol breaks down the rubber, and this contaminates the liquid.

Eugenol is also irritating to the oral mucosa when it

is in direct contact with it. Because of eugenol's disadvantages, some materials that previously contained it are now available in non-eugenol formulations.

ZINC OXIDE–EUGENOL MIXING AND SETTING TIMES

Zinc oxide–eugenol is usually mixed on an oil-resistant (parchment) paper pad. When a slower set is required, a glass slab may be used.

The higher the powder-to-liquid ratio, the faster the set. The normal mixing time ranges from 30 to 60 seconds. The normal setting time in the mouth ranges from 3 to 5 minutes. However, like those of other materials, these specifics depend upon the manufacturer's directions.

When used as a sedative treatment, a thick mix is required. For use in temporary cementation of provisional coverage, a thinner mix is necessary. The thickness of the mix is determined by the powder-to-liquid ratio as recommended by the manufacturer.

Zinc oxide–eugenol is also supplied as a two-paste system. These pastes are dispensed in equal lengths on a paper pad and mixed according to the manufacturer's directions.

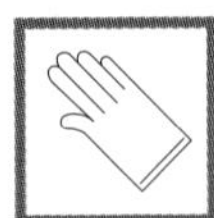
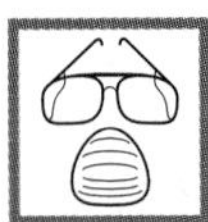
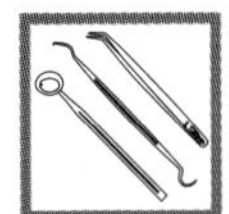

PROCEDURE: **Mixing Zinc Oxide–Eugenol Cement**

The following are general, not brand-specific, instructions for mixing ZOE cement that is supplied as a powder and liquid.

Instrumentation

Parchment paper pad
Spatula (small and flexible)
Zinc oxide powder and dispenser (provided by manufacturer)
Eugenol liquid and dropper (from same manufacturer)
Isopropyl alcohol or oil of orange solvent
Small spoon excavator, explorer, or plastic instrument (for use in placement)

Mixing the Cement

1. Measure the powder and place it on the mixing pad. Replace the cap on the powder container immediately.
2. Dispense the liquid near the powder on the mixing pad (Fig. 23–9). (Do not place the liquid on the powder.) Replace the cap on the liquid container immediately.

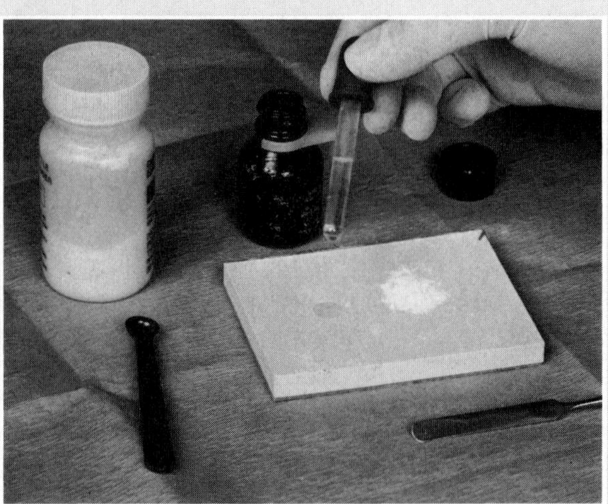

FIGURE 23–9

Dispensing zinc oxide–eugenol powder and liquid.

3. Incorporate the powder and liquid in one or two increments.
4. Mix and strop (wipe vigorously) over a large area of the mixing pad for 5 seconds (Fig. 23–10).
5. For cementation, the mix should be smooth and creamy and completed within the allowed working time. It is placed in the provisional coverage with the same technique as for zinc phosphate cement.
6. For a sedative base, more powder is added to make the mix thicker (Fig. 23–11). It is gathered into a small pellet, and a spoon excavator, an explorer, or a plastic instrument is used to carry it to the base of the cavity preparation.
7. Within the cavity, the mix is placed only on the floor over the pulpal area so that the finished base is even in depth and has a smooth surface.
8. Excess cement is removed with a small spoon excavator.
   □ *RATIONALE:* If too much cement is left in the preparation, there will not be adequate space for the restorative material.

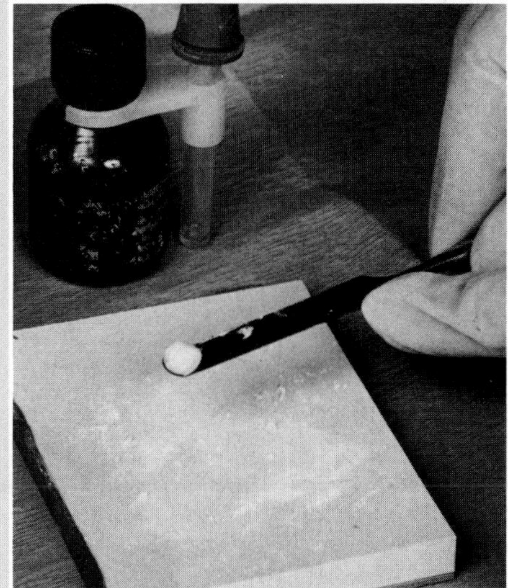

FIGURE 23–11

Zinc oxide–eugenol mixed for a sedative base.

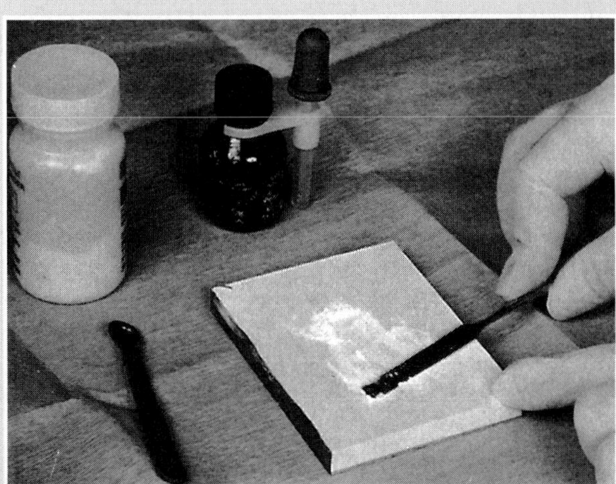

FIGURE 23–10

Mixing zinc oxide–eugenol cement.

CARE OF THE MIXING PAD AND INSTRUMENTS

As soon as possible after mixing, the spatula is wiped free of the mix with a clean tissue or a 2 × 2 inch gauze sponge. The top sheet of the mixing pad is carefully removed and discarded.

If ZOE cement has hardened on the instruments, they may be wiped with alcohol or oil of orange solvent to soften and loosen the cement. Appropriate exposure control measures are then taken.

Ortho-Ethoxybenzoic Acid Cement

The addition of ortho-ethoxybenzoic acid (EBA) to the eugenol liquid and of fillers to the zinc oxide powder results in Type II ZOE cement, which is commonly referred to as EBA cement.

The stronger product is used for permanent cementation of inlays, crowns, and bridges.

The procedures for measuring and mixing EBA cement are similar to those for Type I ZOE cement with these differences:

- The powder is incorporated into the liquid all at once and is mixed for 30 seconds.
- The mix initially is putty-like; additional mixing for another 30 seconds causes the mix to become fluid for loading into the crown.

Intermediate Restorative Material

Intermediate restorative material (IRM) is a reinforced ZOE composition that is used for intermediate restorations that last up to 1 year.

There are many reasons why this type of restoration may be necessary: (1) because of the condition of the tooth, placing a permanent restoration is not advisable at this time; (2) the patient's health does not permit more extensive dental treatment; and (3) when, for financial reasons, more extensive treatment must be postponed.

Intermediate restorative material is available in capsules, which are activated and then triturated. It is also supplied as a powder and liquid that are mixed manually (Fig. 23–12).

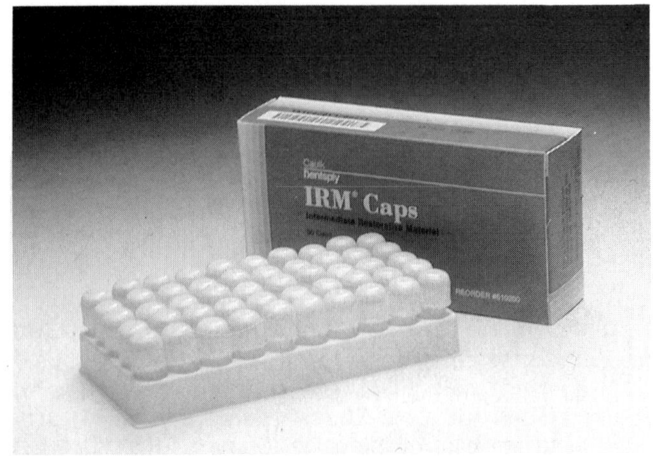

FIGURE 23–12

Immediate restorative material (IRM) capsules are activated and triturated according to the manufacturer's instructions. (Courtesy of Caulk Division, Densply, Milford, DE.)

Polycarboxylate Cement

Polycarboxylate cement differs from the cements previously discussed in that it forms a bond with the tooth. Some formulas also contain crystals that slowly release fluoride. For these reasons, it is used for the cementation of orthodontic bands and cast restorations; however, the tooth surface must be very clean to achieve a good bond with the cement. One means of preparing the tooth is by cleaning it with a pumice slurry (a mixture of pumice and water), followed by thorough rinsing and drying.

Polycarboxylate cement, also known as *polyacrylic cement*, is also used as a nonirritating base under either composite or amalgam restorations and may be used for intermediate restorations.

Polycarboxylate cement is supplied in the form of a powder and liquid. The composition of the powder is similar to that of zinc phosphate cement. The liquid is polyacrylic acid and water. This liquid has a limited shelf life because it thickens as the water evaporates from it. If the liquid has thickened, it should be discarded.

When properly mixed, polycarboxylate cement is similar to zinc phosphate cement in solubility and tensile strength.

The pH of the liquid is quite low (1.7); however, the pH increases rapidly as the material sets, and at 24 hours, it is similar to that of zinc phosphate cement. Polycarboxylate cement is less irritating to pulp than is zinc phosphate cement, and the pulpal reaction is similar to that with ZOE cement.

DISPENSING POLYCARBOXYLATE CEMENT LIQUID AND POWDER

To measure the powder, use the powder measurer supplied by the manufacturer. Press this firmly down into the powder in the bottle. As the measure is removed from the bottle, use the spatula to scrape away excess powder so that the powder is flush with the top of the measuring device.

The liquid may be measured by using either the plastic squeeze bottle or the calibrated syringe-type liquid dispenser supplied by the manufacturer. (Of the two, the calibrated syringe dispenser is more accurate.)

 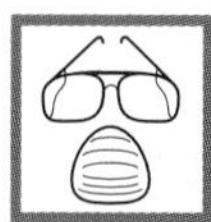 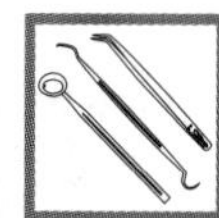 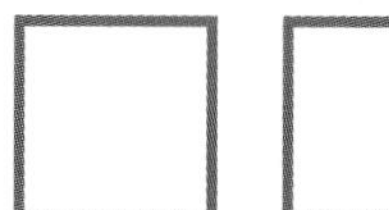

PROCEDURE: **Manually Mixing Intermediate Restorative Material**

Intermediate restorative material is available in capsules, which are activated and then triturated. It is also supplied as a powder and liquid that are mixed manually (Fig. 23–12).

Instrumentation (Fig. 23–13)

Parchment paper pad
Spatula (small and flexible)
Powder and dispenser (provided by manufacturer)
Liquid and dropper (provided by the same manufacturer)

Mixing the Cement

1. Fluff the powder before dispensing, then measure one large scoop of powder onto the mixing pad. Dispense one drop of liquid near the powder on the mixing pad. Recap the containers immediately.
2. Incorporate one-half of the powder into the liquid and mix quickly.
3. Incorporate the remaining powder into the mix in two or three increments, and spatulate thoroughly. The mix will be quite stiff.
4. Vigorously wipe the mix back and forth on the mixing pad for 5 to 10 seconds. The resulting mix should be smooth and adaptable. The mix must be completed within 1 minute.

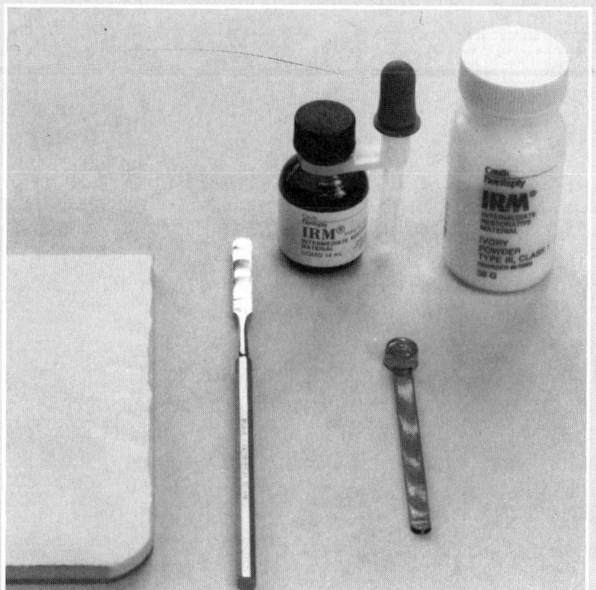

FIGURE 23–13

IRM instrumentation. *Left to right,* Paper mixing pad, small spatula, liquid and dropper, measure for powder, and powder. (From Ehrlich, A., and Torres, H.O.: Essentials of Dental Assisting. Philadelphia, W.B. Saunders Co., 1992, p 361.)

When a calibrated syringe-type liquid dispenser is used, one full calibration of liquid is obtained by moving the plunger from one full calibration mark to the next full calibration mark.

If the plastic squeeze bottle is used, the bottle is held in a vertical position and squeezed as shown in Figure 23–14.

The recommended powder-to-liquid ratio is determined by the manufacturer; the measuring devices are supplied with the following ratios for cementation and bases:

- The ratio for cementation is 1 scoop of powder to 3 drops of liquid (or 1 scoop of powder to 1 full calibration of liquid).
- The ratio for a base is 1 scoop of powder to 2 drops of liquid (or 1 scoop of powder to ⅔ full calibration of liquid).

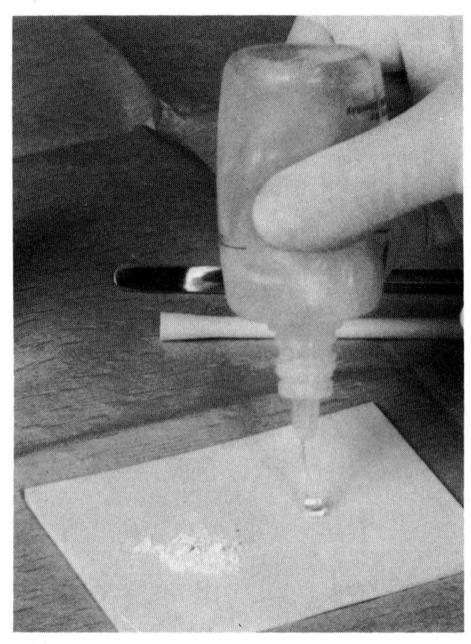

FIGURE 23–14

Dispensing liquid for polycarboxylate cement. (From Ehrlich, A., and Torres, H.O.: Essentials of Dental Assisting. Philadelphia, W.B. Saunders Co., 1992, p 362.)

MANIPULATING POLYCARBOXYLATE CEMENT

Although polycarboxylate cement has many characteristics that are similar to those of zinc phosphate cement, it is *not* mixed in a similar manner.

The following are general instructions for mixing polycarboxylate cement. Before actual mixing, read and follow the manufacturer's instructions.

The material is usually mixed on a nonabsorbent paper pad; however, if it is necessary to increase the working time, a cool (68°F), dry glass slab is used.

The instruments selected for applying the cement depend upon the purpose of the mix and the operator's preference.

CARE OF THE MIXING SLAB AND INSTRUMENTS

Because of the adhesive nature of polycarboxylate cement, the spatula, glass slab, and other instruments should be rinsed clean of cement under running water *immediately* after use. The appropriate exposure control steps are then taken.

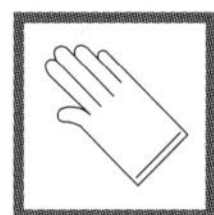 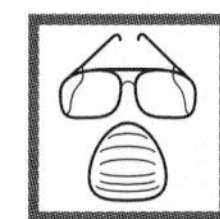 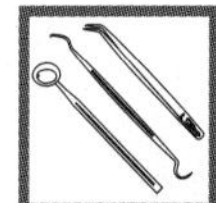  

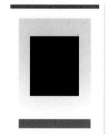

PROCEDURE: Mixing Polycarboxylate Cement

Instrumentation

Nonabsorbent paper pad
Spatula (small, flexible steel)
Powder and measuring device (provided by the manufacturer)
Liquid and measuring device (provided by the same manufacturer)
Operator's choice of placement instrument (usually a small spoon excavator or a ball burnisher)

Mixing the Cement

1. Gently shake the container to fluff the powder, then measure the powder onto the mixing pad. Immediately recap the container.
2. Just before mixing, dispense the liquid. Immediately recap the container.
   □ *RATIONALE:* The water content of this liquid is critical. If left out too long before mixing, water may evaporate from the liquid.

3. Use the flat side of the spatula to quickly incorporate and mix all of the powder into the liquid at one time.
   ☐ *RATIONALE:* The mix *must* be completed within 30 seconds.
4. A correct mix is somewhat thick and has a shiny, glossy surface. It will form a thin strand when picked up by the spatula (Fig. 23–15).
5. Do not over-spatulate. Do not use the mix if it has lost its glossy appearance or reached the stringy (tacky) stage on the slab.
   ☐ *RATIONALE:* A mix that has lost its gloss or is stringy will not form an adhesive bond with the tooth.
7. Dip the end of the placement instrument in cement powder to prevent the cement from sticking to it.

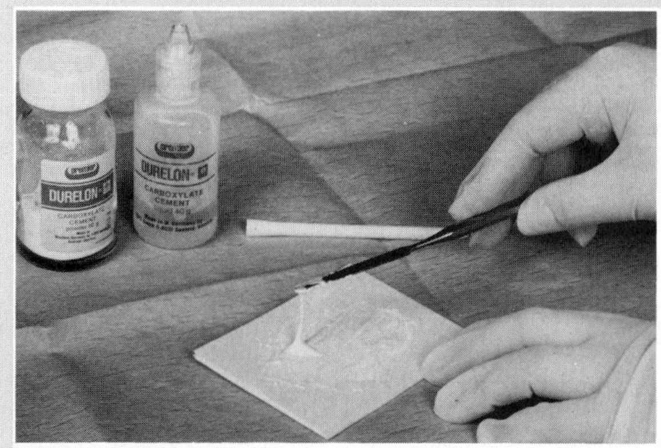

FIGURE 23–15

Polycarboxylate cement mixed for cementation.

Glass Ionomer Cements

Glass ionomers bond to enamel, dentin, and metallic materials. These cements are supplied in the form of a powder and liquid. The powder is an acid-soluble calcium fluoroaluminosilicate glass. The slow release of fluoride from this powder inhibits recurrent decay.

The formulas for the liquid vary. Most are aqueous solutions of polyacrylic acid. (**Aqueous** means containing water.) The water content of the liquid is very important to the setting reaction and the liquids must be protected from water loss or gain. If mixing the material manually, the liquid is dispensed just before use and the container is covered immediately. If the liquid becomes thick, it must be discarded.

These cements have the added advantages of (1) being relatively kind to the pulp; (2) having low solubility in the mouth; (3) adhering to slightly moist tooth surfaces; and (4) leaving a very thin film thickness.

Glass ionomer cements are supplied in special formulations for each specific application (Fig. 23–16):

- **Type I,** for the cementation of metal restorations and direct-bonded orthodontic brackets
- **Type II,** for Class III and Class V cavities as well as restoring areas of erosion near the gingiva
- **Type III,** used as liners and dentin bonding agents
- **Metal-modified glass ionomer,** used for core build-ups and some conservative posterior restorations

BEFORE PLACEMENT

The surface receiving the cement must be clean. This means that the smear layer must be removed from the tooth. When used for cementation, the metal restoration or orthodontic bracket must also be cleaned and etched before the cement is applied.

GLASS IONOMER MIXING AND SETTING TIMES

Each type of glass ionomer cement is mixed and placed in accordance with the manufacturer's directions. These are very specific and must be followed exactly. They include the powder-to-liquid ratio, which must not be altered. Any deviation from the recom-

(Text continues on page 450)

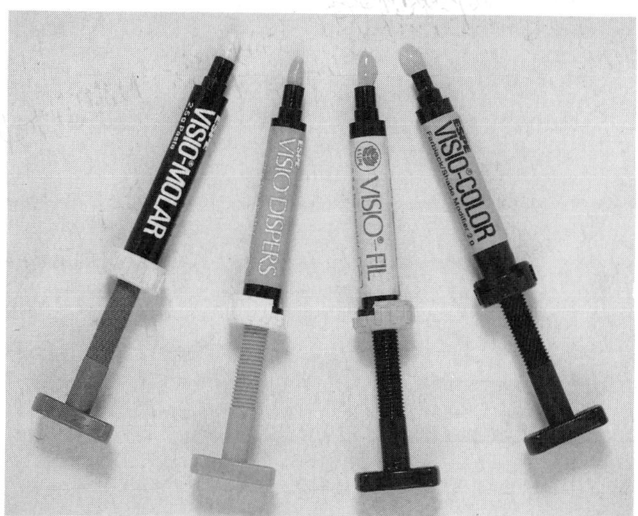

FIGURE 23–16

Glass ionomer cement is supplied in special formulations for each application. (Courtesy of Premier Espe Sales Corp, Norristown, PA.)

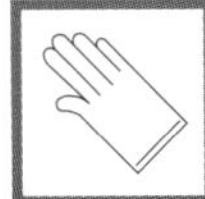
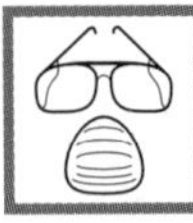
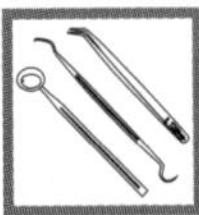

PROCEDURE: **Triturating Glass Ionomer Capsules**

1. Activate the capsule by using the activator provided by the manufacturer (Fig. 23–17).
2. Place the activated capsule in a high-speed amalgamator, and triturate (mix) for the time recommended by the manufacturer.
   ☐ *RATIONALE:* This must be a high-speed amalgamator, and the trituration time is usually 10 seconds.
3. Insert the capsule into the dispenser supplied by the manufacturer and immediately release the sealing pin (Fig. 23–18).
4. Dispense the material by squeezing the dispenser (Fig. 23–19).
5. After use, discard the capsule. Disinfect the activator and dispenser during treatment room cleanup.

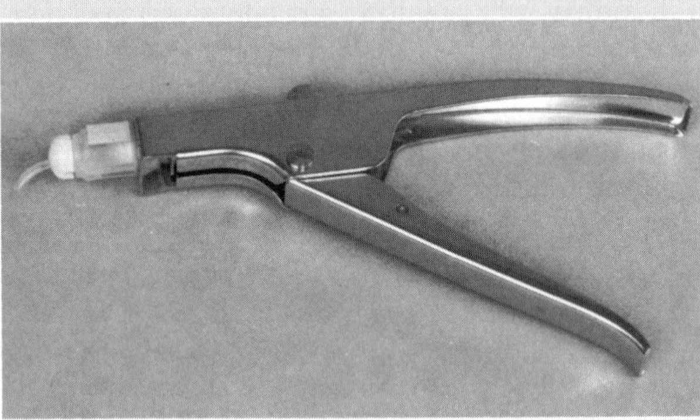

FIGURE 23–18

After the glass ionomer cement capsule has been triturated, it is placed in the dispenser. (From Ehrlich, A., and Torres, H.O.: Essentials of Dental Assisting. Philadelphia, W.B. Saunders Co., 1992, p 364.)

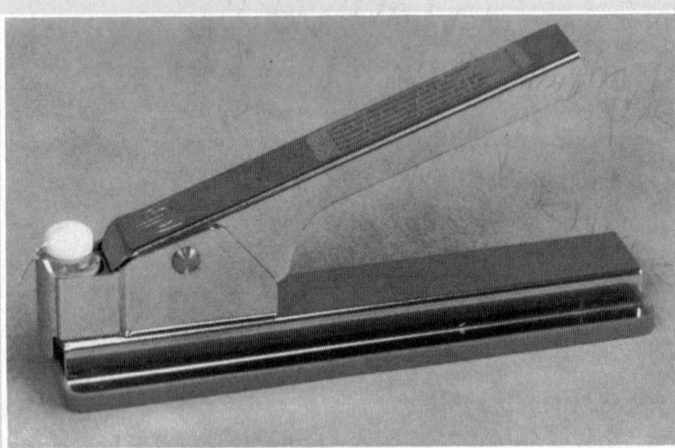

FIGURE 23–17

An "activator" is used to activate the glass ionomer cement capsule. (From Ehrlich, A., and Torres, H.O.: Essentials of Dental Assisting. Philadelphia, W.B. Saunders Co., 1992, p 364.)

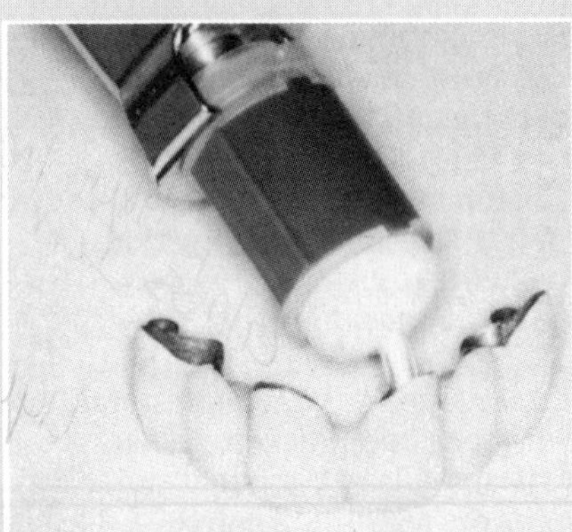

FIGURE 23–19

Glass ionomer cement being dispensed for the cementation of a maxillary anterior fixed bridge. (Courtesy of Premier Espe Sales Corp, Norristown, PA.)

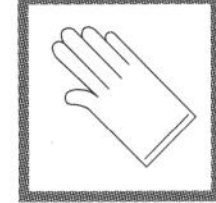
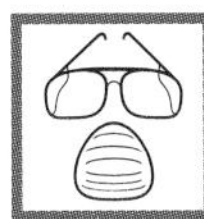
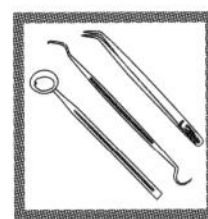
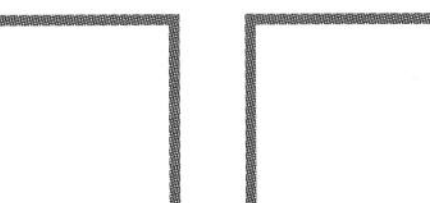

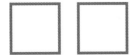

PROCEDURE: **Mixing Calcium Hydroxide Cement**

Instrumentation

Parchment paper pad (small)
Ball-shaped mixer-applicator
Calcium hydroxide base and catalyst paste (from the same manufacturer)
Sterile gauze sponges

Mixing the Cement

1. Extrude very small and equal amounts of the catalyst and base pastes onto the paper pad (Fig. 23–20).
   □ *RATIONALE:* This is approximately ½ to 1 mm., depending on the size of the cavity preparation.
2. Use a circular motion to quickly (10 to 15 seconds) mix the materials over a small area of the mixing pad (Fig. 23–21).
   □ *RATIONALE:* Spreading the material out on the pad wastes it.
3. Use a gauze sponge to wipe the mixer-applicator tip clean. Hold the material near the patient's chin, and hand the mixer-applicator to the operator.
4. Remove and discard the used sheet of the mixing pad.
5. Use a tissue or gauze sponge to wipe the mixer-applicator clean; then return it to the instrument tray.

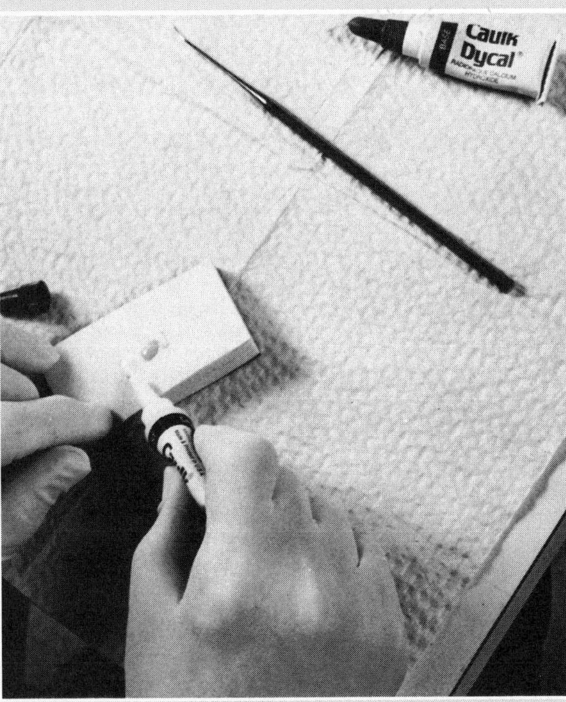

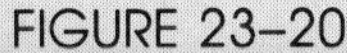
FIGURE 23–20

Dispensing calcium hydroxide catalyst and base.

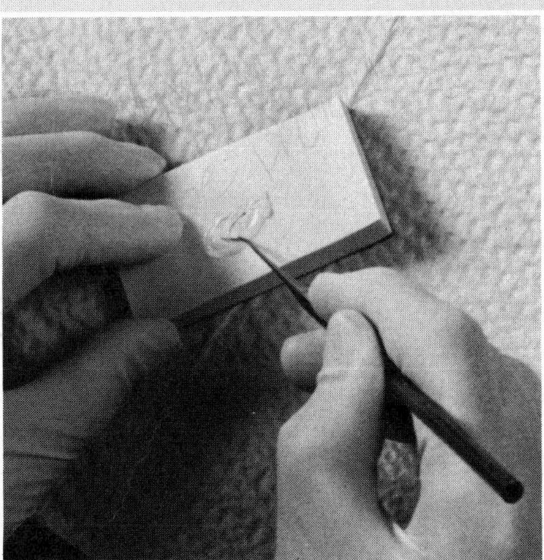

FIGURE 23–21

Mixing calcium hydroxide with a ball-shaped mixer-applicator.

mended ratio changes the characteristics and effectiveness of the cement.

After the powder and liquid are mixed, setting reaction occurs in two steps. The initial hardening occurs very quickly. However, maximum strength and resistance to the oral environment are not developed for 24 hours or longer.

Glass ionomers are available in self-curing and light-cured formulas. They are supplied in bottles of powder and liquid, which are mixed manually, or in capsules, which contain premeasured amounts of powder and liquid. The capsules are more commonly used.

Calcium Hydroxide

Calcium hydroxide protects the pulp by soothing it and may stimulate the production of reparative dentin.

Calcium hydroxide is compatible with all restorative materials, but it is not strong, and a thin layer is placed only over the pulpal floor. If it is also necessary to protect the pulp from thermal shock, an insulating base is placed over the calcium hydroxide.

Calcium hydroxide is available as a two-paste (base and catalyst) system. The catalyst and base pastes *must* be from the same formula and the same manufacturer. The description that follows is of a self-cured mix.

Calcium hydroxide is also available as a light-cured formula, which is frequently selected for use under acid-etched restorations because it is more resistant to the acid-etching process. This material is used according to the manufacturer's directions.

Cavity Liners

Before the placement of the restoration, a cavity liner may be placed to form a barrier that seals the exposed surfaces of the prepared tooth. This step reduces the possibility of postoperative sensitivity or injury to the pulp.

Cavity Varnishes

Varnishes are most commonly used as cavity liners; however, in some situations, dentin bonding material is used instead of a varnish.

COPAL CAVITY VARNISH

Copal cavity varnish consists of copal (a natural gum) dissolved in ether or chloroform (organic solvents). This material is not viscous (thick), and it flows easily. The solvent quickly evaporates and leaves a thin film on the surface. If the material thickens slightly in the bottle, a thinner may be added; however, if the material becomes very thick, it must be discarded.

Copal cavity varnish is used as a cavity liner under an amalgam restoration or on a completed crown preparation to protect the tooth before cementation of the crown.

Because copal cavity varnish interferes with the bonding and setting of composite, resin, or glass ionomer restorations, it *cannot* be used under these materials.

UNIVERSAL CAVITY VARNISH

Universal cavity varnish does *not* contain copal and can be used under several types of restorative materials.

PLACING CAVITY VARNISH

Cavity varnish is placed by a very small disposable brush or a cotton pellet held in cotton pliers. The bottle is uncapped, the applicator is moistened in the liquid, and the bottle is recapped immediately to prevent evaporation. If necessary, excess material is removed from the applicator by blotting it on a 2 × 2 inch gauze sponge.

A thin layer of the varnish is spread on the walls and floor of the cavity preparation, but not on the exterior of the tooth. Varnish that gets on the exterior surface of the tooth is removed with a cotton pellet.

If a second coat of varnish is necessary, a fresh applicator must be used. The applicator is *never* dipped in the varnish a second time because this would contaminate the entire container of solution.

Guidelines for Placement of Cavity Liners

- The liner is placed *over* the calcium hydroxide.
- If a zinc phosphate base is to be placed, the cavity liner is placed *under* this base. (This protects the pulp from irritation by the phosphoric acid in the cement.)
- If a ZOE base is placed, it is not necessary to place a liner under it. (This is because the material is not irritating to the pulp and must be close to the pulp for its soothing effects.)
- The goal is to have a very thin layer of liner covering the walls, floor, and margins of a cavity preparation. (This protects cut tooth surfaces from absorbing restorative material such as amalgam.)
- A tooth that has been prepared for a crown may be coated with a liner before permanent cementation of the crown.

Composite Restorative Materials

The structure and characteristics of composite restorative materials are discussed here. Their application is discussed in Chapter 25.

The Components of Composite Resins

Composites, also known as *resin* restorations, are very important restorative materials. The three major components of dental composites are an organic **resin matrix,** an **inorganic filler,** and a **coupling agent**.

Joining these three materials creates a strong restorative material that can withstand the harsh environment of the mouth, is easily shaped, matches natural tooth color well, and can be bonded directly to the tooth.

THE RESIN MATRIX

Dimethacrylate, referred to as BIS-GMA, is the resin most commonly used in composites. However, urethane dimethacrylate is used in some formulations. Although this is the foundation of the material, this by itself is not strong enough for use as a dental restoration.

FILLERS

The inorganic fillers used in composite resins include quartz, glass, and silica particles. These fillers add the strength and other characteristics necessary for use as restorative materials. The ability of these materials to reflect light aids in creating an esthetically pleasing restoration.

The amount of filler, the particle size, and the type of filler are all important factors in determining the strength and wear resistance characteristics of the material. They also influence the polished finish of the restoration.

Macrofilled Composites. The macrofilled composites, also known as *conventional composites*, contain the largest of filler particles, providing greater strength but a duller, rougher surface. Macrofilled composites are used in areas where greater strength is required to resist fracture.

Microfilled Composites. As the name implies, the inorganic filler in microfilled composites is much smaller in size than that of a macrofilled composite.

Microfilled composite resins are capable of producing a highly polished finished restoration and are used primarily in anterior restorations, in which smoothness is the primary concern.

Hybrid Composites. Hybrid composites contain both macrofill and microfill particles. The hybrids are more polishable than the macrofilled composites and have more strength than the microfilled composites. They also have high wear resistance and excellent shading characteristics.

COUPLING AGENT

The coupling agent is important because it strengthens the composite by chemically bonding the filler to the resin matrix. To achieve this, the filler particles are coated with an organosilane compound.

The silane portion of the molecule bonds to the quartz, glass, and silica filler particles. The organic portion bonds with the resin matrix, thus bonding the filler to the matrix.

Polymerization of Composite Resins

Polymerization is the process in which the resin material is changed from a plastic state (in which it can be molded or shaped) into a hardened restoration. The manner in which polymerization occurs depends upon the type of material used. Composites come in two forms: self-cured and light-cured.

SELF-CURED COMPOSITES

Self-cured composites are supplied as two pastes and polymerization is brought about by a chemical reaction when the pastes are mixed.

The **catalyst**, also known as the *initiator*, contains a benzoyl peroxide. The **base**, also known as the *activator*, contains a tertiary amine. When these pastes are mixed, a chemical reaction begins in which the amine of the base reacts with the benzoyl peroxide of the catalyst to form free radicals that initiate (start) polymerization of the resin material.

Polymerization continues until the cure is complete and the material is hard. The material must be in place for the restoration before it reaches this final cure. When the cure is complete, the restoration can be polished.

Manipulating Self-Cured Composites. Self-cured composites are supplied as two containers of paste. When these materials are removed from the container, it is important not to contaminate the remainder of the contents.

The manufacturer supplies small double-ended plastic mixing sticks and a mixing pad. Use one end of the mixing stick to remove the base material and the opposite end of the mixing stick to remove the catalyst material. These are used in equal quantities.

Use the plastic stick to thoroughly mix the materials within 30 seconds. Follow the manufacturer's instructions, and take care to avoid incorporating air bubbles into the mix.

LIGHT-CURED COMPOSITES

Light-cured composites are supplied as a single paste in a light-proof syringe (Fig. 23–22).

This paste, which contains both the photo initiator and the amine activator, does not polymerize until it is exposed to a curing light that gives off the proper wavelength of light. Exposure to this light for the

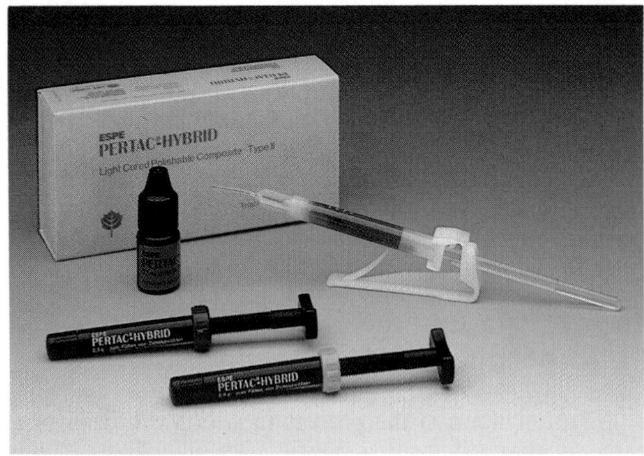

FIGURE 23–22

Light-cured composites are supplied in light-proof syringes. *Bottom,* Two composite syringes. *Upper right,* Acid etchant syringe. *Upper left,* Bonding materials. (Courtesy of Premier Espe Sales Corp, Norristown, PA.)

proper length of time is essential for the successful curing of the restoration.

Manipulating Light-Cured Composites. Light-cured composites do not require mixing and are used directly as they come from the syringe.

After the composite material is in place, it is exposed to the curing light for 20 to 60 seconds. When larger quantities of the material are being placed, each increment is cured before the next is placed.

The exact curing time depends upon (1) the manufacturer's instructions, which must be followed exactly; (2) the thickness and size of the restoration; and (3) the shade of the restorative material used (the darker the shade, the longer the curing time required).

Glass Ionomer as a Restorative Material

Although they are classified as cements, class ionomers are widely used in Class V restorations. Their advantages include (1) the ability to achieve an excellent match with the tooth color, (2) fluoride release to decrease the incidence of secondary caries, and (3) the ability to be placed in the presence of some moisture.

Glass ionomers do not wear well enough to justify their use in occlusal restorations in permanent teeth; however, light-activated glass ionomers are frequently the preferred materials in primary teeth.

Amalgam Restorative Material

Amalgam restorations are used primarily for posterior restorations, in which strength, not appearance, is of primary importance (see Chapter 25). They are also used in core build-ups before restoration of a badly damaged tooth (see Chapter 31).

The Components of Amalgam

Amalgam is a silver-gray metal restorative material. An **alloy** is a mixture of two or more metals. **Amalgam** is an alloy in which mercury is one of the metals. Although the name has not changed, some of the newer "amalgams" are made without mercury.

Amalgam is soft, pliable, and easily shaped when it is first mixed. At this stage, it can be placed and shaped to fit the prepared tooth. Once it hardens, it forms a very strong restoration that can withstand biting forces.

HIGH-COPPER ALLOYS

High-copper alloys, which are now commonly used in dentistry, are so called because they contain a higher percentage of copper than did earlier alloys.

High-copper alloys are classified according to particle shape as **spherical** (round particles), **comminuted** (rough, lathe-cut particles) and **admixed** (a combination of spherical and comminuted particles).

These particle shapes influence the trituration (mixing) and working characteristics (condensing and carving) of the resulting amalgam mixture.

A high-copper alloy is made up of silver (40 to 60 percent), tin (27 to 30 percent), and copper (13 to 30 percent). The percentages are expressed as percentages of the composition by weight.

NON-ZINC ALLOYS

Some alloys also contain a small quantity of zinc, which is added because of its ability to unite with oxygen and other impurities present in the alloy. However, amalgams containing zinc may expand excessively and corrode if moisture is incorporated during manipulation.

Non-zinc alloys may be used to overcome the problems that occur when moisture is present during placement. However, even these alloys may be affected by the presence of moisture during placement.

MERCURY

Pure mercury is a metal that is liquid at room temperature and has a mirror-like appearance. It is also a hazardous substance and must be handled with proper care. (See the "Special Mercury Considerations" section in Chapter 12.)

MERCURY-ALLOY RATIOS

The appropriate mercury-alloy ratio is very important. The ratio must contain just enough mercury to make the mix plastic (workable) without containing

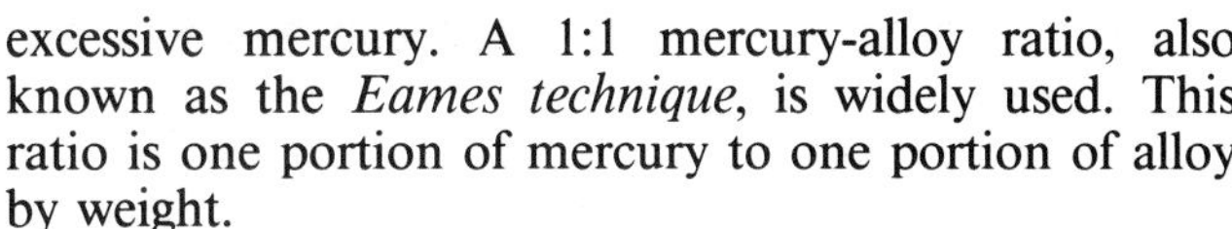

excessive mercury. A 1:1 mercury-alloy ratio, also known as the *Eames technique*, is widely used. This ratio is one portion of mercury to one portion of alloy by weight.

The Manipulation of Amalgam

Single-use capsules are supplied with the proper ratio of mercury and alloy in a sealed capsule. This ensures an accurate mercury-alloy ratio and reduces the possibility of exposure to mercury. Immediately after use, the capsule is reassembled and discarded with nonregulated waste.

A **single capsule** (600 mg. of alloy) is used for small or single-surface restorations. A **double capsule** (800 mg. of alloy) is used for larger restorations. When more than this amount of amalgam is required, additional capsules are mixed as needed.

TRITURATION

Trituration, also known as *amalgamation*, is the process by which the mercury and alloy are mixed together to form the "plastic" mass of amalgam needed to create the dental restoration.

The preloaded capsule of amalgam alloy and liquid mercury contains a **pestle,** which aids in the mixing process. Within the capsule, a thin membrane also separates the mercury and alloy until they are ready to be mixed.

Just before placing the capsule in the amalgamator, an activator is used to break the separating membrane (Fig. 23–23). The activated capsule is placed in the amalgamator, and the cover is closed to prevent mercury vapors from escaping during trituration. (An **amalgamator** is a mechanical device used to triturate amalgam [see Fig. 14–15].)

The amalgamator is set to operate for the length of time specified by the manufacturer's directions. In a proper mix, the plastic mass of amalgam is free of dry alloy particles and does not stick to the sides of the capsule.

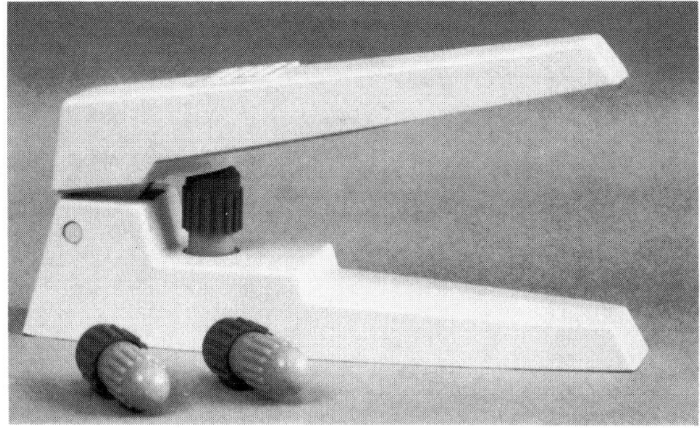

FIGURE 23–23

Just before the capsule is placed in the amalgamator, an activator is used to break the separating membrane. (From Ehrlich, A., and Torres, H.O.: Essentials of Dental Assisting. Philadelphia, W.B. Saunders Co., 1992, p 376.)

The fresh mix is dropped from the capsule into an amalgam well, the pestle is removed, and the mix is loaded into the amalgam carrier.

CONDENSATION

The amalgam is placed in increments in the prepared tooth, and each increment is condensed immediately. The purpose of condensation is to compact the amalgam tightly into all areas of the prepared cavity and to aid in removing any excess mercury from the amalgam mix.

When all of the amalgam has been placed, the surface is smoothed. If excess mercury is present, it is removed with the high-volume evacuator (HVE) before the restoration is carved.

At the end of the procedure, to prevent mercury vapors from escaping, any remaining amalgam scrap is discarded in a sealed container (see Chapter 12).

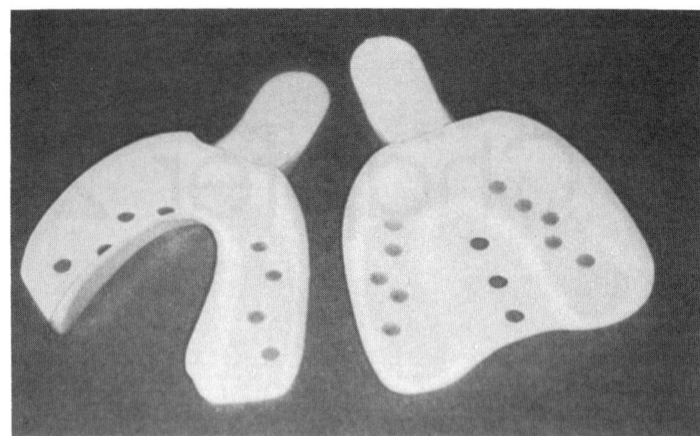

FIGURE 24–1

Stock impression trays. The mandibular and maxillary trays shown here are plastic and have a perforated surface. (Courtesy of 3M Dental Products Division, St. Paul, MN.)

STOCK TRAYS

Stock trays, made of metal or plastic, are available commercially in a range of sizes. They have either a smooth surface or a perforated surface.

Disposable plastic stock trays are discarded after a single use. If a plastic tray is tried in the mouth and not selected for use, it must either be sterilized or discarded. Metal stock trays are cleaned and sterilized before reuse.

CUSTOM TRAYS

A custom tray is constructed by the dental assistant or laboratory technician to fit the mouth of a specific patient. The custom tray is fabricated on a diagnostic cast made from an alginate impression of the arch *before* the teeth were prepared.

Custom trays usually have a solid surface and are painted with an adhesive used to retain the impression material. However, if the dentist prefers a perforated custom tray, an acrylic laboratory bur and a straight handpiece are used to create the perforations.

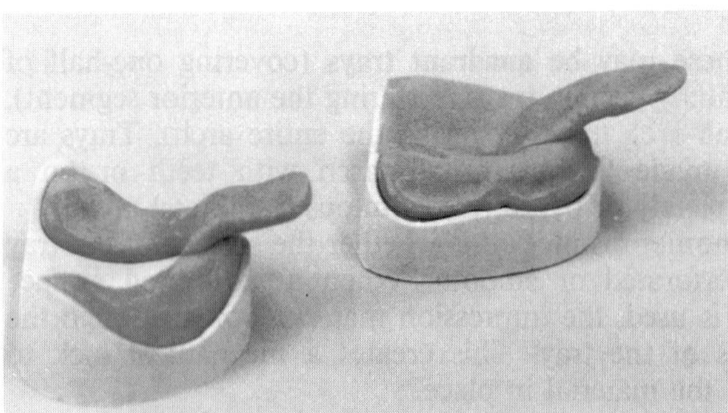

FIGURE 24–2

Custom impression trays for edentulous mandibular and maxillary arches. (From Ehrlich, A., and Torres, H.O.: Essentials of Dental Assisting. Philadelphia, W.B. Saunders Co., 1992, p 402.)

Indications for Use of a Custom Tray

- The dentist prefers a custom tray.
- This is the best way to obtain an accurate impression.
- A stock tray will not fit properly or allow adequate space for the impression material.
- Use of a stock tray will waste impression material and/or result in an inferior impression.

Custom Tray Materials

The following methods or materials are used to construct custom trays: **self-curing acrylic resin**, **light-cured resin**, **thermoplastic material**, and a **vacuum former**.

PROPERTIES OF ACRYLIC RESIN TRAY MATERIALS

A **resin** is a nonmetallic compound, artificially produced (usually from organic compound), that can be molded into various forms and then hardened. Self-curing acrylic resins are the materials most commonly used for creating custom trays.

The major advantage of a self-curing acrylic tray material is that it is strong and is easily adapted to create a custom tray.

The major disadvantages of a self-curing acrylic tray

Criteria for an Acceptable Custom Tray

- It is rigid enough to hold and support the material during tray placement and removal.
- It fits and adapts well to the arch and maintains patient comfort without impinging (pressing uncomfortably) on the surrounding tissues.
- It provides accurate adaptation to an edentulous or partially edentulous arch.
- It maintains an even distribution of 3 to 4 mm. of the impression material between the tray and the teeth.
- The completed maxillary tray covers the teeth and hard palate and extends slightly beyond the gingival margin (but not into the mucobuccal fold).
- The completed mandibular tray covers the teeth and extends beyond the gingival margin (but not into the mucobuccal fold).

material are the hazards of working with the liquid monomer that is very volatile! (**Volatile** means that the material quickly evaporates and forms a vapor.)

This vapor is highly flammable (catches fire easily), is hazardous if inhaled in large concentrations, and may be irritating to the skin. This material must be handled with great care. (This is discussed further in the section "Organic Materials" in Chapter 12.)

Polymerization. Before a resin can be put to its final use, it must be changed from its plastic state and cured into a hardened state. This is accomplished through a process called polymerization. (**Polymerization** is the changing of a material from a plastic to a rigid state.)

Monomers are single particles known as mers. When many of these molecules react or join together, they form a **polymer**. (The prefix *mono-* means one. The prefix *poly-* means many.)

Polymerization, which is also known as *curing,* takes place when the molecules of the catalyst are activated and start to transfer their energy to the monomer molecules. (A **catalyst** is a material that initiates, or starts, a chemical reaction.)

In a self-curing resin, polymerization begins when the **monomer** (a liquid catalyst) and **polymer** (a powder) are mixed together. Once the monomer and polymer are mixed and the polymerization (self-curing) process begins, it cannot be stopped.

These resins are **exothermic,** which means that they give off heat during polymerization. When first mixed, acrylic resin tray is very sticky. It reaches the **initial cure stage** in a matter of minutes, and during this time it begins to harden and to give off heat; however, it can still be shaped.

The material has reached **final set** when it is hard and can no longer be shaped and when the heat has diminished. (The material should not be removed from the cast until it reaches this stage.)

Despite having hardened, the tray material is not dimensionally stable for 24 hours. Therefore, the custom tray should be made 24 hours before the dental appointment. (**Dimensionally stable** means that it will no longer change shape.)

LIGHT-CURED RESIN TRAY MATERIALS

With light-cured resins, a curing light acts as the catalyst to bring about polymerization, and the material remains plastic (workable) until it has been exposed to the curing light. Once exposed, it polymerizes and hardens very quickly.

A specialized form of light-cured resin is used to create custom impression trays. Unlike the other light-cured restorative resins in dentistry, these are cured in a small oven-like appliance that contains a curing light. The design for these trays follows the same principles as for other trays.

THERMOPLASTIC TRAY MATERIALS

Custom trays can also be created with a thermoplastic material. (**Thermoplastic** means that heat causes the material to become soft and workable. When cooled, it is solid.) This material is used according to the manufacturer's guidelines, and the tray design follows the same principles as for other trays (Fig. 24–3).

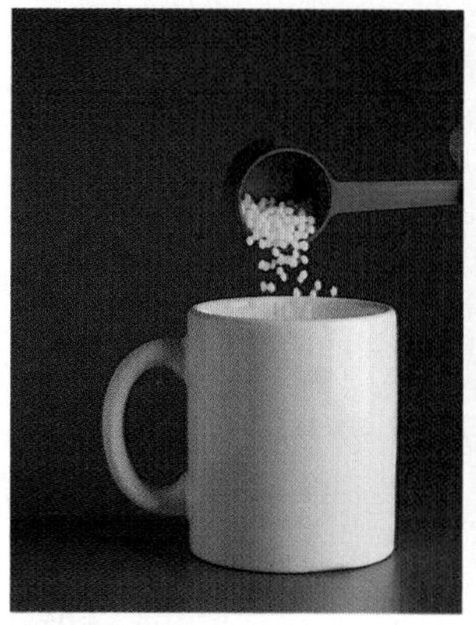
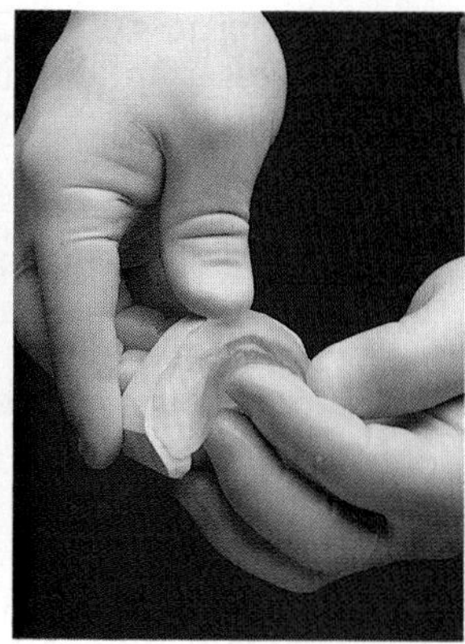

FIGURE 24–3

Thermoplastic tray material. *Left,* Plastic granules are added to a cup of hot water (165°F). *Right,* After 1 minute, the soft mass is removed, kneaded, and shaped to form the tray and handle. (Courtesy of Tak Systems, Wareham, MA.)

Elements of a Custom Impression Tray

No matter what material is used to fabricate the tray, the cast must be prepared and the tray created by using the following technique.

FILLING UNDERCUTS

The first step in cast preparation is to fill all undercuts. (An **undercut** is a recessed area in the surface of the cast or impression.) Undercuts may be caused by air bubbles in cast, the shape of the arch and ridge, carious lesions, fractured teeth, or deep interproximal spaces and malposed teeth.

If undercuts are present on the cast, they may make it impossible to properly seat or remove the tray. These undercuts are filled with wax or other molding material.

OUTLINING THE TRAY

The margins of the finished tray are outlined in pencil on the cast. The outline, which designates the area to be covered by the tray, extends over the attached gingiva to the mucogingival junction and 2 to 3 mm. beyond the last tooth in the quadrant.

THE SPACER

A spacer is placed on the cast to create room in the tray for the impression material. Baseplate wax, a folded moist paper towel, or a commercial nonstick molding material may be used for this purpose.

Room for approximately 2 to 3 mm. of impression material is necessary to obtain a good impression. This is about the thickness of one piece of baseplate wax. The spacer evenly covers the entire area with the finish line marked on the cast.

The spacer is created by cutting a length of baseplate wax, warming it, and placing it on the cast over the area of the tray. A warmed plastic instrument is used to **lute** (secure) the wax to the cast.

SPACER STOPS

Spacer stops are placed to prevent the tray from seating too deeply onto the arch or quadrant. They also allow for an adequate quantity of impression materials around the preparations.

Spacer stops are triangular or round holes that are cut out of the spacer with a laboratory knife or a wax spatula. These cutouts will form bumps on the tissue side of the tray. (The **tissue side** is the inner surface of the completed tray.)

An **edentulous tray** requires a minimum of four stops: one each on the crest of the alveolar ridge in the area of the first or second molar. Additional stops may also be placed on the crest of the ridge in the area of each cuspid.

A tray to take an impression of **prepared natural teeth**, as for a crown or a bridge, has the stops placed near, but not on, the prepared teeth.

SEPARATING MEDIUM

The prepared cast, spacer, and immediate surrounding area are painted with a separating medium so the completed tray can readily be separated from the cast.

THE HANDLE

The tray must have a handle to aid in placing and removing it from the mouth. The handle is *always* placed at the anterior of the tray, as near the midline as possible, facing outward, and parallel to the occlusal surfaces of the teeth.

The handle, which is added after the main portion of the tray has been constructed, must be large and strong enough to provide adequate leverage in removing the tray.

The handle is formed from a piece of scrap acrylic that was just cut away from the tray. The end of the handle and the area where it is to be attached to the tray are moistened with tray resin liquid.

The handle is positioned and pressed firmly in place. It is necessary to hold the handle in place until it is firm enough to stay without support.

REMOVING THE SPACER

After the tray has been formed, it is necessary to remove the spacer and clean the tissue side of the tray.

The heat given off by a self-curing acrylic resin during polymerization causes the wax spacer to adhere to the tray plastic. The tray may be removed from the cast after the resin has reached its initial set (approximately 7 to 10 minutes).

A small stiff brush, such as an old toothbrush, is used to remove most of the wax at this time. The remainder of the spacer is removed, and the interior of the tray is cleaned, after the tray reaches its final set (approximately 30 minutes to an hour).

FINISHING THE TRAY

It is *not* necessary to remove rough areas on the *tissue* side of the tray; this surface will be covered with impression material. However, if the outer edges of the tray are rough, it is necessary to smooth them so they do not injure the tissues of the patient's mouth.

A laboratory knife can be used to smooth minor rough areas. If there are major rough areas, an acrylic bur in a straight hand piece can be used to remove them. An alternative is to use the laboratory lathe to smooth the edges. (Protective eyewear is always worn when the lathe is operated.)

The tray is given a final rinse and disinfected according to the manufacturer's instructions.

TRAY ADHESIVE

The elastomeric impression material is held in place within the tray by a tray adhesive that is painted on the inner surface of the custom tray. This adhesive is specified by the manufacturer and is compatible with the elastomeric impression material.

A tray usually receives two coats of adhesive. The first coat may be applied so that it has time to dry. This may be done in the laboratory or at chairside *before* the preparation of the teeth. The tray is set aside to dry while the teeth are being prepared.

A second coat of tray adhesive is applied to the tray a few minutes before the syringe impression material is ejected around the prepared teeth. This may be done while the dentist is placing the retraction cord.

Vacuum-Formed Custom Trays

The vacuum former utilizes heat and vacuum to shape a sheet of thermoplastic resin to a prepared cast. The vacuum former is discussed in Chapter 14.

In addition to being used for impression trays, the vacuum former has many other uses. The major differences in these applications are the cast preparation and the weight and type of plastic used.

- An **impression tray** uses a rigid heavy gauge plastic and requires a spacer and a handle.
- **Provisional coverage** uses a lighter gauge plastic and does not require a spacer or a handle. (See Chapter 31.)

(text continued on page 464)

PROCEDURE: **Creating an Acrylic Custom Tray**

Instrumentation

Diagnostic cast
Pencil
Tray resin (monomer and polymer from the same manufacturer)
Measurers for liquid and powder (provided by manufacturer)
Baseplate wax
Separating medium with brush
Heat source (alcohol or butane laboratory torch)
Laboratory knife
Laboratory spatula: tapered end and spoon end
Wooden tongue blade
Wax spatula No. 7
Glass jar with lid or smooth-surface paper cup
Petroleum jelly
Tray adhesive and brush (provided by the manufacturer of impression material)

Cast Preparation

1. Fill the undercuts on the diagnostic cast.
2. Outline the tray in pencil (Fig. 24–4).
3. Place the baseplate wax spacer, trim it, and lute the wax to the cast (Figs. 24–5 and 24–6).

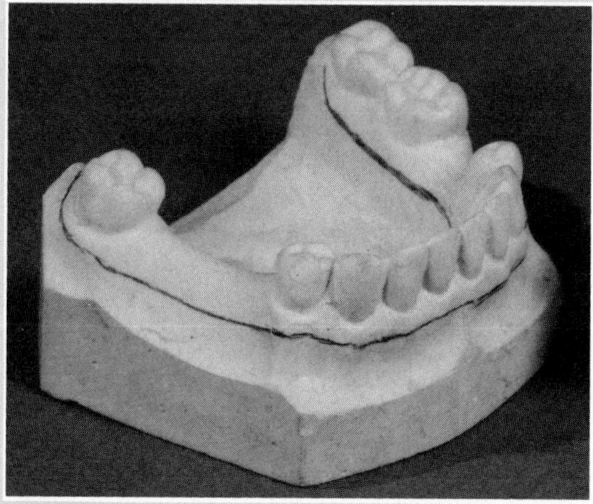

FIGURE 24–4

The tray is outlined in pencil on the cast. This is a mandibular arch with teeth missing in both quadrants.

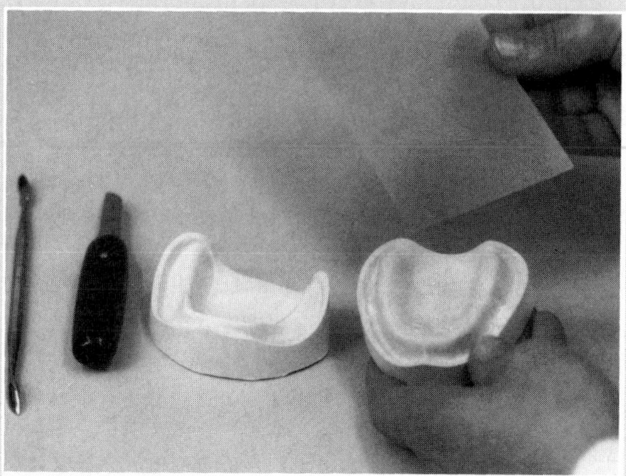

FIGURE 24–5

A sheet of wax is warmed before being shaped to an edentulous maxillary cast. (From Ehrlich, A., and Torres, H.O.: Essentials of Dental Assisting. Philadelphia, W.B. Saunders Co., 1992, p 404.)

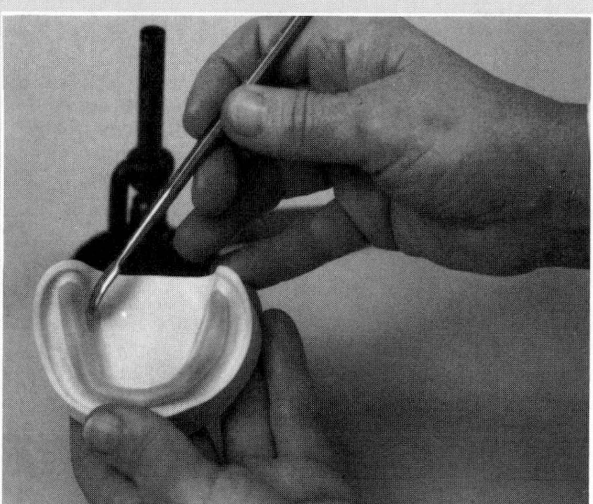

FIGURE 24–6

After the spacer has been fitted and trimmed, a warm instrument is used to lute the edges to the cast. This is an edentulous mandibular cast. (From Ehrlich, A., and Torres, H.O.: Essentials of Dental Assisting. Philadelphia, W.B. Saunders Co., 1992, p 405.)

(continued on following page)

PROCEDURE: **Creating an Acrylic Custom Tray** *(continued)*

4. Cut the appropriate stops in the spacer (Fig. 24–7).
5. Paint the spacer and surrounding area with separating medium (Fig. 24–8).

Mixing the Acrylic Resin

1. Use the manufacturer's measuring devices to measure the powder into the mixing container. Then add an equal part of liquid, and recap the container immediately (Fig. 24–9).
   □ *RATIONALE:* These fumes are toxic.
2. Use the wooden tongue blade to mix the powder and liquid (Fig. 24–10). A homogeneous mix should be obtained within 30 seconds. The mix will be thin and sticky. (**Homogeneous** means the mix has a uniform quality throughout.)
3. Set the mix aside for 2 to 3 minutes to allow polymerization. If the manufacturer specifies a covered container, place the cover during this time.
   □ *RATIONALE:* At this stage, the mix is very sticky.

Forming the Tray

1. When the mix has reached a doughy (not sticky) stage, remove it from the container with the spatula.
2. Lubricate the palms of your hands with petroleum jelly, and knead the resin to form a flat patty that is approximately the size of the wax spacer.
   □ *CAUTION:* Do not knead the dough too much, as it will interfere with working time to adapt and trim the material.

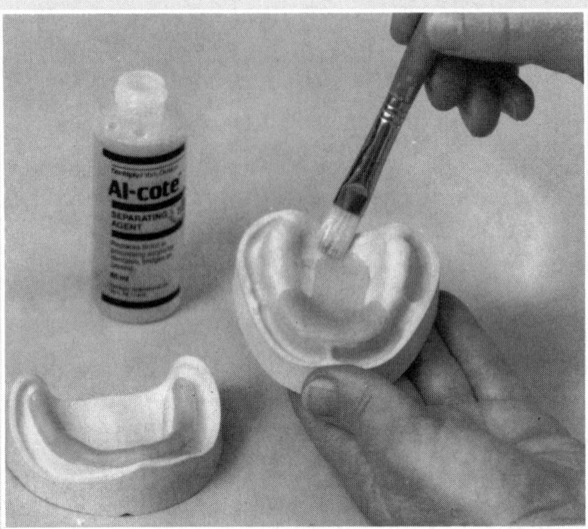

FIGURE 24–8

The completed spacer and cast are painted with separating medium. Note that the spacer is mushroom-shaped in the palatal area of this edentulous maxillary arch. (From Ehrlich, A., and Torres, H.O.: Essentials of Dental Assisting. Philadelphia, W.B. Saunders Co., 1992, p 405.)

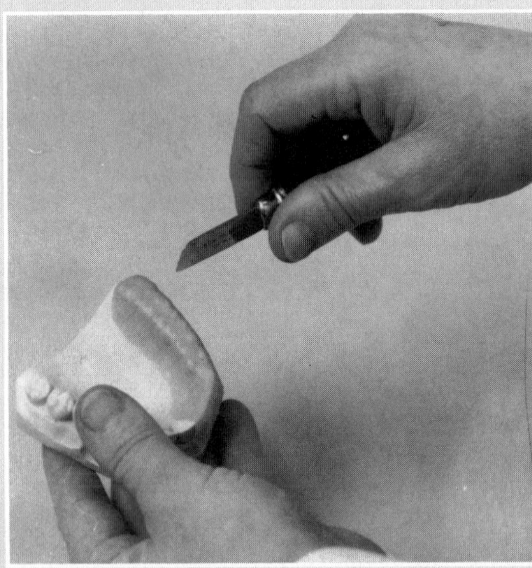

FIGURE 24–7

A laboratory knife is used to cut the stops in the spacer. This maxillary arch cast is being prepared for a quadrant tray. (From Ehrlich, A., and Torres, H.O.: Essentials of Dental Assisting. Philadelphia, W.B. Saunders Co., 1992, p 402.)

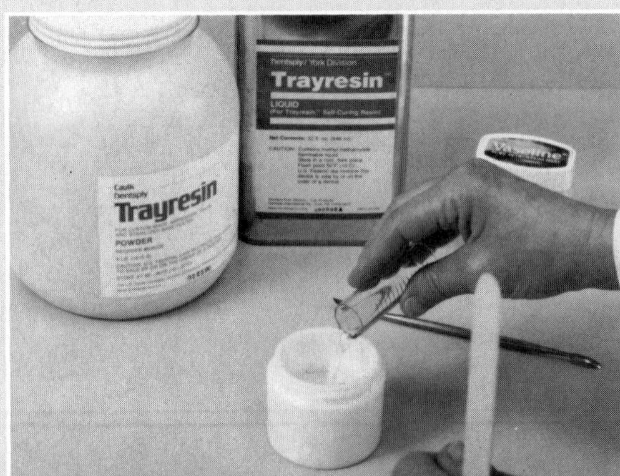

FIGURE 24–9

The tray resin liquid is added to the powder that is already in the mixing container. Both are measured with the use of measuring devices supplied by the manufacturer. (From Ehrlich, A., and Torres, H.O.: Essentials of Dental Assisting. Philadelphia, W.B. Saunders Co., 1992, p 405.)

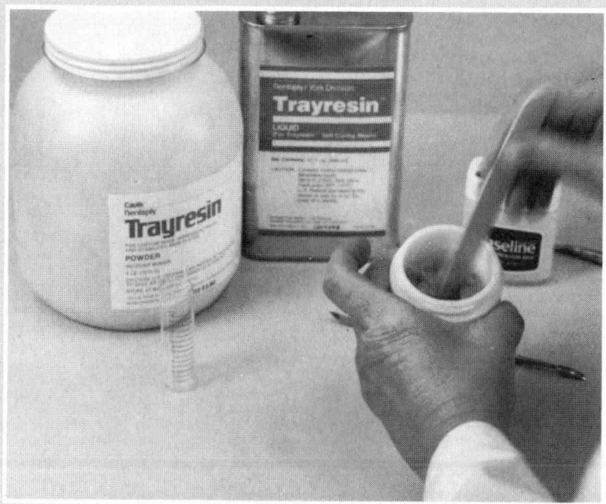

FIGURE 24–10

The tray resin is mixed according to the manufacturer's instructions. (From Ehrlich, A., and Torres, H.O.: Essentials of Dental Assisting. Philadelphia, W.B. Saunders Co., 1992, p 405.)

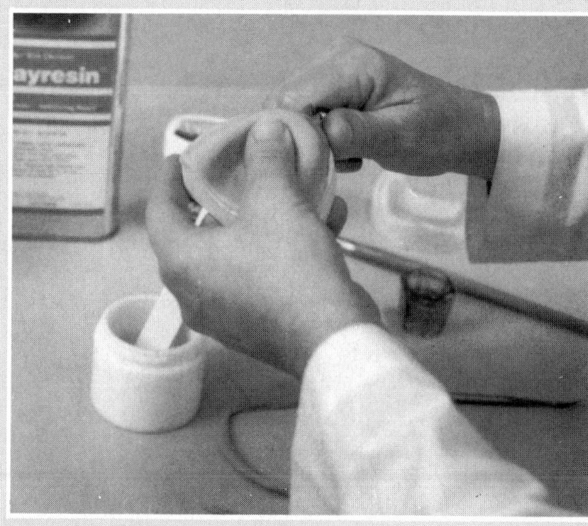

FIGURE 24–12

While the material is still soft, a laboratory knife is used to cut away the excess. (From Ehrlich, A., and Torres, H.O.: Essentials of Dental Assisting. Philadelphia, W.B. Saunders Co., 1992, p 406.)

3. Place the resin dough patty on the cast to cover the wax spacer (Fig. 24–11). Adapt it to extend 1 to 1.5 mm. beyond the edges of the wax spacer.
4. Use a plastic instrument or laboratory knife to quickly trim away the excess tray material while it is still soft (Fig. 24–12).
   ☐ *RATIONALE:* The material is easy to cut at this stage. Trimming now will save time in finishing the tray.

Creating the Handle

1. Use the excess material to shape the handle (Fig. 24–13).

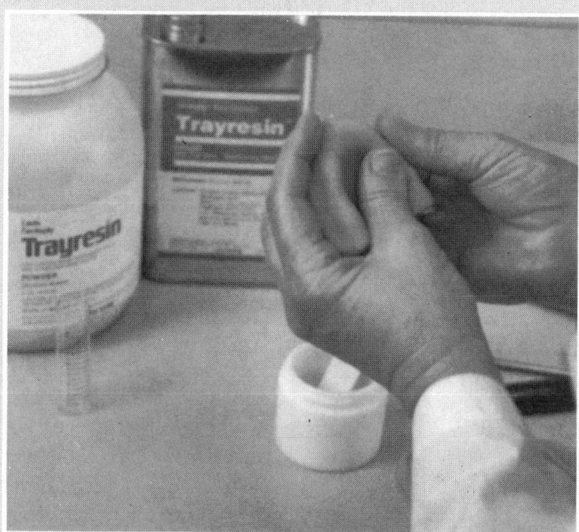

FIGURE 24–11

When the tray resin has reached the doughy stage, it is removed from the container and shaped into a patty. (From Ehrlich, A., and Torres, H.O.: Essentials of Dental Assisting. Philadelphia, W.B. Saunders Co., 1992, p 406.)

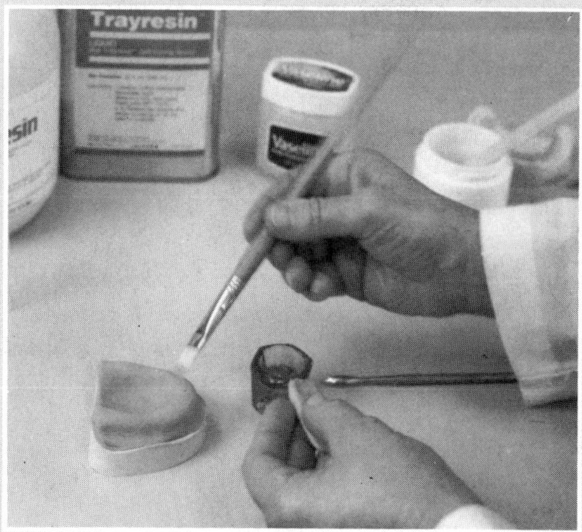

FIGURE 24–13

A handle is formed and attached to the anterior of the tray. (From Ehrlich, A., and Torres, H.O.: Essentials of Dental Assisting. Philadelphia, W.B. Saunders Co., 1992, p 406.)

(continued on following page)

PROCEDURE: **Creating an Acrylic Custom Tray** *(continued)*

2. Place a drop of monomer on the handle and on the tray, where they will join.
3. Attach the handle so it extends out of the mouth and is parallel with the occlusal surfaces of the teeth.
4. Hold the handle in place until it is firm (Fig. 24–14).

Finishing the Tray

1. After the initial set (7 to 10 minutes), remove most of the spacer and return the tray to the cast (Fig. 24–15).
2. Complete cleaning the wax out of the inside of the tray after the tray resin has reached final cure (approximately 30 minutes to an hour).
3. Finish the edges, and then clean and disinfect the tray.
4. Paint the interior of the tray with adhesive (Fig. 24–16).

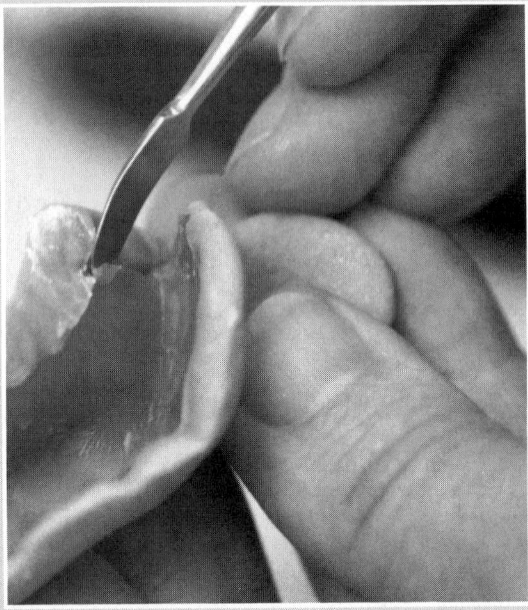

FIGURE 24–15

The spacer is removed from the tray before it reaches its final set. (From Ehrlich, A., and Torres, H.O.: Essentials of Dental Assisting. Philadelphia, W.B. Saunders Co., 1992, p 403.)

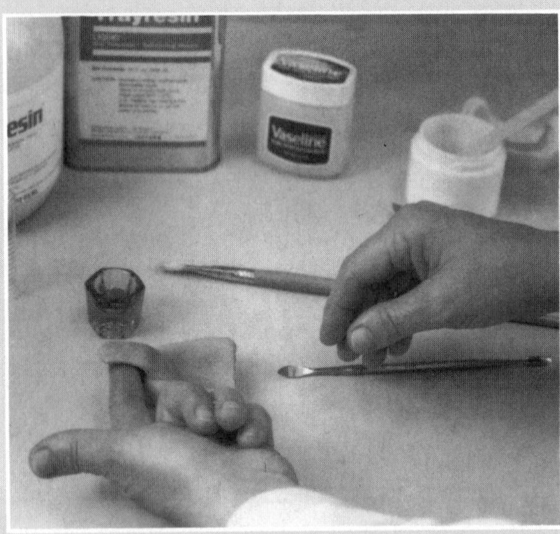

FIGURE 24–14

The handle is held in place until firm. (From Ehrlich, A., and Torres, H.O.: Essentials of Dental Assisting. Philadelphia, W.B. Saunders Co., 1992, p 406.)

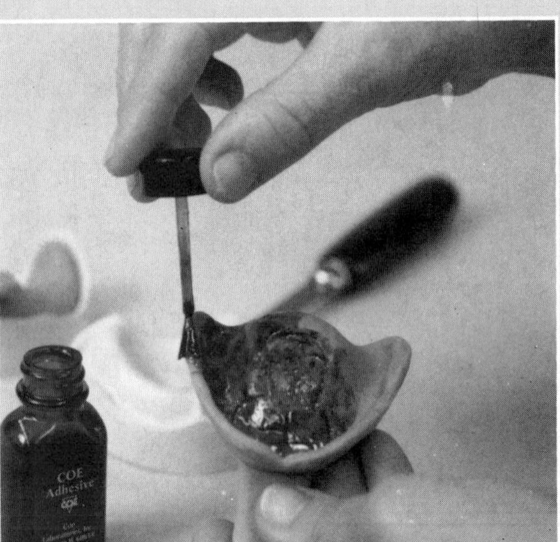

FIGURE 24–16

The prepared tray, including the edges, is painted with tray adhesive provided by the manufacturer of the impression material to be used. (From Ehrlich, A., and Torres, H.O.: Essentials of Dental Assisting. Philadelphia, W.B. Saunders Co., 1992, p 407.)

PROCEDURE: **Creating a Vacuum-Formed Bleaching Tray**

Instrumentation

Diagnostic cast
Pencil
Vacuum former
Acrylic sheets
Laboratory knife
Laboratory scissors

Cast Preparation

1. Soak the prepared cast in warm water for 20 minutes.
   □ *RATIONALE:* This avoids percolation during construction of the tray. (**Percolation** is the process of air bubbles working through the cast to reach the surface. These bubbles may cause spaces to form between the cast and the plastic.)
2. Outline the tray. If a spacer is indicated, it is placed over this area.
3. Place the prepared cast on the platform of the molding unit.

Vacuum Tray Formation

1. Select the thickness of the acrylic sheet to be used, place it in the heater frame of the unit, and turn the heater element on.
   □ *RATIONALE:* The heat will soften the acrylic so that it can be adapted to the cast.
2. Heat the acrylic sheet until it begins to sag slightly or appears to be forming a large drooping bubble.
   □ *CAUTION:* Do not overheat. This will cause multiple air bubbles or pitting in the final product.
3. Turn the heater off, lower the frame over the cast, and fasten it in position.
   □ *CAUTION:* Do *not* touch the hot metal area of the unit.
4. Apply vacuum pressure for 5 to 10 seconds.

Finishing the Vacuum-Formed Tray

1. Allow the acrylic to cool on the cast for approximately 2 to 3 minutes (Fig. 24–17).
2. When it is cool, separate the tray from the cast, and use scissors or a sharp laboratory knife to trim the tray to the desired form (Fig. 24–18).

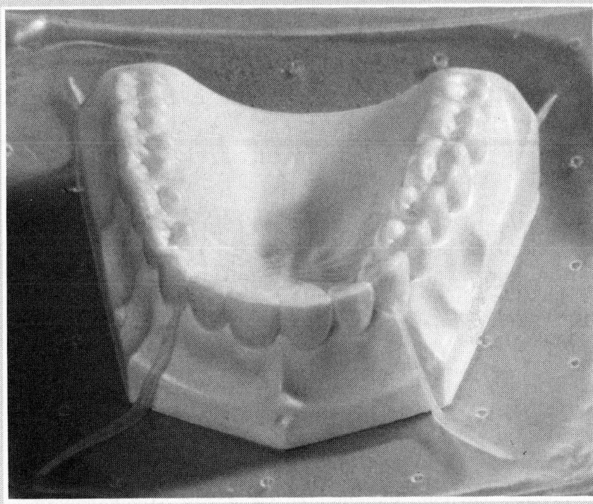

FIGURE 24–17

The acrylic is allowed to cool on the cast before the two are separated.

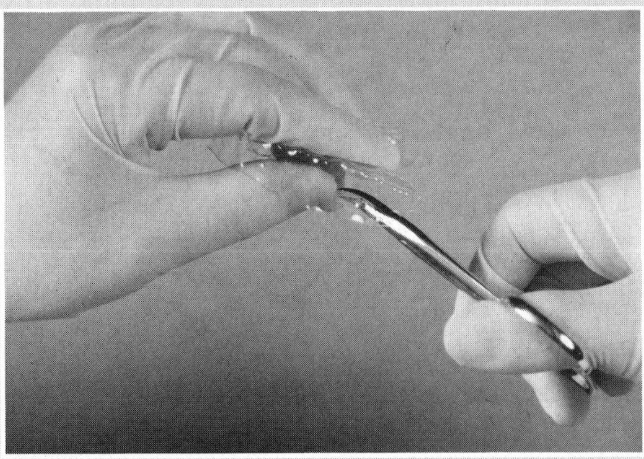

FIGURE 24–18

Scissors are used to trim the tray to the desired shape.

- A **nightguard vital bleaching** uses a lighter gauge plastic and does not require either a spacer or a handle. (See Chapter 25.)
- A **mouth guard** uses a heavier gauge flexible plastic, does not require a spacer, but it does need an attachment for the strap. (See Chapter 27.)
- A splint or habit appliance, such as for bruxism, uses a heavier gauge flexible plastic and does not require a spacer.

Elastomeric Impression Materials

Elastomeric materials are used when an extremely accurate impression is essential. The term **elastomeric** means having elastic or rubber-like qualities, and these materials are frequently referred to as *rubber base impression materials.*

It is this rubber-like quality that makes it possible to remove the impression after it has set without distortion or tearing. (**Distortion** is a change in shape or dimension.)

Types of Elastomeric Impression Materials

Four types of elastomeric impression materials are commonly used in dental practices: **polysulfide**, **polyether**, **condensation silicone**, and **addition silicone**.

Although similar in some aspects, each type has slightly different properties and characteristics. Table 24–1 summarizes the comparative properties of these materials. Of particular concern with these materials are dimensional stability and permanent deformation.

Special Precautions When Using Elastomeric Impression Materials

- The patient's clothing should be protected with a plastic drape before an impression is taken.
  Rationale: Elastomeric impression materials, particularly the polysulfides, stain clothing. (These materials must be handled with care!)
- Each type and brand of elastomeric impression material must be manipulated according to the manufacturer's instructions for that type of material.
- The catalyst and base come packaged together. (Do *not* mix tubes from another package or from another manufacturer.)
  Rationale: This may cause the material to fail to set properly.
- Do *not* interchange caps of the base and catalyst tubes.
  Rationale: This causes contamination of the materials that ruins the contents of the tubes.

TABLE 24–1

Comparative Properties of Rubber Impression Materials

	POLYSULFIDE	POLYETHER	CONDENSATION SILICONE	ADDITION SILICONE
Ease of mix	Fair	Easy	Fair to easy	Easy
Mixing time (sec)	60	30–45	30–60	30–45
Working time (min) at 20°–23°C	3–6	2–3	2–4	2–4
Setting time in mouth (min)	10–20	6–7	6–10	6–8
Cleanup	Difficult	Easy	Easy	Easy
Odor and taste	Unpleasant	Acceptable	Acceptable	Acceptable
Stiffness	Low	Very high	Medium high	High
Dimensional stability after removal from mouth	Moderate	Excellent*	Poor	Excellent
Permanent deformation after removal from mouth	High	Very low	Low	Very low
Wettability by gypsum	Poor	Good	Very poor	Very poor†
Tear resistance	Good‡	Poor	Fair	Poor

* Must be kept dry.
† Material does not fracture easily, but severe distortion occurs.
‡ Hydrophilic silicones that contain wetting agents are available.
From Phillips, R. W., and Moore B. K.: Elements of Dental Materials for Dental Hygienists and Dental Assistants, 5th ed. Philadelphia, W.B. Saunders Co., 1994, p 87.

Dimensional stability refers to the ability of the material to keep its shape after it has been removed from the mouth.

Deformation refers to the ability of the material to resist change caused by stresses during removal from the mouth. **Permanent deformation** means the material was changed and will *not* regain its previous shape.

Characteristics of Elastomeric Impression Materials

Elastomeric impression materials, which are self-curing, are provided as a **base** and a **catalyst**. The base is packaged as a paste in a tube or as a putty in a jar. The catalyst, also known as the *accelerator*, is packaged as a paste in a tube or as a liquid in a bottle with a dropper top.

Curing Stages of Elastomeric Impression Materials

The curing reaction (polymerization), as the elastomeric materials change from a paste into a rubber-like material, begins as soon as the base and the catalyst are brought together. The change occurs in a three-stage process: initial set, final set, and final cure.

INITIAL SET

Initial set is the first stage, and it results in a stiffening of the paste without the appearance of elastic properties. The material may be manipulated only during this first stage. The mix must be completed within the limited working time specified by the manufacturer. (**Manipulated** means mixed or handled.)

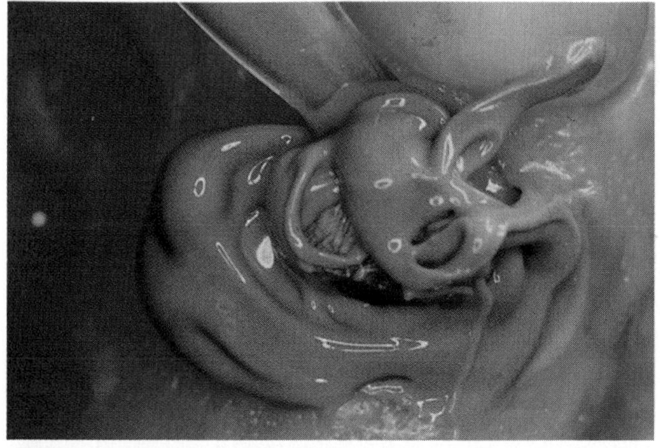

FIGURE 24–19

Use of the syringe material. This material is ejected generously around the prepared teeth and surrounding tissues. (Courtesy of 3M Dental Products Division, St. Paul, MN.)

FINAL SET

Final set is the second stage and begins with the appearance of elasticity and proceeds through a gradual change to a solid rubber-like mass. The material must be in place in the mouth before the elastic properties of the final set begin to develop.

FINAL CURE

Final cure is the last stage, and it occurs from 1 to 24 hours. Only slight dimensional change is noted in the detail of the impression during this time.

Forms of Elastomeric Impression Materials

Elastomeric impression materials are generally supplied in three forms: light-bodied, regular, and heavy-bodied.

LIGHT-BODIED

Light-bodied, or *syringe-type,* material is also sometimes referred to as a *wash.* These materials are used because of their ability to flow in and about the details of the prepared tooth. A special syringe, or extruder gun, is used to place the light-bodied material.

REGULAR AND HEAVY-BODIED

Often referred to as *tray-type* materials, these are much thicker impression materials. As the name implies, they are used to fill the tray. Their stiffness helps to force the light-bodied material into close contact with the prepared teeth and surrounding tissues to ensure a more accurate impression of the details of a preparation.

Basic Impression Technique

There are many different techniques available for use with these impression materials; however, the one most commonly used involves light-bodied and heavy-bodied materials in this sequence.

1. The material selected depends upon the operator's preference and the type of impression that is needed.
2. The operator places the syringe material over and around the prepared teeth and onto the surrounding tissues (Fig. 24–19).
3. The impression tray, loaded with heavy-bodied material, is seated *over* the light-bodied material (Fig. 24–20).
4. When the impression materials have reached final set, the impression is removed and inspected for accuracy (Fig. 24–21).
5. The impression is disinfected, placed in a plastic bag, and taken to the laboratory.

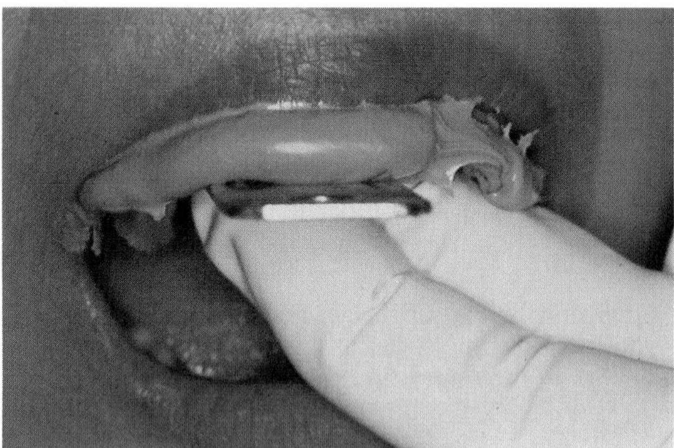

FIGURE 24–20

Use of the tray material. The tray is filled with heavy-bodied material and placed over the arch containing the prepared teeth. (Courtesy of 3M Dental Products Division, St. Paul, MN.)

PREPARING THE EXTRUDER GUN

An extruder gun is used to mix and dispense elastomeric impression materials. (**Extrude** means to force or push out.) The gun itself, which can be used with either syringe-type or heavy body material, is operated with a trigger-like handle.

The extruder gun is loaded with dual cartridges, which consist of a tube of catalyst and a tube of base (Fig. 24–22).

The caps are removed from the tubes, and a small amount of unmixed material is extruded onto a gauze sponge (Fig. 24–23). This is to be certain that there are no air bubbles in the mix and to remove any hardened material that remains at the opening of the tubes.

Next, the mixer tip is attached (Fig. 24–24). The material is mixed and ready to use as it moves through this tip. Tray material can be dispensed directly from the mixer tip.

If this is syringe-type material, one option is to add a small syringe tip and dispense the material directly from the extruder gun (Fig. 24–25).

An alternative is to load an impression syringe from

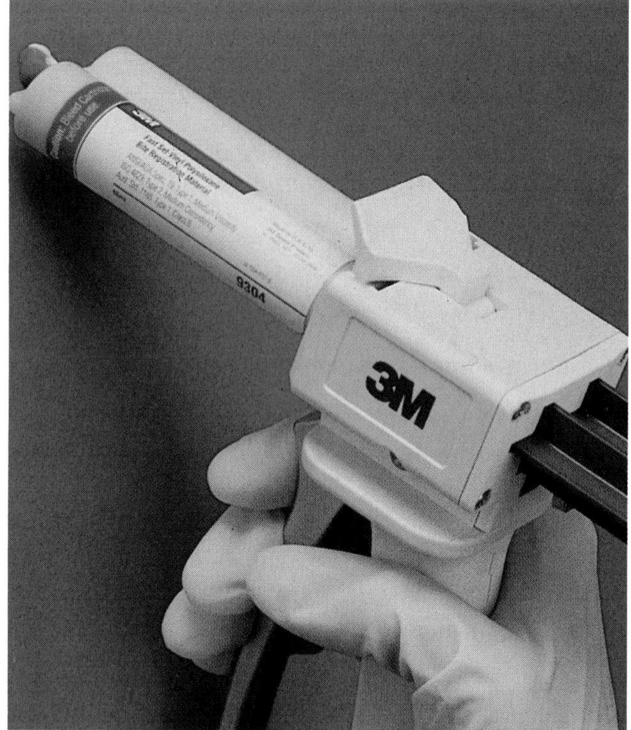

FIGURE 24–22

An extruder gun loaded with cartridges of impression material. (Courtesy of 3M Dental Products Division, St. Paul, MN.)

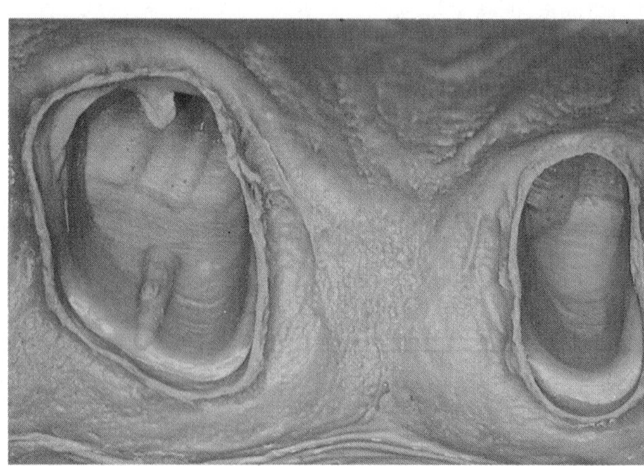

FIGURE 24–21

Details of the completed impression. The details of the prepared teeth are clearly visible in the syringe material. Some tray material can also be seen. (Courtesy of 3M Dental Products Division, St. Paul, MN.)

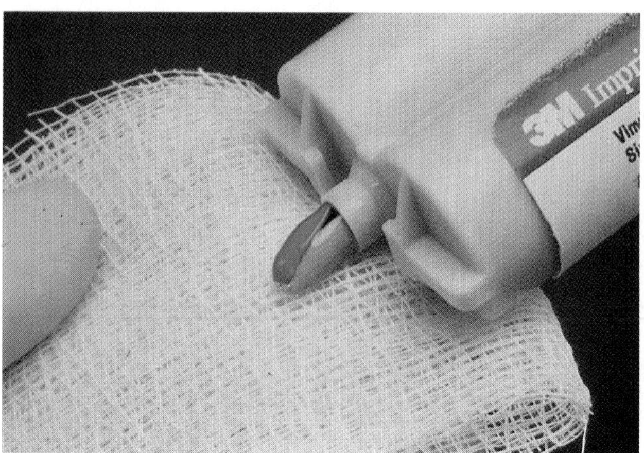

FIGURE 24–23

A small amount of material is dispensed onto a gauze sponge. This is to prevent air bubbles from being trapped in the mix. (Courtesy of 3M Dental Products Division, St. Paul, MN.)

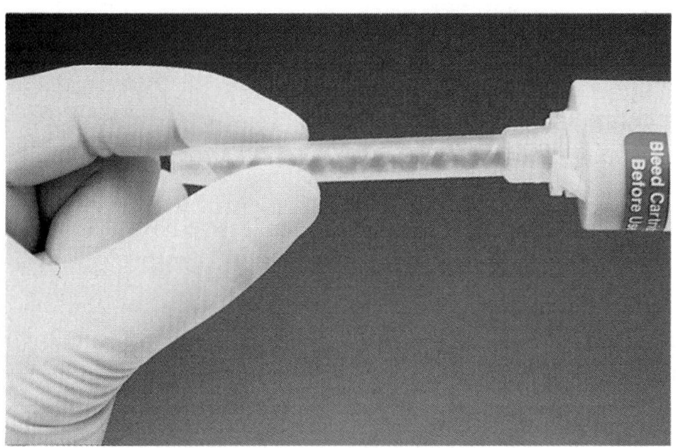

FIGURE 24–24

The mixer tip is attached to the cartridges. (Courtesy of 3M Dental Products Division, St. Paul, MN.)

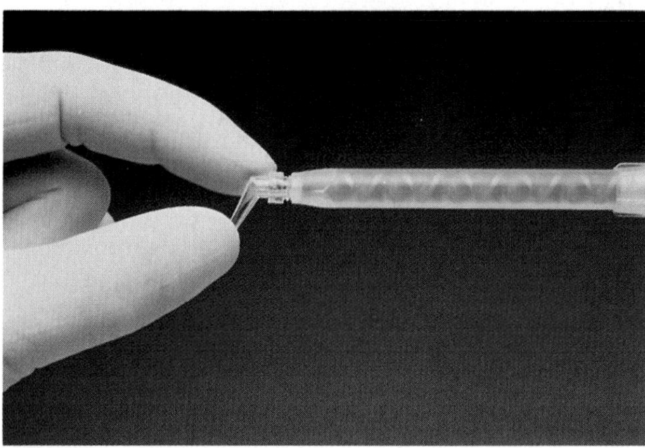

FIGURE 24–25

For syringe-type materials, a syringe tip may be added. (Courtesy of 3M Dental Products Division, St. Paul, MN.)

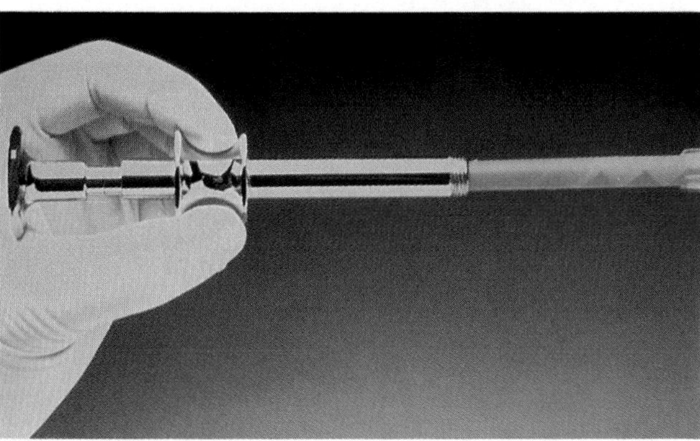

FIGURE 24–26

For syringe-type materials, the mixer tip of the extruder gun may be used to load an impression syringe. (Courtesy of 3M Dental Products Division, St. Paul, MN.)

the mixing tip and use this to dispense the syringe-type material (Fig. 24–26).

BACK LOADING AN IMPRESSION SYRINGE

The following is a commonly used method of loading an impression syringe with material that has been mixed manually.

1. Prepare the syringe by placing the tip and threaded collar. Remove the plunger.
2. Mix the syringe-type impression material and gather it into a mass on the mixing pad.
3. Hold the barrel of the syringe with the plunger end downward and place the plunger end of the barrel into the mass of mix (Fig. 24–27).
4. Use a scraping motion on the pad to force the mix into the chamber to fill it 75 percent full.
5. Place the plunger into the barrel. Slowly force the plunger forward until impression material is extruded from the tip of the syringe.
6. Use a tissue or an alcohol wipe to remove the excess impression material from the syringe surface.
7. Pass the loaded syringe to the dentist.

Equipment Care and Exposure Control

IMPRESSION MATERIAL TUBES

After dispensing material from a tube, the end of the tube must be cleaned immediately. If this is not done, the tube end becomes messy and the cap will stick to it.

To clean the tube end, after dispensing the material, place the opening of the tube flat on the clean surface of the mixing pad. Use a wiping motion of the tube

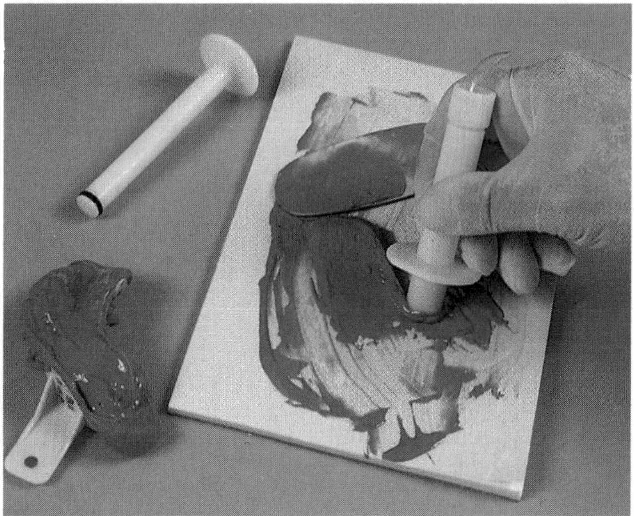

FIGURE 24–27

Back loading an impression syringe. After the barrel is 75 percent full, the plunger is placed and used to force the material out through the tip.

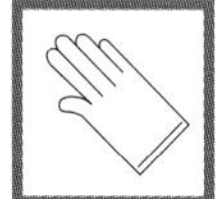 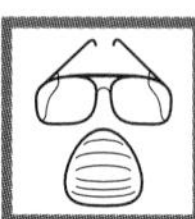 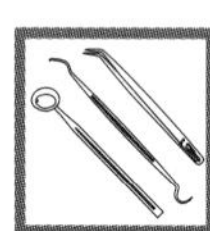 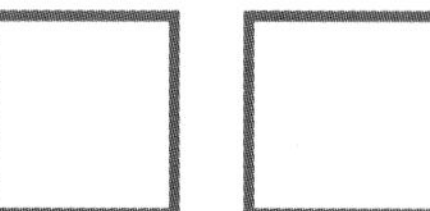

PROCEDURE: **Mixing Polysulfide Impression Materials**

Instrumentation

Custom tray painted with appropriate adhesive
Large, stiff, tapered spatulas (2)
Paper pads (2) (provided by manufacturer)
Polysulfide impression material, light-bodied (base and accelerator from the same manufacturer)
Polysulfide impression material, heavy-bodied (base and accelerator from the same manufacturer)
Impression syringe (with sterile tip in place)

Tray Preparation

1. Determine that the custom tray is ready.
   □ *RATIONALE:* A custom tray is commonly used with polysulfide impression materials to ensure close adaptation around the teeth and to minimize wasting materials.
2. Paint the interior of the tray with the manufacturer-supplied tray adhesive.

Preparation of Syringe-Type Material

1. Dispense approximately 1¼ to 2 inches of the syringe-type base material onto a clean paper pad. Wipe the tube opening clean with a gauze sponge and recap immediately.
   □ *RATIONALE:* Cleaning the top of the tube and the threads prevents a messy cap, which may stick closed.
2. Dispense an equal length of syringe-type accelerator onto the pad near, but not touching, the base material (Fig. 24–28). Wipe the tube opening clean and recap immediately.
3. Place the blade of the spatula into the catalyst so both sides are coated. Then incorporate the catalyst into the base paste.
   □ *RATIONALE:* Having this catalyst on the spatula makes cleanup easier because the catalyst causes the base material to set so it does not stick to the spatula.
4. Spatulate smoothly (wiping back and forth) to produce a homogeneous, streak-free mix within 45 to 60 seconds.
   □ *RATIONALE:* This material is mixed most effectively by spreading it over a wide area of the pad.
5. Load and complete assembly of the syringe in less than 30 seconds, and pass the prepared syringe to the dentist.

Preparation of Tray-Type Material

1. Use a clean mixing pad and clean spatula.
2. Extrude the tray-type base material to the appropriate length (2 to 3 inches). Wipe the tube opening clean and recap immediately.

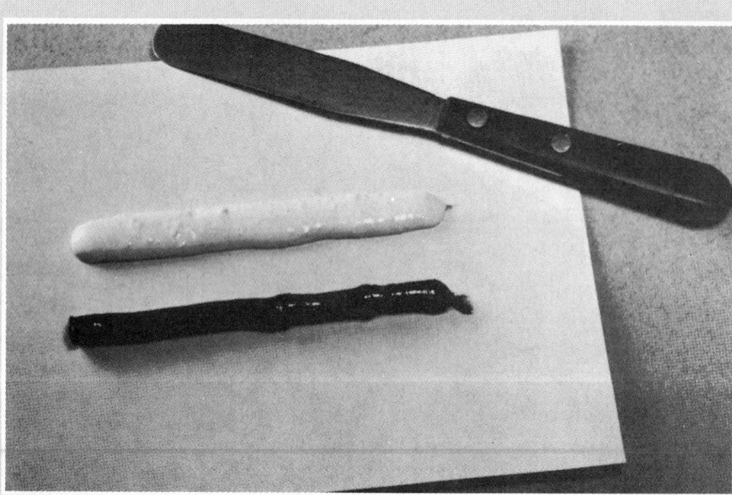

FIGURE 24–28

Dispensing equal lengths of polysulfide base and accelerator on a paper mixing pad. (From Phillips, R.W., and Moore, B.K.: Elements of Dental Materials for Dental Hygienists and Dental Assistants, 5th ed. Philadelphia, W.B. Saunders Co., 1994, p 93.)

3. Extrude an equal length of tray-type catalyst. This is placed on the pad about an inch from the base paste. Wipe the tube opening clean and recap immediately.
4. Place the blade of spatula into catalyst on the mixing pad so that both sides of the blade are covered.
   □ *RATIONALE:* Coating the spatula with catalyst makes cleanup easier because it is not as sticky as the base material.
5. Use the edge of the spatula to scrape the remaining catalyst into the base.
6. Use a flat spreading motion with the spatula to spread the mix in crosswise strokes on the pad.
   □ *RATIONALE:* This material is mixed most effectively by spreading it over a wide area of the pad.
7. Continue to scrape up the mix and spread it smoothly on the pad in even crosswise strokes, to incorporate all material.
   □ *RATIONALE:* The mix must be homogeneous and should appear creamy, of even texture and color, and free of streaks.
8. Complete a homogeneous mix within the time recommended by the manufacturer. (This is usually 45 seconds to 1 minute.)
   □ *RATIONALE:* If the mix is not completed within the recommended working time, the quality of the impression will be compromised.
9. Pick up the bulk of the tray mix with the spatula and load the material into the tray. The mass should flow into the tray.
10. Spread the material until the tray is evenly loaded.
11. Receive the used syringe from the dentist, and pass the loaded tray.

against the pad to clean the opening of the tube. An alternative is to wipe the sides of the tube opening with a moist gauze sponge or a tissue. Then replace the cap (for that tube) immediately.

If any material is found on the side of the tube, wipe it clean with a tissue, a paper towel, or an alcohol wipe. (An **alcohol wipe** is a gauze sponge moistened with alcohol.) Recheck that the tops are tight. After disinfection, return the correct pair of tubes to the same box.

SPATULA CARE

When finished using a spatula, wipe it clean with a tissue, a paper towel, or an alcohol wipe. Discard this wipe carefully.

If it is not possible to clean the spatula immediately, wait until the material has set. Then peel it off the spatula surface and wipe the spatula clean.

If the spatula was handled with contaminated gloves, disinfect it before returning it to storage.

MIXING PADS

Carefully peel off the top sheet of each mixing pad and discard it. Slipping the tip of the spatula under a corner of the soiled sheet makes it easier to remove the paper from the pad.

Return the mixing pad to the box according to its label.

THE IMPRESSION SYRINGE OR EXTRUDER GUN

Once the impression material has set, clean and disinfect the syringe or extruder gun according to the manufacturer's instructions. Discard the used syringe tip.

Polysulfide Impression Materials

Polysulfide impression materials have relatively long working and setting times. However, the curing reaction is accelerated by increased temperature or the presence of moisture (as in the mouth). They also have a very strong odor and will permanently stain clothing.

Polysulfide impression materials are available as three types: light-bodied (syringe-type), regular, and heavy-bodied (tray-type). Each type is supplied as two pastes: the base and the catalyst.

Polyether Impression Materials

Polyether impression materials are available only in regular weight. This material is supplied in tubes as pastes: the base and the catalyst. The tubes are not the same size; however, dispensing equal lengths delivers the correct amount of each material.

Because the set material is quite stiff, a third component called a *thinner* (or *body modifier*) is also included. The body modifier is added to the mix to reduce the thickness of the mix and of the finished impression.

The mixing and impression technique are very similar to that for polysulfide materials (Figs. 24–29 through 24–31).

Silicone Impression Materials

Elastomeric impression materials must be capable of setting in the moist environment of the oral cavity. However, the silicones are **hydrophobic** (do not react favorably to water). These materials have difficulty reaching a set in the presence of moisture.

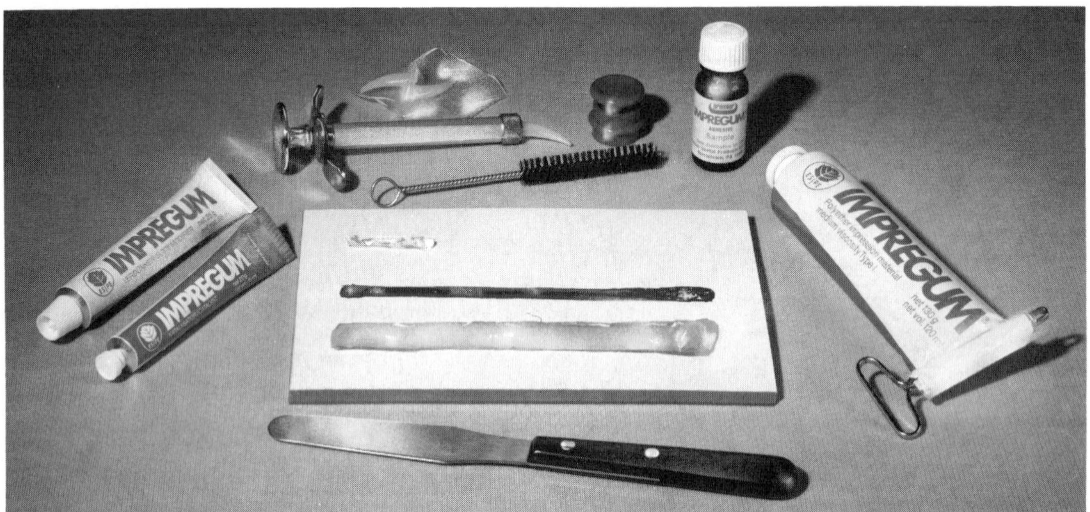

FIGURE 24–29

Polyether impression material and supplies. The third tube is the modifier. (Courtesy of Premier Dental Products Company, Norristown, PA.)

To overcome this disadvantage, some manufacturers have placed surfactants in the paste that make the mix hydrophilic (does react favorably to water). (A **surfactant** is a releasing or separating agent.)

A **hydrophilic** material is able to reach a rubber-like set in the presence of limited moisture. This surfactant also allows the surface of the impression to readily receive the stone mix when the impression is being poured.

Two varieties of silicone impression materials are available. These are named on the basis of the type of polymerization action: condensation silicone impression materials and addition silicone impression materials.

Both types of materials are odor free, not messy to handle, and relatively easy to mix. Their different properties are reviewed in Table 24–1.

CONDENSATION SILICONE IMPRESSION MATERIALS

Condensation silicone impression materials are commonly supplied with the base as a paste in a tube and the catalyst as a liquid in a bottle or smaller metal tube.

The base is a silicone polymer called **polysiloxane,** and the material is frequently referred to by this name (Fig. 24–32).

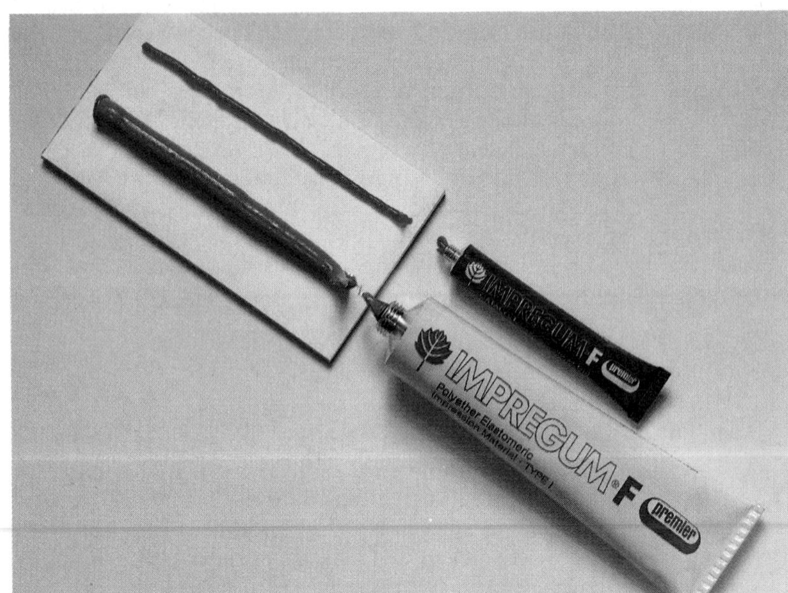

FIGURE 24–30

Dispensing equal lengths of polyether impression material. (Courtesy of Premier Dental Products Company, Norristown, PA.)

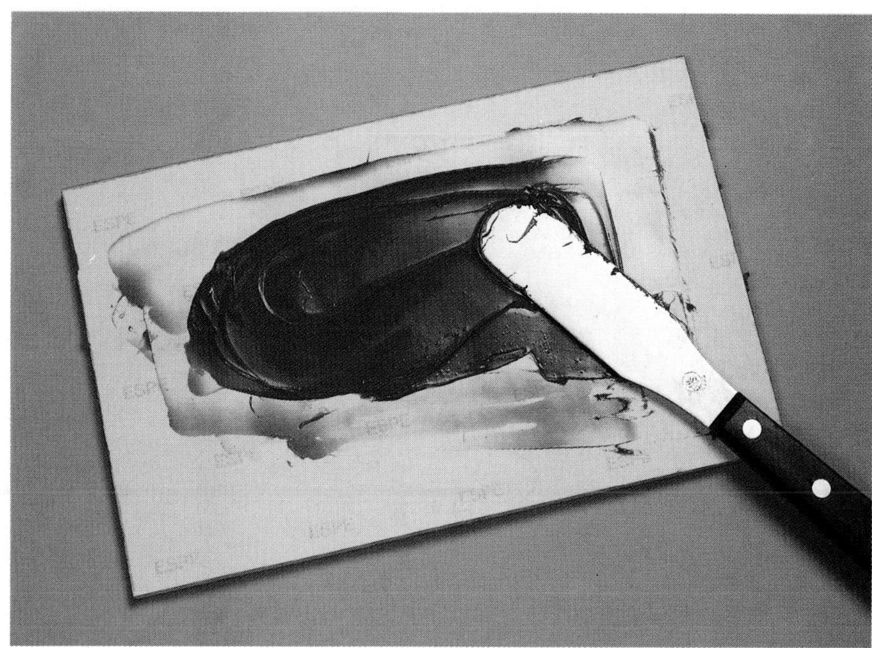

FIGURE 24–31

Polyether is mixed with a wiping motion to avoid incorporating air bubbles into the material. (Courtesy of Premier Dental Products Company, Norristown, PA.)

ADDITION SILICONE IMPRESSION MATERIALS

Addition silicone impression materials, which are frequently referred to as **polyvinyl siloxanes**, are supplied either as a two-paste system or in two jars of putty material.

They are also supplied in a dual-cartridge system for use in an extruder gun that automatically mixes and dispenses the material.

MIXING SILICONE IMPRESSION MATERIALS

Both types come as putties that are mixed with the fingers, with one very important difference:

- Addition silicone impression putty (polyvinyl siloxanes) *is* affected by handling with latex examination gloves. (Contact with latex gloves may severely retard the setting, and vinyl overgloves *must* be worn when these materials are handled and mixed.)
- Condensation silicone impression putty (polysiloxane) is *not* affected by handling with latex examination gloves.

TWO-STEP IMPRESSION TECHNIQUE

Silicone impression materials are commonly used in a two-step impression technique with syringe material and a putty material in a stock tray painted with adhesive.

The putty is used to take a **preliminary impression** *before* the teeth are prepared. After undercuts have been removed from the preliminary impression, it is put aside while the teeth are being prepared. The **final impression**, which is also referred to as a *secondary impression*, is taken, with a syringe material used as a "wash" after the teeth have been prepared.

Light-Cured Impression Materials

Light-cured impression materials are also available. Their primary advantage is that they allow unlimited time for mixing, adapting, loading the tray, and placement *before* the light-curing process is initiated.

These materials *must* be used in a clear plastic tray so that the light can reach all areas of the paste. The curing light is moved over the material and acts as the catalyst to bring about the curing process.

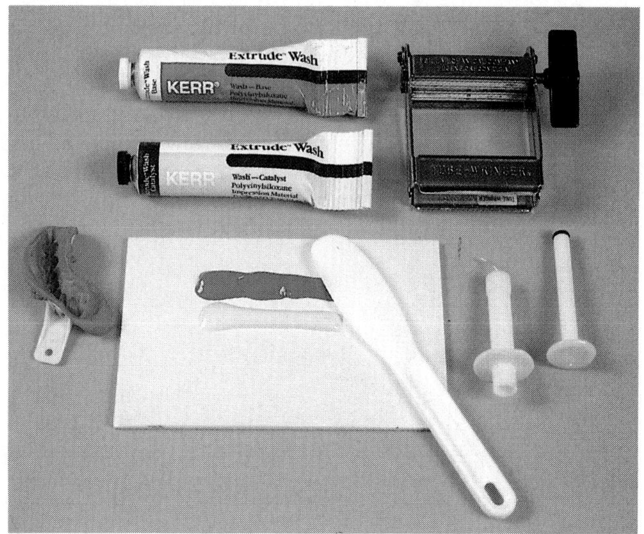

FIGURE 24–32

Polysiloxane dispensed and ready to mix. The "wringer" device at the upper right is used to aid in removing all of the material from the tube.

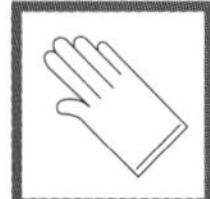 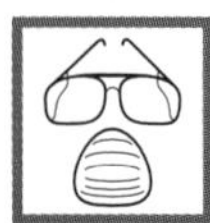 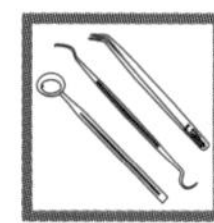 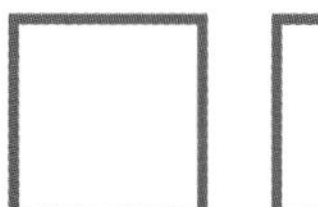

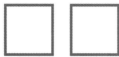

PROCEDURE: **Performing the Two-Step Impression Technique**

Instrumentation

Vinyl overgloves (if polysiloxane is used)
Stock tray (painted with adhesive)
Mixing pad
Spatula
Heavy-bodied putty (base and catalyst)
Measuring scoop for putty (provided by manufacturer)
Plastic sheet spacers
Extruder gun and accessories
Cartridges for extruder gun of light-bodied (wash) material
Disposable scalpel

Preparation of Putty Preliminary Impression

1. If polysiloxane putty is used, the assistant puts on vinyl overgloves.
2. Following the manufacturer's directions, the assistant measures the putty base, places it on the paper mixing pad and scores the surface. (**Score** means to make with criss-cross lines.)
   ☐ *RATIONALE:* These lines help hold the liquid catalyst on the surface of the base.
3. The liquid catalyst is measured by drops onto the base material, and a spatula is used to mix the catalyst into the base with a folding, circular motion until the mix is homogeneous. (This must be completed within the manufacturer's recommended mixing time.)

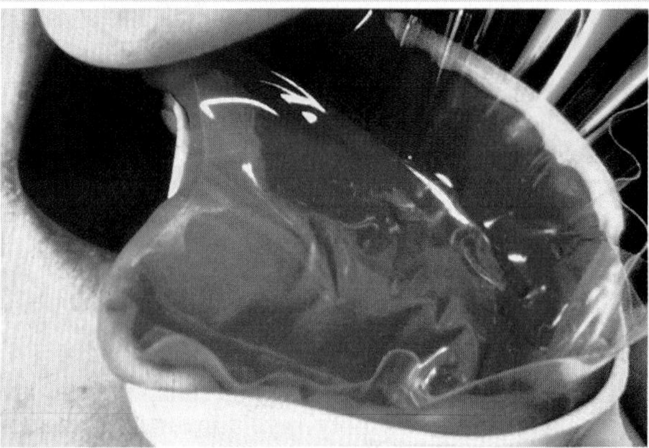

FIGURE 24–33

Tray preparation. The stock tray is filled with impression material, an indentation is made for the teeth, and the spacer is placed over the surface. (Courtesy of 3M Dental Products Division, St. Paul, MN.)

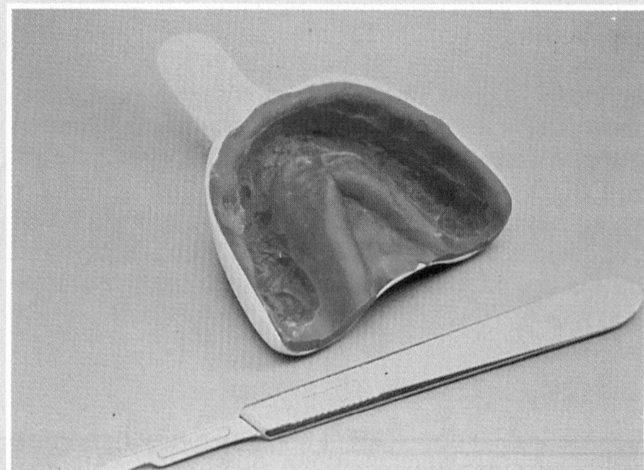

FIGURE 24–34

Impression preparation. The spacer is removed, and excess material is trimmed from the edges of the impression. (Courtesy of 3M Dental Products Division, St. Paul, MN.)

4. The mix is scooped up, kneaded in the fingers, and quickly formed into a patty.
5. The patty is loaded into the prepared tray, and a finger is used to place a slight indentation in tray material where the teeth will be.
6. The tray material is covered with a plastic sheet spacer (Fig. 24–33).
   □ *RATIONALE:* The spacer creates room in the preliminary impression so additional impression material can be added later for the final impression.
7. The assistant hands the prepared tray to the dentist, who positions the tray. It remains in place for 4 minutes and is then removed.
8. The spacer is removed, and the impression is checked for accuracy and freedom from large wrinkles and bubbles.
   □ *RATIONALE:* Large wrinkles or bubbles may cause a void in the finished impression. (Fine wrinkles are acceptable for this putty method.)
9. A scalpel is used to trim away undercuts from the impression.
   □ *RATIONALE:* An undercut is an area that will prevent the impression from seating properly. Trimming also helps to ensure adequate space for the syringe material in the final impression.
10. A scalpel is used to trim away excess from the edges of the impression (Fig. 24–34). The preliminary impression is then set aside for later use after the teeth are prepared.
    □ *RATIONALE:* Trimming away these edges, which are not a critical part of the impression, creates space to seat the tray for the secondary impression.

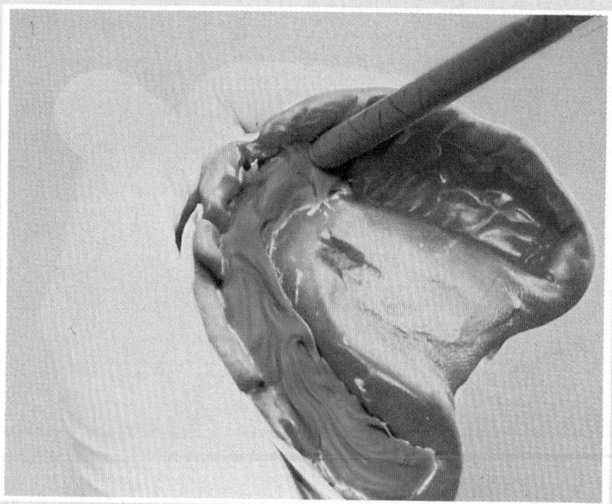

FIGURE 24–35

Preparing to take the final impression. The indentation in the tray is filled with syringe (wash) material. (Courtesy of 3M Dental Products Division, St. Paul, MN.)

The Final Impression

1. The assistant follows the manufacturer's directions and assembles the extruder gun loaded with the wash material.
2. Syringe material is extruded into the indentation in the prepared preliminary impression (Fig. 24–35).
3. The extruder gun is passed to the dentist, who extrudes the material over, into, and around the prepared teeth (Fig. 24–36).
   □ *RATIONALE:* To prevent air bubbles from forming in the material, the operator keeps the tip of the extruder in the mass of the material as it is being placed.
4. The prepared tray is passed to the dentist, who immediately seats it. The tray is held in place until the material has set, usually about 8 minutes, and is then removed.
5. The impression is rinsed, inspected for detail, disinfected, and placed in a plastic bag to be sent to the dental laboratory.

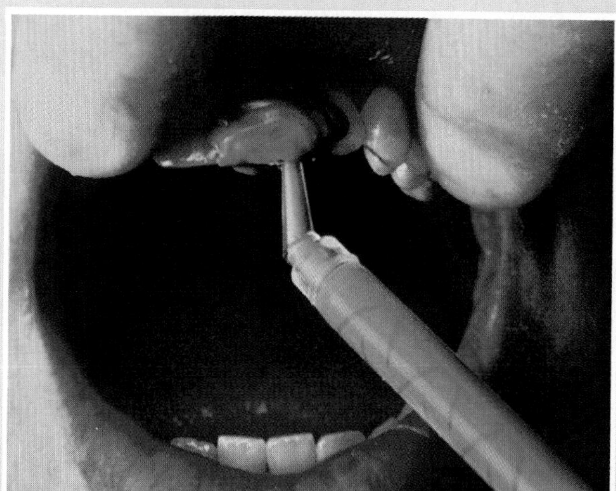

FIGURE 24–36

Taking the final impression. The operator covers the prepared teeth and surrounding tissues with syringe material. Then the tray is placed. (Courtesy of 3M Dental Products Division, St. Paul, MN.)

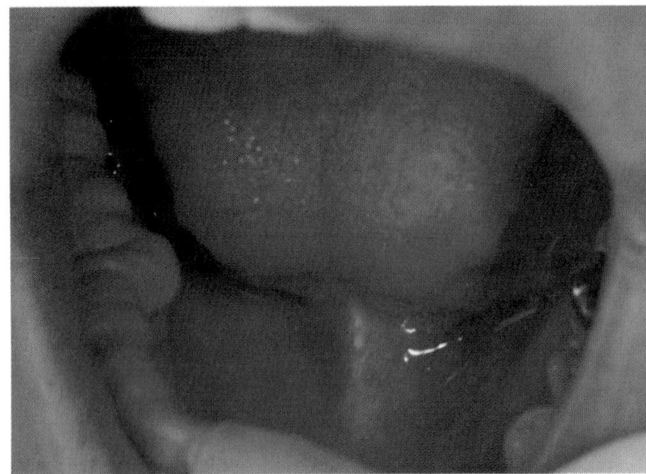

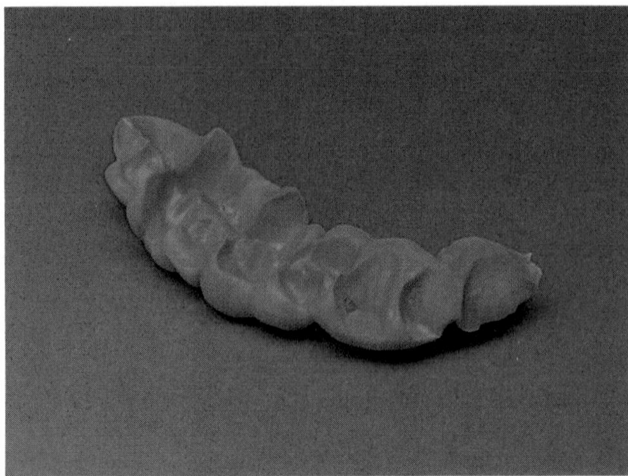

FIGURE 24–37

Open-bite registration method. *Left*, The impression material is dispensed directly on the occlusal surface of the mandibular teeth. The patient closes his teeth into the material. *Right*, The resulting bite registration. (Courtesy of 3M Dental Products Division, St. Paul, MN.)

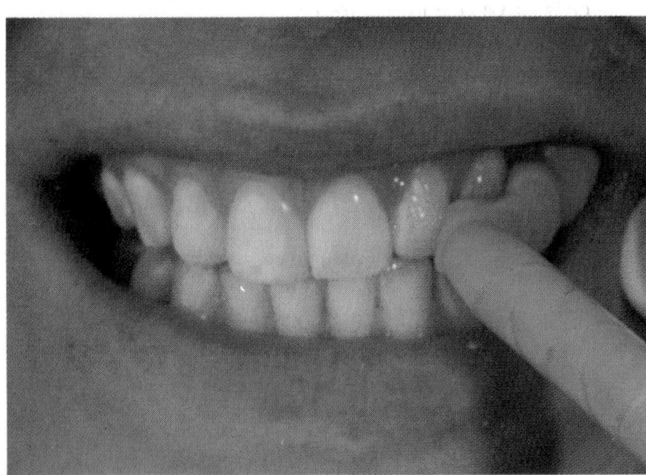

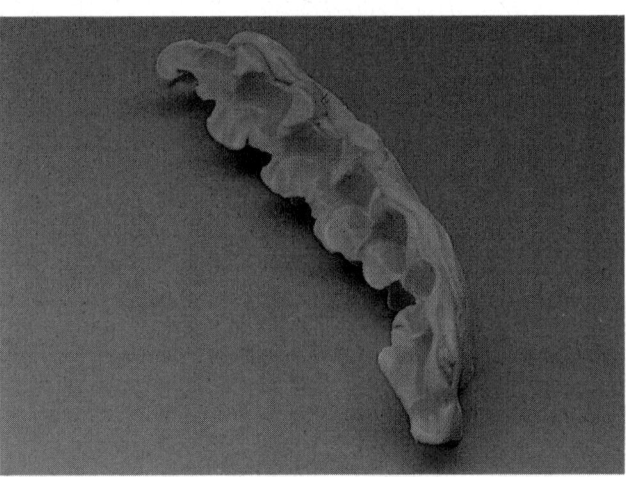

FIGURE 24–38

Closed-bite registration. *Left*, The patient closes his teeth, and the impression material is injected between them. *Right*, The resulting bite registration. (Courtesy of 3M Dental Products Division, St. Paul, MN.)

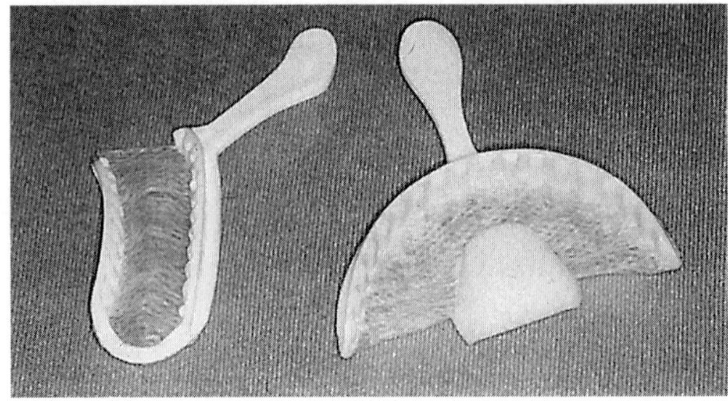

FIGURE 24–39

Disposable plastic bite registration trays. (Courtesy of 3M Dental Products Division, St. Paul, MN.)

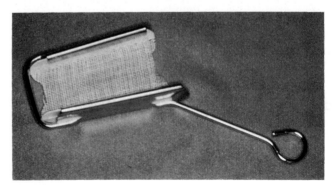

FIGURE 24–40

Metal frame and gauze bite registration tray. (Courtesy of 3M Dental Products Division, St. Paul, MN.)

The Opposing Arch

In addition to the elastomeric impression of the arch containing the prepared teeth, the dental laboratory also needs an impression of the opposite dental arch. Most commonly, an alginate impression is used for this purpose. (Alginate impressions are discussed in Chapter 19.)

Occlusal Registration

In addition to having an accurate impression of the prepared teeth, the dentist and laboratory technician need an accurate registration of the normal centric relationship of the maxillary and mandibular arches. (**Centric** is when the jaws are closed in a position that produces maximal stable contact between the occluding surfaces of the maxillary and mandibular teeth.)

This relationship is recorded as the **occlusal registration**, which is also known as the *interocclusal record* (IOR) but is commonly referred to as the *bite registration.*

When mounting the casts of the upper and lower jaw on the articulator, this "bite" is used to establish the proper centric relationship. (An **articulator** is a device that simulates the movements of the mandible to the maxillary and the temporomandibular joint.)

A wax-bite registration is obtained when the initial impressions for diagnostic casts are obtained (see Chapter 19). However, a more accurate occlusal registration is required for use with the impressions of the prepared teeth discussed as follows.

Silicone Occlusal Registration

A specialized silicone impression material, which is sometimes referred to as *mousse* (because of its soft and creamy texture), is commonly used for this purpose. These materials have very low flow (this means they are stiff). This is an important characteristic because in this technique, the paste is used without a tray.

OPEN-BITE REGISTRATION TECHNIQUE

1. The impression material is mixed and dispensed by an extruder gun.
2. The patient is asked to open his mouth, and the material is extruded directly only the occlusal surface of the mandibular teeth (Fig. 24–37).
3. The patient is instructed to close in proper occlusion.
4. After the material has set (about 1 minute), the impression is removed and checked for accuracy.
5. It is then rinsed, dried, disinfected, and sent to the laboratory with the written prescription and other impressions.

CLOSED-BITE REGISTRATION TECHNIQUE

1. The impression material is mixed and dispensed by an extruder gun.
2. The patient is instructed to close his teeth together in centric occlusion (Fig. 24–38). The patient is also asked to bring his tongue forward, short of going between the teeth.
   ☐ **Rationale**: The tongue acts as the matrix for the lingual aspect of the impression.
3. The impression material is injected between the maxillary and mandibular teeth in the areas where teeth have been prepared.
4. After the material has set, it is removed, checked for accuracy, rinsed, dried, and disinfected before being sent to the dental laboratory.

Triple Tray Occlusal Registration Technique

This occlusal registration technique is so named because it accomplishes three steps with a single tray. At one time, the dentist is able to take (1) the **final impression** of the prepared teeth; (2) the **opposing arch impression,** which is also known as the *counter impression*; and (3) the **bite registration** of the teeth in occlusion.

The technique, in which both syringe and tray type polysiloxane impression material are utilized, is frequently used for crown and bridge preparations.

THE TRIPLE TRAY

A special quadrant tray is used for this technique. The design of the tray must allow the patient to close his teeth normally (in centric occlusion) when the tray is in place. The sides must be high enough to hold the impression material in place, and the tray must have a handle for ease of placing and removal.

One variety is a disposable plastic tray with a thin layer of webbing in the middle (Fig. 24–39). Other varieties have a reusable metal frame with a gauze insert (Fig. 24–40).

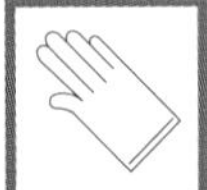
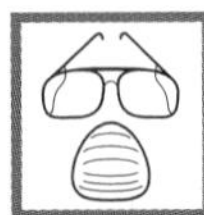
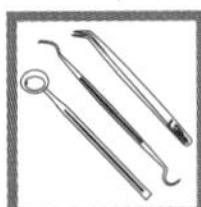

PROCEDURE: **Performing the Triple Tray Impression Technique**

1. The empty tray is tried in the patient's mouth to determine that it fits accurately.
   □ *CAUTION:* A tray that is tried in the mouth but not selected must be discarded or disinfected before reuse.
2. With the tray in place, the patient is asked to close "normally."
   □ *RATIONALE:* This is to determine that the patient is able to close in centric occlusion with the tray in place.
3. The tray is removed, and the walls of the tray, but not the webbing, are painted with an adhesive.
4. The tray material is mixed, and the tray is loaded on both sides of the webbing. The tray should be very full.
5. The syringe material is prepared, and the dentist places it around the prepared teeth (Fig. 24–41).
6. The loaded tray is seated over the teeth, and the patient is asked to close in centric occlusion (Fig. 24–42).
7. When the material is set, the tray is removed, checked for accuracy, and then disinfected before being sent to the laboratory (Fig. 24–43).

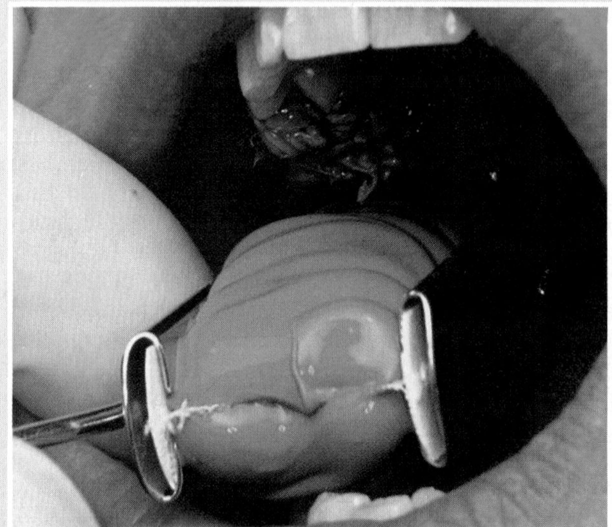

FIGURE 24–42

The tray, which is loaded on both sides, is placed in the patient's mouth. The patient is then asked to close his teeth together. (Courtesy of 3M Dental Products Division, St. Paul, MN.)

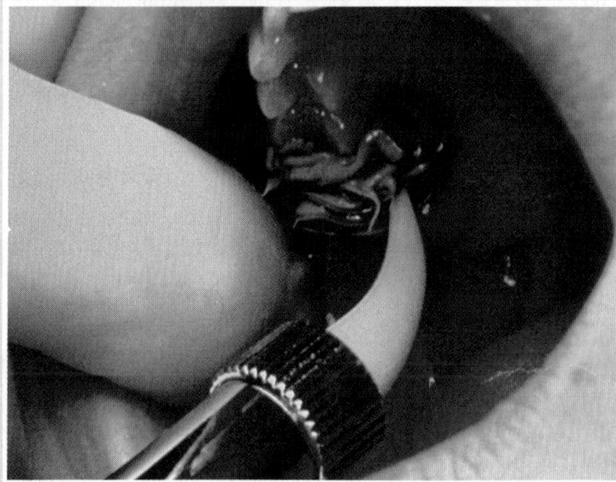

FIGURE 24–41

The dentist places syringe material around the prepared teeth. (Courtesy of 3M Dental Products Division, St. Paul, MN.)

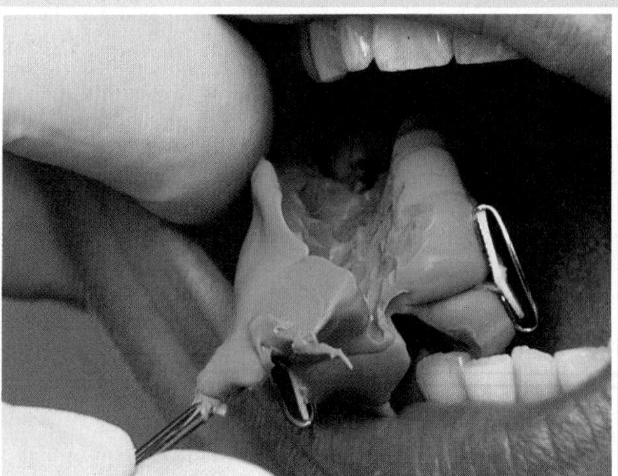

FIGURE 24–43

The completed impression is removed, inspected, and disinfected. (Courtesy of 3M Dental Products Division, St. Paul, MN.)

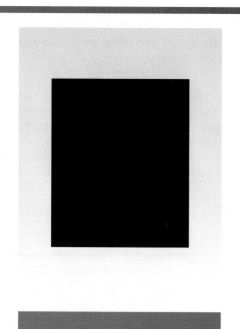

Chapter 25

Restorative and Cosmetic Dentistry

Introduction

Restorative dentistry, also known as *operative dentistry*, is concerned with the restoration of defects or caries in individual teeth. Cosmetic dentistry deals primarily with the improvement of the appearance of the anterior teeth.

The primary goal of restorative dentistry is to return the tooth to full function, in an esthetically pleasing manner, with as little loss of healthy tooth structure as possible. Table 25–1 summarizes the restorative materials of choice of many dentists.

This chapter covers all aspects of restorative dentistry *except* the placement of cast restorations such as inlays, onlays, and single crowns. These are discussed in Chapter 31 with other techniques that require precise impressions and work by a laboratory technician.

Acid etching, dentin bonding, dental cements, and dental restorative materials, which are all key components of restorative dentistry, are introduced in Chapter 23.

Single tooth cast restorations (inlays, onlays, and crowns), which are often included in the definition of restorative dentistry, are discussed in Chapter 31.

Patient Preparation for Restorative Procedures

Before treatment begins, these preparatory steps are taken to ensure patient comfort and safety:

1. The patient is informed of the procedure to be performed and what to expect during the treatment.

   Rationale: The patient must give informed consent before the dentist continues with the procedure.

TABLE 25–1

Preferred Restorative Materials

PERMANENT TEETH	PRIMARY TEETH
Class I	
Sealant (as a preventive measure) Amalgam or composite in a conservative preparation Amalgam in a traditional preparation Laboratory-processed composite or ceramic inlay or onlay Cast metal inlay or onlay	Composite or glass ionomer in a very conservative cavity preparation
Class II	
Amalgam or composite in a conservative preparation Amalgam in a traditional preparation Laboratory-processed composite or ceramic inlay or onlay Cast metal inlay or onlay	Amalgam or composite in a conservative preparation Glass ionomer restoration Amalgam in a traditional preparation Stainless steel crown
Class V	
Composite used with dentin bonding, glass ionomer or light-activated glass ionomers	Composite used with dentin bonding, glass ionomer or light-activated glass ionomers

2. If indicated, a local anesthetic is administered.

   Rationale: Patient comfort and pain control are primary concerns. These topics are discussed in Chapter 20.

3. While the local anesthetic solution is taking effect, the dental dam is placed and secured.

   Rationale: Dental dam is an important part of exposure control, and this is discussed in Chapter 22.

Exposure Control During Restorative Procedures

Restorative dentistry involves the use of the dental handpiece and air-water syringe, which generate a contaminated aerosol spray and spatter. For this reason, it is particularly important that all of the appropriate exposure control protocols be carried out carefully during each restorative visit. This is discussed in Chapter 13.

The Terminology of Cavity Preparation

The involved tooth surfaces and the characteristics of the preparation are discussed in the following sections (Fig. 25–1). You should also know the system of cavity classification, which is discussed in Chapter 18.

CAVITY WALLS

A **cavity wall** is a side of the cavity preparation. Each wall is named for the exterior tooth surface nearest to it. However, there are no occlusal or incisal walls. This is because during the preparation these areas are open and are not enclosed by a wall.

Axial Walls. An axial wall is that portion of the prepared tooth that is vertical and parallel with the long axis of the tooth. The following are the axial walls:

Mesial wall
Distal wall (these mesial and distal walls may also be referred to as *proximal walls*)

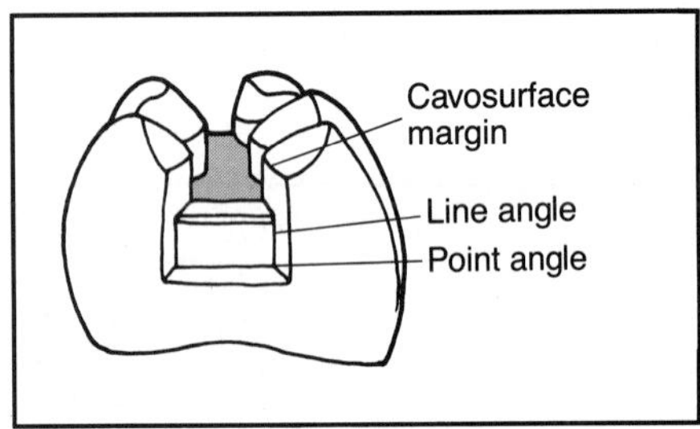

FIGURE 25–1

Terminology of cavity preparation. Shown on a diagrammatic representation of an MOD preparation are a line angle, a point angle, and the cavosurface margin.

- **Lingual wall**
- **Buccal wall**
- **Labial wall** (the buccal and labial walls also may be referred to as *facial walls*)

Pulpal Walls. The pulpal wall, also known as the *pulpal floor*, is the portion of the cavity preparation overlying the pulp. This wall is horizontal and at a right angle to the axial cavity walls.

The **gingival wall** is the wall of the preparation that is nearest the gingiva. Like the pulpal wall, it is horizontal and at a right angle to the other cavity walls.

LINE ANGLES

The junction of two walls in the preparation form a line angle. (This is similar to the angle formed where two walls of a room meet to form a corner.)

To identify a line angle, the names of the two involved walls are combined. For example, the line angle formed by the mesial and lingual walls is called the *mesiolingual line angle*. Note that the suffix "-al" of the word *mesial* is dropped, and the letter "o" is added. Then the two terms can be combined to form the term *mesiolingual*.

It is important not to confuse the names of these angles with the names used to describe the surfaces involved in the restoration itself. (This process is described in Chapter 18.)

POINT ANGLES

A point angle is formed by the junction of two walls and the cavity floor, which makes a corner in the cavity preparation. (This is similar to the angle formed where the walls of a corner join the floor.)

In the identification of a point angle, the names are combined in the same manner as for a line angle. For example, the mesiobuccopulpal point angle is the junction of the mesial, buccal, and pulpal walls of a cavity preparation.

MARGINS

The junction of the walls of the cavity and the exterior tooth surface is known as the **cavosurface margin,** or the *cavosurface angle.*

The Principles of Cavity Preparation

Cavity preparation is a surgical procedure to remove the caries and a limited amount of healthy tooth structure in order to prepare the tooth to receive and retain the restoration.

The principles of cavity preparation describe the steps that the dentist follows to prepare a tooth for an amalgam restoration (Fig. 25–2). Although the preparation is modified for use with other restorative materials, the same principles apply.

The steps are described here separately for teaching

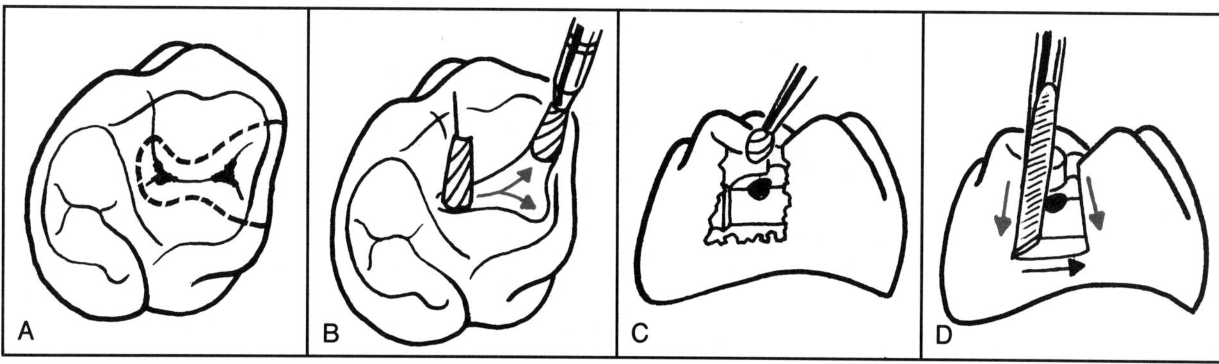

FIGURE 25–2

Steps in cavity preparation. *A*, Planned outline form. *B*, High-speed handpiece used to establish outline, resistance, and retention forms. *C*, Round bur used in a low-speed handpiece to remove caries and unsupported enamel. *D*, An enamel chisel used to refine and finish the enamel walls.

purposes. Actually, the dentist performs several at the same time.

Step 1: Outline form. The outline form is the curved shape and border of the restoration and enamel at the tooth surface.

Step 2: Resistance and retention form. The **resistance form** is the shape and relationship of the cavity walls that protect the tooth structure and restorative material against fracture. (Enamel that is not properly supported will fracture.) **Retention form** is the shape and relationship of the cavity walls that provide mechanical retention necessary to hold the restoration in place.

Step 3: Convenience form. Convenience form is the amount of cavity opening that is necessary so that the dentist can gain access to the cavity preparation for the insertion and finishing of the restorative material.

Step 4: Removal of caries. The removal of caries is the process of removing the decayed and demineralized enamel and dentin.

Step 5: Refinement of the cavity walls and margins. This step, also known as *finishing the enamel walls and margins*, is the process of angling, beveling, and smoothing the walls of the cavity preparation. Because unsupported enamel will fracture, it is removed at this time.

Step 6: Cavity debridement. This is the process of removing debris from the preparation. However, this step does not necessarily include removing the smear layer. (The **smear layer** is the thin film of debris remaining on the dentin after a cavity preparation.)

MATRICES, RETAINERS, AND WEDGES

Frequently after a tooth has been prepared to receive a restoration, one or more walls of that tooth are missing. No matter what type of restorative material is being used, it is necessary to temporarily replace those walls while the restoration is being placed.

A **matrix** is a temporary replacement for the missing wall of a prepared tooth. (*Matrix* is singular. The plural is *matrices.*) The matrix is held securely in place around the tooth with a device called a **retainer.**

A **wedge** is placed to hold the matrix firmly against the interproximal contours of the tooth. This prevents the restorative material from being expressed beyond the gingival margins of the preparation. Specifics about types of matrices, retainers, and wedges are discussed later in this chapter.

Amalgam Restorations

Amalgam is one of the oldest and most serviceable dental restorative materials. Freshly mixed amalgam is pliable (soft) and can be condensed into the cavity preparation. Then it hardens quickly to form a very strong restoration that is capable of withstanding the occlusal forces on the posterior teeth.

For this reason, amalgam is used on all surfaces of the posterior teeth, where strength, rather than appearance, is of major importance. Amalgam is also used to prepare a base or core as a build-up in preparation for a full crown restoration.

Amalgam also has several disadvantages:

- It is not esthetically pleasing because its silver color does not match the tooth color. For this reason, it is not commonly used for restorations of anterior teeth.
- Because it does not bond directly to the tooth, microleakage and recurrent decay may occur. Amalgam bonding aids in overcoming this problem.
- It contains mercury, which is a hazardous substance. Although amalgam containing mercury has a long history of safety, there are questions concerning its continued use. The characteristics of amalgam are discussed in Chapter 23.

The Tofflemire Matrix and Retainer

A metal matrix band is used during the placement of an amalgam restoration requiring the restoration of a wall of the tooth. This band is held snugly in place around the tooth with the matrix retainer (Fig. 25–3). After use, the band is discarded, and the retainer is sterilized for reuse.

The Tofflemire matrix and retainer are frequently used for this purpose during the placement of an amalgam restoration.

To avoid unnecessary delay, the assistant assembles the matrix retainer and band while waiting for the anesthetic to take effect or while the dentist completes the final steps before placement of the restoration. It is *not* assembled at the last minute.

PARTS OF THE TOFFLEMIRE RETAINER

Outer Guide Slots. The outer guide slots, also known as *guide channels*, at the end of the retainer serve as channels to guide the loop of the matrix band. The channel selected is determined by the quadrant being treated.

- The **left** guide channel is used for the maxillary left and the mandibular right quadrants.
- The **straight** guide channel is used for anterior maxillary or mandibular teeth.
- The **right** guide channel is used for the maxillary right and the mandibular left quadrants.

The Diagonal Slot Vise. The diagonal slot vise is a boxlike structure used to position the ends of the matrix band within the retainer. The ends of the matrix

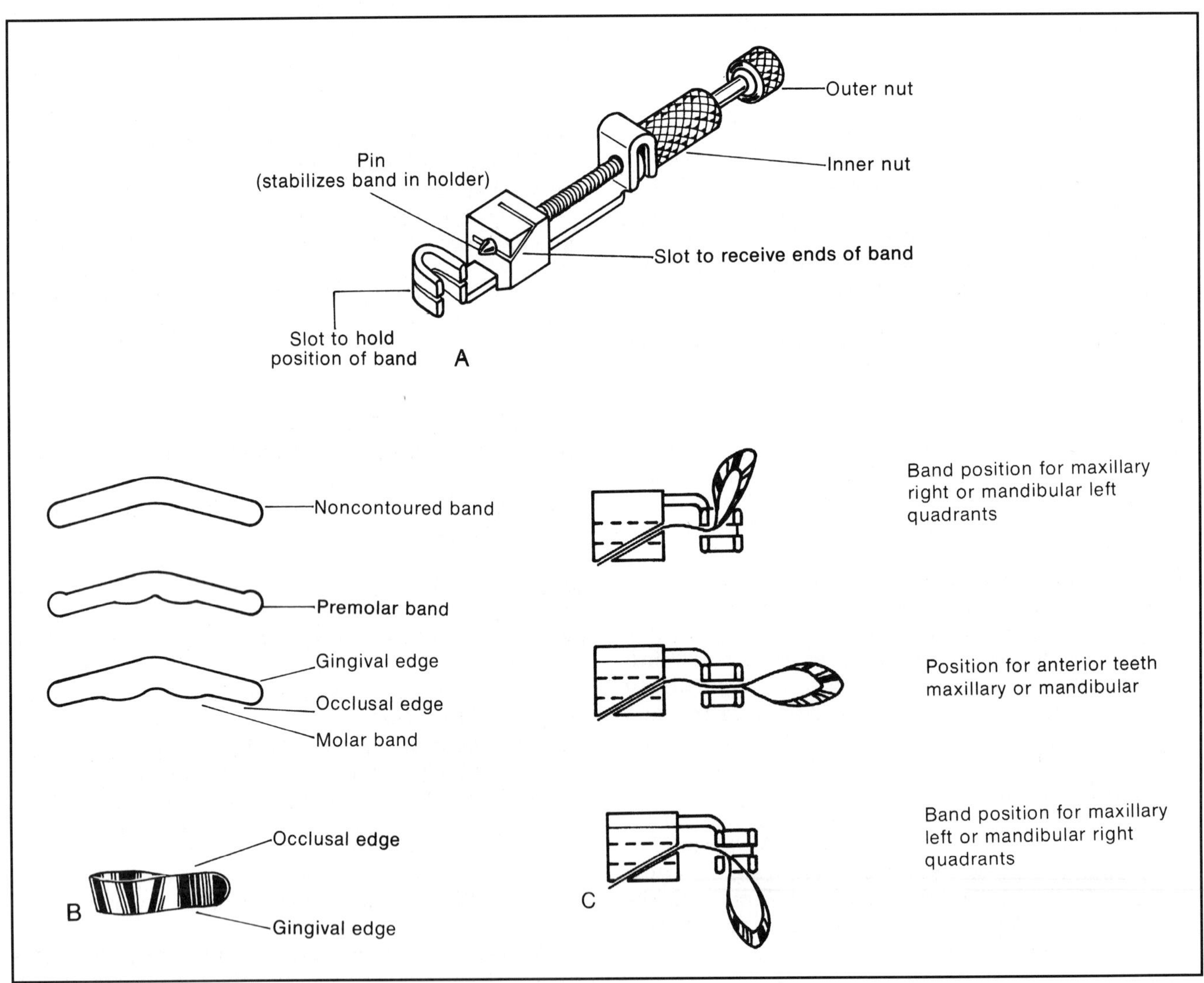

FIGURE 25–3

Tofflemire matrix band and retainer. *A*, The slot is always placed toward the gingiva. *B*, Assorted matrix bands and the shape. *C*, The matrix is placed through the guide slots for different quadrants.

band slip into the diagonal slot that runs all the way across the slot vise.

The Spindle. The spindle, also known as a *pin* or *rod*, is a screw that fits into the diagonal slot vise to hold the ends of the matrix band. When the matrix band is placed into the diagonal slot vice, the spindle point must be clear of the slot.

The **outer knob**, also known as the *outer nut,* is used to tighten or loosen the spindle within the diagonal slot vise. To tighten the spindle, turn the outer nut away from you. To loosen the spindle, turn the outer nut toward you.

Be careful not to turn it too far, or the diagonal slot vise will fall off the spindle. If this happens, insert the end of the spindle into the diagonal slot vise and turn the outer nut away from you.

The **inner knob**, also known as the *inner nut*, is used to adjust the size of the matrix band loop. The size of the loop formed depends upon the tooth to be restored. The loop is made smaller or larger by turning the nut.

MATRIX BANDS

The stainless steel matrix bands that are used with the Tofflemire retainer are available in **premolar**, **molar,** and **universal** sizes and thicknesses.

When the ends of the curved band are brought together, they form a slightly modified "V" shape.

- The **larger** circumference of the band is the *occlusal edge* and is always placed toward the occlusal of the tooth.
- The **smaller** circumference of the band is the *gingival edge* and is always placed toward the gingiva.

Contouring the Band. In preparation for use, the interproximal area of the matrix band must be contoured (shaped) in the proximal contact area so that it will properly contact the tooth next to it.

To contour the band, place the outer surface of the band on a semi-hard surface (such as the back of a mixing pad). Using a small ball- or egg-shaped burnisher, press against the inner surface of the band so that it is bulging slightly outward at the contact area.

Wedges

A triangular wedge of plastic or wood is placed into the embrasure between the matrix band and the adjacent tooth. This adapts the matrix band so that the contours of the finished restoration smoothly match that of the natural tooth structure it replaces.

Improper wedge and band placement can result in an **overhang** (excess restorative material extending beyond the preparation) or in **cupping** (a gap or indentation in the restorative material). Neither condition is acceptable.

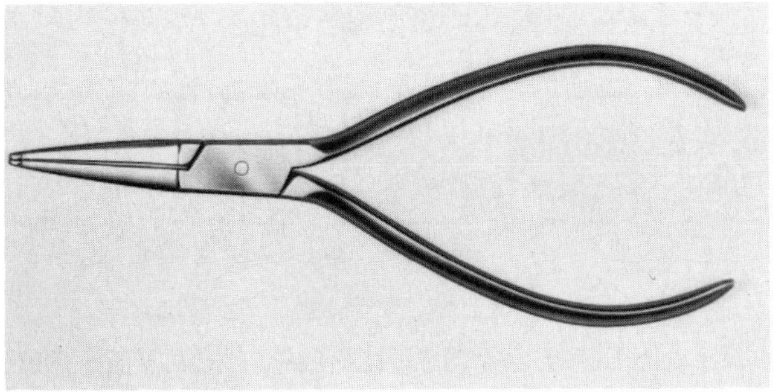

FIGURE 25–4

A number 110 (Howe) pliers may be used to aid in placing and removing the wedge. (Courtesy of Rocky Mountain Orthodontics, Denver, CO.)

Wooden wedges are used for amalgam restorations, and if it is necessary, a knife is used to shape the wedge for a better fit. When a light-cured restoration is placed, a plastic wedge is used.

The matrix is prepared, placed, and wedged *before* the restorative material is mixed and placed. It is removed after the restoration has been placed and before the final finishing steps.

A hemostat, cotton pliers, or No. 110 (Howe) pliers are commonly used to firmly hold the wedge while it is placed and removed (Fig. 25–4). For posterior restorations, the wedge is placed firmly from the lingual side so that the adjacent teeth are slightly separated and the wedge will not be easily dislodged.

Placement of the Matrix, Tofflemire Retainer, and Wedge

CRITERIA FOR A MATRIX RETAINER AND BAND PLACEMENT

- The slotted surface of the retainer is always positioned toward the gingiva.
- The retainer is positioned at the facial surface of the tooth.
- The handle extends out from the oral cavity at the corner of the lips.
- The seated band extends approximately 1 mm. below the gingival margin of the preparation.
- The seated band extends no more than 1½ to 2 mm. above the occlusal surface of the tooth.

Automatrix Retainerless Matrix System

An alternative to the use of a retainer is the automatrix system, which has the advantage that there is no retainer to get in the way (Fig. 25–5). The major disadvantage is that it is more difficult to create the proper proximal contours.

The bands, which are already formed as a circle, are

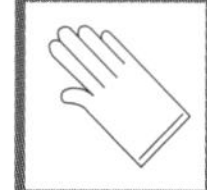 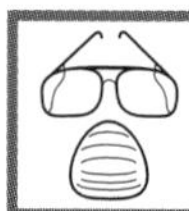 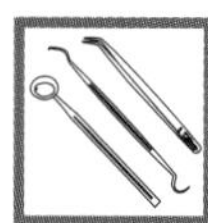  

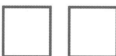

PROCEDURE: **Assembling, Placing, and Removing the Matrix, Tofflemire Retainer, and Wedge**

Instrumentation

Tofflemire matrix retainer
Matrix bands (premolar and molar)
Burnisher (egg- and ball-shaped)
Number 110 (Howe) pliers
Wooden wedge
Optimal: Knife (to shape wedges)

Assembling the Matrix and Retainer

1. Determine the tooth to be treated and select the appropriate matrix band.
   □ *RATIONALE:* The tooth being treated influences every step in preparing the retainer and band.
2. If necessary, use the burnisher to contour the band.
3. Bring the ends of the band evenly together. With ends touching, place the occlusal edge (larger circumference) of the band into the diagonal slot vise.
   □ *RATIONALE:* This creates the loop that goes around the tooth and places the occlusal edge in the appropriate position.
4. Turn the outer knob clockwise to secure the spindle on the matrix band.
   □ *RATIONALE:* This holds the band securely in the retainer.
5. Guide the loop through the appropriate guide channel.
   □ *RATIONALE:* The guide channel selected depends on the quadrant being treated.
6. If necessary, use the handle of an instrument to open (fully extend) the loop of the band.
   □ *RATIONALE:* This makes it easier to slip the loop over the tooth.
7. Turn the inner knob slightly to close the band.
   □ *RATIONALE:* This alters the size of the loop.
8. Return the assembled matrix and retainer to the instrument tray until it is needed.

Placing the Matrix and Retainer

1. Try the band, in the retainer, on the tooth. If necessary, adjustments are made so it fits snugly around the tooth.
2. If additional adaptation is needed, remove the band and retainer, and contour the contact area of the band.
3. Reassemble and reposition the band and retainer so that the band is properly seated on the tooth.
4. Place the index finger of one hand on top of the band to hold it securely. With the other hand, slowly tighten the inner nut to tighten the band around the tooth.
5. Use an explorer to check the adaptation of the band to determine that it is firm and provides proper contour and contact.

Placing the Wedge

1. Place the wedge at right angles to the beaks of the pliers so the "flat side" is down (toward the gingiva).
2. Before placing the wedge, use the fingers of the other hand to retract the patient's cheek and tongue near the prepared tooth.
3. Use firm pressure to insert the wedge from the lingual side between the band and proximal surface of the adjacent tooth. During this step, use the fingers of the other hand to steady the band.
4. *Optimal:* Occasionally it is necessary to place a second wedge from the lingual side.
5. If both the mesial and distal surfaces are being restored, place a wedge between each proximal area.

Removing the Wedge, Retainer, and Matrix

1. After the amalgam is initially carved, use the pliers to firmly grasp and remove each wedge.
   □ *RATIONALE:* Careful removal of each wedge is necessary to avoid fracture or displacement of the freshly placed restoration.
2. Hold the matrix band firmly in place with the fingers of one hand. Use the other hand to slowly turn the outer nut of the retainer in a counterclockwise direction.
   □ *RATIONALE:* This releases the ends of the band from the retainer.
3. Carefully lift the retainer upward and off the tooth. The band remains in place.
4. Use cotton pliers to straighten the ends of the matrix *away* from the tooth crown. Then gently, and very carefully, lift the band free of the tooth.

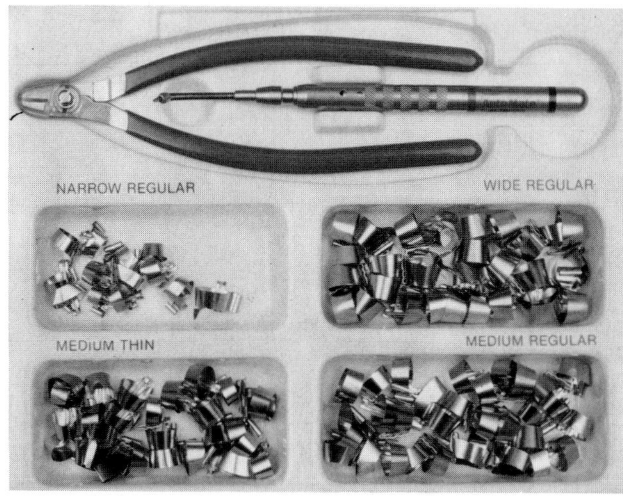

FIGURE 25–5

Automatrix system. *Top left*, Removal pliers. *Top right*, Tightening wrench. *Bottom*, Bands in assorted sizes.

available in assorted sizes in both metal and plastic. Each band has a coil-like autolock loop. The tightening wrench is inserted into the coil and turned clockwise to tighten the band. No additional retainer is necessary, and wedges are placed as indicated.

When the procedure is finished, the wedges are removed, and the tightening wrench is inserted into the coil and turned counterclockwise to loosen the band. The removing pliers are used to cut the band. The band is removed and discarded with the sharps. The tightening wrench and the removing pliers are sterilized or disinfected in accordance with the manufacturer's directions.

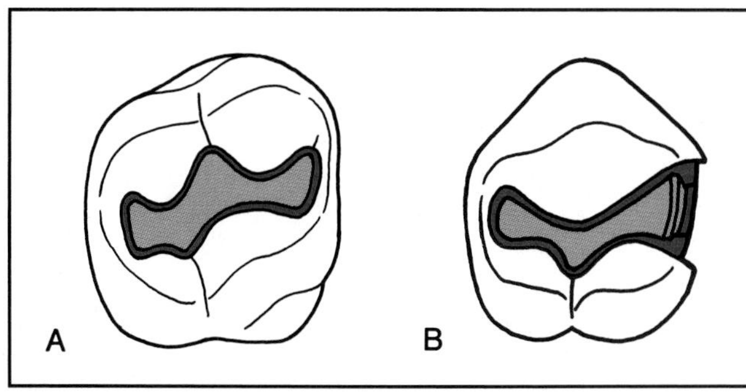

FIGURE 25–6

Cavity preparations. *A*, A Class I preparation on a maxillary molar. *B*, A Class II preparation on a maxillary premolar.

Placing a Class I Amalgam Restoration

A Class I amalgam restoration involves only one surface of the tooth. These restorations are most commonly placed on the occlusal surface of a posterior tooth (Fig. 25–6*A*).

Placing a Class I restoration does *not* involve the replacement of a missing wall of the tooth. For this reason, a matrix band, retainer, and wedge are not necessary. Aside from this, the preparation steps are very similar to those of a Class II restoration, and the details are described in the next section.

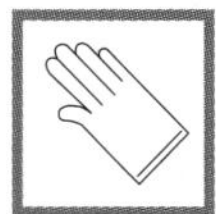
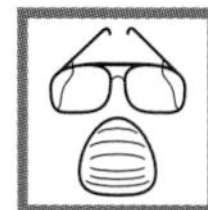
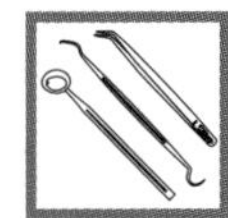
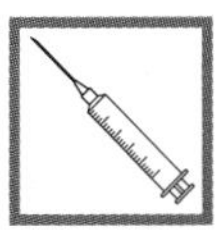
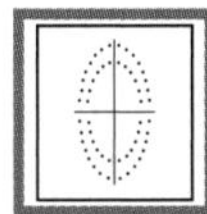

PROCEDURE: **Placing a Class II Amalgam Restoration**

Instrumentation (Fig. 25–7)

High-speed handpiece
Low-speed handpiece
Burs (dentist's choice)
Spoon excavators (small and medium)
Enamel hatchets (mesial and distal)
Other hand-cutting instruments (dentist's choice)
Cotton pellets, cotton rolls, and gauze sponges (2 × 2 inch)
Calcium hydroxide setup
Ball burnisher
Metal matrix band, holder, and wooden wedge
Number 110 (Howe) pliers (for wedge placement)
Premeasured amalgam capsules

(continued on following page)

PROCEDURE: **Placing a Class II Amalgam Restoration** *(continued)*

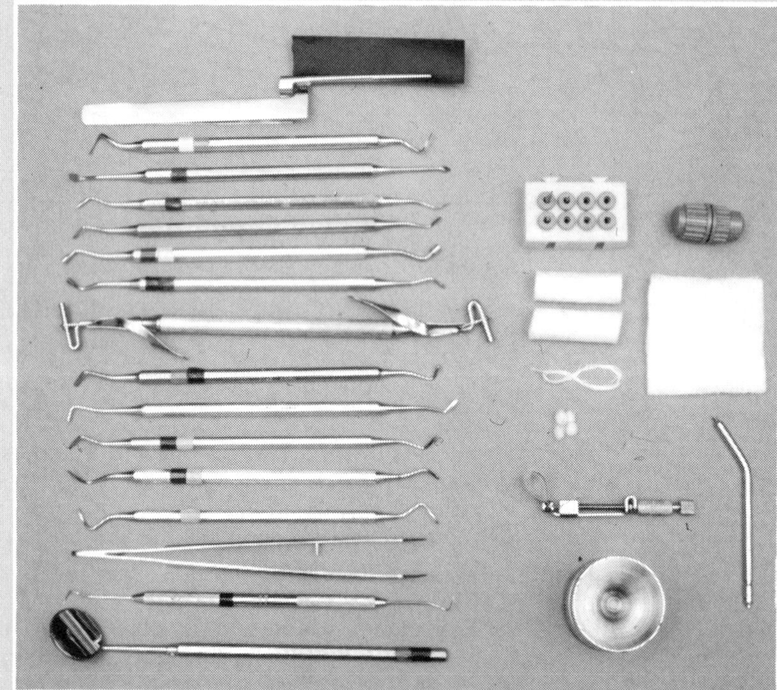

FIGURE 25–7

Amalgam instrumentation setup. *Left, bottom to top,* Mirror, explorer, cotton pliers, spoon excavators (2), binangle chisel, plastic instrument, burnisher, amalgam carrier, amalgam condensers (2), amalgam carvers (3), interproximal finishing knife, articulating forceps with articulating paper. *Right, bottom to top,* Amalgam well, Tofflemire retainer (assembled), cotton pellets and wedges, dental floss, cotton rolls, and bur block. *Far right,* Air-water syringe tip, gauze sponges, and premeasured amalgam capsule.

Amalgam well
Amalgam carrier
Amalgam condensers (large and small, smooth and serrated)
Carvers (discoid-cleoid, Hollenback)
Articulating forceps with articulating paper
High-volume evacuator (HVE) tip

Preparing the Cavity

1. The local anesthetic is administered, and the dental dam is placed.
2. The assistant transfers the mouth mirror and explorer to the dentist. The dentist examines the tooth to be restored.
3. The assistant prepares the high-speed handpiece with the first bur (many dentists use a No. 245 bur for this purpose). The assistant receives the used explorer and transfers the handpiece.
4. During the preparation of the tooth, the assistant uses the HVE and retracts the patient's cheek and tongue as needed to maintain a clear operating field.
5. As necessary, the assistant also

   a. Changes the bur in the high-speed handpiece
   b. Prepares the low-speed handpiece with a large, round bur
   c. Transfers and receives hand instruments (such as the spoon excavator, enamel chisel, and gingival margin trimmer)

6. Upon completion of the cavity preparation, the assistant uses the water syringe to remove all debris from the cavity preparation.
7. Warm air or cotton pellets are used to gently dry the tooth preparation.

Placing the Sedative Base and Cavity Liner (See Chapter 23)

1. The calcium hydroxide is mixed and placed over the dentin near the pulp.
2. The cavity varnish is placed on the walls of the preparation.

Placing the Matrix Band, Retainer, and Wedge

This procedure is described earlier in this chapter.

Mixing the Amalgam

1. The assistant activates the capsule (according to the manufacturer's directions), then places it in the amalgamator, and closes the cover.
2. The amalgamator is set for the number of seconds recommended by the manufacturer.

3. At a signal from the operator, the amalgamator is turned on to triturate the amalgam.
4. Immediately after the amalgamator stops, the assistant opens the cover and removes the capsule.
5. The capsule is opened, and the amalgam is emptied directly into a dry amalgam well. Cotton pliers are used to remove the pestle.
   □ *RATIONALE:* Amalgam must not be allowed to be contaminated with moisture; therefore, it is never touched by the gloved hands.
6. As soon as possible, the used capsule is reassembled.
   □ *RATIONALE:* This minimizes the possibility that mercury vapor will escape into the air.

Placing and Condensing Amalgam

1. With one hand, the assistant passes the smallest condenser to the operator. With the other hand, the assistant loads the small end of the amalgam carrier.
2. The assistant dispenses the amalgam firmly into the cavity preparation as directed by the operator. The operator condenses each increment of amalgam after it has been placed.
3. At a signal from the operator, the assistant begins using the large end of the carrier. Also at a signal from the operator, the assistant passes the operator's choice of a larger condenser. When a new condenser is passed, the assistant receives the used one.
4. This process of placing and condensing amalgam is repeated until the cavity is overfilled with condensed amalgam.
   □ *RATIONALE:* The excess mercury-rich material is carved away and removed with the HVE tip.
5. The assistant receives the last condenser and hands the explorer to the operator.
6. The assistant empties the amalgam carrier and discards any excess amalgam in the scrap amalgam container as described in Chapter 12.

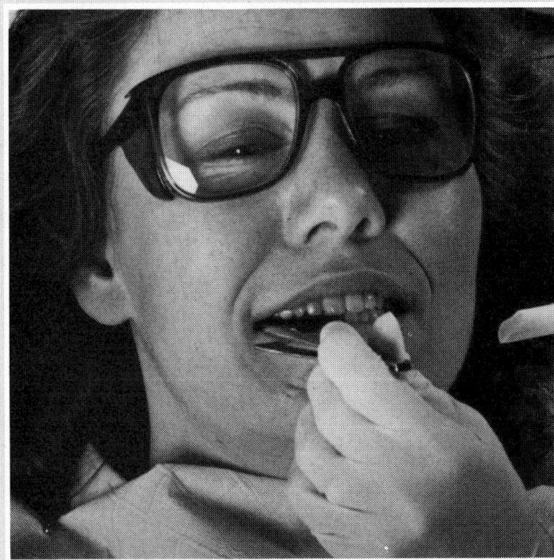

FIGURE 25–8

Articulating paper is placed, and the patient is instructed to close gently.

Carving the Amalgam Restoration

1. The operator receives the explorer and uses it to remove the amalgam near the marginal surface of the matrix band.
2. The wedge, matrix retainer, and matrix band are then removed.
3. The assistant passes the carver of choice to the operator. While the operator is carving the restoration, the assistant uses the HVE to remove any scrap material.
4. The previous step is repeated until initial carving of the restoration is complete.

Adjusting the Occlusion

1. The assistant receives the last carver, passes the rubber dam forceps, and aids in the removal of the dental dam.
2. The assistant places articulating paper in the articulating paper holder and passes it to the operator. (During the transfer, this is positioned so that the operator can grasp the handle.)
3. The operator places the articulating paper on the occlusal surface of the opposing arch teeth, and the patient is instructed to cautiously close the teeth together (Fig. 25–8).
   □ *CAUTION:* Sudden closure on a freshly placed amalgam will fracture the restoration.
4. The assistant passes a carving instrument to the operator for use in reducing any high spots.
   □ *RATIONALE:* The articulating paper will leave colored marks on high spots of the freshly placed restoration.
5. The surface of the new restoration is again checked with articulating paper and carved until clear of indicator marks when in light occlusion.
6. After light carving to relieve the occlusion, a moist cotton pellet is used to gently rub the surface of the amalgam to smooth the finish.
7. A further check of the occlusion is made with articulating paper, and the final carving is completed.
8. After the final carving, the air-water syringe and HVE are used to rinse the patient's mouth.
9. The patient is cautioned not to chew on the restoration for a few hours.
   □ *RATIONALE:* Amalgam does not achieve its final strength for several hours. Biting on it before that time could cause the restoration to fracture.

Bonded Amalgam Restorations

Amalgam bonding creates a bond between the material, the bonding agent, and the tooth structure (Fig. 25–9). This reduces the possibility of microleakage and enhances the retention of the restoration. However, not all amalgam restorations require bonding.

Bonding is best suited for use with very large restorations in which supplemental retention (such as pins) is required, and in some situations, bonding may eliminate the need for such retention.

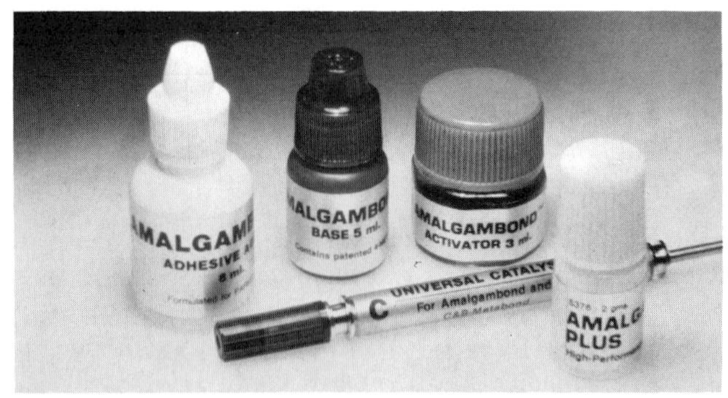

FIGURE 25–9

Amalgam bonding materials. (Courtesy of Parkell, Farmingdale, NY.)

Amalgam Restorations with Retention Pins

When there has been extensive decay, it is occasionally necessary to use pins as an additional means of retaining and supporting the restoration: for example, when the tooth has extensive caries of the distolingual cusp that has undermined the enamel and dentin.

Pins are available in several diameters (widths) and styles (Fig. 25–10). However, all pins are *very small* and easily dropped. For this reason, it is essential that the dental dam be in place during the process of preparing and placing the pins.

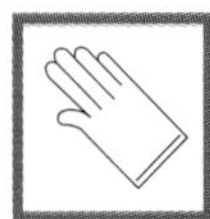
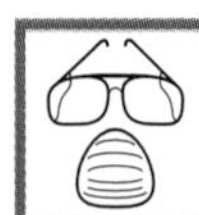
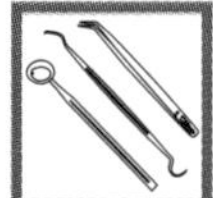
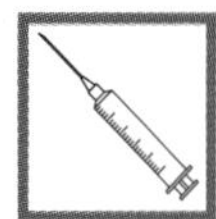
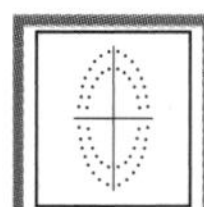

PROCEDURE: **Applying Amalgam Bonding**

1. The dentist completes a traditional cavity preparation that provides mechanical retention.
   ☐ *RATIONALE:* Bonding is a supplemental means of retaining the restoration.
2. If the cavity preparation is near the pulp, a small calcium hydroxide base is placed over the affected area. An additional base is *not* indicated because it may interfere with the bonding.
3. A metal matrix band is used; however, before placement, the band is coated with cavity varnish. This prevents the bonding resin and amalgam from adhering to its surface. No varnish should contact the tooth, as this will negate the bonding effects of the resin primers.
4. The matrix band is placed before the tooth is conditioned and the bonding resins and the amalgam are placed. The band should be properly adapted and wedged as in any traditional amalgam restorative procedure.
5. The entire dentin surface of the preparation and the enamel margins should be properly conditioned with the appropriate acid conditioner. Etching times range from 15 to 30 seconds, depending upon the conditioner used.
6. The conditioning acid is thoroughly rinsed with water from the air-water syringe; then the excess water is removed with a light puff of air from the air-water syringe.
7. The primer is applied to the entire preparation in one or multiple coats, depending upon the manufacturer's directions. The properly primed surfaces should appear damp after drying with air.
8. After primer placement, the dual-cured adhesive resin is mixed, painted in the entire cavity preparation, and lightly air-thinned.
9. The amalgam is immediately mixed and condensed into the cavity preparation before the adhesive resin has had a chance to polymerize.
10. The amalgam is compressed against the floors and walls of the cavity preparation as soon as possible to integrate the resin into the amalgam. Remaining condensation, carving, and finishing of the amalgam follow the conventional format.

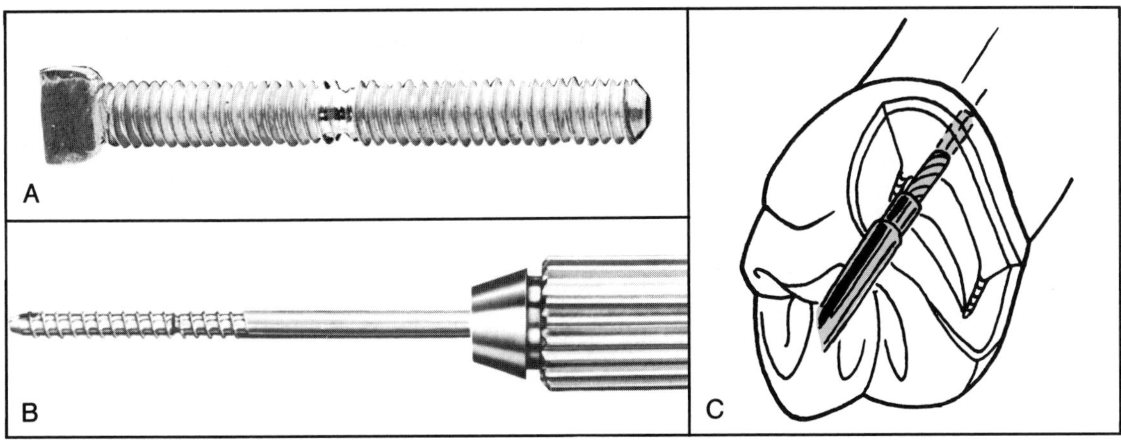

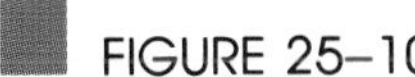

FIGURE 25–10

Retention pin placement. *A*, Close-up of a self-treading snap-off retention pin. (Courtesy of Whaledent International, New York, NY.) *B*, Close-up of a retention pin with holder. (Courtesy of Syntex Dental Products, Valley Forge, PA.) *C*, Threading a retention pin into the dentin.

 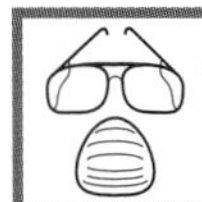 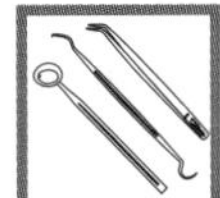 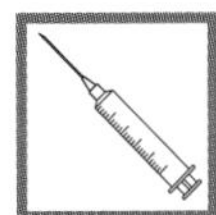 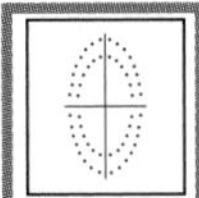

PROCEDURE: **Placing Amalgam Retention Pins**

Preparing the Retention Pins

1. The tooth is prepared, and the liner and base are placed. The dentist determines the type of pins to be used and where they are to be placed.
   □ *RATIONALE:* These decisions are influenced by the location of the caries and the amount of remaining sound dentin.
2. A twist-drill is used in the low-speed handpiece to prepare the pin holes.
3. Each pin is cut to fit into the hole and extend for the desired length above the dentin. The prepared pins are tried in the holes and then removed before cementation.
4. *Alternative:* A self-shearing pin is threaded into place with the low-speed handpiece. When the pin approaches the bottom of the hole, the head of the pin shears off, leaving a length of pin extending from the dentin.

Cementing the Retention Pins

1. The assistant mixes zinc phosphate cement to cementing consistency.
2. A Lentulo spiral instrument is used in a low-speed handpiece to convey the cement to the full depth of the pin hole.
3. The end of the wire pin is coated with cement and pressed into place.
4. After the initial set, any excess cement is removed with an explorer.
5. The matrix is positioned, and the amalgam restoration is placed and finished.

Composite Restorations

Composites resins have the major advantage as restorative materials in that they match the tooth color and are esthetically pleasing. They are also capable of bonding directly to the tooth structure, and this reduces the possibility of microleakage (Fig. 25–11).

Their major disadvantage is that they are not as strong as amalgam or other metal restorations and cannot withstand the chewing forces in Class II restorations as well as these other materials.

Composites are widely used for Class III, Class IV, and Class V restorations in which appearance is very important and in which they are *not* subjected to the heavy chewing forces placed on the posterior teeth.

In the posterior teeth, composites are used in Class I restorations in which they are surrounded and supported by natural tooth structure. They are used in Class II restorations when appearance is of primary concern.

The physical characteristics of composite resins and the details of enamel and dentin bonding are discussed in Chapter 23.

Characteristics of Placing Composite Restorations

The tooth preparation steps for placing a composite restoration are similar to those described for amalgam with several important exceptions:

- The dentist is usually able to do a more conservative preparation that requires less removal of healthy tooth structure. Sometimes this does not require the administration of a local anesthetic.
- Before bonding and placement of a composite, the tooth must be cleaned of all calculus, plaque, and debris. Either pumice and water or a fluoride-free and oil-free polishing paste is used for this purpose.
- The tooth being treated must be isolated to keep it free of contamination such as blood, moisture, or debris. Dental dam aids in maintaining a clean, dry environment.
- The air and water supply used to dry an etched tooth must be free of oil or debris. (Oil and debris interfere with the bonding process.)
- When indicated, a calcium hydroxide cavity liner is applied. A liner containing eugenol is *not* used because it would interfere with the polymerization of the composite.
- Because composite may stick to metal and/or metal may leave black marks on the material, special placement instruments are used in placing and working with the material. These are made of a nonstick plastic or highly polished stainless steel.

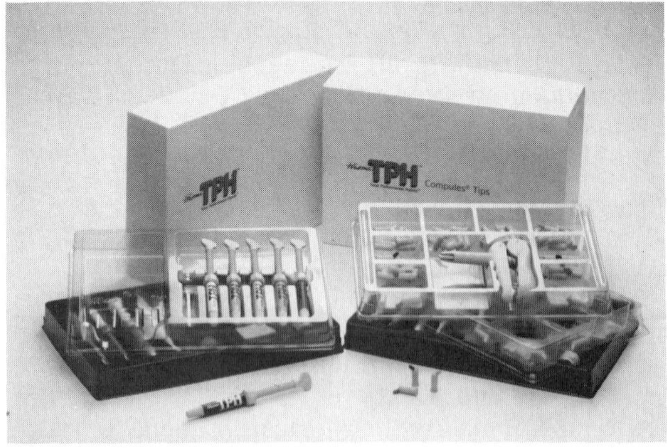

FIGURE 25–11

Light-cured composite restorative material. *Left*, Composite in light-proof syringes. *Right*, Composite in premeasured capsules with centrix syringe and disposable tips. (Courtesy of L.D. Caulk Co., Milford, DE.)

SHADE SELECTION

It is possible to select a shade of composite that will very closely match the natural tooth. To achieve an accurate match, this shade must be selected in excellent light, with the natural tooth wet. Some dentists select the shade before the dental dam is placed and before preparing the tooth. Other dentists select the shade just before placement of the restoration.

A shade guide, which is provided by the manufacturer, contains a tooth-shaped sample of each color available in that material. This guide aids in the selection of a color to exactly match the patient's natural dentition.

During the shade selection process, the shade piece is moistened and held next to the natural tooth. At the end of the treatment visit, the entire shade guide is sterilized or disinfected according to the manufacturer's directions.

Self-curing composites are mixed to the correct shade. Light-cured composites are supplied in light-proof syringes of individual shades.

MATRICES FOR COMPOSITE RESTORATIONS

A clear plastic matrix is used with a composite resin or glass ionomer. (A metal band would leave black marks on the restoration and would interfere with light-curing.) If a wedge is necessary, a plastic wedge is used.

A clear plastic strip is used as a matrix for a Class III restoration in which the proximal wall of an anterior tooth is missing. Should contouring (shaping) of the band be necessary before placement, the plastic strip is shaped by pulling it lengthwise over the rounded back end of the cotton pliers.

The strip is eased between adjacent teeth. Immediately after the restoration material has been placed, the strip is pulled tightly around the tooth to reconstruct the natural contours.

For a self-curing composite material, the matrix can be held in place with a retainer clip until the restoration has cured. A metal clip is *not used* with a light-cured material.

A crown former may be used for a Class IV restoration in which both the proximal wall and incisal angle of an anterior tooth are involved. (A **crown former** is a thin clear plastic form shaped like the crown of the tooth being restored.)

After the restoration material has reached its final set, the matrix is removed or the crown former is cut away and discarded.

Anterior Composite Restorations

PLACING CLASS III COMPOSITE RESTORATIONS

A Class III cavity involves the proximal surface of an anterior tooth. Because the appearance and finish of the restoration are so important, and since the restoration is supported by tooth structure, the dentist may select a microfilled composite that is noted primarily for its ability to finish smoothly.

If the carious lesion is very deep, calcium hydroxide or a glass ionomer base is placed only over the deepest area of the preparation. Otherwise, bases and liners are not commonly used in these restorations.

PLACING CLASS IV COMPOSITE RESTORATIONS

A Class IV restoration involves the proximal surface and incisal edge of an anterior tooth. Preparation and placement of this type of restoration are very similar to those for a Class III restoration with these major differences:

- A Class IV restoration is subjected to some biting and chewing stress. For this reason, the dentist may select a composite that has greater strength and the ability to take a smooth finish.
- This restoration involves restoring either the mesioincisal or distoincisal corner of the tooth. A shaped matrix, such as an incisal angle or a crown former, is used for a Class IV restoration.
- Instead of being placed directly into the cavity preparation, the restorative material is loaded into the matrix former. Then the former is pressed into place, and the material is forced into the preparation.

Before use, a hole may be made at the incisal-proximal angle of the crown form. This allows excess material to escape and aids in placement of the form on the prepared tooth.

Posterior Composite Restorations

Composite materials used must be able to withstand the wear and stress factors placed on it by the biting and chewing forces. The strength of the composite used in this area, particularly for Class II restorations, is very important. In this area, the ability of the material to be highly polished is less important than it is in an anterior tooth.

PLACING CLASS I COMPOSITE RESTORATIONS

A Class I composite restoration involves only one surface of the tooth. The preparation and placement steps are similar to those for a Class II restoration except that no matrix is used.

PLACING CLASS V RESTORATIONS

A Class V restoration is placed on the facial surface at the cervical third of the clinical crown. Damage to the tooth may have been caused by root caries, erosion, or abrasion.

Glass ionomer cement or a composite restoration, which will bond to the tooth and match the tooth color, are the materials of choice for this type of restoration.

The steps in the placement of a Class V restoration are similar to those of other anterior restorations with glass ionomer or composites with the following exceptions:

- Care must be taken to maintain a clean and dry field. (This is particularly difficult because the restoration is near the gingiva.)
- Frequently this type of restoration requires very little preparation of the tooth, and many patients are comfortable without local anesthesia.
- The prepared tooth is etched and bonded according to the manufacturer's directions.
- A clear plastic preformed facial surface matrix may be used. (This is precontoured to fit the facial surface of the tooth.)
- The restorative material may be placed directly into the prepared tooth, *or* it may be loaded into the contoured matrix and then forced into the preparation.
- The material is light-cured, the matrix is removed, and the restoration is finished.

COMPOSITE-IONOMER LAMINATED RESTORATIONS

Glass ionomer cements may be used as restorations in which minimal preparation of the tooth is desired (such as where there is root abrasion) or in which the fluoride release from the cement is desired to resist recurrence of caries.

When a composite resin or glass ionomer restoration is indicated for esthetic purposes, a laminated restoration may be placed. (**Laminated** means layered.)

After the tooth has been prepared, if necessary, a light-cured calcium hydroxide is placed near the pulpal area and cured. Then ionomer cement is prepared and placed over the floor and walls of the cavity.

(text continues on page 493)

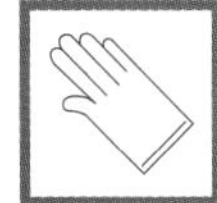 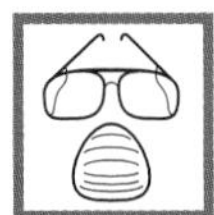 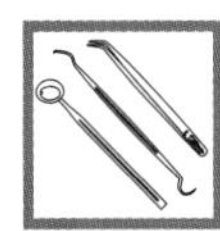 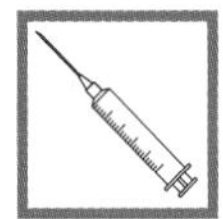 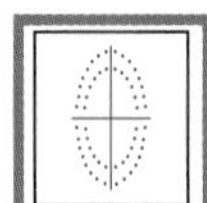

PROCEDURE: **Placing a Class III Composite Restoration**

Instrumentation (Figs. 25–12, 25–13)

Composite shade guide
High-speed handpiece
Low-speed handpiece (straight or right-angle)
HVE tip
Instruments for cavity preparation (operator's choice)
Calcium hydroxide and mixer/applicator
Syringes of composite material (light-cured)
Etchant gel and applicator
Dentin etchant solution or gel
Primer for dentin and enamel
Plastic composite placement instrument
Plastic matrix
Wedge and pliers (optional)
Curing light with protective shield
Finishing burs or diamonds
Abrasive strips
Articulating paper
Polishing kit (disks and mandrels)
Polishing paste
Petroleum jelly
Dental floss

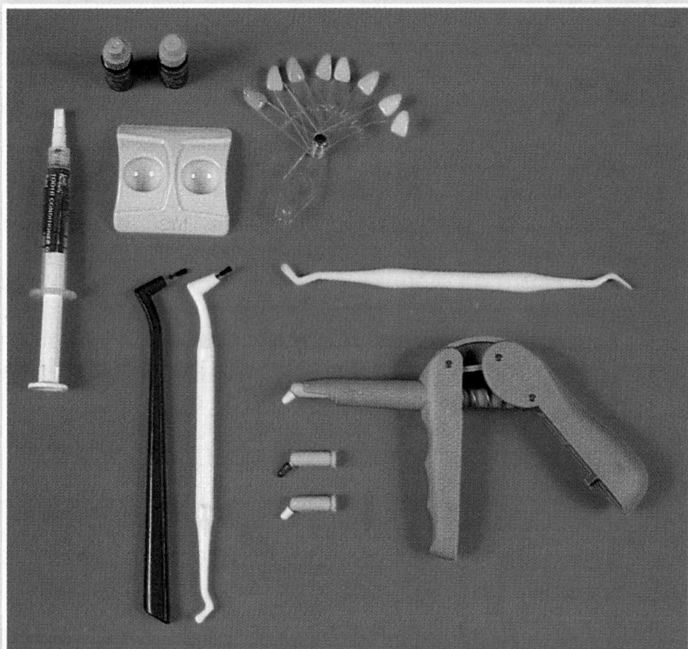

FIGURE 25–12

Composite instrumentation setup. *Left,* Acid etchant (blue syringe), primer materials A and B (gray- and orange-capped bottles), double plastic mixing wells (for use with primer), and brushes with color-coded handles (one for the etchant, one for the primer). *Top right,* A shade guide and plastic composite instrument (white). *Bottom right,* Two premeasured capsules of composite materials (color-coded to indicate different shades). This material is dispensed through the centrix syringe (beige) shown above them.

Preparing the Tooth

1. If indicated, local anesthetic solution is administered. While it takes effect, the shade is selected and the dental dam is applied.
2. The dentist prepares the tooth. If possible, the preparation is from the lingual surface.
   □ *RATIONALE:* This preserves the appearance of the facial surface of the tooth.
3. Throughout the procedure, the assistant uses the HVE to maintain a clear operating field. The assistant also passes and receives hand instruments as needed.
4. The cavity is rinsed and dried. If indicated, a calcium hydroxide base is placed.

Etching, Bonding, and Composite Placement

1. The enamel and dentin are etched, rinsed, and dried in accordance with the manufacturer's directions.
2. The matrix strip is placed. If indicated, a plastic wedge is also placed.
3. The bonding resin is applied and light-cured in accordance with the manufacturer's directions.
4. The syringe-type composite material is dispensed directly into the preparation.
5. The matrix is pulled and held tightly around the tooth to restore the contour.
6. The composite is light-cured from the lingual and facial surfaces.

Finishing the Restoration

1. The matrix and wedge are removed.
2. Finishing burs or diamonds are used in the high-speed handpiece to contour the restoration.
3. If indicated, the interproximal surface is smoothed with abrasive strips.
4. The dental dam is removed, and articulating paper is used to check the occlusion. Adjustments are made as necessary.
5. Polishing discs, points, and cups are used in the low-speed handpiece to polish the restoration.
6. A final coating of the sealing material or a neutral substance, such as petroleum jelly, is placed over the finished restoration.

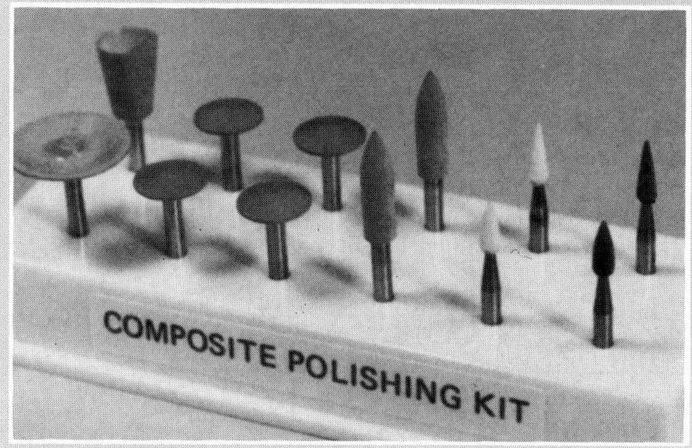

FIGURE 25–13

Composite finishing kit. (Courtesy of Shofu Dental Corp., Menlo Park, CA.)

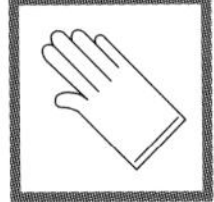 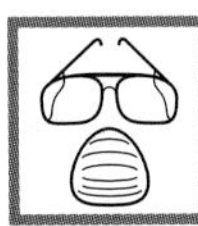 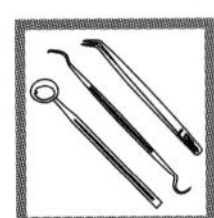 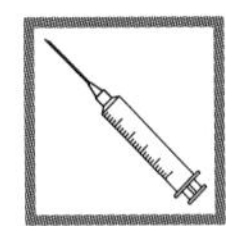 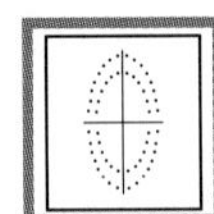 

PROCEDURE: **Placing a Class II Composite Restoration**

Instrumentation

High-speed handpiece
Low-speed handpiece (right-angle)
Instruments for cavity preparation (operator's choice)
HVE tip
Calcium hydroxide setup
Etchant gel and applicator
Matrix band, holder, and wedges
Bonding agent, mixing dish, and applicators
Light-cured composite (supplied in a preloaded syringe)
Condensable composite (supplied as pastes with mixing supplies)
Plastic amalgam carrier
Condensers (smooth)
Ball burnisher
Articulating paper in holder
Finishing burs (operator's choice)
Polishing discs and points
White webbed-type rubber polishing cup
Polishing paste
Petroleum jelly
Curing light with protective shield

Preparing and Etching the Cavity

1. Local anesthetic solution is administered, and the dental dam is placed.
2. The tooth is prepared, and calcium hydroxide is placed to protect the pulp.
3. The gel etchant is placed, and the tooth is etched in accordance with the manufacturer's directions.
4. The tooth is thoroughly rinsed to remove all traces of gel etchant. The air-water syringe is used to dry the tooth until the surface appears frost white and dry.
   □ *IMPORTANT:* Do not overdry the tooth.
5. The matrix band is placed and wedged.

Bonding

1. The bonding agent is dispensed according to the manufacturer's instructions.
2. The bonding agent is applied with a disposable applicator to all of the dentin and etched enamel surfaces.
3. A gentle air stream is used to spread the bonding agent.
4. The entire bonding agent surface is light-cured if so directed.

Placing the Restorative Material

1. The tip of the preloaded composite syringe is used to place the restorative material into the deepest portion of the prepared tooth. This layer is light-cured.
   □ *NOTE:* Some dentists place the composite in layers. Each layer is cured before the next is placed.
2. The condensable material is placed with either a plastic amalgam carrier or a plastic placement instrument. This is condensed with a smooth surface condenser.
3. Before curing, the occlusal anatomy is formed by using a ball burnisher or waxing-instrument.
4. The occlusal layer is light-cured, and the matrix band is removed.
5. The restoration is light-cured from the facial and lingual surfaces.
6. The restoration is contoured and finished with 12- and 30-bladed finishing burs or a diamond bur in a high-speed handpiece.
7. The dental dam is removed, and the occlusion is adjusted.

Finishing and Polishing the Restoration

1. Polishing discs, stones, and points are used in a low-speed handpiece with water spray.
2. The polishing paste is applied with a white webbed polishing cup in a low-speed handpiece, and the surface is polished lightly for approximately 60 seconds.
   □ *RATIONALE:* A dark-colored rubber polishing cup would stain the restoration.

Depending upon the type of material, this is light-cured or is allowed to self-cure (harden by polymerization).

Excess material is trimmed away from the enamel margins. The preparation, including the glass ionomer, is etched and bonded before the placement of the composite restorative material.

Direct Bonded Composite Veneers

A veneer may be placed on one or more anterior teeth to improve their appearance. (A **veneer** is a layer of tooth-colored material that is attached to the facial surface of a prepared tooth.)

A composite veneer that is bonded directly to the tooth surface is created by using the **direct technique.** A composite or porcelain veneer prepared in the dental laboratory and then cemented to the tooth surface is known as the **indirect technique**. This technique is discussed in Chapter 31.

Veneers are used to improve the appearance of teeth that are slightly abraded, eroded, discolored with intrinsic stains, or darkened after endodontic treatment.

Veneers may also be used to slightly improve the alignment of the teeth or to close a diastema. (A **diastema** is an unusually large separation between the maxillary central incisors.)

Regardless of the type of veneer that is applied, the patient is advised of the following:

- Composite veneers have a limited life span and need to be reapplied when wear, chipping, or discoloration occurs.
- Good oral hygiene is important to keep the surfaces and margins free of plaque and food debris.
- Biting on hard substances, such as ice, bones, and crusts of bread, could fracture the veneer.

INSTRUMENTATION

The instrumentation is similar to that required for the preparation of a Class II composite restoration. Usually the dentist removes a thin layer of enamel equal to the thickness of the composite to be placed. This avoids overcontouring of the tooth or having it look and feel thicker than the adjacent teeth.

In some situations, little or no enamel reduction is needed. When enamel must be removed, special diamond burs in the high-speed handpiece are used for this purpose.

MATRIX SELECTION

A special plastic matrix is used for this purpose. This form, which is constructed of Mylar, consists of an anatomic facial form flanked by two very thin, high-strength matrix strips. (**Mylar** is a trade name for a polyester made in extremely thin sheets of high tensile strength.)

The strips placed mesially or distally, when held around the tooth, hold the composite in place while the material is being cured.

The matrix has a tab on the incisal edge. This is used to grasp the form while scissors are being used to trim the gingival edge. After the matrix has been trimmed to shape, the tab is removed.

Bleaching of Teeth

Bleaching is often desirable because it is the least invasive method of lightening the color of dark or discolored teeth.

Indications for Bleaching Teeth

- The removal of intrinsic stains (intrinsic and extrinsic stains are discussed in Chapter 21)
- Discoloration after injury to the tooth that has caused a hemorrhage of the pulpal tissues into the dentin (this hemorrhage reflects through the enamel and the tooth appears darker)
- Discoloration due to a metallic restorative material
- Tetracycline stains (bleaching may lighten these stains; however, it cannot remove them)
- Mottled enamel caused by fluorosis (brown fluorosis stains generally respond; fluorosis white spots are unaffected)
- The patient's dissatisfaction with the current color of otherwise sound teeth
- Persons whose teeth were originally lighter but have been darkened by age, coffee, tea, smoking, or other stain-producing habits (when extrinsic stains can be removed by coronal polishing, this is the treatment of choice; see Chapter 21)
- Before placement of a veneer, lightening the underlying tooth base and making the subsequent veneer more esthetically pleasing
- Lightening natural teeth to match existing ceramic crowns or similar restorations

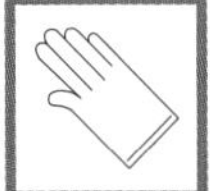
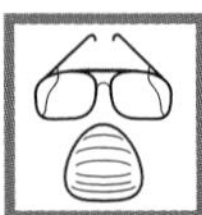
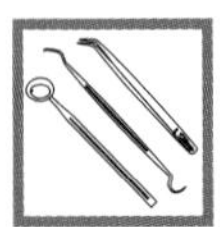

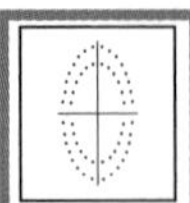

PROCEDURE: **Placing a Composite Veneer**

1. Local anesthesia is not usually required for this procedure.
2. At the beginning of the visit, the shade is selected. Dental dam placement is optimal.
3. The tooth is measured to determine the appropriate crown form size. If necessary, the form is trimmed to fit the gingival contour.
4. The required amount of enamel is removed, then the tooth is etched and bonded.
5. If the veneers are being placed to cover dark stains, an opaque material may be placed to block out the stains (Fig. 25–14). (**Opaque** means to block light or not allow light through.)
6. The composite is placed on the inner surface of the form. The form is placed on the tooth with the interproximal strips between the teeth (Fig. 25–15). With one hand, the form is slowly pushed into place. With the other hand, the interproximal strips are pinched together at the lingual of the tooth (Fig. 25–16).
7. An explorer is used to trim away excess composite material that has extruded beyond the crown form.
8. With the matrix properly positioned, the strips are held tightly while material is light-cured for the time recommended by the manufacturer. When curing is complete, the form is removed and discarded (Fig. 25–17).
9. The operator uses sandpaper discs to adjust the tooth to the proper length. Finishing burs are used to trim and smooth the veneer (Fig. 25–18).
10. These steps are repeated for each tooth to receive a veneer (Fig. 25–19).

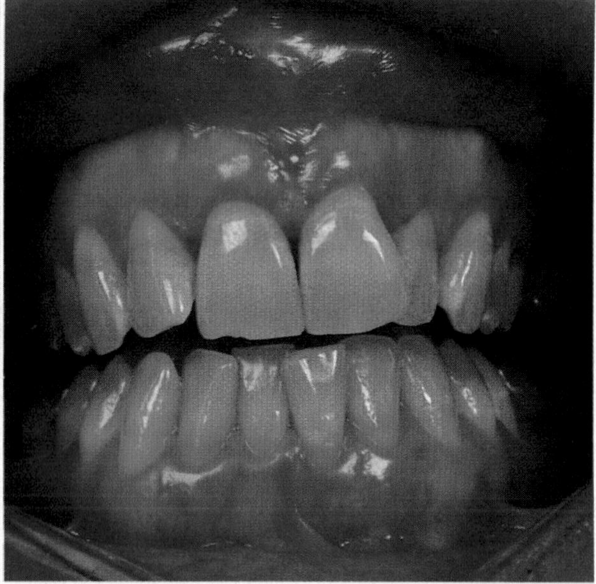

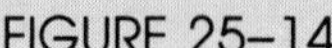

FIGURE 25–14

Patient's teeth before placement of bonded composite veneers. Notice the tetracycline stains. (Courtesy of Plastodontics, Flint, MI.)

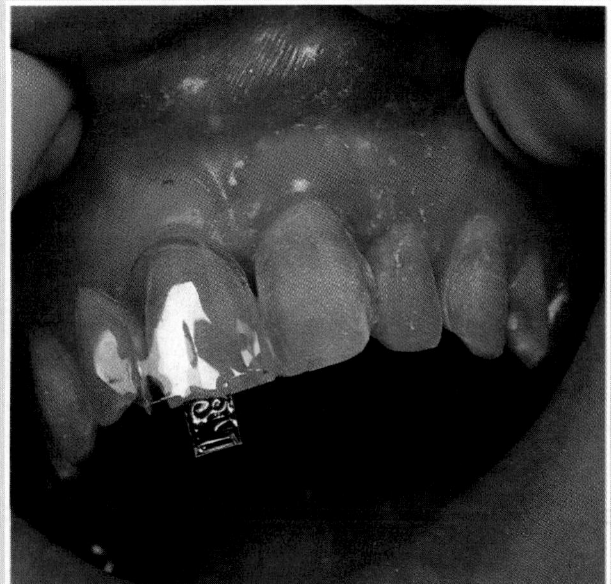

FIGURE 25–15

The clear plastic former is tried for size. (Courtesy of Plastodontics, Flint, MI.)

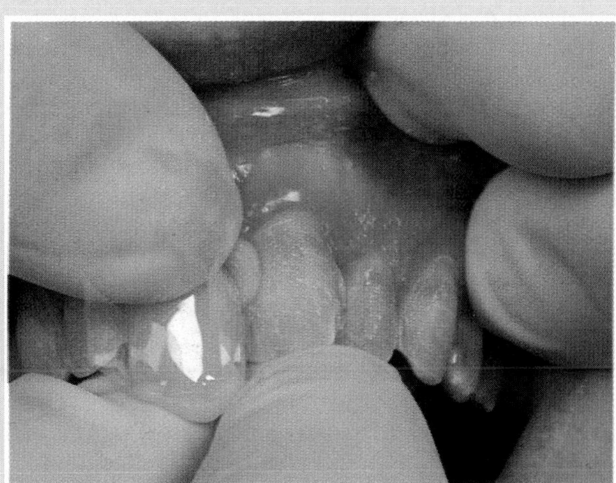

FIGURE 25–16

The former is filled with composite and then placed on the tooth. (Courtesy of Plastodontics, Flint, MI.)

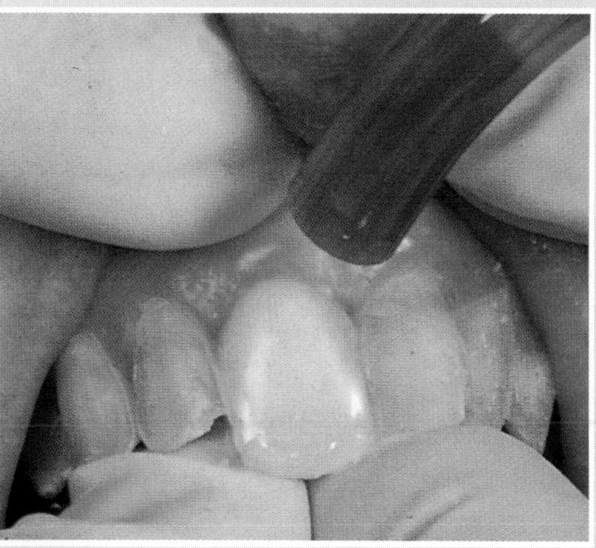

FIGURE 25–17

Excess material is removed, and the composite is light-cured. (Courtesy of Plastodontics, Flint, MI.)

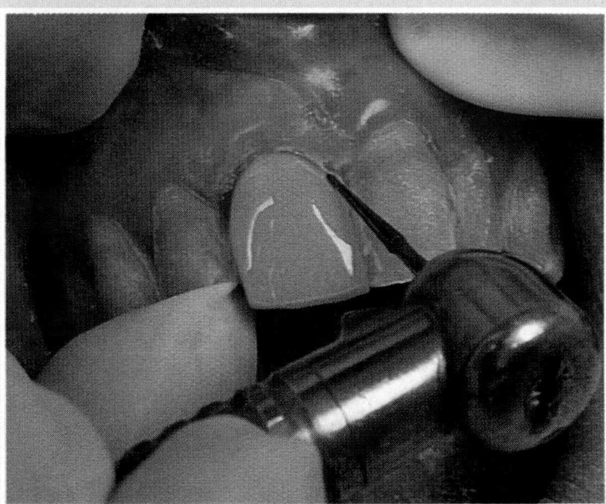

FIGURE 25–18

The former is removed, and the veneer is finished. (Courtesy of Plastodontics, Flint, MI.)

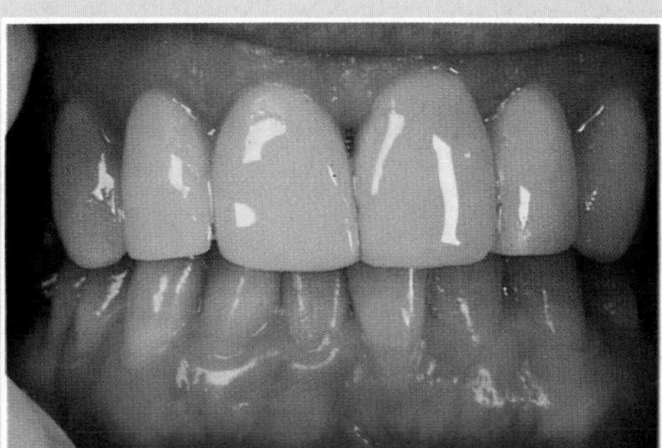

FIGURE 25–19

The completed placement of four bonded anterior veneers. (Courtesy of Plastodontics, Flint, MI.)

Contraindications for Bleaching Teeth

- Results are not predictable.
- It is impossible to tell how long it will take to get results.
- It is impossible to tell how long the results will last.
- Some stains will not respond to bleaching.
- Some stains, such as those from foods, will recur.
- Bleaching is not usually indicated for children because of the large pulp chambers in the teeth.

Bleaching Techniques

The three most widely accepted bleaching techniques are non-vital bleaching, in-office bleaching, and night-guard vital bleaching. Non-vital teeth are those that have been treated endodontically. Vital teeth are healthy, normal, intact teeth.

NON-VITAL BLEACHING

If there has been bleeding within the crown of the tooth before endodontic treatment, the crown may become discolored after the endodontic treatment has been completed. If this happens in an anterior tooth, non-vital bleaching may be indicated to lighten the tooth.

The most commonly used non-vital bleaching technique is called **walking bleach technique**. It is so named because the bleaching process takes place as the patient continues with his normal activities. Walking bleaching is performed after the endodontic treatment has been completed and *before* the tooth is restored. After the bleaching, the restoration is placed.

A mixture of 35 percent hydrogen peroxide and sodium perborate in a thick paste is sealed in the pulp chamber with cotton and a cavity sealer. The bleaching effect occurs out of the office. The paste is changed every 2 to 7 days (depending on the operator's preference) until the maximum result has been achieved.

IN-OFFICE BLEACHING

The advantages of in-office bleaching of vital teeth are that results can be seen quickly and the technique is under the control of the dentist. The disadvantages are that it is costly (because it is time consuming and may require four to six treatments) and that it is not possible to accurately predict the results.

Commonly used in-office bleaching techniques involve 35 percent hydrogen peroxide. Heat or a light

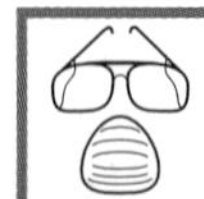
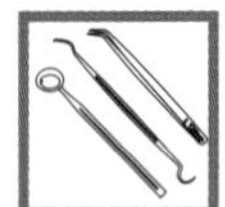

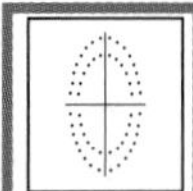

PROCEDURE: **Performing In-Office Bleaching, Using a Curing Light**

1. Dental dam is placed before the treatment. A ligature of waxed dental floss is placed around the cervix of each tooth to be bleached.
   □ *RATIONALE:* This is essential because this solution is caustic and the soft tissues must be protected. Waxed floss must be used so that it will *not* absorb the bleaching solution.
2. Selective coronal polishing may be recommended for the teeth to be treated.
   □ *RATIONALE:* It is important that as much stain as possible be removed before bleaching. As with all materials, it is important to follow the manufacturer's instructions.
3. The bleaching solution is a gel that is mixed just before use. It is painted on the teeth with the brush applicator.
4. The composite curing light is used for approximately 3½ minutes to activate the bleaching solution.
5. After treatment is complete, the teeth are rinsed and the dam is removed.

source may be used to enhance the action of the peroxide. Some systems do not use either light or heat.

When heat is used, it is accomplished without anesthesia to allow the patient's pain threshold to determine the appropriate heat level. (Excessive heat can damage the pulp.)

SUPERVISED NIGHTGUARD VITAL BLEACHING

A primary indication for nightguard vital bleaching is for patients who are dissatisfied with the natural color of their otherwise sound teeth. Another indication is for persons whose teeth have been darkened by age, coffee, tea, smoking, or other stain-producing habits.

This bleaching process is carried out by the patient at home. There are home bleaching kits available for patient use without the supervision of a dentist. However, to ensure patient safety and maximum results, dentist-supervised nightguard bleaching is recommended.

Before starting treatment, the patient must be aware that the results are not guaranteed and are not permanent.

Nightguard bleaching involves the use of a bleaching gel that is placed in a custom tray. This is commonly called nightguard because the patient wears the tray while he sleeps.

Nightguard bleaching takes from 2 to 6 weeks to achieve optimum results. During this period the dentist sees the patient periodically to review progress and to detect any tissue irritation.

The bleaching gel is 10 percent carbamide peroxide, which is approximately one-tenth the concentration of the solutions used during in-office bleaching. The custom tray, which may be fabricated by the assistant, must fit properly. This protects the patient's soft tissues from irritation and prevents the patient from swallowing excessive amounts of the solution.

These trays are constructed by using the vacuum former technique described in Chapter 24.

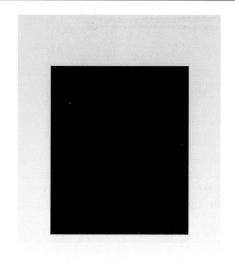

Chapter 26

Periodontics

Introduction

Periodontal diseases, which involve the bone and ligaments that support the teeth, are the leading causes of tooth loss in adults. Fortunately, with early detection and treatment of periodontal disease, it is now possible for most people to keep their teeth for a lifetime (Fig. 26–1).

To prepare for this chapter, you should review the following:

- Chapter 4: normal features of the periodontium
- Chapter 6: plaque and preventive care
- Chapter 11: periodontal case types and periodontal diseases

Instrumentation for Periodontics

Periodontal therapy requires the use of specialized instruments to remove local irritants, measure periodontal pockets, and perform periodontal surgery.

These instruments must be sharp in order to scale, root plane, or perform periodontal procedures. In general, the registered dental hygienist who uses these in-

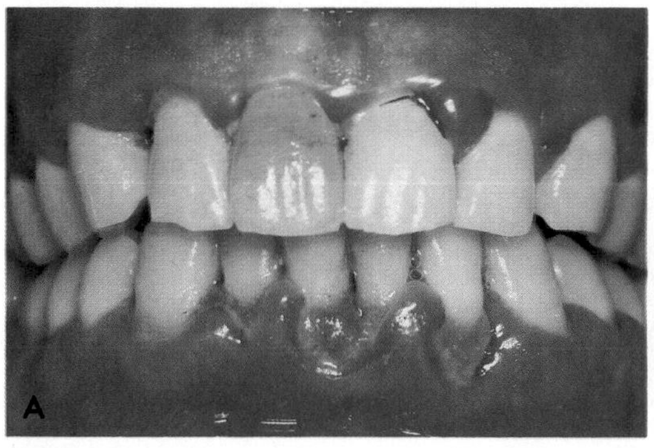

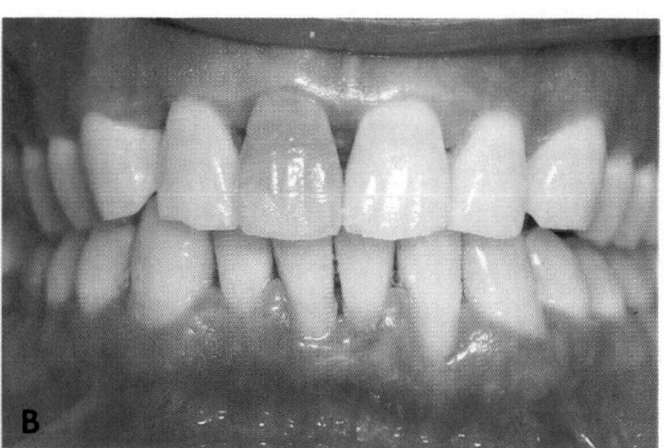

FIGURE 26–1

Periodontal therapy, combined with good home care, can be very effective. *A*, Heavy calculus deposits and severe gingival inflammation. *B*, Three weeks after elimination of irritants, gingival healing has resulted. (From Carranza, F.A.: Glickman's Clinical Periodontology, 7th ed. Philadelphia, W.B. Saunders Co., 1990, p 674.)

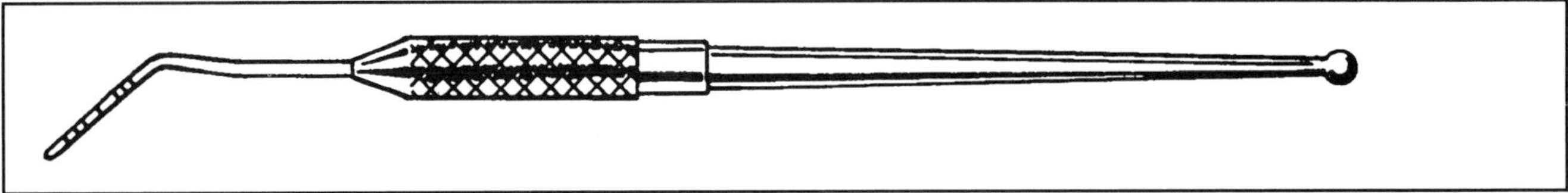

FIGURE 26–2

Gradations on the tip of a periodontal probe are marked in millimeters.

struments takes responsibility for maintaining the sharpness of these instruments.

Because periodontal procedures routinely involve blood, these instruments are classified as critical instruments and must be sterilized before use.

Periodontal Probes

Periodontal probes, which are calibrated in millimeters, are used to locate and measure the depth of periodontal pockets (Fig. 26–2). On some, the tips are color-coded to make the measurements easier to read.

The **manual probe** is tapered to fit into the gingival sulcus and has a blunt or rounded tip. This probe is available in many designs, and selection depends on personal preference of the operator (Fig. 26–3).

Automated computerized probes are extremely accurate electronic devices used to measure the depth of periodontal pockets. With the probe, a thin wirelike device is inserted into the sulcus, and data are recorded by a microcomputer.

Explorers

Explorers are used in periodontics to locate calculus deposits and provide tactile information to the operator about the roughness or smoothness of the root surfaces.

There are many types of explorers used in periodontal treatment. These are longer and more curved than explorers used for caries detection. (Explorers are discussed in Chapter 15.)

The working ends of periodontal explorers are thin, fine, and easily adapted around root surfaces. They are also capable of reaching to the base of deep pockets and furcations. (A **furcation** is the point at which the roots of a multi-rooted tooth diverge.)

Scalers

Sickle scalers are used primarily to remove large deposits of supragingival calculus. A sickle scaler with a long, straight shank is used to remove calculus from the anterior areas of the mouth (Fig. 26–4). A contra-angle sickle scaler, which is angled at the shank, is designed to remove calculus from the posterior teeth.

Chisel scalers are used to remove supragingival calculus in the contact area of anterior teeth. The blade on the chisel scaler is curved slightly to adapt the tooth surfaces (Fig. 26–5).

Hoe scalers are used to remove heavy supragingival calculus. Hoes are most effective when used on buccal and lingual surfaces of the posterior teeth (Fig. 26–6).

Files are used to crush or fracture very heavy calculus. The fractured calculus is then removed from the tooth surface with curettes (Fig. 26–7).

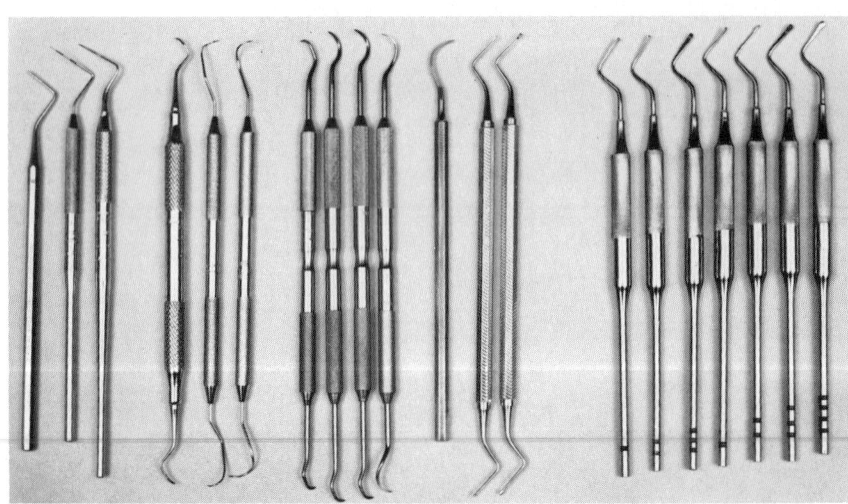

FIGURE 26–3

Periodontal probes and scalers. The three instruments on the left are periodontal probes. The remaining instruments are scalers.

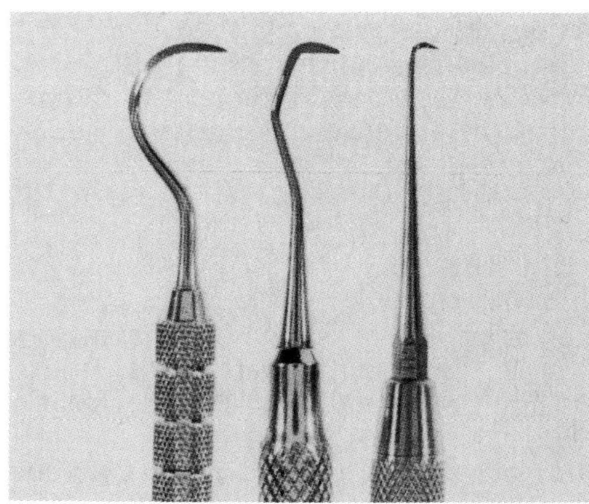

FIGURE 26–4

The working ends of anterior sickle scalers. (From Perry, D.A., Beemsterboer, P., and Carranza, F.A.: Techniques and Theory of Periodontal Instrumentation. Philadelphia, W.B. Saunders Co., 1990, p 132.)

Curettes

Curettes are used after scalers to complete calculus removal and to smooth root surfaces (root planing).

Universal curettes are designed so one instrument is able to adapt to all tooth surfaces. There are *two cutting edges,* one on each side of the blade. Universal curettes resemble the spoon excavators used in restorative dentistry (Fig. 26–8).

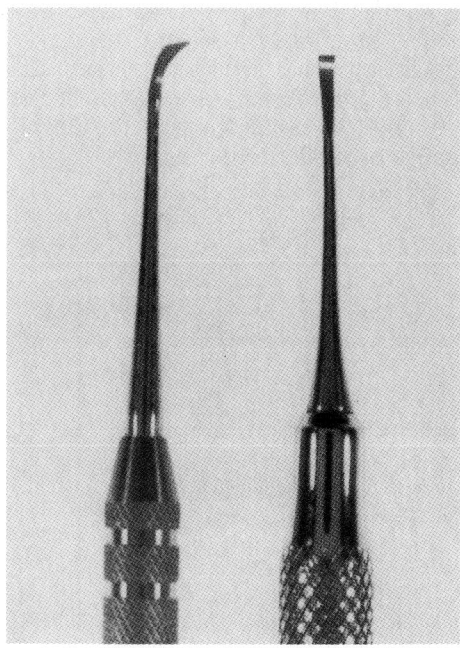

FIGURE 26–5

The working ends of chisel scalers. (From Perry, D.A., Beemsterboer, P., and Carranza, F.A.: Techniques and Theory of Periodontal Instrumentation. Philadelphia, W.B. Saunders Co., 1990, p 298.)

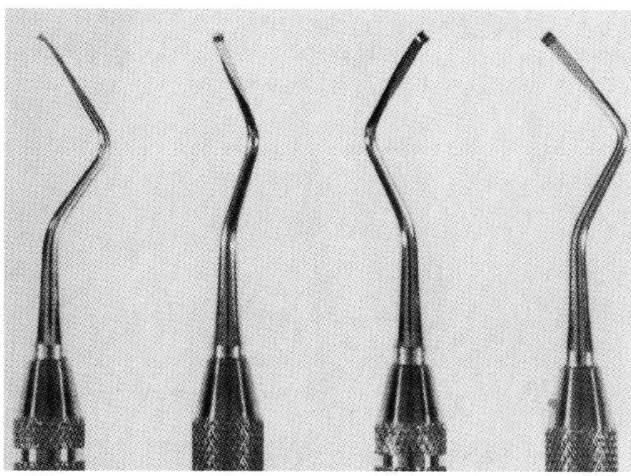

FIGURE 26–6

The working ends of hoe scalers. (From Perry, D.A., Beemsterboer, P., and Carranza, F.A.: Techniques and Theory of Periodontal Instrumentation. Philadelphia, W.B. Saunders Co., 1990, p 299.)

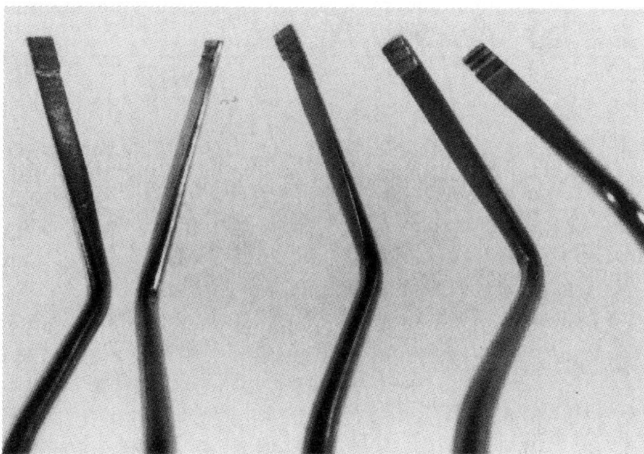

FIGURE 26–7

Set of files designed for access to all areas. (From Perry, D.A., Beemsterboer, P., and Carranza, F.A.: Techniques and Theory of Periodontal Instrumentation. Philadelphia, W.B. Saunders Co., 1990, p 299.)

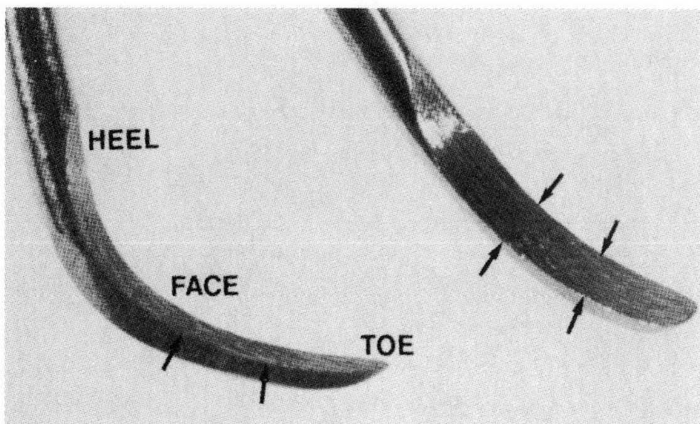

FIGURE 26–8

The universal curette. This instrument has a rounded toe, the face of the blade curves from heel to toe, and the back is rounded. The universal curette has two parallel cutting edges, indicated by arrows. (From Perry, D.A., Beemsterboer, P., and Carranza, F.A.: Techniques and Theory of Periodontal Instrumentation. Philadelphia, W.B. Saunders Co., 1990, p 149.)

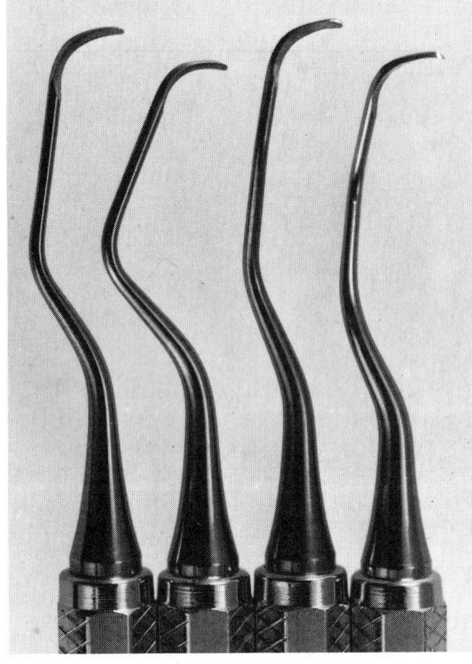

FIGURE 26–9

Gracey curettes. This is a reduced set and shown here from the left are No. 5-6, No. 7-8, No. 11-12, and No. 13-14. (From Carranza, F.A.: Glickman's Clinical Periodontology, 7th ed. Philadelphia, W.B. Saunders Co., 1990, p 601.)

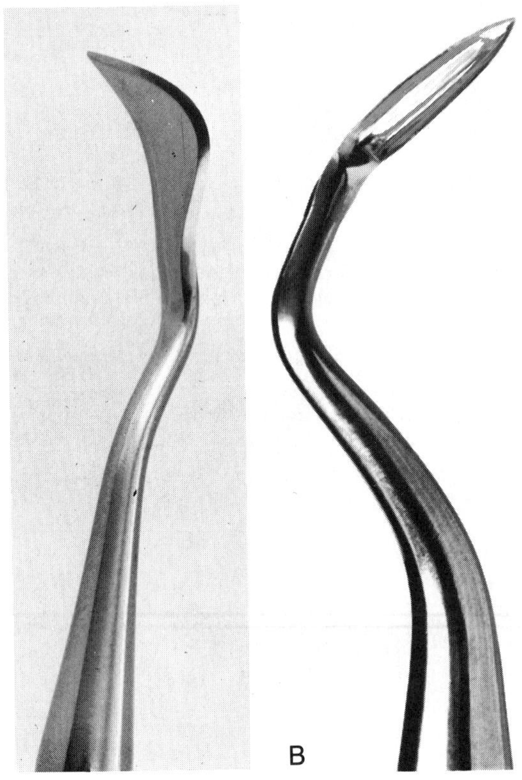

FIGURE 26–10

Periodontal knives. *Left*, Kirkland knife. *Right*, Orban interdental knife. (From Carranza, F.A.: Glickman's Clinical Periodontology, 7th ed. Philadelphia, W.B. Saunders Co., 1990, p 608.)

Gracey curettes, which have only *one cutting edge,* are area specific. This means that they are designed to adapt to specific tooth surfaces. Treatment of the full dentition requires the use of several curettes (Fig. 26–9).

Periodontal Knives

Kirkland knives are one of the most common types of knives used in periodontal surgery. These instruments are usually double-ended with kidney-shaped blades (Fig. 26–10, left).

Orban knives are used to remove tissue from the interdental areas. These knives are shaped like spears and have cutting edges on both sides of the blades (see Fig. 26–10, right).

Pocket Markers

Pocket markers are similar in appearance to cotton pliers; however, the tips are pointed and designed to make pinpoint perforations in the gingival tissue (Fig. 26–11). These perforations, which are referred to as bleeding points, are used to outline the area for a gingivectomy.

Ultrasonic Scalers

Ultrasonic scalers may be used for scaling, curettage, and root planing. In periodontal instrumentation, ultrasonic tips are thinner than the regular type and produce up to 29,000 vibrations per second.

Periodontal tips are available in various shapes, depending on the type of procedure to be performed. See Chapter 28 for a complete explanation of the operation and maintenance of the ultrasonic scaler.

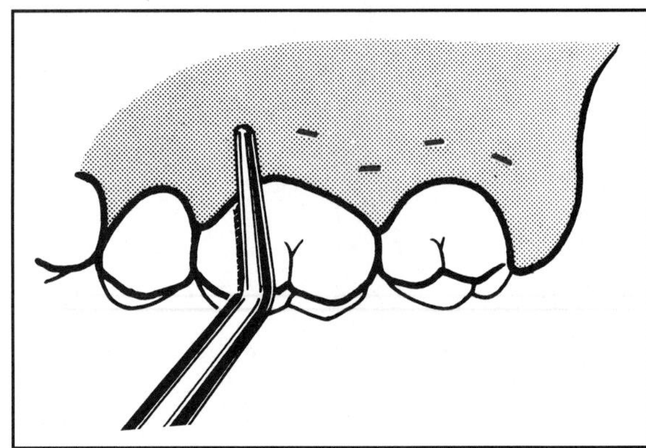

FIGURE 26–11

Periodontal pocket marker makes pinpoint perforations that indicate pocket depth. (From Carranza, F.A.: Glickman's Clinical Periodontology, 7th ed. Philadelphia, W.B. Saunders Co., 1990, p 783.)

The Periodontal Examination

Periodontal screening and recording (PSR), which is part of every dental examination, is discussed in Chapter 18. However, in addition to a thorough dental examination, specialized procedures are necessary to diagnose periodontal disease and to determine the proper treatment.

These procedures include medical and dental histories, dental and periodontal examinations, and a radiographic evaluation.

Medical and Dental Histories

The dentist reviews the medical history to detect any systemic conditions that may influence periodontal treatment. Systemic diseases, such as acquired immunodeficiency syndrome (AIDS) or diabetes, can lower tissues' resistance to infection. Lowered resistance makes periodontal disease more severe.

The dental history is used to gather information about conditions that could indicate periodontal disease. For example, patients with periodontal disease often complain of bleeding gums, loose teeth, or a bad taste. They may describe a dull pain after eating, or a burning sensation in the gums.

Dental Examination

The dental examination focuses on the teeth for indications of periodontal disease. These would include the following:

- **Sensitivity** in the teeth to changes in temperature can be caused by gingival recession over the roots.
- **Pathologic migration**, which is a shift in the position of the teeth, can be caused by a loss of periodontal support.
- **Clenching or grinding**, which are habits that place excessive biting forces on the teeth, may accelerate bone loss.
- **Defective restorations or bridgework** are areas that may retain plaque and increase the risk of periodontal disease.

MOBILITY

Mobility is the movement of the tooth within its socket, and all teeth have a very small degree of mobility. However, increased mobility is an indication of periodontal disease (Fig. 26–12). Mobility is recorded with the Dental Mobility Scale, shown in the right column.

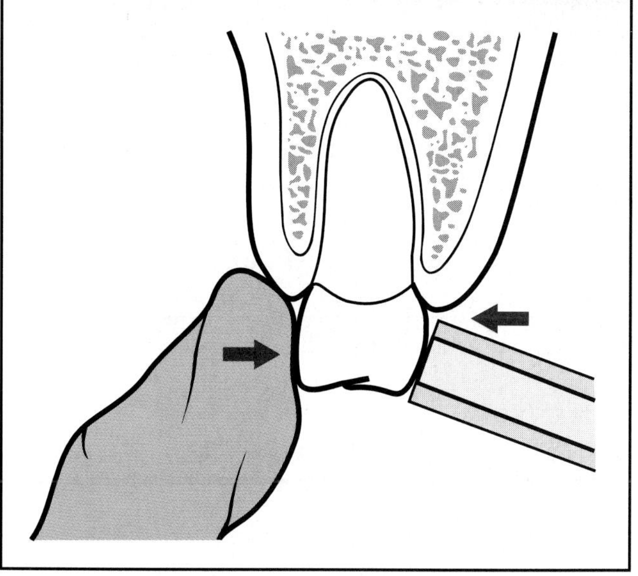

FIGURE 26–12

Tooth mobility is checked with a metal instrument and one finger. (Modified from Carranza, F.A., and Perry, D.A.: Clinical Periodontology for the Dental Hygienist. Philadelphia, W.B. Saunders Co., 1986, p 131.)

Periodontal Examination

The periodontal examination includes an assessment of the amount of plaque and calculus, changes in the gingiva, signs of bleeding, presence of periodontal pockets, presence of bleeding, and signs of improper occlusion.

PLAQUE AND CALCULUS

Plaque is the cause of gingival inflammation and most other forms of periodontal disease. (Plaque is discussed in Chapter 6.)

Calculus is hardened, mineralized plaque that adheres to the surfaces of natural teeth, crowns, bridges, and dentures. Calculus cannot be removed by brushing or using other plaque control methods. Calculus is a factor in periodontal disease because it is always covered by plaque (Fig. 26–13).

Plaque and calculus accumulate **supragingivally** (above the gingival margin) and **subgingivally** (below the gingival margin). Supragingival calculus is easily

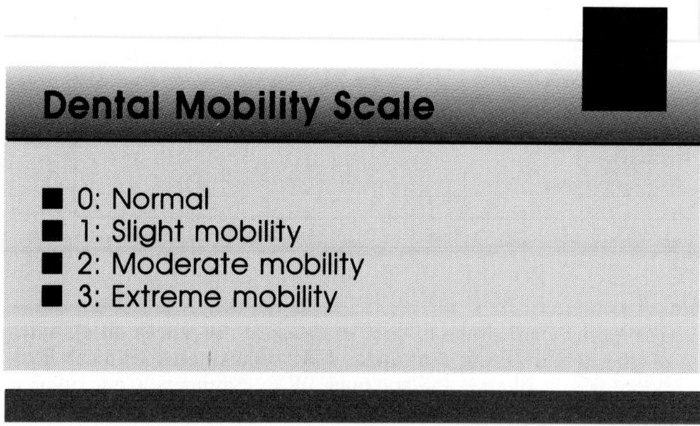

Dental Mobility Scale

- 0: Normal
- 1: Slight mobility
- 2: Moderate mobility
- 3: Extreme mobility

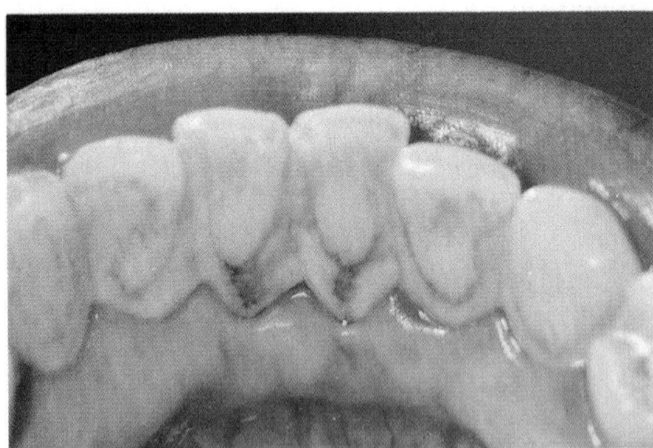

FIGURE 26–13

Calculus deposits on lingual surfaces of lower incisors. (From Carranza, F.A.: Glickman's Clinical Periodontology, 7th ed. Philadelphia, W.B. Saunders Co., 1990, p 390.)

seen on the tooth surfaces. Subgingival calculus is detected by checking each tooth surface, to the level of the gingival attachment, with a sharp explorer.

GINGIVA

The gingiva is examined for changes in color, size, contour, consistency, surface texture, and bleeding.

PERIODONTAL PROBING

A **periodontal pocket** occurs when disease causes the gingival sulcus to become deeper than normal (a nor-

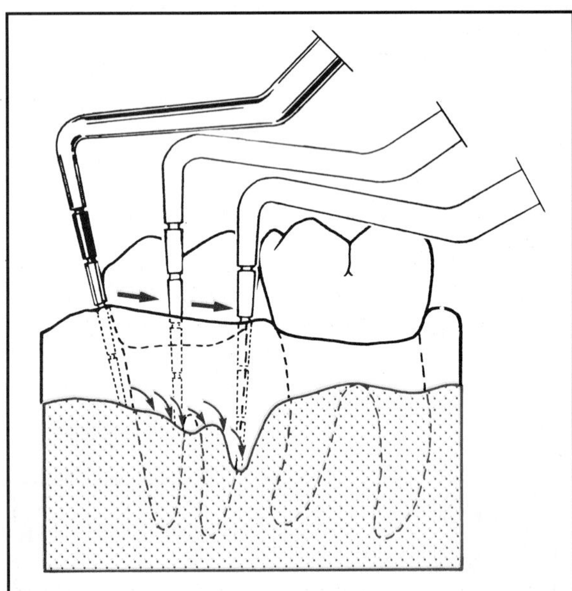

FIGURE 26–14

The periodontal probe is used to measure the sulcus on all sides of the tooth. (From Carranza, F.A.: Glickman's Clinical Periodontology, 7th ed. Philadelphia, W.B. Saunders Co., 1990, p 494.)

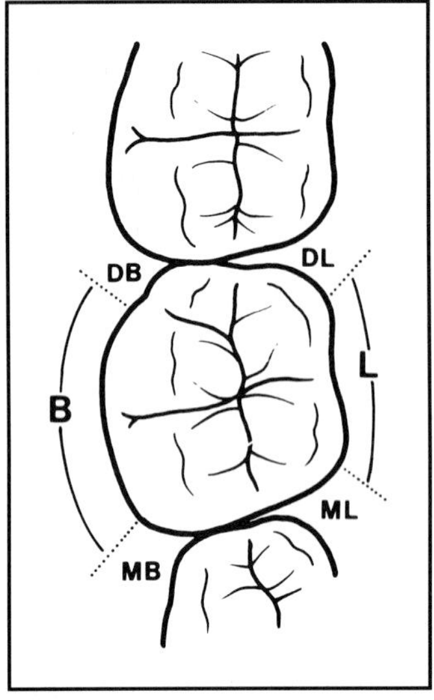

FIGURE 26–15

Six probing depth measurements are taken for each tooth. DB, distobuccal; B, buccal; MB, mesiobuccal; DL, distolingual; L, lingual; ML, mesiolingual. (From Perry, D.A., Beemsterboer, P., and Carranza, F.A.: Techniques and Theory of Periodontal Instrumentation. Philadelphia, W.B. Saunders Co., 1990, p 35.)

mal sulcus is 3 mm. or less). The depth of the pocket is measured by using a periodontal probe.

Six measurements are taken for each tooth (Figs. 26–14 and 26–15). The deepest measurement on each surface is recorded on the patient's chart (Fig. 26–16). The surfaces measured are

- Mesiofacial
- Facial
- Distofacial
- Mesiolingual
- Lingual
- Distolingual

BLEEDING INDEX

The severity of gingival inflammation can be measured by the amount of bleeding observed during probing. Several different systems of bleeding scores are used. Each system is based on the principle that healthy gingiva does not bleed.

Occlusal Analysis

The periodontium requires some occlusal force (pressure) for stimulation to remain healthy. However, if there is excessive force, occlusal trauma (injury) can result. The patient's occlusion is evaluated for signs of excessive force on the teeth.

Occlusal trauma does not cause periodontal pocket formation; however, it can cause tooth mobility, destruction of bone, migration of teeth, and temporomandibular joint pain.

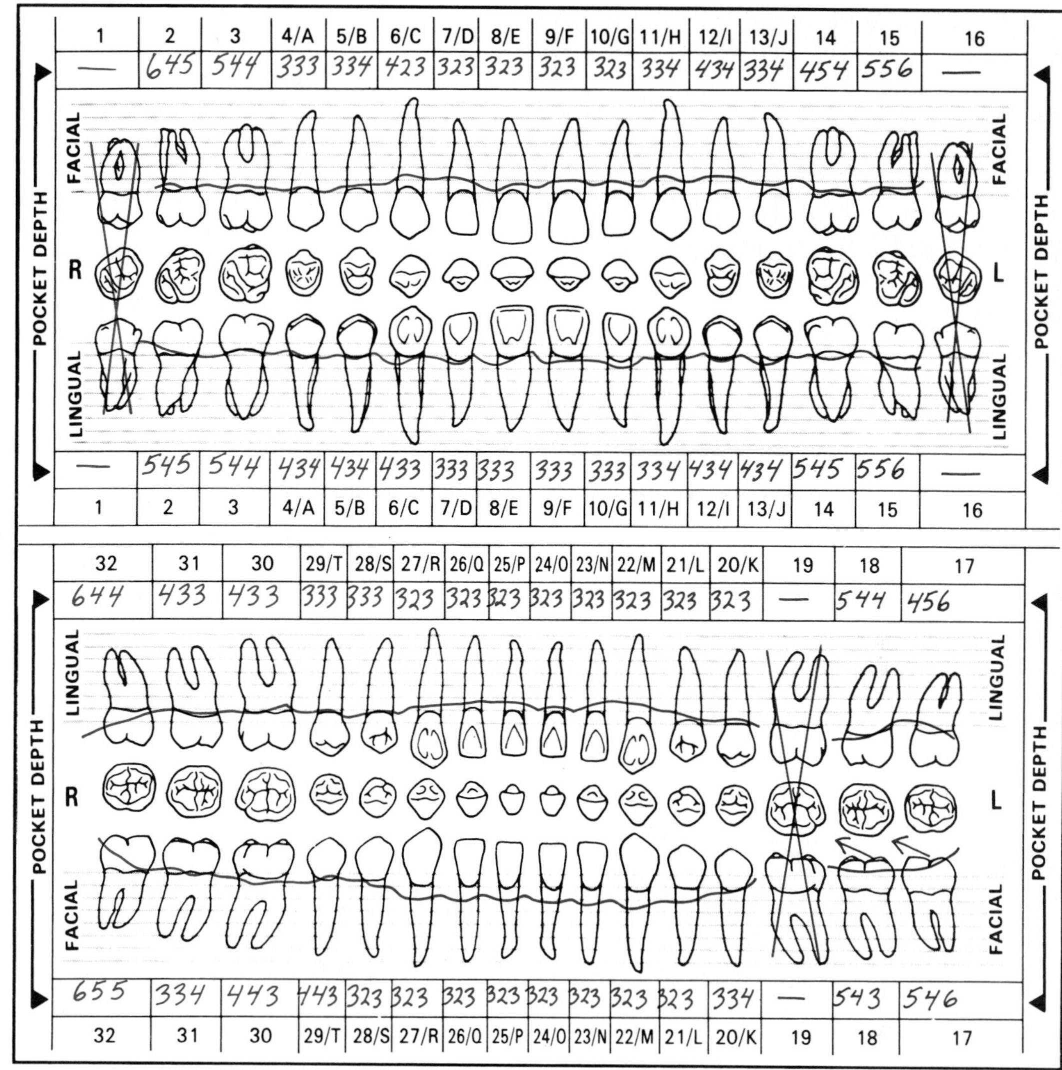

FIGURE 26–16

Periodontal charting for a 40-year-old patient. (Form courtesy of Colwell Systems, Champaign, IL.)

Articulating paper and occlusal wax are used to identify occlusal interferences, which may require removal by occlusal equilibration. (An **occlusal interference** is an area on a tooth that prevents the teeth from occluding properly.)

Radiographic Evaluation

Radiographs are a valuable aid for evaluating periodontal disease. The accuracy of the radiographs is *critical* in the diagnosis of periodontal disease, because a distortion can result in a diagnostic error. Radiographs are used to

- Detect interproximal bone loss
- Show the changes in the bone as periodontitis progresses
- Locate furcation involvements
- Measure the crown-to-root ratio (the length of the clinical crown compared with the length of the root of the tooth)
- Show signs of traumatic occlusion

Periodontal Treatment Procedures

The method of periodontal treatment depends on the severity of the disease and the amount of tissue destruction that has occurred. Regardless of the treatment plan, ongoing good daily oral hygiene is essential for the success of any type of periodontal therapy.

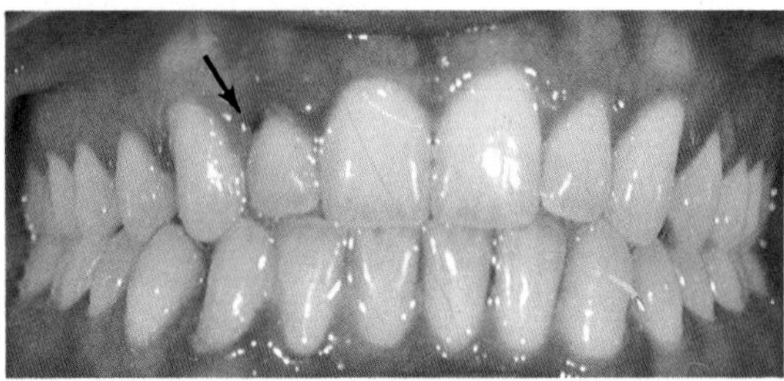

FIGURE 26–17

Gingivitis, case type I. Note slight puffiness and bleeding (arrow) around upper right lateral incisor. (From Carranza, F.A.: Glickman's Clinical Periodontology, 7th ed. Philadelphia, W.B. Saunders Co., 1990, Plate XI, *A*, p 492.)

Dental Prophylaxis

A dental prophylaxis, commonly referred to as a *prophy*, is the complete removal of calculus, soft deposits, plaque, and stain from all unattached supragingival and subgingival tooth surfaces. The dentist and dental hygienist are the only members of the dental health team licensed to perform this procedure.

A prophylaxis is indicated for patients with healthy gingiva as a preventive measure and is most commonly performed during recall appointments. A dental prophylaxis is also the primary treatment for gingivitis, case type I (Fig. 26–17).

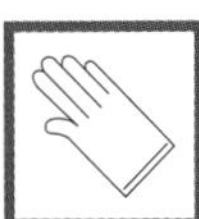
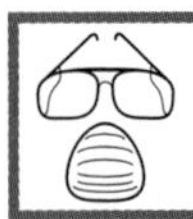
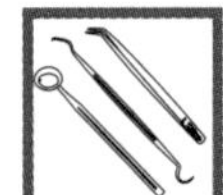

PROCEDURE: **Performing a Dental Prophylaxis**

Instrumentation (Fig. 26–18)

High-volume evacuator (HVE) tip or saliva ejector
Scalers, universal curette
Prophy angle
Rubber polishing cup and brushes
Polishing agent
Dental floss and/or tape

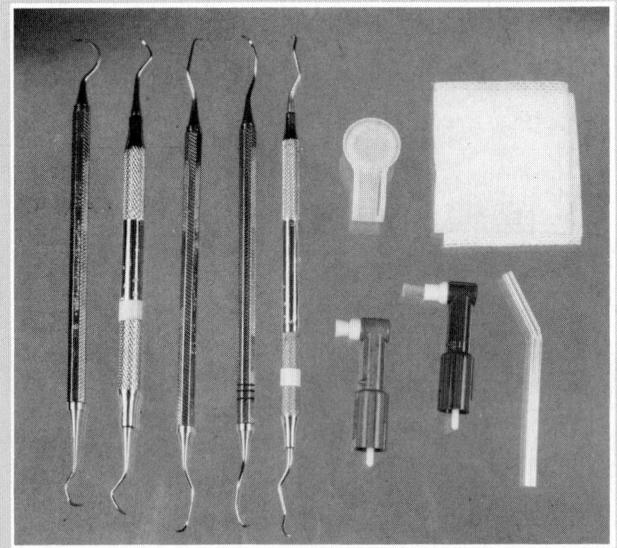

FIGURE 26–18

Instrumentation for a dental prophylaxis. Not shown here are the basic setup and dental floss.

Prophylaxis Steps

1. The operator uses an explorer to locate interproximal and subgingival calculus.
   □ *NOTE:* It is important for the operator to have good access and visibility during this procedure.
2. The operator uses scalers and curettes to remove all calculus and plaque.
   □ *NOTE:* Visibility and access can be improved by an assistant through oral evacuation and retraction of the lips and cheeks.
3. The operator checks for and removes any remaining calculus.
4. The operator polishes the teeth, using polishing paste, a rubber cup, and bristle brushes.
5. The operator removes any remaining interproximal debris with dental floss or tape.
6. Oral hygiene instructions are provided as needed by the patient.

Scaling, Root Planing, and Gingival Curettage

Scaling and root planing are indicated as the initial treatment for case types II and III and before periodontal surgery. In some cases, gingival curettage is also indicated (Fig. 26–19).

SCALING

Scaling is the removal of calculus from the tooth surface with sharp periodontal instruments. After subgingival calculus is scaled off, there may be areas on the root surface that remain rough. This is because the cementum has become necrotic (dead) or because the scaling has produced grooves and scratches. The root surface must be planed until it is smooth.

ROOT PLANING

Root planing is the removal of calculus and necrotic cementum embedded in the root. After root planing, the surfaces are smooth and glasslike. Smooth root surfaces resist new calculus formation and are easier for the patient to keep clean.

GINGIVAL CURETTAGE

In addition to scaling and root planing, which involve treatment of the surfaces of the tooth, some patients also require gingival curettage. (**Curettage** means scraping or cleaning with a curette.)

Gingival curettage, also referred to as *subgingival curettage*, is the scraping of the gingival wall of a periodontal pocket. This is performed to remove necrotic (dead) tissue from the pocket wall.

Postoperative Instructions After Scaling and Curettage

Discomfort. There may be mild discomfort for a few hours after the local anesthetic has worn off. Usually a mild analgesic such as aspirin is adequate for relieving this discomfort.

Diet. A normal diet is recommended; however, it is best to avoid very spiced foods, citrus fruits, and alcoholic beverages.

Smoking. The patient is advised not to smoke. Smoking irritates the tissues and delays healing.

Home Care. Good home care is essential for the success of this therapy. Normal home care should be resumed the following day.

Antimicrobial and Antibiotic Agents

Antimicrobial agents and nonsteroidal anti-inflammatory agents (NSAIDS) may be prescribed by the dentist for use in conjunction with pocket treatment.

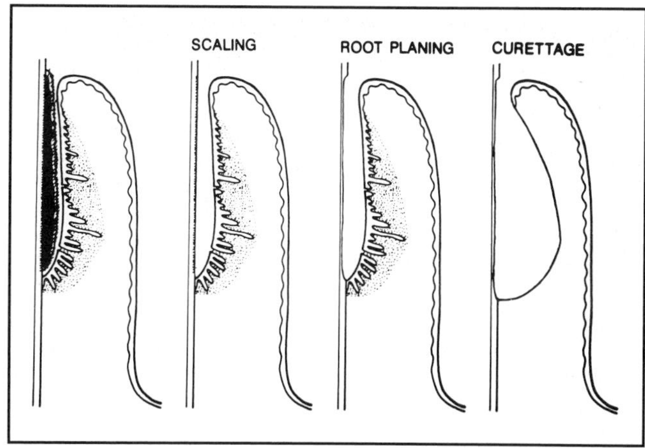

FIGURE 26–19

Scaling, root planing, and curettage. On the left is a periodontal pocket with calculus on the root of the tooth. *Scaling* removes the calculus. *Root planing* smooths the surface of the root. *Curettage* removes the infected tissue from the interior of the periodontal pocket. (From Perry, D.A., Beemsterboer, P., and Carranza, F.A.: Techniques and Theory of Periodontal Instrumentation. Philadelphia, W.B. Saunders Co., 1990, p 4.)

These agents can be taken orally or can be applied directly to the diseased tissue.

Nonsteroidal anti-inflammatory agents, such as flurbiprofen, are inhibitors of the bone loss common in periodontal disease.

Tetracycline currently appears to be the best antibiotic for the treatment of periodontitis, juvenile periodontitis, and rapidly destructive periodontitis. The recommended administration is 250 mg. four times per day for 1 to 2 weeks.

Fluorides have bactericidal effects against plaque bacteria. Use of a solution of 1.64 percent stannous fluoride to irrigate periodontal pockets delays bacterial growth. Mouth rinses containing fluoride have been shown to reduce bleeding by delaying bacterial growth in the periodontal pockets.

Chlorhexidine is the most effective agent available to reduce plaque and gingivitis. Two daily rinses with a 0.12 percent chlorhexidine mouthwash almost completely inhibit the development of dental plaque and gingivitis. Chlorhexidine can cause some temporary brown staining of the teeth, tongue, and resin restorations.

Types of Periodontal Surgery

Gingivectomy

A gingivectomy is the surgical removal of diseased gingival tissue from the soft tissue wall of the periodontal pocket (Fig. 26–20). This procedure is indicated for the removal of (1) deep gingival pockets, (2) gingival enlargements, or (3) suprabony periodontal abscesses.

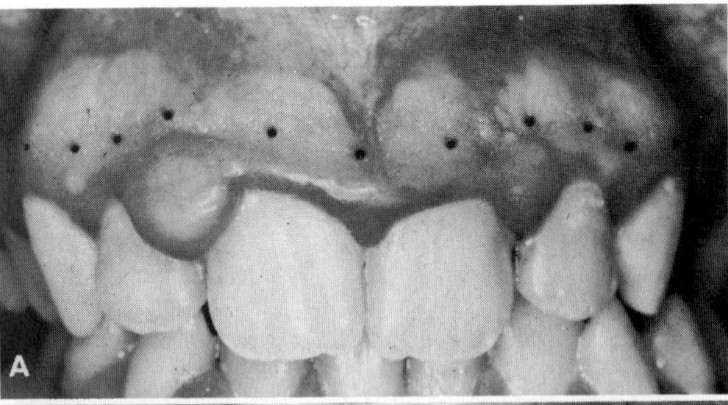

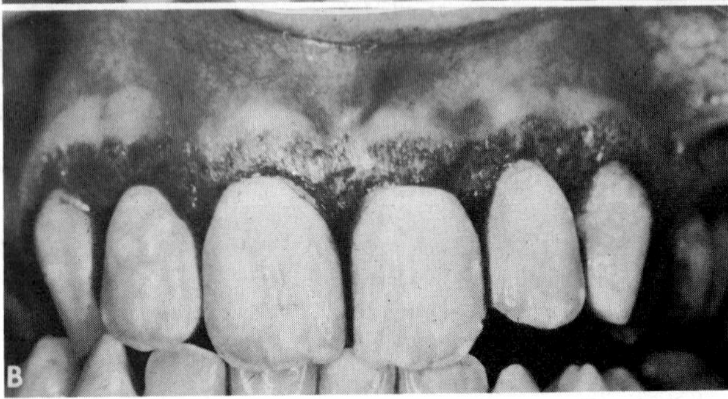

FIGURE 26–20

Gingivectomy incision for gingival enlargement. *A,* Pinpoint markings outline extent of the enlargement to be removed. *B,* Enlarged gingiva removed. (From Carranza, F.A.: Glickman's Clinical Periodontology, 7th ed. Philadelphia, W.B. Saunders Co., 1990, p 909.)

A gingivectomy is contraindicated when (1) the pocket is complicated by extension into the underlying bone, (2) osseous (bone) surgery is needed, and (3) the bottom of the pocket is apical to (below) the mucogingival junction.

POSTGINGIVECTOMY INSTRUCTIONS

The postoperative instructions should be given to the patient in written form. The instructions should include information about the following:

Discomfort. Mild to moderate discomfort can be expected, especially during the first 24 hours. If indicated, pain medication will be prescribed.

Periodontal Dressing. If bleeding is apparent under the dressing, call the dental office immediately.

Small pieces of the dressing may break off, and if there is no pain or bleeding, the dressing usually does not have to be replaced.

Rinsing. Do not rinse your mouth for the first 24 hours. After 24 hours, you may use a warm salt water rinse (1 teaspoon of salt in 8 oz. of warm water).

Diet. A normal diet is recommended. Avoid hard foods, alcoholic beverages, citrus fruit, and spicy foods.

Activity. Avoid excessive exercise for the first few days. This allows a firm clot to form in the surgical area.

Home Care. The areas of the mouth that were not involved in the surgery should be brushed and flossed normally. Gently clean the areas of the periodontal dressing using a toothbrush.

Postoperative Visit. Approximately 1 week after surgery, the dressing will be removed for a postoperative check. Usually after the dressing is removed, it is not necessary to replace it.

Gingivoplasty

A gingivoplasty is a surgical procedure that corrects gingival deformities, particularly enlargements. The technique for a gingivoplasty is similar to the gingivectomy technique. However, the purposes for these two techniques are different.

A **gingivectomy** is performed only when periodontal pockets *are present.* A **gingivoplasty** is performed only when periodontal pockets are *not present.* In the absence of periodontal pockets, a gingivoplasty includes

- Tapering the gingival margins
- Creating a scalloped marginal outline
- Shaping the interdental papillae

A

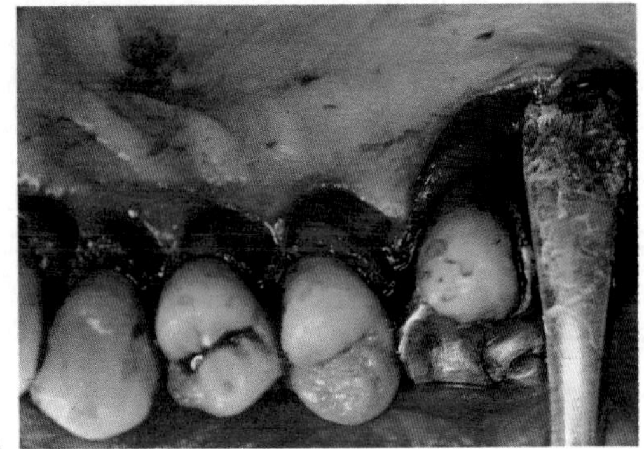

B

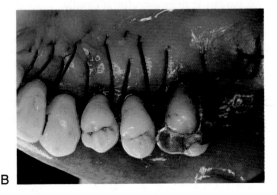

FIGURE 26–21

Periodontal flap technique. *A,* After the initial incisions, the flap shown here is elevated. *B,* At the end of the procedure, the flap is sutured in place. (From Carranza, F.A.: Glickman's Clinical Periodontology, 7th ed. Philadelphia, W.B. Saunders Co., 1990, p 793.)

 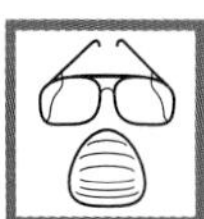 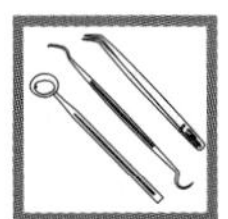 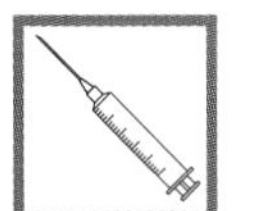 

PROCEDURE: **Performing a Gingivectomy**

During the gingivectomy, the dental assistant provides retraction and evacuation. Proper oral evacuation is critical for the comfort of the patient and the visibility by the dentist.

The following steps are performed by the *dentist.*

Instrumentation

HVE tip and surgical aspirating tip
Scalpel
Surgical periodontal knives
Surgical tissue retraction forceps
Pocket marker
Tissue tweezers
Scalers and curettes
Suture needle and sutures
Periodontal surgical dressing
Sterile gauze sponges

Gingivectomy Steps

1. Mark the pockets on both the facial and lingual surfaces, using the periodontal pocket marker.
2. Use either a scalpel or a periodontal knife to incise the gingiva, following along the bleeding spots. The incision is beveled to create a normally contoured free gingival margin.
3. Remove the gingival tissue along the incision line, using surgical knives.
4. Scale and root plane the root surfaces to remove any residual calculus.
5. Irrigate the surgical site and then cover it with a periodontal surgical dressing.
   □ *NOTE:* In some states, placing periodontal surgical dressing is delegated to the dental assistant.

The same types of periodontal surgical instruments are used for both techniques, and the postoperative home care instructions are the same.

Periodontal Flap Surgery

In periodontal flap surgery, a flap of the gingiva and/or adjacent oral mucosa is separated from the underlying tissues (Fig. 26–21, *left*). When the flap is elevated (lifted up), the dentist may perform one or more of the following procedures:

- Thorough scaling and root planing of the exposed root surfaces
- Moving the flap laterally (to the side) to cover the root surfaces of an adjacent tooth that does not have adequate tissue coverage (this procedure is called a "*laterally sliding flap*")
- Recontouring (reshaping) of the underlying bone

After the procedure is completed, the flap is closed and sutured into place (see Fig. 26–21, *right*). A periodontal pack is usually placed after flap surgery.

Osteoplasty

Osteoplasty, the surgical reshaping of bone, is performed to remove defects and to restore normal contours in the bone. This may be in the form of subtractive osseous surgery or of additive osseous surgery.

Both types of osteoplasty require surgically exposing the bone and recontouring it with a rotary diamond stone or a bone chisel.

SUBTRACTIVE OSSEOUS SURGERY

Subtractive osseous surgery, in which bone is removed, is performed when the patient has large exostoses (bony growths) that must be removed in order to restore the normal contour. This is most commonly necessary before the placement of a prosthesis that may rest on and irritate the area.

ADDITIVE OSSEOUS SURGERY

Additive osseous surgery, in which bone is added, is accomplished through bone graft procedures. This may be necessary for patients with bone defects (missing bone).

Periodontal Abscess

A periodontal abscess, which may be acute or chronic, is the accumulation of pus within a periodontal pocket.

The patient with an **acute periodontal abscess** may complain of symptoms such as throbbing, radiating pain, extreme tenderness of the area, tooth sensitivity, and even tooth mobility. The **chronic periodontal abscess** is usually *asymptomatic* (without symptoms).

The goal of treatment is to eliminate the infection. Treatment includes

- Draining the exudate from the pocket (an **exudate** is pus containing matter discharged from an infected area)
- Cleaning the inside of the pocket by gingival curettage
- Scaling and root planing the tooth
- Prescribing antibiotics and pain medication if necessary

Pericoronitis

Pericoronitis is an inflammatory process that occurs when the gingiva surrounding a partially erupted tooth becomes infected (Fig. 26–22). Because food debris is easily trapped under the tissue covering the partially erupted tooth, this occurs most frequently in the mandibular third molar area.

Pericoronitis may be acute or chronic. The patient may complain of severe pain, a foul taste in the mouth, swelling of the cheek, and fever. Upon examination, the tissue appears very red and swollen.

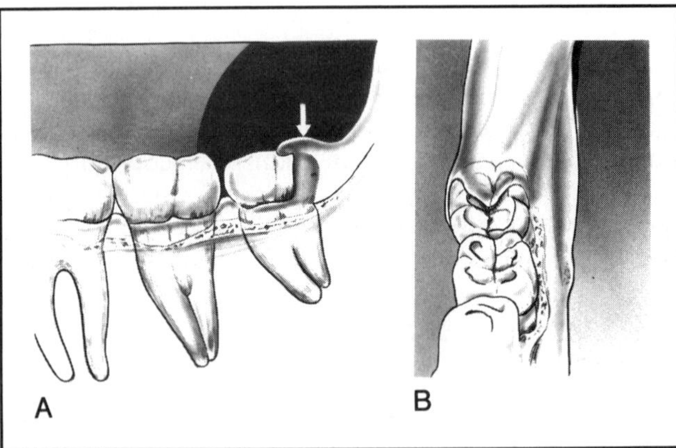

FIGURE 26–22

Acute pericoronitis. *A*, Inflamed pericoronal flap (arrow) partially covers the mandibular third molar. *B*, Anterior and topical view of the flap and third molar. (From Carranza, F.A.: Glickman's Clinical Periodontology, 7th ed. Philadelphia, W.B. Saunders Co., 1990, p 665.)

The initial goal of the treatment is to control the infection. This includes

- Irrigating under the gingival flap with warm saline solution
- Placing a drain under the gingival flap
- Prescribing antibiotics and pain medication

Because of the danger of spreading the infection during surgery, the infection must be controlled before further treatment can be undertaken.

Depending upon the circumstances, the tooth may be extracted. It the tooth is to be retained (not extracted), the gingival flap is surgically removed after the infection is cleared.

Acute Necrotizing Ulcerative Gingivitis

Acute necrotizing ulcerative gingivitis (ANUG) is a very painful, destructive, infectious disease of the gingiva. The clinical symptoms are described in Chapter 12. Treatment includes

- Improved nutrition (because the mouth is sore, nutrition is often poor): the patient is advised to follow a mild, but nutritionally sound diet
- Avoidance of tobacco products, carbonated beverages, and alcohol
- Plenty of rest, because stress and overactivity are contributing factors in this condition

Once the acute inflammation has subsided, the patient should have a thorough prophylaxis and be placed on a program of preventive home care.

Lasers in Periodontics

The term **laser** is an acronym for "light amplification by simulated emission of radiation." (An **acronym** is a word created from the initial letters of a name or compound term.)

A laser beam is a highly concentrated beam of light. The power of this beam can be adjusted to enable it to cut, vaporize, or cauterize tissue.

The use of lasers is a promising new technology for dentistry. Research that may lead to more widespread uses of lasers in clinical dentistry is continuing. At this time, the periodontal applications of lasers on soft tissue include

- Removing tumors and lesions
- Vaporizing excess tissues, as in gingivoplasty, gingivectomy, and frenectomies
- Removing or reducing hyperplastic tissues
- Controlling bleeding of vascular lesions

Advantages of Laser Surgery

Lasers offer a number of advantages over conventional surgical techniques:

- Laser incisions heal faster than incisions made with electrosurgery. (However, incisions made with scalpels heal faster than those made with lasers.)
- Hemostasis (control of bleeding) is rapid.
- The surgical field is relatively dry.
- The opportunity for bloodborne contamination is reduced.
- There is less trauma to adjacent tissues.
- There is less postsurgical swelling, scarring, and pain.
- Some procedures can be performed more quickly.
- Patients who are afraid of "surgery" may accept this method.

Laser Safety

Precautions must be taken to protect both the patient and the dental staff during laser procedures (see Guidelines for Laser Safety). Any person who operates a laser or assists during a laser operation must be thoroughly trained in the use of this powerful instrument.

Guidelines for Laser Safety

Shielded eyeglasses: Special shielded eyeglasses must be worn by the dental staff and the patient to protect the eyes.
Matte-finished instruments: Reflective surfaces such as instruments, mirrors, and even polished restorations can reflect laser energy. Matte-finished (not shiny) instruments are recommended in order to avoid this reflection.
Protection of nontarget tissues: Nontarget oral tissues (tissues not being treated with laser) should be shielded with wet gauze packs.
High-volume evacuation: High-volume evacuation (HVE) should be used to draw off the plume (cloud) created when tissue vaporizes. This plume should be considered infectious.

Periodontal Surgical Dressings

A periodontal surgical dressing serves much like a bandage over a surgical site. Periodontal dressings (perio packs) are used to

- Protect the newly forming tissues
- Minimize postoperative pain, infection, and hemorrhage
- Protect the surgical site from trauma during eating and drinking
- Support mobile teeth during the healing process

Types of Periodontal Dressings

Materials for periodontal dressings are available in three types: (1) those that contain zinc oxide and eugenol; (2) those that do not contain eugenol (non-eugenol); and (3) light-cured material.

ZINC OXIDE–EUGENOL DRESSING

Zinc oxide–eugenol dressings are supplied as a powder and liquid that are mixed before use. The material may be mixed ahead of time, wrapped in wax paper, and frozen for future use.

This type of dressing has a slow set, which allows for longer working time. It sets to a firm and heavy consistency and provides good support and protection for tissues and flaps.

Some patients are allergic to the eugenol and experience redness and burning pain in the area of the dressing.

NON-EUGENOL DRESSING

Non-eugenol dressing is the most widely used type of periodontal dressings. This material is supplied in two tubes: one of base material and the other of accelerator.

This material is easy to mix and place and has a smooth surface for patient comfort. This material has a rapid setting time if exposed to warm temperatures, and it *cannot* be mixed in advance and stored.

LIGHT-CURED DRESSING

Light-cured dressing is supplied in a single-dose syringe-type dispenser. The material can be injected directly onto the surgical site, molded into place, and light-cured. When the material is cured, it is almost the same color as the gingivae.

Another technique is to dispense the appropriate amount of material onto a mixing pad, roll it into a rope shape, and then place over the surgical site, mold into place, and light cure.

(text continued on page 516)

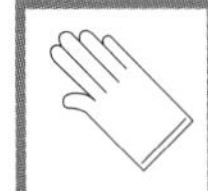
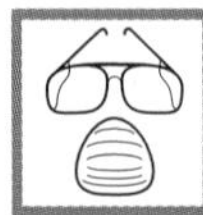
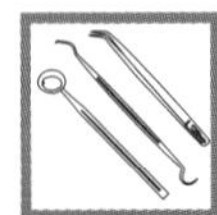

PROCEDURE: Preparing and Placing Non-Eugenol Periodontal Dressing

Instrumentation (Fig. 26–23)

Paper mixing pad (supplied by manufacturer)
Wooden tongue depressor
Non-eugenol dressing (base and accelerator)
Paper cup filled with room-temperature water
Saline solution
Plastic-type filling instrument

Mixing

1. Extrude equal lengths of the two pastes on paper pad.
2. Mix the pastes with a wooden tongue depressor until a uniform color has been obtained (2 to 3 minutes) (Fig. 26–24).
3. When the paste looses its tackiness, place it in the paper cup filled with room-temperature water (Fig. 26–25).
4. Lubricate gloved fingers with saline solution.
   □ *RATIONALE:* This prevents the material from sticking to the gloves.
5. Roll the paste into strips approximately the length of the surgical site (Fig. 26–26).

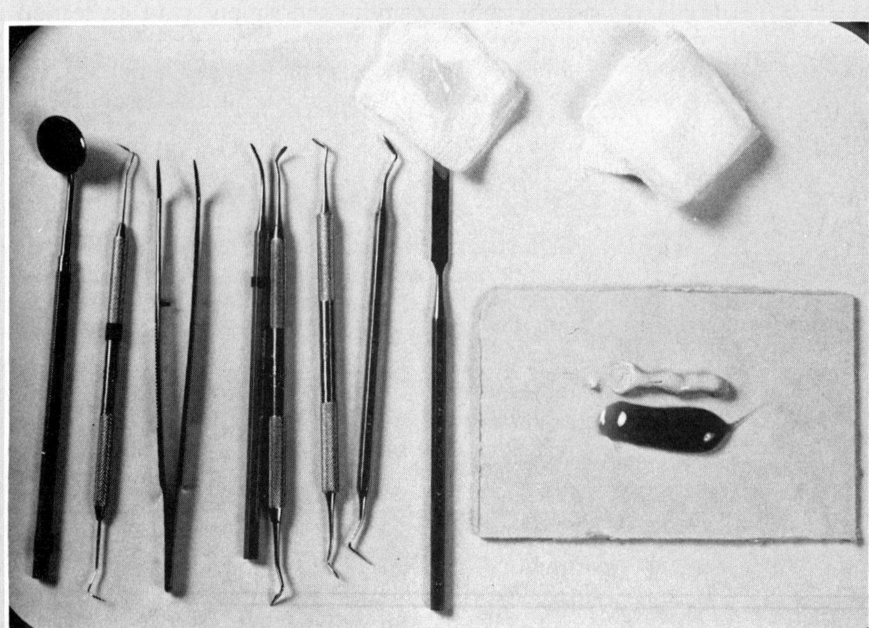

FIGURE 26–23

Instrumentation for periodontal dressing placement.

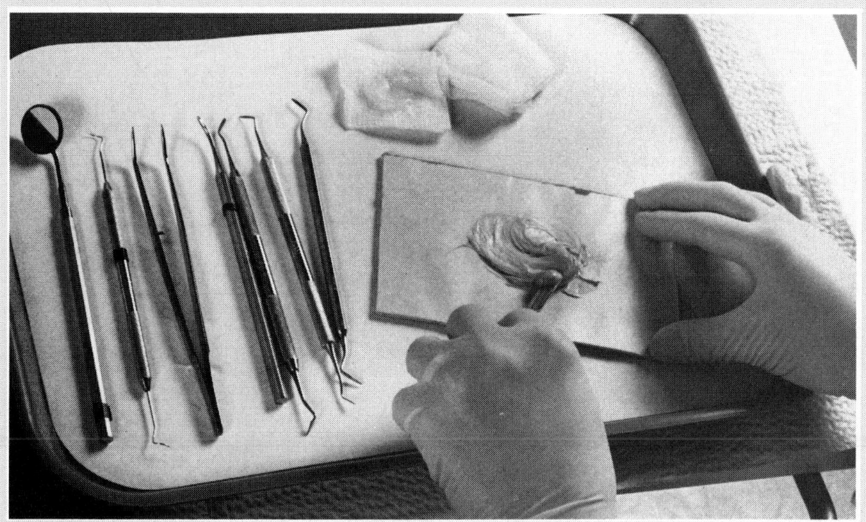

FIGURE 26–24

Mixing periodontal surgical dressing.

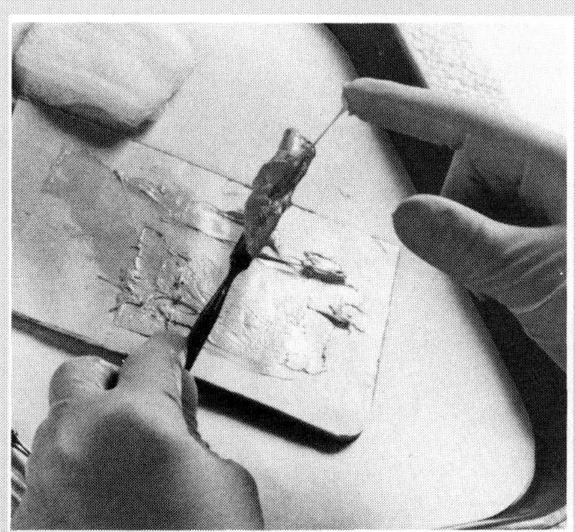

FIGURE 26–25

Testing mix for tackiness.

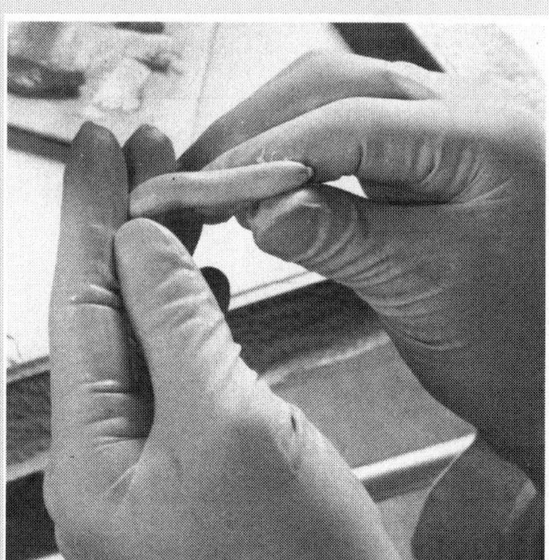

FIGURE 26–26

Forming a roll of dressing material.

(continued on following page)

PROCEDURE: **Preparing and Placing Non-Eugenol Periodontal Dressing** *(continued)*

Placement

1. Place the strip over the facial surface of the surgical site (Fig. 26–27).
2. Adapt one end of the strip around the distal surface of the last tooth in the surgical site.
3. Bring the remainder of the strip forward along the facial surface, and gently press the strip along the incised gingival margin.
4. Gently press the strip into the interproximal areas.
5. Apply the second strip in the same manner from the lingual surface.
6. Join the facial and lingual strips at the distal surface of the last tooth at both ends of the surgical site.
7. Apply gentle pressure on the facial and lingual surfaces.
   □ *RATIONALE:* This joins the two strips interproximally.
8. Check the dressing for overextension and interference with occlusion.
   □ *RATIONALE:* Excess pack irritates the mucobuccal fold and floor of the mouth.
9. Remove any excess dressing, and adjust the new margins to remove any roughness (Fig. 26–28.)
   □ *RATIONALE:* If the pack is not adapted properly, it will probably break off.

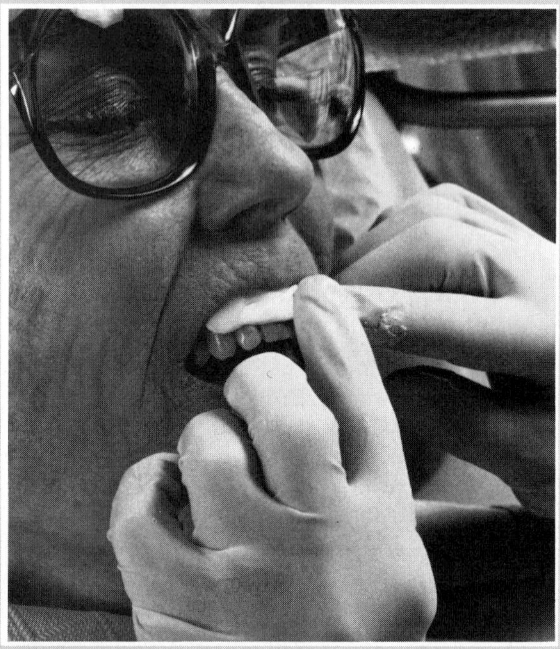

FIGURE 26–27

Placement of the roll of dressing material.

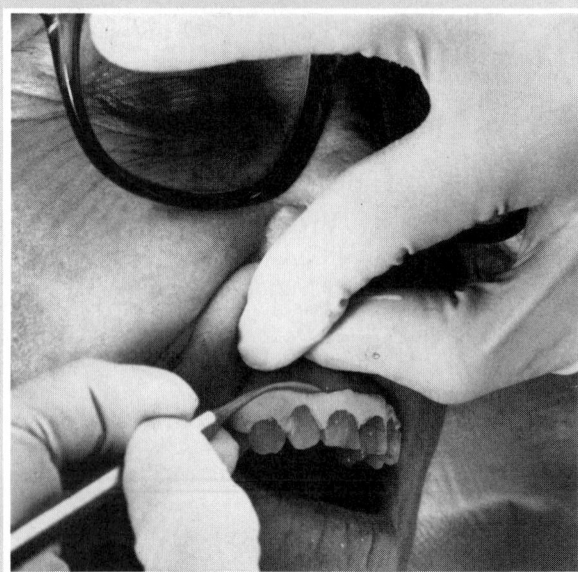

FIGURE 26–28

Removing excess and adjusting contours of the dressing material.

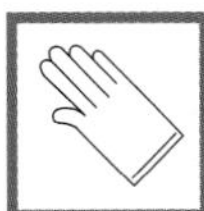
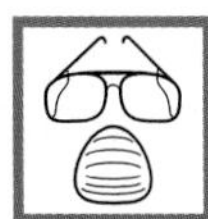
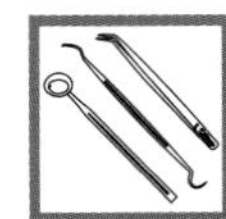
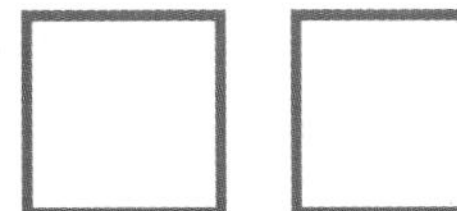

PROCEDURE: **Removing Periodontal Dressing**

Instrumentation

Spoon excavator
Suture scissors (for sutures if present)
Dental floss
Warm saline solution
Irrigating syringe
HVE tip or saliva ejector

Removal Steps

1. Gently insert the spoon excavator under the margin.
2. Use lateral pressure to gently pry the dressing away from the tissue.
   □ *RATIONALE:* The area may still be sensitive, and the newly healed tissue is delicate and easily injured.
3. If sutures are embedded in the dressing material, cut the suture material free. Remove the sutures from the tissue.
4. Gently use dental floss to remove all fragments of dressing material from the interproximal surfaces (Fig. 26–29).
5. Irrigate the entire area gently with warm saline to remove superficial debris.
6. Cautiously use the HVE tip or saliva ejector to remove the excess fluid from the patient's mouth.

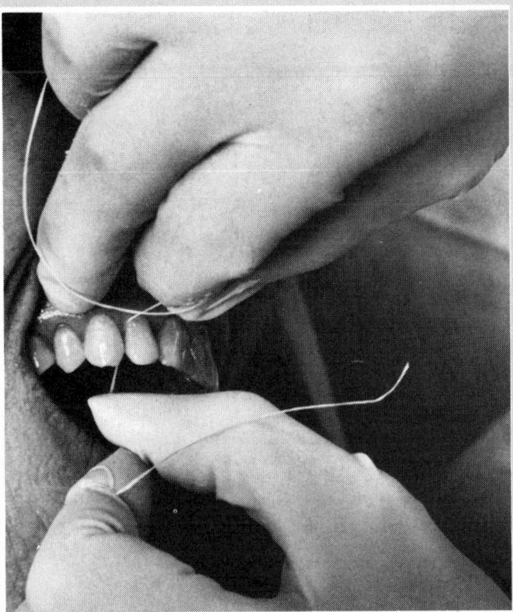

FIGURE 26–29

Using dental floss to remove any dressing material that may remain in the interproximal spaces.

Splinting

Splinting is used in periodontics to stabilize mobile teeth to enable the patient to chew more comfortably. Splints may be temporary or permanent.

Temporary splints, made from acrylic, are placed before periodontal surgery to immobilize the teeth.

Permanent splints are placed as part of the final restorative phase of treatment. Permanent splints are made by using inlays, onlays, and crowns soldered together to form a rigid appliance (Fig. 26–30). This design distributes the chewing forces over all the teeth in the arch equally.

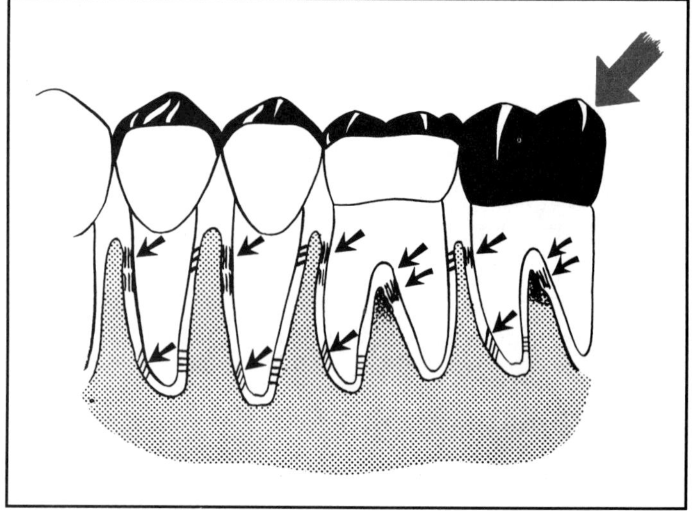

FIGURE 26–30

A splint helps to distribute the stress of mastication over all the teeth in the arch. The occlusal stress is indicated by the large red arrow. Distribution of the stress to all four of the splinted teeth is indicated by the smaller arrows. (Modified from Carranza, F.A.: Glickman's Clinical Periodontology, 7th ed. Philadelphia, W.B. Saunders Co., 1990, p 952.)

Maintenance Recall Therapy

Periodic maintenance recall visits are critical for the long-term success of any type of periodontal treatment. The initial maintenance recall visit is usually set for 3 months, but the time may be varied according to the needs of the patient. At each periodontal maintenance recall visit, the patient receives

- An examination and evaluation of his current oral health, including full mouth periodontal probing
- An assessment of home care for plaque control
- Recommendations for any necessary changes in home care (if good oral hygiene is not maintained, periodontal disease will recur or become worse)
- Scaling, root planing, and polishing, if indicated
- If pockets remain, irrigation with antimicrobial agents, such as stannous fluoride or chlorhexidine

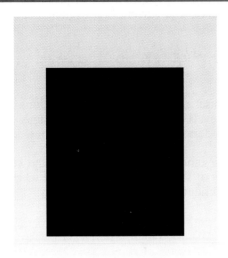

Chapter 27

Pediatric Dentistry

Introduction

Pediatric dentistry is the treatment of children from infancy through adolescence. The emphasis of the pediatric dental practice is on the early detection and prevention of dental diseases, and the following services are also routinely provided:

- Restorative procedures
- Pulpal therapy
- Surgical procedures
- Space maintenance
- Interceptive orthodontics

Although many of the procedures performed for children are similar to those for other patients, children have special needs (Fig. 27–1).

The Pediatric Dental Office

The decor of a pediatric dental office must be cheerful, pleasant, and nonthreatening to a child. Many pediatric dental offices have a "theme" in the overall decor, such as a circus tent, a space adventure, or popular cartoon characters.

Some pediatric dental offices have computer/video equipment available with programs intended for both patient education and entertainment.

Reading material such as magazines and patient education brochures should be available for both the child patient and the parent. There should be a variety of reading materials selected to be of interest to various age groups.

Many pediatric dental offices are designed with the "open concept." This means that several dental chairs

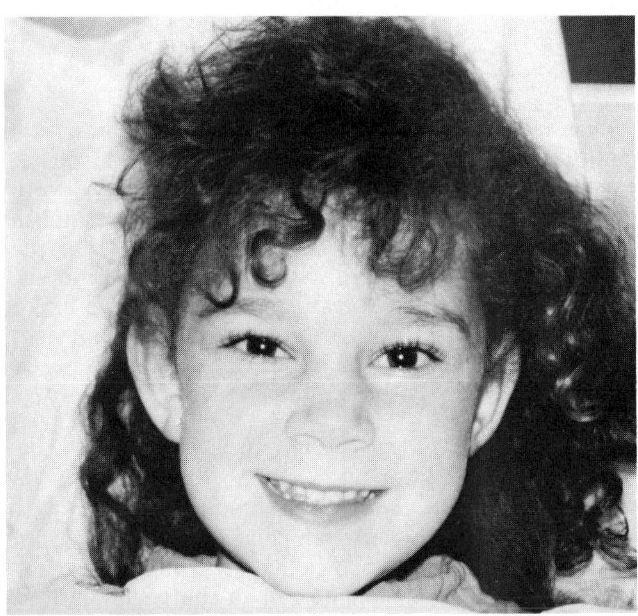

FIGURE 27–1

Providing dental care for children can be a happy experience for the child and the staff.

are arranged in one large area. The advantage of this design is that it provides reassurance to the child to see other children being treated. This is psychologically effective, because children are often hesitant to express fear or to misbehave in the presence of other children.

Some pediatric offices have a "quiet room." This treatment room is separate from the open area and is used for children whose behavior may upset the other children.

Behavioral Management Techniques

Children have to be managed differently than adult patients, and the techniques of management selected by the dentist depend on the age of the child.

Also, the assistant must know when basic assisting skills need to be modified because of the age, size, or behavior of the child patient.

Preventive Dentistry

When children adopt good oral health behaviors early in life, most dental disease can be prevented. This includes learning and practicing the preventive techniques that are discussed in Chapter 6.

Helping teach these techniques is one of the important roles of the assistant in a pediatric practice. To do this, the assistant must have a thorough understanding of preventive dentistry, nutrition, and both systemic and topical fluorides. (These are discussed in Chapter 6.)

Examination of the Pediatric Dentistry Patient

The initial examination is important for both the child and the dental team. It is often the first dental experience for the child. The rapport developed with the child during the initial examination can establish an attitude toward dental health that will last for the child's lifetime.

The child's parent or legal guardian must give his or her consent (permission) before any dental treatment can be provided for the child.

Medical and Dental History

Before the examination, the parent or guardian provides the **medical history,** which includes information about the child's general health background. Two examples that are often mentioned in the health history are heart murmurs and allergies. The dentist may choose to contact the child's pediatrician to obtain a more complete medical history.

The **dental history** includes information about the eruption pattern of the teeth, past dental problems and care, fluoride intake, and current oral hygiene habits.

General Appraisal and Behavioral Assessment

General appraisal addresses physical conditions and developmental levels. It also includes vital signs and baseline health data for emergency situations. (See Chapter 9.)

Behavioral assessment is used to evaluate the communication skills of the patient and determine whether behavior management techniques are necessary.

Head, Neck, and Facial Examinations

The head and neck examination provides a nonthreatening environment and enables the dentist to establish a rapport with the child. (**Rapport** means a feeling of ease or comfort.) The examination is similar to that of an adult and includes palpation of the lymph nodes and observation of any speech disorders.

The facial examination evaluates the patient's profile to determine skeletal characteristics. Also, any facial deviations or asymmetry of the eyes, ears, or nose may be symptoms of an undiagnosed syndrome. In this case, the child would be referred to an appropriate professional for a complete evaluation.

Intraoral Examination

The intraoral examination requires the use of a mouth mirror, an explorer, and gauze sponges. Very young children may be uncooperative and may allow "only fingers" in their mouths. Other young children may allow only a mirror.

Ideally, each of the 20 primary teeth should be explored and examined. Also, the occlusion is analyzed to determine spacing and crowding and the presence or absence of teeth.

Radiographic Examination

A radiographic examination is necessary to make a complete diagnosis in children. Young children often have difficulty with the radiographic procedure, and the radiographic examination may have to be deferred until the behavior improves or can be managed. (Specific radiographic procedures are discussed in Chapter 17.)

When radiographs are possible, the following steps are a helpful way to introduce the child to the procedure:

1. Obtain parental permission to perform dental procedures.

2. Use a "big camera" analogy to explain the procedure. This works only if the child is old enough to understand.
3. Use the "tell-show-do" introduction. By "practicing" positioning the film and x-ray machine, you can determine whether the child will sit for the exposure.
   ☐ **Rationale**: This prevents unproductive irradiation as a result of faulty exposures.
4. Match the size of the film to the level of comfort for the child. In some cases, bending the anterior corners helps for bite-wing placement.
5. Perform the easiest procedures first. Usually occlusal projections are the most comfortable for the child.
6. If a parent *must* be used to stabilize film placement, both the parent and child must be adequately shielded with a lead apron.

Topical Application of Fluorides

Fluorides have had a major role in bringing about the decline in dental caries; however, for many children, caries are still a major health problem. Often these children are those who have not had the benefits of fluoride from birth. (Fluorides are discussed in Chapter 6.)

The professional topical application of fluoride is very important in controlling dental disease in these children. It also plays an important role in controlling caries in high-risk adults.

Methods of Application

Two methods are used in the topical application of fluoride. **Tray application**, the more commonly used technique, involves the use of a foam or a viscous (thick) gel. This material adheres (sticks) to the tray and teeth and is transferred easily into the mouth with minimal leakage.

The **rinse technique** is used with concentrated fluoride solutions. The concentration of fluoride in professional rinses is greater than the concentration used in the over-the-counter fluoride rinses. The concentrated solutions have a consistency similar to that of syrup.

The patient is given a paper cup containing the proper amount of fluoride and is told to rinse and swish the fluoride around his mouth. This technique should be used only with children who are old enough to understand the instructions "Do not swallow this."

Tray Application of Fluoride Gels

When applying fluoride gels, it is important to use a minimal amount of the gel. The American Academy of Pediatric Dentistry recommends no more than 2 ml. per tray or 5 ml. total.

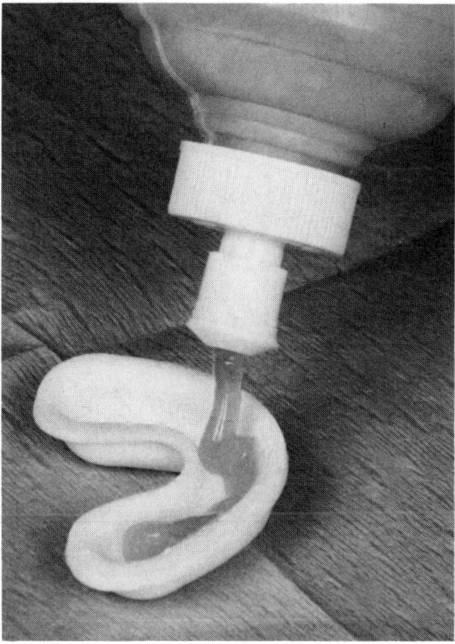

FIGURE 27–2

Dispensing topical fluoride gel into the disposable tray.

Commercially prepared gels are dispensed directly from the bottle into the tray (Fig. 27–2). Containers that are handled with gloved hands during the appointment should be surface disinfected during treatment room cleanup.

PREPARATION OF THE TEETH

Fluoride diffuses through pellicle and bacterial plaque without being inhibited; therefore, "rubber cup polishing" is not required before topical application of fluoride. However, calculus and heavy stains could prevent the fluoride from reaching the enamel of the tooth, and these should be removed. Selective polishing, which is discussed in Chapter 21, is used for those teeth with heavy stain.

TRAY SELECTION FOR FLUORIDE GEL APPLICATION

A wide variety of trays are commercially available for application of fluoride gels. Listed as follows are factors to consider when deciding on the type of tray to use. The tray should

- Be available in a variety of sizes to fit primary, mixed, and adult size dentition
- Be long enough to completely cover all erupted teeth without extending beyond the distal of the most posterior tooth
- Be wide and deep enough to cover the tooth surfaces when it is in place
- Have closed ends so that the fluoride does not spill into the mouth

These trays are discarded after a single use. If a tray is tried in the mouth but not selected, it too is discarded.

Concentrated Fluoride Rinse Technique

When the "concentrated rinse" method of applying topical fluoride is used, it is very important to instruct the patient not to swallow the fluoride. The amount of fluoride used in the rinse technique is not enough to cause harm to the patient, but fluoride is acidic, and swallowing it can cause nausea in some children. Should nausea occur, the dentist may recommend that an antacid be given to the child.

Before the treatment, check the fluoride manufacturer's instructions as to the exact rinse time and any post-treatment instructions. Some types of fluoride rinse do not require the patient to refrain from drinking water after the fluoride application.

Pit and Fissure Sealants

Systemic fluorides are most effective in reducing caries on smooth tooth surfaces (facial, lingual, and interproximal). They are the least effective on occlusal surfaces, pits, and grooves.

In addition, the occlusal surfaces are particularly difficult to clean because the bristles of a tooth brush cannot reach into the deep pit and fissure areas, and plaque may remain even after brushing. These factors combined make the occlusal surfaces particularly prone to caries.

Dental caries on occlusal tooth surfaces are best prevented by the application of pit and fissure sealants. A **sealant** is a clear or tinted plastic-like material applied to the occlusal surfaces, buccal pits, and lingual grooves of molars and premolars.

This material bonds to the tooth surface and acts as a barrier, protecting the pit and fissure areas of the tooth. Sealants can also be placed on the lingual pits of anterior teeth.

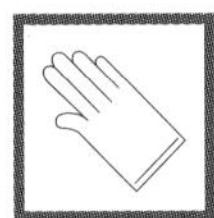
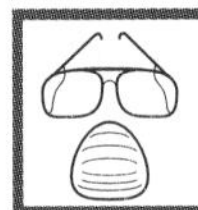
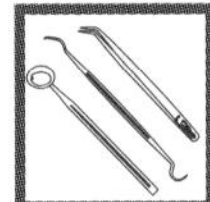

PROCEDURE: **Applying Topical Fluoride Gel**

Instrumentation

Fluoride gel
Disposable trays of appropriate size
Saliva ejector
High-volume evacuator (HVE) tip
Timer

Application

1. Explain the procedure and seat the patient in an upright position.
   □ *RATIONALE:* Having the patient upright prevents the gel from going into the throat.
2. Instruct the patient not to swallow the fluoride.
3. Select the appropriate tray and load it.
4. Dry the teeth, using air from the air-water syringe.
5. Insert the tray, and promptly place the saliva ejector. Tilt the patient's head forward.
   □ *RATIONALE:* This helps prevent the patient from swallowing the gel.
6. Press the tray gently against the teeth, starting from the occlusal surfaces and on the sides to force the gel between the teeth.
7. Set the timer for the appropriate amount of time based on the manufacturer's instructions (usually 4 minutes).
8. Do not leave the patient unattended.
9. On completion, remove the tray.
10. Do not allow the patient to rinse or swallow.
11. Use the saliva ejector or HVE tip to remove excess saliva and solution.
12. Instruct the patient not to rinse, eat, drink, brush the teeth, or perform any other activity that could disturb the action of the fluoride for at least 30 minutes.

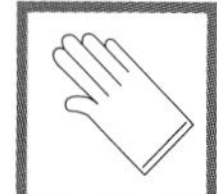 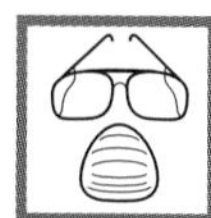 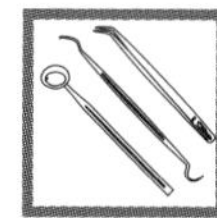 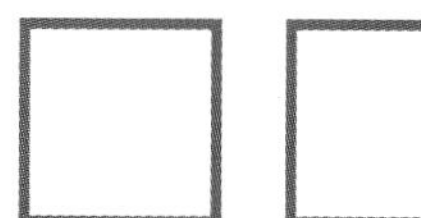

PROCEDURE: **Applying Concentrated Fluoride Rinse**

Instrumentation

Concentrated fluoride solution
Disposable paper cup
Measuring device
Timing device
Saliva ejector and/or HVE tip

Technique

1. Explain the procedure, and seat the patient in an upright position. An alternative is to have the patient stand at a sink.
   □ *RATIONALE:* The goal is to prevent the solution from going down the patient's throat.
2. Instruct the patient not to swallow the fluoride.
3. Dispense the amount of fluoride into the paper cup.
4. Instruct the patient to rinse with one half of the fluoride through the mouth, usually for 1 minute.
5. After 1 minute, instruct the patient to spit out the fluoride into the sink, saliva ejector, or HVE tip.
6. Instruct the patient to swish with the remaining half of fluoride for an additional minute.
7. After 1 minute, instruct the patient to spit out the remaining fluoride in the same manner as the for the first rinse.
8. Give the patient post-treatment instructions as recommended by the manufacturer.

Sealant Materials

Sealants are made from several types of materials. The major difference between the materials is the method of polymerization (self-curing or light-cured). Both types are safe and effective.

Self-cured materials are supplied as a two-part system (base and catalyst). When these pastes are mixed together, they quickly polymerize (harden). This usually occurs within 1 minute, and the material must be in place before this happens.

Light-cured sealants do not require mixing. After the material has been placed, it hardens after exposure to a curing light (Fig. 27–3).

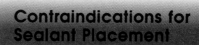

Indications for Sealant Placement

- Deep pits and fissures are present.
- The tooth is recently erupted (less than 4 years ago).
- Sealant placement is to be used in conjunction with a preventive program, such as fluoride therapy.

Contraindications for Sealant Placement

- The pit and fissures are well-coalesced and self cleansing.
- The occlusal surface is decayed. (A restoration must be placed to repair this damage.)
- The proximal surfaces are decayed. (The occlusal surface will be included in the restoration of the involved proximal surfaces.)
- A restoration is already in place.

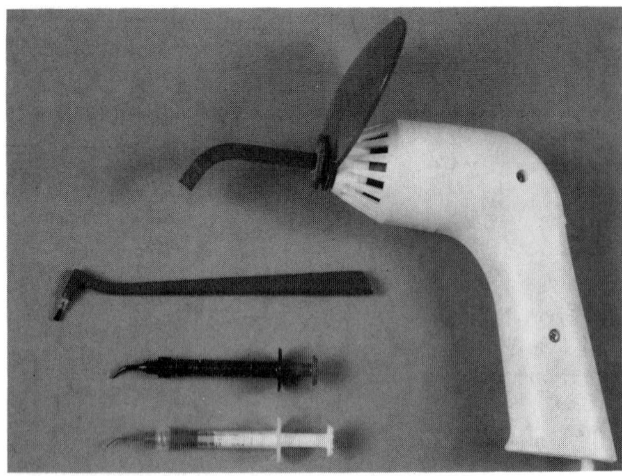

FIGURE 27–3

Equipment used with light-cured sealants. The curing light is to the right. Also shown are the placement instrument, sealant syringe, and etching syringe.

Careful handling is necessary with these materials. It is important to

- Store the material according to the manufacturer's instructions.
  Rationale: Some products must be refrigerated.
- Recap the tube immediately after use, and protect the sealant material from exposure to air during storage.
  Rationale: Exposure to air causes evaporation. This makes the material less fluid and reduces penetration into the pits and fissures.
- Store visible light-cured materials in darkness.
  Rationale: These materials begin to set when exposed to light.
- Do not use if the material has passed the expiration date printed on the package.
  Rationale: If the material has passed the expiration date, it may not flow or cure properly.
- Keep applicator devices clean and free from debris.
  Rationale: Debris contaminates the material.
- Provide special protective eye wear for both patient and operator when the curing light is in use. An alternative for the operator is a protective shield on the curing light. The patient may be instructed to close his eyes.

Guidelines for Sealant Placement

The ultimate success of placing any sealant product is determined by the following four points.

STRICT MAINTENANCE OF A DRY TOOTH SURFACE

Saliva contamination can interfere with the adhesion of the sealant to the surfaces of the teeth. Therefore, the tooth must be isolated to keep it dry.

Dental dam is most effective for this purpose. It isolates the teeth being treated and protects the patient against accidental contact with the etching solution.

Isolation of the teeth with cotton rolls and adequate suction is an alternative technique, although it is not ideal because of the difficulty in maintaining a dry field.

Also, the air supply must be free of moisture and/or oil contamination. To check the air lines for moisture and/or oil contamination, spray air across the surface of a mouth mirror. If the air is free of contamination, the surface of the mirror should not reveal any moisture or oil.

ACCURATE TIMING FOR ETCHING AND RINSING

If the enamel is not etched properly, the sealant cannot bond well to the tooth. Therefore, accurate timing for etching and rinsing is essential.

If salivary contamination does occur during etching, it is necessary to rinse the tooth surface, dry it thoroughly, and repeat the etching process for the full time period. Saliva contamination can interfere with the adhesion of the sealant to the tooth surface.

PROPER SEALANT MATERIAL PLACEMENT

Sealant is placed in adequate amounts to cover all fissures on the occlusal surface. Then a thin layer of sealant should be carried up the buccal and lingual inclines of the occlusal surface in order to seal supplementary fissures. Finally, sealant is also placed in the lingual grooves and buccal pits. (Remember, each of these areas must have been etched before placement of the sealant.)

When placing the sealant, be careful not to apply excess or to allow the sealant to flow into the contact area.

FOLLOW THE MANUFACTURER'S DIRECTIONS

It is essential that the manufacturer's directions be followed for placement and polymerization of the material. If the material is not properly cured, the sealants may be defective and will not wear well.

Sealant Application

The products used for sealants vary according to the manufacturer, but the basic steps in sealant application are similar. The procedure described here is for light-cured sealants.

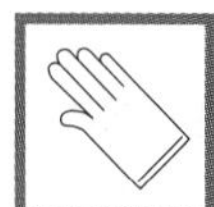
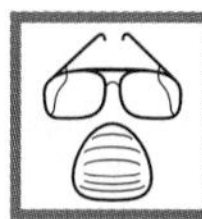
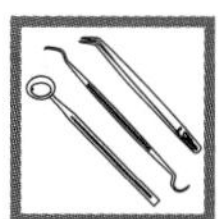

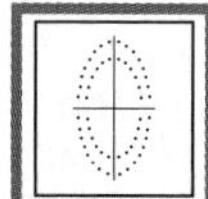

PROCEDURE: **Applying Sealants**

Instrumentation

Etching (conditioning) agent (liquid or gel)
Sealant material
Applicator device (manufacturer supplied or recommended)
Cotton pellets
Low-speed handpiece with contra-angle attachment
Bristle brush or rubber cup
Fluoride-free abrasive (pumice slurry)
HVE tip
Curing light
Articulating paper
Round white mounted stone, latch type
Dental floss

Preparing and Etching the Teeth

1. Place the dental dam to isolate those teeth receiving sealants (Fig. 27–4).
   □ *RATIONALE:* The teeth must be kept free of moisture or contamination.
2. Using a bristle brush, or rubber cup, polish the tooth. Polish with either pumice and water or a fluoride-free paste.
   □ *RATIONALE:* Fluoride interferes with the etching process.
3. Rinse thoroughly to remove all particles of abrasive. Use the HVE tip to remove water and debris.
4. Use the air syringe to dry the tooth thoroughly.
   □ *RATIONALE:* The working area must be dry.

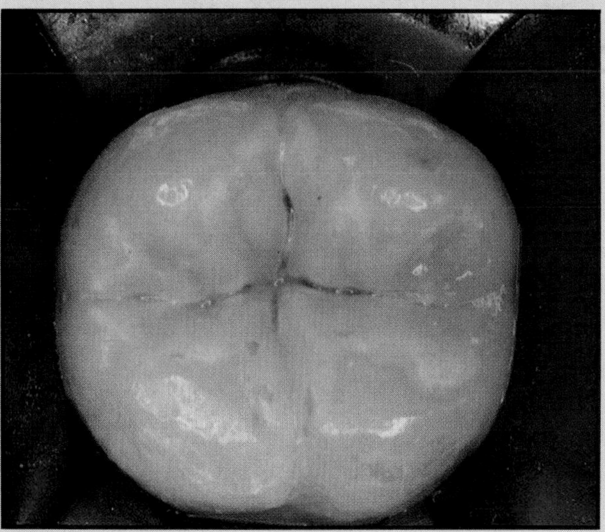

FIGURE 27–4

Dental dam is in place, and the tooth is prepared for pit and fissure sealant placement. (Courtesy of 3M Dental Products Division, St. Paul, MN.)

(continued on following page)

PROCEDURE: **Applying Sealants** *(continued)*

5. In accordance with the manufacturer's directions, apply the etching agent to the occlusal surfaces, buccal pits, and lingual grooves (Fig. 27–5).
6. Leave the etching agent on the tooth for the amount of time recommended by the manufacturer. (This is usually 60 seconds.)
7. Use water, from the air-water syringe, to rinse the tooth and remove all etching material.
8. Use air, from the air-water syringe, to dry the tooth.
9. Check the appearance of the etched enamel. A properly etched tooth surface appears dull and chalky (Fig. 27–6).
10. If the enamel does not have this appearance, repeat the etching step.

Applying and Curing the Sealant

1. Apply the sealant material, using the applicator supplied or recommended by the manufacturer (Fig. 27–7).
2. Trace the fissures with an explorer tip to enable air bubbles to rise and the sealant to penetrate.

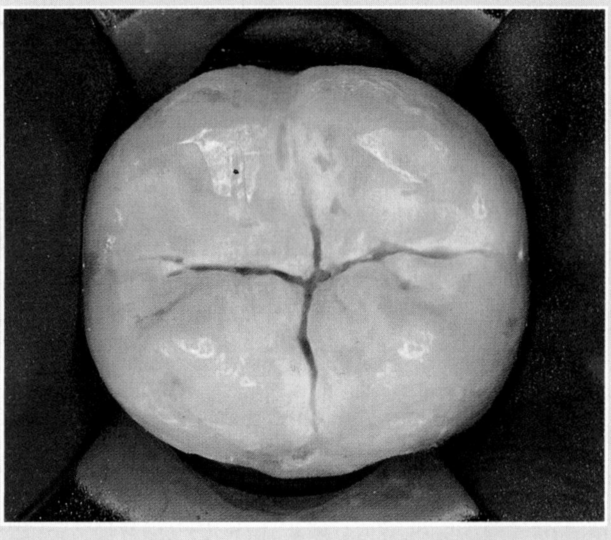

FIGURE 27–6

Areas of the tooth that have been etched now have a dull, chalky appearance. (Courtesy of 3M Dental Products Division, St. Paul, MN.)

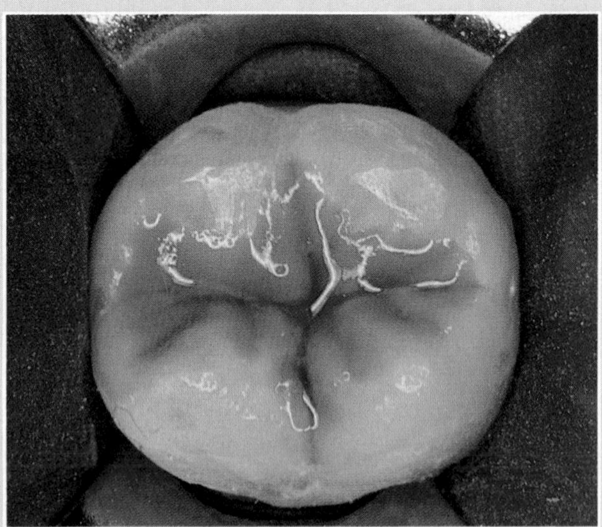

FIGURE 27–5

Acid etching gel is applied in accordance with the manufacturer's instructions. (Courtesy of 3M Dental Products Division, St. Paul, MN.)

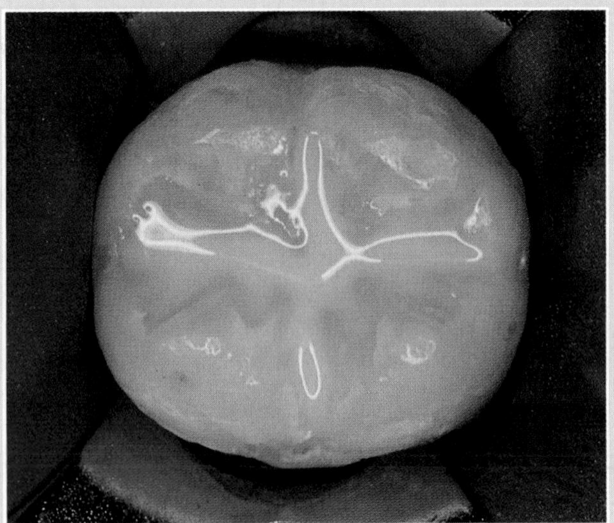

FIGURE 27–7

The sealant is applied and is ready to be light-cured. (Courtesy of 3M Dental Products Division, St. Paul, MN.)

3. Follow the manufacturer's directions for placement of the curing light wand and for correct exposure time (approximately 20 seconds per tooth).
4. Evaluate the sealed surfaces with an explorer to be certain that the surface is smooth and hard. Check for voids and incomplete coverage. Repeat the entire process in areas with voids or incomplete coverage.
5. After the sealant material has been cured, rinse with water and wipe the sealed surfaces with a moist cotton pellet.

☐ *RATIONALE:* This removes any sticky sealant material that has failed to polymerize.
6. Check the occlusal relationship with articulating paper. If the sealant has high spots, use a round stone in the low-speed handpiece to reduce the sealant. (**High spots** are areas where the sealant material is too thick and interferes with occlusion.)
7. Use dental floss to make certain that the contact areas are free from sealant material.

Stainless Steel Crowns

Stainless steel crowns are commonly used in the treatment of badly broken down primary teeth. They are generally considered superior to large multisurface amalgam restorations (Fig. 27–8).

Stainless steel crowns are available in a variety of sizes for the various primary and permanent teeth. In many states, the assistant is permitted to select the correct size of stainless steel crown.

However, a stainless steel crown is considered to be a permanent restoration, and the *trimming and adaptation* of the crown are *not* delegated to the dental assistant.

Indications for Use of Stainless Steel Crowns

- Restoration of primary or young teeth with extensive carious lesions
- Restoration of primary teeth after pulpotomy or pulpectomy procedures (a discussion of these procedures follows in this chapter)
- Permanent restoration after accidental fracture of the tooth
- Temporary restoration of a fractured tooth
- Restorations for patients who have difficulty maintaining good oral hygiene, such as disabled children
- As an abutment for space maintainers or prosthetic appliances

Types of Stainless Steel Crowns

There are two types of stainless steel crowns commonly used in pediatric dentistry:

Pre-Trimmed Crowns. These crowns have straight sides but are festooned to follow a line parallel to the gingival crest. They must be trimmed and contoured to fit the tooth. (**Festooned** means trimmed. **Contoured** means shaped to fit.)

Pre-Contoured Crowns. These crowns are already festooned and contoured. Some additional trimming and contouring may be necessary before placement but are usually minimal.

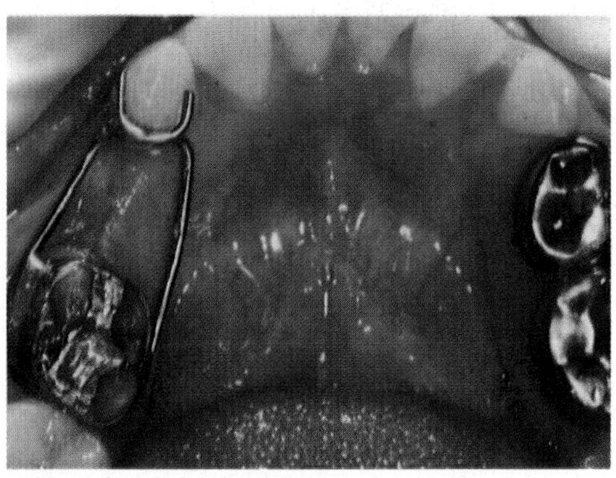

FIGURE 27–8

Stainless steel crowns and a space maintainer on primary teeth. As viewed in a mirror, on the right side of the photo there are two stainless steel crowns on the molars. On the left, the first molar is replaced with a space maintainer, which is held in place by a band on the second molar, which also has an amalgam restoration.

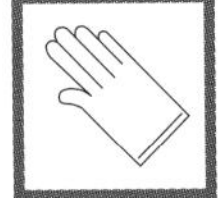
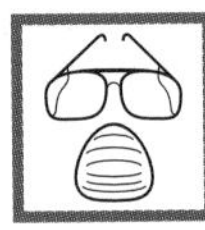
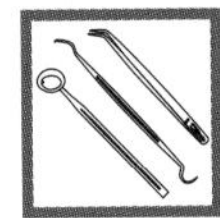
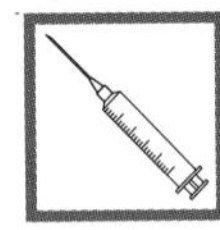

PROCEDURE: **Placing a Stainless Steel Crown**

Instrumentation

Low- and high-speed handpieces
Friction grip burs (dentist's choice of diamond or carbide burs)
Spoon excavator
Selection of stainless steel crowns
Crown scissors
Contouring and crimping pliers
Mandrel
Finishing and polishing discs
Mounted green stones
Cotton rolls
Gauze 2 × 2 sponges
Cementation setup
Dental floss
Articulating paper and holder

Tooth Preparation

1. After the local anesthetic has been administered, the dentist prepares the tooth in a method similar to that for a cast-gold crown, using either a tapered diamond or carbide bur. (See Chapter 31.)
2. The dentist reduces the entire circumference of the tooth, as well as the height of the tooth.
3. All dental caries are removed with conventional methods. (See Chapter 25.)

Sizing the Stainless Steel Crown

In some states, it is legal for the assistant to perform this function. In all other states, this step is performed by the dentist.

1. Select a crown of approximately the proper size, and try it on the prepared tooth for fit.
2. The stainless steel crown is properly sized when it fits snugly on the prepared tooth and has *both* mesial and distal contact.
3. Crowns that are tried in the mouth but not selected must be sterilized before being returned to storage.

Trimming and Contouring the Stainless Steel Crown

These steps are *always* performed by the dentist.

1. Use contouring scissors to reduce the height of the crown until it is approximately the same height as the adjacent teeth.
2. Use a green stone to smooth the rough edges of the crown along the cervical margin.
3. Polish the cervical margin with a rubber abrasive wheel.
4. Check the occlusion and adjust it as needed.
5. Crimp the cervical margins of the crown toward the tooth to obtain a tight fit and a proper cervical contour.

Cementing the Crown

1. The tooth is dried thoroughly.
2. The crown is filled with permanent cement (zinc phosphate or a polycarboxylate) and seated into place.
3. The excess cement is removed from around the tooth.
4. Dental floss is used to check the interproximal areas for remaining cement.
5. The air-water syringe and the HVE tip or saliva ejector are used to rinse the patient's mouth before he is dismissed.

Pulpal Therapy for Primary and Young Permanent Teeth

Young permanent teeth are recently erupted teeth with the apex still wide open because apical development of the root is not yet complete. The two most common factors that affect the pulpal health of young teeth are deep caries and traumatic injuries.

Deep caries is much more likely to affect the posterior teeth, especially the first molars. Trauma is much more likely to affect the anterior teeth, especially the maxillary incisors.

Pulpal therapy is an attempt to stimulate pulpal regeneration. When pulpal therapy is not effective, the tooth must be treated endodontically or extracted.

Indirect Pulp Capping

Indirect pulp capping is indicated when the pulp has *not yet* been exposed but there is the chance that the pulp will become exposed when the very deep caries near the pulp are removed.

In performing an indirect pulp cap on a *young permanent tooth,* the dentist uses burs and spoon excavators to remove as much of the caries as possible from the coronal portion of the tooth. To avoid accidental pulp exposure, a very thin layer of caries is allowed to remain.

A calcium hydroxide material is applied over the remaining caries, and then the tooth is sealed with a zinc oxide–eugenol temporary restoration (Fig. 27–9). The goals are to promote pulpal healing by removing the majority of caries and to stimulate the production of reparative dentin through the action of calcium hydroxide.

After approximately 6 weeks to allow for healing, if the treatment is successful, the dentist can then reenter the tooth and remove the remaining caries without a pulp exposure.

Direct Pulp Cap

A direct pulp cap is indicated when the pulp of a *young permanent tooth* has been slightly exposed. With a direct pulp cap, the tooth is still vital; however, it may become infected and require additional treatment, or it may die and require endodontic treatment.

When a direct pulp cap is performed, it is necessary to inform the patient and parent that problems (such as an abscess) may develop later and that periodic monitoring is necessary.

A calcium hydroxide material is applied directly onto the exposed pulpal tissue. In some instances, the dentist may choose to place an additional protective base under the final restoration.

Pulpotomy

A **pulpotomy** is indicated for a vital *primary tooth* whose pulp has been exposed. This procedure involves the *partial removal* of the dental pulp, and the tooth remains vital.

A **pulpectomy** is a procedure that involves the *complete removal* of the dental pulp, and the tooth is no longer vital. Pulpectomy is discussed in Chapter 29.

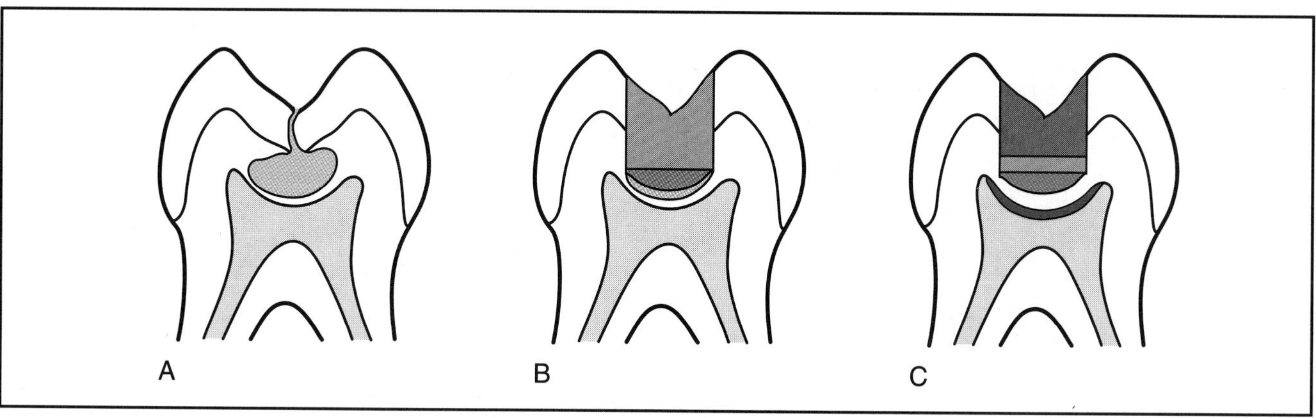

FIGURE 27–9

Indirect pulp cap. *A,* Carious lesion (black area) progressing through enamel and dentin toward the pulp. *B,* A small layer of soft dentin is left over the pulp, over which a calcium hydroxide preparation is placed. Then the tooth is sealed with a temporary restoration. *C,* Reparative dentin has formed across the pulp chamber roof. When the final amalgam restoration is placed, some of the temporary restoration is left in place. (Modified from Pinkham, J.R.: Dentistry: Infancy Through Adolescence. Philadelphia, W.B. Saunders Co., 1988, p 403.)

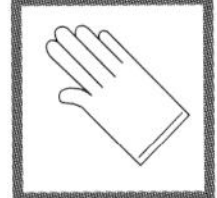
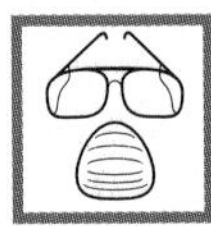
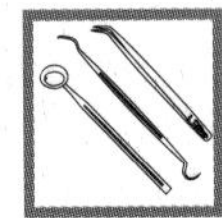
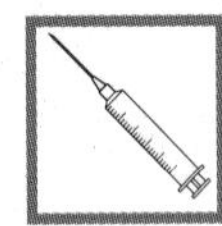
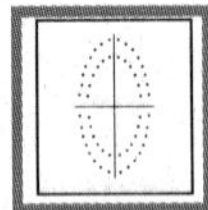

PROCEDURE: **Performing a Pulpotomy**

Instrumentation

Radiographs of the involved tooth or teeth
Low-speed handpiece
Round burs
Spoon excavators (various sizes)
Sterile cotton pellets
Formocresol (one-fifth dilution)
Zinc oxide–eugenol base
Final restorative material

Pulpotomy Steps

1. With a dental dam in place, the dentist removes the dental caries and exposes the pulp chamber.
2. Using a large spoon excavator, the dentist removes all pulp tissue inside the coronal chamber (Fig. 27–10).
3. The dentist places a sterile cotton pellet moistened with formocresol in the chamber for approximately 5 minutes to control hemorrhage.
4. After the hemorrhage is controlled, the pulp chamber is filled with a zinc oxide–eugenol paste, to which a drop of formocresol is added.
5. The zinc oxide–eugenol base and the final restoration are placed.

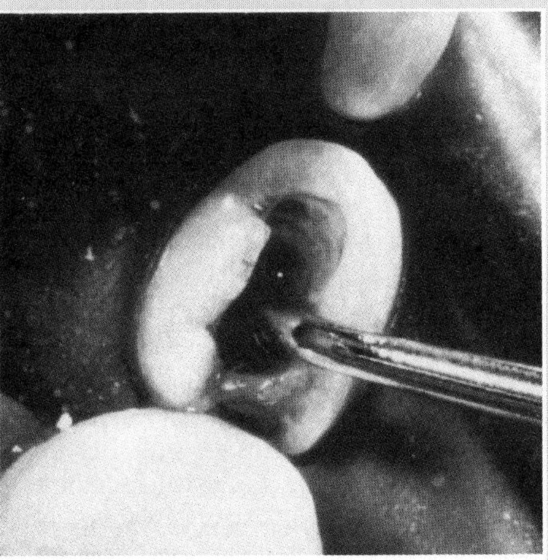

FIGURE 27–10

Pulpotomy. Through an access opening, a spoon excavator is used to remove the coronal pulp tissue. (From Pinkham, J.R.: Dentistry: Infancy Through Adolescence. Philadelphia, W.B. Saunders Co., 1988, p 261.)

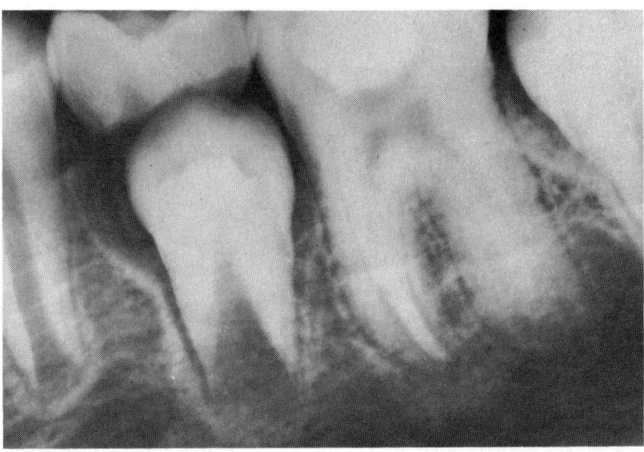

FIGURE 27–11

Open apices of developing mandibular teeth shown on a radiograph of mixed dentition. Shown left to right are a permanent first premolar, a permanent second premolar that will erupt after the second primary molar is shed, and a permanent first molar.

Apexogenesis and Apexification

When a tooth first erupts, the root tip is not fully formed and the apex (root tip) is still wide open (Fig. 27–11). If a young permanent tooth is severely damaged or the pulp is infected, there is danger that the tooth will lose its vitality (die) before the normal narrowing of the apex occurs.

The term **apexogenesis** refers to the treatment of a *vital pulp* either by pulp capping (direct or indirect) or by pulpotomy in order to give the young root enough time to continue to develop and close normally (Fig. 27–12).

If the procedure is successful, a permanent restoration will be placed at a later date. However, the patient and parent must be informed that the procedure may not stimulate the permanent closure of the apex and that the tooth may be lost.

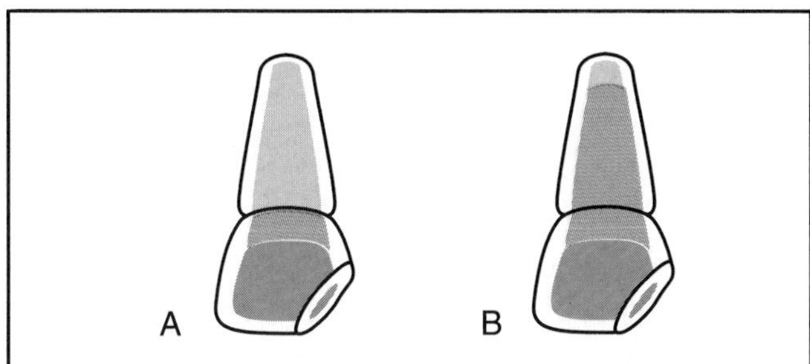

FIGURE 27–12

Apexogenesis and apexification. If the pulp is vital, as shown on the left, the tooth can be treated by apexogenesis. If the pulp is nonvital (dead), as shown on the right, it can be treated by apexification. The arrow indicates the level where calcium hydroxide is placed. This is covered with a temporary restoration. (Modified from Pinkham, J.R.: Dentistry: Infancy Through Adolescence. Philadelphia, W.B. Saunders Co., 1988, p 404.)

Unlike apexogenesis, in which at least part of the pulp is still vital, **apexification** refers to the treatment of a young permanent tooth when it is *no longer vital* and when the development of the root is incomplete.

The goal of apexification is to stimulate closure of the apex by stimulating the formation of a cementum bridge at the apex. This may take anywhere from many months to over a year to occur.

Apexification involves the complete removal of the pulp in the chamber and canals. The canals are irrigated with sodium hypochlorite or a nonirritating saline solution.

In contrast to traditional endodontic treatment, the canals are not filled. Instead, calcium hydroxide (used to stimulate the formation of the cementum bridge) is placed at the apex of the canal, covered with a sterile cotton pellet, and sealed with an interim restoration. After the root has closed, the tooth may be filled endodontically and then restored.

Traumatic Injuries

An injury to the teeth of a young child can have serious and long-term consequences, including discoloration and possible loss. Many injuries to primary teeth occur at 1½ to 2½ years of age, the toddler stage. The teeth most frequently injured in the primary dentition are the maxillary central incisors. These injuries may also damage the permanent teeth that are forming near the roots of the primary teeth.

Causes of dental injuries to children include automobile accidents, bicycle accidents, sports injuries, and child abuse. (Child abuse is discussed in Chapter 8.)

Fractured Anterior Teeth

Fractures of anterior teeth are common emergencies in a pediatric dental practice. Fractures of anterior teeth are classified according to the degree of severity (Table 27–1; Figs. 27–13 and 27–14).

Children with fractured teeth should be seen by the dentist as soon as possible. A complete documentation of the accident, clinical examination, vitality testing, and radiographs are almost always part of the emergency visit.

The dentist often prefers to delay restorative treatment that might involve further trauma to the pulp of an injured tooth for 3 to 6 weeks. This gives the delicate pulp a greater opportunity to recover without additional injury.

In the meantime, the dentist provides temporary relief by covering all exposed dentin with calcium hydroxide to prevent thermal sensitivity and places an interim covering of resin material. Radiographs and vitality tests are taken at subsequent appointments to determine the status of the injured tooth.

If the pulp is still vital, more definitive restorative procedures can be performed on the injured tooth.

TABLE 27–1

Classification and Treatment of Fracture of Young Anterior Teeth

CLASS	DESCRIPTION	TREATMENT
1	Enamel only is fractured Little, if any, dentin involved	Smooth sharp edges Reaccess at 6-month intervals
2	Fracture is into dentin, but *no* pulp exposure	Cover exposed dentin with a zinc oxide–eugenol type paste
3	Extensive fracture Pulp *is* exposed	Pulpotomy or pulpectomy, depending on degree of injury Place temporary crown until the pulp matures for a permanent crown placement
4	Crown is fractured off	Pulpectomy must be performed Post and crown are placed after endodontic treatment is completed

- Class I and II fractures can be restored with composite restorations involving the use of acid etch techniques.
- Class III and IV fractures may eventually necessitate permanent crowns, but treatment will have to be postponed until the apex of the root is completely developed.

TRAUMATIC INTRUSION

Traumatic intrusion results from an injury during which the tooth is forcibly driven *into* the alveolus so that only a portion of the crown is visible. (**Intrude** means to thrust inward.)

Traumatic intrusion can occur to either primary or permanent dentition. Teeth that are intruded should be allowed to re-erupt on their own. These teeth often require endodontic treatment later.

Damage to the developing permanent tooth can occur when a primary tooth is intruded. There is no way to determine the extent of damage to the permanent tooth until it erupts.

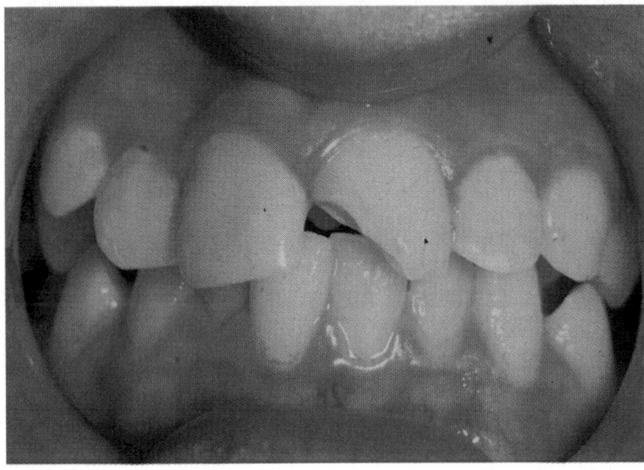

FIGURE 27–13

Fractured permanent central incisor with no pulp exposure.

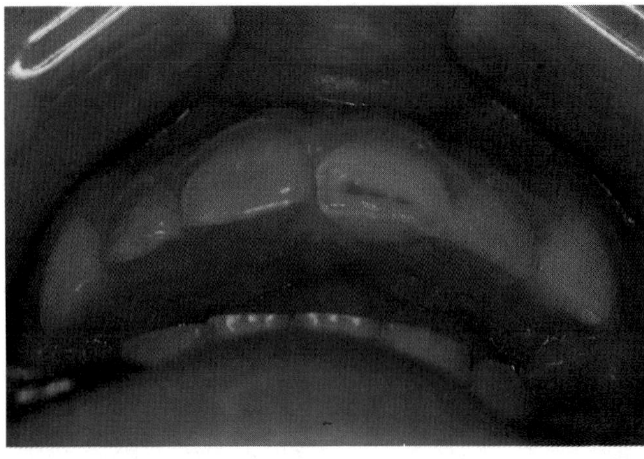

FIGURE 27–14

Fractured permanent central incisor with pulp exposure.

EXTRUSION AND LATERAL LUXATION INJURIES

Extrusion and lateral luxation are injuries in which the teeth are actually displaced from their position. In injuries of this type, severe damage to the periodontal ligaments usually occurs (Fig. 27–15). (**Extrusion**

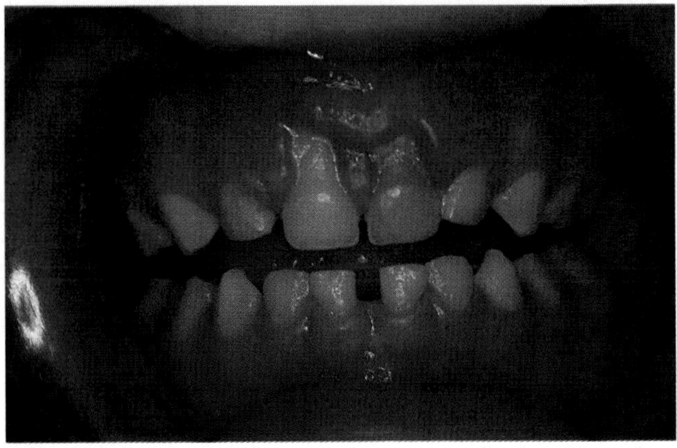

FIGURE 27–15

Gingiva healing after trauma to the primary central incisors.

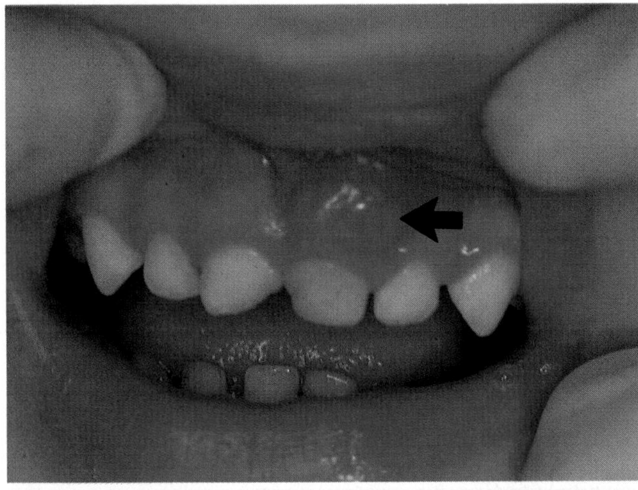

FIGURE 27–16

An abscess formed after injury to the right primary central incisor.

means thrust outward. **Luxate** means to dislocate, bend, or put out of joint.)

The dentist repositions the displaced teeth as soon as possible. The repositioned permanent teeth will be stabilized by a temporary splint of self-curing acrylic resin or wire ligature.

Endodontic treatment is often required in the future for these teeth. Primary teeth tend to undergo root resorption more quickly after injuries of this type and tend to become mobile. They should be observed for signs of infection and removed if that is indicated (Fig. 27–16).

AVULSED TEETH

Permanent teeth that have been avulsed—that is, knocked completely out of the mouth—can be replanted with varying degrees of success. Primary teeth are not usually replanted. (**Avulsed** means torn away or removed by force.)

The more quickly a tooth can be replanted, the greater the chance for success. Therefore, when an injury of this type occurs, parents should be instructed to

- Recover the tooth immediately
- Wrap the tooth in a moistened gauze
- Come immediately to the dentist's office

Treatment of the Avulsed Tooth. The highest success rate for replantation of permanent teeth occurs when the tooth is replanted within 30 minutes of the accident. The procedure for replantation is as follows:

1. A local anesthetic is administered.
2. Radiographs are taken. Often both periapical and occlusal radiographs are indicated, to reveal any fragments of tooth or bone.
3. Clotted blood is removed from the alveolus (socket) with a surgical curette.
4. The avulsed tooth is washed in saline solution and inserted into the alveolus.
5. The tooth is splinted in place with wire, acrylic, or orthodontic splints.
6. Postoperative radiographs are taken.
7. Endodontic treatment is carried out 6 to 8 weeks after replantation (see Chapter 29).

Sports Injuries

Many states have regulations that require all athletes in school contact sports to wear protective mouth guards to help prevent traumatic injuries to the teeth. Professional athletes in sports in which oral injuries may occur are also required to wear mouth guards.

Two types of mouth guards are used: commercial mouth guards and custom-fitted vacuum-formed mouth guards. Custom-fitted mouth guards are easily fabricated in the dental office.

COMMERCIAL MOUTH GUARDS

There are a variety of commercial "do-it-yourself" types of mouth guard kits (Fig. 27–17). These products may be purchased in assorted sizes to approximate the arch size. The material is heated in warm water and placed in the individual's mouth and molded to fit the arch.

This type of mouth guard is less accurate in fit than the custom type, but it is used by many athletes and is certainly better than no mouth guard at all.

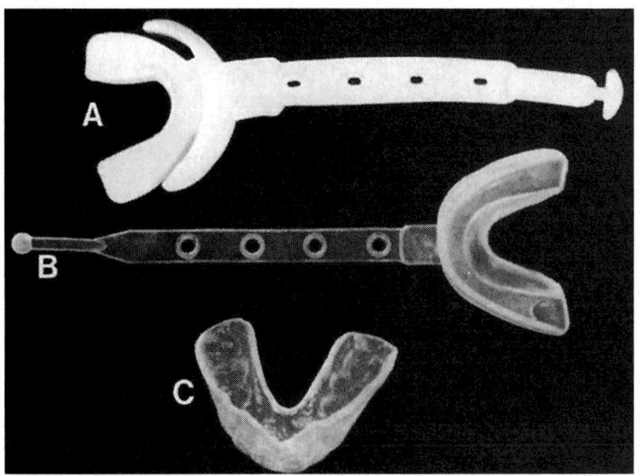

FIGURE 27–17

Three types of mouth guards. *A*, Stock mouth guard. *B*, Mouth-formed protector. *C*, Custom-fit mouth guard. (From Pinkham, J.R.: Dentistry: Infancy Through Adolescence. Philadelphia, W.B. Saunders Co., 1988, p 499.)

PROCEDURE: **Vacuum-Forming Custom Mouth Guards**

Instrumentation

Maxillary cast
Pencil
Vacuum former
3-mm. sheet clear plastic material
Strap holder attachment
Scalpel or sharp laboratory knife

Steps (Fig. 27–18)

1. Select the trimmed cast of the patient's maxillary arch.
   □ *RATIONALE:* A maxillary guard is more comfortable to wear. The only time a mandibular guard is constructed is when the patient has a class III malocclusion (see Chapter 5).
2. Use an indelible pencil to mark a finish (trim) line on the model at the junction of the attached gingiva and the oral mucosa.
3. Soak the cast in water for 10 minutes.
4. Attach the strap holder to the anterior teeth on the cast.
5. Heat the vacuum unit.
6. Place a sheet of 3-mm. clear plastic material in the heating section of the vacuum former.
7. Lower the heated plastic over the occlusal surfaces of the moist cast, and apply vacuum as recommended by the manufacturer. This is usually 4 to 5 pounds per square inch (psi).
8. Allow the machine to cool for a few minutes with the cast and material in place. When the plastic mouth guard is cool, strip it from the cast.
9. Use a scalpel or a heated, sharp laboratory knife to trim the plastic to the finish line marked on the cast.
10. *Optional:* To smooth the edges of the mouth guard, buff them with a chamois wheel on the bench lathe.

Preventive and Interceptive Orthodontics

It is common practice for pediatric dentists and general practitioners to provide preventive and interceptive orthodontic services for their patients.

Preventive orthodontic procedures are designed to prevent or minimize the degree of severity of future orthodontic problems. **Interceptive orthodontic** procedures are designed to intercept orthodontic problems that may worsen if left untreated.

It is important to recognize that not all orthodontic problems can be prevented (see Chapter 28). However, there are procedures that can prevent entirely, or at least minimize the degree of severity of, future orthodontic problems. Following are some of the common interceptive orthodontic services:

- Correcting oral habits
- Maintaining space
- Regaining space
- Correcting crossbites

Correcting Oral Habits

Thumb sucking and tongue thrusting are habits that involve abnormal muscle behavior. This can have a damaging effect on jaw growth, the occlusion, facial contour, and even speech.

THUMB SUCKING

Thumb sucking can cause serious malocclusions in some children, yet other children experience mild effects or none at all. The most common form of malocclusion is the anterior open bite.

There is varied opinion on treatment of a thumb-sucking problem. Some psychologists tend to favor a "let it run its course" approach, at least until the permanent maxillary anterior teeth erupt. It is hoped that the habit will disappear by then.

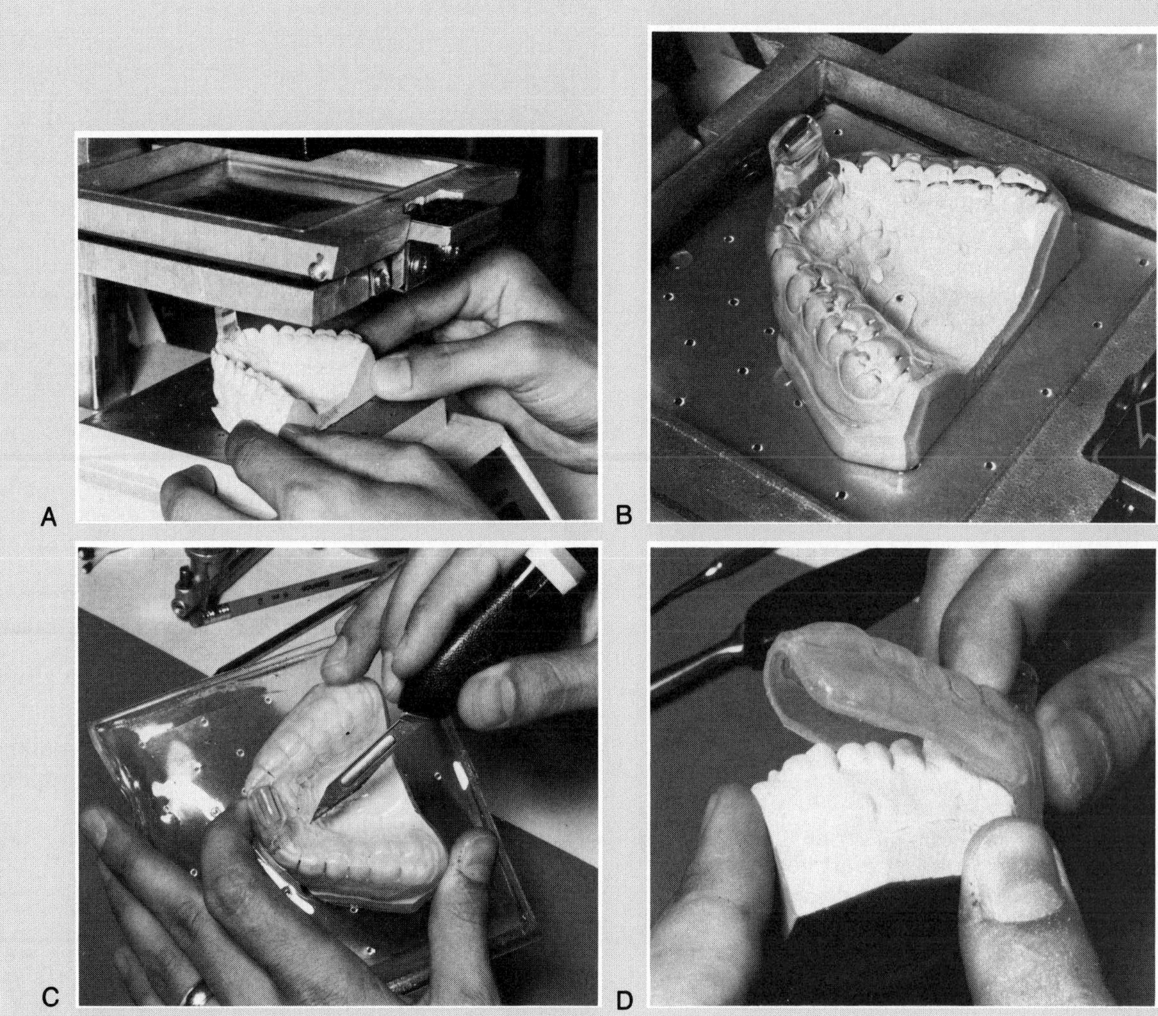

FIGURE 27–18

Use of the vacuum former to construct a custom mouth guard. *A*, The prepared cast is placed on the vacuum former. Notice that the plastic is beginning to sag from the heat. *B*, The heater element is lowered, and the vacuum is applied. *C*, A laboratory knife is used to carefully cut away the excess plastic. *D*, The edges are smoothed, and the fit of the guard is tried again on the cast. (Courtesy of Regina Dreyer, RDH, MPH.)

Most dentists feel that once the thumb-sucking habit extends beyond 4 years of age, some corrective action should be taken. This is the age when the habit can affect the permanent dentition. Many pediatric dentists suggest the following approach to treatment of thumb sucking:

1. Talk to the child about the problem, without the parents present.
2. Teach the child about the problems that thumb sucking can cause to the teeth.
3. Do not embarrass or shame the child.
4. Encourage the child to try to end the habit on his own.
5. Ask the parents to avoid discussing the habit with the child during treatment.
6. If this approach is unsuccessful, habit-correction appliances can be inserted in the patient's mouth as a reminder to keep the thumb out (Fig. 27–19).
7. Work in cooperation with a child psychologist for severe cases.

TONGUE THRUSTING

Tongue thrusting is a habit in which the patient pushes his tongue forcefully against the anterior teeth during swallowing. (The normal and infantile swallow patterns are discussed in Chapter 3.)

Tongue thrusting can result in an anterior open bite (Fig. 27–20). There is varying opinion on the treatment of tongue thrusting. Some believe that the prob-

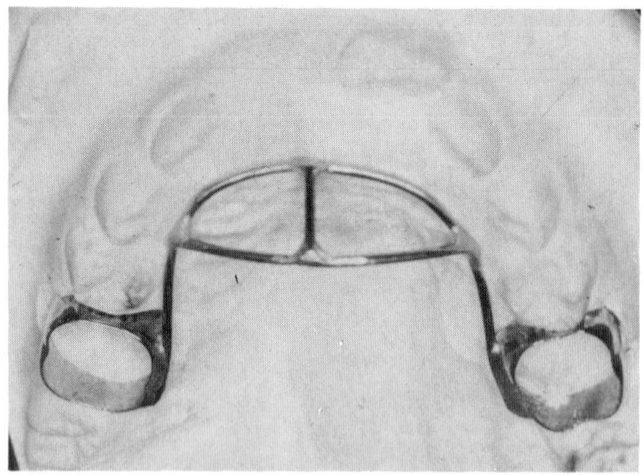

FIGURE 27–19

A fixed appliance to help break a thumb-sucking habit.

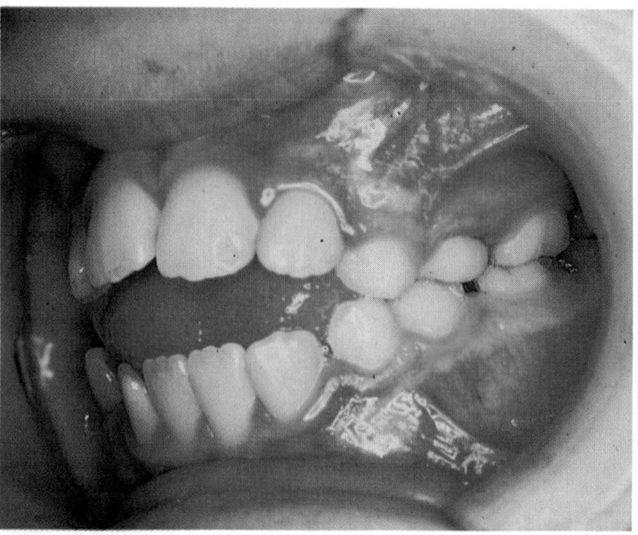

FIGURE 27–20

An open bite as the result of a tongue-thrusting habit. The spot on the lower portion of the maxillary central incisor is an enamel defect. Mamelons are visible on the mandibular incisors.

lem can be eliminated by training the patient to position the tongue properly through myofunctional therapy (exercises).

Others view myofunctional therapy as futile and prefer to use appliances on a long-term basis to counteract the forces put on the teeth by tongue thrusting.

Maintaining Space

After the premature loss of a primary tooth, a space maintainer is often used to keep the space in the arch until the permanent tooth erupts (see Fig. 27–8).

The space maintainer appliance is designed according to the needs of the individual patient. This may be either fixed or removable.

Fixed space maintainers, which are cemented in place, give more precise control, because the patient cannot remove the appliance.

Removable space maintainers, which can be placed and removed by the patient, are effective only if the patient wears them according to the dentist's directions.

Regaining Space

It is often necessary to regain lost space when teeth have drifted out of position. These malposed teeth can be returned to their proper position and held there until the permanent teeth erupt. The space-maintaining appliance can also be used as a space-regaining appliance.

Correcting Crossbites

In normal occlusion, the facial aspects of the maxillary teeth are located labial to the mandibular teeth when the jaws are brought together. (See Chapter 5.) A crossbite exists when the maxillary teeth are located lingual to the mandibular teeth.

Simple crossbites in children with normal jaw relationships can often be easily treated without extensive orthodontic treatment. One method is with the use of an acrylic **bite plane** that is cemented onto the mandibular anterior teeth. (A **bite plane** is a fixed appliance made of acrylic that is used to treat crossbites.)

When the jaws are closed, only the teeth in crossbite contact the bite plane. The force applied to these teeth when they close on the bite plane guides them into the proper position. This process may require only a few days to a few weeks to accomplish. Once the teeth are in normal occlusion, the bite plane is removed.

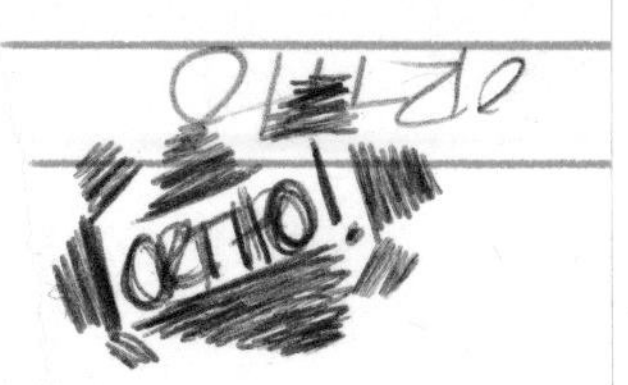

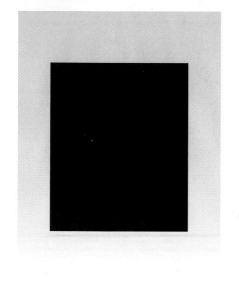

Chapter 28

Orthodontics

Introduction

Orthodontics is the specialty in dentistry concerned with the supervision, guidance, and correction of the growing and mature dentofacial structures. (The **dentofacial structures** are the jaws and surrounding facial bones.)

Orthodontics includes those conditions that require movement of teeth and correction of malrelationships and malformations. These adjustments between and among teeth and facial bones are made by the application of forces and/or the stimulation and redirection of the functional forces within the dentofacial structure.

The responsibilities of the orthodontic practice include the diagnosis, prevention, interception, and treatment of all forms of malocclusion of the teeth and surrounding structures. (**Malocclusion** is an occlusion and positioning of the teeth that are not in accordance with the usual rules of anatomic form.)

Benefits of Orthodontic Treatment

Orthodontic treatment may aid in eliminating or reducing three types of problems for the patient: psycho-social function, oral function, and dental disease.

PSYCHO-SOCIAL FUNCTION

Severe malocclusion can be a social handicap. The impact of this type of problem on individuals strongly influences their self-esteem and the extent of their positive feelings about themselves.

ORAL FUNCTION

Malocclusion may compromise all aspects of oral function:

- There can be difficulty in chewing if only a few teeth come together.
- Jaw discrepancies can force changes in the manner of swallowing.
- Malocclusion can make it more difficult to produce certain speech sounds.
- Temporomandibular joint (TMJ) pain may come from minor imperfections in occlusion that may trigger clenching and grinding activities.

DENTAL DISEASE

Malocclusion can contribute to both dental decay and periodontal disease because the teeth and tissues do not receive the benefits of normal occlusion and natural cleansing. Of equal importance is the difficulty the patient encounters in caring for the teeth properly.

Indications for Orthodontic Treatment

Orthodontic treatment may be necessary as a result of any combination of the following conditions:

- Impaired mastication
- Abnormal appearance due to malocclusion
- Dysfunction of the TMJ
- Susceptibility to dental caries

- Susceptibility to periodontal disease
- Impaired speech caused by malposition of the teeth and/or jaws

Contraindications for Orthodontic Treatment

Orthodontic treatment is not recommended under the following conditions:

- Lack of bony support for the dentition
- Rampant caries activity
- Poor general or mental health
- Poor oral hygiene and lack of patient cooperation
- Lack of patient interest in treatment to correct malalignment of the teeth
- Lack of financial support

Exposure Control for Orthodontics

As with any dental treatment, it is important that all appropriate exposure control measures be carried out during all patient care and while laboratory procedures are performed.

Factors Affecting Malocclusion

According to Angle's classification, which is described in Chapter 5, Class I occlusion is considered to be the ideal normal. Any deviation from this norm is considered to be malocclusion.

The most common orthodontic problems are

- **Crowded malaligned teeth** (this is the most common single contributor to malocclusion)
- **Overjet**, which is excessive protrusion of maxillary incisors
- **Overbite**, which is an increased vertical overlap
- **Open bite,** in which there is *no* vertical overlap (Fig. 28–1).

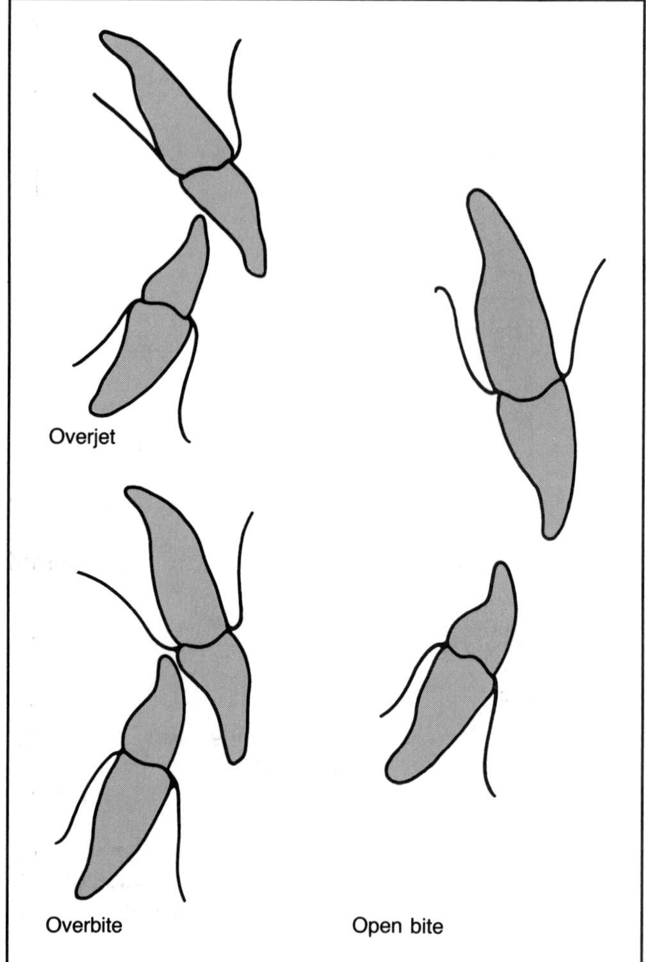

FIGURE 28–1

Abnormal overjet, overbite, and open bite.

In most cases, malocclusion and dentofacial deformity result from moderate distortions of normal development as described in Chapter 4. The orthodontic problems of most patients seem to arise from an interaction among developmental, genetic, environmental, and functional influences.

Developmental Causes

Disturbances of dental development may accompany major congenital defects; however, more frequently they occur as isolated findings. The most commonly encountered developmental disturbances include

- Congenitally missing teeth
- Malformed teeth
- Supernumerary teeth
- Interference with eruption (this may be an impaction in which eruption is blocked or the tooth may be forced to erupt into an abnormal position)
- Ectopic eruption (**ectopic** means located away from normal position)

Genetic Causes

Genetic causes are responsible for malocclusion when there are discrepancies in the size of the jaw and the size of the teeth. This happens more commonly when the child inherits a small jaw from one parent and large teeth from the other.

Environmental Causes

BIRTH INJURIES

Injuries at birth come under two major categories: fetal molding and trauma during birth.

Fetal molding occurs when a limb of the fetus is pressed against another part of the body, for example, when an arm is abnormally pressed against the mandible. This pressure can lead to distortion of rapidly growing areas.

Trauma during birth, such as an injury to the jaw, may occur during the birth, particularly from the use of forceps in delivery.

INJURIES THROUGHOUT LIFE

There can also be trauma to the teeth throughout life. Dental trauma can lead to the development of malocclusion in three ways:

1. Damage to permanent tooth buds when an injury to primary teeth has occurred
2. Movement of a tooth or teeth as a result of the premature loss of a primary tooth
3. Direct injury to permanent teeth (this is discussed in Chapter 27)

Functional Causes

As a general rule, **sucking habits** such as thumb, tongue, lip, or finger sucking during the primary dentition years are considered to be normal, and these habits have little if any long-term effect past mixed dentition; however, if they persist beyond this stage, it may be necessary to eliminate the habit if orthodontic treatment is to be successful. (These habits are discussed in Chapter 27.)

Phases of Orthodontic Treatment

Orthodontic treatment may be arbitrarily divided into three broad categories: preventive, interceptive, and corrective.

Preventive

Preventive orthodontics is the phase of orthodontic treatment involving the recognition and elimination of irregularities and malposition in the developing dentofacial complex. Preventive orthodontics includes

- Control of caries to prevent the premature loss of primary teeth that may result in the loss of space for the eruption of permanent teeth
- Use of a space maintainer to save the space for the permanent tooth
- Correction of oral habits that may be damaging to the permanent dentition
- Early detection of genetic and congenital anomalies that may influence dental development
- Supervision of the natural exfoliation of the primary teeth (primary teeth retained too long may cause the permanent teeth to erupt out of alignment or to be impacted)

Interceptive

Interceptive orthodontics consists of steps taken to prevent or correct problems as they are developing, including

- The removal of primary teeth that may be contributing to malalignment of the permanent dentition
- The serial extraction of teeth

The **serial extraction** of primary or permanent teeth to correct a critical overcrowding of teeth in the allotted space in the arch is performed *only* when more conservative methods of treatment will not be effective.

When extractions are required, the orthodontist refers the patient to a general dentist or to an oral maxillofacial surgeon.

Corrective

Corrective orthodontics refers to the use of

- Fixed appliances (a fixed appliance is cemented in place and cannot be removed by the patient)
- Removable appliances (a removable appliance can be placed and removed by the patient)
- Orthognathic surgery when the orthodontic problem is too severe to be corrected by other means

Records Visit and Treatment Planning

The first orthodontic appointment is scheduled to obtain records required by the orthodontist in order to make a diagnosis and create a treatment plan. There is an initial fee for this appointment.

The patient's diagnosis is based on information from three major sources:

- Interviewing the patient
- A clinical examination of the patient
- Evaluation of diagnostic records

Interview Information

The orthodontist requires information that is gathered by interviewing the patient and/or accompanying adult.

MEDICAL AND DENTAL HISTORY

A careful medical and dental history is necessary to provide a comprehensive understanding of the physical

HARRY W. HUMPHREYS, D.D.S., M.S. ORTHODONTICS

Date ______

Name of Patient ______ Age ____ Date of Birth ______
*Address ______ City ______ Phone ______
Name of Parent ______ Occupation ______
Business Address ______ Business Phone ______
Patient's Dentist ______ Who Referred You? ______
School ______ Grade ______
No. children in family ______ Orthodontic Insurance ? ______
*Zip Code ______ Physician ______
Medical History: ______
Tonsils: in ____; out ____. If out, what age? ______
Any complications or high fever with childhood diseases? Which ______
Scarlet Fever? ______ Rheumatic Fever? ______ Tonsillitis? ______ Mastoid or Ear Infection? ______ Chronic Sinus? ______
Chronic Allergy? ______ Normal Birth? ______ Surgery? ______ Fractured Bones? ______ Asthma? ______
Difficulty Chewing? ______ Swallowing? ______ Injuries to face or teeth? ______ Thumb or finger sucking? ______
Additional, Not Listed Above: ______
Menstrual Cycle: Yes ____ No ____ When ______
Other Orthodontic Consultations? ______ When? ______
Other Orthodontic Treatment? ______ When? ______

Exam ______ Study Casts and Orthodontic Analysis ______ Consultation ______

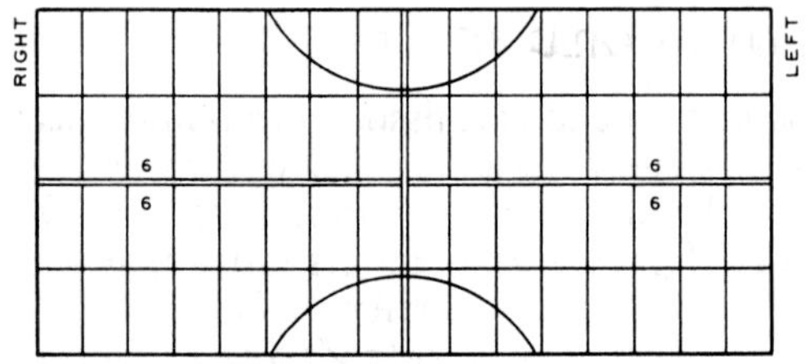

RIGHT 6 6 6 6 LEFT

EXAMINATION CARD

CASE NO. ______
NAME ______ DATE ______
AGE ______ BIRTHDAY ______ SEX ______
ADDRESS ______ (ZIP) PHONE ______
PARENT ______ OCCUPATION ______
BUSINESS ADDRESS ______ PHONE ______
DENTIST ______ PHONE ______
REFERRED BY ______
SCHOOL ______ GRADE ______

DESCRIPTION ______

TYPE FACE ______ TYPE HEAD ______ HABITS ______ SPEECH ______
HYGIENE ______ CARIES RATE ______ MUSCLE TONE ______ TISSUE ______
CLASSIFICATION ______ MUTILATION ______

	MODELS	CEPH	PHOTO	TRACING	FMX	ORTHO ANAL	RX RECORD
INITIAL	☐	☐	☐	☐	☐	☐	☐
FINAL	☐	☐	☐	☐	☐	☐	☐

ESTIMATED TIME ______
FEE - TOTAL ______ INITIAL ______ MONTHLY ______ RETENTION ______
OTHER ARRANGEMENTS ______
ADVISED ______ RECORDS: ______ NOTE TO REFERRING DOCTOR: ______
RECALL IN: ______
POSSIBLE TREATMENT: ______
DISPOSITION ______ MISCELLANEOUS ______

FIGURE 28–2

Combination of medical history and examination form for an orthodontic patient. (Courtesy of Harry W. Humphreys, DDS, San Rafael, CA.)

condition and to evaluate specific orthodontically related concerns (Fig. 28–2). (See also Chapter 18.)

PHYSICAL GROWTH EVALUATION

Because orthodontic treatment in children is closely related to growth stages, it is necessary to evaluate the child's physical growth status. Questions are asked about how rapidly the child has grown recently and signs of sexual maturation.

SOCIAL AND BEHAVIORAL EVALUATION

Motivation for seeking treatment is very important. What does the patient expect as a result from treatment? How cooperative or uncooperative is the patient likely to be?

A major motivation for orthodontic treatment of children is the parents' desire for treatment; however, it is essential that the child be willing and cooperative. The typical child accepts orthodontic treatment in the same manner as he or she accepts going to school.

Adults, however, seek orthodontic treatment for themselves for other reasons. These reasons include the need to improve personal appearance or the function of the teeth. Whichever the reason, it is important to explore why the patient seeks treatment at this time.

The Clinical Examination

The purpose of the orthodontic clinical examination is to document and evaluate the facial aspects, the occlusal relationship, and the functional characteristics of the jaws. At the records visit, the orthodontist decides which diagnostic records are required for the patient.

EVALUATION OF FACIAL ESTHETICS

A reasonable goal for orthodontic treatment is to improve facial symmetry by correcting disproportions.

Frontal Evaluation

From the front, the face is examined for

- Bilateral symmetry
- Size proportions of midline to lateral structures
- Vertical proportionality

Profile Evaluation

Analysis of the profile relationships must be evaluated in greater depth (Fig. 28–3). Skeletal proportions revealed in this view affect both anteroposterior and vertical tooth relationships in addition to facial esthetics.

During the profile examination, the orthodontist

- Determines whether the jaws are proportionately positioned
- Evaluates lip protrusion (excessive lip protrusion is most often caused by protrusion of the incisors)
- Evaluates the vertical facial proportions and the mandibular plane angle

Facial form analysis carried out in this manner takes only a few minutes but provides information that cannot be gathered from dental radiographs and diagnostic casts.

EVALUATION OF ORAL HEALTH

A thorough hard and soft tissue examination, as well as an oral hygiene assessment and prophylaxis, must be completed before any orthodontic treatment begins. Any charting of periodontal pockets must be noted.

If necessary, the patient is referred for the treatment of these problems before orthodontic treatment is started.

EVALUATION OF JAW AND OCCLUSAL FUNCTION

The orthodontist examines the patient's occlusion and palpates the TMJ to evaluate its function. Of spe-

Maxilla:	☐ Retrusive	☐ Normal	☐ Protrusive
Mandible:	☐ Retrusive	☐ Normal	☐ Protrusive
Ant. Face Ht.:	☐ Decreased	☐ Normal	☐ Increased
Post. Face Ht.:	☐ Decreased	☐ Normal	☐ Increased
Nose:	☐ Small	☐ Medium	☐ Large
Nasolabial Angle:	☐ Obtuse	☐ Average	☐ Acute
Lips:	☐ Retrusive	☐ Normal	☐ Protrusive
Lip Proportions:	☐ Thick	☐ Normal	☐ Thin
Lip Incompetence:	☐ No	☐ Yes If yes, interlabial gap at rest: _____ mm.	
Mentolabial Fold:	☐ Deep	☐ Average	☐ Shallow
Neck/Chin Angle:	☐ Obtuse	☐ Average	☐ Acute
Throat Length:	☐ Short	☐ Average	☐ Long

FIGURE 28–3

Facial profile diagnostic record form.

cial interest for orthodontic purposes are any lateral or anterior shifts of the mandible on closure.

Diagnostic Records

Before the clinical evaluation can be completed, diagnostic records in the form of photographs, radiographs, and diagnostic casts are required. When possible, it is best to have these available at the time of the intraoral examination. Diagnostic records document features such as tooth angulation, dental crowding, and the presence of unerupted teeth.

DIAGNOSTIC CASTS

Evaluation of the occlusion requires impressions for diagnostic casts and a record of the occlusion so the casts can be articulated. Alginate impressions and diagnostic casts are covered in Chapter 19.

Diagnostic casts for orthodontic purposes are usually trimmed so that the bases have a symmetrical shape. When the casts are trimmed in this manner, the symmetrical base is oriented to the midline of the palate, thus making it much easier to detect asymmetry within the dental arches.

The casts are also polished so that they will be more acceptable for presentation to the patient (Fig. 28–4).

PHOTOGRAPHS

Photographs capture the color, shape, texture, and characteristics of intraoral and extraoral structures. Photography is also useful as an aid in patient identification, treatment planning, case presentation, case documentation, and patient education and instruction.

Two standard **extraoral photographs** are taken: (1) the frontal view, with lips in a relaxed position, and (2) a profile view of the patient's right side, with lips in a relaxed position (see Fig. 28–4).

Three standard **intraoral photographs** are also required: (1) the full direct view, which includes all teeth in occlusion; (2) the maxillary occlusal view, which includes the palate and all maxillary occlusal surfaces; and (3) the right buccal view, which includes the distal of the cuspid to distal of last molar views.

When intraoral photographs are taken, it is important that the cheeks and lips are retracted sufficiently to show all of these structures.

RADIOGRAPHS

The **panoramic film** has two advantages over a series of intraoral radiographs: (1) it gives a broader view that will show any pathologic lesions and supernumerary or impacted teeth, and (2) the radiation exposure is much lower (Fig. 28–5). The panoramic film is supplemented with periapical and bite-wing radiographs only when greater detail is needed. (See Chapter 17.)

The orthodontist needs to know how the major functional components of the face are related to each other. **Cephalometric films** make it possible to evaluate dentofacial proportions and clarify the anatomic basis for a malocclusion (Fig. 28–6).

Serial cephalometric radiographs taken at intervals before, during, and after treatment can be superimposed to study changes in jaw and tooth positions. It is very important to place the patient in the same posi-

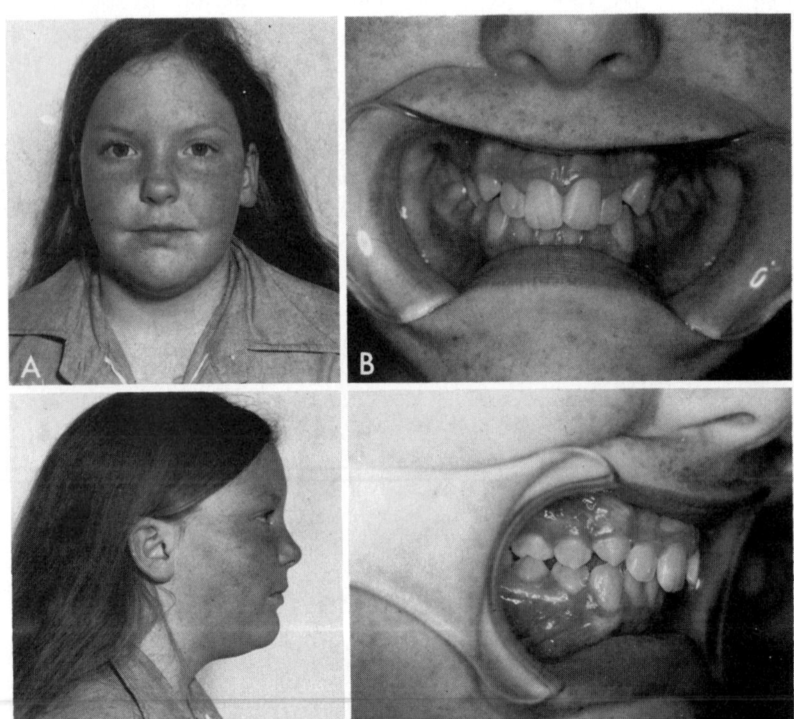

FIGURE 28–4

Pretreatment photographs and diagnostic casts of a patient with Class I malocclusion with bimaxillary crowding. (Courtesy of James M. Miller, DDS, San Anselmo, CA.)

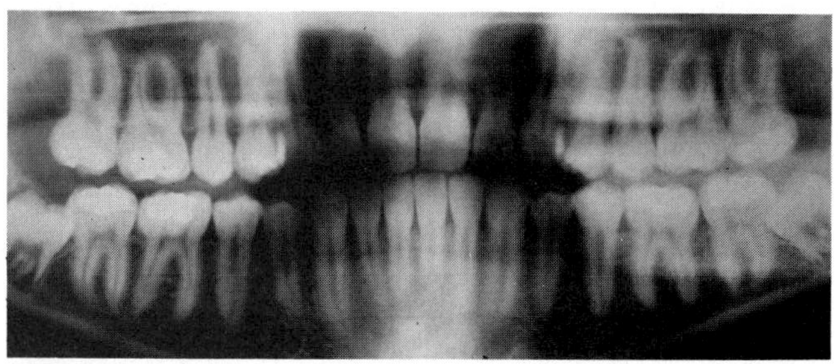

FIGURE 28–5

Panoramic post-treatment radiograph of a 17-year-old male.

tion each time, in order to evaluate these changes (see Fig. 17–43).

CEPHALOMETRIC ANALYSIS

Cephalometric analysis is carried out, not on the radiograph itself, but on a tracing that emphasizes the relationship of selected points. Cephalometric landmarks can be represented as a series of points whose coordinates are specified, making it possible to compute a means of mathematical descriptions and measurements of the status of the skull.

An additional responsibility for the dental assistant may be the preparation of a cephalometric tracing for use by the orthodontist in the cephalometric study (Fig. 28–7).

The orthodontist identifies the points needed in a cephalometric tracing and the manner in which the tracing must be completed. An understanding of the anatomic landmarks identified on a lateral view of the skull is necessary for an exact cephalometric radiographic technique.

Cephalometric Landmarks and Points

- **Articulare** (Ar): the point of intersection between the shadow of the zygomatic arch and the posterior border of the mandibular ramus
- **Anterior nasal spine** (ANS): the median bony process of the maxilla at the lower margin of the anterior nasal opening
- **Basion** (Ba): the most forward and lowest point on the anterior margin of the foramen magnum
- **Bolton point** (Bo): the highest point in the upward curvature of the retrocondylar fossa of the occipital bone
- **Gnathion** (Gn): the center of the inferior contour of the chin
- **Gonion** (Go): the center of the inferior contour of the mandibular angle
- **Menton** (Me): the most inferior point on the mandibular symphysis (the bottom of the chin)
- **Nasion** (Na): the anterior point of the intersection between the nasal and frontal bones
- **Orbitale** (Or): the lowest point on the inferior margin of the orbit
- **Point A:** the innermost point on the contour of the premaxilla between the anterior nasal spine and the incisor

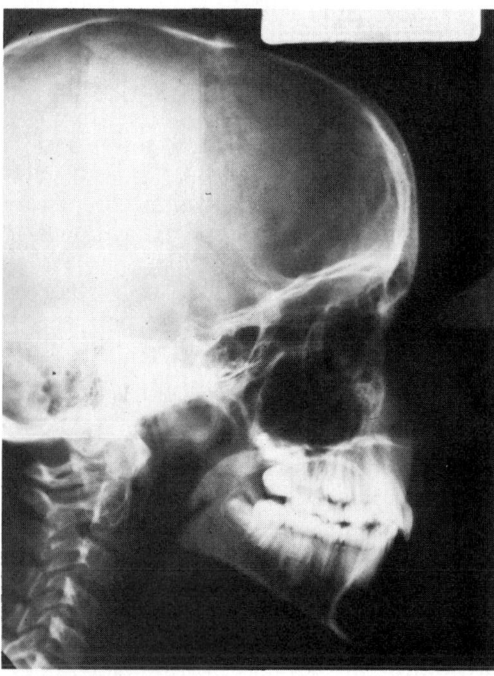

FIGURE 28–6

Cephalometric radiograph. (Courtesy of James M. Miller, DDS, San Anselmo, CA.)

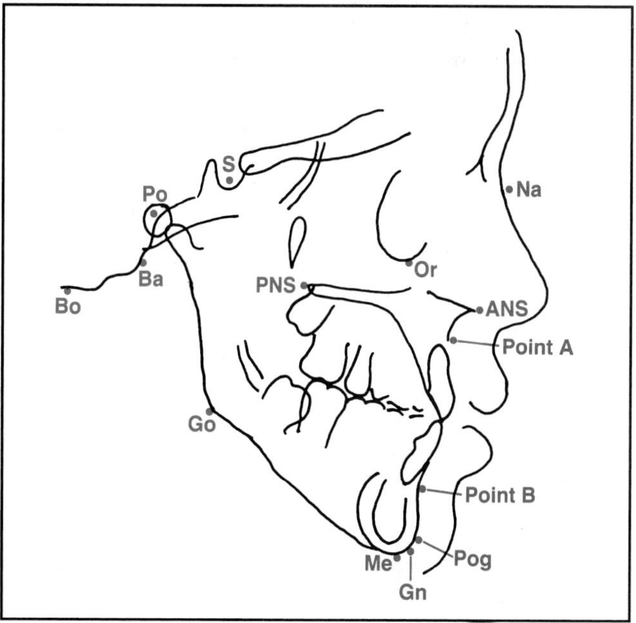

FIGURE 28–7

Cephalometric tracing points and landmarks. *Abbreviations:* Bo, Bolton point; Ba, basion; Po, porion; S, sella; Go, gonion; PNS, posterior nasal spine; Na, nasion; Or, orbitale; ANS, anterior nasal spine; Pog, pogonion; Gn, gnathion; Me, menton.

PROCEDURE: Creating a Cephalometric Tracing

Instrumentation (Fig. 28–8)

Cephalometric lateral skull film (facing to the right)
Table top light source
Tracing template
Sharp pencil
Clear tape
Protractor with straight edge
Acetate tracing paper
Transparent millimeter ruler
Art gum eraser

Cephalometric Tracing

1. Place the acetate paper, rough side up, exactly over the film and tape them together, making sure the top and right sides of the film and plastic coincide.
2. Trace the outline of sella (S). Determine the midpoint, and place a dot.
3. Trace the ethmoid triad. The lower line represents the top of the hard palate. (This can be seen in Fig. 28–7 running from the lingual surface of the maxillary anterior tooth back to the PNS point and then forward again.)
4. Trace the outline of the frontal and nasal bones. This is Point Na. Where these two lines cross should be the most anterior point of the frontonasal suture.
5. Draw the outline of the bony orbit. The lowest point on this curve is Or.
   □ *IMPORTANT:* Because this is a bilateral structure, two images may be seen. When this happens, split the difference between the two and draw it.
6. Use the middle circle of the template and draw in Po. If more than one point is seen, split the difference and trace it.
7. Draw in the cross-section of the palate; this represents Point A.
8. Use the template and draw in the most prominent upper incisor.
   □ *IMPORTANT:* This is a key landmark; be very careful to represent the angular position of this tooth accurately.

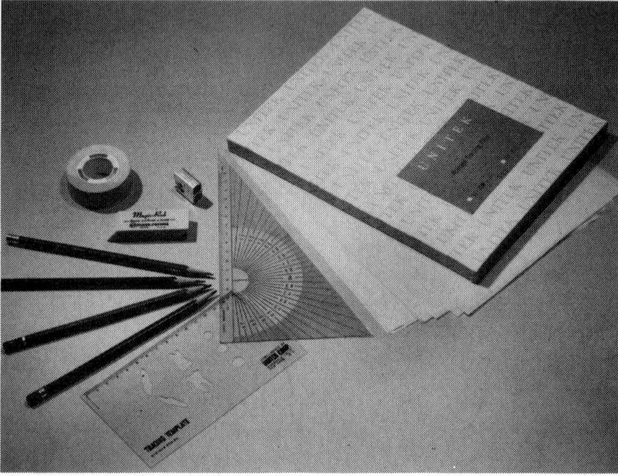

FIGURE 28–8

Cephalometric tracing supplies. (Courtesy of Unitek Corp, Monrovia, CA.)

9. Use the template and trace in the maxillary first molar.
10. Draw the mandibular symphysis and lower and inferior borders of the mandible. Be careful to represent Point B accurately as it is the deepest point of the curve of the border of the symphysis and also Pg, the most anterior point on the bony chin.
11. Use the template and draw the most prominent lower incisor.
   □ *IMPORTANT:* This too is a key landmark that must be accurate.
12. Trace the inferior alveolar nerve canal and the unerupted third molar crypt.
13. Use the template and trace in the mandibular molars.
14. Draw in the outline of the soft tissue profile.
15. Label any points not already marked.
16. Identify the tracing by patient's name, date, age, and record number.
17. Place the completed tracing in the patient's record.

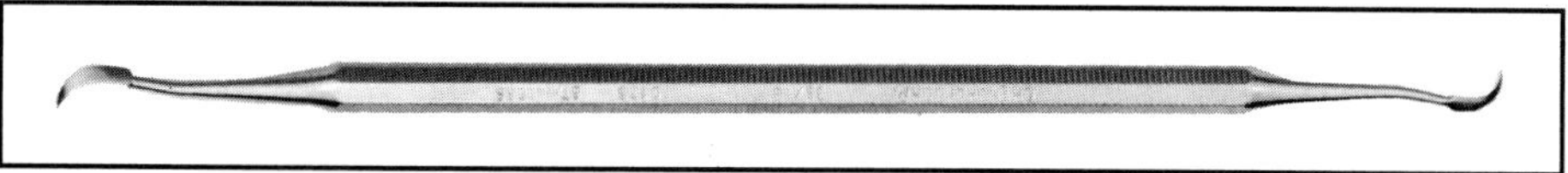

FIGURE 28–9

Orthodontic scaler. (Courtesy of Orthopli Corp., Philadelphia, PA.)

- **Point B**: the innermost point on the contour of the mandible between the incisor and the bony chin
- **Pogonion** (Pog): the most anterior point on the contour of the chin
- **Porion** (Po): the midpoint of the upper contour of the external auditory canal
- **Posterior nasal spine** (PNS): the tip of the posterior spine of the palatine bone, at the junction of the hard and soft palates
- **Sella** (S): the midpoint of the cavity of sella turcica

The Case Presentation

The orthodontist studies the information gathered and develops a treatment plan and cost estimate for the patient in preparation for the case presentation.

Approximately 1 hour is reserved for the case presentation visit, and the patient, and a responsible adult if the patient is a child, should be present. At this visit, the dentist uses the photographs, radiographs, cephalometric tracing, diagnostic casts, and any other aids to present the diagnosis and treatment plan.

This presentation includes the approximate length of treatment and a clear statement of the responsibility of the patient in helping ensure successful completion.

Once treatment has been accepted, a consent form is signed by the adult or legal guardian. (A minor cannot legally give consent.) This consent form clearly states the information presented during the case presentation.

Financial Arrangements

In addition to the case presentation and consent form, a formal contract for payment of the treatment fee is presented and discussed with the individual responsible for the finances.

The most frequently used payment plan involves divided payments. Once the patient and responsible person are in agreement that treatment should proceed, the contract is signed by the person legally responsible for the account.

Some dental insurance plans cover part of the cost of orthodontic treatment. When there is insurance coverage, it is usually the responsibility of the subscriber, not the orthodontic practice, to submit periodic progress claims for reimbursement.

Specialized Instrumentation for Orthodontics

Orthodontics requires the use of highly specialized instruments. Listed as follows are the most commonly used types of instruments and pliers.

Double-Ended Instruments

The **orthodontic scaler** is an instrument with several uses, including as an aid in direct bracket placement, removing elastomeric rings, and removing excess cement or bonding material (Fig. 28–9).

The **ligature director** allows the operator to guide the ligature tie once cut and twisted under the arch wire (Fig. 28–10).

The **band plugger** has a small, round, serrated end to help seat a molar band for a fixed appliance (Fig. 28–11).

The **bite-stick**, which consists of a molded plastic handle with either a triangular or rounded stainless steel serrated working area, is used to assist in seating a molar band for a fixed appliance (Fig. 28–12).

Bracket placement tweezers are long-tipped, reverse-action tweezers with finely serrated beaks. This instrument is used to assist in placing direct bonding brackets (Fig. 28–13).

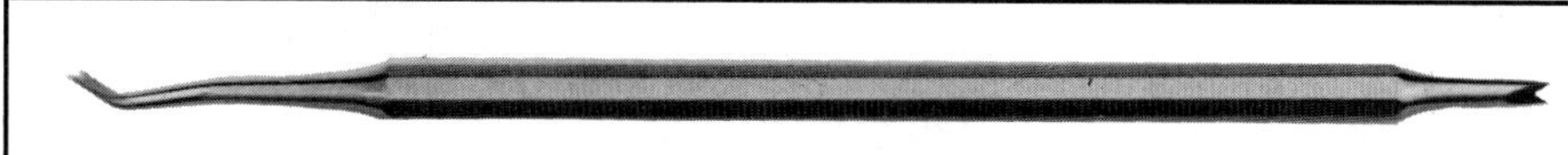

FIGURE 28–10

Ligature director. (Courtesy of Orthopli Corp., Philadelphia, PA.)

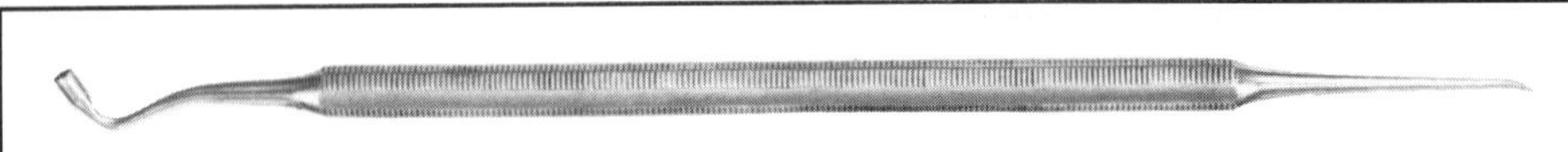

FIGURE 28–11

Band plugger. (Courtesy of Orthopli Corp., Philadelphia, PA.)

FIGURE 28–12

Bite stick. (Courtesy of Orthopli Corp., Philadelphia, PA.)

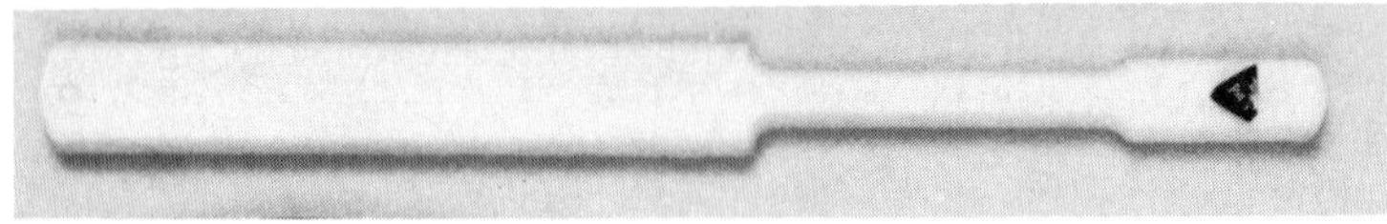

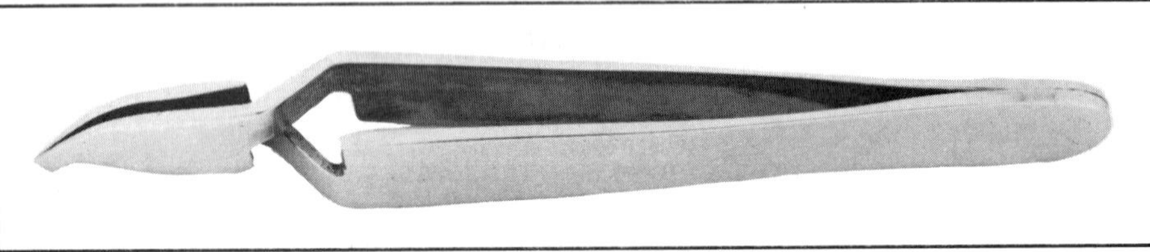

FIGURE 28–13

Bracket placement tweezers. (Courtesy of Orthopli Corp., Philadelphia, PA.)

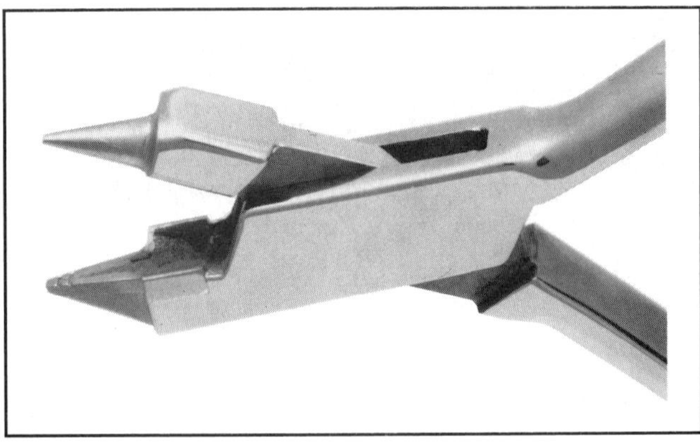

FIGURE 28–14

Bird-beak plier. (Courtesy of Orthopli Corp., Philadelphia, PA.)

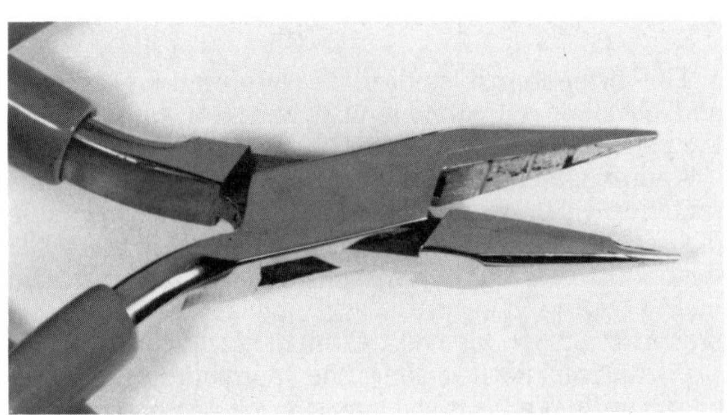

FIGURE 28–15

Jarabak plier. (Courtesy of Orthopli Corp., Philadelphia, PA.)

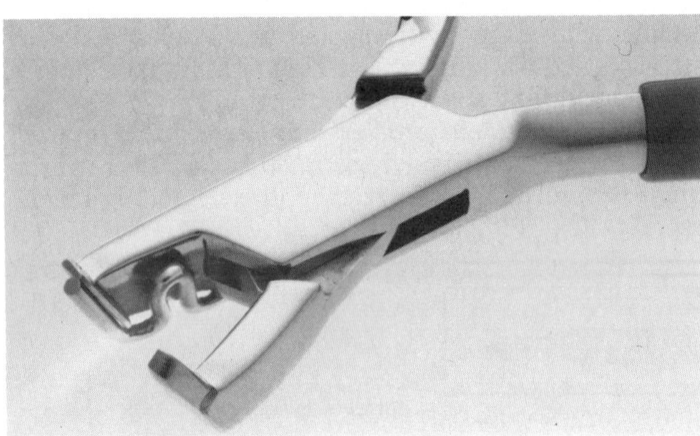

FIGURE 28–16

Distal end cutter. (Courtesy of Orthopli Corp., Philadelphia, PA.)

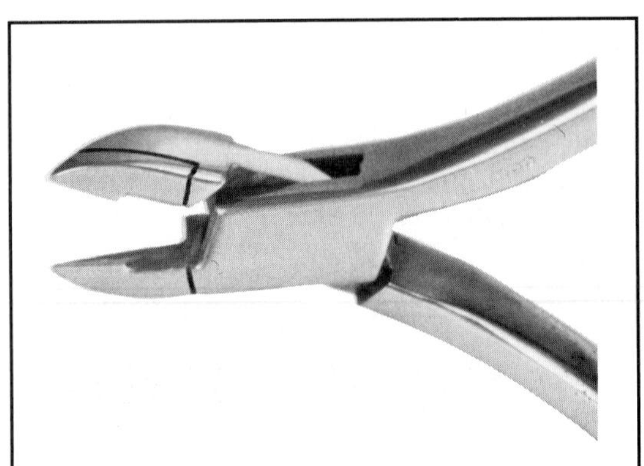

FIGURE 28–17

Pin-and-ligature cutter. (Courtesy of Orthopli Corp., Philadelphia, PA.)

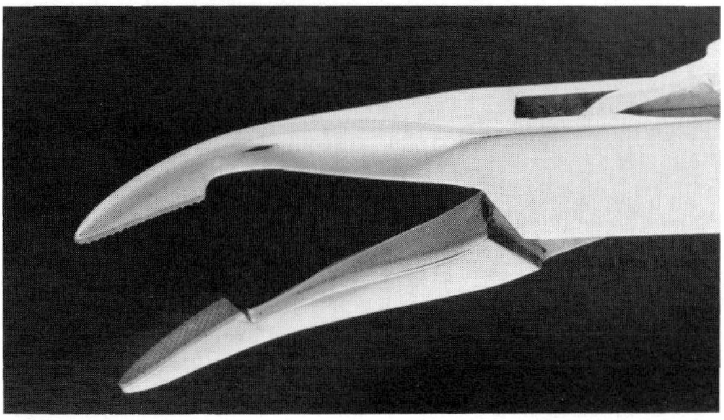

FIGURE 28–18

Weingart utility plier. (Courtesy of Orthopli Corp., Philadelphia, PA.)

Pliers

A **bird-beak plier** is useful in forming and bending wires for either fixed or removable appliances (Fig. 28–14).

The **Jarabak plier**, which is sometimes referred to as a *Tweed loop plier*, has grooves to allow bending and closing of loops for fixed or removable appliances (Fig. 28–15).

A **distal end cutter** is designed to cut and hold the distal end of the arch wire once it has been placed into the buccal tube of a fixed molar band (Fig. 28–16).

A **pin-and-ligature cutter** is designed to cut the ligature wire once it has been ligated (fastened) around the bracket (Fig. 28–17).

The **Weingart utility plier** has finely serrated narrow beaks, allowing accessibility to all areas. It is utilized in placing arch wires (Fig. 28–18).

A **posterior band remover** is used to remove bands without stress on the tooth or discomfort to the patient (Fig. 28–19).

The **Coon ligature tying plier** has finely serrated narrow beaks to allow ease in ligature tying and also the placement of elastics (Fig. 28–20).

A **light wire forming plier** is used to form various loop designs in wires, to make minor adjustment bends in the arch wires, and to place metal spring separators (Fig. 28–21).

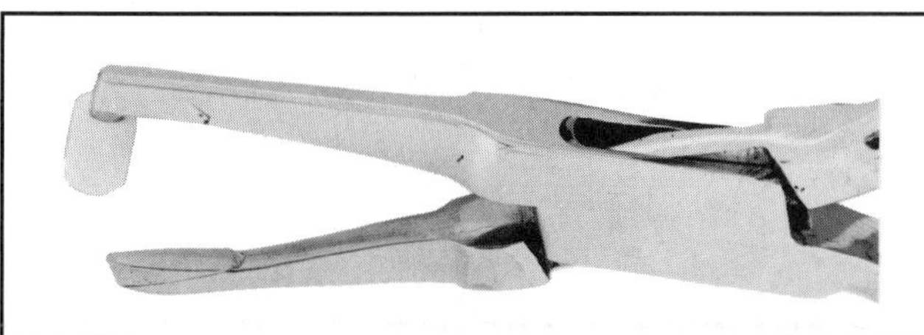

FIGURE 28–19

Posterior band remover. (Courtesy of Orthopli Corp., Philadelphia, PA.)

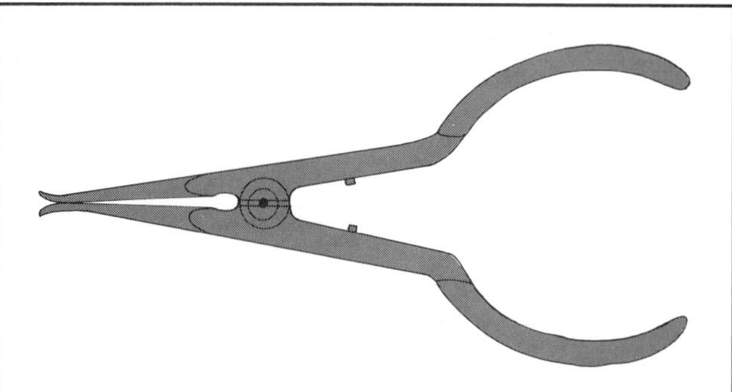

FIGURE 28–20

Coon ligature tying plier.

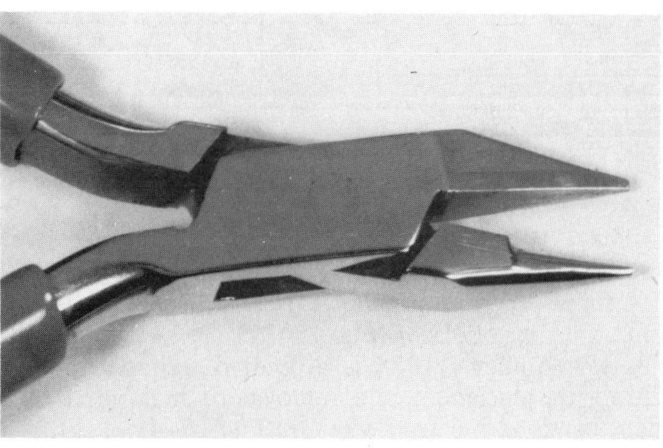

FIGURE 28–21

Light wire forming plier. (Courtesy of Orthopli Corp., Philadelphia, PA.)

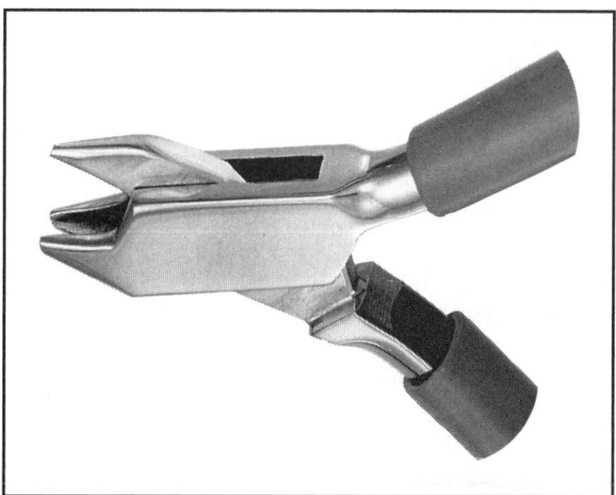

FIGURE 28–22

Three-prong plier. (Courtesy of Orthopli Corp., Philadelphia, PA.)

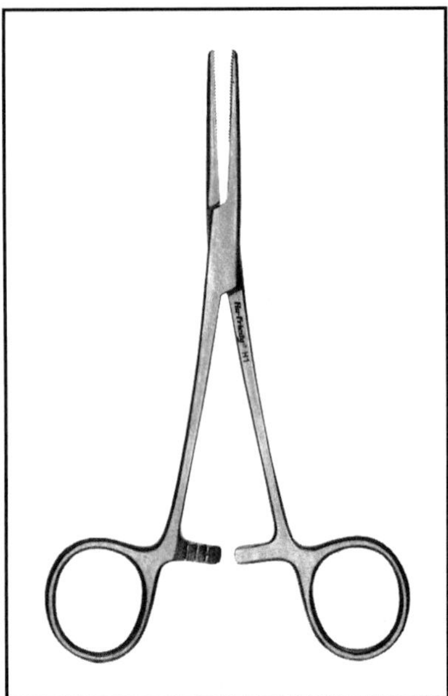

FIGURE 28–23

Hemostat. (Courtesy of Hu-Friedy Manufacturing, Inc., Chicago, IL.)

A **three-prong clasp plier** is used primarily in closing and adjusting of clasps (Fig. 28–22).

A **Howe plier (110)** has a pointed serrated tip that allows for placement and removal or making adjustment bends in the arch wire (see Fig. 25–4).

A **hemostat** has narrow serrated beaks and handles that can be clasped together. This makes it possible to hold something, such as a separator, securely between the beaks (Fig. 28–23).

An **arch torquing and bending plier,** also known as an *edgewise plier,* is used for holding and adjusting arch wires, usually those with rectangular cross sections (Fig. 28–24).

Types of Orthodontic Appliances

Orthodontic treatment utilizes fixed and removable appliances to aid in the mechanical movement of the teeth and/or jaw. The remodeling of the bone that takes place during tooth movement is discussed in Chapter 4.

Removable appliances are used primarily as retainers or in tipping teeth. (**Tipping** is the movement of a tooth into a more upright position.) They are not used to produce major tooth movement. These appliances are discussed in Chapter 27 and at the end of this chapter.

Fixed appliances, commonly known as *braces*, are attached to the teeth and assist in tooth movement. These appliances are discussed in this chapter.

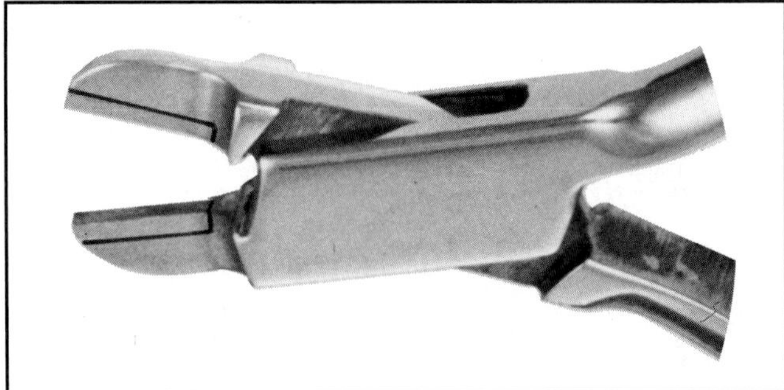

FIGURE 28–24

Arch torquing and bending plier. (Courtesy of Orthopli Corp., Philadelphia, PA.)

Fixed Appliances

Through the use of fixed appliances, a tooth can be moved in six directions: mesially, distally, lingually, facially, apically, and occlusally. It can also be rotated on its axis. (**Rotation** is the force of turning a tooth to the left or right within its socket.)

The principal components of fixed appliances are attachments, auxiliaries, and arch wires.

Attachments are bands, which circle the tooth and are cemented in place, and brackets, which are bonded directly to the enamel of the tooth. Most commonly, bands are placed on the first and second molars, and brackets are cemented to the anterior teeth and premolars.

Auxiliaries are attachments to the brackets and bands, such as tubes and hooks that make it possible to attach the arch wire to the tooth and to give strength in movement of the tooth.

The **arch wire** is attached to the brackets and bands and serves as a pattern for the dental arch. By bending the arch wire, force and pressure are created, and these cause the tooth or teeth to move in the desired direction.

SEPARATION BEFORE PLACEMENT OF ORTHODONTIC BANDS

Bands are preformed stainless steel rings fitted around the teeth and cemented in place (Fig. 28–25). The bands are divided into upper (maxillary) and

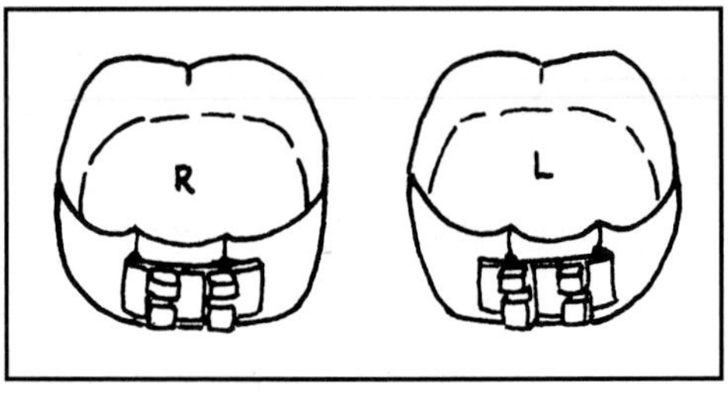

FIGURE 28–25

Right and left first mandibular molar bands.

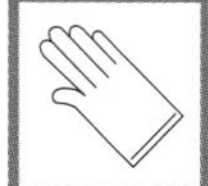 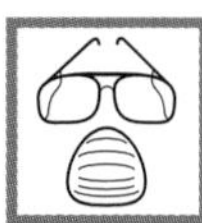 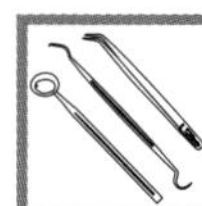 

PROCEDURE: **Placing and Removing Brass Wire Separators**

Placement of Brass Wire Separators

1. Bend a 20 mil soft brass wire into an open hook shape (Fig. 28–26*A*).
2. Use a hemostat to pass the wire beneath the contact from the lingual side (see Fig. 28–26*B*).
3. Bring the wire back over the contact and twist it slightly (see Fig. 28–26*C*).
4. Use a ligature wire cutter to cut the twisted pigtail to 3 mm. in length. Tuck the pigtail into the gingival crevice between the teeth (see Fig. 28–26*D*).
5. This type of separator is normally left in place 5 to 7 days.

Removal of Brass Wire Separators

1. Use a ligature wire cutter to carefully cut the twisted pigtail (see Fig. 28–26*E*).
2. Use a hemostat to carefully remove the wire from under the contact from the facial side.

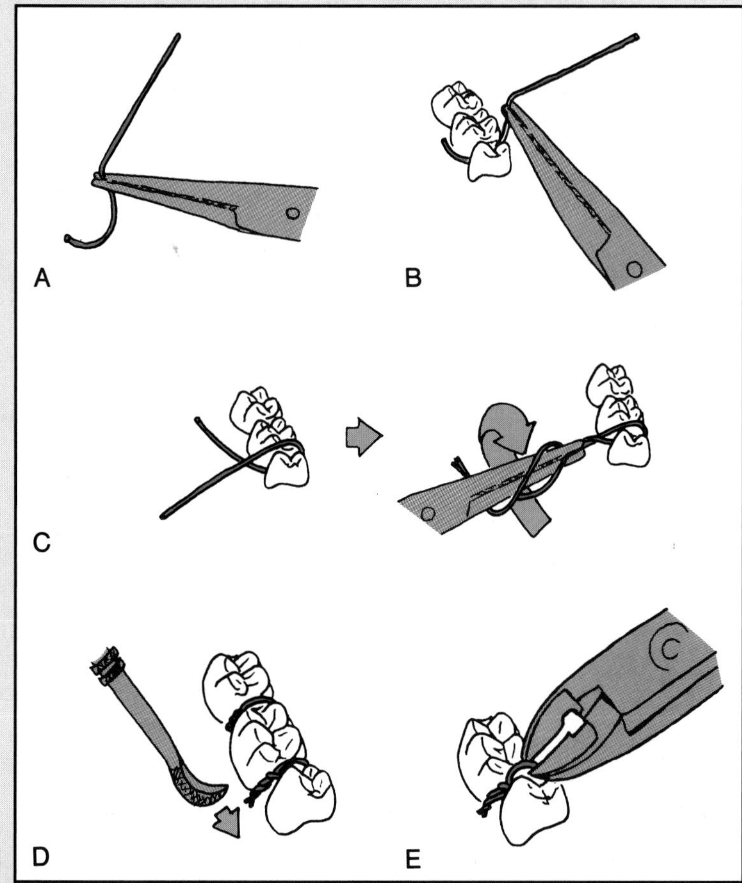

FIGURE 28–26

Placement and removal of a brass wire separator.

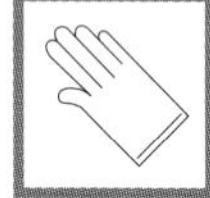
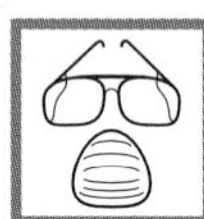
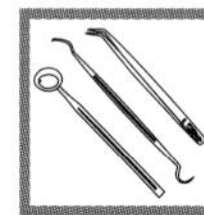
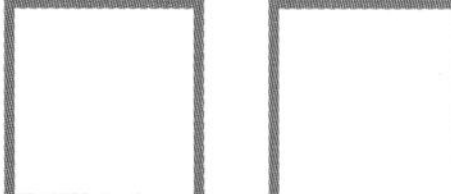

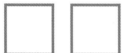

PROCEDURE: **Placing and Removing Steel Separating Springs**

Placement of Steel Separating Springs

1. Grasp the spring with a bird-beak plier at the base of its shorter leg (Fig. 28–27*A*).
2. Place the bent-over end of the longer leg in the lingual embrasure. Pull the spring open so the shorter leg can slip beneath the contact from lingual to facial.
3. Slip the spring into place with the helix to the facial side.
4. This type of separator is normally left in place 3 to 5 days.

Removal of Steel Separating Springs

1. During this procedure, keep the fingers of the other hand over the separator to prevent it from coming off the tooth unexpectedly (see Fig. 28–27*B*).
   □ *RATIONALE:* If it springs off the tooth, it may injure the operator or the patient.
2. Use an orthodontic scaler to engage the helix of the separator (see Fig. 28–27*C*). Lift upward until there is space between the upper arm and the occlusal aspect of the marginal ridge.
3. Support the separator on the helix with the index finger. Disengage the upper arm from the lingual embrasure and pull the separator toward the facial surface.

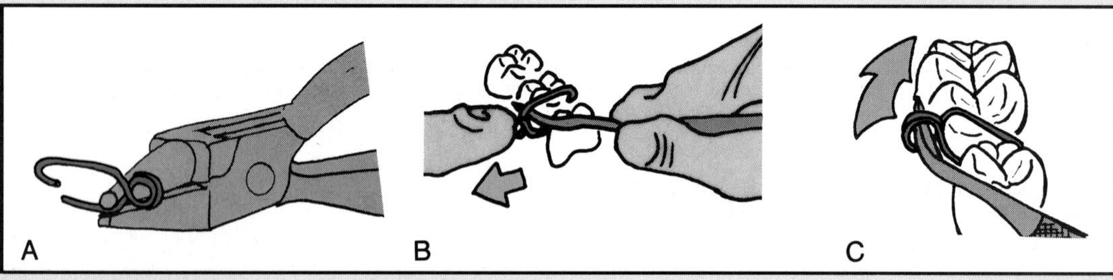

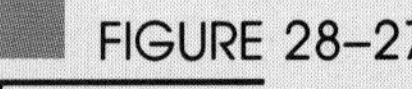

FIGURE 28–27

Placement and removal of a steel spring separator.

 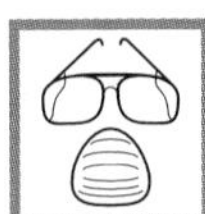 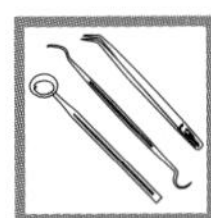 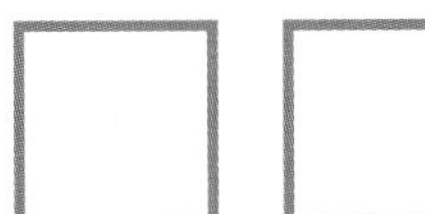

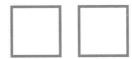

PROCEDURE: Placing and Removing Elastomeric Ring Separators

Placement of Elastomeric Ring Separators

1. Place the separator over the beaks of a separating plier.
2. Stretch the ring, then use a see-saw motion to gently force it through the contact (Fig. 28–28).
3. An alternative method is two loops of dental floss to stretch the ring and guide it into place.
4. This type of separator can be left in place for up to 2 weeks.

Removal of Elastomeric Ring Separators

1. Slide an orthodontic scaler into the doughnut-shaped separator.
2. Use slight pressure to remove the ring from under the contact.
   □ *CAUTION:* Be careful with the instrument so that it does not slip and injure the patient or operator.

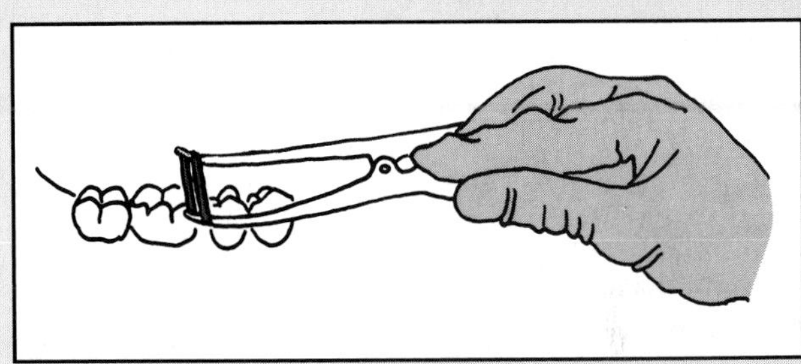

FIGURE 28–28

Placement of an elastic separator.

lower (mandibular) and, right and left to compensate for individual tooth differences. The occlusal edge of the band is slightly rolled or contoured, whereas the gingival edge is straight and smooth. Buttons, tubes, and cleats may also be attached for the arch wire and power products. (A **power product** is anything that is elastic and is used to create tooth movement.)

Tight interproximal contacts can make it impossible to properly seat a band; therefore, the teeth must be separated before fitting and placement of the bands. A separator is used for this purpose.

Although separators are available in many varieties, the principle is the same in each case: a device is placed to force or wedge the teeth apart long enough for initial tooth movement to occur, so the teeth are slightly separated before the appointment at which bands are to be fitted.

It is important to instruct the patient to call the office promptly if a separator comes out and to schedule an appointment to have it placed again.

The three main methods of separation used for posterior teeth are brass wire, steel separating springs, and elastomeric separators.

PLACEMENT OF ORTHODONTIC BANDS

Bands to be fitted are selected from the manufacturer's tray with sterile cotton pliers. At chairside, bands can be selected by visual inspection and estimating the size of the tooth and then fitted.

An alternative is to select, adapt, and fit the bands on the patient's diagnostic cast. This method eliminates the lengthy process at chairside, and minor alterations can be accomplished at chairside as necessary.

Preformed bands are designed to be fitted in a certain sequence, and it is important to follow the manufacturer's instructions.

Fitting Molar Bands

Initially, the **maxillary molar band** is forced over the tooth by finger pressure on the mesial and distal surfaces. This brings the band down close to the height of the marginal ridges. Then a **band pusher** is used on the mesiobuccal and distolingual edges to drive the band into place.

Mandibular molar bands are designed to be seated initially with finger pressure on the proximal surfaces.

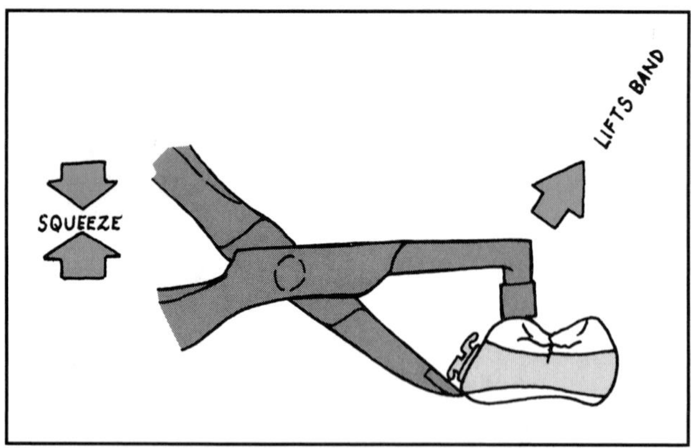

FIGURE 28–29

Removal of a fitted band.

Then a **band seater** is placed along the buccal margins, and the patient's heavy biting force is utilized to drive the band into place.

The Removal of Fitted Bands

Bands are removed with the **band-removing plier** (Fig. 28–29). The cushioned tip of the plier is placed on the distobuccal cusp of the occlusal surface. The blade edge of the plier is used against the buccogingival margin of the band, and the band is gently lifted upward.

If necessary, this process is repeated on the mesial and lingual aspects. Take care to avoid scratching the band or bending the gingival margins, which may require recontouring before cementation.

Cementation of Orthodontic Bands

Cementing orthodontic bands is similar to cementing cast restorations; the difference is that the cementation is exclusively to enamel.

A relatively acid cement such as zinc phosphate is needed for orthodontic purposes, so that an acid etch of the enamel surface is produced to aid in retention. In addition, orthodontic cement is mixed to be thicker than the cement for an inlay or a crown, because the escape of excess from the margins of a band is not the same problem as it is from beneath a cast restoration.

An alternative is the use of a glass ionomer cement. This tends to be chosen because the potential fluoride release over the months aids in preventing decay under the band.

The cement to be used is determined by the orthodontist. Whichever type is selected must be mixed in accordance with the manufacturer's directions. The

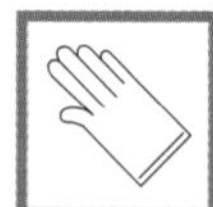 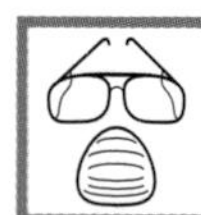 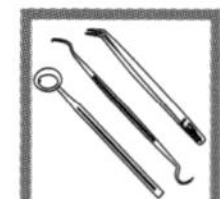  

PROCEDURE: Cementing Orthodontic Bands with Zinc Phosphate Cement

Instrumentation

Basic setup
Gloves
High-volume evacuator (HVE) tip
Orthodontic bands
Zinc phosphate cement (powder and liquid)
Chilled glass slab
Spatula, stainless steel
Gauze sponges
Band pusher
Band seater
Isopropyl alcohol
Masking tape (cut into small squares)
Lip balm

Advance Preparation

1. Place each preselected orthodontic band on a small square of masking tape with the occlusal surface on the tape and the gingival margin of the band upright.
   □ *RATIONALE:* This keeps the bands in order and prevents the cement from flowing out the other side.

2. Wipe any buccal tubes or attachments with lip balm.
   □ *RATIONALE:* This prevents cement from getting into or around those areas.
3. Chill the glass slab in a refrigerator or cool it under cold water.
   □ *RATIONALE:* A chilled slab retards the set and allows more mixing time for the cement.
4. Dry the slab before use.

Mixing the Cement

1. At a signal from the orthodontist, the assistant dispenses the cement according to the manufacturer's directions.
2. The assistant quickly spatulates the cement to obtain a homogeneous mix.
3. The assistant holds the orthodontic band by the margin of the masking tape. The gingival surface is upright, and the cement spatula is placed on the margin of the band.
4. The assistant wipes the spatula over the margin, and cement flows into the circumference of the band (Fig. 28–30).
5. The assistant passes the cement-filled band to the orthodontist, who inverts the band over the tooth.
6. The assistant transfers the band seater, and the orthodontist places it on the buccal margin of the band.
7. The patient is instructed to bite gently on the band. This action forces the band down onto approximately the middle third of the tooth crown.
8. Excess cement is forced out from under the gingival and occlusal margins of the bands and is allowed to harden.
9. This process is repeated until all of the bands have been seated.

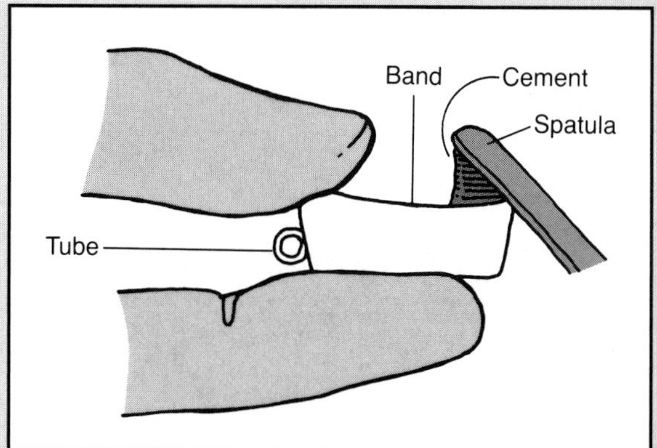

FIGURE 28–30

Placing cement in the orthodontic band.

Removing Excess Cement

1. After the cement has reached its final stage of setting, the assistant uses a scaler or explorer to remove the excess cement on the enamel surfaces.
   □ *CAUTION:* Proper fulcrums must be used to avoid injury to the gingiva.
2. The patient's mouth is rinsed, flossed, and checked to determine that all of the excess cement has been removed.

procedure described here utilizes zinc phosphate cement.

BONDED BRACKETS

The most commonly used type of attachment is the bonded edgewise bracket (Fig. 28–31). This bracket is attached to a stainless steel backing pad that is bonded to the enamel of the tooth.

The bonded bracket is designed with four tie wings so the arch wire is placed horizontally in the bracket and ligated (attached) to it.

This initiates tooth movement by transmitting forces from the arch wire to the tooth. This technique allows more control of each individual tooth in relationship to the complete treatment.

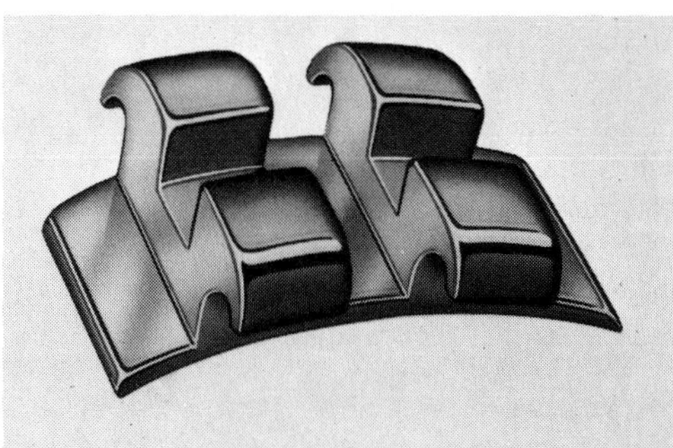

FIGURE 28–31

Edgewise bracket. The arch wire is placed in the central groove and is held in place with a ligature secured around the four tie wings. (Courtesy of Unitek Corp, Monrovia, CA.)

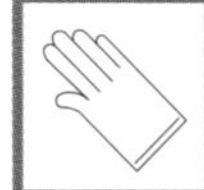
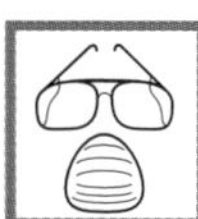
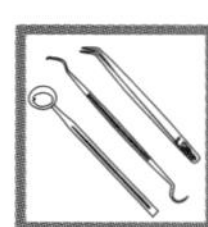

PROCEDURE: **Performing Direct Bonding of Orthodontic Brackets**

Instrumentation

Brackets (type specified by the orthodontist)
Coronal polishing setup
HVE tip
Bonding setup
Cotton rolls or retractors
Bracket placement tweezers
Orthodontic scales

Preparing the Teeth

1. If stain or plaque is present, the tooth surface is cleaned with a rubber cup and pumice slurry.
2. The teeth are isolated by using either cotton rolls or retractors.
3. Acid etchant gel is placed only on the area to be bonded (Fig. 28–32). This is left in place for the time specified in the manufacturer's instructions.
4. The etching material is rinsed away, and the tooth surface is dried.
5. After proper etching, the enamel surface should appear dull and chalky or frosted.

Bonding the Brackets

1. The orthodontist applies a liquid sealant, usually the monomer of the bonding agent, to the prepared tooth surface.
2. The assistant mixes a small quantity of bonding material so that it will set in 30 to 60 seconds.
   □ *RATIONALE:* To avoid premature setting, a separate mix of bonding material is used for each tooth.
3. The assistant places bonding material on the back of the bracket (Fig. 28–33). Bracket placement tweezers are used to transfer the bracket to the orthodontist.
4. The assistant prepares to transfer an orthodontic scaler. The orthodontist places the bracket and moves it into final position with a scaler.
5. The orthodontist presses the bracket to place against the enamel surface. This causes excess bonding material to extrude around the edges.
6. A scaler is used to immediately remove the excess bonding material before it sets (Fig. 28–34).

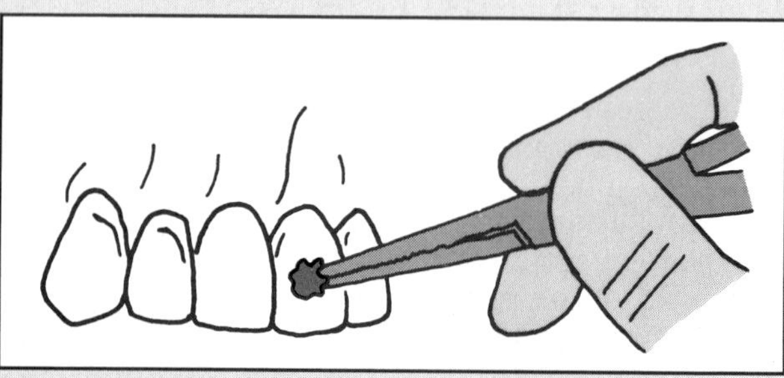

FIGURE 28–32

Applying etchant to the surface of the tooth.

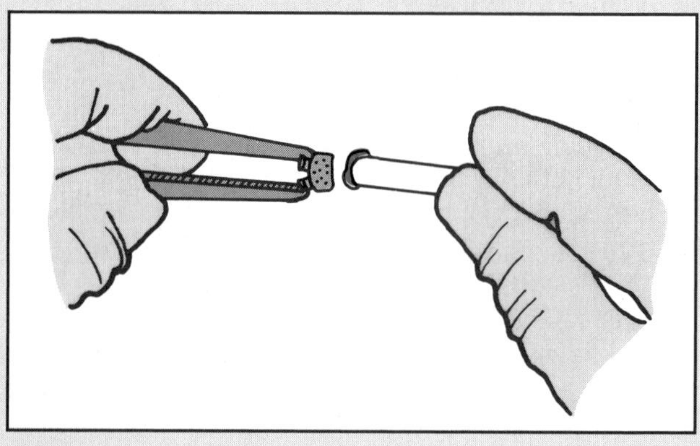

FIGURE 28–33

Applying bonding material to the back of the bracket.

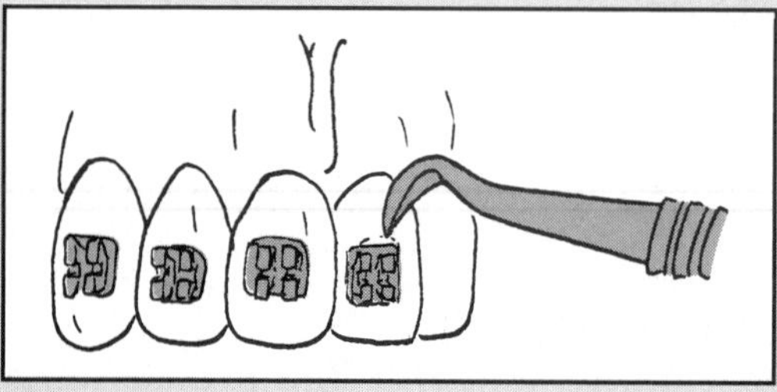

FIGURE 28–34

Excess cement is removed immediately with a scaler.

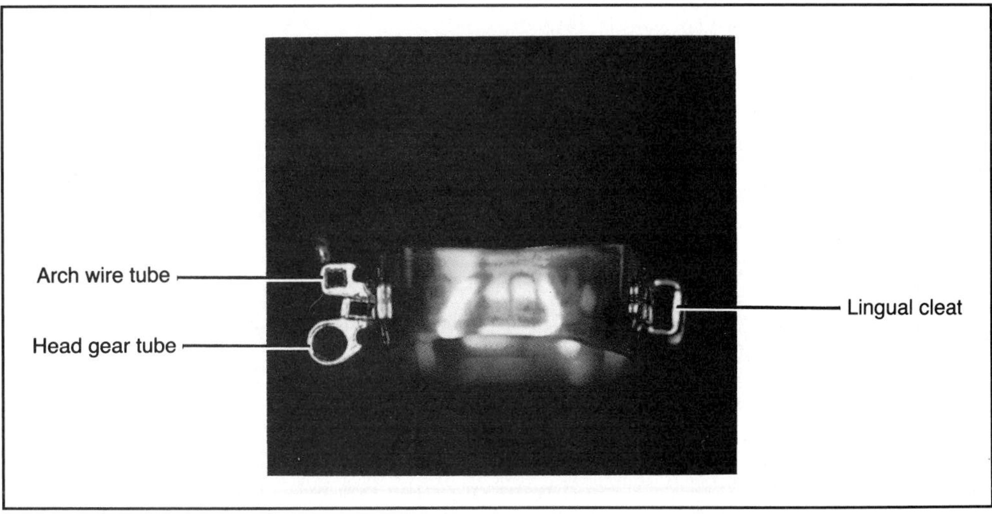

FIGURE 28–35

Soldered attachments on a maxillary molar band. (From Viazis, A.D.: Atlas of Orthodontics: Principles and Applications. Philadelphia, W.B. Saunders Co., 1993.

AUXILIARY ATTACHMENTS

Auxiliary attachments are an integral part of the contemporary edgewise appliance. They can be attached to the molar bands or to single brackets (Fig. 28–35).

Headgear tubes are round tubes placed routinely on maxillary first molar bands. They are used for the insertion of the inner bow of a facebow appliance.

Edgewise tubes are rectangular tubes placed gingivally to the plane of the main arch wire. These tubes should be present on the facial surfaces of the upper and lower first molars to receive the arch wire.

Labial hooks are hooks located on the facial surfaces of the first and second molar bands for both arches. These hooks hold the interarch elastics.

Lingual arch attachments are a sheath or bracket located on the lingual portion of the bands for stabilization of the arch, to reinforce anchorage and tooth movement.

THE ARCH WIRE

The preformed arch wire, which is shaped like a horseshoe, is a very important part of orthodontic treatment. When the arch wire is tied into the brackets, it provides enough force to mold in the arch form. It also serves as a guide to slide the teeth along.

There are several types of arch wire used in treating a case. Each type has properties that are unique to a particular application (Fig. 28–36).

Nickel titanium is utilized during the initial stages of tooth movement for very crooked and/or crowded teeth. This type of wire is flexible and resists permanent deformation.

Round wires are normally used in the initial and intermediate stages of treatment. Their main function is to correct crowded and crooked teeth and to level the arch. They can also be used in opening a bite and sliding teeth along to close spaces.

Square or rectangular wires are used during the final stages of treatment to position the crown and root in the correct maxillary and mandibular relationship. These wires also give the tooth more stability and apply more force. These wires are sometimes referred to as *edgewise wires,* because they fill the dimensions of an edgewise bracket.

Stainless steel wire, which is stiffer and stronger than the other wires, is used to apply more force and give better stability to control the teeth. It can withstand greater forces and is called the **working arch wire**.

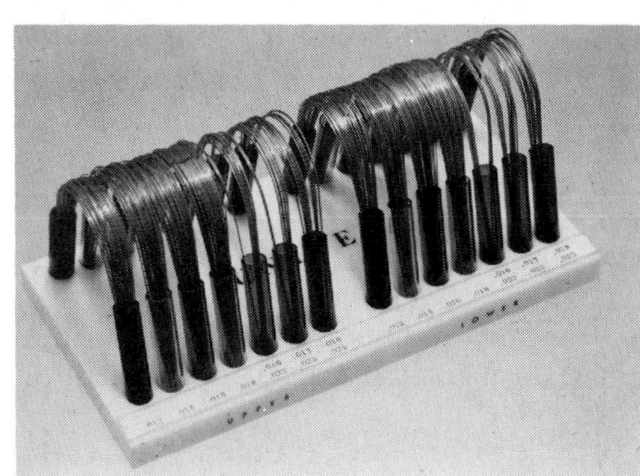

FIGURE 28–36

Assorted arch wires in a dispenser-holder. (Courtesy of Unitek Corp., Monrovia, CA.)

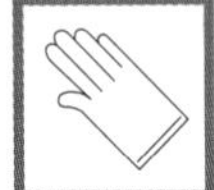
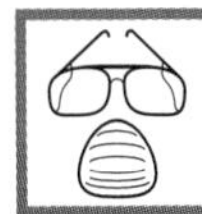
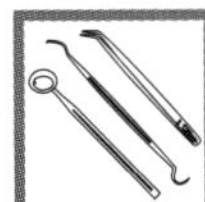

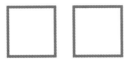

PROCEDURE: **Placing Arch Wires**

Instrumentation

Preformed arch wire
Patient's diagnostic casts (or previously used arch wire)
Weingart plier
Bird-beak plier
Torquing plier (edgewise)
Distal end cutter

Measuring the Arch Wire

1. Preformed wires are measured before they are placed in the mouth. The wire should be long enough to extend past the end of the buccal tube on the molar band, but not so long that it injures the patient's tissue.
2. Measure the wire by trying it on the patient's diagnostic cast.
3. *Alternative:* If available, it can be measured against the arch wire that was just removed from the patient's mouth.
4. If the orthodontist will place bends in the wire, additional length must be allowed for the length and number of the bends.
   □ *RATIONALE:* These bends in the wire are important in guiding the teeth into exactly the correct position.

Positioning the Arch Wire

1. Locate the mark at the center of the arch wire.
   □ *RATIONALE:* This is placed on most preformed arch wires to indicate midline or center of the arch form.
2. Position the wire in the mouth with the mark between the central incisors.
3. Place the arch wire in the main arch wire slot of the buccal tube.
4. Use a Weingart plier to slide the wire in on either side of the arch and to position the wire in the bracket slots.
5. Check the distal ends to determine that they are securely positioned and are neither too long or too short.

Once the arch wire has been positioned, it must be ligated (tied) to be held in place. The four types of ligatures used are wires, elastomeric ties, elastic chain, and continuous wire ties.

- **Wire ligatures** are thin wires that are twisted around the bracket to hold the arch wire in place
- **Elastomeric ties** are made of a plastic or rubber-like material and are available in many colors
- **Elastic chain ties** are continuous "O's" that form a chain. They are used to close space between teeth or to correct rotated teeth
- **Continuous wire ties** are used primarily to close spaces and where two or more teeth are ligated together

In some states, placing ligatures is the responsibility of the chairside assistant. When doing this, it is important to establish a routine to ensure that all steps are completed. One effective method is working left to right in both arches.

Kobyashi Hooks

Kobyashi hooks are ligature ties that have been spot welded at the tip to form a hook for the attachment of elastics. These hooks are ligated on a bracket as necessary to attach elastics.

ELASTICS

Elastics, commonly referred to as *rubber bands*, are placed between the maxillary and mandibular arches to bring about tooth movement. On the basis of the movement required, the orthodontist determines where and when the elastics are to be placed.

Patients are instructed in how to place and remove these elastics and are encouraged to wear them regularly as directed.

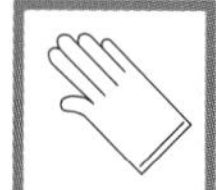 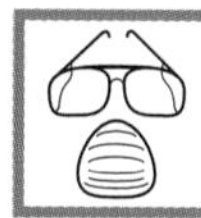 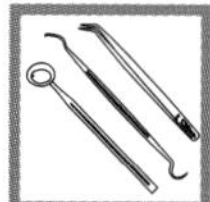 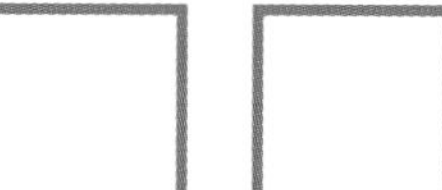

PROCEDURE: **Placing and Removing Wire Ligatures**

Placement (Fig. 28–37)

1. Hold the ligature between the thumb and index finger, and slide the wire between these fingers so that only the section that wraps around the bracket is exposed. Push this up at a slight angle.
2. Slide the ligature around the bracket, and use the ligature director to push the wire against the tie wing (see Fig. 28–37*A*).
3. Twist the ends of the ligature together. Always place the ligature so that it is twisted on the side farthest from the arch wire (see Fig. 28–37*B*).
4. Place the hemostat about 3 to 5 mm. from the bracket, and twist the wire snugly against the bracket (see Fig. 28–37*C*).
5. Repeat the procedure until all brackets are ligated.
6. After all teeth have been ligated, use a **ligature cutter** to cut the excess wire, leaving a 4- to 5-mm. pigtail.
7. Use the **ligature wire pusher** to tuck the pigtails under the arch wire toward the gingiva at the interproximal space.
8. Repeat this procedure until all ligatures have been cut and tucked away.
9. Run a finger along the wires to determine that none are protruding and might injure the patient.
10. Check the distal end of the arch wire, to make sure of its length.
    □ *RATIONALE:* It must be positioned properly, yet not injuring the patient's tissues.

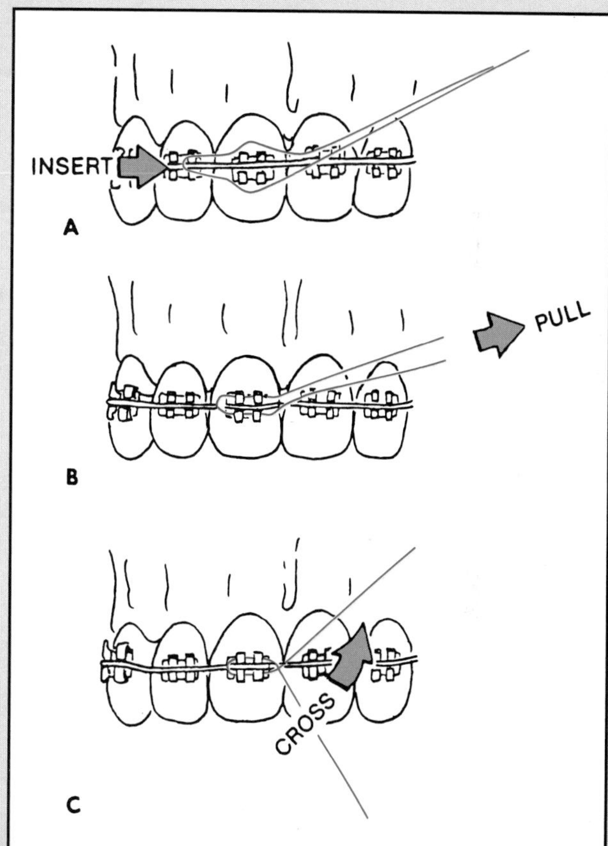

FIGURE 28–37

Placement of ligature wires. *A*, The wire is slipped under the edges of the tie wings. *B*, The wire is pulled tight around the bracket. *C*, The wire is crossed, pulled tight, and then twisted.

Removal

1. Hold the **ligature cutter** in your palm, with the thumb and index finger on the handle and the middle finger between the handles.
2. Use the beaks of the plier to cut the wire at easiest access. Then carefully unwrap the ligature and remove it.
3. Do not twist or pull as you cut and remove the ligatures.
4. Continue cutting and removing until all brackets have been untied.

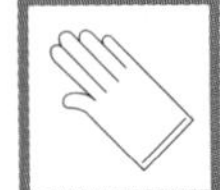
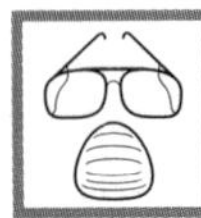
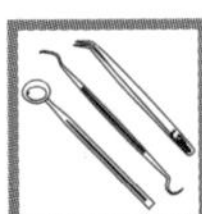

PROCEDURE: **Placing and Removing Elastomeric Ties**

Placement

1. Use a hemostat to place the plier beak on a tie, and close the plier.
2. Do not place the beaks too closely to the center of the "O" or you will not be able to stretch the tie around the bracket.
3. Place the tie on the occlusal portion or one tie wing, and slide the tie under the edge of the bracket.
4. To get the tie started, support it with your finger.
5. Pull the tie up and over the tie wing and then over and down the other tie wing.
6. Release the plier.

Removal

1. Use an orthodontic scaler held in a pen grasp.
2. Support the teeth and tissue with your other hand.
3. Place the scaler tip in between the bracket tie wings, and pull the tie at the occlusal position with a rolling motion.
4. Remove the tie in a gingival direction.

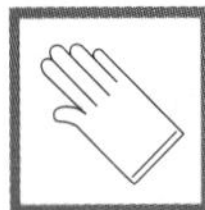
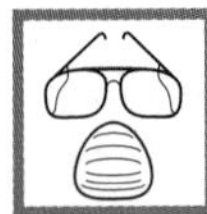
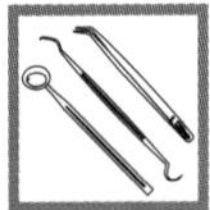

PROCEDURE: **Placing and Removing Elastic Chains**

Placement

1. Count the number of teeth to be ligated, and cut the appropriate number of links from the spool.
2. Place the same way you would place the elastomeric ties.

Removal

1. Place the scaler between the bracket tie wings, pull off at the occlusal end, and roll the elastic toward the gingiva.
2. Remove each link until the whole chain has been removed.

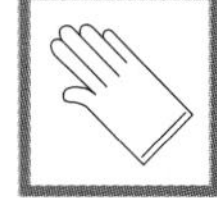 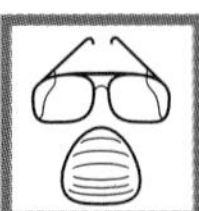 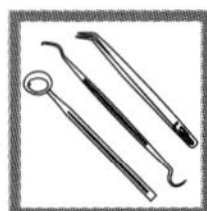 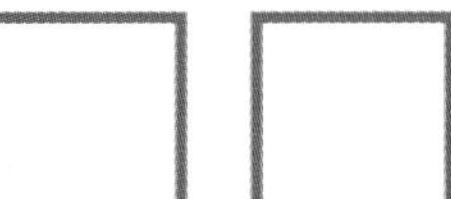

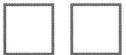

PROCEDURE: **Placing and Removing Continuous Wire Ties**

Placement

1. Begin as you would with a wire ligature tie.
2. Push the wire against the tie wing with the ligature director.
3. Wrap the wire around the bracket and twist.
4. Use the hemostat to twist the wire to fill the space between each bracket.
5. With firm pressure, wrap the entire wire around the next bracket.
6. Repeat until all teeth are tied together.
7. Place the hemostat on the last tie and twist.
8. Use the ligature cutter to cut the excess, and then tuck the "pigtail" under the arch wire.

Removal

1. Cut continuous ties in the same manner as ligature ties.
2. Cut each tie individually and remove them one at a time, or cut each tie at the occlusal surface and carefully unwrap the entire tie at one time.
3. Be careful not to injure the soft tissues when removing the ligature.

ADJUSTMENT VISITS

Throughout active orthodontic treatment, the patient must return regularly for adjustments. At these appointments, the orthodontist reviews the patient's progress and makes adjustments as necessary.

Although these visits are brief, each is extremely important, and the necessity of keeping each appointment should be stressed to the patient.

Checking the Appliance

At each adjustment appointment, it is the responsibility of the chairside assistant to check the patient's appliance to determine that there is nothing bent, broken, loose, or missing. Things to look for include

- Broken or missing arch wires
- Loose brackets and bands
- Loose, broken, or missing ligature
- Loose, broken, or missing rubber bands

Bands. Loose bands can result from a break in the cement seal or from poor eating habits, or they could involve the use of elastics, headgear or other types of power products.

A loose band can be spotted by its appearance. Bands are checked with either an explorer or scaler, and a loose band slides up and down on the tooth. Unless the band has been distorted, it can be cleaned and recemented.

Bonded Brackets. There are two main problems with bonded attachments: (1) they can be loose and off the surface of the tooth, or (2) on rare occasions, the bracket may break loose from the pad of the bond.

Most bonds are replaced, unless the orthodontist elects to leave the attachment off because it is not necessary for the current phase of treatment.

Arch Wires. Poor eating habits and the patient's picking or playing with the appliance can bend the arch wire. Bent or broken wires must be reshaped or replaced.

The patient should be advised to call the office if a problem develops between appointment times. The orthodontist should make repairs promptly without waiting for the regular adjustment appointment.

When checking for bends in the arch wire, also look for broken wires. Some breaks are hard to see. A tooth that moves out of alignment or a complaint of a sore tooth is an indication of a problem and must be investigated.

HEADGEAR

Another aspect of the treatment phase in fixed appliances is the headgear. The headgear is an orthopedic device used to control growth and tooth movement. It is made up of two parts: the facebow and the traction device.

Facebow

The facebow is used to stabilize or move the maxillary first molar distally and create more room in the arch (Fig. 28–38).

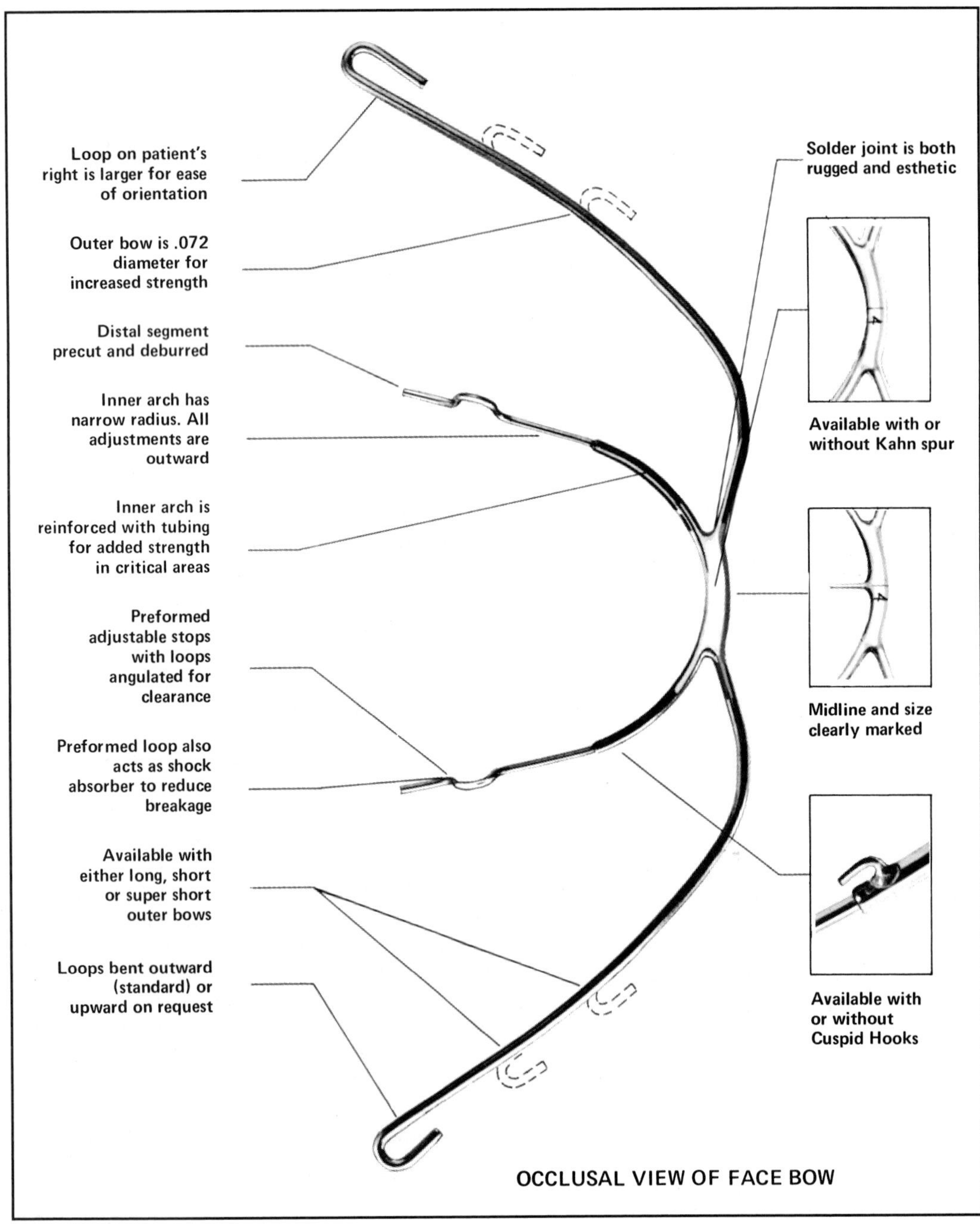
Loop on patient's right is larger for ease of orientation
Outer bow is .072 diameter for increased strength
Distal segment precut and deburred
Inner arch has narrow radius. All adjustments are outward
Inner arch is reinforced with tubing for added strength in critical areas
Preformed adjustable stops with loops angulated for clearance
Preformed loop also acts as shock absorber to reduce breakage
Available with either long, short or super short outer bows
Loops bent outward (standard) or upward on request
Solder joint is both rugged and esthetic
Available with or without Kahn spur
Midline and size clearly marked
Available with or without Cuspid Hooks
OCCLUSAL VIEW OF FACE BOW

FIGURE 28–38

Orthodontic facebow for use with extraoral traction devices. (Courtesy of Unitek Corp., Monrovia, CA.)

The intraoral part of the facebow that fits into the buccal tubes of the maxillary first molars. The outer part of the bow attaches to the traction device.

Traction Devices

The traction device applies the extraoral force used to achieve the desired treatment results. There are four types: high-pull, cervical, combination, and chip cap.

High-Pull Traction. This is a caplike device that fits around the top of the patient's head and hooks perpendicular to the occlusal plane (Fig. 28–39*A*). It can be used in controlling the growth of the maxilla or retraction of anterior teeth.

Cervical Traction. Cervical traction fits around the patient's neck (see Fig. 28–39*B*). (**Cervical** means neck.) The exerted force is parallel to the occlusal plane of the patient's teeth. This type of traction is used when the maxillary first molars are stabilized or moved distally.

Combination. This device is a combination of the

high-pull and the cervical traction devices. It exerts a force along the occlusal plane and upward (see Fig. 28–39*C*).

Chin Cap. This type of device is a combination of a high-pull strap and a chin cup that fits on the mandible. This helps control the growth of the mandible in patients with Class III malocclusions.

Oral Hygiene and Dietary Instructions

Oral Hygiene

Orthodontic appliances offer areas for food and plaque to be trapped and hidden, and they make brushing more difficult.

Good oral hygiene during orthodontic treatment is imperative! If the patient does not take care of his mouth properly, the results can be disastrous, including rampant caries and periodontal disease.

- The procedure of tooth brushing, flossing, using an interproximal brush, and a fluoride mouth rinse *must* be completed daily.
- Many patients find that they have more time available at bedtime to perform this entire oral care routine.
- Flossing with braces is not easy, but it can be accomplished by using bridge threaders, short pieces of dental floss, and a well-lighted area with a mirror.
- The toothbrush should be held at an angle to avoid stabbing the bristles into the tissue, thereby causing irritation.
- An interproximal brush is used for cleaning under the arch wire but does not take the place of flossing.
- Rinse thoroughly to remove any remaining food particles.

Dietary Instructions

Another concern with patients in orthodontic treatment is poor eating habits. The patient should be urged to use good sense in selecting foods and to avoid those that can break bands and bonds or bend arch wires.

Examples of foods to be avoided are ice, hard foods (such as popcorn and nuts), and sticky foods (such as caramel candy and chewing gum).

Completed Treatment

Once the patient has completed the treatment phase of orthodontics, the bands and bonded attachments are removed.

- Band removal is accomplished by simply breaking the cement attachment and then lifting the band off the tooth.
- Bonded brackets must be removed *without* damaging the enamel surface. This can be done by creating a fracture within the resin bonding material or between the bracket and the resin, and then removing the residual resin from the enamel surface.
- Any cement left on the teeth after debanding can be removed easily by scaling with a hand instrument or with an ultrasonic scaler.

The Removal of Cement

Some states permit the trained extended-functions dental assistant (EFDA) to remove excess cement *only* from the crown of the tooth, using a hand instrument. This is strictly limited to the supragingival surfaces of the dentition.

In some states, an EFDA who is trained in the operation of the ultrasonic unit is permitted to use the ultrasonic scaler to remove excess cement *only* from the crown of the tooth. This too is strictly limited to the supragingival surfaces of the dentition.

Before performing either of these procedures, the EFDA must check with the Board of Dental Examiners to determine whether this is legal in the state in which he or she is employed.

THE ULTRASONIC SCALER

An ultrasonic scaler converts very high-frequency sound waves into mechanical energy in the form of rapid vibrations at the tip of the instrument. These vibrations are able to fracture and remove hardened

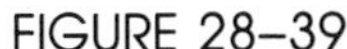

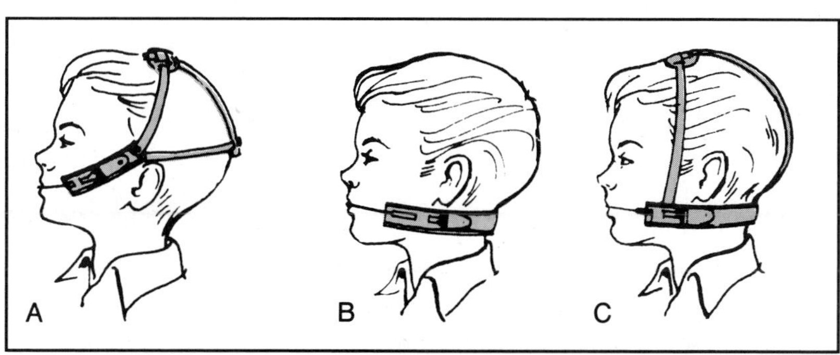

FIGURE 28–39

Extraoral orthodontic appliances. *A*, High-pull headgear. *B*, Cervical band. *C*, Combination headgear and cervical band. (Courtesy of Unitek Corp., Monrovia, CA.)

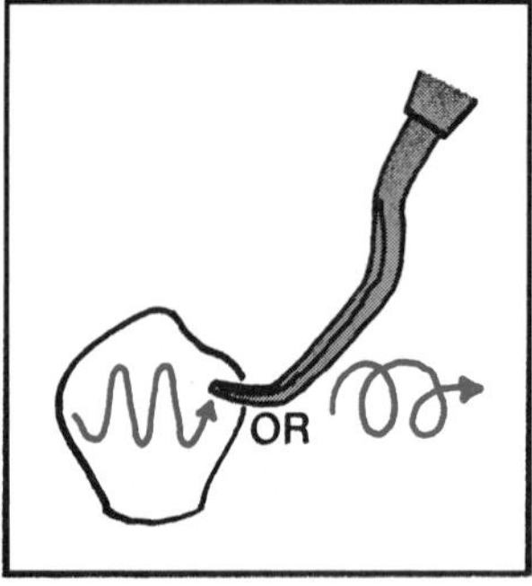

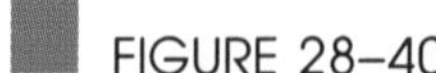

FIGURE 28–40

Position and motion of the ultrasonic scaler. The tip is held parallel to the long axis of the tooth and is brushed lightly over the cement to be removed.

cement without injuring the teeth or surrounding tissues. The ultrasonic scaler is discussed further in Chapter 15.

Parts of the Ultrasonic Unit

The ultrasonic scaler must always be assembled, adjusted, and used in accordance with the manufacturer's directions. The parts of the ultrasonic unit include

- Handpiece (to hold tip)
- Scaler tip (blunted)
- Water nozzle
- Tip guard (some manufacturers)
- Knob to lock tip into handpiece
- Retainer knob
- Connected body (connects handpiece to electric and water supply)
- Rheostat (foot control for water and compressed air)

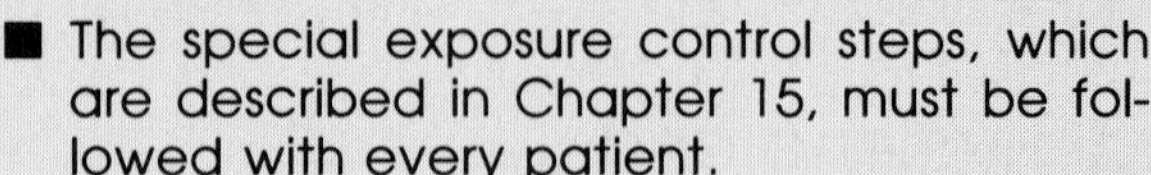

Guidelines for Use of the Ultrasonic Scaler

- The special exposure control steps, which are described in Chapter 15, must be followed with every patient.
- To avoid removing small amounts of enamel, the tooth is *never* touched with the ultrasonic scaler tip.
- The operator holds the tip parallel to the long axis of the tooth and brushes it lightly over the cement to be removed (Fig. 28–40).
- A generous flow of water is directed from the handpiece to rinse and cool the tooth surface.
- If a chairside assistant is available, water and debris are removed with the HVE tip.
- If an assistant is not available, a saliva ejector is placed and the HVE tip is applied intermittently by the operator.

CARE OF THE ULTRASONIC UNIT

Exposure Control. The scaler tip is removed and taken to the sterilization center to be cleaned, wrapped, and sterilized in preparation for reuse.

 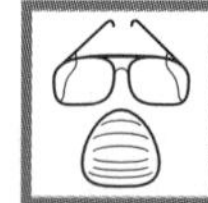 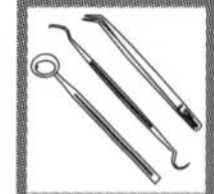  

PROCEDURE: **Removing Excess Cement with an Ultrasonic Scaler**

Instrumentation

Ultrasonic unit (with pressure gauge)
Handpiece (with unit)
Scaling tips (blunted)
HVE tip
Saliva ejector

Preparation

1. The patient is seated, covered with a plastic drape and patient towel, and given protective eyewear to put on. The back of the dental chair is reclined at a 45-degree angle.

2. The operator and assistant wear plastic face shields in addition to their other personal protective equipment.
3. The operator is seated at the 9 o'clock position.
4. If an assistant is present, he or she is seated at the 3 o'clock position.

Adjustment of the Ultrasonic Unit

1. The water pressure is adjusted to approximately 15 pounds per square inch (psi) with water flow of approximately 25 ml. per minute.
   □ *NOTE:* In most ultrasonic handpieces, the water flow is adequate if the water fills the receptacle of the handpiece to the brim *before* the blunted scaling tip is inserted.
2. The blunted scaling tip is placed into the handpiece and the water adjustment is checked again (Fig. 28–41).
   □ *NOTE:* In most ultrasonic handpieces, the water adjustment is correct when a slight halo of water mist shows around the scaler tip.
3. If the air pressure is measured with a simulator gauge, it is adjusted to approximately 40 psi at the scaler tip.

Application of the Scaler Tip

1. As necessary, ask the patient to turn his head slightly from right to left.
   □ *RATIONALE:* This provides visible access to areas of the lingual and facial surfaces of the teeth.
2. Retract the patient's tongue, cheeks, or lips with the mouth mirror or the fingers of one hand.
3. Obtain a fulcrum near the teeth to be cleaned of cement, using the fourth or ring finger of the other hand placed on the occlusal or incisal tooth surfaces within the quadrant.
4. Hold the ultrasonic handpiece firmly in a pen grasp, using the index finger, third finger, and thumb.
5. Place the tip at a 15-degree angle with the surface of the tooth under treatment. Turn the end of the tip slightly on its side, using only ⅛ inch of the tip (Fig. 28–42).
6. Direct the tip toward the occlusal or incisal surface. Place the tip angle lightly against the surface of the excess cement, not directly on the the surface of the enamel.
   □ *CAUTION:* Avoid touching the cement near the band, as the vibrations could loosen the cement *under* the band.

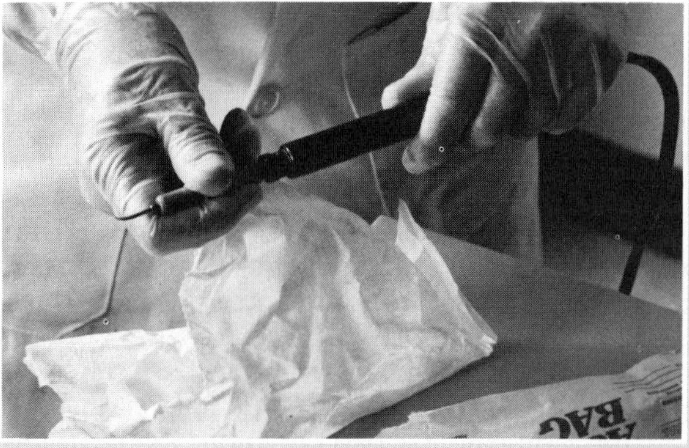

FIGURE 28–41

The scaling tip is inserted into the ultrasonic handpiece.

7. Move the tip constantly by applying short and rapid vertical strokes to the cement on the tooth surface.
   □ *RATIONALE:* The ultrasonic vibrations (pulsations) of the tip will fracture the mass of the cement.
8. As needed, use the HVE tip to remove the debris and water.
9. When finished with the scaler, turn off the compressed air-water supply to the handpiece and lay the scaler aside.
10. Carefully pass dental floss through the contact areas to remove any remaining cement.
11. Rinse the patient's mouth and examine it for remaining cement. If no further treatment is indicated, dismiss the patient.

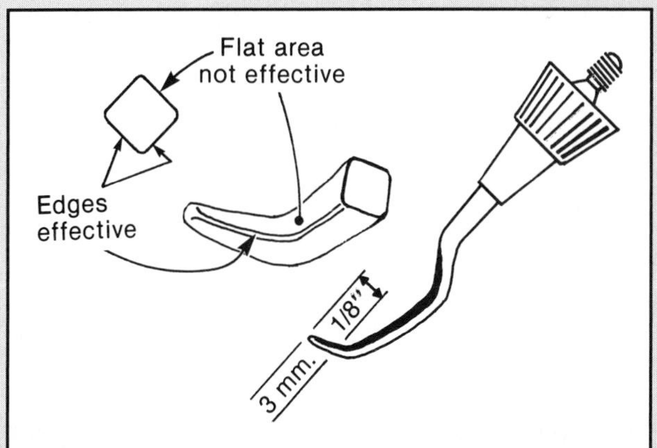

FIGURE 28–42

The effective area of the tip of the ultrasonic scaler.

The water tube of the unit is cleared after each use by blowing air from the air-water syringe through the line.

The surfaces of the ultrasonic scaler unit are covered with protective barriers during use. Any surface that was potentially contaminated during use must be cleaned and disinfected with a high-level EPA-registered disinfectant.

Lubrication and Maintenance. The unit is cared for in accordance with the manufacturer's instructions. If the unit is to be lubricated, this function is performed daily.

Also, the seals and gaskets are checked and replaced as needed. The suspension rings and muffler may be replaced on a semiannual basis or more frequently as needed.

Retention

A patient may feel that treatment is complete when the fixed appliances are removed, but an important stage in orthodontic treatment lies ahead. Orthodontic control of tooth position and occlusal relationships must be withdrawn gradually, not abruptly, if excellent long-term results are to be achieved.

Retention is necessary to

- Allow gingival and periodontal tissues the required time for reorganization
- Support the teeth that are in an unstable position, so that the pressure of the cheeks and tongue do not cause a relapse
- Control changes caused by growth

Orthodontic Positioner

The positioner is a custom appliance made of rubber or pliable acrylic that fits over the patient's maxillary dentition after orthodontic treatment (Fig. 28–43). The positioner is designed to

- Retain the teeth in their desired position
- Permit the alveolus to rebuild support around the teeth before the patient wears a retainer
- Massage the gingiva

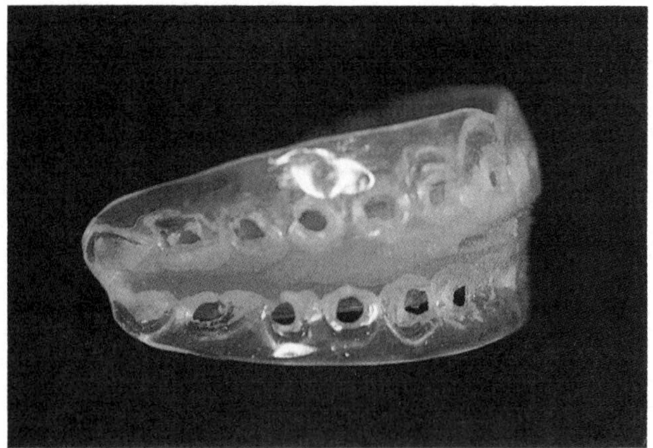

FIGURE 28–43

Orthodontic positioner. (From Viazis, A.D.: Atlas of Orthodontics: Principles and Applications. Philadelphia, W.B. Saunders Co., 1993, p 335.)

The patient is directed to bite into the positioner with the lower teeth, chewing it into place. This should be worn at least 12 hours per day, usually at night, thus permitting the patient to speak and to perform other daily activities.

The patient is usually advised to exercise his jaws with the positioner in place, chewing up and down, thus stimulating the teeth and the alveolar bone.

Hawley Retainers

The Hawley retainer, which is the most commonly used removable retainer, is worn to passively retain the teeth in their new position after the removal of the orthodontic bands. The retainer also encourages some tooth movement to close band spaces and provides control of the incisors (Fig. 28–44).

A Hawley retainer is constructed of clear, self-polymerizing acrylic that is designed to hold wire clasps on molar teeth. On a maxillary retainer, the plastic portion is placed over the palate. On a mandibular retainer, the plastic portion is placed on the anterior floor of the mouth.

The anterior facial wire of the retainer should rest lightly on the facial surfaces at the midline of the anterior maxillary teeth and the lingual surface of the anterior mandibular teeth. The wire should fit lightly between the contact areas of the cuspids and first premolars.

PLACEMENT AND CARE OF THE RETAINER

The patient removes the retainer by placing the thumbnails under each side of the arch wire simultaneously, near the cuspids, and lifting up slightly.

The patient may remove the retainer while brushing his teeth. Using soap and cool water, he may scrub the appliance with a denture brush. After rinsing it thoroughly, the patient reinserts the retainer into his mouth.

Care should be taken to avoid changing the contour of the appliance during removal and insertion, thus altering the fit of the appliance and eventually the alignment of the teeth. If the retainer is left out of the mouth for a period of time, it should be placed in a moist sealed container to prevent warpage of the acrylic.

The Hawley retainer should be worn for approximately 6 to 12 months according to the patient's need. The patient should maintain a record of the time the removable retainer is worn and should report back to

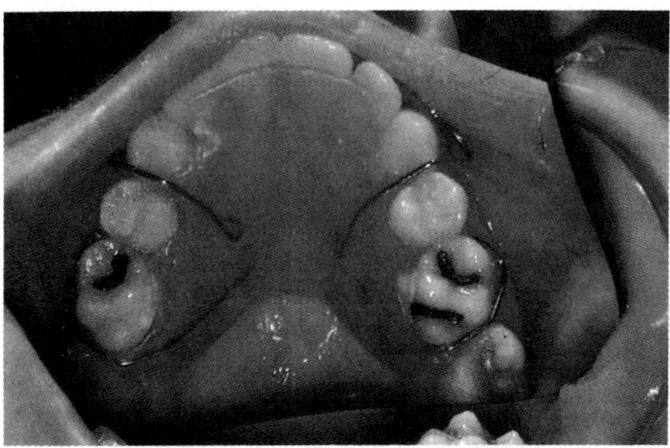
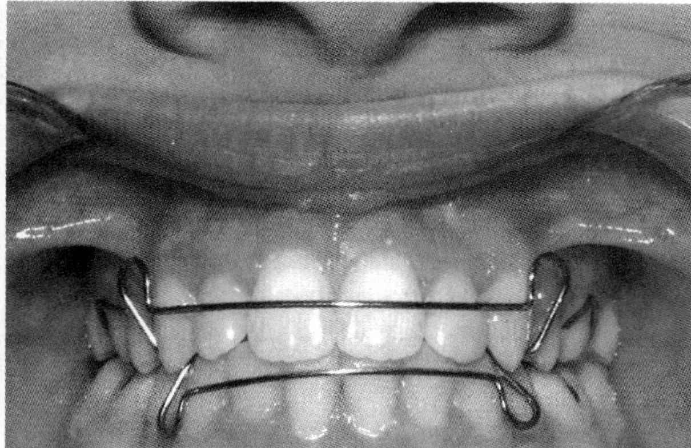

FIGURE 28–44

Hawley appliance. (From Morris, A.L., et al: The Dental Specialties in General Practice. Philadelphia, W.B. Saunders Co., 1983, p 283.)

the orthodontist at prescribed intervals to monitor progress.

Lingual Retainers

A fixed lingual cuspid-to-cuspid retainer can be designed to be banded from cuspid-to-cuspid or most commonly to be bonded to the lingual surfaces of the cuspids. This will provide lower incisor position during late growth.

The fabrication is of a light steel wire bent so that it rests against the flat part of the lingual surface of the incisors with a long loop over the cingulum of the cuspids.

Active Retainer

This type of retainer is unique because it can actively move teeth as well as serve as a retainer at the same time (Fig. 28–45). A relapse or growth change after orthodontic treatment can lead to a need for minor tooth movement during retention. This is usually accomplished with a removable appliance that continues as a retainer after it has repositioned the teeth.

Specialized Types of Fixed Appliances

Lingual Arch

A lingual arch is a fixed appliance that is used to hold existing teeth in their place while the patient waits for the permanent teeth to erupt (Fig. 28–46). The appliance is attached by cementing bands on the mandibular first molars with the lingual arch wire extending from molar to molar, keeping the teeth in place.

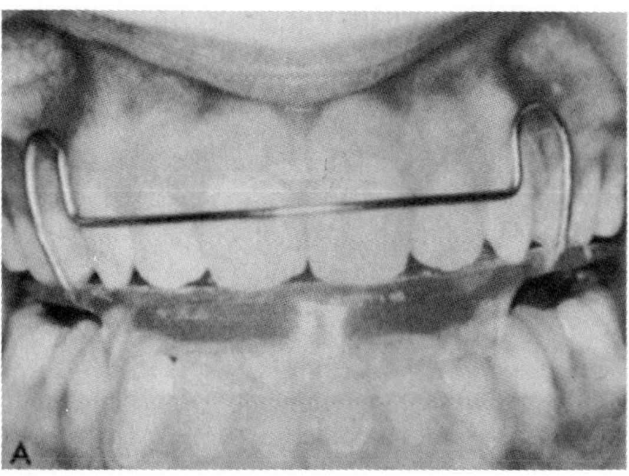

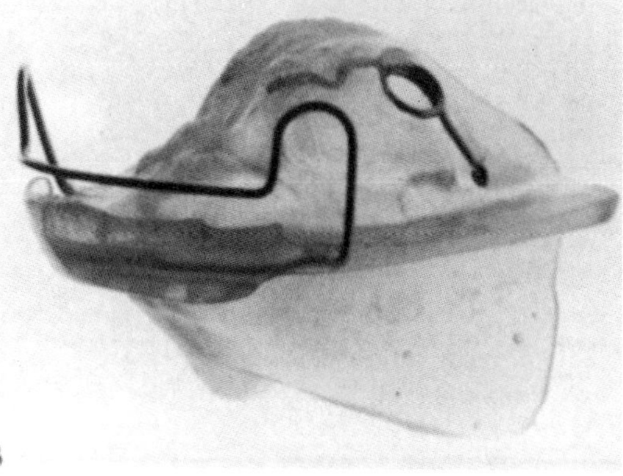

FIGURE 28–45

Active retainer. (From Morris, A.L., et al.: The Dental Specialties in General Practice. Philadelphia, W.B. Saunders Co., 1983.)

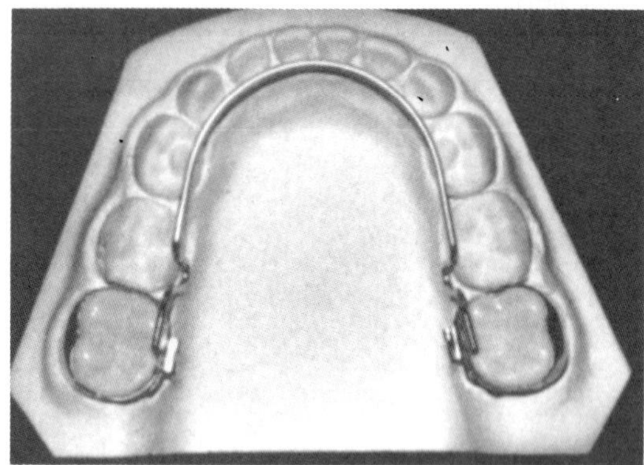

FIGURE 28–46

Lingual arch fixed retainer. (From Morris, A.L., et al.: The Dental Specialties in General Practice. Philadelphia, W.B. Saunders Co., 1983.)

Nance Appliance

A Nance appliance is cemented to the maxillary first molars. This is most commonly used during the mixed dentition stage to keep the molars from moving forward or tilting mesially. This allows the permanent teeth room for eruption.

Palatal Expansion

A palatal expansion appliance is used to correct crossbites and allow expansion of the maxilla. It is normally cemented to the maxillary first molars and first premolars.

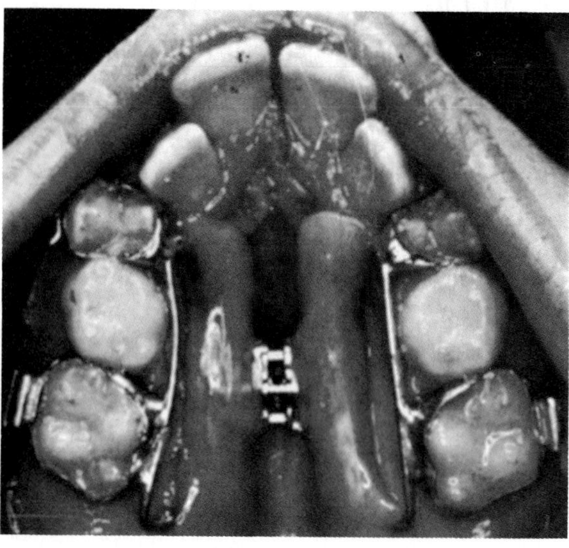

FIGURE 28–47

Palate expansion appliance. (From Morris, A.L., et al.: The Dental Specialties in General Practice. Philadelphia, W.B. Saunders Co., 1983.)

The expansion part of the appliance extends across the palate with a screw-type device that is activated by a key according to the doctor's instructions. Each turn of the key causes the arch to widen. Once the desired results have been achieved, the appliance remains on until stabilization occurs (Fig. 28–47).

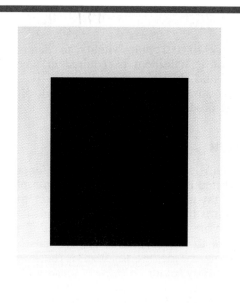

Chapter 29

Endodontics

Introduction

Endodontics is the specialty of dentistry that deals with the prevention, diagnosis, and treatment of disorders of the dental pulp. Endodontic treatment, which is often called *root canal treatment* (RCT), provides an effective means of saving teeth that might otherwise require extraction.

The pulp pathology, which frequently makes endodontic treatment necessary, is discussed in Chapter 11.

Anterior teeth usually have one canal, and posterior teeth may have up to four canals. There are anatomical variations between patients. Some patients have additional canals, or a tooth may be so calcified that it is difficult to locate the canal.

A general dentist is qualified to perform endodontic treatment; however, some dentists refer patients in need of this treatment to an endodontist (a dentist with advanced training in endodontics).

Endodontic treatment does *not* include the placement of a final restoration to return the tooth to full function. After the endodontic treatment has been completed, the patient is referred back to the general dentist for placement of this restoration.

Indications for Endodontic Treatment

- The pulp is non-vital or necrotic. (**Vital** means alive. Both **necrotic** and **non-vital** mean dead.)
- Irreversible pulpitis is present. (**Irreversible pulpitis** is an inflammation of the pulp in which the pulp cannot be healed. **Reversible pulpitis** is an inflammation of the pulp in which the pulp may be able to heal itself.)
- The apical third of the tooth has been fractured.
- The tooth has been irreversibly damaged by trauma. (Injury due to impact is the most common cause.)
- The tooth was accidentally avulsed and has been successfully replanted. (This procedure is described in Chapter 27.)

Contraindications for Endodontic Treatment

- Inflammation of the pulp is reversible. (The tooth may heal, and endodontic treatment will not be required.)
- The tooth has a poor periodontal prognosis.
- The patient has a medical condition that contraindicates dental treatment.
- The patient chooses to have the tooth extracted instead of having endodontic treatment.

Endodontic Diagnosis

To avoid misdiagnosis, a step-by-step systematic approach to endodontic diagnosis must be followed. The diagnosis is made from an examination that has both subjective and objective components.

The **subjective** portion of the examination includes evaluation of symptoms or problems described by the patient. These include the patient's description of the *location*, *intensity*, and *duration* of the pain.

The location of the pain may be very specific, or it may be vague and difficult to locate exactly. Terms such as *dull*, *sharp*, *aching*, and *piercing* may be used to describe the intensity of the pain.

The patient may state that the pain "lasts for long periods," "comes and goes quickly," or occurs at specific times such as when lying down or upon exposure to hot or cold.

The **objective examination** includes the patient's medical and dental histories, radiographs, clinical examination, and pulp vitality tests.

The **medical history** may provide information about conditions that could contribute to the toothache that the patient is experiencing. For example, a diabetic patient may experience an otherwise unexplained dental pain.

The **dental history** may provide information concerning injury to the tooth or recent dental treatment that might help explain the pain that the patient is experiencing.

The dentist will require **radiographs** showing the full length of the tooth and the periapical tissues immediately surrounding it (Fig. 29–1). Radiographs and specialized endodontic radiography techniques are discussed in Chapter 17.

In addition to the usual **clinical examination** procedures, which are discussed in Chapter 18, the dentist will perform specialized tests to determine the vitality of the pulp.

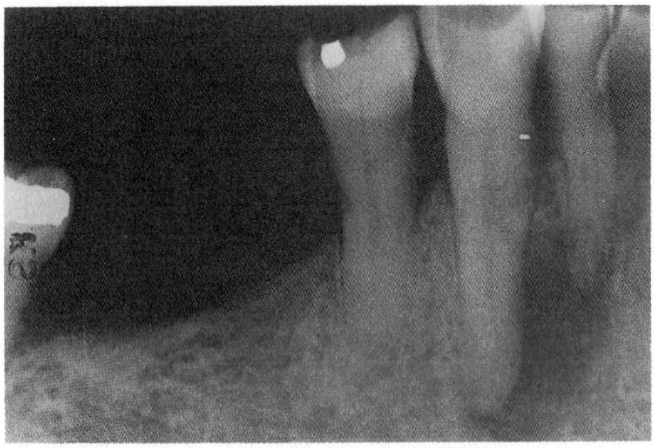

FIGURE 29–1

A mandibular premolar with a necrotic pulp. Notice the area of infection surrounding the apex of the root. (From Walton, R.E., and Torabinejad, M.: Principles and Practice of Endodontics, Philadelphia, W.B. Saunders Co., 1989, p 72.)

Testing Pulp Vitality

It is necessary to test pulp vitality to determine whether endodontic treatment is required or whether the pulp is vital and able to repair itself.

Pulp vitality testing is accomplished through one or more diagnostic procedures.

CONTROL TEETH

A healthy tooth (of the same type) in the opposite quadrant is selected as a control tooth. For example, if the maxillary right first premolar is the suspect tooth, the control tooth is the maxillary left premolar.

Control teeth are used during each type of pulp testing procedure to let the patient know what to expect and to allow the dentist to observe the level of response on a healthy tooth.

The use of a control tooth also shows whether the stimulus, such as hot or cold, is capable of getting a response. For example, posterior teeth in adults may be unresponsive to thermal tests, or the patient may have a very high tolerance and not respond.

PERCUSSION AND PALPATION TESTS

Percussion (tapping) and palpation (pressure) tests are done to determine whether the inflammatory process has extended into the periapical tissues. Positive test results indicate that there is inflammation in the periodontal ligament.

The **percussion** test is performed by tapping on the incisal or occlusal surface of a tooth with the end of a mirror handle held parallel to the long axis of the tooth.

The **palpation** test is performed by applying firm pressure to the mucosa above the apex of the root. The pressure is usually applied by the tip of the gloved index finger.

Both types of tests involve the use of at least one control tooth in addition to the suspect tooth.

THERMAL SENSITIVITY TESTS

Tests with temperature extremes are another method of determining the status of the pulp.

Cold Test. In the cold test, ice, dry ice, or ethyl chloride is used to determine the response of a tooth to cold. The suspected tooth is isolated and dried, and the source of cold is applied first to the cervical area of the control tooth and then to the suspect tooth. (Fig. 29–2).

The necrotic pulp will *not* respond to cold. Irreversible pulpitis is suspected when the cold relieves the pain. However, cold can also initiate severe, lingering pain in teeth with irreversible pulpitis.

Heat Test. The heat test is generally the least useful of the vitality tests. This is because a painful response to the heat could indicate *either* reversible pulpitis or

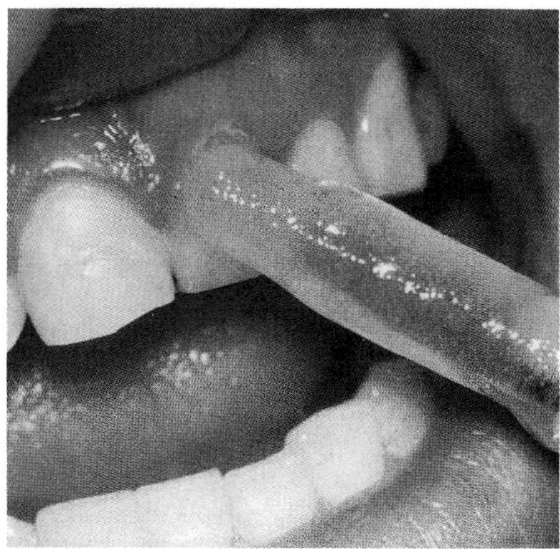

FIGURE 29–2

The reaction of the tooth to cold is tested by the application of an ice stick to the facial surface. (From Walton R.E., and Torabinejad, M.: Principles and Practice of Endodontics, Philadelphia, W.B. Saunders Co., 1989, p 61.)

irreversible pulpitis. The necrotic pulp will not respond to heat.

A small (pea-sized) piece of gutta-percha is heated in a flame and applied to the facial surface of the tooth. Another method is to heat the end of an instrument and place the heated end on the tooth.

MOBILITY TEST

The tooth is tested for mobility with the standard technique as described in Chapter 26. Teeth with large periapical lesions or severely inflamed periodontal membranes may have some mobility. If there is adequate periodontal support, the mobility usually diminishes dramatically after successful endodontic treatment.

SELECTIVE ANESTHESIA TEST

Sometimes the patient may not be able to tell which tooth is causing the pain or even whether the pain is on the maxillary or mandibular arch. In these cases, **selective anesthesia** is used.

The dentist administers a local anesthetic beginning from anterior to posterior. For example, if the source of the pain is suspected to be in the maxillary molar or premolar region, the maxillary premolars are anesthetized first and then the molars.

Selective anesthesia is not used as a diagnostic aid on the mandible because the mandibular nerve block usually anesthetizes all teeth in the quadrant.

TRANSILLUMINATION TEST

This test is used to identify vertical crown fractures. A small, intense light source (usually fiber optic) is directed (from the lingual side) through the tooth. Transillumination produces shadows at the fracture site.

DEPTH OF DECAY TEST

This is often the final, definitive test to determine the status of the pulp in a tooth with a carious lesion. This may be necessary when radiographs indicate deep caries but the patient has no symptoms and the tooth responds in a positive manner to other clinical tests.

The dentist gently removes the decay from the tooth to determine how far the caries extends into the tooth. If the decay has penetrated into the pulp, bacteria have entered the pulp and irreversible pulpitis exists, making endodontic treatment (or extraction) necessary.

If the decay has not penetrated the pulp, the condition is *usually* reversible pulpitis. In this situation, the dentist may place a sedative treatment and wait to determine how the tooth responds. However, the patient should be warned that the pulp may be irreversibly damaged without pulpal exposure. The patient is then informed of the treatment options.

ELECTRIC PULP TESTING

Electric pulp testing is helpful in endodontic diagnosis in attempting to determine whether a pulp is vital or non-vital (Fig. 29–3).

However, like other testing devices, this one can produce false-positive and false-negative responses. Therefore, the test results must be supported by other diagnostic findings.

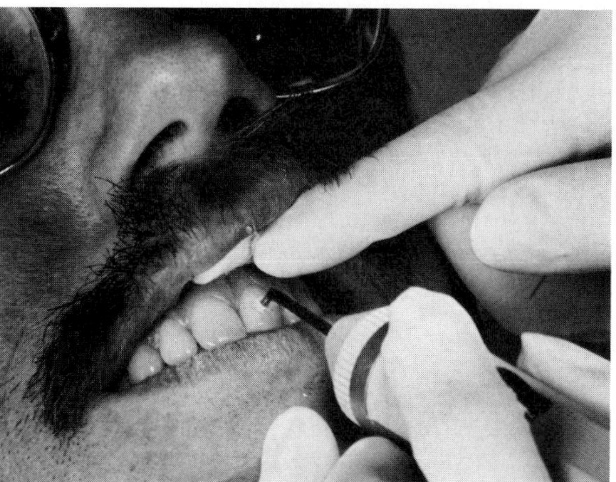

FIGURE 29–3

Electric pulp tester. The tip is placed on the cervical third of an anterior tooth.

 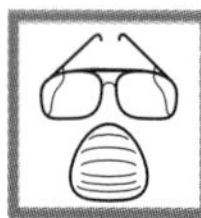 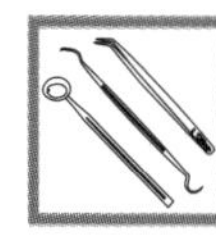 

PROCEDURE: **Performing Electric Pulp Testing**

Instrumentation

Electric pulp tester
Small amount of toothpaste

Electric Pulp Testing

1. Describe the procedure to the patient and explain that he may feel a tingling or warm sensation.
2. Isolate the teeth to be tested and dry them thoroughly.
3. Test the control tooth first.
4. Set the dial (current level) at zero.
5. Place a thin layer of toothpaste on the tip of the pulp tester electrode.
   □ *RATIONALE:* This is to establish an adequate contact to conduct the current from the pulp tester to the tooth.
6. Place the tip of the electrode on the facial surface of the tooth at the cervical third.
   □ *IMPORTANT:* Never place the tip on any type of restoration. This causes an abnormal response.
7. Gradually increase the level of the current until the patient feels a response. Record the response on the patient's chart.
8. Repeat the procedure on the tooth to be diagnosed.

Most electric pulp testers are battery operated and deliver a current of high-frequency electrical stimulus directly to the pulp. Factors that can influence the reliability of the pulp tester include the following:

- Batteries weaken over time.
- Teeth with extensive restorations can vary in response.
- In molars with several canals, one canal may be vital but the others are non-vital.
- Control teeth may not respond as anticipated.
- Dying pulps can produce a variety of responses.
- Moisture on the tooth during testing produces an inaccurate reading.
- If the tip of the tester touches the gingiva, this causes a sensation in the gingiva but not necessarily in the tooth.

Case Presentation to the Patient

The patient must be provided with enough information to give informed consent for endodontic treatment. Informed consent is discussed in Chapter 2.

Many people are very apprehensive about endodontic treatment, and good patient education helps to relieve this uneasiness. Table 29–1 lists hints that are useful in discussing the treatment with the patient.

Instrumentation for Endodontic Treatment

Broaches

Broaches, which have tiny fishhook-like barbs along the shaft, are used to remove the bulk of the pulp tissue (Fig. 29–4*A*). They are also useful for removing fragments of paper points that become lodged in the canal. They are *not* used to shape or enlarge the canal.

Broaches are discarded after a single use because they can fracture after repeated sterilization.

Endodontic Files

Endodontic files are tapered instruments with sharp cutting edges. These files are fitted into the canal and worked with a short up-and-down, twisting motion to smooth and enlarge the canal so it can be filled (see Fig. 29–4*B*).

The **K-type file** has a twisted design and is used in the initial debridement (cleaning) of the canal and in the later stages of shaping and contouring the canal.

TABLE 29–1

Never Promise the Patient That . . .

THE PROMISE	WHY NOT
All root canal treatments are successful	There are too many variables to make such promises
There is no discomfort	This can cause him to panic if there is even mild pain
Once the root canal is completed, the tooth will last forever	Remind the patient that a 6-month recall is necessary to check healing
There may be extreme pain and swelling	Do not inject unnecessary fear into the patient; give him a reasonable idea of what to expect

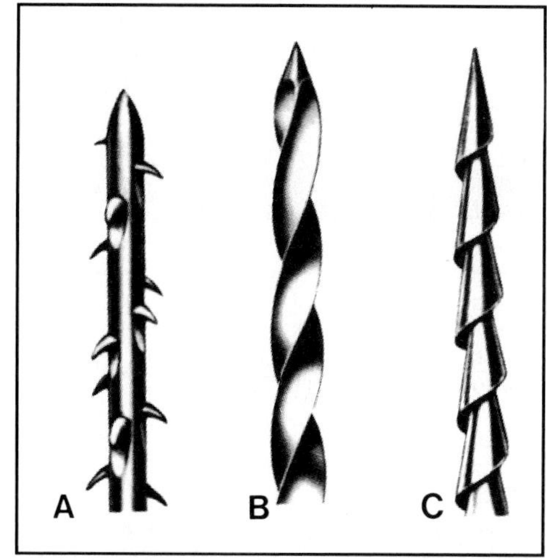

FIGURE 29–4

Details of endodontic broaches and files. *A*, Barbed broach. *B*, Standard file. *C*, Hedström file. (From Ehrlich, A and Torres H.O.: Essentials of Dental Assisting. Philadelphia, W.B. Saunders Co., 1993, p 492.)

The conventional K-type file has a "stiff" feel and is very effective for straight canals. For narrow canals and curved canals, some dentists prefer the flexible K-type file (Fig. 29–5).

The **Hedström file** provides greater cutting efficiency because of the design (see Fig 29–4*C*). The Hedström file can be for final enlargement of the canal after a Gates-Glidden or Pesso bur has been used. This makes the dentinal walls smoother and easier to fill.

Both K-type and Hedström files are available in stainless steel or the newer nickel-titanium ("Ni-Ti") alloy. Although these nickel-titanium files are more expensive than the stainless steel, they have the advantages of (1) extreme flexibility, which enables them to follow the contour of the canal better; (2) good strength, which is an important safety factor to keep the instrument from breaking while in the canal; and (3) a longer working life.

SIZES AND COLOR CODES

To provide uniformity between manufacturers, the American Dental Association (ADA) has standardized the numbering and color-coding system for intracanal instruments. Files are supplied in different diameters ranging from size 08 (the smallest) to size 140 (the largest).

Files are available in various lengths as well as diameters. Table 29–2 shows how colors are used to code handles of the instruments according to diameter.

RUBBER STOPS

These are small, round pieces of rubber or plastic that prevent the files from perforating the apex of the

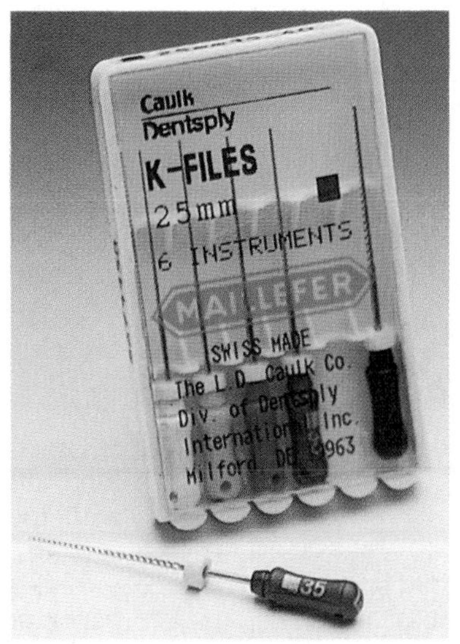

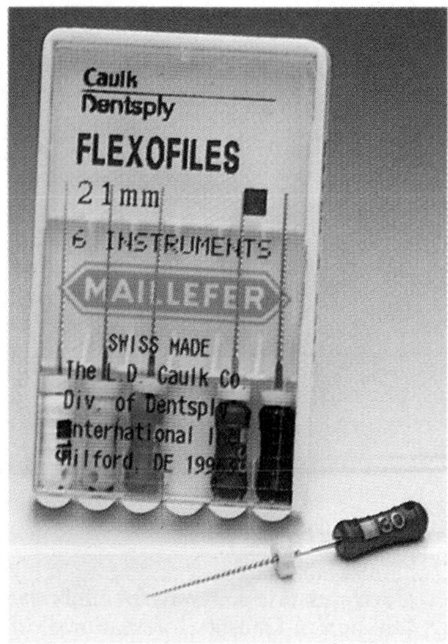

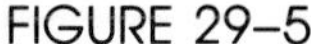

FIGURE 29–5

K-type endodontic files. On the left is the traditional file. On the right is the flexible K-type file. (Courtesy of LD Caulk, Division of Densply International, Milford, DE.)

TABLE 29–2

Color Coding of Endodontic Files

HANDLE COLOR	DIAMETER
Gray	08
Purple	10
White	15-45-90
Yellow	20-50-100
Red	25-55-110
Blue	30-60-120
Green	35-70-130
Black	40-80-140

tooth during instrumentation (Fig. 29–6). The length of the files is carefully measured, and the stop is placed precisely at the predetermined working length of the canal.

Endodontic Explorer

The endodontic explorer is a double-ended instrument that is long and straight (Fig. 29–7*A*). The working ends are at an angle to the handle. The unique design of this explorer facilitates locating canal openings.

Endodontic Spoon Excavator

The double-ended endodontic spoon excavator is very similar to other spoon excavators except that the endodontic spoon has a very long shank to allow the instrument to reach far into the tooth and canal to remove deep coronal pulp tissue, temporary cements, and caries (see Fig. 29–7*B*).

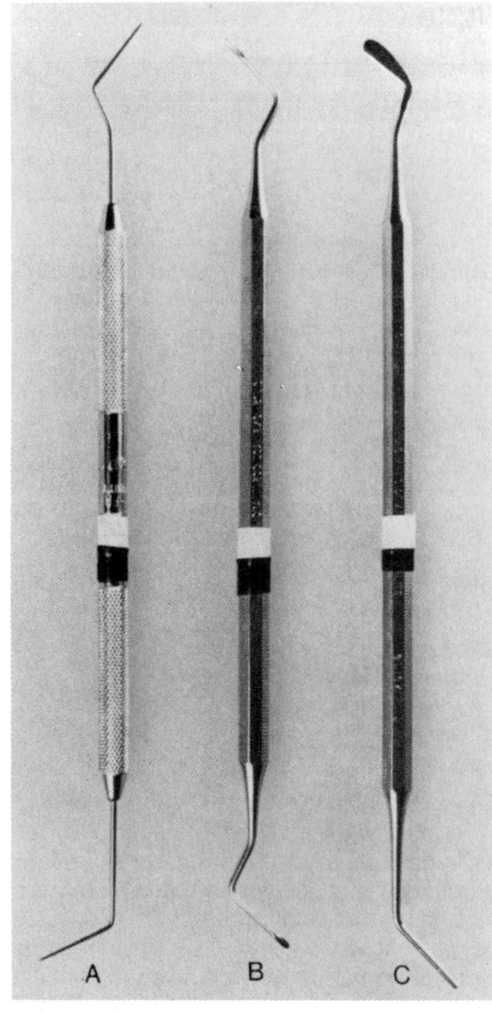

FIGURE 29–7

Specialized endodontic instruments. *A*, Explorer. *B*, Spoon excavator. *C*, Glick #1. (From Walton, R.E., and Torabinejad, M.: Principles and Practice of Endodontics, W.B. Saunders Co., Philadelphia, 1989, p 152.)

Irrigation Solution

Sodium hypochlorite, which is household bleach diluted with equal parts of water, is used as an irrigation solution to flush debris from the canal during treatment. A 5- to 6-ml. disposable plastic syringe with a special 27-gauge needle is used for this irrigation.

Sodium hypochlorite has excellent antibacterial qualities and dissolves necrotic tissue; however, it must be used with caution, because a bleach solution causes skin irritation and can ruin the patient's clothing if it drips or splashes.

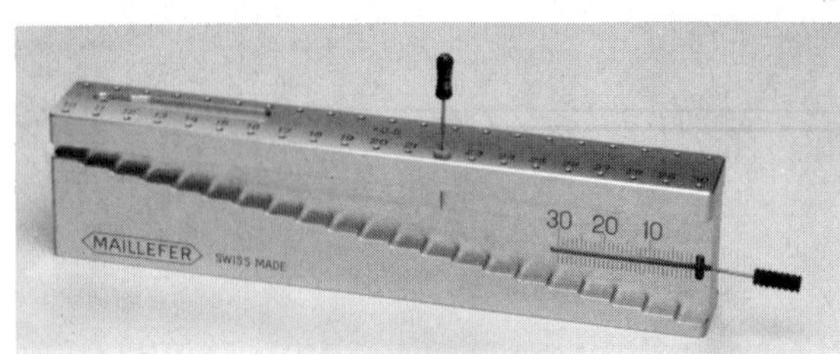

FIGURE 29–6

Device used to measure for rubber stops. (Courtesy of LD Caulk, Division of Densply International, Milford, DE.)

Paper Points

Paper points are made of absorbent paper rolled into long, narrow points (Fig. 29–8). A paper point is held with locking pliers and inserted into the canal to absorb the irrigating solution and dry the canals.

This procedure is repeated several times until the paper point is completely dry when removed from the

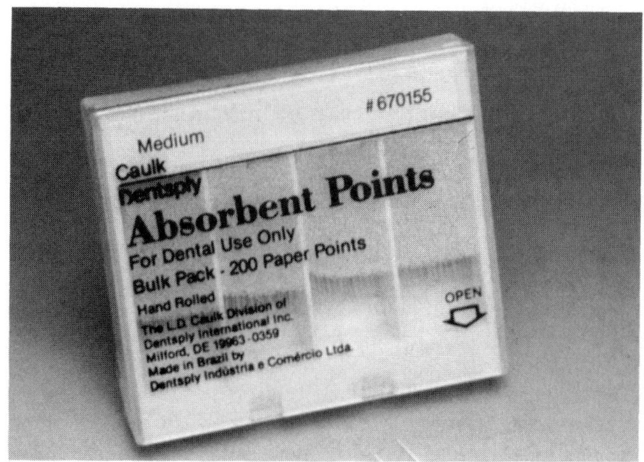

FIGURE 29–8

Paper points. (Courtesy of LD Caulk, Division of Dentsply International, Milford, DE.)

canal. Sterile paper points are available in a variety of sizes ranging from fine to coarse.

Glick #1

The paddle-shaped end of this instrument is specifically designed for placement of temporary restorations, and the rod-shaped plugger at the opposite end is ideal for removal of excess gutta-percha (see Fig 29–7*C*). The plugger end is graduated at 5-mm. increments and can be heated for placement or removal of gutta-percha.

Spreaders and Pluggers

These instruments are used to obturate (fill) the canal. They condense and adapt gutta-percha points to the canals. Pluggers and spreaders look similar but differ at the tip (Fig. 29–9). The pluggers are flat at the end, and the spreaders are have a pointed tip.

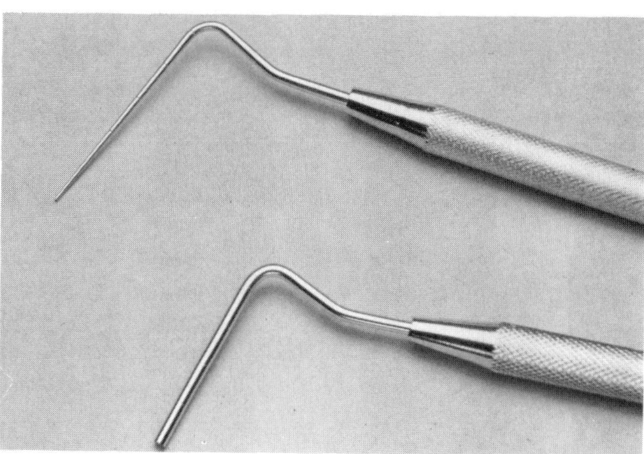

FIGURE 29–9

Working end of an endodontic spreader (top) and endodontic plugger (bottom). (Courtesy of LD Caulk, Division of Dentsply International, Milford, DE.)

Gutta-Percha Points

Gutta-percha points are the most frequently used material to obturate the canal after treatment has been completed (Fig. 29–10). Gutta-percha is solid at room temperature and becomes soft and plastic when heated.

Handpiece-Driven Instruments

Techniques for endodontic instrumentation sometimes involve using slow-speed rotary instruments to facilitate the preparation of the coronal portion of the canal. The following are the most commonly used devices.

GATES-GLIDDEN BURS

These are elliptically shaped (oval) burs with a very long shank. The cutting end looks like a football (Fig. 29–11*A*). They are always used in a low-speed handpiece, with a latch-type attachment, and operated in a clockwise direction. These burs are *not* end cutting. This means the cutting edge is only on the sides of the bur.

PESSO FILES

These are basically similar to the Gates-Glidden burs, but they have parallel cutting sides rather than an

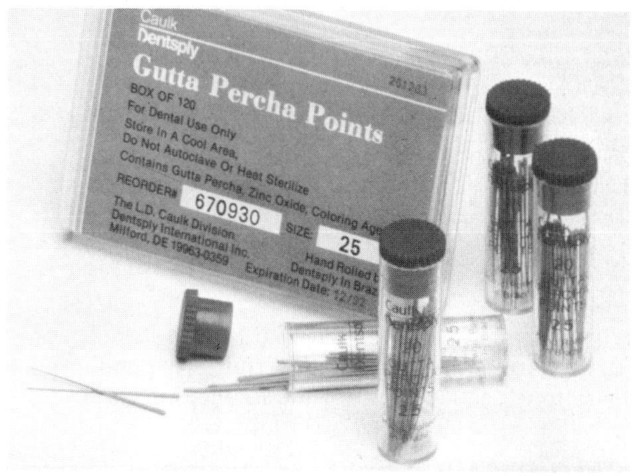

FIGURE 29–10

Gutta-percha points. (Courtesy of LD Caulk, Division of Dentsply International, Milford, DE.)

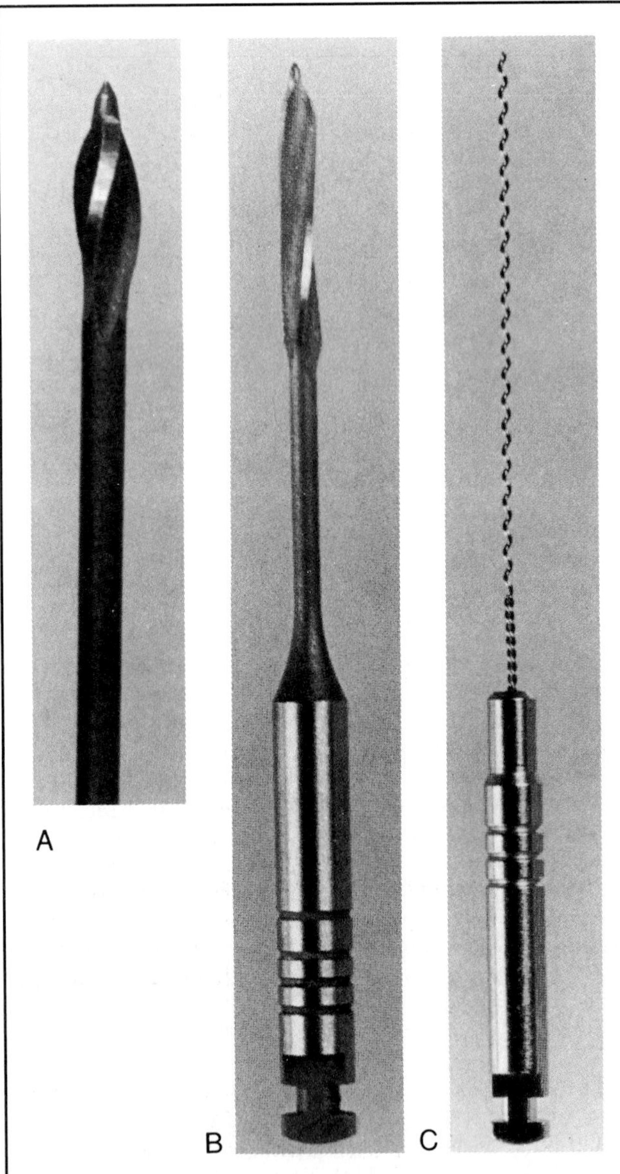

FIGURE 29–11

Handpiece-driven endodontic instruments. *A*, Tip of a Gates-Glidden drill. *B*, Pesso file. *C*, Lentulo spiral. (From Walton, R.E., and Torabinejad, M.: Principles and Practice of Endodontics, Philadelphia, W.B. Saunders Co., 1989, pp 150 and 151.)

elliptical shape (see Fig. 29–11*B*). The Pesso file is used primarily when the tooth requires a parallel post preparation for placement of the final restoration.

LENTULO SPIRALS

The Lentulo spiral is a twisted wire instrument used in the low-speed handpiece (see Fig. 29–11*C*). It is used to spin sealer, cements, or calcium hydroxide pastes into the canal or canals.

Specialized Instrument Sterilization

The packages of files and broaches are *not* sterilized by the manufacturer, and new instruments must be sterilized before use. Because of their fragile nature, files and broaches are not sterilized for reuse. They are discarded as sharps at the end of the patient visit.

Endodontic Instrumentation Setup

- High-speed handpiece with burs of dentist's choice
- Low-speed handpiece with latch attachment
- 5- to 6-ml. syringe with 27-gauge needle
- Broaches, Hedström files, and K-type files (assorted sizes and lengths)
- Rubber instrument stops
- Paper points
- Gutta-percha points
- Sealer material (to seal the apex of the tooth)
- Endodontic spoon excavator
- Endodontic explorer
- Glick #1
- Millimeter ruler
- Locking cotton pliers (for holding paper points)
- Sodium hypochlorite solution (for irrigation)
- Hemostat (for holding x-ray film during working length and master cone radiographs)
- High-volume evacuator (HVE) tip

Overview of Endodontic Treatment

There are five phases of treatment in endodontic therapy: (1) administration of local anesthetic; (2) isolation with the dental dam; (3) access preparation (opening the tooth); (4) cleaning and preparing the canal or canals; and (5) filling and sealing the canal or canals.

Anesthesia and Pain Control

The anesthesia techniques of choice for endodontic treatment are infiltration for maxillary teeth and nerve blocks for mandibular teeth (see Chapter 20).

A local anesthetic is administered any time there is vitality (life) remaining in the tooth to be treated. If the tooth is non-vital, the dentist may decide not to use a local anesthetic.

After the pulp has been removed, local anesthetic may or may not be administered during subsequent visits, depending on the preference of the patient.

Inflamed and infected tissues are difficult to anesthetize. Since endodontic treatment procedures gener-

The Role of the Dental Assistant

Those steps with an asterisk can be performed by the dental assistant in some states.

- Administer local anesthetic.
- Apply and disinfect the dental dam.*
- Cut the access preparation.
- Locate the canal or canals with an endodontic explorer.
- Remove the pulp with a broach.
- Irrigate the canals with sodium hypochlorite solution.*
- Determine the working length of the tooth.
- Place rubber stops on files.*
- Clean and shape the canals, using endodontic files.
- Frequently irrigate the canals during the cleaning and shaping process.*
- Dry canals after irrigation.*
- Mix the sealing material.*
- Seal the apex of the tooth with the sealing material.
- Condense gutta-percha points into the canal, using the pluggers and spreaders.
- Seal the tooth with a temporary cement.*
- Take a post-treatment radiograph.*

ally involve inflamed pulp and/or periapical tissues, obtaining adequate anesthesia can sometimes be a problem.

When this occurs, it may be necessary to inject additional local anesthesia directly into the pulp. In addition, sedation (intravenous, oral, or inhalation) is sometimes used for those patients who are extremely apprehensive.

Isolation and Disinfection of the Operating Field

The standard of care (established by the ADA) for endodontic treatment requires the use of a dental dam. Legal ramifications make use of the dental dam *mandatory in endodontic treatment.*

Before treatment begins, it is important to remove all bacterial contaminants from the tooth, clamp, and surrounding dental dam material.

Access Preparation

Using a high-speed handpiece and round bur, the dentist makes an opening in the tooth. This step is called an **access preparation.** The purpose of this preparation is to make a large enough entrance in the coronal portion of the tooth to allow the endodontic instruments to pass through.

The access preparation is made through the occlusal surface on posterior teeth and through the lingual surface on anterior teeth.

The Estimated Working Length

It is very important to know what the length of the completed canal preparation and root canal filling should be. Problems that result from inaccurate measurement of length include

- Perforation of the apex
- Over- or under-instrumentation of the canal length
- Overfilling the canal
- Underfilling the canal
- Increased incidence of postoperative pain

Because exact apex locations vary, and because it is not always possible to see these variations on radiographs, the length is determined by estimate and is called the **estimated working length** (Fig. 29–12).

The estimated working length is determined by selecting a reference point on the tooth. (This is usually the highest point on the incisal or occlusal surface.) Then, on the diagnostic radiographic, a millimeter en-

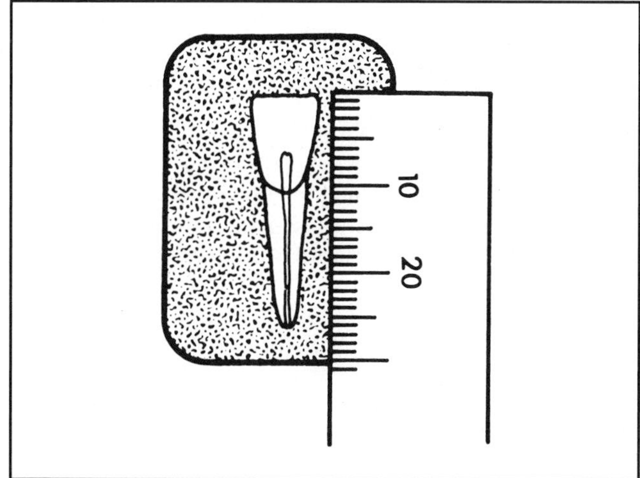

FIGURE 29–12

Estimated working length determination with a millimeter ruler. (From Walton, R.E., and Torabinejad, M.: Principles and Practice of Endodontics, Philadelphia, W.B. Saunders Co., 1989, p 189.)

dodontic ruler is used to measure the distance from the reference point to the apex of the tooth.

ELECTRONIC APEX LOCATORS

These are electronic devices that determine the canal length by sensing when the file tip has reached the apical foramen. They work on a simple principle of electrical resistance.

An electrode is clipped to the endodontic file, and the file is placed into the canal. When the electrical current (which is flowing through the file) reaches the tissue at the apex, the resistance is decreased, and the device signals the operator. Depending on the brand, the signal may be a beep, a buzz, a flashing light, or a digital read-out. These devices are especially useful if the radiograph is distorted.

Cleaning and Shaping the Canal

The purposes of cleaning (debridement) and shaping the canal are (1) to remove irritants such as bacteria, bacterial by-products, necrotic tissue, and organic debris from the root canal and (2) to smooth and shape the canal so that the filling material can be completely adapted to the walls of the canal.

Filling the Canal (Obturation)

After the canal has been filed to the desired size and shape, it is cleaned and dried. The canal is now ready to be filled by the dentist. If the tooth has more than one canal, each canal is filled individually, and each one requires a properly fitted and sealed gutta-percha point.

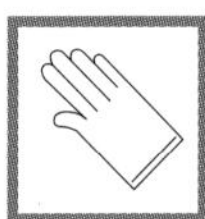
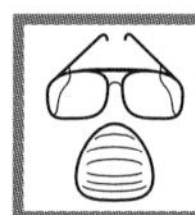
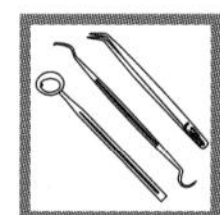
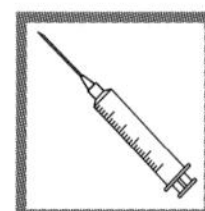
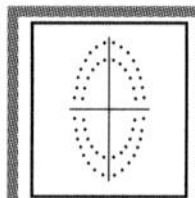

PROCEDURE: **Providing Endodontic Treatment**

Cleaning and Disinfecting the Field of Operation

1. Before the dam is placed, coronal polish is used to remove plaque from the surfaces of the tooth to be exposed (see the section "Selective polishing" in Chapter 21).
2. The dental dam is placed so only the tooth being treated is exposed.
   □ *RATIONALE:* The dental dam should prevent saliva and blood from reaching the pulp space.
3. A cotton-tip applicator dipped in sodium hypochlorite solution is used to wipe and disinfect the tooth surface, clamp, and surrounding dental dam.
   □ *RATIONALE:* This is the same solution that is used for irrigation. It is household bleach mixed with equal parts of water.

Removing the Pulp

1. After locating the canals with the endodontic explorer, the dentist removes the pulp tissue, with a barbed broach.
2. The assistant irrigates the canals gently with a solution of sodium hypochlorite.
3. The assistant uses the HVE tip to catch the excess solution.
4. The dentist uses a small endodontic file to rub the irrigation solution against the walls of the canal and pulp chamber.
   □ *RATIONALE:* The solution acts as a disinfectant to destroy bacteria in the canal and to wash away debris. This step is called **biochemical** cleaning.

Cleaning and Shaping the Canals

1. Small-size files are inserted into the canal and moved up and down with short strokes.
   □ *RATIONALE:* During this motion, the cutting edges of the instruments remove dentin and debris from the walls of the canal.
2. The size of the files is increased as cleaning and shaping continues.
   □ *RATIONALE:* This is done to enlarge the diameter of the canal.
3. The rubber stop must be placed at the desired working length for that canal. In teeth with more than one canal, *each* canal is filed to the predetermined length.

4. The canals must be thoroughly irrigated at frequent intervals during filing.
   □ *RATIONALE:* This prevents the dentin shavings from clogging the cutting edges of the instruments.

Preparing to Fill the Canals

1. Select the appropriate size gutta-percha point and cut it to the predetermined length. (This is called the **trial-point**.)
2. Take a periapical radiograph of the tooth with the trial point in the canal. (This is called the **trial-point radiograph**.)
3. If the radiograph does not show the tip of the trial point within 1 mm. of the apex of the root, the point is repositioned, and another radiograph is taken.
4. At a signal from the dentist, prepare a thin mix of endodontic sealer on a sterile glass slab.
   □ *RATIONALE:* The sealer is used to ensure a perfect seal at the apical foramen.

Filling the Canals

1. Dip a file or Lentulo spiral into the cement and pass it to the dentist.
2. The dentist inserts the file into the canal (1 mm. short of working length). The file is rotated counterclockwise to spread the sealer around the canal.
3. Dip the tip of the gutta-percha point into the sealer and pass it to the dentist.
4. The dentist inserts the gutta-percha point to the length established in the final trial-point radiograph.
5. The dentist uses an endodontic spreader and applies lateral (sideways) pressure to condense the points against the walls of the canal.
6. The dentist adds smaller gutta-percha points to the canal.
7. The dentist uses a heated Glick #1 to remove the excess ends of the gutta-percha points.
8. The dentist uses an endodontic plugger to vertically condense the warm gutta-percha. This continues until the canal is completely filled.
9. The dentist seals the tooth with a temporary cement. (See Chapter 23.)
10. Take a post-treatment radiograph (Fig. 29–13).
11. The dentist checks the occlusion and adjusts it as needed (Fig. 29–14).
12. Provide post-treatment instructions to the patient.
    □ *RATIONALE:* Post-treatment instructions to the patient emphasize the importance of returning for the post-treatment evaluation and permanent restoration.

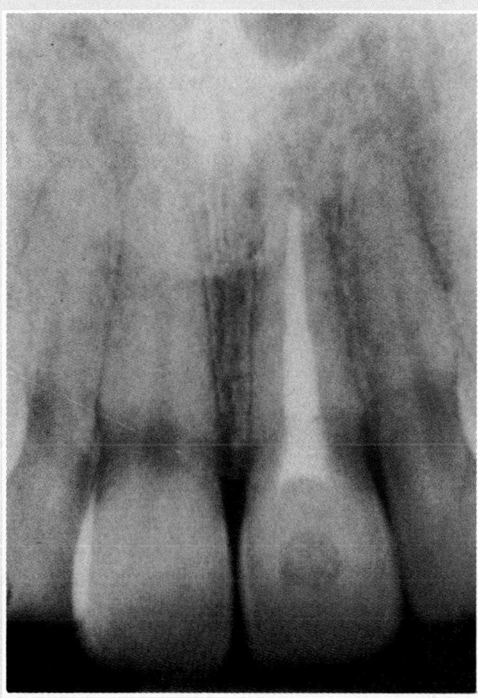

FIGURE 29–13

A radiograph showing gutta-percha in the pulp canal of a maxillary central incisor. (From Haring, J.I., and Lind, L.J.: Radiographic Interpretation for the Dental Hygienist. Philadelphia, W.B. Saunders, 1993, p 90.)

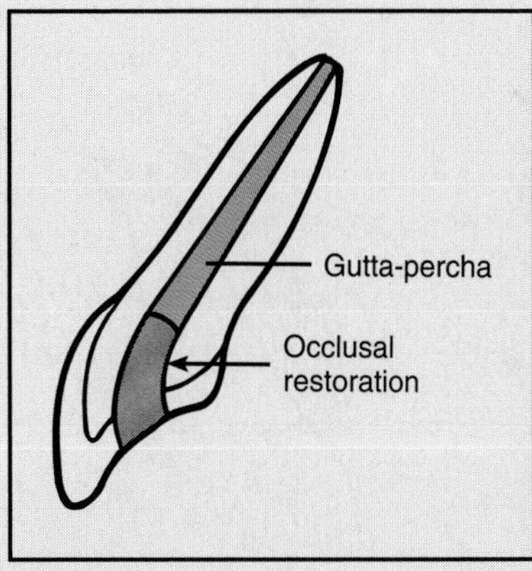

FIGURE 29–14

After the canal has been completely filled, the excess material is removed from the clinical crown. A restoration is then placed by the general dentist. (From Levine, N.: Current Treatment in Dental Practice. Philadelphia, W.B. Saunders Co., 1986, p 193.)

Postoperative Follow-Up

After the endodontic treatment, the patient must have a permanent restoration placed. Depending upon the condition of the tooth, this may be a simple composite or an amalgam restoration. If the tooth is badly broken down, it may be necessary to place a core and crown. (These are discussed in Chapter 31.)

To be certain that the endodontic treatment was successful, the patient is instructed to return to the endodontist for follow-up at intervals ranging from 3 to 6 months.

Surgical Endodontics

Routine endodontic treatment, which does not involve surgery, is successful approximately 90 to 95 percent of the time. There are, however, situations when surgical endodontic techniques must be used to save a tooth from extraction. Indications for surgical intervention include the following:

Endodontic Failure. Failure of nonsurgical endodontics may be caused by persistent infection, severely curved roots, perforation of the canal, fractured roots, extensive root resorption, pulp stones, or accessory canals that cannot be treated.

Exploratory Surgery. This may be necessary to determine why healing has not occurred after endodontic treatment. Sometimes this is caused by canal medications' having extended beyond the apex and into the periapical tissues.

Biopsy. A tissue sample for a biopsy may be required. This is described in Chapter 30.

Apicoectomy

An apicoectomy is the surgical removal of the apical portion of the root with the use of a tapered fissure bur in a high-speed handpiece (Fig. 29–15*A*). The dentist can then examine the apex for signs of

- Inadequate sealing of the canal
- Accessory (additional) canals
- Fractures of the root
- Other causes of endodontic treatment failure

Apical Curettage

Inflamed tissue around the root tip may delay the healing process. If required, apical curettage is performed to remove the pathological soft tissue around the root apex (see Fig. 29–15*B*). (**Curettage** means the removal of diseased tissue by scraping with an instrument called a curette.)

Retrograde Restoration

A retrograde restoration (filling) is placed when the apical seal is not adequate. A small class I preparation is made at the apex and is sealed with filling materials such as gutta-percha, amalgam, or composite (see Figs. 29–15*C* and 29–15*D*).

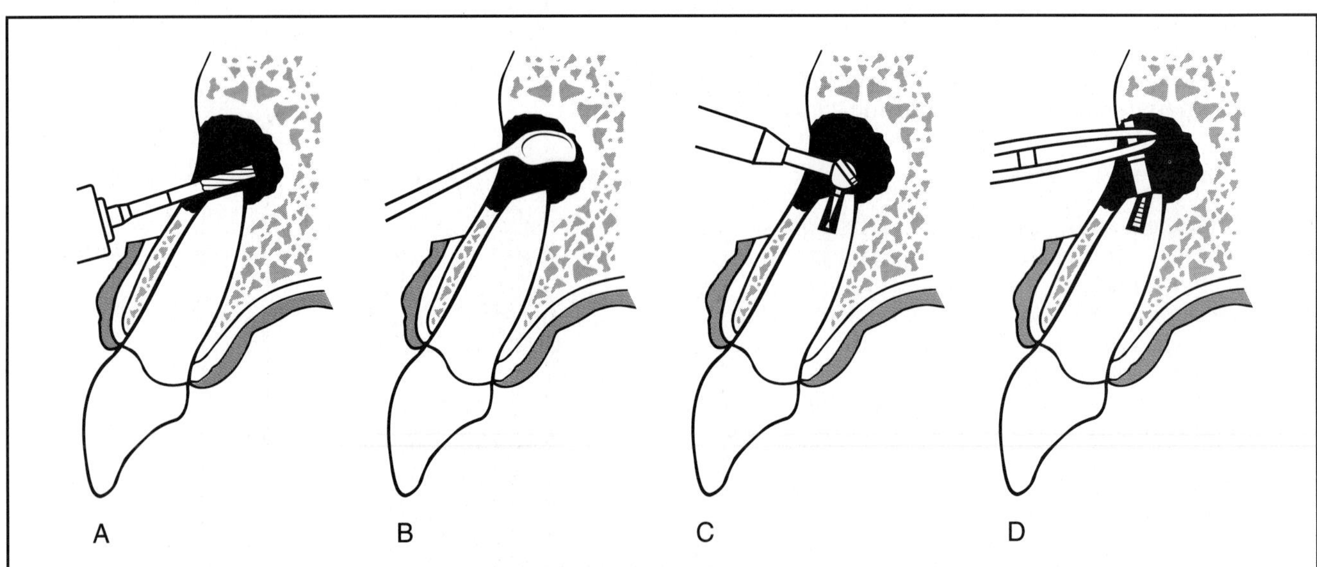

FIGURE 29–15

Surgical endodontics. *A*, Apicoectomy. *B*, Curettage. *C*, Preparation for a retrograde restoration. *D*, Placement of a retrograde restoration. (From Walton, R.E., and Torabinejad, M.: Principles and Practice of Endodontics, Philadelphia, W.B. Saunders Co., 1989, pp 408 and 409.)

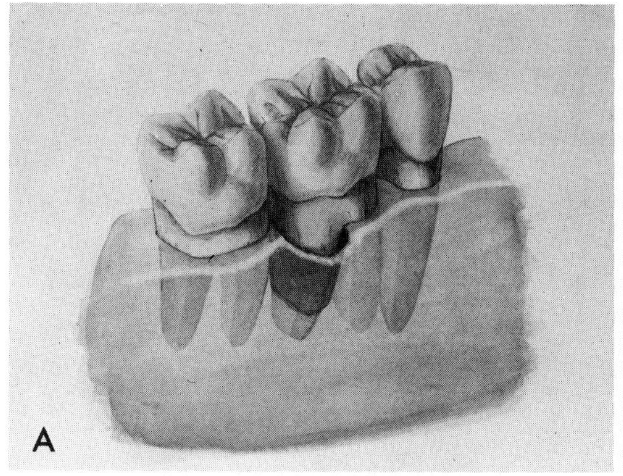

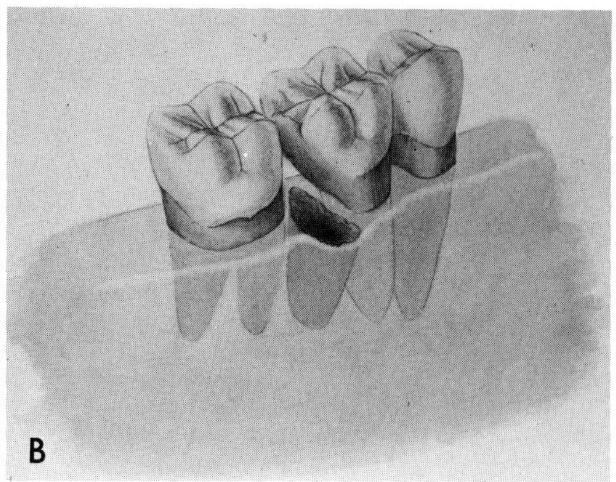

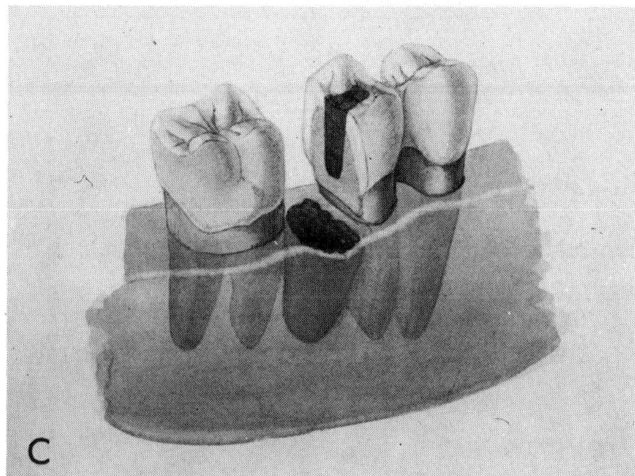

FIGURE 29–16

Diagrammatic view of furcation involvement in a mandibular first molar. *A*, Vertical lesion around distal root. *B*, After resection of distal root. *C*, Another approach with the use of hemisection of the distal half of the tooth (root and crown). (From Carranza, F.A.: Glickman's Clinical Periodontology, 7th ed. Philadelphia, W.B. Saunders Co., 1990, p 868.)

Root Amputation and Hemisection

Root amputation and **hemisection** are surgical procedures in which one or more roots of a multirooted tooth are removed while the other roots are saved through endodontic treatment (Fig. 29–16).

Root amputation is the removal of one or more roots of a multirooted tooth *without* the removal of the crown. The amputation occurs at the point where the root joins the crown. Root amputation is most commonly performed on maxillary molars.

A **hemisection** is a procedure in which the root and the crown are cut lengthwise and removed. Hemisections are most often performed on mandibular molars.

INDICATIONS FOR ROOT AMPUTATION OR HEMISECTION

- When there is severe periodontal involvement in which the tooth has untreatable bone loss around one of the roots or at the furcation (this is the most common indication, and these conditions are discussed in Chapter 26)
- When one or more roots are untreatable by endodontic therapy
- When one of the roots is fractured
- When the remaining part of the tooth can be treated with endodontic therapy and then restored

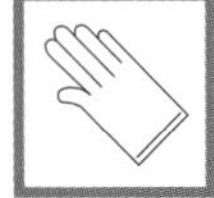 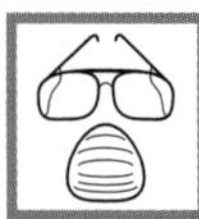 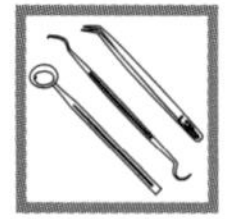 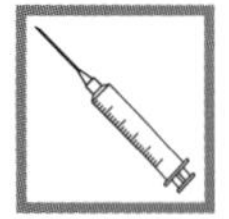 

PROCEDURE: **Performing Apical Surgery**

Apical surgery is a term used to group together the specific procedures described earlier. It is performed when there is a need to gain direct access to the apical area of a tooth.

Instrumentation

Scalpel
Periosteal elevator
Tissue retractors (operator's choice)
Rongeurs
Surgical curette (operator's choice)
Saline solution and irrigating syringe
Surgical HVE aspirator tips
Surgical burs
Suture setup (material, needle, holders)
Handpiece (operator's choice) or ultrasonic handpiece with special retro-tips (these are tips that fit easily into the apex of the tooth)
Sterile gauze sponges

Apical Surgery Steps

1. Local anesthetic is administered.
2. To gain access to the apex, the dentist makes the incision and reflects the flap (Fig. 29–17). (As used here, **reflect** means to lay back out of the way.)
3. The dentist performs the necessary apical procedure and then replaces the flap and sutures it in place.
4. As necessary, the assistant aspirates and maintains a clear operating field.
5. The patient is provided with postoperative care instructions.

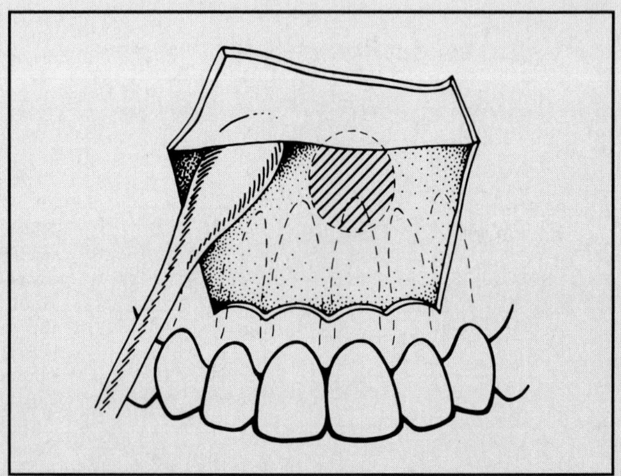

FIGURE 29–17

At the beginning of apical surgery, the dentist makes the incision and reflects the tissue. At the end of the procedure, the tissue is replaced and sutured in place. (From Walton, R.E., and Torabinejad, M.: Principles and Practice of Endodontics. Philadelphia, W.B. Saunders Co., 1989, p 407.)

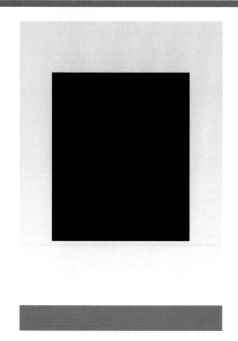

Chapter 30

Oral and Maxillofacial Surgery and Dental Implants

Introduction

An oral and maxillofacial surgeon (OMFS), commonly referred to simply as an *oral surgeon,* is a dentist who has had 3 to 5 years of postgraduate training in oral and maxillofacial surgery. In addition to simple and complex dental extractions, the OMFS performs reconstructive surgery, treats fractures of the bones of the face and jaws, performs implant surgeries, and performs other surgical procedures that involve the orofacial region.

The general dentist receives training in surgical dental procedures, and some general dentists perform less complex surgical procedures as a routine part of their practice. However, other general dentists prefer to refer all surgery patients to an oral and maxillofacial surgeon.

Indications for Oral and Maxillofacial Surgery

- Extraction of carious teeth that cannot be restored or that the patient does not choose to have restored
- Surgical removal of impacted teeth
- Extraction of non-vital teeth when endodontic treatment is not indicated
- Preprosthetic surgery to smooth and contour the ridges so the prosthetic appliance will fit better
- Removal of teeth before orthodontic treatment to provide more room in the dental arch
- Removal of root fragments
- Removal of cysts and tumors
- Biopsy procedures
- Treatment of fractures of the mandible or maxilla
- Surgery to alter the size or shape of the facial bones (these patients are co-treated by an orthodontist)
- Surgery of the temporomandibular joint (TMJ)
- Reconstructive surgery
- Salivary gland surgery
- Surgical implant procedure

Contraindications for Oral and Maxillofacial Surgery

- Bleeding and clotting disorders
- Uncontrolled or poorly controlled diabetes
- Local or systemic infection (the infection should be eliminated before the surgery to prevent the infection from spreading to other parts of the body; in addition, total local anesthesia may be difficult to achieve in the presence of infection)
- Medications that can have an adverse effect on healing (these include immunosuppressive drugs and anticoagulants)

Specialized Needs

Oral surgery, even when performed in the dental office, is just as much a surgical procedure as one performed in a hospital operating room. Before under-

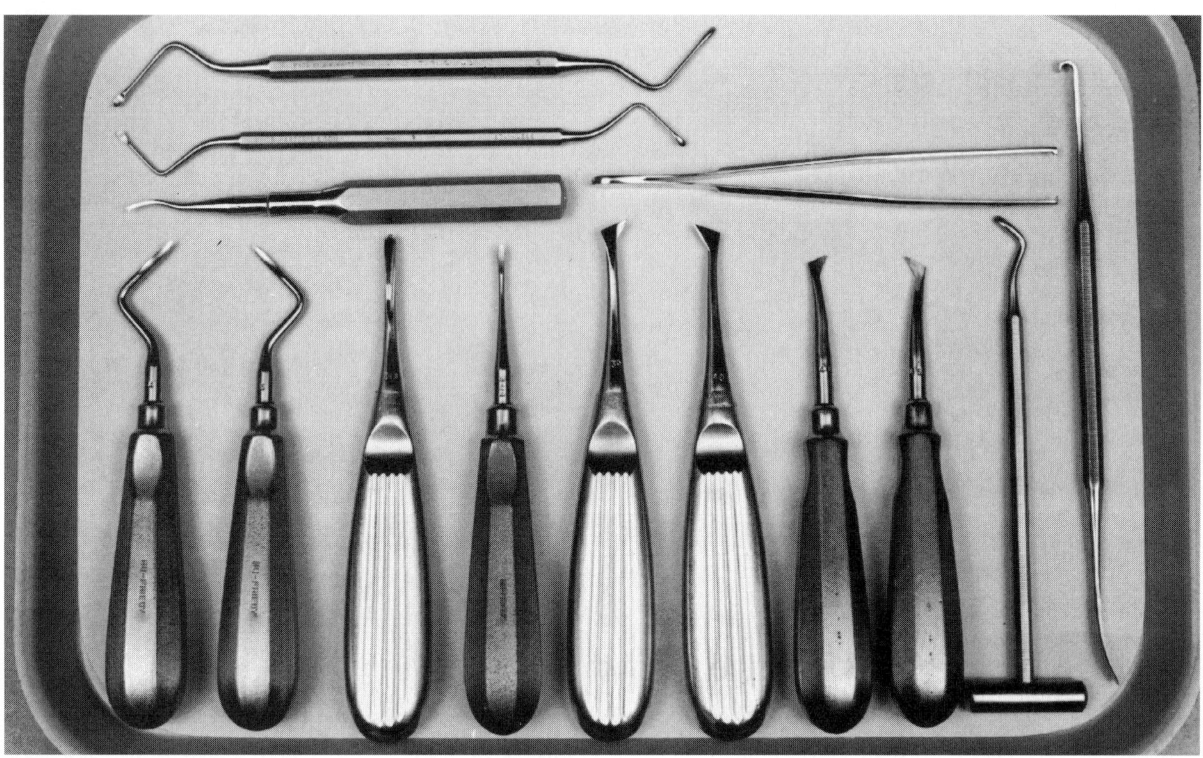

FIGURE 30–1

Surgical instruments. *Top left,* Two curettes and a root pick. *Top right,* Tissue forceps. *Bottom left to right,* Apical elevators (left and right pair), large straight elevator, small straight elevator, Cryer elevators (left and right pair), smaller Cryer root elevators (left and right pair), Potts elevator with crossbar handle, double-ended instrument (the top is a tissue retractor, the bottom is a periosteal elevator).

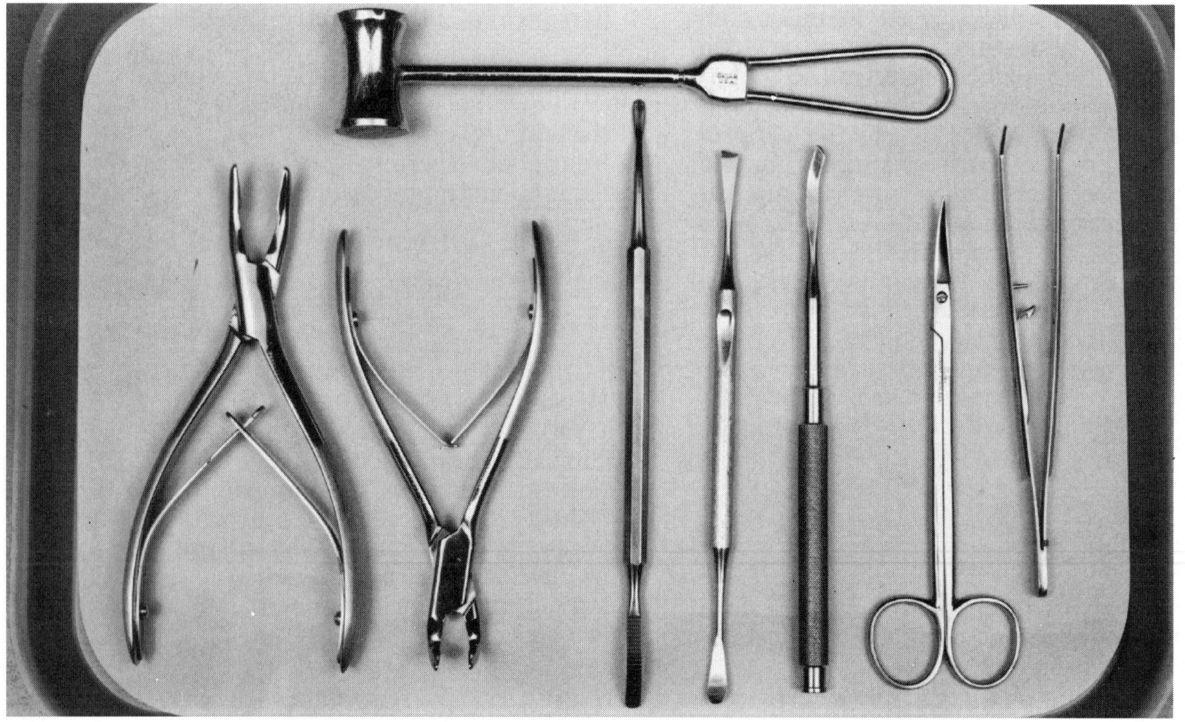

FIGURE 30–2

Assorted surgical instruments. *Top,* Surgical mallet. *Bottom left to right,* Straight rongeur, curved rongeur, bone file, periosteal elevator, bone chisel, tissue scissors, tissue forceps.

taking this procedure, both the oral surgeon and patient have specialized needs.

MEDICAL HISTORY

The oral surgeon must have a complete medical history for the patient. If extensive surgery is planned or if general anesthesia is to be used, a physical examination by a physician also may be required.

RADIOGRAPHS

The type of radiographs and the number of exposures necessary for a surgical procedure depend on the surgical procedure to be performed. For example, if an impacted tooth is to be removed, the OMFS requires specialized radiographs to "locate" the tooth that is covered by bone.

The radiographs most commonly used are periapical views. In addition the oral surgeon may require occlusal, panoramic, specialized extraoral, and TMJ views. More extensive surgeries may necessitate computerized tomography (CT). These techniques are discussed in Chapter 17.

PAIN CONTROL

Pain control methods are discussed in Chapter 20. These are of particular importance to the oral surgery patient. In addition, a longer duration and a more profound (deeper) level of local anesthesia may be required in oral maxillofacial surgery than is required for most restorative procedures.

For this reason, additional injections may be made to block peripheral nerves in the surrounding tissues. Also, the oral surgeon may select a local anesthetic formula that has a longer duration.

At the end of the surgical procedures, some oral surgeons give their patients an additional injection of a long-acting local anesthetic to aid in the immediate postoperative pain control.

Oral Surgery Instrumentation

Oral surgery instruments are used to penetrate soft tissue or bone. They are designated as critical instruments, which means they *must* be sterilized after each use.

ELEVATORS

Periosteal elevators are manufactured in a variety of designs, yet they all have the same basic function. They are used to reflect (separate) and retract the periosteum from the surface of the bone. (The **periosteum** is the fibrous covering of the bone.)

Before the placement of the surgical forceps, the dentist uses a periosteal elevator to detach the gingival tissues from around the cervix (neck) of the tooth (Figs. 30–1 to 30–3).

Extraction elevators, also known as *straight elevators*, are used to apply leverage against the tooth to

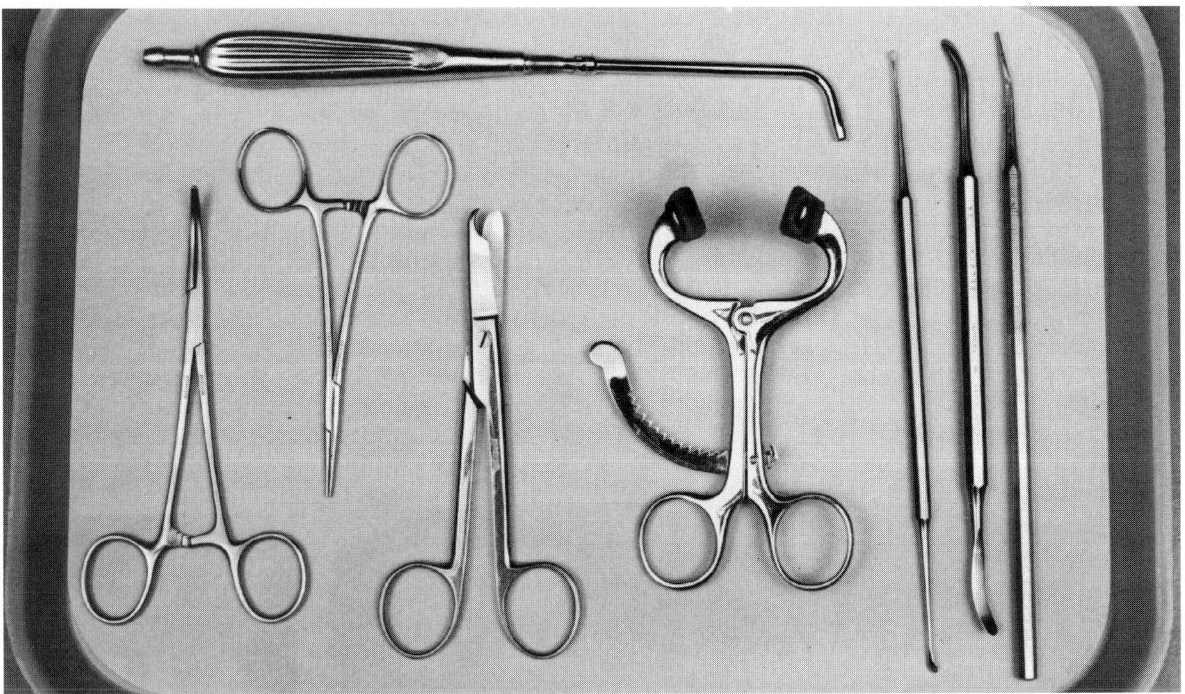

FIGURE 30–3

Surgical instruments and accessories. *Top,* Surgical aspirating tip. *Bottom left to right,* Curved hemostat, straight hemostat, suture scissors, mouth prop, double-ended curette and periosteal elevator, double-ended periosteal elevator, bone chisel.

loosen it from the periodontal ligament and ease the extraction. Other uses of extraction elevators include the removal of residual root fragments and removing teeth that have been sectioned by a surgical handpiece and bur.

Elevator tips are available in a variety of styles to accommodate the intended area of use and the amount of leverage required. The handle of the elevator is large enough to fit comfortably into the dentist's hand, and it is passed to the dentist in a palm grasp. Some elevators are available with a T-shaped handle.

Some elevator styles are paired as right and left. This refers to the patient's right and left (see Fig. 30–1).

Root tip picks, also known as *root tip teasers*, are delicate instruments for the removal of root tips or fragments that may break away from the tooth during the extraction procedure (see Fig. 30–1). Some designs have a slightly heavier tip for greater leverage.

SURGICAL CURETTES

The surgical curette is a double-ended, scoop-shaped instrument with sharp edges that resembles a large spoon excavator and is used with a scraping motion. Curettes come in varying sizes, and the shanks are straight or angled to reach different areas of the mouth (see Figs. 30–1 and 30–3).

Some dentists use a curette to sever the epithelial attachment of the gingiva around the tooth before the application of the extraction forceps. Curettes are used after extractions to scrape the interior of the socket to remove diseased tissue and/or abscesses.

RONGEUR

The rongeur is similar in size to forceps, and the design resembles finger nail clippers. It has a spring between the handles and blades with sharp cutting edges. The blades of the rongeur may be end-cutting or side-cutting, depending on the design (see Fig. 30–2).

The rongeur is used to trim alveolar bone. It is widely used after multiple extractions to eliminate sharp projections and to shape the edentulous ridge. The beaks of the rongeur must be kept clean during the procedure. As necessary, the dentist holds the instrument toward the assistant with the beaks open. The assistant then carefully removes the debris by wiping the beaks with a sterile gauze sponge.

BONE FILE

The working ends of bone files are very rough and are available in a variety of shapes and sizes (see Fig. 30–2).

The bone file is used with a push-pull motion to smooth the surface of the bone after the rongeur has removed the majority of undesirable bone. Bone files can also be used to smooth rough margins of the alveolus after an extraction.

SCALPEL

The scalpel is a surgical knife used to make a precise incision into soft tissue with the least amount of trauma to the tissue. The size and shape of the blade selected depend on the procedure being performed and on the dentist's preference (Fig. 30–4).

Disposable scalpels are supplied in sterile sealed packages. They have plastic handles with metal blades. These instruments are designed to be used once and then discarded into the sharps container.

Reusable scalpels have metal handles that are sterilized after each use. Sterile disposable metal blades are attached to these handles before use. After use, the blade is removed and discarded in the sharps container. Care must be taken to avoid injury while the blades are attached and removed. Use of a mechanical scalpel blade remover helps avoid injury while scalpel blades are removed.

HEMOSTAT AND NEEDLE HOLDERS

Hemostats, which were originally designed for use in general surgery to clamp off blood vessels, are multipurpose instruments that are used to grasp and hold things. During oral surgery, a hemostat is used to grasp soft tissue, bone, and tooth fragments that have been removed during the procedure.

In addition to surgical applications, hemostats are commonly used in a variety of situations in which is it necessary to hold and lock small or thin items such as wedges and matrix bands.

A hemostat somewhat resembles scissors; however, the beaks are not sharp. Instead, the beaks have serrations or grooves for grasping and holding. Also, the handles have a mechanical lock to make it possible to securely hold an object or tissue in the beaks.

These instruments are available in a variety of sizes,

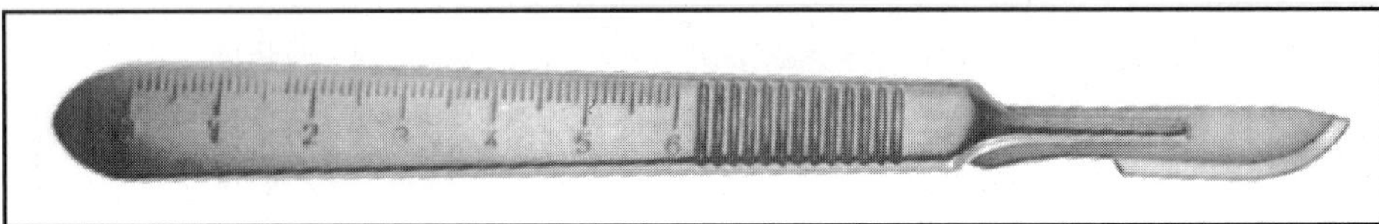

FIGURE 30–4

Reusable scalpel handle with disposable blade in place. The centimeter marks on the handle are used to measure the length of a surgical incision or pathological lesion. (Courtesy of Hu-Friedy Manufacturing, Inc., Chicago, IL.)

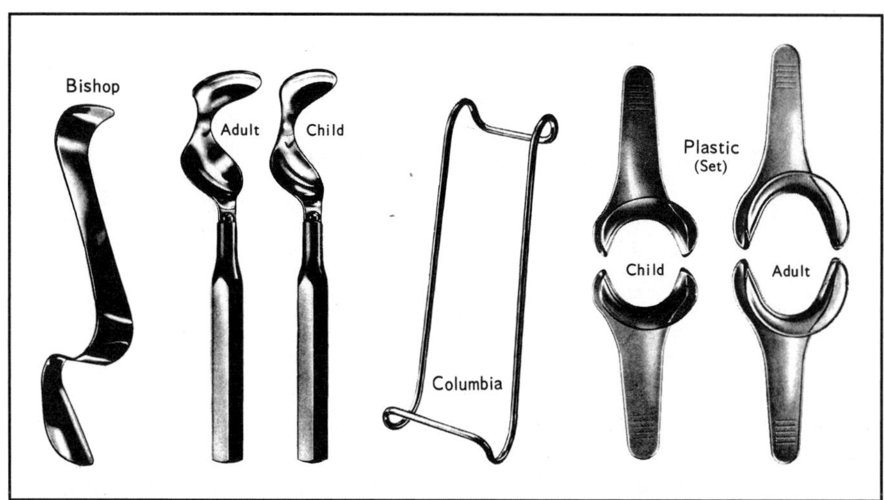

FIGURE 30–5

Tongue and cheek retractors. The plastic retractors at the right are commonly used when intraoral photographs are taken. (Courtesy of Hu-Friedy Manufacturing, Inc., Chicago, IL.)

with straight and curved beaks and with different handle lengths (see Fig. 30–3).

The **needle holder** looks and operates much like a hemostat. The beaks are straight with fine serrations; however, there is a groove on the serrated surface to firmly grasp a suture needle.

The handles of the needle holder and hemostat are held in place by ratchet action that holds an object until the dentist releases it. This handle design allows the dentist to tie the suture material by using the needle holder without snagging it in the joint of the instrument.

SCISSORS

Surgical scissors are available with straight or curved blades that have smooth or serrated cutting edges. The handles range in length from approximately 3½ inches to 6¼ inches.

These delicate scissors are used to trim soft tissue, and maintaining their sharpness is essential. For this reason, surgical scissors should never be used for nonsurgical tasks that would dull the cutting surfaces.

Suture scissors are designed to cut only suture material. They are similar in design to surgical scissors; however, they are sturdier, and many have a small notch on the cutting edge of one blade (see Fig. 30–3).

TISSUE RETRACTORS

During surgical procedures, it is important to handle soft tissue as carefully as possible to prevent trauma that may delay healing. Tissue retractors are used to hold soft tissue during surgical procedures.

These instruments resemble cotton pliers that have notched tips (see Fig. 30–1). Tissue retractors must always be used with care to avoid undue trauma or damage to the delicate tissue.

CHEEK AND TONGUE RETRACTORS

These retractors are designed to hold and retract the cheeks and tongue during surgical procedures. They are large, curved, angled instruments made of metal or plastic. If plastic retractors are used during surgery, they must be able to withstand heat sterilization (Fig. 30–5).

MOUTH PROPS

During a surgical procedure performed with local anesthetic, a rubber mouth prop (also known as a *bite-block*) allows the patient to rest and relax the jaw muscles (Fig. 30–6).

During general anesthesia, a mouth prop (also

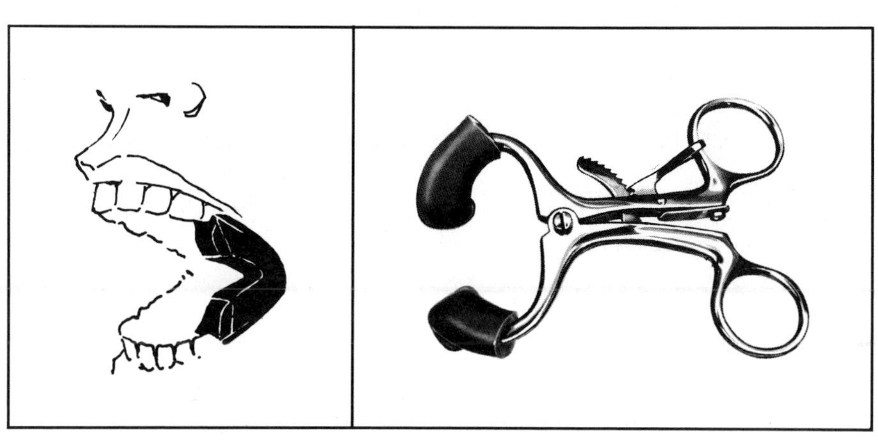

FIGURE 30–6

Mouth props. *Left,* This type of prop is used to aid a conscious patient in keeping his mouth open. *Right,* A mouth gag is used to hold open the mouth of an unconscious patient during general anesthesia. (Courtesy of Hu-Friedy Manufacturing, Inc., Chicago, IL.)

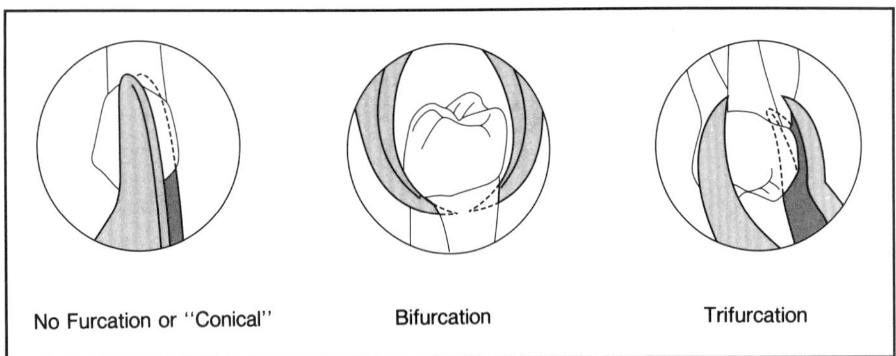

FIGURE 30–7

The tips of surgical forceps are designed to fit the crown and root structure of the tooth. (Courtesy of Hu-Friedy Manufacturing, Inc., Chicago, IL.)

known as a *mouth gag*) must be used to prevent involuntary closure of the patient's mouth.

The mouth prop is placed on the side of the mouth opposite the area being treated. These rubber blocks are available in sizes for children and adults. Care should be taken to select a bite-block that provides access to the oral cavity for the dentist and yet is comfortable for the patient.

SURGICAL CHISELS AND MALLETS

When there is a need to remove bone to facilitate the removal of a tooth or to reshape bone, surgical chisels and a mallet can be used (see Figs. 30–2 and 30–3). Surgical chisels can also be used when it is necessary to split teeth before surgical removal.

Surgical chisels are available in either a single bevel or bi-bevel design. The single-bevel type (bevel on one side of the edge) is used for removing bone. The bi-bevel type (bevel on both sides of the edge) is used for splitting teeth.

Some chisels are designed for use with a hand mallet. Another type is driven by a surgical handpiece driven by an electrical surgical system.

SURGICAL ASPIRATING TIPS

The primary objective of surgical aspiration is to provide a clear field of vision for the surgeon. The aspirator tips used in oral surgery are much smaller than those used in restorative dentistry. The smaller tips fit easily into the socket or surgical site (see Fig. 30–3).

Because the surgical aspirator tip is small and often slightly curved, it tends to clog easily with clotted blood, bone, and tooth fragments. To prevent this

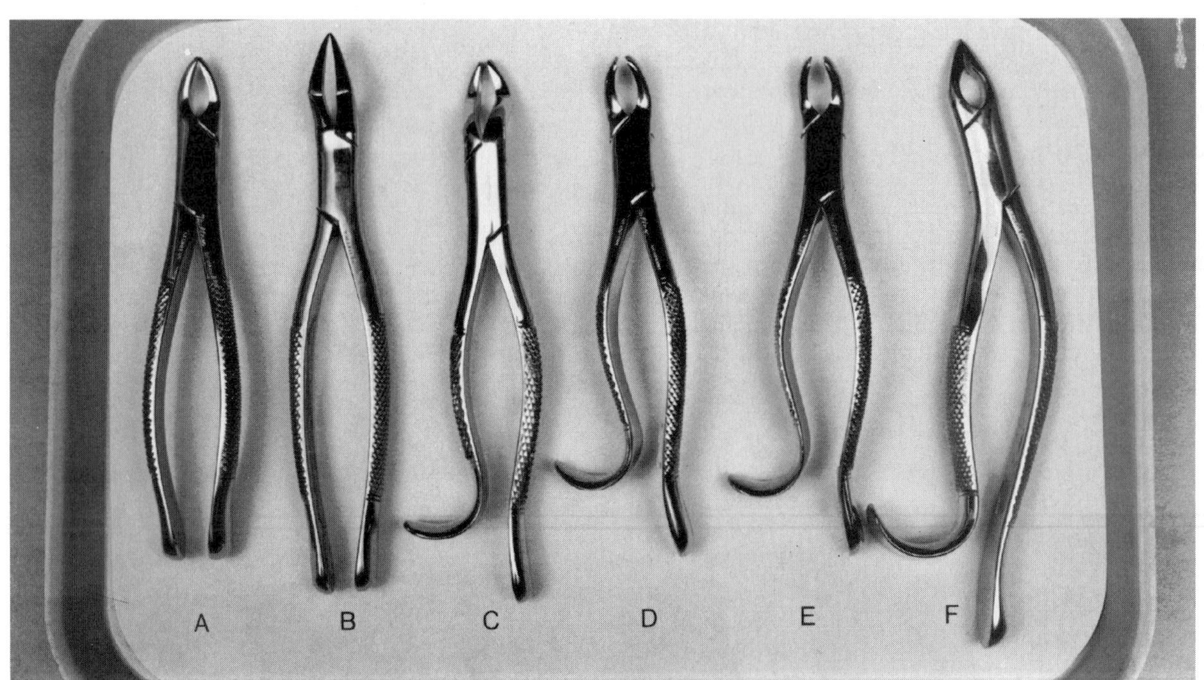

FIGURE 30–8

Maxillary extraction forceps. *A*, Maxillary No. 150 forceps (universal). *B*, Maxillary anterior forceps. *C*, Maxillary molar forceps. *D*, Maxillary molar forceps. *E*, Maxillary molar forceps. *F*, Maxillary premolar forceps.

from occurring, the aspirator tip is dipped into a container of sterile saline solution periodically during the procedure. This flushes the tip and cleans the line.

FORCEPS

Extraction forceps are available in many different shapes and designs to accommodate the oral surgeon's needs in grasping teeth with different crown shapes, root configurations, and location in the mouth (Figs. 30–7 to 30–9).

The beaks are shaped to grasp the crown of the tooth firmly at or below the cervical line. The inner surface of the beaks may be either plain (smooth finish) or serrated (rough) to provide additional grasping power when a tooth is extracted.

The handles are either horizontal (side by side) or vertical. The vertical design, which is used only in mandibular forceps, is referred to as a bird-beak forceps (see Fig. 30–9). The bayonet-type design, with horizontal handles, is used only on maxillary forceps.

Another variable is the angulation in the beaks of the forceps. As a rule, mandibular forceps have a greater angle to provide better access to the mandibular teeth.

The handles, which are held firmly in a palm grasp, provide the dentist with the leverage necessary to remove the tooth. Some handles are straight. Others have a hook on one handle to provide a better grasp.

The operator holds the forceps with the palm of the hand facing *upward* for maxillary extractions (see Fig.

TABLE 30–1

Commonly Used Forceps for Each Area of the Mouth

MAXILLARY FORCEPS

Anterior

Forceps No. 1 is a universal forceps that is used for incisors and cuspids

Complete Maxillary

Forceps No. 150 is a universal forceps that is used for maxillary premolars and molars and can also be used for cuspids and incisors

First and Second Molars

Forceps No. 18R and 18L (notice that these are supplied in right and left pairs)

Third Molars

Forceps No. 210 (the bayonet design assists in gaining access to the third molar area)

MANDIBULAR FORCEPS

Universal Mandibular

Forceps No. 151 is a universal mandibular forceps

First and Second Molars

Forceps Nos. 16 and 17 (the No. 16 forceps is often referred to as the "cowhorn" because of the unique design of the beaks, which are designed to fit into the bifurcation area of the tooth)

Third Molars

Forceps No. 222 (because of the lack of space in this area of the arch, these teeth are frequently extracted with a variety of forceps and elevators)

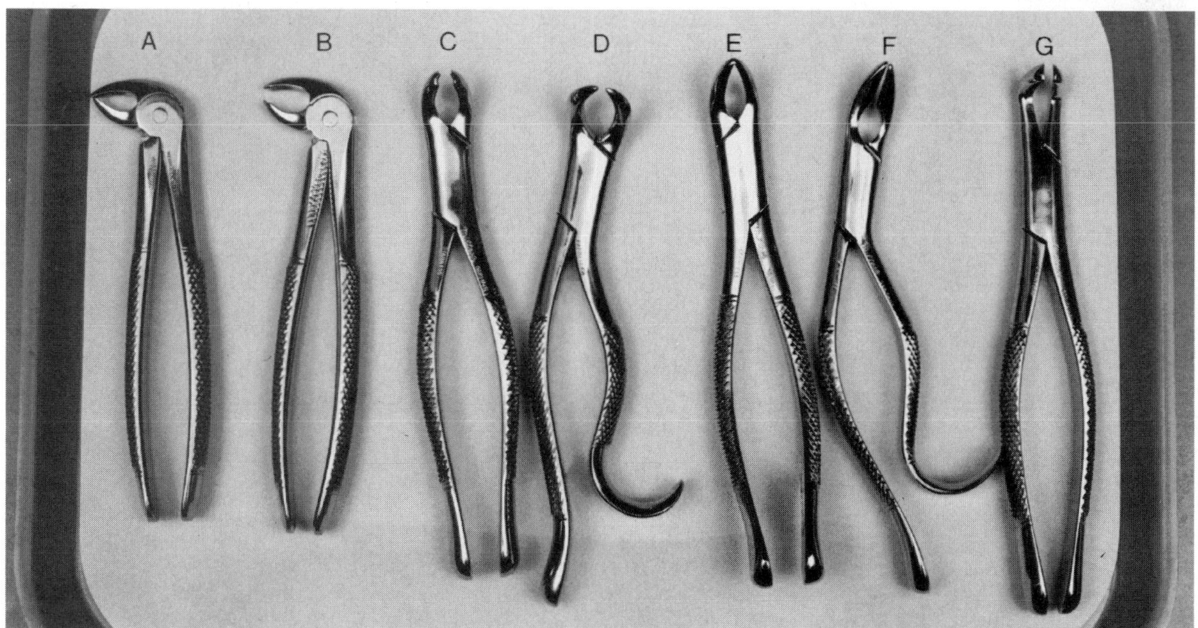

FIGURE 30–9

Mandibular extraction forceps. *A*, Bird-beak mandibular universal forceps. *B*, Bird-beak mandibular universal forceps. *C*, Mandibular universal forceps. *D*, Cowhorn mandibular molar forceps. *E*, Mandibular No. 101 forceps (universal). *F*, Mandibular posterior forceps. *G*, Mandibular third molar forceps.

30–14) and the palm of the hand facing *downward* for mandibular extractions (see Fig. 30–15).

Forceps are used to remove teeth from the alveolar bone after they have been slightly loosened with the elevators. Each dentist has his or her preferences in forceps designs. These preferences must be taken into consideration when the forceps to be used for an extraction are selected.

Forceps are divided into two basic types. One type, called **universal forceps**, are designed to be used on either the left or right side of the same arch. The other type is designed for use on specific teeth, and these

PROCEDURE: Performing a Surgical Scrub

1. Wet hands and forearms up to the elbows with warm water; then dispense about 5 ml. of antimicrobial soap (i.e., chlorhexidine gluconate) into cupped hands (Fig. 30–10).
2. Use a surgical scrub brush to scrub hands and forearms for 3 minutes.
3. Rinse thoroughly with warm water.
4. Dispense about 5 ml. of antimicrobial soap into cupped hands.
5. Wash for an additional 3 minutes without using a brush. Then rinse so that the contaminated water runs down the arms and off the elbows.
6. Dry hands and arms with a sterile, disposable towel.
7. Place surgical gloves on the hands, using sterile technique (Fig. 30–11).
   □ *RATIONALE:* The sterility of gloves used in surgical procedures must be maintained.

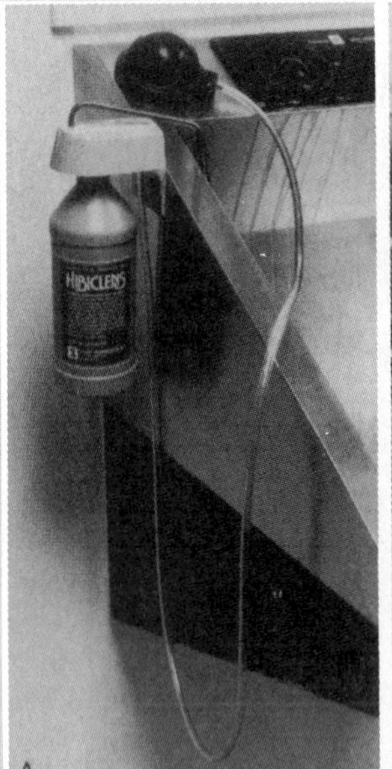

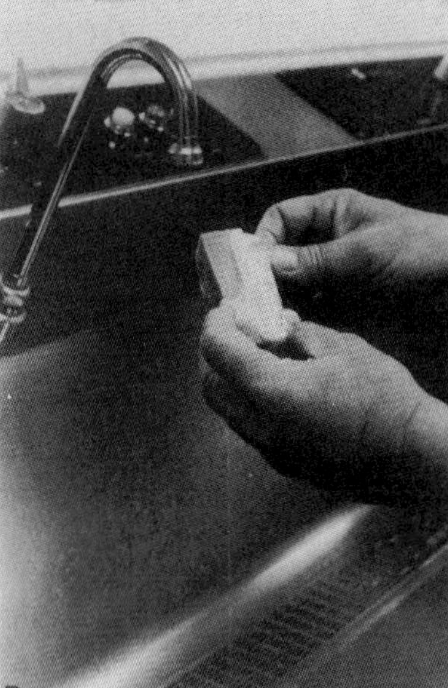

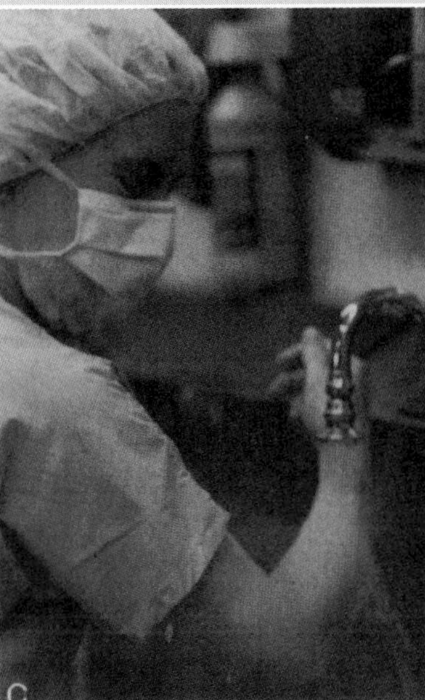

FIGURE 30–10

Surgical scrub. *A*, Antimicrobial surgical soap is dispensed with a foot-operated dispenser. *B*, A disposable sponge/brush is used to scrub the hands and forearms for 3 minutes. *C*, After the second scrub, the water used for rinsing is allowed to drain from the elbows so as not to recontaminate the hands. (From Pedersen, G.W.: Oral Surgery. Philadelphia, W.B. Saunders Co., 1988, p 7.)

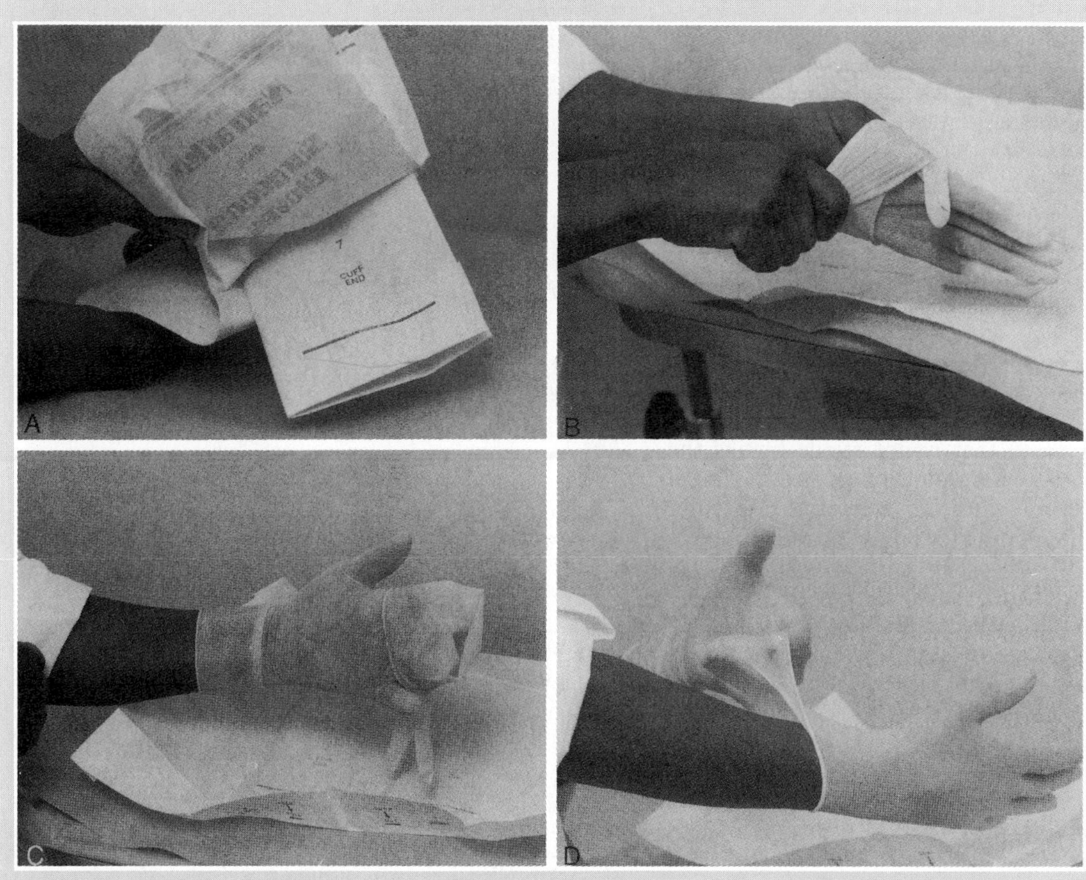

FIGURE 30–11

Gloving with sterile surgical gloves. *A*, The outer packaging is opened. The gloves remain on the surface of the inner pack when it is opened. *B*, The left glove is grasped by the inside of the cuff and the hand inserted. (This is the side that will be toward the hand.) *C*, The gloved left hand engages the outer surface of the right glove. (This is the side of the glove that remains sterile.) *D*, The right hand is inserted into the glove without touching the outer surface. (From Pedersen, G.W.: Oral Surgery. Philadelphia, W.B. Saunders Co., 1988, p 7.)

forceps are supplied as left and right pairs. The R in the forceps number indicates that the forceps is used on the patient's right. The L in the forceps number indicates that the forceps is used on the patient's left side.

Table 30–1 lists commonly used forceps for each area of the mouth. Additional forceps are shown in Figures 30–8 and 30–9. (Be aware that forceps names and numbering may vary by manufacturer.)

Forceps for Pediatric Dentistry. The forceps used in pediatric dentistry are smaller than those used on the permanent teeth. They are also designed to fit the shape of the primary teeth.

MAINTENANCE OF SURGICAL INSTRUMENTS

Surgical instruments require the following care to maintain proper function and appearance:

- Surgical instruments that cannot be cleaned immediately are placed in a holding solution.
  ☐ **Rationale:** Dried blood is very difficult to remove, and this solution prevents the blood from drying on the instruments.
- Hinged surgical instruments, such as forceps and hemostats, are placed in the ultrasonic cleaner with the hinge in an open position.
  ☐ **Rationale:** This allows the ultrasonic solution and action to reach the hinge and blade areas for cleaning.
- Thoroughly dry the forceps before sterilization.
  ☐ **Rationale:** This helps prevent rusting.
- Lubricate hinges of forceps with a silicone-type lubricant before sterilization.
  ☐ **Rationale:** This provides protection from rust and deposits that could interfere with the working action of the hinge.
- Remove forceps from the sterilizer while they are still hot.
  ☐ **Rationale:** This prevents moisture condensation that could cause rusting.

- Do not allow forceps to remain in water or steam for long periods.
  □ **Rationale:** This may cause rusting or corrosion.
- Never close a hinged instrument during sterilization.
  □ **Rationale:** Closing prevents adequate exposure to the sterilizing conditions, steam, or chemical vapors.

Chain of Asepsis

Asepsis means the absence from pathogenic microorganisms. Establishing and maintaining the chain of asepsis means that the instruments, surgical drapes, and gloved hands of the operating team must be sterile. Once established, the chain of asepsis must *not* be broken.

Contact with anything that is not sterile breaks the chain of asepsis and contaminates the surgical area. For example, if after gowning and gloving the assistant touches anything that is not sterile, the chain of asepsis is broken.

For this reason, the assistant does not perform the surgical scrub until all preparatory duties have been completed. Also, during oral surgery, sterile surgical gloves are worn. It is *not* acceptable to wear the examination gloves used for other procedures because these gloves are not sterile.

The Role of the Assistant

Every surgical procedure requires preparation and planning by the dental assistant. Following is a list of the dental assistant's responsibilities and when they need to be performed.

THE DAY BEFORE SURGERY

1. Check that all patient records and radiographs are complete and ready for use.
2. Verify that any information requested from the patient's physician has been received.
3. If a surgical stent or template is to be used, check that it has been returned by the dental laboratory and is properly sterilized.
4. If a prosthesis is to be placed, check that it has been returned by the dental laboratory sterilized and in a sealed pouch.
5. *Alternative:* If the prosthesis is not sterile, place it in a container and cover it with an appropriate high-level EPA-registered disinfectant.
6. Determine that the appropriate surgical setups have been prepared and sterilized.

JUST BEFORE SURGERY

1. Prepare the treatment room. This include disinfecting surfaces and placing protective barriers on anything that might be touched during the procedure.
2. Keep surgical instruments in their sterile wraps until they are set up on a sterile towel for the procedure. The surgical setup should be kept covered with a sterile towel until the procedure begins (Fig. 30–12).

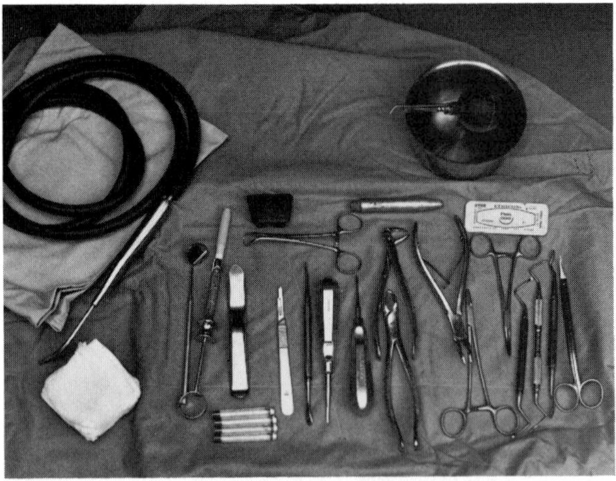

FIGURE 30–12

Sterile surgical tray ready for use. The inside of the cloth wrapping forms a sterile field for the instruments. (Courtesy of University of the Pacific School of Dentistry, San Francisco, CA.)

PATIENT PREPARATION

1. Check with the patient to determine that prescribed premedication was taken as directed. If not, the surgeon should be alerted immediately.
2. Ask the patient to empty his bladder before proceeding to the treatment room.
3. Seat the patient, and place a full-length patient drape.
4. Place a sterile towel over the patient's chest on top of the drape.
5. Adjust the dental chair to the proper position.

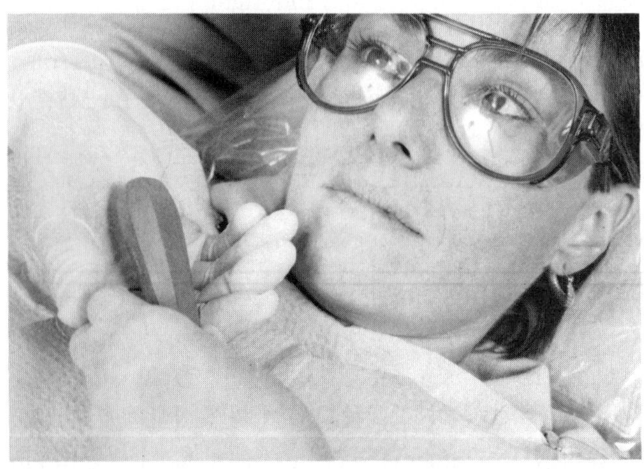

FIGURE 30–13

Transfer of the straight elevator to the surgeon.

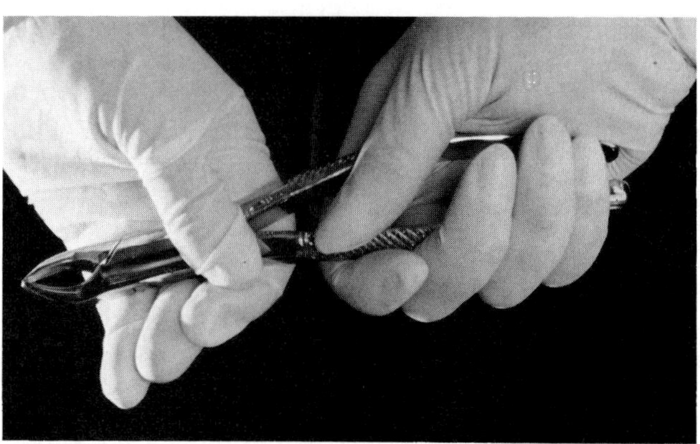

FIGURE 30–14

Transfer of No. 150 maxillary forceps. The surgeon, whose hand is shown on the right, receives the forceps in the position of use for a maxillary extraction.

6. Stay with the patient until the surgeon enters the treatment room.
   □ **Rationale**: It is essential to monitor the patient if premedication has been administered. Also, having someone present may help to ease the patient's apprehension.
7. Scrub and put on gloves just before the start of the procedure.

DURING SURGERY

1. Maintain the chain of asepsis.
2. Pass and receive instruments (Figs. 30–13 to 30–15.)
3. Aspirate and retract as needed.
4. Maintain a clear operating field with adequate light and irrigation.
5. Steady the patient's head and mandible if necessary.
6. Observe the patient's condition and anticipate the surgeon's needs.

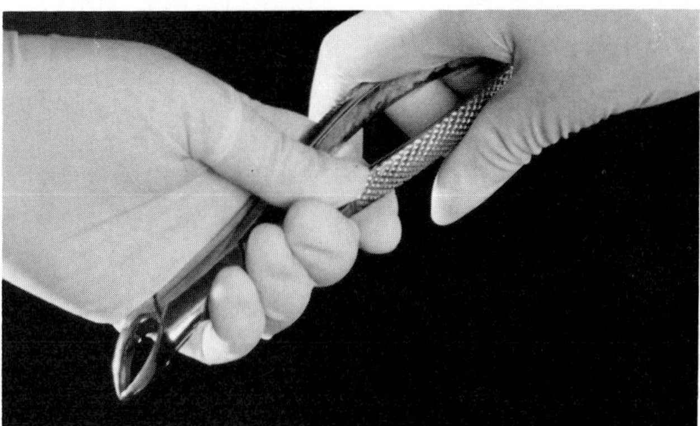

FIGURE 30–15

Transfer of No. 151 mandibular forceps. The surgeon, whose hand is shown on the right, receives the forceps in the position of use for a mandibular extraction.

Immediate Postoperative Care

INSTRUCTIONS TO AND DISMISSAL OF THE PATIENT

In accordance with the directions of the surgeon, the assistant provides the postoperative instructions to the patient. Instructions for home care should be provided in both written and verbal forms.

If the patient is non–English-speaking, the assistant should be certain that the person accompanying the patient understands the instructions and is also given a copy of the written instructions.

Control of Bleeding

The patient is given the following instructions regarding the control of bleeding:

- A pressure pack made of folded sterile gauze sponges has been placed over the socket to control bleeding and to encourage clot formation and healing.
- Keep the pack in place for at least another 30 minutes. If the pack is removed too soon, this will disturb clot formation and may increase bleeding.
- If bleeding continues, moisten a tea bag, place it over the surgical site, and bite firmly for about 20 minutes to apply pressure. Tea contains tannic acid, which aids in clotting.
- If bleeding increases or does not stop, call the dental office.
- It is recommended that strenuous work or physical activity be restricted for a few days. (This is to avoid hemorrhage at the site of the surgery.)

Control of Swelling

The patient is given the following instructions regarding the control of swelling:

- Because ibuprofen has anti-inflammatory qualities, the dentist may recommend that the patient take one or two doses before the surgery and then continue taking the medication as instructed after the surgery. (Taking the drug before the surgery aids in preventing the swelling after the surgery.)
- During the first 24 hours, a cold pack (an ice bag covered with a towel or commercially prepared cold packs) is usually placed in a cycle of 20 minutes on and 20 minutes off. (Cold slows the circulation in these tissues and controls swelling.)
- After the first 24 hours, external heat may be applied to the face to promote healing. (Heat increases circulation and promotes healing.)
- After the first 24 hours, gently rinse the oral cavity with warm saline solution (salt water) every 2 hours. (The percentage of salt in the solution should be approximately 1 teaspoon of salt to 8 ounces of warm water. A stronger solution will irritate the tissue.)

Control of Pain

Analgesics, most commonly in the form of aspirin or ibuprofen, are used to control minor discomfort after surgery.

If the patient is in extreme discomfort, stronger analgesics such as codeine and aspirin may be prescribed by the dentist. All prescriptions are recorded in the patient's chart.

Control of Infection

Antibiotics are administered to control any infection expected to arise after surgery. Each prescription is recorded in the patient's chart.

Penicillin is frequently used for gram-positive infections of the oral cavity. Penicillins G and V are the most commonly prescribed.

Precaution: Many patients have an allergic reaction to any form of penicillin. The dentist always reviews the patient's allergies before prescribing any medication.

Erythromycin is effective against gram-positive organisms, and 250 mg. every 6 hours is the usual adult dose.

Precaution: Gastrointestinal disturbances may be noticed in some patients who are given erythromycin.

Diet and Nutrition

A soft diet may be recommended for a few days after surgery. Good nutrition is especially important during the healing process. It is important for the patient to take in more than the usual quantities of water and fruit juices. Some surgeons prescribe vitamin supplements, particularly vitamins C and B complex for patients after surgery.

POSTOPERATIVE VISIT

A postoperative visit may be scheduled so that the surgeon can check on healing and, if necessary, remove the sutures.

After extensive surgery, the surgeon may request postoperative radiographs to ascertain the removal of the pathological condition and the extent of healing.

Within 6 to 8 weeks after surgery, the formation of regenerative bone may be detected on the radiograph.

ALVEOLITIS (DRY SOCKET)

After a tooth is extracted, healing begins immediately with blood oozing into the socket and forming a clot. The clot is later replaced by granulation tissue and ultimately by bone as healing progresses.

Failure of the normal healing process may result in alveolitis, which is also known as a *dry socket*. If the blood clot does not remain in the socket or is disturbed, this very painful condition may occur 2 to 4 days after the removal of a tooth.

The patient complains of severe pain and a foul odor and taste in his mouth. When the socket is inspected, there is no blood clot, and the bone is exposed to the oral environment.

The exact cause of this complication is not clear; however, several factors seem to be involved, including

- Inadequate blood supply to the socket as a result of individual anatomic deficiencies
- Excessive trauma to the alveolus (socket) during the extraction process
- Diminished blood supply to the socket as a result of the vasoconstriction action of the local anesthetic
- Preoperative or postoperative infection interfering with the normal healing process
- Accidental dislodging of the clot by the patient from vigorous rinsing, smoking, or sucking on a straw to drink liquids
- Existing nutritional deficiencies in the patient
- Foreign debris contaminating the alveolus either during the surgery or immediately afterward

Treatment of this condition is palliative; that is, it is intended to make the patient comfortable while the wound heals. The healing process can take from 10 to 40 days.

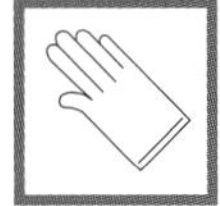 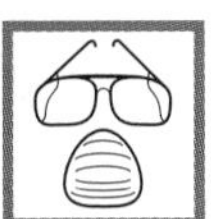 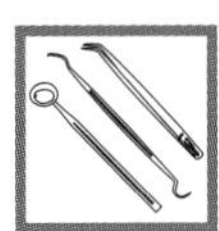 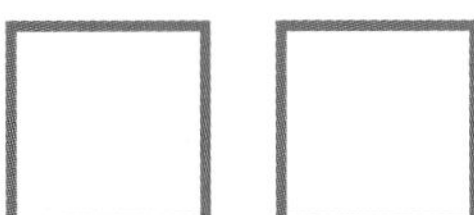

PROCEDURE: **Treating Alveolitis**

Although exact treatment varies between dentists, the typical sequence is as follows:

Instrumentation

Scissors
Irrigation syringe
Warm saline solution
Iodoform gauze
Medicated dressing such as Bipps paste (Bipps paste is a combination of benzocaine, subnitrate, iodoform, and petrolatum)
High-volume evacuator (HVE) tip

Treatment

1. The alveolus (socket) is gently irrigated with warm saline solution.
   □ *RATIONALE:* This removes accumulated debris from the alveolus. Some surgeons also curette the socket to stimulate the formation of a new clot.
2. A narrow strip of iodoform gauze is cut to a length that fills the alveolus.
   □ *RATIONALE:* The iodoform in the gauze is a topical antiseptic that helps prevent infection. The gauze prevents food from being packed into the alveolus.
3. The gauze is dipped in the medication and gently packed into the alveolus.
   □ *RATIONALE:* The medication soothes nerve endings in the exposed bone.
4. The dentist often prescribes analgesics to relieve the pain until the exposed bone is covered sufficiently by a layer of granulation tissue as healing progresses.
   □ *RATIONALE:* Analgesics make the patient more comfortable until the pain diminishes as healing progresses.
5. The patient is dismissed. As needed, the patient is asked to return every 1 to 2 days to repeat this procedure.

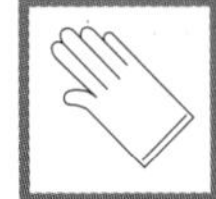 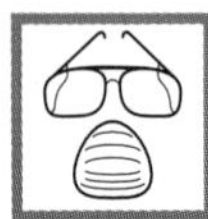 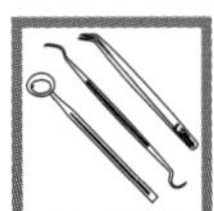 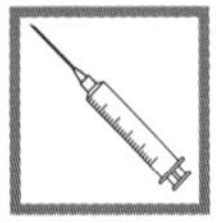  

PROCEDURE: **Performing a Forceps Extraction**

Forceps extractions are often described as "routine" or "simple" extractions. These terms are misleading because all extractions are surgical procedures. These terms are meant to imply that the extraction can be done without extensive instrumentation or complication during the procedure.

A forceps extraction is usually performed on a tooth that is (1) at least partially erupted and (2) has a solid, intact crown.

Instrumentation

Sterile surgical gloves
Periosteal elevator
Elevator (of operator's choice)
Forceps (of operator's choice)
Surgical curette
Sterile gauze sponges
Surgical aspirator tip

The Forceps Extraction

1. The local anesthetic is administered. More than one injection may be required to provide adequate anesthesia.
2. Using a sharp instrument, such as an explorer, the surgeon gently probes the gingiva surrounding the tooth to be extracted.
   □ *RATIONALE:* This is to be certain that there is adequate anesthesia.
3. The patient is advised that it is normal to feel some pressure during the extraction. The patient is also advised that is normal to hear grating or cracking sounds during the extraction.
4. Using a periosteal elevator, the surgeon gently loosens the gingival tissue and compresses the alveolar bone surrounding the neck of the tooth.
5. If it is indicated, the surgeon may use the elevator to loosen the tooth before placement of the forceps.
6. The beaks of the forceps are placed on the tooth and seated firmly to grasp the tooth around the cementoenamel junction.
7. The tooth is luxated in the socket to compress the bone and enlarge the socket. When this is complete, the tooth can be freely lifted, not pulled, from the socket. (**Luxate** means to rock back and forth.)
8. The extracted tooth is examined to be certain that the root has not been fractured and a fragment left in the socket.
   □ *NOTE:* If the root tip has fractured, the surgeon uses root picks and apical elevators to remove the fragments. The assistant suctions the socket frequently to keep the tip visible. If the suction loosens the root tip, it is removed from the aspirating tip and examined to be certain that all fragments have been removed.
9. The suction tip is used to debride the surgical site. Tooth fragments, carious tooth structure, and broken pieces of restorative material may have been left in the open alveolus after the tooth has been removed.
   □ *RATIONALE:* It is important to remove any debris so that it does not become embedded in the tissue because this may cause irritation or infection.
10. If indicated, sutures are placed to close the surgical site. Most forceps extractions do not require suturing.
11. Several moistened sterile gauze sponges are folded into a tight pad to form a pressure pack. The cheek is retracted, and the folded gauze is placed over the extraction site and toward the cheek.
    □ *RATIONALE:* Positioning the pressure pack toward the cheek minimizes gagging and patient discomfort.
12. The patient is instructed to bite on the pack for at least 30 minutes.
    □ *RATIONALE:* This pressure pack aids in control of bleeding and in the formation of the clot.
13. The dental chair is slowly moved to an upright position, and the patient is given postoperative instructions.
    □ *RATIONALE:* The patient is most comfortable in this position and is better able to communicate.

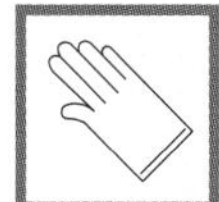
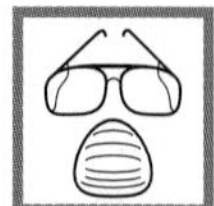
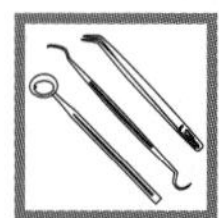
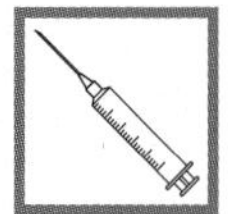

PROCEDURE: Performing Multiple Extractions and an Alveoloplasty

When several teeth are to be extracted at the same time, the basic extraction procedure is essentially the same as for a single extraction. However, when several teeth are to be extracted, the surgeon must also surgically contour the remaining bone and soft tissue.

This procedure, called an **alveoloplasty**, is the surgical reduction and reshaping of the alveolar ridge. It is performed to provide a properly contoured edentulous ridge on which to fit a denture.

Instrumentation

Single extraction setup
Additional forceps (as indicated)
Rongeur
Bone file
Suture placement setup
Sterile saline solution

Performing Multiple Extractions and Alveoloplasty

1. After the teeth have been extracted, the rongeur is used to trim the alveolus. After each cut with the rongeur, the assistant uses a sterile gauze sponge to carefully remove any debris from the blades.
2. After use of the rongeur, the bone file is used to finish smoothing rough edges.
3. The surgical site is irrigated to remove any bone fragments.
4. The mucosa is repositioned over the ridge and sutured into place.
5. Pressure packs made of sterile gauze sponges are positioned as needed.

Complex Extractions

The term **complex extraction** is used when conditions exist that require additional skill, effort, and instrumentation to remove the tooth. A complex extraction may also involve one or more of the following procedures during or after the extraction:

- Removal of impacted teeth
- Ostectomy (removal of bone)
- Tooth sectioning (dividing the tooth into parts for removal)
- Recovery of fractured roots
- Mucoperiosteal flap removal
- Soft tissue resection

Dental Surgical Procedures

BONE REMOVAL AND SPLITTING TEETH

A surgical mallet and chisel, as shown in Figures 30–1 and 30–2, are designed for use when it is necessary to remove bone or split a tooth before its extraction.

An alternative method is the use of a surgical system, as shown in Figure 30–16, that consists of

- High- or low-speed micro motors
- Irrigating system for cooling and debridement
- RPM digital display
- Foot-operated control
- Surgical handpiece (various types)
- Electric motor
- Assorted dental burs

When the handpiece is used, irrigation with sterile water is necessary to reduce frictional heat from the bur, remove tooth and bone fragments, and maintain visibility for the operator.

SUTURES

As a rule, if a scalpel has been used, sutures are needed to control bleeding and promote healing. The suture material is threaded into a curved suture needle. The threaded needle is held in a hemostat or needle holder as the surgeon guides it through the tissue. Most commonly used are suture needles that are supplied already threaded and in a sterile pack.

Suture material is available in both **absorbable** and **nonabsorbable** varieties. The absorbable sutures include gut, collagen, and polydioxanone. These sutures are readily absorbed by the body and do not have to be removed.

The nonabsorbable suture materials include silk, nylon, and polypropylene. Black silk suture material is popular because of its easy manipulation, durability, visibility and strength.

Silk sutures are usually removed approximately 5 to 7 days after surgery, provided adequate healing has taken place. The number of sutures placed is noted on the patient's chart. An accurate count is important because the sutures must be counted again at the time of removal. This is to be certain that all of the sutures have been removed and that none remain.

Suture Placement Instrumentation. When sutures are to be placed, add the following to the instrument tray: sterile prethreaded suture needle, suture scissors, and a hemostat or needle holder.

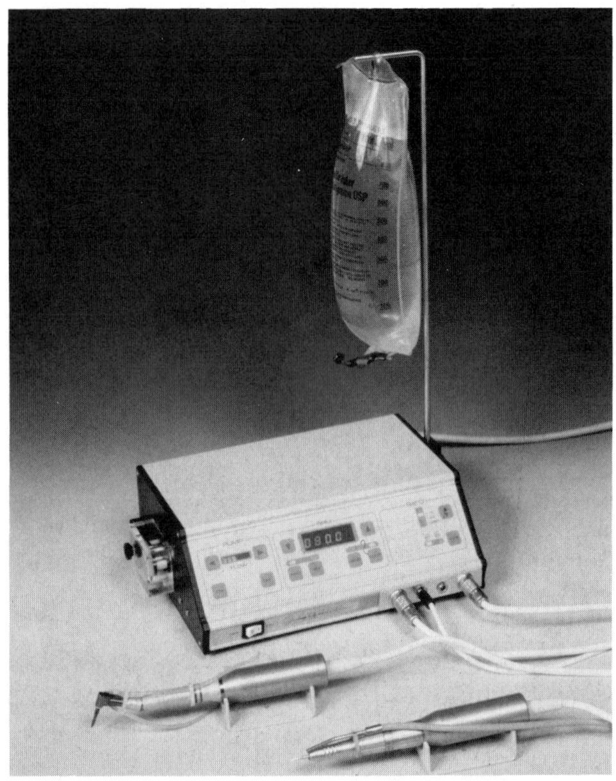

FIGURE 30–16

Surgical handpiece system. (Courtesy Aspetico, Kirkland, WA.)

Biopsy Procedures

A biopsy is a process in which tissues are removed and examined to distinguish malignancies (cancers) from other nonmalignant (noncancerous) lesions in the oral cavity.

The three most common biopsy procedures used in dentistry are incisional biopsy, excisional biopsy, and exfoliative cytology.

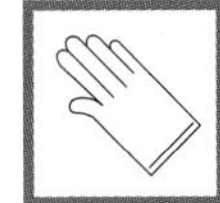
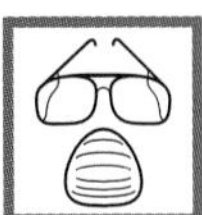
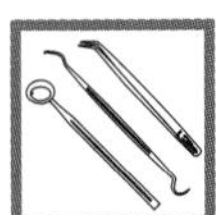
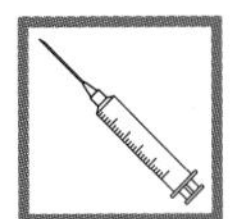

PROCEDURE: **Removing an Impacted Third Molar**

The extraction of an impacted mandibular third molar is an example of a complex extraction. It can involve several of the aforementioned conditions.

Instrumentation

Sterile surgical gloves
Scalpel, No. 15 blade
Periosteal elevator
Extraction elevators
Extraction forceps
Rongeur forceps
Bone file
Surgical curette
Root tip picks
Conventional handpiece with surgical bur or mallet and chisels
Irrigating syringe
Sterile saline solution
Surgical evacuator tip
Sterile suture material and needle
Needle holder or hemostat
Suture scissors
Sterile gauze sponges

Reaching the Tooth

1. The surgeon determines that adequate anesthesia has been achieved.
2. The surgeon makes the initial incision along the ridge distal to the second molar. The incision is made through both the gingival mucosa and the periosteum that covers the underlying bone.
3. The mucoperiosteum (combination of mucosa and periosteum) is lifted from the bone with the periosteal elevator.
4. Once the incision is made, the assistant must constantly evacuate blood from the surgical site.
5. The surgeon removes the bony covering from the impacted tooth with either a surgical mallet and chisels or a surgical handpiece with surgical burs.
6. The surgical site is irrigated with sterile saline solution and evacuated to remove bone fragments and improve visibility.

Removing the Tooth

1. When the surgeon has uncovered the impacted tooth, it can be luxated and lifted from the alveolus with extraction elevators or forceps.
2. In some cases, an impacted third molar is lodged between the ramus of the mandible and the distal surface of the second molar. This may necessitate sectioning the crown of the impacted teeth with either the mallet and chisel or the surgical bur.
   □ *RATIONALE:* Sectioning involves dividing the tooth into two or more parts to facilitate removal.
3. After the tooth has been removed, the surgical site is curetted, irrigated, and evacuated to remove all debris.
4. After thorough debridement, the surgeon returns the mucoperiosteal flap to its normal position over the wound and sutures it into place.
5. The patient is slowly returned to the upright position and allowed to remain seated until he feels comfortable enough to move.
6. Some surgeons provide the patient with a cold pack to apply immediately to the face over the surgical site.
   □ *RATIONALE:* This aids in minimizing postoperative swelling.
7. Postoperative instructions are given.

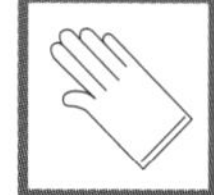
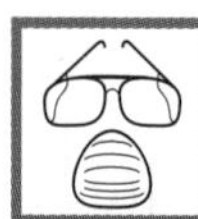
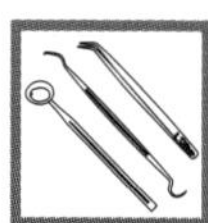
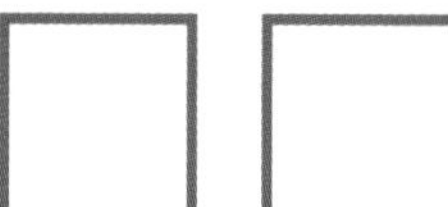

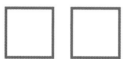

PROCEDURE: **Removing Sutures**

In some states, suture removal is delegated to the dental assistant. However, this procedure is performed only *after* the dentist has inspected the surgical site for adequate healing.

Suture Removal Instrumentation

Cotton-tipped applicators
2 × 2 inch gauze sponges
Solution for disinfecting surgical site
Suture scissors
Cotton pliers

Suture Removal

1. Locate and account for all the sutures placed during the surgical appointment (Fig. 30–17*A*).
2. Use antiseptic solution on a cotton-tipped applicator to swab the wound (see Fig. 30–17*B*).
   □ *RATIONALE:* This removes any debris that might contaminate the wound.
4. Use the cotton pliers to lift the suture by the knot. With the other hand, use the scissors to cut the suture as close as possible to the tissue (see Fig. 30–17*C*).
   □ *RATIONALE:* Contaminated suture material must *not* be passed through the tissue.
5. Use the cotton pliers to gently pull the suture material from the tissue (see Fig. 30–17*D*).
   □ *RATIONALE:* The knot is never pulled through because it would injure the tissues.
6. Repeat these steps until all sutures have been removed.
7. Recheck the wound to make sure all sutures have been removed.
8. If there is any bleeding, a compress may be held briefly on the surgical site to encourage clotting.

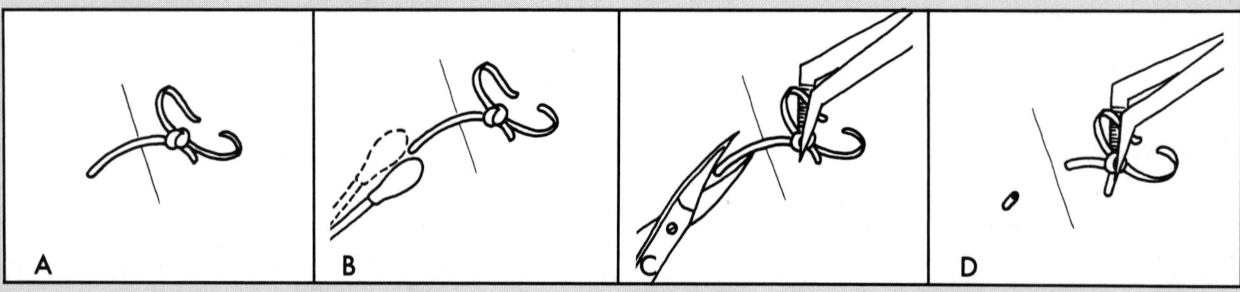

FIGURE 30–17

Suture removal steps. *A*, Suture site. Note the location of the knot. *B*, The suture and tissue are swabbed with antiseptic solution. *C*, The knot is grasped with sterile pliers, the blade of suture scissors is slid under the suture, and then the suture is cut. *D*, The suture is gently pulled through the tissue.

EXCISIONAL BIOPSY

Excisional biopsy involves the removal of the entire lesion plus some adjacent normal tissue (Fig. 30–18). This procedure is ideal for small lesions in which complete removal would not create esthetic or functional problems. For example, a small, nonhealing sore on the labial mucosa may be completely removed during the biopsy.

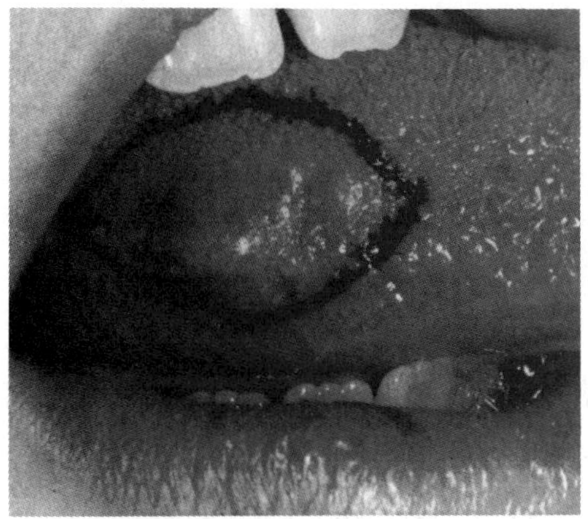

FIGURE 30–18

The planned incision for an excisional biopsy. (From Pedersen, G.W.: Oral Surgery. Philadelphia, W.B. Saunders Co., 1988, p 160.)

INCISIONAL BIOPSY

When a lesion is located in an area that would be cosmetically or functionally impaired by surgery, an incisional biopsy is often indicated.

An incisional biopsy is also indicated when the lesion is larger than 1 cm. in all dimensions. In this technique, the surgeon cuts a wedge of tissue from the lesion, along with some normal tissue to be used for comparison. Complete surgical removal of the lesion is not performed until a final diagnosis of the type of lesion is made.

EXFOLIATIVE CYTOLOGY

This is a nonsurgical technique that is helpful in diagnosing oral lesions. The surface of the lesion is scraped or wiped to gather a sample of the cells. The cells are spread onto a glass slide for microscopic examination. This procedure has limitations and is considered an adjunct to the surgical techniques mentioned earlier.

RESULTS OF BIOPSIES

The pathology report indicates whether the lesion is malignant or benign (noncancerous).

Nonmalignant tumors and cysts are removed if their size and location interfere with appearance and normal function. If they do not interfere and do not pose a threat to the patient, removal may be postponed. However, the situation must be reviewed regularly to determine whether the tumor has changed in size or shape.

Informing the patient of a **malignant tumor** requires kindness, empathy, and special tact. In general, this is never done by telephone; the ideal situation is for the dentist to tell the patient in person with a close family member present. A malignant tumor dictates immediate treatment by a qualified specialist.

Dental Implants

When natural teeth are lost, it is very difficult to duplicate their function and appearance; however, dental implants are a step closer to providing artificial teeth that look natural and feel secure in the mouth.

Dental implants attach artificial teeth to anchors (similar to posts) that have been surgically embedded into the bone (Fig. 30–19). The implant process involves several steps and may take from 6 to 9 months to complete. Depending upon the type of implant, the steps may vary. Many dental implant surgeries are done in the dental office. Depending on the type of implant and the patient's general health, the dentist may prefer to perform the implant surgery in a hospital.

Placing dental implants, which involves both surgery and the placement of a prosthesis, may require the services of several specialists. Dental implants are placed by periodontists, maxillofacial surgeons, prosthodontists, and implantologists (general dentists with specialized training).

The category of the clinician placing the implants is less important than the ability, experience, and education of the clinician involved. It is important for the

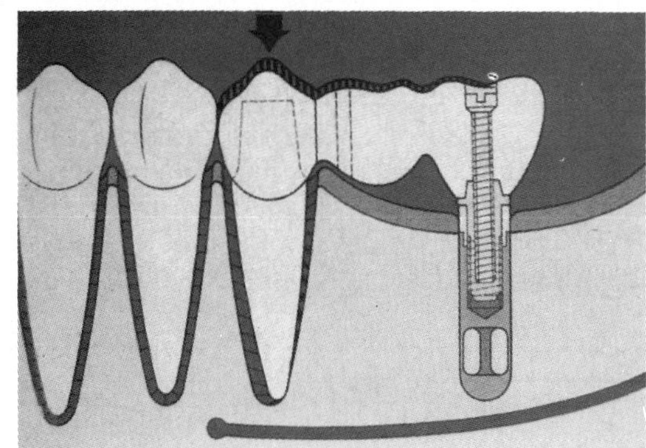

FIGURE 30–19

Diagram of an endoseous implant used as the posterior abutment for a three-unit fixed bridge. (From Babbush, C.A.: Dental Implants: Principles and Practice. Philadelphia, W.B. Saunders Co., 1991, Fig. 5-4.)

clinician to have an in-depth knowledge about both surgical and prosthodontic aspects of implants.

Advantages of Dental Implants

Dental implants are most often indicated when traditional dentistry is the least adequate. For example, lower full dentures have a very low rate of patient satisfaction, and implant dentistry has a very good chance of solving the problems associated with a mandibular denture. On the other hand, the placement of a three-unit fixed bridge has a very high success rate, so consideration of implants in these cases is less likely.

When properly placed, dental implants have a success rate of over 90 percent. With effective home care and regular dental visits, dental implants have lasted as long as 20 years and may last a lifetime.

Dental implants can

- Replace one or more teeth as single units with crowns
- Provide support for a partial denture
- Increase support, stability, and patient satisfaction for a full lower denture
- Increase patient comfort in chewing
- Increase patient confidence in smiling and speaking

Disadvantages of Dental Implants

As with any dental procedure, dental implants involve some risk. Because each patient is unique, implant success cannot be guaranteed. The following should be considered when implant options are discussed:

- The financial investment is greater than that for a conventional bridge or denture.
- Treatment can take up to 9 months to complete.
- As with any surgical procedure, there is a risk of infection and other complications.
- Occasionally, an implant may loosen and require replacement.
- Patients with certain medical complications are not good candidates for dental implants. These conditions include leukemia, severe valvular heart disease, a seriously compromised immune system, and any other chronic conditions that impede healing.

Selection of the Dental Implant Patient

Dental implants are not for everyone. The ideal candidate has good general health, has adequate alveolar bone, and is willing to commit to conscientious oral hygiene and regular dental visits.

A comprehensive evaluation is essential to determine whether the patient is likely to benefit from dental implants. This includes psychological, dental, and medical evaluations. The patient also requires specialized radiographs and impressions for the creation of diagnostic casts and the surgical stents.

PSYCHOLOGICAL EVALUATION

The psychological evaluation takes place at the initial visit. The dentist assesses the patient's attitude, ability to cooperate during complex procedures and overall outlook on dental treatment. The dentist also determines that the patient has realistic expectations about dental implants.

DENTAL EXAMINATION

During the dental examination, the dentist evaluates the condition of the teeth and soft tissues, areas of attached and unattached tissue, and the height and width of edentulous areas. This information is necessary in determining the best location to place the implants.

MEDICAL HISTORY AND EVALUATION

The purpose of the medical history and evaluation is to assess any existing medical conditions that could worsen as a result of the stress of implant surgery. Any medical conditions that could interfere with normal healing must be carefully evaluated.

SPECIALIZED RADIOGRAPHS

Diagnostic aids such as panographic x-rays, lateral cephalometric x-rays, and tomograms are needed to evaluate the height, width, and quality of the bone.

These films are also useful in locating the exact position of anatomic structures such as the inferior alveolar nerve, mental foramen, maxillary sinus, and nasal floor.

DIAGNOSTIC CASTS AND SURGICAL STENTS

Diagnostic casts, which are discussed in Chapter 19, also help the dentist in planning the implants. In addition, the cast is used to make a surgical stent.

A **surgical stent**, which covers the area of surgery, is made from clear acrylic. Also known as a *template*, it acts as a guide during surgery to place the implants in their proper location (Fig. 30–20). The stent *must* be sterilized before use.

Types of Dental Implants

There are several types of implants. Two types of implants that the American Dental Association (ADA) considers to be safe are **endosteal implants** and **subperiosteal implants**. One factor in determining the type of implant to use is whether or not there is adequate bone to support the implant.

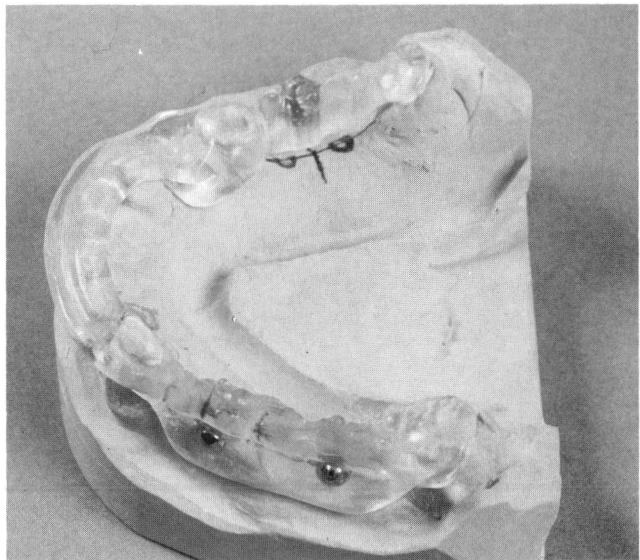

FIGURE 30–20

Custom stent is used to aid the dentist in placing the implants. The metal ball bearings serve as radiographic markers.

ENDOSTEAL IMPLANTS

Endosteal implants, also known as *osseointegrated integrated implants*, are surgically placed *into* the bone (Fig. 30–21). (**Endosteal** means within the bone.) These implants have three components:

- The **titanium implant,** which is surgically embedded into the bone during the stage I surgery
- The **titanium abutment screw,** which is screwed into the implant after osseointegration of the implant has occurred; the abutment screw is placed during the stage II surgery
- The **abutment post or cylinder,** which attaches to the artificial teeth or denture

The implants and abutment screws are frequently made from a metal called titanium because it is very compatible with bone and oral tissues.

The titanium implants can be coated with hydroxyapatite (HA), a ceramic substance that rapidly osseointegrates the implant to the bone. (**Osseointegration** is the attachment of healthy bone to the dental implant.)

After the osseointegration process has occurred (which can take from 3 to 6 months), the abutment screw is screwed into the implant, and the artificial teeth are then attached to the abutment post.

An adequate amount of alveolar bone is required for this type of implant to be successful. Two surgeries are required: in the first surgery, the implant is placed into the bone, and in the second surgery, the abutment screw is screwed into the anchor.

After both surgeries are complete and the tissues have healed, the patient begins the restorative phase in which the final crown, bridge, or partial denture is fabricated. The entire process can require from 3 to 9 months to reach completion.

MANDIBULAR SUBPERIOSTEAL IMPLANTS

A mandibular subperiosteal implant is a metal frame that is placed under the periosteum and *on top* of the bone. In contrast to an endosteal implant, it is *not* placed into the bone (Fig. 30–22). These implants are indicated for patients who do not have enough ridge remaining in the mandible to support the endosteal type implant. Subperiosteal implants are used most frequently to support a mandibular complete denture (Fig. 30–23).

Two surgeries are required. During the first, the alveolar ridge is exposed and impressions are taken of the alveolar ridge. After the impressions are taken, the tissue is repositioned over the ridge and sutured back into place. The impression is sent to a dental laboratory, where a metal frame with posts is constructed.

After the frame has been constructed, the second surgery is performed. The alveolar ridge is again surgically exposed and the metal frame is placed over the ridge. When the frame is in place, the tissues are repositioned and sutured in place.

Techniques that are still experimental are being developed with the use of computer analysis and imaging in place of the first surgery and impression.

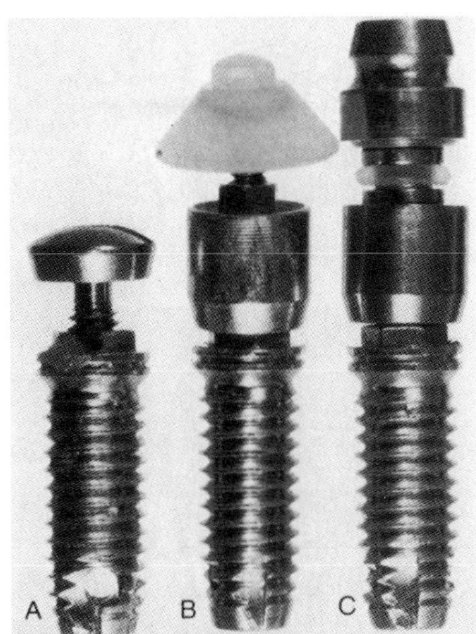

FIGURE 30–21

Treatment stages in the placement of osseointegrated implants. *A*, Stage I surgery consists of preparation of bone and insertion of a screw-shaped titanium implant and a titanium cover screw. *B*, At Stage II surgery, the cover screw is removed, and a titanium abutment is secured. A plastic healing cap is also placed. *C*, In the prosthodontic phase of treatment, a prosthesis is designed and constructed. It will be retained by the implant assembly by means of a gold screw. (From Babbush, C.A.: Dental Implants: Principles and Practice. Philadelphia, W.B. Saunders Co., 1991, p 112.)

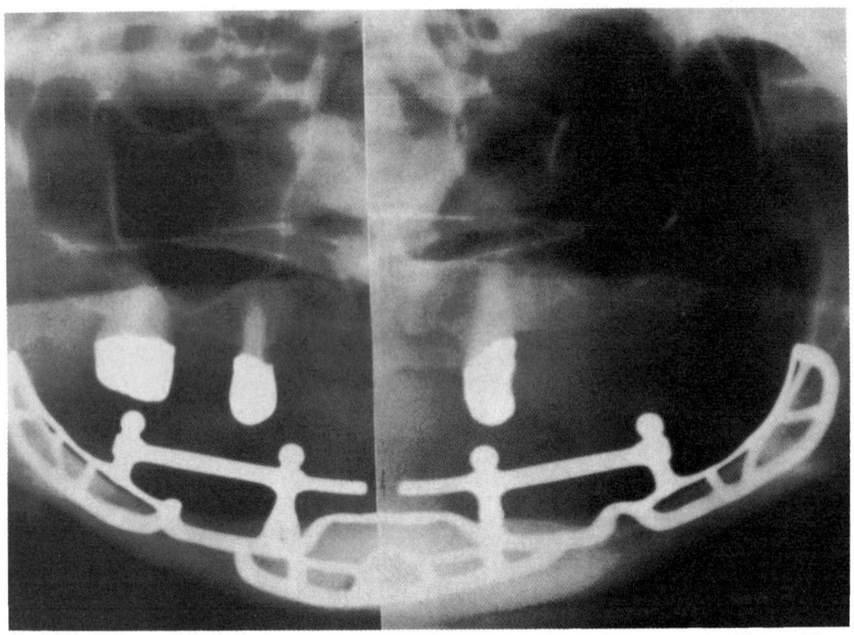

FIGURE 30–22

Panoramic radiograph view of mandibular subperiosteal implant. (From Babbush, C.A.: Dental Implants: Principles and Practice. Philadelphia, W.B. Saunders Co., 1991, p 225.)

Surgical Procedures for Standard Implants

PREOPERATIVE GUIDELINES

Written informed patient consent is required before treatment of the implant patient begins. The consent form should advise the patient of the expected results and of the associated risks involved with the surgical procedure. The patient should be informed that there is no guarantee of success and, if successful, the implants may not last forever.

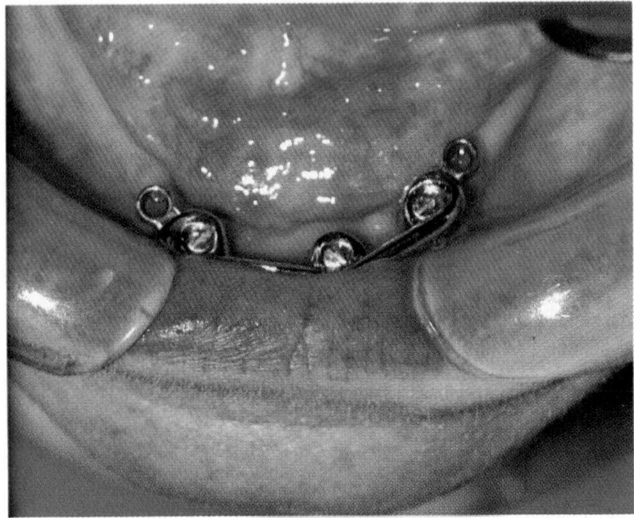

A

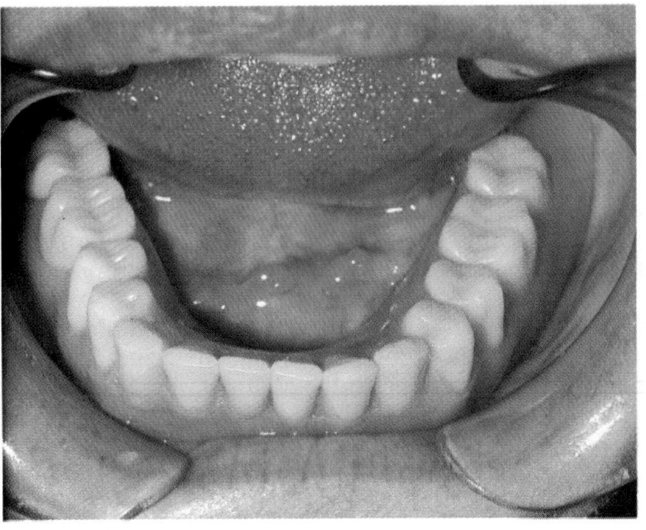

B

FIGURE 30–23

Subperiosteal implant to support a mandibular complete denture. *A*, Healed implant attachments. *B*, Denture in place.

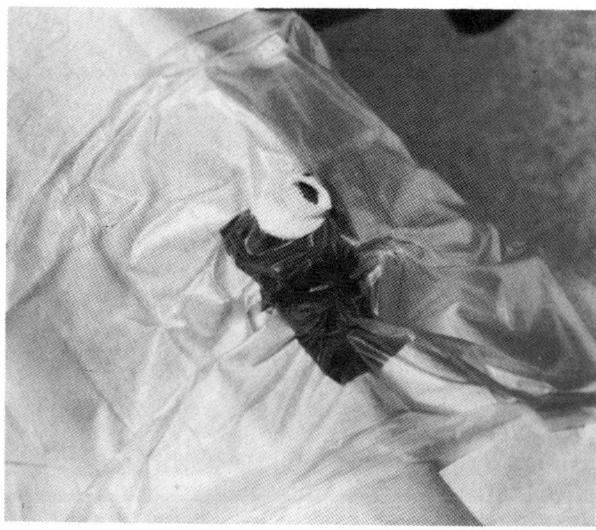

FIGURE 30–24

The head is draped, and a sterile drape is applied to the immediate circumoral area. (From Babbush, C.A.: Dental Implants: Principles and Practice. Philadelphia, W.B. Saunders Co., 1991, p 110.)

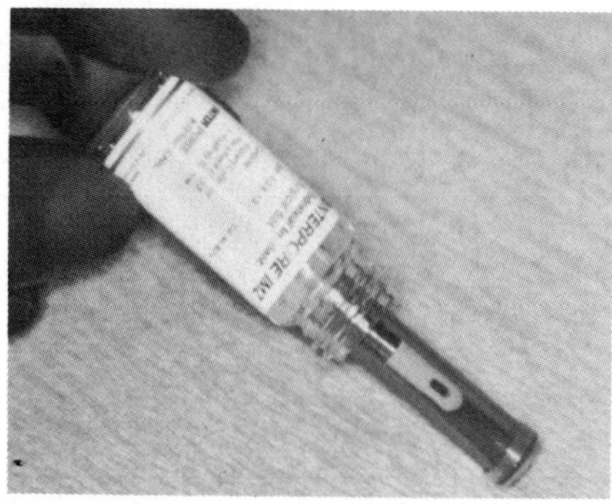

FIGURE 30–25

The implant is slid out onto a sterile surface. (From Babbush, C.A.: Dental Implants: Principles and Practice. Philadelphia, W.B. Saunders Co., 1991, p 87.)

SURGICAL PREPARATION

Implant surgery must be done under strict, surgically clean conditions with sterile instrumentation. The patient's mouth is rinsed with 0.1 percent chlorhexidine. Then the head is draped and a sterile surgical drape is applied to the circumoral area, leaving only the mouth exposed (Fig. 30–24). (**Circumoral** means surrounding the mouth.)

It is recommended that the implant team consist of at least three people: the clinician, surgical dental assistant, and nonsterile circulating assistant. The clinician and surgical dental assistant should be gowned and masked and should wear talcum-free *sterile* gloves.

The implants come in double aseptic packaging. They must remain in this packaging until the actual time of placement. Just before placement, the inner vial is opened and the implant is allowed to slide (untouched) onto a sterile surface (Fig. 30–25).

 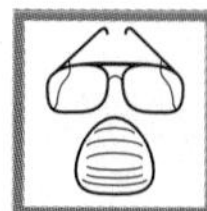 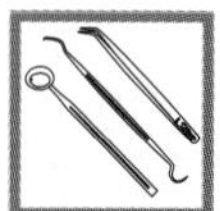 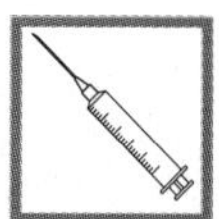 

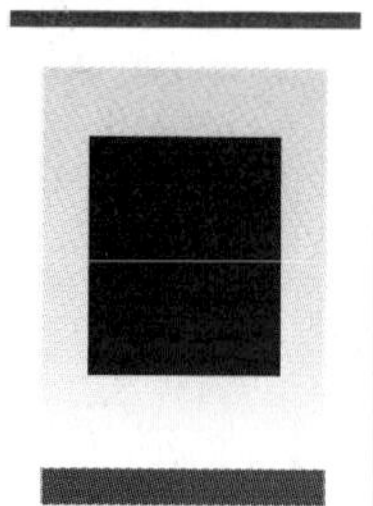

PROCEDURE: **Performing Implant Surgery**

Depending on the type of implant to be placed, the surgical technique may vary slightly. The following describes the surgical components of a two-stage standard osteointegrated implant system for a single tooth.

Instrumentation (Fig. 30–26)

Sterile surgical gloves
Sterile surgical drilling unit
Surgical irrigation tip
Scalpel
Periosteal elevator
Implant instrument kit
Implant kit
Low-speed handpiece
Inserting mallet
Suture setup
Electrosurgical unit and tips (or tissue punch)
Hydrogen peroxide
Sterile cotton pellets
Sterile gauze sponges

Text continued on page 604

PROCEDURE: **Performing Implant Surgery** *(continued)*

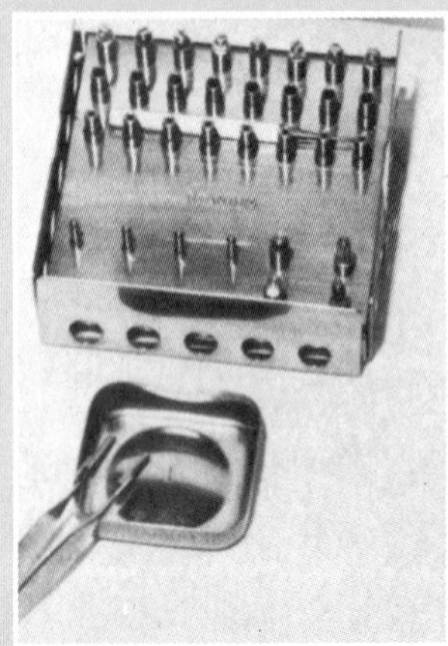

FIGURE 30–26

Setups for Stage I surgery and close up view of its components. (From Babbush, C.A.: Dental Implants: Principles and Practice. Philadelphia, W.B. Saunders Co., 1991, p 111.)

Stage I Surgery: Implant Placement

1. The surgical stent (template) is placed in position in the patient's mouth.
2. After achieving adequate anesthesia, the surgeon uses a "pilot drill" (similar to a long fissure bur) to drill through the stent and into the soft tissue on the ridge. This creates a target point on the bone for the implant site.
   □ *IMPORTANT:* All drilling of the bone is accomplished with generous amounts of sterile saline irrigation.
3. The surgeon removes the surgical stent and makes the incision at the implant site (Fig. 30–27).
4. The mucoperiosteal tissues are reflected. To keep the mucoperiosteal flap out of the field of operation, the flap is temporarily tied to the natural teeth with silk sutures.
5. The surgeon smoothes any sharp edges on the crest of the ridge. The crest should be at least 2 mm. wider than the implant being used.
6. A variety of drill tips (similar to burs) are used to prepare the osseous receptor site (Fig. 30–28).
7. The implant cylinder (with a plastic cap over the top of it) is partially inserted into the osseous receptor site.
8. The plastic cap is removed, and the implant is tapped into its final position with the inserting mallet.
9. The sterile sealing screw (also called a healing collar) is placed into the implant cylinder with the contra-angle screwdriver. The final tightening of the sealing screw is accomplished with the hand-held screwdriver.
10. The retraction suture is removed, and the mucoperiosteal flaps are repositioned and sutured in place. The implant receptor is now covered by the tissue and is not visible in the mouth.

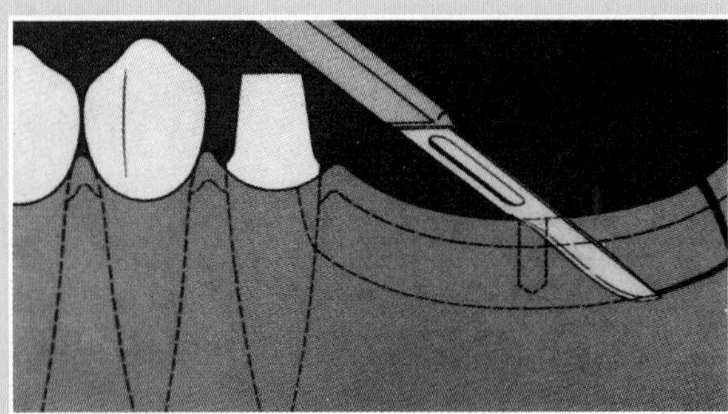

FIGURE 30–27

An incision is made to expose the receptor site. (From Babbush, C.A.: Dental Implants: Principles and Practice. Philadelphia, W.B. Saunders Co., 1991, Fig. 5–41.)

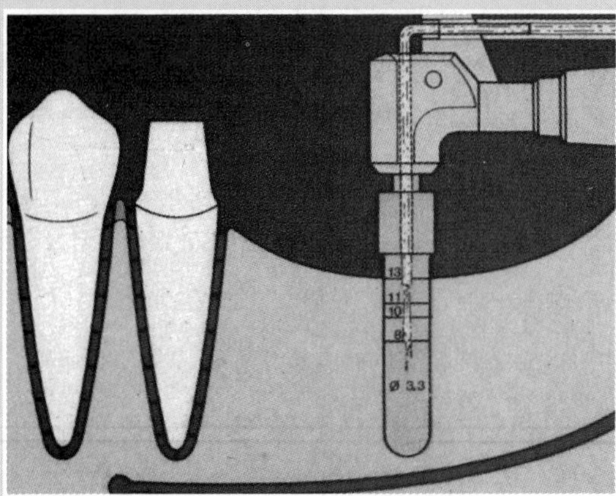

FIGURE 30–28

Special burs are used for the final preparation of the osseous receptor site. (From Babbush, C.A.: Dental Implants: Principles and Practice. Philadelphia, W.B. Saunders Co., 1991, Fig. 5–46b.)

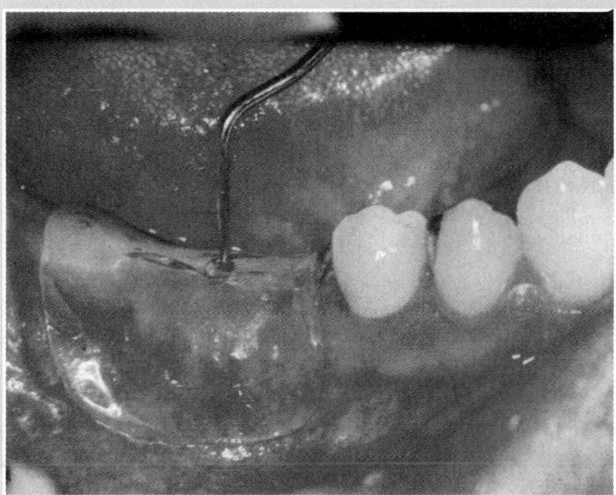

FIGURE 30–29

At Stage II, the surgical template is repositioned after anesthesia is accomplished, and a sharp instrument is lowered through the opening in the template to mark the soft tissues. (From Babbush, C.A.: Dental Implants: Principles and Practice. Philadelphia, W.B. Saunders Co., 1991, Fig. 5–59.)

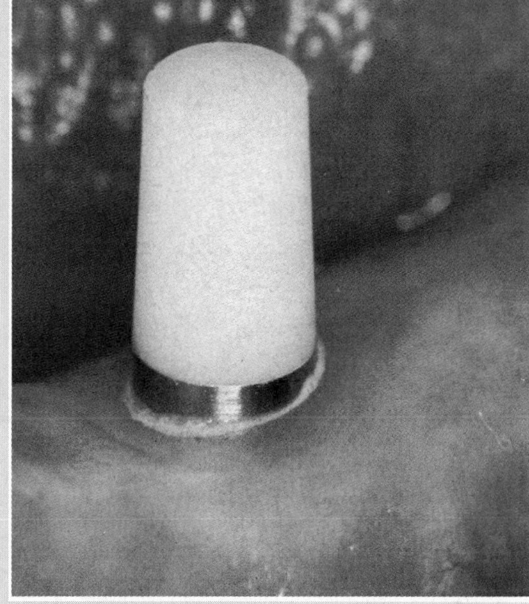

FIGURE 30–31

The impression post extends above the gingiva. (From Babbush, C.A.: Dental Implants: Principles and Practice. Philadelphia, W.B. Saunders Co., 1991, Fig. 5–67.)

Stage II Surgery: Implant Exposure

1. After local anesthesia is accomplished, the surgical stent (template) is repositioned (Fig. 30–29).
2. A sharp instrument, such as a periodontal probe, is lowered through the opening in the stent to make bleeding points.
3. The stent is removed, and the mark on the soft tissue shows the position of the previously placed implant.
4. An electrosurgical loop is used to remove the soft tissue over the implant site by peeling it back a layer at a time until the titanium sealing screw is located (Fig. 30–30). A special tissue punch can also be used to remove the tissue from over the implant.
5. The implant is uncovered, and the sealing screw is removed.
6. The inside of the implant cylinder is cleaned with sterile cotton soaked in hydrogen peroxide.
7. An impression post is screwed into the implant (Fig. 30–31). This attachment now extends above the mucosa.
8. The soft tissues are allowed to heal for 10 to 14 days before the fabrication of the crown.

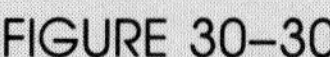

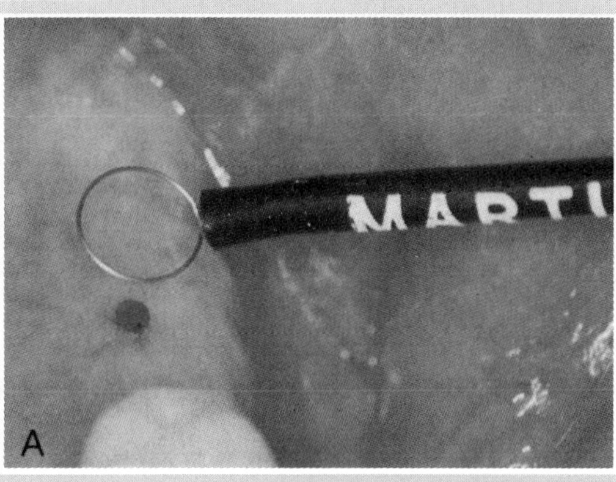

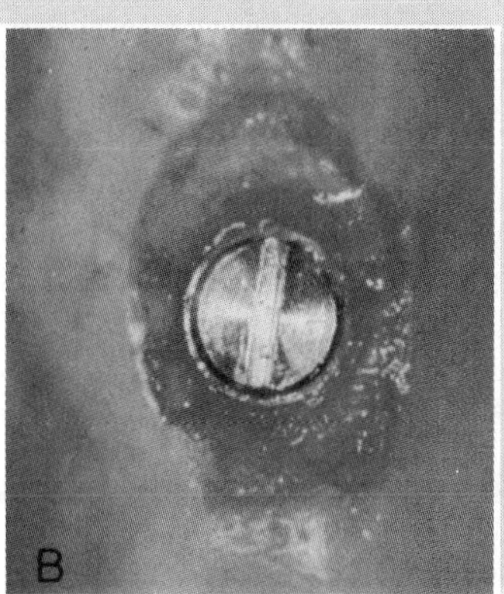

FIGURE 30–30

The electrosurgical loop is used to remove the soft tissue over the implant by peeling it back a layer at a time until the implant is seen. (From Babbush, C.A.: Dental Implants: Principles and Practice. Philadelphia, W.B. Saunders Co., 1991, Fig. 5–61.)

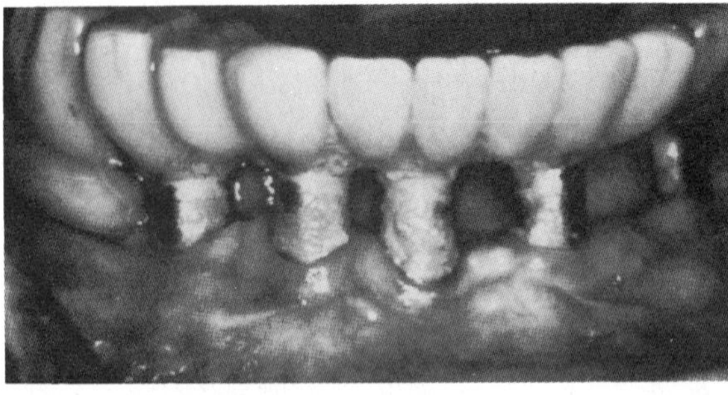

FIGURE 30–32

Calculus formed on the implant and fixed superstructure. (From Perry, D.A., Beemsterboer, P., and Carranza, F.A.: Techniques and Theory of Periodontal Instrumentation. Philadelphia, W.B. Saunders Co., 1990, p 322.)

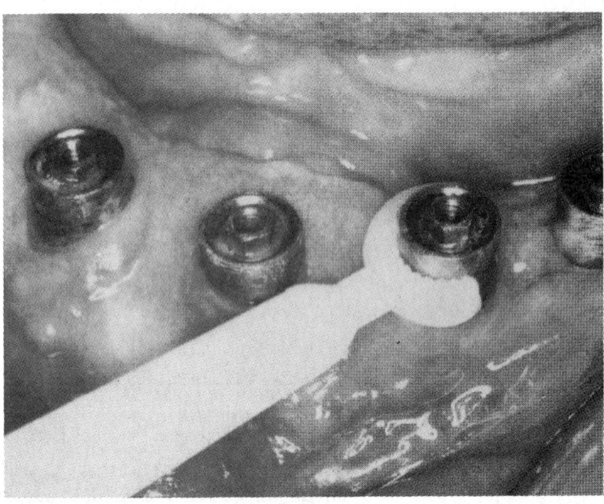

FIGURE 30–33

Plastic scaling instruments adapted to implant abutments. (From Perry, D.A., Beemsterboer, P., and Carranza, F.A.: Techniques and Theory of Periodontal Instrumentation. Philadelphia, W.B. Saunders Co., 1990, p 323.)

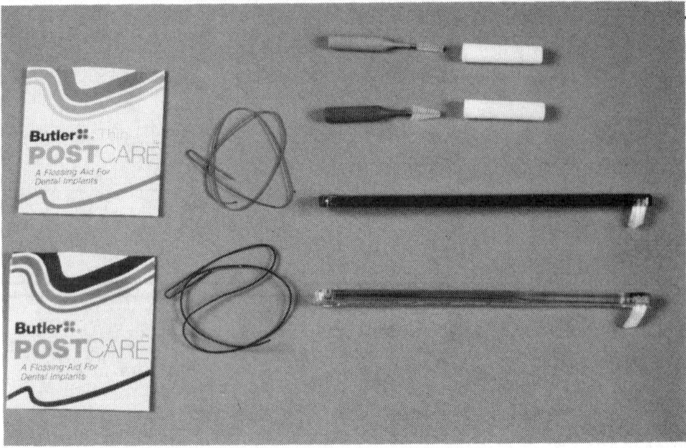

FIGURE 30–34

A variety of home care products for patients. *Left,* Implant floss. *Right top,* Interdental brushes. *Right bottom,* End tuft tooth brushes.

Maintenance of Dental Implants

Long-term maintenance for dental implant patients is an integral part of treatment. This includes home care by the patient and periodic maintenance visits to the dental office.

The health of the peri-implant tissue is a critical factor in the success of dental implants. (**Peri-implant tissue** is the gingival sulcus surrounding the implant. It is similar to the gingival sulcus surrounding a natural tooth.)

The peri-implant tissue responds to bacterial plaque with inflammation and bleeding, in much the same way as the gingival tissues around a normal tooth.

Many implant patients lost their natural teeth because of chronic periodontal disease. This was caused, in part, by poor oral hygiene. The task of educating and motivating these persons to practice proper home care is difficult but critical to the long-term success of the implants.

Dental plaque and calculus form on implants just as they do on natural teeth (Fig. 30–32). Because the surface of implants are very smooth, plaque is less adherent and more easily removed from the implants than from natural teeth.

Calculus is relatively easy to remove from the implants because it cannot become embedded in the titanium surface. However, it is critical to remove plaque and calculus from the implant in such a way that the implant surface is not scratched (Fig. 30–33).

HOME CARE TECHNIQUE

The following devices can be very helpful in plaque removal for implant patients (Fig. 30–34):

- Toothbrushes, manual or powered
- Single-tufted toothbrushes
- Partial denture clasp brushes
- Interproximal brushes
- Floss (thick, thin, or fuzzy)
- Dental implant floss, with a stiff, curved end

As with all home care, the goal is to remove all plaque and debris at least once daily. Patients are instructed in the use of these aids, and their progress is monitored regularly.

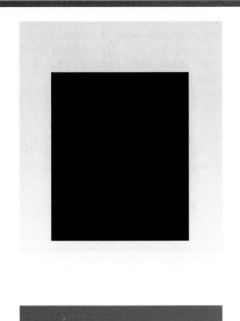

Chapter 31

Fixed Prosthodontics

Introduction

A **prosthesis** is a replacement for a missing body part. (The plural is *prostheses.*) Fixed prosthodontics, commonly known as *crown and bridge*, is the area of dentistry specializing in the replacement of missing teeth with cast prostheses that are cemented in place and cannot be removed by the patient.

The discussion in this chapter also covers the fabrication and placement of other cast restorations, including veneers, single crowns, inlays, and onlays.

Removable prosthodontics, which involve appliances that the patient can place and remove for cleaning, are discussed in Chapter 32.

The benefits of a fixed prosthesis to replace missing teeth include

- Prevention of drifting of adjacent teeth caused by missing teeth and providing support to the remaining teeth in the arch
- Prevention of the extrusion of teeth in the opposing arch
- Providing the dentition needed to masticate food properly
- Providing acceptable esthetics for the patient

Indications for Fixed Prosthodontics

- One or two adjacent teeth are missing in the same arch.
- The supportive tissues are healthy.
- Suitable abutment teeth are present.
- The patient is in good health and wants to have the prosthesis placed.
- The patient has the skills and motivation to maintain good oral hygiene.

Contraindications for Fixed Prosthodontics

- Necessary supportive tissues are diseased or missing.
- Suitable abutment teeth are not present.
- The patient is in poor health or is not motivated to have the prosthesis placed.
- The patient has poor oral hygiene habits.
- The patient cannot afford the treatment.

Exposure Control and Fixed Prosthodontics

Fixed prosthodontics involves extensive chairside procedures, obtaining and handling impressions, and sending and receiving cases to and from the dental laboratory.

The appropriate exposure control protocols must be followed at each step in these procedures. (See Chapter 13.)

The Role of the Dental Laboratory Technician

A cast restoration is very precise and must, with only minor adjustments, fit the prepared tooth exactly.

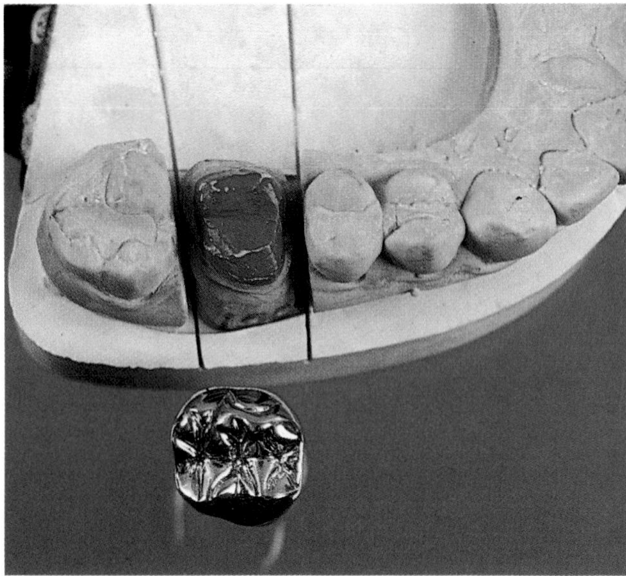

FIGURE 31–1

A cast gold crown and master cast. The die is the blue portion of the master cast.

Usually these cases are sent to a commercial dental laboratory, where they are fabricated by a trained dental laboratory technician who carefully creates a casting that meets these requirements.

The following is an overview of what happens to the case (final impression, opposing arch, and occlusal registration) after it has been received and disinfected in the laboratory.

1. The final impression is poured to create the master casts. In the **master casts**, the prepared teeth are poured as dies (Fig. 31–1). (A **die** is an exact replica of the prepared portion of the tooth. The die is constructed so that it can be taken in and out of the master cast.)
2. The occlusal registration is used to position the casts properly on an articulator to simulate the patient's normal occlusion. (An **articulator** is a dental laboratory device that replicates the movements of the temporomandibular joint.)
3. Working on the die of the prepared tooth, the laboratory technician very carefully creates a wax pattern for the casting (Fig. 31–2).
4. The completed wax pattern is removed from the die, and a wax or plastic sprue is attached. In the casting process, the sprue forms a channel that allows the molten metal to flow into the mold.
5. The completed pattern and sprue are placed in a casting ring and invested (encased) in investment material. (**Investment material** is a specialized gypsum product that is able to withstand extreme heat.)
6. The casting ring is placed in a very hot burn-out oven. During the burn-out process, the wax of the pattern and sprue are lost (burned away), and a negative pattern of the casting remains in the investment material.
7. The metal alloy is heated until it melts. Then centrifugal force is used to cause the molten metal to flow through the sprue opening and into the pattern. This creates the casting.
8. The cooled casting ring is placed in water. This aids in removing the investment material, and the casting remains.
9. The sprue button (created when molten metal filled the sprue opening) is removed, and the casting is polished and completed.

The Laboratory Prescription

The laboratory technician can fabricate a prosthesis only on the basis of a written prescription from the dentist (Fig. 31–3).

Also known as a *work order* or *requisition*, a copy of this prescription is included with the case, and a copy is retained with the practice records. The prescription contains the information concerning

- Identification of the patient (name or case number)
- Type of prosthesis requested
- Type of alloy or other materials to be used
- Exact shade
- Date when the case is expected back in the dental practice
- Dentist's name, license number, address, telephone number, and signature

The amount of time needed by the laboratory to construct each type of prosthesis is expressed in terms of "working days," and the try-in visit is scheduled to

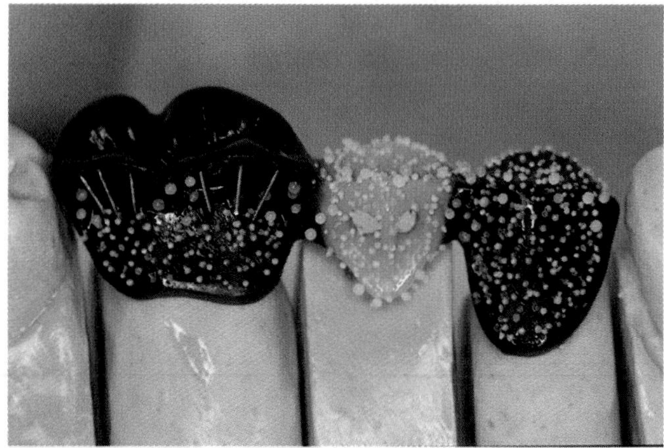

FIGURE 31–2

Wax pattern for a three-unit porcelain-fused-to-metal bridge. When completed, the smooth surfaces will be gold. The rough surfaces will be covered with tooth-colored ceramic. (Courtesy of Williams-Ivoclar, Amherst, NY.)

TRUE IMAGE BUSINESS FORMS 313377

PRECISION CERAMICS DENTAL LABORATORY

9591 Central Avenue • Montclair, CA 91763
(909) 625-8787 • (800) 223-6322
FAX: (909) 621-3125

™ FROM: DATE ____________

DR. ______________________ PHONE (____) ____________

ADDRESS ______________________ ACCT. NO. ____________

CITY ____________ STATE ________ ZIP ________

PATIENT'S NAME ______________________ AGE ____ SEX M F ____

TYPE OF CASE

☐ DICOR ☐ **DICOR PLUS**
☐ RENAISSANCE
☐ PORCELAIN ON METAL
☐ LAMINATE VENEER
☐ FULL CAST METAL
☐ MARYLAND BRIDGE
☐ ONLAY / INLAY
☐ PORCELAIN JACKET
☐ ACRYLIC JACKETS
☐ ACRYLIC ON METAL

TYPE OF METAL

☐ PREMIUM GOLD
☐ ECONOMY GOLD
Hard ☐ CLASS 4
☐ SEMI-PRECIOUS
☐ TITANIUM

GINGIVAL BANDS

☐ LINGUAL ONLY
☐ LINGUAL & FACIAL

CONTACTS

☐ NONE ☐ MEDIUM
☐ HEAVY

RIDGE RELIEF

☐ SLIGHT ☐ NONE
☐ MEDIUM ☐ SOCKET

☐ METAL TRY-IN ☐ BISQUE BAKE TRY-IN ☐ FINISH

	IN	OUT
DOCTOR'S MODELS (OPP)		
WORKING MODEL		
DIES		
IMPRESSIONS		
BITE		
ARTICULATOR		
SHADE GUIDE		
CROWN		
PARTIAL		
STUDY MODEL		
OTHER		
CHECK		

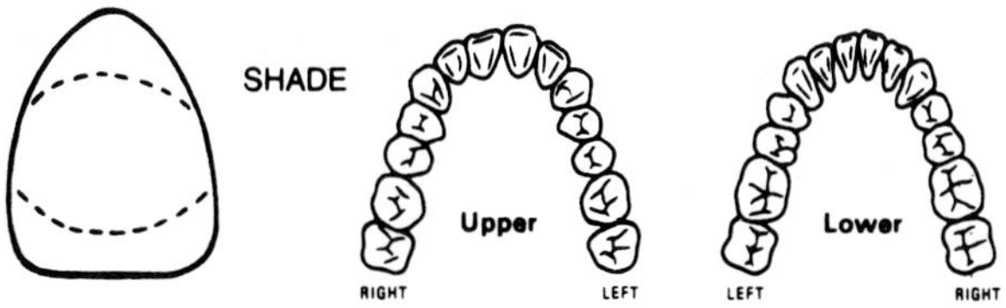

SHADE

Upper — RIGHT / LEFT

Lower — LEFT / RIGHT

☐ OCCLUSAL STAIN Due In Your Office ____________

PLEASE SEND: ☐ **BOXES** ☐ **Rx FORMS** ☐ **MAILING LABELS**
PLEASE CALL: ☐ ☐ **PARTIAL & DENTURE FORMS** ☐ **PRICE LIST**
CHECK NO: ________ **VISA** ☐ **MC** ☐

Signature ______________________ Lic. # ____________

TERMS: Customer agrees to company policy as stated on reverse.

LAB COPY

FIGURE 31–3

A laboratory prescription for a fixed prosthesis. (Courtesy of Precision Ceramics Dental Laboratory, Montclair, CA.)

allow adequate working days for construction of the case.

Before the patient's appointment, the assistant must determine that the case has been returned to the practice. If it has not been returned, it may be necessary to reschedule the patient's appointment.

Types of Cast Restorations

Amalgam and composite restorations, also known as *direct restorations*, are created in the mouth while the material is soft and can be adapted to fit the tooth.

Cast restorations, are also known as *indirect restorations*, are created in the dental laboratory from precise impressions of the prepared tooth. This casting is hard and cannot be reshaped. Therefore the prepared tooth must be shaped to permit the casting to slide into place with only minor adjustments. The finished casting is bonded and luted (cemented) in place.

Inlays and Onlays

Inlays and onlays are cast restorations that are designed to fit snugly into a preparation *within* a tooth. An **inlay**, like a Class II restoration, covers a portion of the occlusal and proximal surfaces. An **onlay** usually covers the proximal surfaces and most, or all, of the occlusal surface (Fig. 31–4).

Gold is the strongest material available for these cast restorations; however, it does not match the color of the tooth. When esthetics are of primary importance, inlays and onlays that exactly match the tooth color are fabricated from porcelain or composite resin.

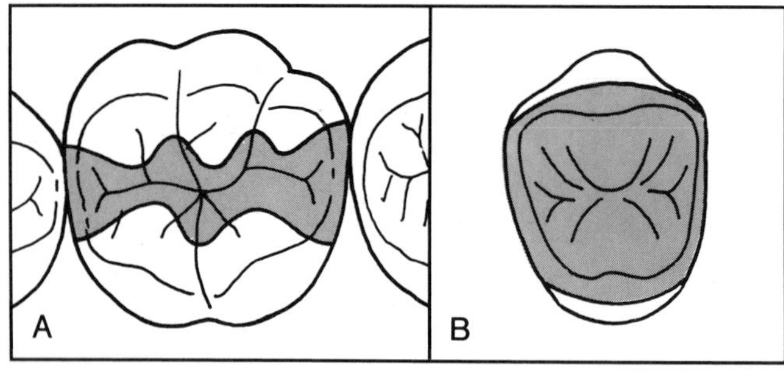

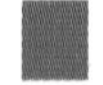

FIGURE 31–4

Occlusal view of an inlay and an onlay. *A*, A class II MOD gold inlay on a mandibular first molar. *B*, A gold onlay covering the occlusal surfaces of a maxillary second molar.

Veneers

A veneer is a thin shell of tooth-colored material. The types of veneer discussed here are placed on the prepared facial surface of an anterior tooth. A **direct veneer**, also known as a *bonded veneer*, is created directly in the patient's mouth (see Fig. 25–19).

An **indirect veneer** is fabricated in the dental laboratory on the basis of an impression taken of the prepared tooth. The completed veneer is returned to the dental office and bonded in place on the prepared tooth (see Figs. 31–23 to 31–26).

Crowns

A **full crown**, also known as a *cast crown*, completely covers the anatomic crown of an individual tooth to restore the tooth to its original contour and function (see Fig. 31–1). Crowns are also used as abutments to support a fixed bridge. (Fixed bridges are discussed later in this chapter.)

Usually a full crown is placed only if the tooth is too badly decayed or fractured to be reconstructed with a more conservative restoration. If a tooth is very badly broken down, additional retention is required, and this is discussed later in the chapter.

The **three-quarter crown** differs from the full crown in that it does not cover the entire anatomic crown. Instead, the tooth is prepared so that the facial surface of the tooth is unchanged. When the crown is placed, the natural enamel on the facial surface is visible, and the prepared portion is covered by the crown.

A **porcelain-fused-to-metal** (PFM) crown, also known as a *veneer crown*, is a full metal crown with outer surfaces covered with a veneer (thin layer) of tooth-colored substance. This resulting restoration has the strength of a metal crown and the esthetic appeal of matching the natural tooth color.

Porcelain jacket crowns (PJCs) are constructed with a *very* thin metal shell covered by layers of porcelain build-up to resemble the shading and translucence of the enamel of a natural tooth. These restorations are esthetically very pleasing and are used on anterior teeth; however, they lack the strength of a PFM crown.

Fixed Bridges

A **fixed bridge** is a prosthesis used to replace one or more adjacent teeth in the same arch (Figs. 31–5 and 31–6). The bridge is cemented in place and cannot be removed by the patient. With the proper oral hygiene, a fixed bridge will provide many years of excellent service.

Materials for Cast Restorations

Metals for Cast Restorations

Gold in its pure form has the ability to resist tarnish and etching when exposed to the harsh conditions in

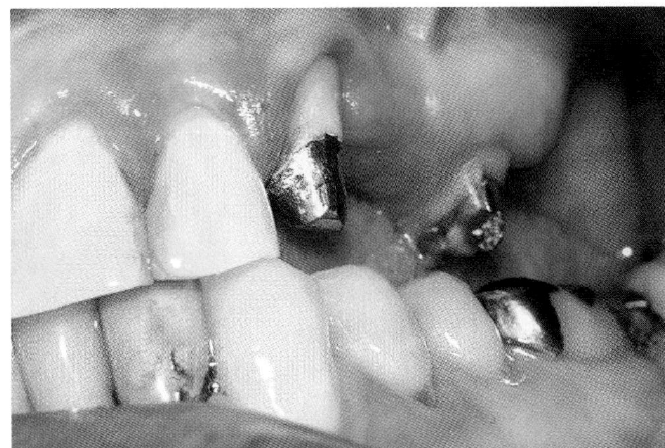

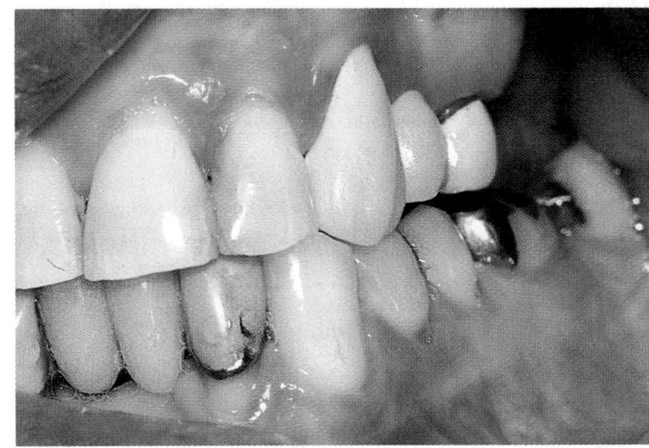

FIGURE 31–5

Three-unit posterior bridge. *Left,* The prepared abutment teeth. *Right,* The bridge cemented in place.

the mouth; however, in its pure form, it is too soft for use in cast dental restorations.

By combining gold with other metals to form an alloy, it acquires the characteristics and hardness required for this purpose. (An **alloy** is a substance consisting of two or more metals.)

NOBLE METAL ALLOYS

One way of describing the alloys used in dentistry is on the basis of their noble and base metal content.

The **noble metals** used in dentistry are **gold** (Au), **palladium** (Pd), and **platinum** (Pt). All other metals in the alloy that are not classified as noble metals are considered to be base metals.

A **base metal** is a metal of relatively low value and with inferior properties such as lack of resistance to corrosion and tarnish. Iron, tin, and zinc are examples of base metals.

High noble alloys consist of at least 60 percent noble metals. Of this noble metal portion, at least 40 percent *must* be gold, and the other 20 percent consists of the other noble metals. The remaining 40 percent of the alloy is made up of base metals.

Noble alloys consist of at least 25 percent noble metals. The percentage of required gold is not fixed, and the noble alloys portion may be made up of any combination of the three noble metals. The remaining 75 percent of the alloy is of base metals.

Predominantly base alloys are made up of less than 25 percent of the noble metals. The remaining portion of the alloy consists of base metals.

DENTAL GOLD-CASTING ALLOYS

Gold alloys are also described according to their hardness, malleability, and adaptability. (**Malleability** is the ability to be shaped or formed.) According to this descriptive system, there are four types of gold alloys:

- **Soft, type I alloys** are used for casting inlays subject to slight stress during mastication.
- **Medium, type II alloys** can be used for practically all types of cast inlays and possibly posterior bridge abutments.
- **Hard, type III alloys** are acceptable for inlay, full crowns, three-quarter crowns, and anterior or posterior bridge abutments.
- **Extra hard, type IV alloys**, also known as *partial denture alloys*, are designed for cast-removable partial dentures. (These are discussed in Chapter 32.)

The mechanical properties of these alloys are described by these characteristics:

- **Yield strength:** Amount of stress on an alloy at which deformation begins
- **Tensile strength:** Amount of stress before the fracture of the alloy
- **Elongation:** Amount of stretching before deformation occurs
- **Hardness:** Amount of resistance of a solid to penetration

Tooth-Colored Materials for Cast Restorations

Porcelain, which is the type of ceramic used most commonly in dentistry, combines strength with translucence and the ability to match the natural tooth color. (A **ceramic** is a material composed of a metal chemically bonded to a nonmetal.) Porcelain is used to create

- **Inlays** that match the tooth color
- **Bonded veneers** to improve the appearance of anterior teeth
- **Porcelain-fused-to-metal** (PFM) crowns and bridges

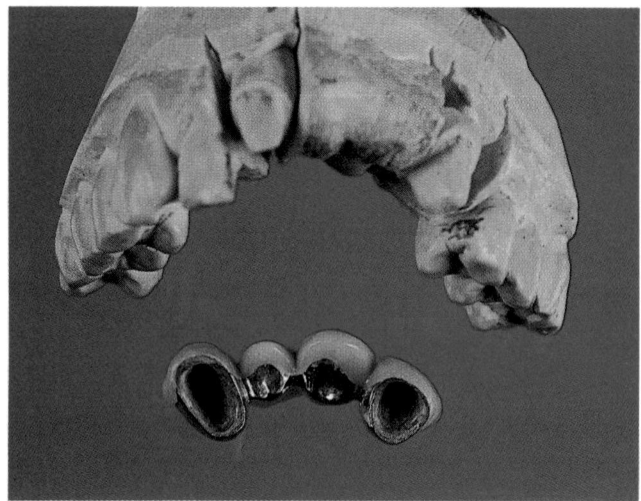

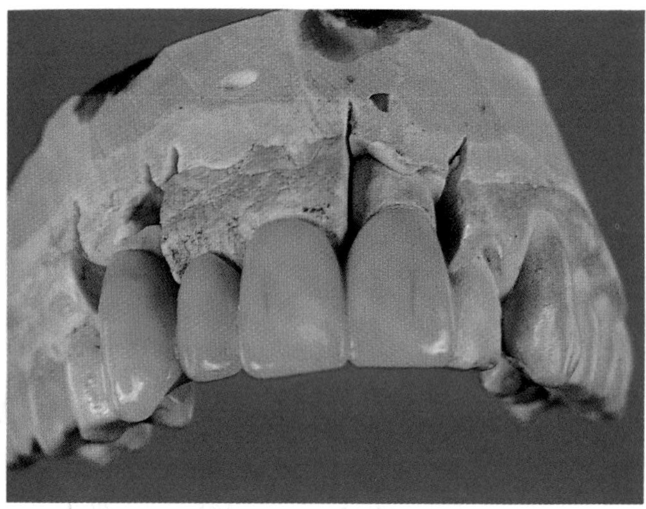

FIGURE 31–6

A four-unit anterior porcelain-fused-to-metal bridge. *Left*, The metal, which provides strength, is visible on the underside. *Right*, In place, the bridge is esthetically pleasing because none of the metal is visible.

that are esthetically pleasing, yet have the strength of metal (see Fig. 31–6).

Cast composite restorations created in the dental laboratory by the *indirect technique*, include inlays, onlays, and veneers. Because laboratory fabrication techniques incorporate heat and pressure, these restorations are stronger than those created in the mouth.

Instrumentation

Two basic crown and bridge preset trays are used in fixed prosthodontics: the preparation tray and the delivery tray (Figs. 31–7 and 31–8).

Preparation Instrumentation

- Large spoon excavator
- Additional hand instruments (operator's choice)
- Burs, diamond stones, and discs (operator's choice)
- Gingival retraction setup
- Cotton rolls and gauze sponges
- High-volume evacuator (HVE) tip

In addition to these preparation instruments, setups are also required at this visit for

- Elastomeric impressions, which may include a custom tray
- Occlusal registration
- Alginate impression for opposing arch
- Provisional coverage fabrication, adjustment, and cementation supplies (these are discussed later in this chapter)

Delivery Instrumentation

- Cast restoration
- Backhaus towel forceps (to remove temporary coverage)
- Large spoon excavator
- Cavity varnish and applicator (optional)
- Bonding supplies (operator's choice)
- Cementation supplies (operator's choice)
- Cotton rolls
- Saliva ejector (optional)
- Bite-stick
- Articulating paper and holder
- Polishing points and stones (operator's choice)
- Dental floss
- Scaler (to remove excess cement)

Preparation and Placement of a Cast Crown

The following is an overview of the steps in the preparation and placement of a cast crown; however, these steps are very similar for all cast restorations. The placement of a cast restoration usually requires two visits: one for the preparation and impressions and a second for cementation and finishing of the restoration.

The Preparation Appointment

During the preparation, the height and contour of the tooth are reduced to provide space for a casting thick enough to have the necessary strength without

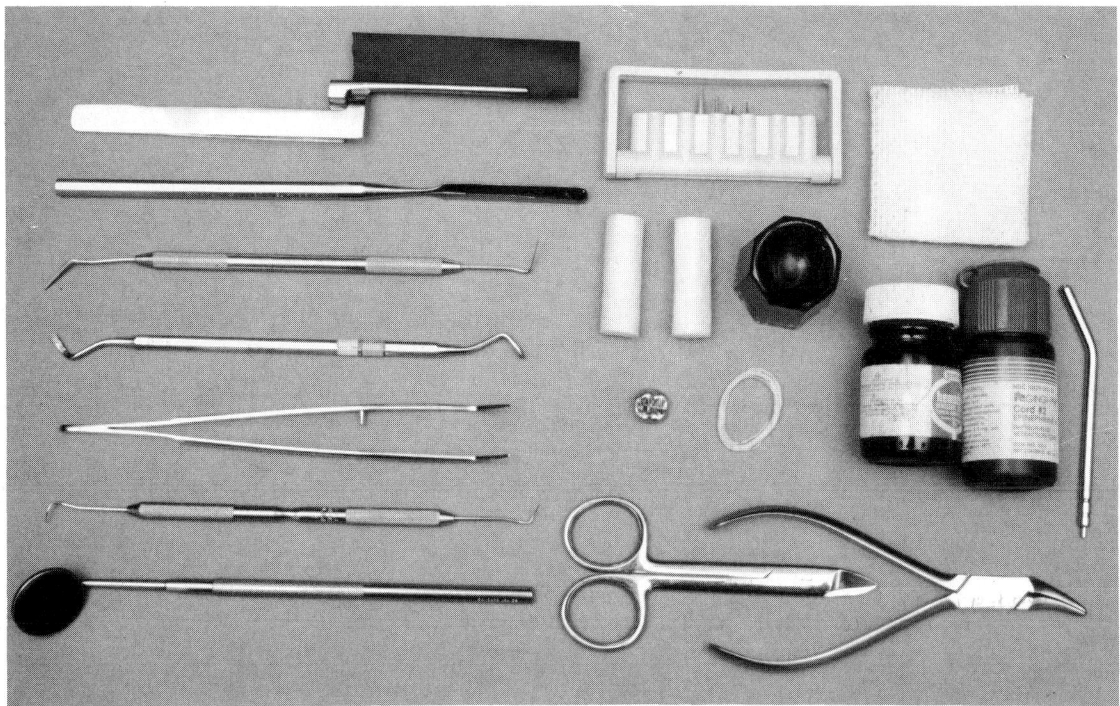

FIGURE 31–7

Crown and bridge preparation tray. *Left, bottom to top,* Mouth mirror, explorer, cotton pliers, large spoon excavator, cord-packing instrument, cement spatula, articulating forceps, and articulating paper. *Right, bottom to top,* Crown and bridge scissors, curved contouring pliers, temporary crown, dental floss, hemostatic solution, retraction cord, air-water syringe tip, cotton rolls, dappen dish, bur block, and gauze sponges.

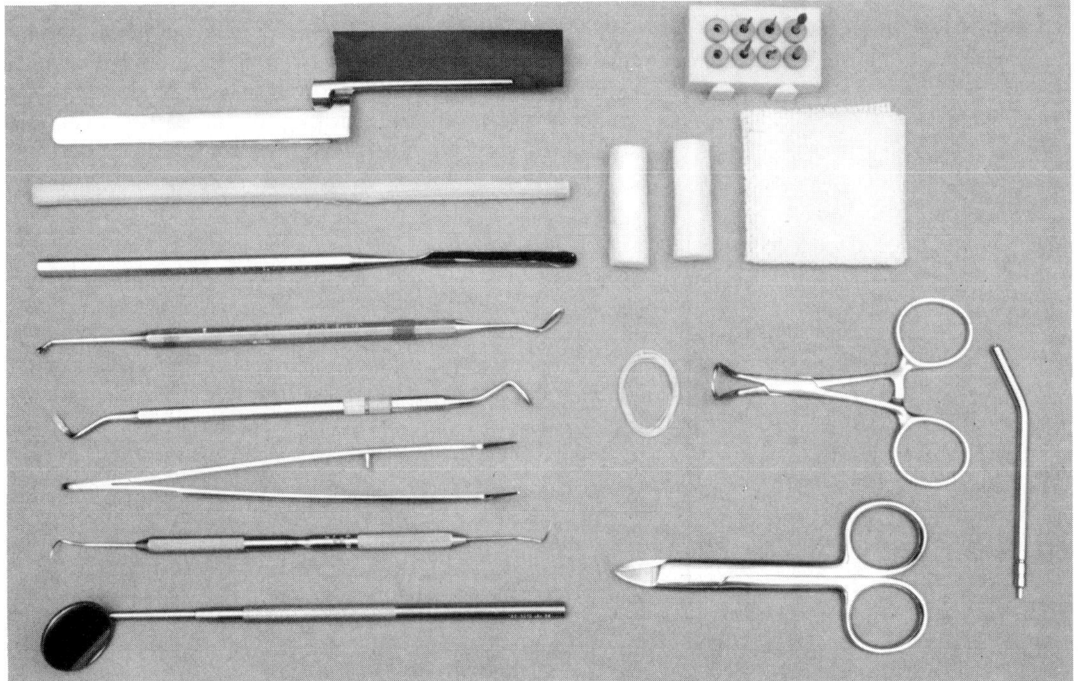

FIGURE 31–8

Crown and bridge cementation tray. *Left, bottom to top,* Mouth mirror, explorer, cotton pliers, large spoon excavator, plastic instrument, cement spatula, wooden bite-stick, articulating forceps, and articulating paper. *Right, bottom to top,* crown and bridge scissors, dental floss, Backhaus towel forceps, air-water syringe tip, cotton rolls, gauze sponges, and bur block.

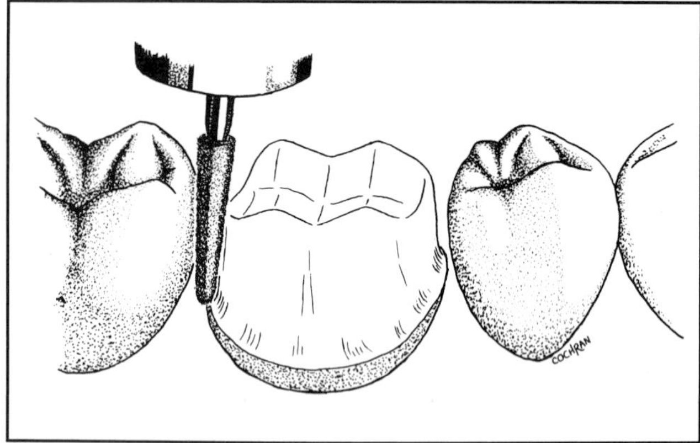

FIGURE 31–9

A crown preparation requires reducing the height and bulk of the tooth. (From Baum, L., Phillips, R.W., and Lund, M.R.: Textbook of Operative Dentistry, 2nd ed. Philadelphia, W.B. Saunders Co., 1985, p 433.)

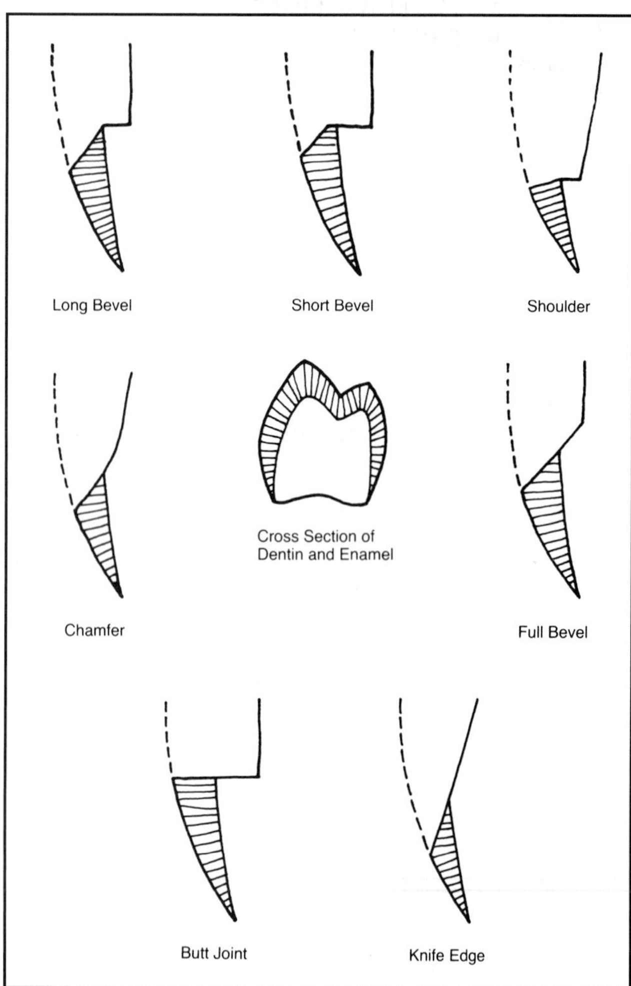

FIGURE 31–10

Types of bevels and gingival margins for crown preparations. The shaded portions represent enamel. The dotted lines indicate where enamel has been removed.

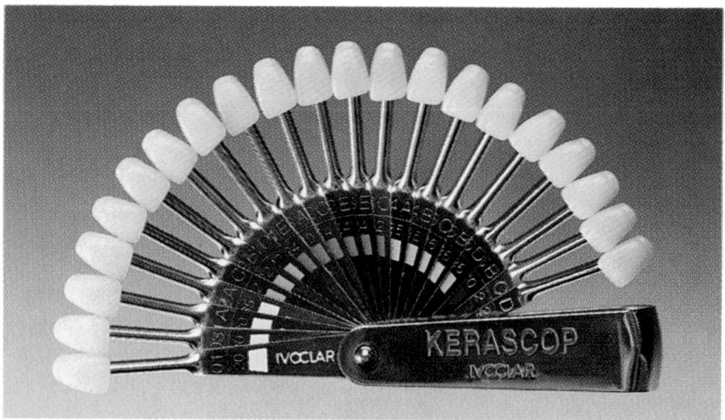

FIGURE 31–11

A shade guide is used to match the exact shade of the natural tooth. (Courtesy of Ivoclar Vivadent, Amherst, NY.)

increasing the overall size of the restored tooth (Fig. 31–9; also see Fig. 31–1).

The prepared tooth must also be shaped so that the cast restoration can slide into place and be able to withstand the forces of occlusion.

The gingival margins of the preparation are designed to provide a smooth, strong junction of the edges (margins) of the casting with the surface of the tooth. These margins are known by several terms, including the *bevel, chamfer,* and *shoulder* (Fig. 31–10).

SHADE SELECTION

If this is to be a tooth-colored restoration, matching the shade of the natural teeth is very important and is usually done before the tooth is prepared. A **shade guide**, which contains samples of all of the available shades, is used to match the natural tooth color (Fig. 31–11).

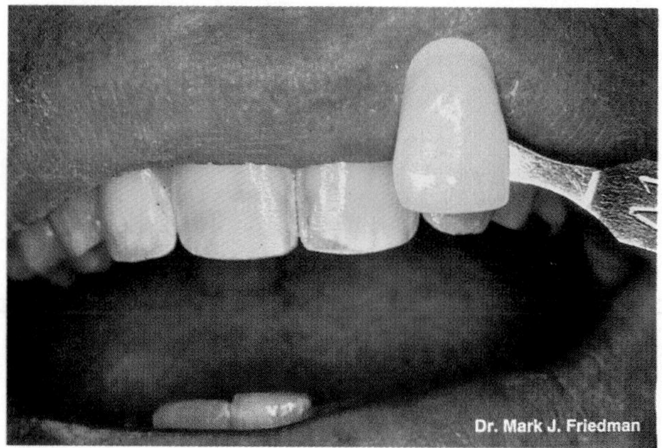

FIGURE 31–12

The shade guide piece is moistened and held near the natural tooth. (Courtesy of 3M Dental Products Division, St. Paul, MN.)

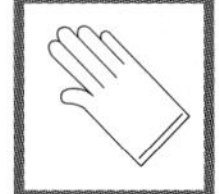
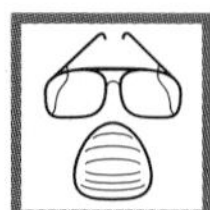
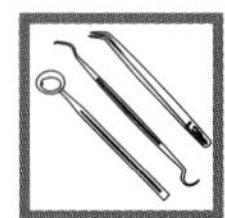
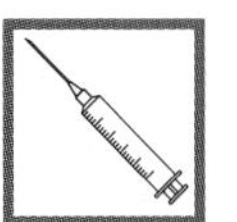
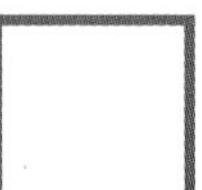

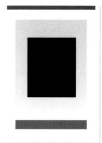

PROCEDURE: **Preparing a Tooth for a Cast Restoration**

Preliminary Steps

1. Local anesthetic is administered.
2. If an alginate impression is required for use in fabricating temporary coverage, it is obtained at this time. (See Chapter 19.)
3. If a silicone two-step impression method is to be used, the first impression is obtained at this time.
4. If this is to be a tooth-colored restoration, the shade is selected at this time.

Tooth Preparation

1. Throughout the preparation, the assistant maintains a clear operating field by using the HVE to retract the lips and tongue and to remove water and debris.
2. The dentist uses diamond stones in the high-speed handpiece to remove all caries or fractured portions of the tooth.

☐ *RATIONALE:* Diamond stones are used during crown preparation because of their ability to rapidly remove tooth structure.

3. The dentist reduces the bulk of the tooth and completes the preparation. Different-shaped burs are used during this process, and the assistant aids in bur changes as necessary.
4. When the preparation is complete, gingival retraction is placed, and the final impressions and occlusal registration are obtained. (These are discussed later in this chapter.)
5. Temporary coverage is placed to protect the prepared teeth. (This is discussed later in this chapter.)
6. The patient is scheduled for a return visit and then dismissed.
7. The dentist writes the prescription, and then the case is prepared and sent to the laboratory.

Most dentists prefer to make the shade selection while waiting for the local anesthetic to take effect and before the tooth has been prepared.

The color sample is moistened and held close to the tooth to be restored (Fig. 31–12). Since the teeth are normally wet, this moisture helps to achieve a more accurate match.

To accurately determine the shade, the match is checked in good light. For best results, many dentists prefer to use natural sunlight light coming from a northern direction.

The shade selected is identified by number from the shade guide and noted on the patient's chart and on the laboratory prescription.

The shade guide is a semicritical item that cannot withstand the heat of sterilization. After use, it is disinfected with a high-level Environmental Protection Agency (EPA)–registered disinfectant.

Characterization

To achieve a truly natural look on anterior restorations, the dentist may instruct the laboratory technician to add characterization to the finished surface. These fine lines and small areas of slight discoloration resemble the stains or cracks that are present on the natural tooth (see Fig. 31–6, *right*).

The Delivery Appointment

When the casting has been fitted and is acceptable, the dentist lutes (cements) it to the tooth with a permanent cement. Great care must be taken during this step, because once a cast restoration has been permanently cemented to the tooth, it is almost impossible to remove it without damaging the casting and/or tooth. In contrast, if the casting is not cemented properly, the margins may leak, there can be recurrent decay, or the crown could come off.

The cement selected for luting is the operator's choice. Proper mixing of this cement, in accordance with the manufacturer's directions, and the placement of cement on only the interior surface of the crown are very important steps that are the assistant's responsibility. These steps are explained in Chapter 23.

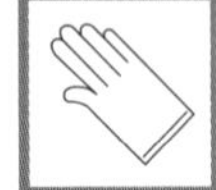
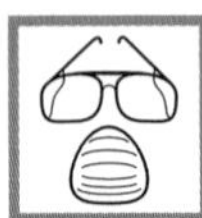
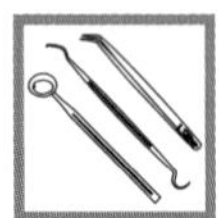
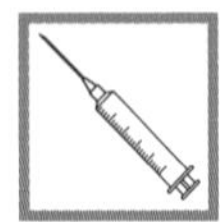

PROCEDURE: **Trying-In and Adjusting a Casting**

1. Before the patient's return visit, the assistant determines that the completed case has been returned from the laboratory.
2. Local anesthetic is administered, and the temporary coverage and any remaining temporary cement are removed from the tooth.
   □ *NOTE:* If the tooth is not sensitive, local anesthetic may not be required at this visit.
3. The crown is seated, the occlusion is checked, and minor adjustments are made. If necessary, the crown is polished again in the office laboratory. If taken to the laboratory, the crown is disinfected before it is returned to the treatment room.
   □ *IMPORTANT:* Examination gloves are always worn when anything that has been in the patient's mouth is handled.
4. Cotton rolls are placed to isolate the quadrant and to keep the area dry.
5. Before cementation, cavity varnish or a protective lining may be placed.
   □ *RATIONALE:* These protect the tooth and reduce postoperative sensitivity.
6. The tooth and the interior of the casting are prepared by etching and bonding.

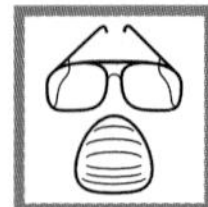
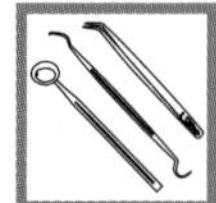
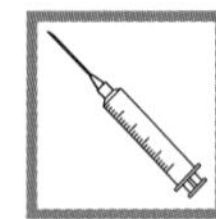

PROCEDURE: **Cementing a Casting**

1. At a signal from the dentist, the assistant mixes the cement, covers the internal surface of the casting with cement, and passes the prepared crown to the dentist.
2. The dentist places the crown on the prepared tooth, presses it into place, and then asks the patient to bite down on a wooden bite-stick to completely seat the restoration.
3. The patient continues this biting pressure until the cement reaches the initial set (approximately 8 to 10 minutes).
4. *Optional:* Once the casting is firmly seated, a saliva ejector may be placed in the floor of the patient's mouth.

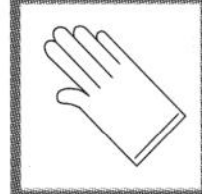 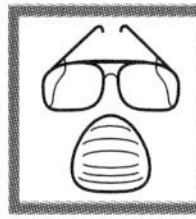 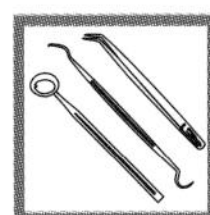 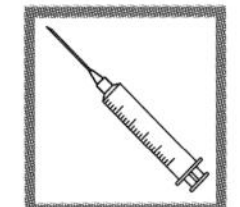 

PROCEDURE: **Removing Excess Cement from a Casting**

1. After the cement has set, the cotton rolls are removed.
2. An explorer is used to carefully remove the excess cement from the crowns of the teeth.
   □ *IMPORTANT:* This is done very carefully so as not to scratch the newly placed crown or injure the gingiva.
3. Dental floss, with knots tied in it, is passed between the teeth to remove excess cement from the interproximal areas.
   □ *RATIONALE:* The knots in the floss provide added bulk to remove the cement.
4. After the excess cement has been removed, the crown may be polished by using polishing points in the low-speed handpiece (Figs. 31–13 and 31–14).

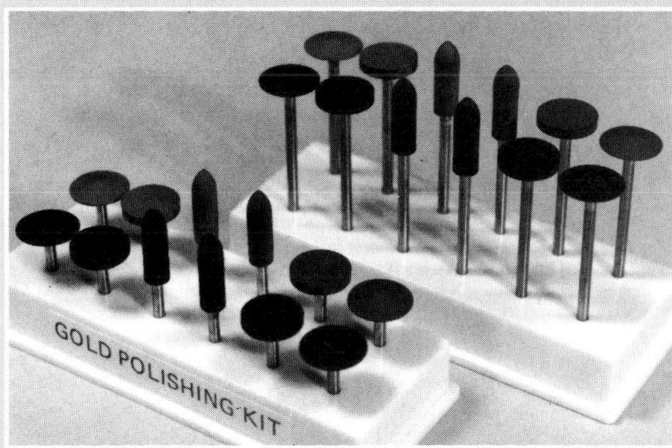

FIGURE 31–13

Polishing kits for gold restorations. These kits contain Brownie points for finishing, Greenie points for polishing, and Supergreenie points for final polishing. (Courtesy of Shofu Dental Corp., Menlo Park, CA.)

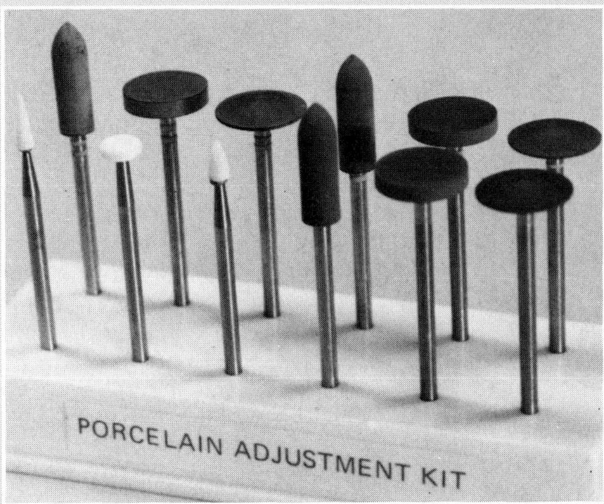

FIGURE 31–14

Polishing kit for porcelain adjustments. This kit contains the points and stones required for polishing and adjusting porcelain restorations. White points, which do not discolor the restoration, are used for the final polish. (Courtesy of Shofu Dental Corp., Menlo Park, CA.)

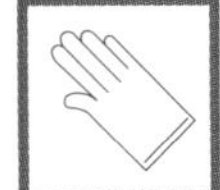
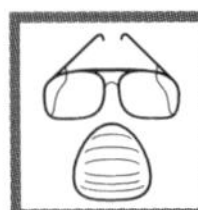
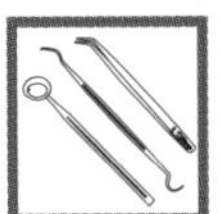
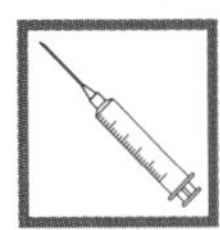

PROCEDURE: Creating a Self-Curing Composite Core Build-Up

1. The self-curing composite is prepared. When the composite is mixed, a small amount of a contrasting color, such as blue, is added.
   □ *RATIONALE:* This distinguishes the core material from the dentin of the tooth.
2. The composite is placed in a lubricated celluloid anatomic crown form and placed on the tooth.
3. After the initial set of the composite material, the crown form is slit and peeled away. The initial set is generally only a few minutes.
4. After the final set (approximately 10 minutes), the composite tooth material is reduced to provide the foundation of the crown preparation.

Before the permanent restoration can be placed, the temporary coverage must be removed. A large spoon excavator, a scaler, or a Backhaus towel forceps may be used for this purpose. The temporary coverage should be placed aside, just in case there is a problem with the crown and it is needed again.

PROVISIONAL PLACEMENT OF A PERMANENT RESTORATION

Once a cast restoration has been permanently cemented, it *cannot* be removed without damaging the casting. In special situations, such as when a tooth is very sensitive, the dentist may choose to initially place the casting with a temporary cement such as the one used for provisional coverage.

This provisional placement makes it possible to remove the casting without damage if there is a problem with the tooth. If there are no problems, within a few weeks the crown is luted into place with a permanent cement.

Retention Aids for Crowns

If the coronal portion of the tooth is extensively decayed, fractured, or badly broken down or has been treated endodontically, it may be necessary to provide additional support for the crown.

CORE BUILD-UPS

If the tooth is vital, a core build-up is used. This core supports the cast and crown and provides a larger area of retention for cementation of the crown.

If an amalgam restoration is already in place in the tooth, this may be shaped and prepared (just like natural tooth structure) for use as the core. If this is not the case, either a self-curing or light-cured composite material or reinforced glass ionomer cement is used for the build-up.

Pin Retention

Pin retention may be necessary to add strength to the core build-up for the crown. The exact location of the pin holes and placement of the pins are determined by the type of crown and the location of the pulp.

When pins are used, they are placed before the core build-up and are then incorporated into the build-up material. The steps in the preparation and placement of these pins are very similar to those in the placement of pins in an amalgam restoration, which is discussed in Chapter 25.

POSTS AND CORE

If the tooth is non-vital (has been treated endodontically), a post is placed into the pulp canal. Prefabricated posts made of titanium and titanium alloy are available. If one of these fits accurately, a preformed post may be used.

To provide strength and stability to the post and crown, the post is usually placed deep into the canal, and a portion of the post extends out of the canal to the height of the core build-up. After the post has been cemented in place, a core build-up is placed to support the crown (Fig. 31–15).

A post channel, which is the opening where the post will be cemented, is created by enlarging the treated

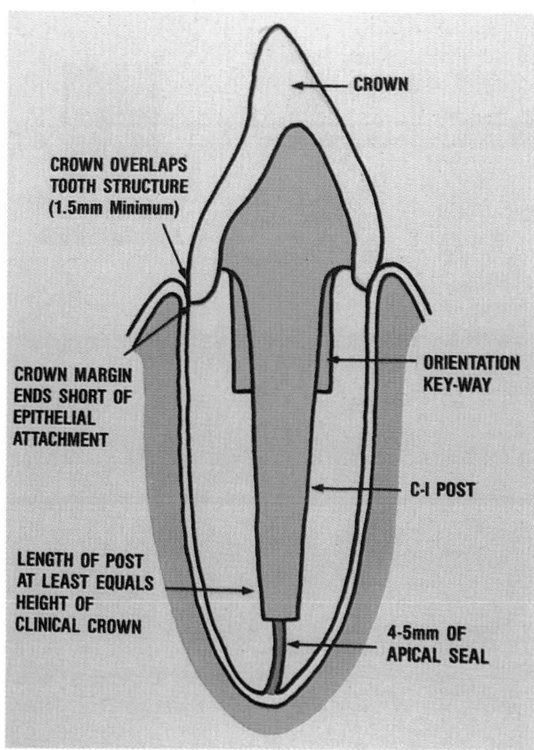

FIGURE 31–15

Post and core placement in an endodontically treated tooth. Highlights of the design are noted as labels on the diagram. (Courtesy of Parkell, Farmingdale, NY.)

pulp canal. Keyway slots, which hold the post steady in the canal, are created in the adjacent dentin.

After the opening has been prepared, a preformed post is selected and fitted. A Lentulo spiral, of the type used in endodontic treatment, is used to place the bonding system materials down the post channel. Once bonding of the post is complete, the dentist may proceed with the composite core build-up and tooth preparation.

Gingival Retraction

The final impression must include detail of the preparation that extends slightly below the finish line. Obtaining this detail is possible through the use of gingival retraction, which temporarily displaces the gingival tissue and widens the gingival sulcus so that the impression material can flow around all parts of the preparation.

Gingival retraction takes place *after* the preparation is complete and *just before* the final impression is taken. Chemical retraction, through the use of retraction cord, is the most commonly used method. However, in special situations, surgical or mechanical retraction may be required.

In some states the extended function dental assistant (EFDA), with the appropriate training, is delegated the task of placing and removing the retraction cord. These tasks are performed under the direct supervision of the dentist.

Gingival Retraction Cord

Chemical retraction involves placing **gingival retraction cord,** also known as *packing cord,* into the sulcus surrounding the tooth. The mechanical action of the cord forces the tissues away from the tooth. The chemicals on the cord also cause the tissues to contract (shrink), and this temporarily widens the sulcus.

STYLES OF RETRACTION CORD

Gingival retraction cords are available as untwisted (plain), twisted, or braided. Untwisted cords must be twisted just before placement. Twisted and braided cords do not require additional twisting.

NON-IMPREGNATED AND IMPREGNATED RETRACTION CORD

Non-impregnated retraction cord does not contain chemicals and retracts the tissues only by mechanical action.

Impregnated retraction cord contains an astringent-vasoconstrictor chemical that controls bleeding and causes the desired temporary shrinkage of the tissues.

Cords impregnated with epinephrine are potentially hazardous to the patient with cardiovascular disease. For this reason, the patient's updated medical history is reviewed before the impregnated forms are used.

When the use of epinephrine is contraindicated, a cord impregnated with aluminum chloride may be used instead. Aluminum chloride is a mineral astringent that does not produce undesirable cardiovascular effects.

A hemostatic solution may also be used to control bleeding in the area. This is dispensed into a dappen dish and applied by dabbing the area of bleeding lightly with a cotton pellet moistened with the solution. Any solution that is dispensed but not used is discarded.

RETRACTION CORD PACKING INSTRUMENT

Retraction cord is placed with the use of a blunt cord-packing instrument (see Fig. 31–7, upper left). This has a straight handle with a broad, rounded working end that is used to gently place the retraction cord in the sulcus.

Some operators use a plastic instrument with a blunted tip for this purpose. No matter what instrument is used, the goal is to place the retraction cord *without* damaging the gingival tissues.

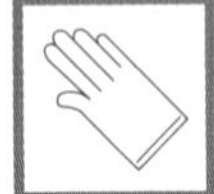
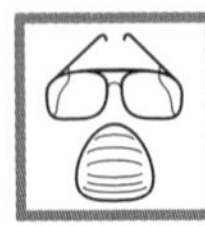
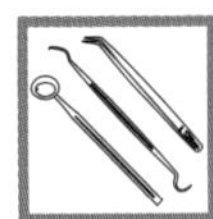
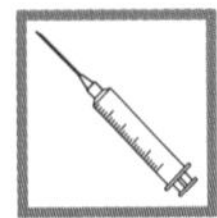

PROCEDURE: **Placing and Removing Retraction Cord**

Preparation

1. The prepared tooth is rinsed and gently dried, and the quadrant is isolated with cotton rolls.
   □ *RATIONALE:* Dry tissue makes it easier to see the details of the gingival tissue and to place the retraction cord.
2. The assistant cuts a piece of retraction cord 1 to 1½ inches in length, depending on the size and type of tooth under preparation.
   □ *RATIONALE:* The length is determined by the circumference of the prepared tooth and the placement technique to be used.
3. The assistant uses cotton pliers to form a loose loop of the cord. The cord, in the cotton plier, is passed to the operator along with the blunt packing instrument.
   □ *IMPORTANT:* This loop makes the cord easy to slip over the tooth; however, the loop is *not* tied or knotted.

Placement

1. The loop of the retraction cord is slipped over the tooth and laid in the sulcus around the prepared tooth (Fig. 31–16).
2. The operator uses the packing instrument and, working in a clockwise direction, packs the cord very gently into the sulcus surrounding the prepared tooth so that the ends are on the facial aspect (Fig. 31–17).
   □ *RATIONALE:* The ends in this position are easiest to reach for removal of the cord.

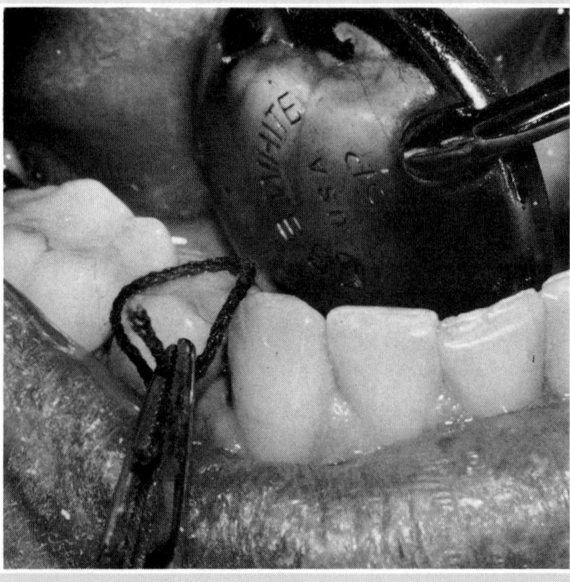

FIGURE 31–16

A loop of twisted retraction cord is placed over the prepared tooth.

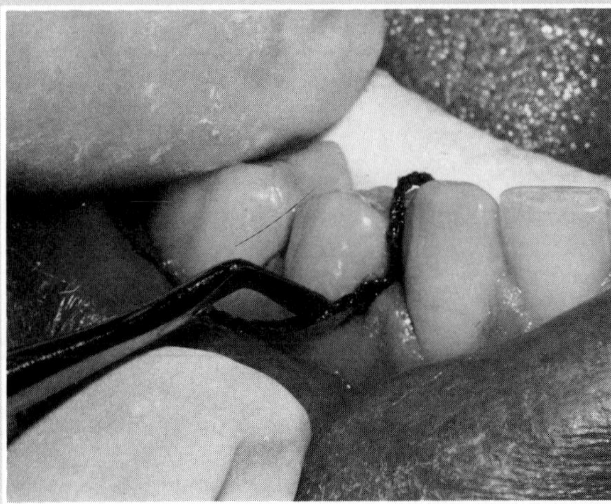

FIGURE 31–17

A blunt packing instrument is used to gently force the cord into the sulcus. The cord is packed in a clockwise direction.

3. The operator packs the cord into the sulcus by gently rocking the instrument slightly backward as the instrument is moved forward to the next loose section of retraction cord. This action is repeated until the length of cord is packed in place.
4. The cord is overlapped where it meets the first end of the cord. The ends may be tucked into the sulcus on the facial aspect.
   □ *ALTERNATIVE:* Leave a short length of the cord sticking out of the sulcus. This makes it easier to grasp and quickly remove the cord (Fig. 31–18).
5. *Optional:* When a wider and deeper sulcus is required, two retraction cords may be placed with one on top of the other. *Before* the impression material is taken, the top cord is removed. *After* the impression has been completed, the second retraction cord is removed.
6. The cord is left in place for 5 to a maximum of 7 minutes. During this time, the patient is advised to remain still, and the area is kept dry.
   □ *RATIONALE:* The exact time depends on the type of chemical retraction used.

Removal

1. The retraction cord is removed just before the impression material is placed (Fig. 31–19). Usually the operator removes the cord while the assistant prepares the syringe-type impression material.
2. The end of the retraction cord is grasped with cotton pliers and is removed in a counterclockwise direction. (This direction is the reverse of that used in the method of packing.)
3. The area is gently dried, fresh cotton rolls are placed, and the impression is taken immediately.

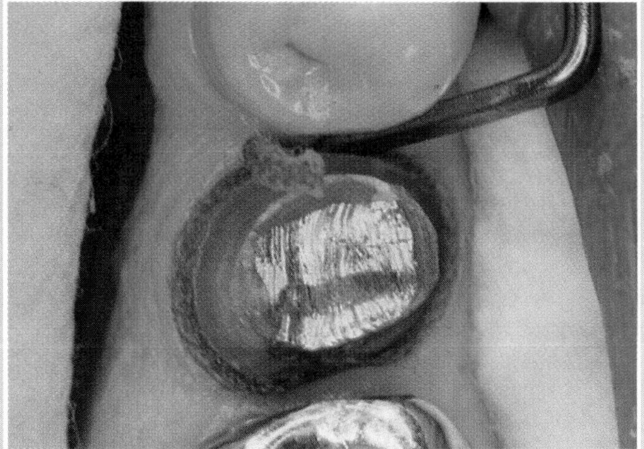

FIGURE 31–18

Completed placement of the gingival retraction cord. (Courtesy of 3M Dental Products Division, St. Paul, MN.)

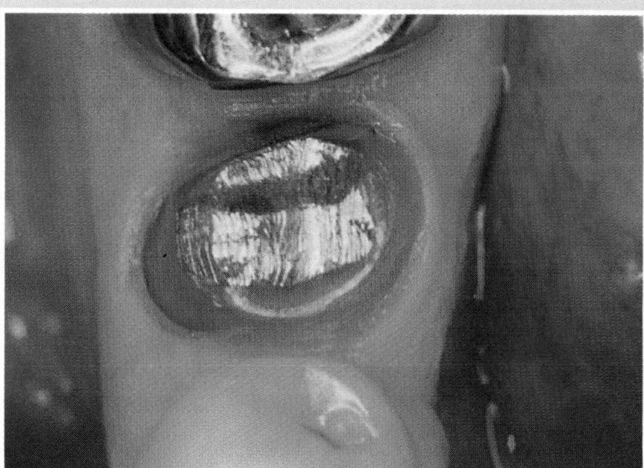

FIGURE 31–19

The retraction cord is removed just before the impression is taken. The gingiva is retracted, and the area is ready for the impression. (Courtesy of 3M Dental Products Division, St. Paul, MN.)

Surgical Retraction

Surgical retraction may be necessary if there is hypertrophied (overgrown) tissue that interferes with preparing and placing the restoration. This excess tissue may be removed surgically by using electrosurgery or a surgical knife.

Electrosurgery, the most commonly used method, is performed with a special electric tip that quickly cuts away the excess tissue and controls the bleeding.

With a **surgical knife**, the operator cuts the excess gingiva and frees it from the area. Bleeding may be profuse, and pressure or hemostatic material must be applied.

Mechanical Retraction

If other retraction methods are not suitable for the patient, the dentist may use mechanical retraction to force the tissue away from the tooth. A temporary crown, one that extends into the sulcus, is placed and worn by the patient for several days. It is removed just before the impression is taken. The use of mechanical retraction requires an extra patient visit in order to take the final impressions. At the end of that visit, normal temporary coverage is placed.

The Final Impression

The final impression, also referred to as the *master impression*, for a cast restoration must be accurate and detailed. If the impression is defective, the casting will also be defective. Elastomeric impression materials are used to create these extremely accurate impressions.

It is also necessary at this time to obtain an occlusal registration and an opposing arch registration. All of these materials and techniques are discussed in Chapter 24.

Temporary Coverage

After the tooth has been prepared, and before the cast restoration is ready, the patient wears **temporary coverage,** which is also known as *provisional coverage.* This coverage

- Reduces sensitivity and discomfort in the prepared tooth
- Maintains function and esthetics of the tooth
- Protects the margins of the preparation
- Prevents shifting of the adjacent or opposing teeth

Temporary coverage may be a preformed acrylic crown, a preformed metal crown, or custom-constructed temporary coverage (Fig. 31–20) (see Criteria for Temporary Coverage). In some states, the construction and seating of custom temporary coverage are delegated to the EFDA.

Preformed Acrylic Crown

Preformed acrylic crowns, also known as *stock crowns*, are available in a variety of sizes, shapes, and shades. If a preformed crown is tried in the mouth and *not* selected for use, it must be sterilized before reuse.

Preformed Aluminum Temporary Coverage

A prepared posterior tooth may be protected by placement of a preformed aluminum temporary crown. Like other preformed crowns, these are available in a range of sizes. Those tried in the mouth but not selected for use must be sterilized before reuse.

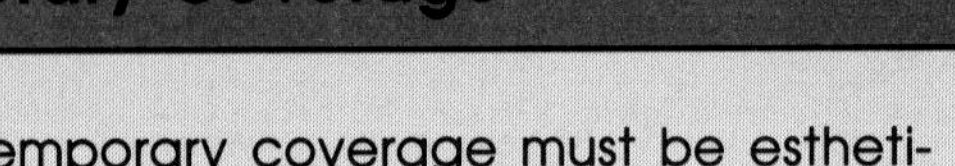

Criteria for Temporary Coverage

- The temporary coverage must be esthetically acceptable to the patient.
- The contours of the temporary coverage are similar to those of the natural tooth, with adequate interproximal contacts and appropriate alignment within the arch.
- The cervical margin of the temporary coverage is smooth and fits snugly, with no more than 0.5 mm. of space between the crown margin and the finish line of the preparation.
- The occlusal surface of the temporary coverage is aligned with the occlusal plane of the adjacent teeth.
- To avoid trauma to the prepared tooth, the crown may be intentionally taken out of occlusion by making the occlusal surface slightly lower than the adjacent teeth.
- When cemented, the temporary crown remains stable, stays in place, and is comfortable for the patient.
- The temporary coverage can be readily removed without damage to the tooth or adjacent tissues.

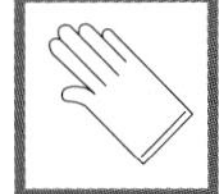
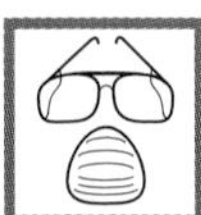
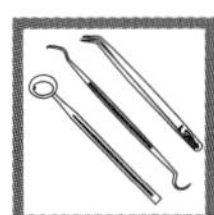
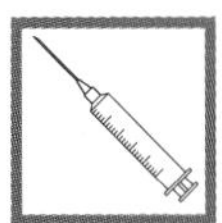
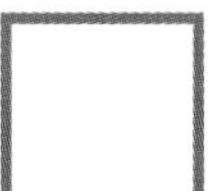

PROCEDURE: **Placing a Preformed Acrylic Crown**

Preparation of a Preformed Acrylic Crown

1. The appropriate-shape and -size crown is selected and checked for width, length, and adaptation at the margins.
2. If necessary, crown scissors are used to reduce the height (length) of the crown by trimming the cervical margin.
3. Rough edges are smoothed with an acrylic trimming stone or acrylic bur and polished with a Burlew wheel or a brush with pumice.

Cementation of a Preformed Acrylic Crown

1. Temporary cement is used to hold the crown in place. Intermediate restorative material (IRM) powder mixed with a small amount of petroleum jelly may be used.
   □ *RATIONALE:* The petroleum jelly facilitates removal of the crown.
2. Excess cement is carefully removed with an explorer or scaler.
3. The occlusion is checked. If indicated, a stone in the low-speed handpiece is used lightly to adjust the occlusion.

Custom Acrylic Temporary Coverage

Custom acrylic temporary coverage for crowns and bridges is prepared with self-curing acrylic (methylmethacrylate) placed in an alginate impression or vacuum-formed tray of the arch taken before the preparation of the teeth. (Methylmethacrylate, a hazardous material, is discussed in Chapter 12.)

This material is supplied as a liquid (monomer) and a powder (polymer) (Fig. 31–21). The polymer is supplied in a variety of shades, and one can be selected to approximate the color of the adjacent teeth.

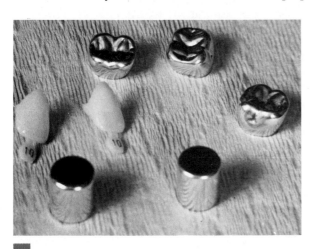

FIGURE 31–20

Preformed temporary coverage. *Top,* Three posterior crowns with anatomic features. *Center,* Two anterior acrylic temporary crowns. *Bottom,* Two aluminum crowns with no anatomic features.

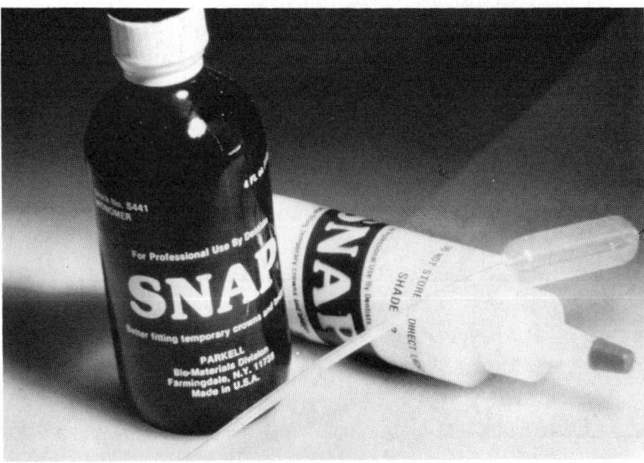

FIGURE 31–21

A self-curing acrylic used to fabricate custom temporary coverage. (Courtesy of Parkell, Farmingdale, NY.)

 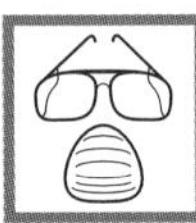 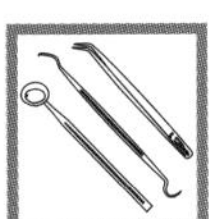 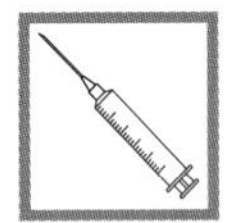 

PROCEDURE: **Fitting and Cementing an Aluminum Temporary Crown**

Preparation

1. In the mouth, a millimeter ruler is used to measure the mesial-to-distal space available for the temporary crown.
   □ *RATIONALE:* This mesial-to-distal measurement is taken so that the crown selected will maintain contact with the adjacent teeth.
2. *Optional step:* The temporary aluminum crown may be lined with methylmethacrylate (self-curing acrylic) for a better internal fit to the preparation.
3. To determine the crown length, the crown is placed on the prepared tooth and aligned with the other teeth.
   □ *RATIONALE:* Initially, the crown will be seated high on the tooth and must be trimmed to fit.
4. Using an explorer, the operator scribes (marks) a trim line on the lingual and facial surfaces of the crown near the gingiva. Then the crown is removed.
   □ *RATIONALE:* This line represents the length of the completed crown. It also follows the contour of the gingival margin.
5. Curved crown scissors are used in a continuous cut action to trim the crown to length and contour in a smooth, gently curved line.
   □ *RATIONALE:* A snipping action in trimming the crown results in sharp or uneven edges that can irritate the gingiva.
6. Contouring pliers are used to crimp the marginal edge of the crown *inward* on itself. (Contouring pliers Nos. 112, 114, and 115 are commonly used for this purpose.)
   □ *RATIONALE:* This aids in adapting the circumference of the crown to the finish line of the preparation.
7. The edges of the crown are smoothed by using various discs (coarse/medium garnet, sandpaper) on a mandrel and a rubber wheel mounted in the straight handpiece.
   □ *CAUTION:* To avoid creating a rough area, these are placed at an angle, not perpendicular, to the edge of the crown.
8. The crown is seated on the prepared tooth, and the patient is requested to close his teeth together normally.
   □ *RATIONALE:* This biting action impresses the preliminary occlusal anatomy onto the soft aluminum crown.
9. The occlusion is checked with articulating paper, and adjustments are made if necessary.
10. Dental floss is passed through the interproximal areas to determine that the crown provides contact with the adjacent teeth.
11. If the crown needs additional contour at the mesial-distal contact, it is removed from the tooth and placed on a paper pad, and the inside of the crown is burnished at contact areas with a ball burnisher.

Cementation

1. The prepared tooth is rinsed and dried carefully. Cotton rolls are placed to maintain dry conditions.
2. The crown is filled with temporary cement and then forced onto the prepared tooth.
3. Intermediate restorative material (IRM) powder mixed with petroleum jelly or zinc oxide–eugenol (ZOE) may be used for this purpose.
4. The patient is requested to close his teeth together to complete the seating of the crown. The cement is permitted to set for approximately 8 to 10 minutes.
5. When the cement has set, excess cement is removed with an explorer or scaler. The contacts are checked with dental floss to determine that all excess cement has been removed.
6. The crown is inspected to determine that it fits snugly and that the cement seals the margins.
7. The occlusion of the tooth is rechecked with articulating paper. If the crown is too high, the occlusion is reduced.

 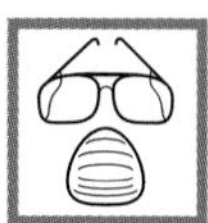 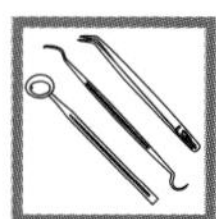 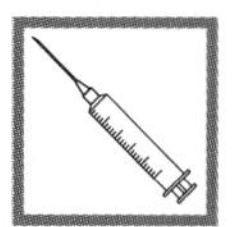 

PROCEDURE: **Fabricating Custom Acrylic Temporary Coverage**

Instrumentation

Alginate impression (obtained *before* the preparation of the teeth)
Separating medium
Self-curing acrylic resin (liquid and powder)
Spatula (small, cement-type)
Mixing container
Scissors
Surgical knife (optional)
Burnisher (beavertail or ball)
Mandrel and discs (garnet and sandpaper)
Greenstone acrylic trimming bur
Articulating paper
Straight handpiece
Pumice paste
Lathe and sterile white rag wheel
Safety goggles

Obtaining the Alginate Impression

1. Obtain an alginate impression of the arch *before* the teeth are prepared.
2. Check the impression to be sure it is free of debris and tears in the area selected for the construction of the temporary crown or bridge covering.
3. Disinfect the impression and keep it moist until needed.
   □ *RATIONALE:* If allowed to dry, the impression will be distorted and the temporary coverage will not fit.

Laboratory Preparation

These laboratory steps are performed just a few minutes before it is time to fit the temporary coverage in the patient's mouth.

1. Place a small amount of the selected shade of self-curing powder in the mixing container. Dispense just enough monomer to saturate the polymer.
   □ *IMPORTANT:* Cover the monomer container immediately. This material is very volatile.
2. Use a small spatula to blend the powder and liquid to a homogeneous mix.
3. Set the mixed material aside for 2 to 3 minutes until the resin reaches a doughy stage.
   □ *IMPORTANT:* Do not let the resin cure beyond this point.
4. Unwrap the alginate impression, and gently dry the area of the teeth to receive temporary coverage.
   □ *REMINDER:* Always wear gloves when handling an impression.
5. Remove the resin dough from the mixing container with the spatula or burnisher and immediately place it *within* the initial alginate impression in the area of the prepared teeth.

Treatment Room Preparation

1. Coat the prepared teeth with petroleum jelly or a liquid separating medium to facilitate separating the acrylic dough from the preparations.
2. Place the acrylic-loaded impression back into the patient's mouth on the prepared teeth.
3. Allow the material to reach an initial set (approximately 3 minutes) and remove the tray from the patient's mouth.
4. Carefully remove the temporary covering from the alginate impression and replace it back onto the patient's teeth.
   □ *RATIONALE:* This avoids excess shrinkage during the final curing stage.
5. Gross excess acrylic can be cut with scissors during the doughy stage. After the final setting, fine adjustments are made with an acrylic bur or stone. The acrylic resin should be trimmed to within 1 mm. of the gingival shoulder of the prepared tooth.
6. The occlusion, accuracy, and completeness of the temporary covering are checked and adjusted as necessary.
7. The temporary covering is removed and taken to the laboratory, where it is polished with a sterile, white rag wheel and pumice on the laboratory lathe.

(continued on following page)

PROCEDURE: **Fabricating Custom Acrylic Temporary Coverage** *(continued)*

☐ *CAUTION:* Safety goggles *must* be worn throughout the trimming and polishing procedure. Also, be aware that the rag wheel could remove a large bulk or could overheat and cause warpage of the temporary covering.

Cementation of Temporary Coverage

1. The occlusion is checked with articulating paper. If necessary, the temporary is removed and the marked areas are reduced with an acrylic trimming bur.
2. The covering is seated with a temporary cement such as ZOE or IRM with a little petroleum jelly added to the mix (Fig. 31–22).

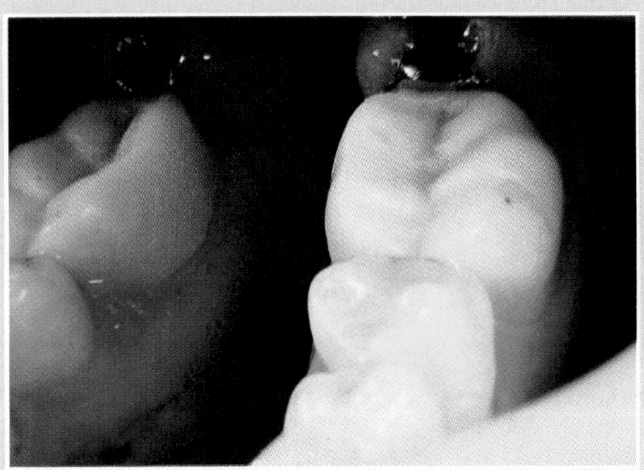

FIGURE 31–22

Temporary coverage placed on a mandibular molar. The sides of the coverage can be seen to the left reflected in a mirror. (Courtesy of Parkell, Farmingdale, NY.)

Home Care Instructions for the Patient with Temporary Coverage

1. Bite and chew carefully on the temporary coverage and avoid sticky foods.
2. Clean interproximally by pulling the floss down through the contact and then pull one end out of the contact (to either the lingual or facial side). This avoids dislodging the temporary by pulling the floss up through the contact.
3. If the temporary covering is loose or lost, contact the office immediately to have it replaced.

Porcelain and Composite Inlays and Onlays

The clinical preparation and placement steps for porcelain or composite inlay and onlay fabrication in the dental laboratory are very similar and are summarized here.

At the first visit, the shade is selected, the teeth are prepared, and the impressions and occlusal registration are taken. Self-curing acrylic (methylmethacrylate) temporary coverage is placed to protect the prepared tooth between visits.

At the delivery appointment, the temporary coverage is removed, dental dam is placed, and the cast restoration is tried for fit and occlusion. Adjustments are made as necessary.

The restoration is removed, rinsed, and dried, and the internal surface (tooth side) of the casting is painted with a thin coating of bonding material. The entire interior surface of the prepared tooth (dentin and margins) is prepared for bonding according to the manufacturer's directions.

The restoration is seated and held in place with a flat-ended instrument, such as a small condenser. Excess bonding agent around the occlusal and interproximal margins of the preparation is removed. Removal from the interproximal areas is particularly important because these areas are less accessible for polishing once the bonding material is cured and hardened.

In accordance with the manufacturer's instructions, the curing light is used to cure around the edges (margins) of the restoration.

After curing, any excess bonding material is removed with a curette, and the restoration is polished with a fine finishing bur in the high-speed handpiece.

The completed restoration is rinsed, dried, and coated with a thin film of light-cured, unfilled resin.

Porcelain Veneers

Porcelain veneers are placed to improve the appearance of the anterior teeth. Figures 31–23 to 31–26 show the placement of six veneers to improve the appearance of a patient with enamel hyperplasia.

An important factor in the creation and placement

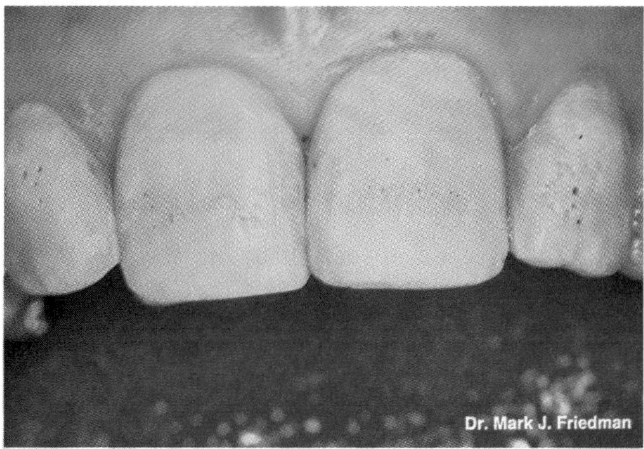

FIGURE 31–23

The patient's teeth before the placement of porcelain veneers. Notice the hyperplasia of the enamel. (Courtesy of 3M Dental Products Division, St. Paul, MN.)

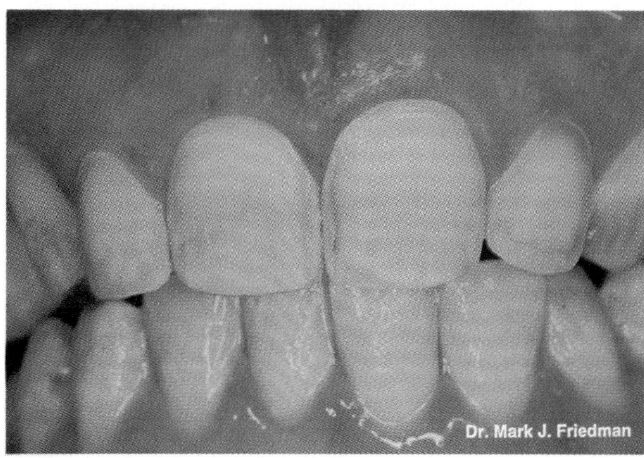

FIGURE 31–25

The completed preparations for six porcelain veneers. (Courtesy of 3M Dental Products Division, St. Paul, MN.)

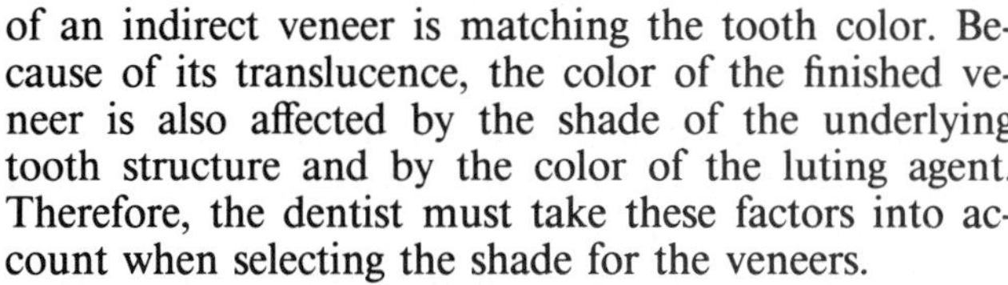

of an indirect veneer is matching the tooth color. Because of its translucence, the color of the finished veneer is also affected by the shade of the underlying tooth structure and by the color of the luting agent. Therefore, the dentist must take these factors into account when selecting the shade for the veneers.

The dentist uses specialized burs and discs to cut the preparation as conservatively as possible. After the preparations have been completed, gingival retraction is performed and the impressions are taken. Because the preparations remove only a thin layer of enamel on the facial surface and do not penetrate the dentin, temporary coverage is not required.

At the cementation visit, the dentist tries the veneers for fit and color match. Before cementation, an **opaquer** may be placed on the tooth surface to block out underlying color and structural defects.

The cement is also selected in a shade that will enhance the color match. After etching and bonding of the teeth, the veneers are cemented in place. Any excess cement is removed, and final adjustments are made.

Fixed Bridge Preparation and Placement

The construction of a fixed bridge, which is commonly referred to as *crown and bridge*, requires preci-

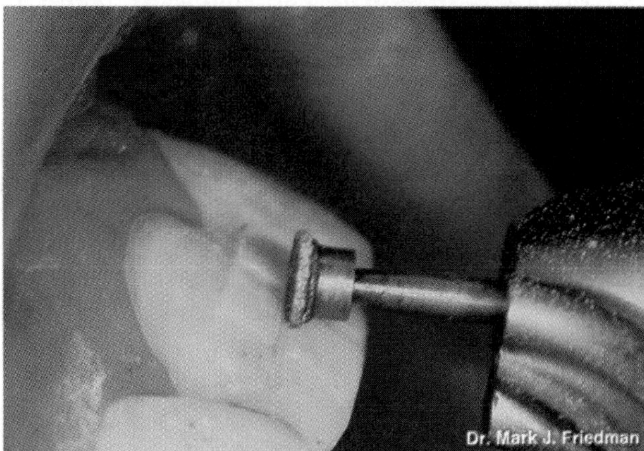

FIGURE 31–24

A depth-cutting diamond bur is used to ensure even reduction of the enamel. (Courtesy of 3M Dental Products Division, St. Paul, MN.)

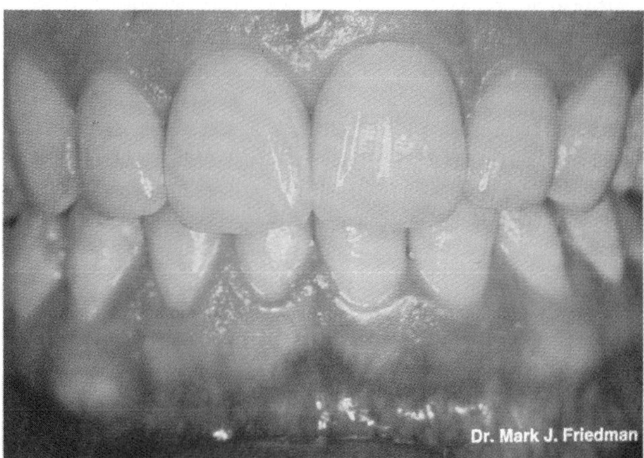

FIGURE 31–26

The completed case with six porcelain veneers in place. (Courtesy of 3M Dental Products Division, St. Paul, MN.)

sion and close cooperation on the part of the dentist and the dental laboratory technician.

The Components of a Fixed Bridge

A fixed bridge consists of a series of units joined together for greater strength. A **solder joint** is that point where two adjacent units of the bridge are joined together.

PONTICS

A pontic is an artificial tooth, or part of the dental appliance, that replaces a missing natural tooth. When a bridge replaces more than one tooth, there is a pontic for each tooth being replaced. The bridge shown in Figure 31–6 has two pontics.

ABUTMENTS

An abutment, also known as a *retainer*, is a natural tooth that serves as the support for the replacement tooth or teeth in a fixed bridge. There is at *least* one abutment at each end of the bridge. When a longer bridge is constructed to replace several teeth, there may be two abutment teeth at either end.

The abutment tooth is usually prepared with an onlay or a cast crown. Because the completed bridge is placed in the mouth as a single piece, the preparations of the abutment teeth must be in parallel alignment to allow the bridge to slide into place without adding excessive width or length.

UNITS

A bridge is described by the number of units involved. For example, a bridge to replace a single missing tooth is called a three-unit bridge because it consists of three parts (two abutments and a pontic).

Depending upon the abutments available, a four- to six-tooth span is the maximum advised for a fixed bridge. Where there is a long span without adequate natural abutments, an implant may be used to provide additional support. (Implants are discussed in Chapter 30.)

Crown and Bridge Appointments

The preparation for a fixed bridge is usually completed in three appointments.

THE PREPARATION APPOINTMENT

The first appointment is very similar to that for a crown; however, this involves the preparation of at least two or more teeth, and a longer appointment is required.

Depending on the case, the abutment teeth are usually prepared for either a full crown or an onlay. After the preparations are complete, final impressions, occlusal registration, and the opposing arch impression must be taken. Then a custom provisional or temporary bridge is placed. This is prepared according to the same technique as for coverage for an individual tooth.

THE TRY-IN APPOINTMENT

Before the second appointment, the assistant determines that the case has been returned from the laboratory. At this stage, the case consists of the castings for the abutment teeth without their tooth-colored covering.

Local anesthetic is administered, and the temporary coverage is carefully removed, cleaned, and placed aside to be used again.

The castings are tried on the abutment teeth and checked carefully to determine their accurate fit. If the castings do not fit properly, final impressions must be retaken and the try-in steps must be repeated at the next appointment.

If the castings fit, they are left in place, and a vinyl polysiloxane impression is taken. When the impression is removed, the castings come off in the impression. The impression and castings are disinfected and returned to the dental laboratory for finishing.

The temporary coverage is replaced, and the patient is scheduled for the final appointment.

In the laboratory, the technician uses this impression to assemble the bridge exactly as it will fit in the mouth. The units are soldered together, and the tooth-colored porcelain covering is added.

THE CEMENTATION APPOINTMENT

Before the patient's appointment, the assistant checks to determine that the finished bridge has been returned by the laboratory.

A local anesthetic is administered, and the temporary coverage is removed. The completed bridge is

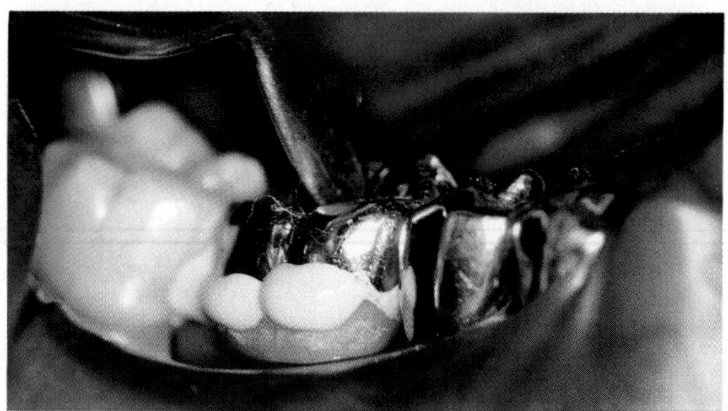

FIGURE 31–27

Cementation of a three-unit gold bridge. Notice the excess cement near the gingival margin. (Courtesy of Parkell, Farmingdale, NY.)

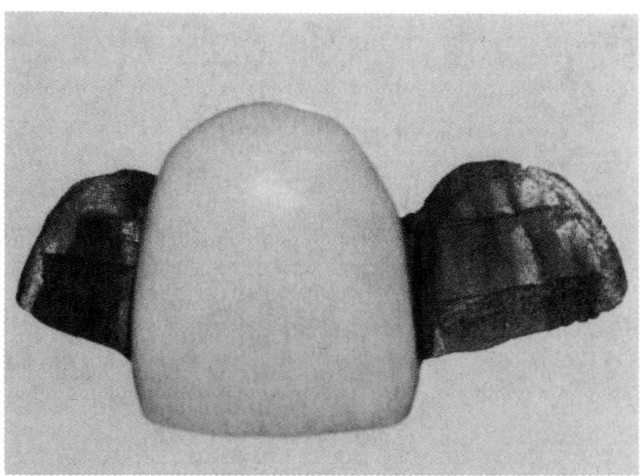

FIGURE 31–28

A resin-bonded bridge ready for placement. The cast metal abutments have been etched for retention. (From Phillips, R.W., and Moore, B.K.: Elements of Dental Materials for Dental Hygienists and Dental Assistants, 5th ed. Philadelphia, W.B. Saunders Co., 1994, p 270.)

tried on the prepared teeth. Adjustments are made as necessary, and the bridge is cemented in place (Fig. 31–27).

Resin-Bonded Bridges

A resin-bonded bridge, also known as a *Maryland bridge*, consists of a pontic with winglike extensions coming from the mesial and distal sides (Fig. 31–28). The pontic is supported by bonding these extensions to the lingual surfaces of the adjacent teeth.

In selected situations, such as the replacement of a single missing anterior tooth or the replacement of congenitally missing lateral incisors, a bonded bridge is an attractive alternative to a traditional bridge.

A traditional bridge requires extensive preparation of the abutment teeth, and the completed restoration is cemented in place. In contrast, a bonded bridge requires very little preparation of the abutment teeth, and the completed restoration is bonded in place.

The lingual surfaces of the adjacent teeth require only enough preparation to accommodate the bridge supports. Some bonded bridges have very thin metal mesh extensions. Others have cast or porcelain-fused-to-metal extensions. These require more extensive tooth preparation so that the natural contours of the abutment tooth are maintained when the completed bridge is bonded in place.

Dental dam is applied before placement of a bonded bridge to protect the adjacent tissues from the acid etchant. The surfaces to receive the bridge are etched and then bonded in accordance with the manufacturer's directions.

Home Care for the Patient with a Fixed Prosthesis

1. Good home care is essential to the maintenance of a fixed prosthesis.
2. The fixed prosthesis and supporting tissues must be brushed carefully each day.
3. A bridge threader is used to pass dental floss under the pontic and down into the sulcus at both abutments of the bridge.
4. Other teeth are flossed normally.

Chapter 32

Removable Prosthodontics

Introduction

Removable prosthodontics is the area of dentistry dealing with replacement of missing teeth with a prosthesis that the patient is able to remove and replace. There are two major types: removable partial dentures and removable complete dentures.

A **removable partial denture**, commonly referred to simply as a *partial*, replaces one or more teeth in one arch (Fig. 32–1).

A **removable complete denture**, commonly referred to simply as a *denture*, replaces most or all of the teeth in one arch (Fig. 32–2).

The laboratory technician plays an important part in the construction of these prostheses. The technician follows the dentist's written prescription and works in close cooperation with the dentist in the fabrication of each prosthesis.

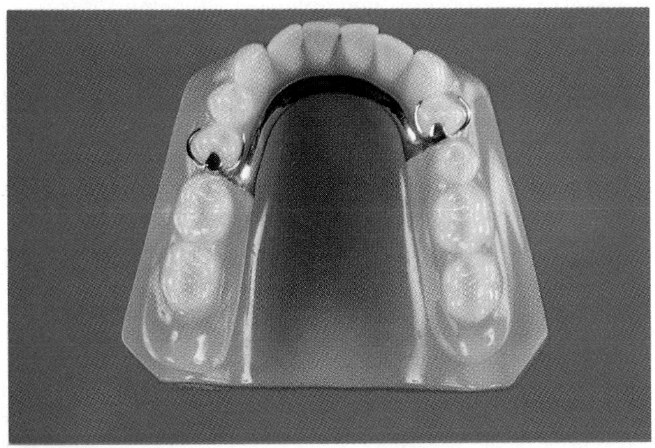

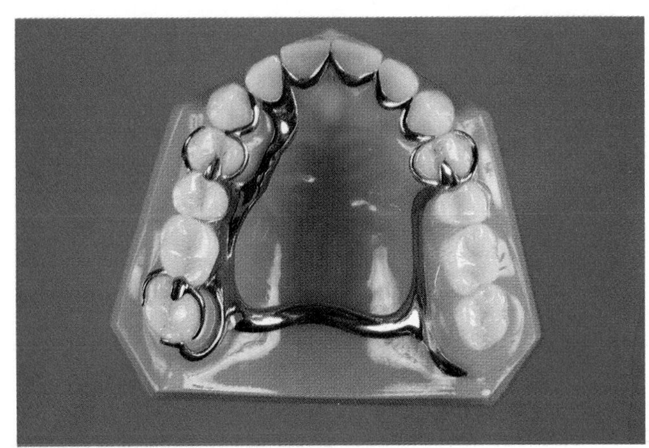

FIGURE 32–1

Removable partial dentures shown on typodonts. *Left*, Mandibular partial. *Right*, Maxillary partial.

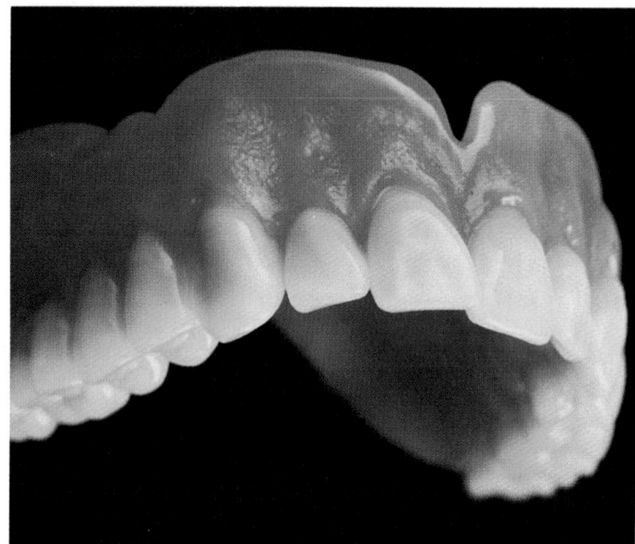

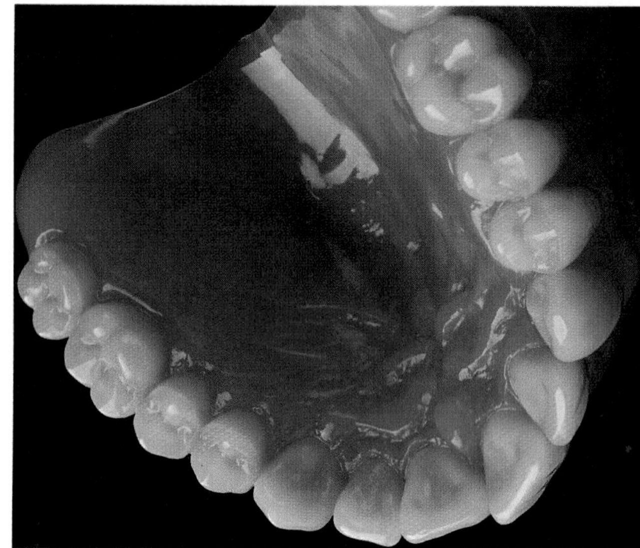

FIGURE 32–2

A complete maxillary denture. *Left*, Profile view. *Right*, Palatal view. (Courtesy of Ivoclar Williams, Amherst, NY.)

Examination and Case Presentation Visits

The examination and case presentation visits are similar for both a removable partial denture and a removable complete denture. They include a thorough clinical examination, a medical history, a complete radiographic survey, impressions for the diagnostic casts, and photographs of the full face and profile (if indicated).

The examination visit is discussed in Chapter 18. The chairside assistant may produce some of the diagnostic aids. (Radiographs are discussed in Chapter 17. Diagnostic casts are discussed in Chapter 19.)

If the prosthesis is to be supported by an implant, treatment planning is completed in cooperation with the oral surgeon, who will perform the surgical portion of treatment. (See Chapter 30.)

At the consultation visit, the dentist explains the diagnosis, presents the recommended treatment plan, and answers the patient's questions. If the patient is satisfied and agrees to the proposed treatment, the administrative assistant makes financial arrangements and schedules the necessary appointments.

The appointments required for partial and complete dentures are summarized in Tables 32–1 and 32–2.

TABLE 32–1

Appointments Required for Partial Dentures

APPOINTMENT NO.	BETWEEN APPOINTMENTS
Appointment 1: Preliminary impressions are taken for diagnostic casts	If indicated, custom trays are constructed on the diagnostic casts
Appointment 2: Final impressions are taken	The framework and occlusal rims are constructed
Appointment 3: Try-in of framework is made; occlusal registration is taken	Artificial teeth are set, and the partial is finished
Appointment 4: The completed partial denture is delivered	
Appointment 5: Adjustments are made as needed	

TABLE 32–2

Appointments Required for Complete Dentures

APPOINTMENT NO.	BETWEEN APPOINTMENTS
Appointment 1: Preliminary impressions are taken for diagnostic casts	Custom trays are constructed on the diagnostic casts
Appointment 2: Final impressions are taken	Baseplates and occlusal rims are constructed
Appointment 3: Try-in of baseplates and occlusal rims is made; occlusal registration is taken	Artificial teeth are set as prescribed by the dentist
Appointment 4: Try-in of the completed wax-up is made	The dentures are finished and polished
Appointment 5: The completed dentures are delivered	
Appointment 6: Adjustments are made as needed	

The number of days between appointments depends on the number of "working days" required by the laboratory for each step in the fabrication.

If the treatment plan involves restorative, periodontal, endodontic, or surgical treatment before the preparation for the prosthesis, this treatment must be completed and healing must have taken place *before* the prosthodontics treatment begins. The exception is immediate dentures, and these are discussed later in this chapter.

Factors Influencing the Choice of a Removable Prosthesis

The dentist advises all patients who are considering a removable prosthesis that, no matter how well constructed and fitted a prosthesis may be, it can never function as well as the natural dentition it is to replace.

The dentist takes the following extraoral and intraoral factors into consideration before recommending a treatment plan for the patient.

EXTRAORAL FACTORS

Although extraoral factors are usually beyond the control of the dentist, they cannot be ignored. These include the patient's physical and mental health, age, and occupation.

Physical Health. Certain physical conditions, such as diabetes, affect the ability of the tissues to tolerate the pressure of a removable prosthesis. Also, if the patient is in extremely poor health, he may be unable to cooperate during the fabrication of a new prosthesis or to adapt to wearing it.

Mental Health. An individual who is not in good mental health may be irritated by, and overly concerned about, the denture in his or her mouth.

Also, patients with severe mental retardation or advanced senility may not be able to keep the appliance in place or to maintain adequate oral hygiene.

Occasionally a patient's major reason for having teeth extracted and replaced with a prosthesis is esthetic—that is, only to improve appearance. When this happens, the dentist explores all other acceptable alternative treatment options before giving serious consideration to the request.

Age. The design of a prosthesis for a young person must allow for growth and accommodate new teeth as they erupt. If the patient is very active or plays contact sports, the strength of the appliance is also an important factor.

Chronological age alone is not a factor in determining whether a fixed or removable prosthesis is placed. Instead, the decision must be based on all of the other factors combined.

A different problem is found in the attitude of an older patient who associates the loss of teeth with age and has an unrealistic desire to retain teeth that are structurally unsound.

Social and Economic Factors. Social and economic factors are also important. These include the patient's attitude toward the importance of replacing lost teeth and his ability to pay for this treatment.

Occupation. A patient whose daily activities involve meeting the public is concerned about the possible change in his or her appearance during or after the transition to partial or full dentures.

Appointments for surgery and the delivery of the prosthesis should be scheduled without seriously disrupting the patient's social and occupational activities.

INTRAORAL FACTORS

The condition of the tissues of the patient's mouth is a key factor in determining whether a removable partial or a complete denture can be recommended.

Musculature. Facial muscles contribute to the retention and functional control of the prosthesis. For these reasons, strong muscle attachments with good muscle tone are important.

Conversely, a large or very active tongue may cause difficulty in retention and wearing of the prosthesis. A patient with severe nervous, eccentric facial habits may have difficulty retaining and adjusting to a prosthesis. Extreme facial contortions will displace the denture by breaking the suction holding the denture in place, particularly the maxillary denture.

Salivary Flow. A new object in the oral cavity, such as a prosthesis, may stimulate an excessive flow of saliva. This response usually diminishes and is controlled as the patient becomes accustomed to wearing the prosthesis.

However, the denture may aggravate a condition in which the patient cannot control salivation, such as paralysis of the facial muscles in a stroke victim.

In contrast, a patient with a problem that severely inhibits the flow of saliva may find a prosthesis uncomfortable and difficult to wear. Lack of adequate salivary flow may be caused by physical conditions, medications, or radiation treatment.

Residual Alveolar Ridge. The prosthesis depends mainly upon the quality of the residual alveolar ridge for support. The **residual alveolar ridge** is the bony ridge remaining *after* the teeth have been extracted.

If the alveolar ridge is high and evenly contoured, it provides good support and even distribution of the stress of mastication. If the alveolar ridge has been resorbed so that it is narrow or irregular in formation, it does not provide adequate support, and the denture causes sore spots where it rests on the mucosa.

In some cases, before the placement of a prosthesis it is necessary to surgically recontour the ridge to minimize such problems. This procedure, known as an alveoloplasty, is discussed in Chapter 30.

It is a normal ongoing process that the alveolar ridge will continue to decrease in size and change in shape after the teeth are lost. A well-fitted prosthesis minimizes these changes. An ill-fitting prosthesis accelerates the process. Because of these changes, it is important that the patient return periodically for an oral examination and reevaluation of the fit of the prosthesis.

Oral Mucosa. If the attached mucosa covering the residual ridge is altered by the patient's physical condition, the prosthesis may cause friction and irritation and be difficult for the patient to wear.

Likewise, an ill-fitting prosthesis may cause irritation and sore spots, known as **pressure points**, on the oral mucosa. When this occurs, the patient should be seen promptly so that the dentist can relieve these sore spots.

Oral Habits. Because they cause extreme stress on the ridges and remaining teeth, oral habits such as clenching or grinding must be taken into account when a prosthesis is planned.

Mouth breathing may also affect the patient's ability to hold the appliance in place.

Tori. If either mandibular or maxillary tori are present, they will impact the patient's ability to wear a prosthesis in that arch. (A **torus** is a benign bulging bony projection. *Tori* is the plural.)

Depending upon the type of prosthesis required, it may be necessary to have the tori surgically removed before fabrication of the appliance is begun.

Exposure Control and Removable Prosthodontics

The appropriate exposure control protocols must be followed throughout prosthodontics treatment in the treatment room, while laboratory work is performed, and whenever laboratory cases are handled. (See Chapter 13.)

- Examination gloves are always worn when laboratory work that has been tried in the mouth is handled.
- Laboratory work is always disinfected before it is sent to the laboratory.
- Laboratory work is always disinfected when it is returned from the laboratory.
- The prosthesis is always disinfected and rinsed before it is placed in the patient's mouth.

These cases are disinfected by spraying them with an Environmental Protection Agency– (EPA-) registered disinfectant.

Physical Properties of Removable Prosthodontics Materials

Removable prostheses involve primarily the use of castings made of base metal alloys and denture resins.

Base Metal Alloys

These alloys are used primarily in the construction of removable partial dentures. A base metal alloy contains at least 85 percent of nickel, cobalt, and chromium. These alloys are shiny silver in color and have special qualities that make them well suited for this application.

The **elastic modulus** of these alloys is about twice that of gold-based alloys. This results in the ability to construct thinner, lighter restorations. (**Elastic modulus** is a measure of the rigidity or stiffness of a material at stresses below its elastic limit. **Elastic limit** is the maximum stress that a structure or material can withstand without being permanently deformed.)

The **hardness** of base metal alloys is greater than that of gold-based alloys, but these alloys have low ductility. (**Ductility** is the ability of a material to withstand permanent deformation under tensile stress without fracture. **Tensile stress** is the force that tends to stretch, or elongate, an object.)

Low ductility means that they are somewhat brittle, and patients should be cautioned about bending the retainers on a partial denture framework because this could cause them to break.

Base metal alloys have the advantage in that they do not corrode in the oral environment. However, chlorine, as found in sodium hypochlorite bleaches, is very destructive and causes rapid corrosion. For this reason, an appliance with a metal frame is never immersed in a chlorine-containing disinfectant.

Occasionally, a patient is sensitive to the nickel content of the base metal alloy. In these cases, an alternative alloy, such as a strong gold alloy, would be recommended.

Denture Resins

The material for the base of complete or partial removable dentures is gingiva-tinted polymethyl-methacrylate resin. Unlike the other resins previously discussed, these are cast into shape in a rigid mold and are polymerized under heat and pressure.

Partial Dentures

A **removable partial denture** receives its support and retention from the underlying tissues and some of the remaining teeth that serve as abutments. The prosthesis is designed to distribute the forces of mastication between these abutments and the supporting tissues.

Indications for a Partial Denture

- To replace several teeth in the same quadrant or in both quadrants of the same arch
- As a temporary replacement for missing teeth in a child (as necessary, a new appliance is constructed to compensate for the child's growth)
- To avoid reducing tooth structure on primary or permanent dentition of children and adolescents

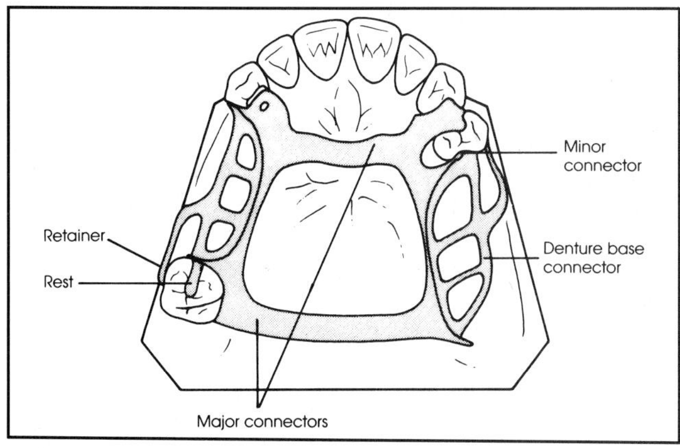

FIGURE 32–3

The parts of a maxillary partial denture. (Modified from Kratochvil, F.J.: Partial Removable Prosthodontics. Philadelphia, W.B. Saunders Co., 1988, p 8.)

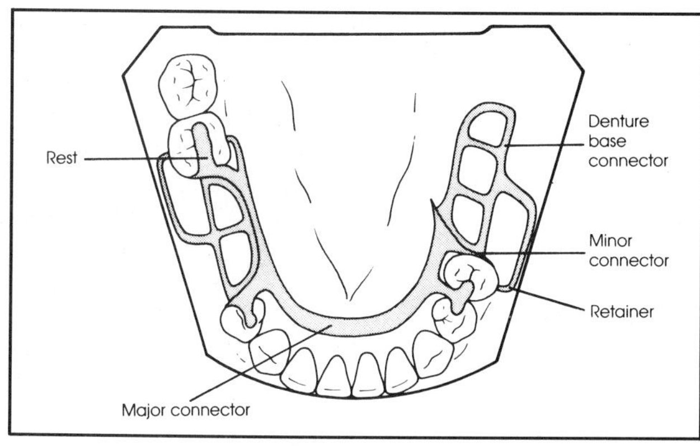

FIGURE 32–4

The parts of a mandibular partial denture. (Modified from Kratochvil, F.J.: Partial Removable Prosthodontics. Philadelphia, W.B. Saunders Co., 1988, p 8.)

- Preparation and placement of the appliance usually requires only a few patient visits.
- Because the appliance is removable, the patient may find it easier to maintain good oral hygiene
- The removable prosthesis may be designed to serve also as a splint to support periodontally involved teeth

Contraindications for a Partial Denture

- A lack of suitable teeth in the arch to support, stabilize, and retain the removable prosthesis
- Rampant caries and/or severe periodontal conditions that threaten the remaining teeth in the arch
- A lack of patient acceptance and/or chronic poor oral hygiene

Components of a Partial Denture

The basic components of a removable partial denture are the framework, major connector, saddle, retainers, rests, and artificial teeth (Figs. 32–3 and 32–4; also see Fig. 32–1).

FRAMEWORK

The framework is the cast metal skeleton that provides support for the saddle and the connectors of the partial denture (Fig. 32–5). Instead of a metal framework, some partials are made with an acrylic resin base.

MAJOR CONNECTOR

The major connector, also known as a *bar,* is the piece of rigid metal that joins the right and left quadrant framework of the partial denture. The connector also helps to form support for the remaining teeth so that the stress is evenly distributed.

A maxillary partial denture has a **palatal connector,** and a mandibular partial denture has a **lingual connector.**

A **stress-breaker** is a metal device built into a partial denture design that relieves the abutment teeth from excessive occlusal loads and stresses during mastication. A stress-breaker is advised for abutment teeth that have limited support in the alveolar ridge.

SADDLE

The saddle is a metal mesh extension of the connector that is covered with the acrylic. Resting on the oral mucosa covering the alveolar ridge, the saddle holds the artificial teeth and provides some support for the prosthesis.

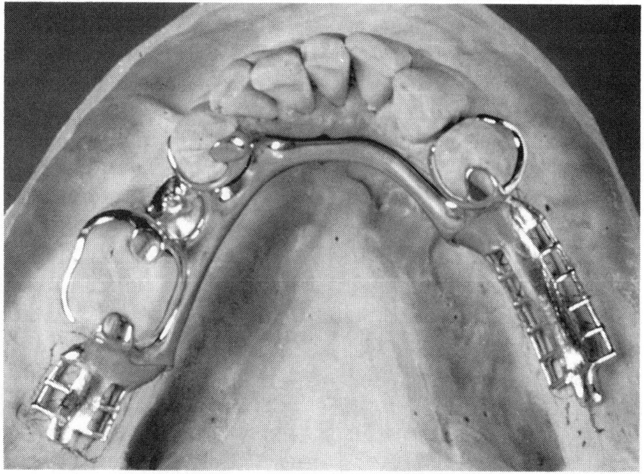

FIGURE 32–5

The framework for a mandibular partial denture. Notice the retainers around the teeth and the rests on the teeth. The mesh will be covered with denture resin to support the artificial teeth and form the saddle.

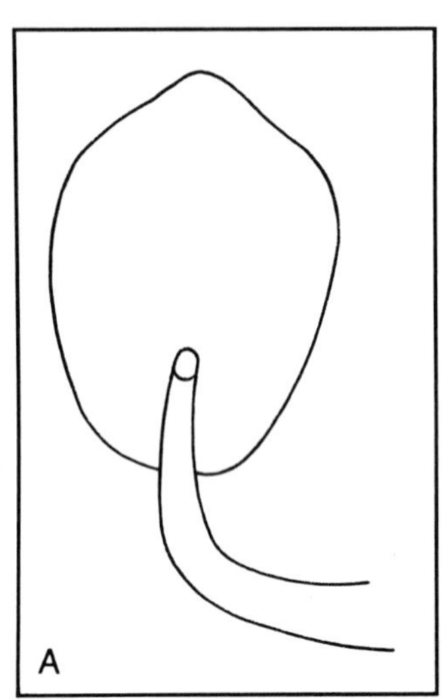

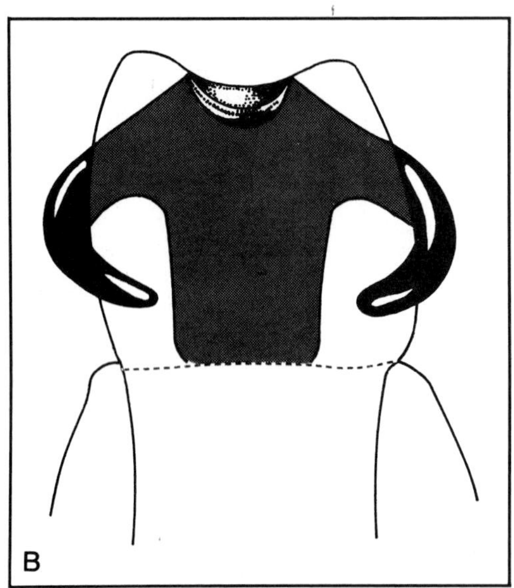

FIGURE 32–6

Types of retainers. *A*, Diagram of an I-bar retainer. *B*, Diagram of a circumferential retainer. (Modified from Kratochvil, F.J.: Partial Removable Prosthodontics. Philadelphia, W.B. Saunders Co., 1988, pp 42 and 8.)

RETAINERS

A retainer, also known as a *clasp*, is the portion of the framework that directly supports and provides stability to the partial denture by partially encircling an abutment tooth.

An **I-bar retainer** approaches the tooth in a straight line from the apical direction and extends upward against the tooth (Fig. 32–6*A*).

A **circumferential retainer** originates at the occlusal surface of the tooth and extends downward so that it partially encircles the tooth (see Figs. 32–1, 32–5, and 32–6*B*.)

RESTS

A rest is a metal projection on or near the clasp. The rest is designed to control the extent of the seating of the prosthesis as it is inserted into the oral cavity and placed on the teeth. (**Seating** describes placement of the partial removable denture and lowering it into position as far as possible in the space allotted.)

Rests prevent the partial denture from moving gingivally, thus preventing abnormal stress and wear on the abutment tooth.

They also aid in distributing the retention load of the partial denture to several teeth, not just a single tooth, and prevent passage of food between the abutment tooth and the retainer.

The Placement of Rests. Rests are designed to lie in a prepared recess on the occlusal or lingual surface of a tooth. The recess is usually prepared in a cast restoration such as an onlay or a crown. This cast restoration protects the tooth structure against wear caused by movement of the rest.

Although the rest fits into the casting, it is not attached to it. Two common types of rests are the occlusal and lingual rests.

The recess for an **occlusal rest** is on the occlusal surface of the tooth. This placement minimizes trauma to the tooth by transmitting stress along the long axis of the tooth.

The recess for a **lingual rest** is placed on the cingulum of the lingual surface of the tooth where it has good support but is not visible.

PRECISION ATTACHMENTS

A precision attachment is a **retainer,** sometimes used in removable partial denture construction, consisting of a metal receptor and a closely fitting part.

The **receptor** (the "female" portion) is contained in a cast restoration in the abutment tooth. The **fitted part** (the "male" portion) is attached to the framework of the partial denture.

This precision attachment is made to prevent lateral motion and to provide vertical movement of the saddle. If the attachment is designed correctly, the long axis of the abutment teeth supports the load of stress of the occlusal force.

ARTIFICIAL TEETH

Artificial teeth are constructed from acrylic or porcelain. Acrylic teeth may be selected because they do not produce a clicking sound during mastication. However, acrylic teeth have a tendency to wear under occlusion. Placing acrylic teeth with natural or porcelain teeth in the opposing arch is often a satisfactory compromise.

Anterior teeth made of porcelain are designed with gold pins in the back of the tooth. These pins are embedded in the resin that forms the gingiva of the partial denture.

Tube teeth are artificial posterior teeth (porcelain or acrylic) prepared with a recessed hole in the base of the crown. The tube tooth is fixed in position when the acrylic of the saddle material flows into the hole and hardens there during processing.

Abutment Teeth

A partial denture is supported and stabilized primarily by the abutment teeth. The abutments may be remaining natural teeth or surgical implants.

THE SELECTION OF ABUTMENT TEETH

Because of the stress placed on them, abutments must have strong roots and strong bone support. The cuspids and molars, which have strong roots, are the teeth best suited for this purpose. Because of the differences in their root structure, maxillary premolars are more acceptable for abutments than are the mandibular premolars.

Because of their relatively weak root structure, individual maxillary and mandibular anterior teeth are the least acceptable teeth for use as abutments. However, if they are splinted together so that the stress is distributed evenly over several teeth, the anterior teeth make adequate supports.

THE PREPARATION OF ABUTMENT TEETH

Preparation of abutment teeth is determined by the type of rest selected. A recessed area is prepared to receive the rest so that it is held securely and yet does not interfere with occlusion or normal function. This preparation may involve one of these options:

- A slight modification of the tooth itself
- The modification of an amalgam restoration if present
- Placement of a cast metal restoration with a recessed area to receive the rest or precision attachment (see Chapter 31)

Preliminary Impressions

A preliminary impression is required so a custom tray may be fabricated for use in taking the master impression. The diagnostic casts, which were created at the patient's first visit, are frequently used for this purpose.

Final Impressions for Working Casts

A precise **final impression**, also known as the *master impression*, is required for the creation of the working casts. These **working casts**, also known as *refractory casts*, are used during the construction of the partial denture.

FINAL IMPRESSION MATERIALS AND TECHNIQUES

Because this *must* be an exact impression, an elastomeric impression material is used. The type of material and the impression technique are the dentist's choice. These materials and their use are discussed in Chapter 24.

At the time of the final impression, accuracy is extremely important; however, in contrast to the impression procedure for a fixed prosthesis, the use of gingival retraction is not required.

This is because when the final impression for a removable prosthesis is taken, none of the teeth are prepared below the gingival margin. If cast restorations are required, these are completed and cemented in place *before* the final impression is taken.

ADDITIONAL RECORDS

In addition to the final impression, it is also necessary to take an impression of the opposing arch and obtain an occlusal registration. Most commonly, this is a silicone occlusal registration, and this technique is described in Chapter 24.

ALGINATE-HYDROCOLLOID IMPRESSION TECHNIQUE

This impression system, known as the *Cohere technique*, combines alginate and hydrocolloid impression materials. Some dentists prefer this specialized technique for taking the final impressions for a partial denture.

Reversible and Irreversible Hydrocolloids

As discussed in Chapter 19, alginate (which is an irreversible hydrocolloid) is changed from a sol (solution) into a gel (solid) through chemical action. Once the reaction has started, it cannot be stopped or reversed. Alginate is used for impressions where extreme accuracy is not necessary.

Reversible hydrocolloids, known simply as hydrocolloids, can be changed repeatedly. When heated, the material forms a sol (solution). When cooled, it becomes a gel (solid). These hydrocolloids create very accurate impressions.

To use traditional hydrocolloid impression material, a conditioner is required to (1) liquify the material by heating it, (2) condition the material so that it is cool enough to be safely placed in the mouth, and (3) hold the material so that it is ready to use.

A special water-cooled impression tray is used to place the hydrocolloid material in the mouth and to cool it so it hardens again.

Materials for Alginate-Hydrocolloid Technique

This technique involves the use of a special formula of alginate that creates a bond with the hydrocolloid impression material. This is slower setting than regular

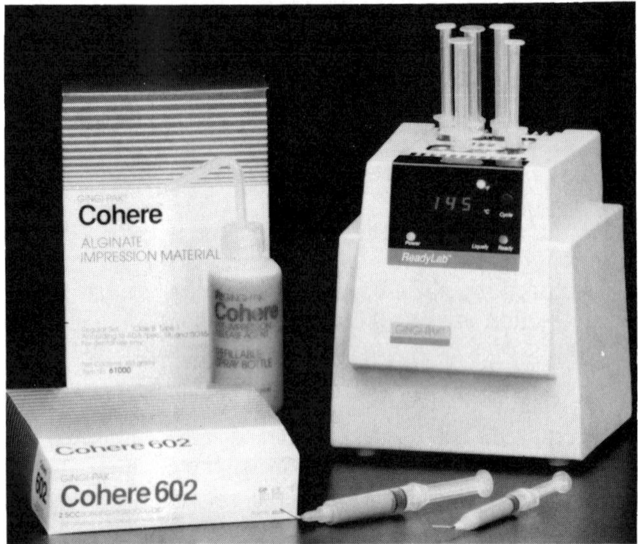

FIGURE 32–7

Hydrocolloid conditioning unit and syringes. (Courtesy of Gingi-Pak, Camarillo, CA.)

alginates (about 3 minutes), so that the alginate and hydrocolloid set at the same time.

A special formula of syringe-type hydrocolloid is used for this technique, and the hydrocolloid is supplied in single-use cartridges. A specialized hydrocolloid conditioning unit is also used (Fig. 32–7).

Selecting the Artificial Teeth

After the final impression, the **shade** (color) and **mold** (shape) of the teeth are selected. The manufacturer of the artificial teeth provides a shade guide. To identify the teeth, the mold and shade number are imprinted by the manufacturer on the back of each tooth in the shade guide.

When choosing the tooth shade and mold, the dentist considers the age and the body size of the patient, the length of the lip, and the space to be occupied by the artificial tooth or teeth. The goal is to match as closely as possible the color, size, and shape of the patient's natural teeth.

A sample is removed from the shade guide holder. It

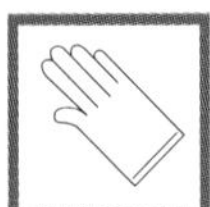
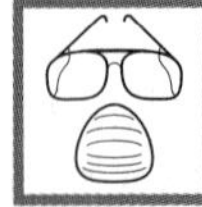
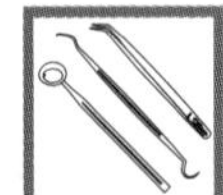

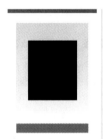

PROCEDURE: **Obtaining an Alginate-Hydrocolloid Impression**

Preparation

1. The hydrocolloid is heated in the conditioning unit to 212°F (100°C) for 10 minutes.
   □ *RATIONALE:* This liquifies the hydrocolloid.
2. Then it is cooled in the conditioning unit to 150°F (65°C) for 20 minutes.
   □ *RATIONALE:* This makes it cool enough to place in the patient's mouth.
3. When the hydrocolloid is ready, the alginate is mixed and is loaded in a nonperforated (solid) tray.
   □ *RATIONALE:* A solid tray is necessary to provide the support required by the materials in this technique.
4. The prepared hydrocolloid cartridge is slipped into a special impression syringe with a disposable tip.

The Impression

1. The dentist wipes the teeth with a wetting agent provided by the manufacturer and then uses the syringe to extrude the warm hydrocolloid around the prepared teeth.
2. The tray filled with alginate is placed over the hydrocolloid on the prepared teeth.
3. The completed impression is removed after the alginate has set.
4. The impression is disinfected in the same way as for other alginate materials. The used cartridge and the syringe tip are discarded. The syringe is sterilized for reuse.

is moistened with saliva or water to approximate the moist surface of the natural teeth in the oral cavity.

The shade of the artificial teeth is checked by natural light (preferably northern light) to determine an accurate shade. When the selection has been made, the mold and shade of the artificial teeth are written on the patient's chart.

This information, plus the name of the manufacturer and the material of the teeth, is also noted on the laboratory prescription so that the technician will select the correct artificial teeth.

The shade guide, which is a semicritical item, cannot be heat sterilized because the plastic will warp. Therefore, after use the entire shade guide is disinfected by using a high-level EPA-registered disinfectant.

The Laboratory Prescription

Before the case is sent to the laboratory, the dentist prepares a written prescription. This includes all details concerning the construction of the prosthesis (Fig. 32–8). This prescription must be signed by the dentist, and a copy is retained in the practice records.

Wax Setup Try-In Appointment

An appointment is scheduled for the initial "try-in" of the prosthesis in the patient's mouth. At this point, the appliance consists of the cast framework and the artificial teeth set in wax.

At this visit the dentist evaluates the fit, comfort, and function of the appliance. The shade, mold, and arrangement of the teeth are reviewed so that their appearance is acceptable to the patient. If necessary, the dentist may alter the alignment of the teeth in the wax.

When the appliance is acceptable, another bite registration may be required to reflect any changes made during the try-in. This may be a wax-bite registration, and this is discussed in Chapter 19.

Any changes in the partial denture design are noted

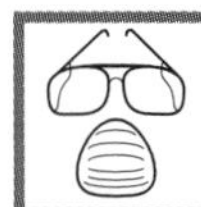
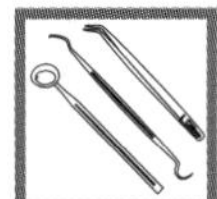

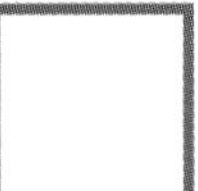

PROCEDURE: **Delivery of a Partial Denture**

1. The assistant seats the patient. If the patient is wearing a prosthesis, he is asked to remove it.
   □ *IMPORTANT:* The assistant always wears examination gloves when handling a prosthesis that has been in the patient's mouth.
2. The dentist places the new partial denture in the patient's mouth, and the patient is instructed to close his teeth together.
   □ *IMPORTANT:* Before being placed in the patient's mouth, the prosthesis must be disinfected and rinsed with water.
3. To check the occlusion, articulating paper is placed on the occlusal surface of the mandibular teeth, and the patient is requested to simulate chewing motions. If the occlusion is too high, the artificial teeth are reduced with a small, round carbide bur.
4. To detect pressure points (high spots) that could cause the patient discomfort, pressure indicator paste is sprayed on the tissue surface of the prosthesis, and the prosthesis is placed again in the patient's mouth. As necessary, these high spots in the prosthesis are adjusted.
5. The retainers are checked for tension on the natural abutment teeth. Pliers are used to very carefully adjust the tension on the retainers.
6. After the adjustments, the assistant polishes the partial denture on the laboratory lathe, using the appropriate pastes and sterile buffing wheels.
   □ *IMPORTANT:* The assistant must wear examination gloves while handling the appliance that has been in the patient's mouth.
7. The partial is scrubbed with soap, water, and a brush; is disinfected and rinsed; and is returned to the treatment room for delivery to the patient.
8. The patient is given instructions on how to place and remove the partial denture and how to care for it.

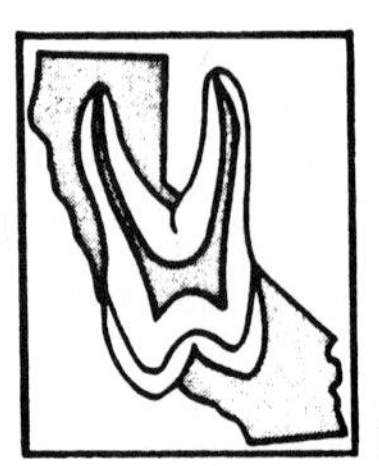

PRECISION CERAMICS DENTAL LABORATORY
9591 Central Avenue / Montclair, CA 91763
(909) 625-8787 / (800) 223-6322
FAX (909) 621-3125

FROM: DATE ______

DR. ______ PHONE (____) ______

ADDRESS ______ ACCT. NO. ______

CITY ______ STATE ______ ZIP ______

PATIENT'S NAME ______ AGE ____ SEX M F ____

	Shade	Mould
❑ BIOBLEND •		
❑ BIOFORM • IPN •		
❑ BIOFORM •		
❑ NEW HUE • V.F.		
❑ NEW HUE •		
❑ BIOTONE •		

❑ BIOFORM • 20° PLASTIC
❑ BIOFORM • IPN • 20° PLASTIC
❑ IPN • ANATOLINE •
❑ IPN • MONOLINE ™ 0°

	IN	OUT
DOCTOR'S MODELS (OPP)		
WORKING MODEL		
DIES		
IMPRESSIONS		
BITE		
ARTICULATOR		
TEETH		
CROWN		
PARTIAL/DENTURE		
STUDY MODEL		
OTHER		

• NO SUBSTITUTIONS OF MOULD SHADE, MATERIAL, OR BRAND WITHOUT APPROVAL.
PLEASE RETURN EMPTY TOOTH CARD(S) WITH TRY-IN.

TYPE OF METAL ❑ CHROME ❑ GOLD ❑ TITANIUM

DESIGN FRAME HERE

TRY-IN ❑ WAX ❑ METAL ❑ BITE RIM / BLOCKS ❑ FINISH   DUE DATE ______

PLEASE SEND: ❑ BOXES ❑ Rx FORMS ❑ MAILING LABELS
PLEASE CALL: ❑ ❑ C + B FORMS ❑ PRICE LIST

Signature ______ Lic. # ______

TERMS: Customer agrees to company policy as stated on reverse.

FIGURE 32–8

Laboratory prescription form for a removable prosthesis. (Courtesy of Precision Ceramics Dental Laboratory, Montclair, CA.)

on the laboratory prescription. The wax-up is disinfected and forwarded to the dental technician along with the prescription.

The laboratory technician proceeds to finish the partial denture as prescribed by the dentist. The completed prosthesis is delivered to the dental office in a sealed, moist container. The acrylic must be kept moist at all times to prevent warpage.

In the office, the prosthesis is stored in this sealed container. The appliance is disinfected and rinsed before it is inserted into the patient's mouth.

Delivery of the Partial Denture

A 20- to 30-minute appointment is usually adequate for delivery of the partial denture. The day before the appointment, the assistant verifies that the case has been returned from the laboratory.

Home Care Instructions to the Patient

Because the acrylic saddle will warp if it is allowed to get dry or too hot, the patient is instructed to store the prosthesis in water or a moist, airtight container when it is not in use.

Patients with removable partials must maintain good oral hygiene. The importance of this cannot be overemphasized. After the patient has eaten, the removable partial denture is removed from the mouth and brushed or rinsed so that the retainers, rests, and saddles are clean.

The patient should also carefully brush and floss the abutment teeth and the remaining natural teeth to keep them free of food debris and plaque.

Appointment for Post-Delivery Check

The patient is given an appointment to return within a few days after the delivery of the partial denture. A 10- to 20-minute appointment is usually adequate for this post-delivery visit.

At this time the dentist removes the partial denture and checks the mucosa for pressure areas and sore spots. If necessary, minor adjustments are made to the denture. When the dentist and patient are satisfied that the prosthesis is functioning correctly, the patient is given a recall appointment for several months later.

It is important that the patient return regularly for these recall visits, so that the dentist may evaluate the fit, changes to the mucosa, the function of the prosthesis, and the effectiveness of the patient's oral hygiene.

As time passes, changes in the alveolar ridge and surrounding tissues may make it necessary to reline the partial denture. (Relining procedures are discussed later in this chapter.)

Complete Dentures

Complete dentures, also known as *full dentures*, are designed to restore function and esthetics of the natural dentition when all or most of the natural teeth are missing. A complete denture receives all of its support and retention from the underlying tissues, the alveolar ridges, the hard and soft palates (maxillary), and the surrounding oral mucosa.

Indications for a Complete Denture

- The patient is totally edentulous (without teeth).
- The remaining teeth cannot be saved.
- The remaining teeth cannot support a removable partial denture, and there are no acceptable alternatives available.
- The patient refuses alternative treatment recommendations.

Contraindications for a Complete Denture

- When any other acceptable alternative is available
- Physical or mental illness that affects the patient's ability to cooperate during the fabrication of the denture and to accept and/or wear the denture
- Hypersensitivity to denture materials (in these cases, a hypoallergenic denture material may be indicated)
- The patient is not interested in replacing missing teeth.

Components of a Complete Denture

The **base** is designed to fit over the residual alveolar ridge and surrounding gingival area. The base is usually constructed from denture acrylic; however, to provide additional strength, it may be reinforced with a metal mesh embedded in the acrylic.

The **flange** is the part of the base that extends over the attached mucosa from the cervical margin of the teeth to the border of the denture. (The **border** is the circumferential margin of the denture.)

The flange of the **mandibular denture** base extends over the residual ridge and attached mucosa, down to the oblique ridge and mylohyoid ridges, and over the genial tubercles and the retromolar pads.

The flange of the **maxillary denture** base extends beyond the residual ridge and over the attached mucosa to the tuberosities and the junction of the hard and soft palates.

THE POST DAM

Retention of a maxillary denture depends on the suction seal known as the post dam or the *posterior palatal seal.* The base of a maxillary denture covers the entire hard palate, and the seal is formed at the junction of the tissues and the posterior border of the denture.

The post dam extends across the entire posterior of the denture from one buccal space across the back of the palate behind the maxillary tuberosity to the opposite buccal space.

RETENTION OF A MANDIBULAR DENTURE

Retention for a mandibular denture depends upon the support of the remaining alveolar ridge and the suction that can be achieved between the prosthesis and the tissues covering the ridge.

Achieving good retention of a mandibular denture can be difficult. It lacks the broad suction area found in a maxillary denture, and there is constant action of the tongue, which may dislodge the prosthesis. For these reasons, retained teeth or implants are desirable to help hold the appliance in place. (Overdentures are discussed later in this chapter.)

ARTIFICIAL TEETH

The denture teeth are fabricated from acrylic or porcelain and are designed to be retained in the acrylic base of the denture (Fig. 32–9). Third molars are not included on dentures because of the need to provide space in the posterior region to allow the patient to close, chew, swallow, and speak normally.

The **anterior denture teeth** simulate the form and landmarks of the natural tooth crown. Small gold pins extending from the back of the tooth in the cingulum area retain the anterior tooth in the acrylic of the denture base.

A natural tooth functions as an individual unit, whereas 14 artificial teeth for one arch attached to each denture base constitute a single unit. For this reason, the posterior teeth are designed in two major mold types: anatomic and nonanatomic.

Anatomic posterior teeth are designed with normal cusps and ridges reproduced on the occlusal surface to aid in the chewing of food. During fabrication, the acrylic of the base flows into a hole in the bottom of the tooth, and this holds the tooth in place on the denture.

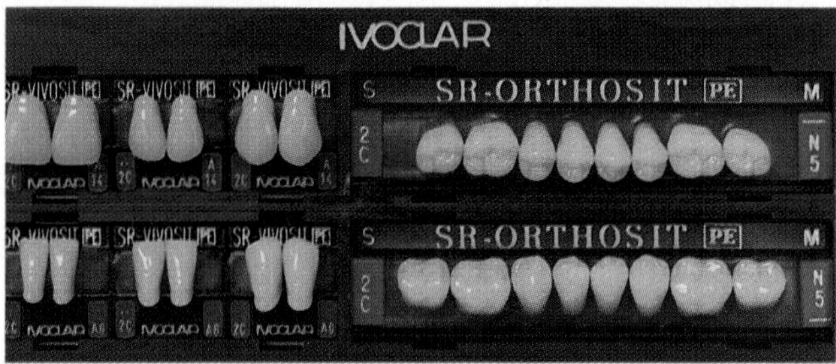

FIGURE 32–9

Anterior and posterior denture teeth. Notice that there are no third molars included here. (Courtesy of Ivoclar Williams, Amherst, NY.)

Nonanatomic posterior teeth, also known as *zero-degree* or *rational teeth,* are so named because they do not have extensive anatomic detail. Instead, the occlusal surface is rounded and somewhat concave or flat. The design of these teeth is modified to reduce the effects and pressures of occlusion that are transmitted through the denture to the oral mucosa and the residual alveolar ridge.

Impressions for Diagnostic Casts of Edentulous Arches

Taking an alginate impression of an edentulous arch differs from taking other alginate impressions in two ways: (1) the height of the teeth is missing, and (2) it is important to include more extensive tissue details.

An edentulous tray is used to take this impression. This tray is not as deep as other trays used for alginate impressions. In addition, the borders of the tray are modified by attaching soft beading wax, or a similar material, to the edges.

This modification allows **border-molding,** also known as *muscle-trimming,* to achieve closer adaptation of the edges of the impression of the tissues in the mucobuccal fold.

Border-molding is performed after the impression tray is in place. The dentist uses his or her fingers to gently massage the area of the face over these borders. This shapes the wax-covered edges of the tray so these edges more closely approximate the tissues.

Custom Trays for the Final Impression

Because of the shape of the edentulous arch, custom trays are usually required for the final impression. These are constructed on the diagnostic casts and are prepared before the patient's appointment for the final impression. The basic construction of custom trays is discussed in Chapter 24.

The edges of the custom tray for an edentulous arch are modified with beading wax to allow border-molding. The edges of the tray should extend to 2 mm. *short* of the mucobuccal fold.

Final Impressions for Complete Dentures

Because accuracy is essential, an elastomeric impression material is used for the final impressions that will be used for the creation of the working casts (Fig. 32–10).

ESSENTIALS OF THE FINAL IMPRESSION

1. The material should be free of bubbles and distributed evenly over the tray and its margins so the

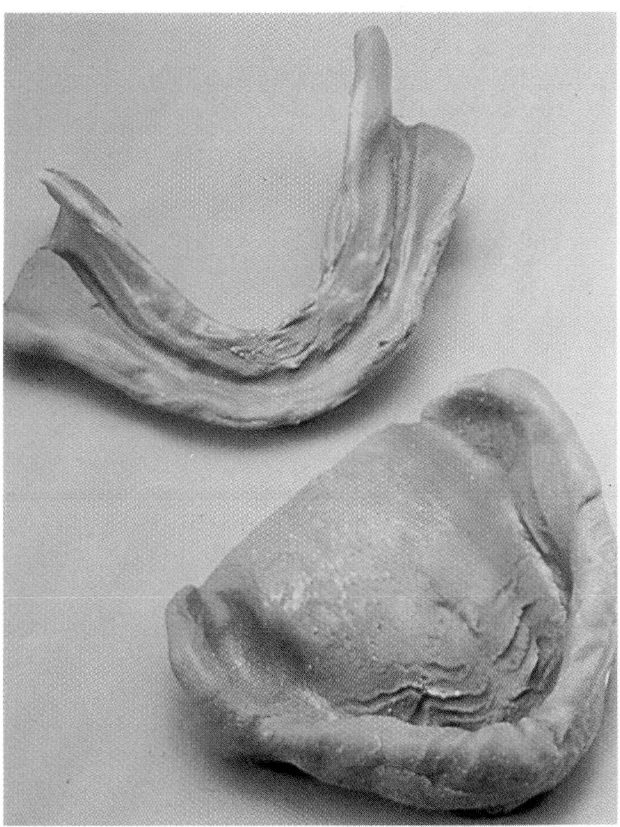

FIGURE 32–10

Completed polyvinyl siloxane maxillary and mandibular edentulous impressions. (Courtesy of 3M Dental Products Division, St. Paul, MN.)

landmarks of the dental arches are accurately reproduced in the impression.

2. The maxillary impression should include the hamular notches, post dam, tuberosities, and frenum attachments.
3. The mandibular impression should include the retromolar pads, oblique ridge, outline of the mylohyoid ridge, and the genial tubercles, plus the lingual, labial, and buccal frena.

Baseplates and Occlusal Rims

The baseplate and occlusal rims are used while (1) bite relationship records are made; (2) the casts are articulated; (3) the artificial teeth are arranged; and (4) the prosthesis is tried in the mouth.

The **baseplate**, which is constructed on the master casts, is made of a semi-rigid material such as shellac and self-curing or heat-cured resins. If necessary for added stability, acrylic baseplates may be reinforced with wires or mesh metal sheets embedded in the material at the time of processing.

The **occlusal rims** are built of wax on the alveolar crest of the baseplate and are high and wide enough to occupy the space of the missing dentition.

Try-In of Baseplate–Occlusal Rim Assembly

The baseplate–occlusal rim assembly is returned to the dental office on an articulator. (An **articulator**, as shown in Fig. 32–11, is a laboratory device that simulates the movements of the mandible and the temporomandibular joint.)

Before it is tried in the patient's mouth, the baseplate–occlusal rim is removed from the articulator, disinfected, and rinsed. On the occlusal rims, the dentist records

- The **vertical dimensions** of the arches (this is the space occupied by the height of the teeth is normal occlusion)
- The **occlusal relationships** of the arches (these include centric, protrusive, retrusive, and lateral excursion)
- The **smile line** (this represents the amount of teeth that normally shows when the patient is smiling)
- The **cuspid eminence** (this vertical line indicates the location of the cuspids)

Selecting the Artificial Teeth

At this appointment, the mold, shade, and material of the artificial teeth to be placed in the denture are selected. These factors are determined in the same way as for the teeth of a partial denture.

When placing the teeth in the denture, the laboratory technician is able to modify the arrangement as requested in order to produce a more natural appearance for the patient: for example, slightly overlapping the mesial incisal margin of the maxillary lateral over the distal margin of the central incisor.

Also, the technician may set (position) the teeth to expose less or more of the cervical area of the teeth to emulate the natural setting of the teeth according to the age of the patient. Less cervical area is shown in a younger patient; more is visible in an older patient to simulate gingival recession.

Occlusal Registration

During the construction of a complete denture, the laboratory technician must have an accurate and extensive record of the patient's occlusion. The technician uses this information to articulate the casts so that the completed prosthesis will replicate these normal motions.

The measurements most frequently used are the patient's bite registered in the following positions:

- **Centric relation** with the jaws closed, relaxed, and comfortably positioned
- **Protrusion** with the mandible placed as far forward as possible from the centric position
- **Retrusion** with the mandible placed as far posterior as possible from the centric position

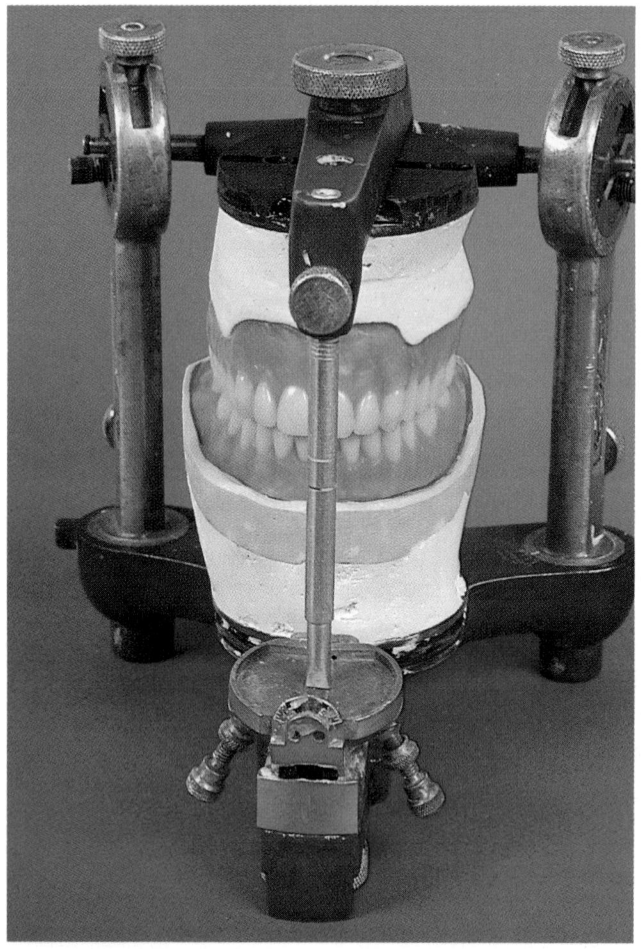

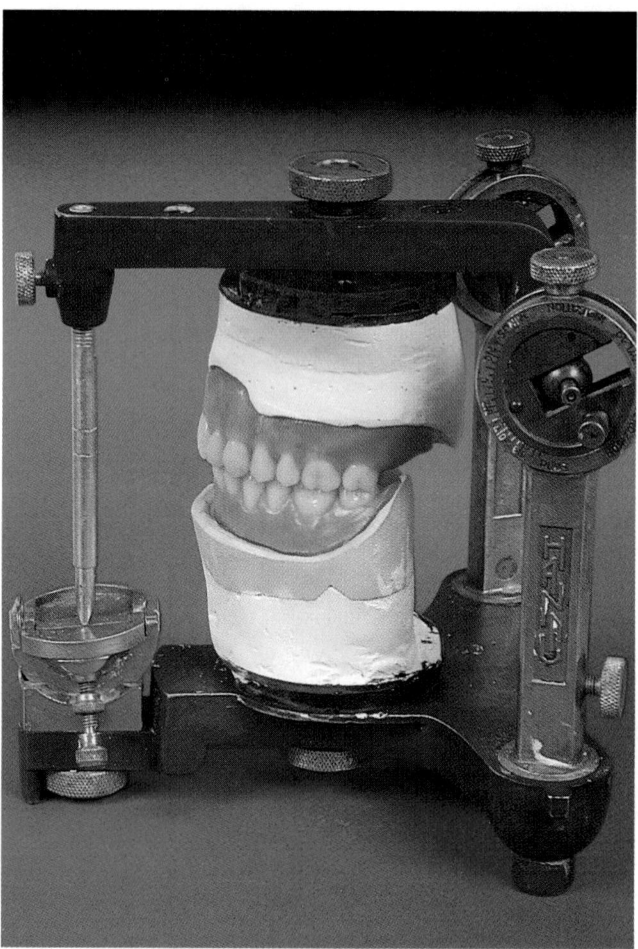

FIGURE 32–11

Wax-up of complete denture on an articulator.

- **Lateral excursion,** which is sliding the mandible to the left or right of the centric position

These exaggerated motions simulate the actual movements of the mandible as it functions in the acts of mastication, biting, yawning, and speaking. Various measuring devices are used to obtain these measurements.

FUNCTIONALLY GENERATED PATH TECHNIQUE

The functionally generated path technique uses the patient's ability to create his own occlusal relationship by tracing, in wax, the movements of the mandible on the maxilla.

To establish a functionally generated path, the baseplates and occlusal rims for the new prosthesis are placed in the mouth. A double thickness of specially formulated bite wax is prepared in a horseshoe shape and laid over the occlusal surface of the mandibular teeth.

The patient is instructed to close firmly into the wax and to simulate the act of chewing as accurately as possible. The wax bite is removed approximately 20 to 30 seconds later.

In the treatment room, the wax bite is disinfected and put aside. In the laboratory, it is poured with stone immediately after the dismissal of the patient.

Wax Setup Try-In Appointment

The **wax setup** consists of the baseplate with the artificial teeth set in wax that resembles gingival tissue (see Fig. 32–11). The shaping of the wax to simulate normal tissue contours, grooves, and eminences is known as **festooning.**

The teeth are articulated according to the bite registration of the patient's occlusion, established on the articulator through functional arch tracing.

The complete denture try-in, which has been fabricated in wax by the laboratory technician on an articulator, is returned to the dental office before the patient's appointment. The wax setup is removed from the articulator and disinfected before it is tried in the patient's mouth.

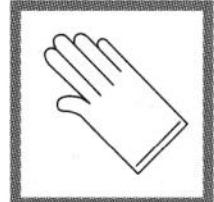 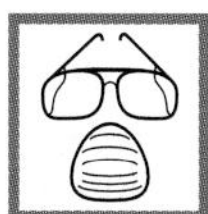 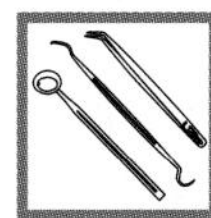 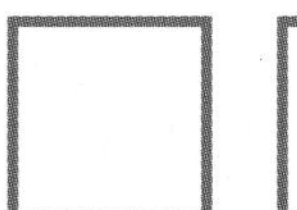 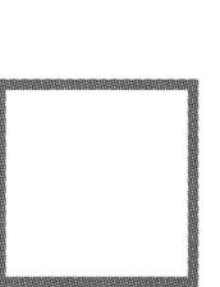  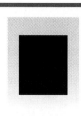

PROCEDURE: **Evaluating the Wax Setup**

1. The wax setup of the denture is evaluated for fit, comfort, and stability.
2. The patient's acceptance of the appearance of the denture, including the shade, mold, and alignment of the teeth, is verified.
3. The retention of the denture setup is checked as the patient verbalizes the *f, v, s,* and *th* sounds; swallows; and yawns.
4. The occlusion of the denture is checked with the teeth of the opposing arch.
5. The dentist prepares the laboratory prescription for completion of the denture. The case is disinfected, returned to the articulator, packed, and returned to the laboratory.

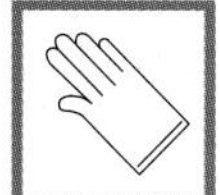 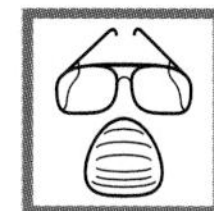 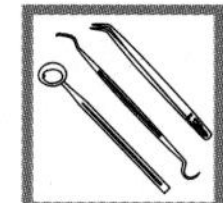   

PROCEDURE: **Delivering the Complete Denture**

1. The completed dentures are delivered to the dental office in a sealed moist container. The dentures must be disinfected before they are placed in the patient's mouth.
2. The patient is seated. If applicable, the previously worn denture is removed by the patient.
3. The new denture is inserted into the patient's mouth, and the shade and mold of the artificial teeth are checked for natural appearance.
4. The patient is requested to perform the facial expressions and the actions of swallowing, chewing, and speaking, using *s* and *th* sounds. These sounds also are appropriate for exercises to help the patient learn to speak normally with his new denture.
5. The occlusion is checked by using carbon articulating paper.
   □ *RATIONALE:* Cusps that are too high in contact will be marked with the color of the articulating paper.
6. If the cusps are too high, the denture is removed from the mouth and adjusted with a heatless stone mounted on a straight handpiece.
7. The denture is replaced in the mouth, and the procedure is repeated until the cusps appear to be in occlusion with the opposing arch.
   □ *NOTE:* If the denture must be taken into the laboratory for adjustment, it must be disinfected again before it is returned to the patient.
8. When the patient is pleased with the appearance, function, and comfort of the denture, another appointment is made for the post-delivery checkup.
9. Before dismissal, the patient is warned that learning to wear a new denture will take several days or weeks.

Home Care Instructions to the Patient

With the denture removed, the patient should thoroughly rinse the oral tissues at least once daily. At this time, all surfaces of the denture should be thoroughly cleaned. A special denture brush may be recommended for this purpose, and harsh abrasives, such as toothpaste, should be avoided.

During cleaning, the denture is carefully held over a sink half filled with cool water. The denture must not be soaked in either hot water or a strong solution such as undiluted bleach because these will damage the denture.

As a precaution to minimize damage if the denture is dropped, a wash cloth may be placed in the bottom of the sink.

When dentures are not in the mouth, they must be stored in a moist, airtight container to prevent drying and warpage. Also, if the prosthesis is not stored in a safe container, it may be accidentally knocked to the floor, stepped on, or broken.

Immediate Dentures

Most commonly, an immediate denture is one that is placed immediately after the extraction of the patient's remaining anterior teeth. During the healing process, the denture serves as a compress and bandage to protect the surgical area.

Although an immediate denture may be placed in either arch, placement of a maxillary immediate denture is more common because it restores function and spares the patient the embarrassment of being without any teeth in that arch.

The Provisional Denture

When the anterior teeth are extracted, they are replaced by a complete provisional denture. (A **provisional prosthesis** is designed for use over a limited period of time and is then to be replaced.)

Before agreeing to an immediate denture, the patient must be aware that normal healing and resorption cause changes in the alveolar ridge. Because of these changes, the denture that is placed immediately after surgery must be replaced or relined within 3 to 6 months.

Construction of the Denture

The patient has previously had the posterior teeth extracted, and healing is complete. Before surgery, the try-in of the wax setup includes only the posterior teeth. These are aligned in the occlusal rims and checked for their ability to occlude with the opposing teeth.

The denture, complete with the anterior teeth, is constructed, sterilized, and ready for placement at the time of surgery.

The Surgical Template

In addition to the denture, a surgical template is prepared by the laboratory. (The **surgical template** resembles a clear plastic impression tray of the anterior area as it should appear *after* the teeth have been extracted.) The denture and template must be sterilized before the surgery.

After the anterior teeth have been extracted, the oral surgeon uses the surgical template as a guide in properly contouring the remaining alveolar ridge. (See Chapter 30.)

Placement of the Immediate Denture

When the resulting alveolar ridge is satisfactory, the tissues are sutured in place. Then the sterilized denture is rinsed with saline solution and positioned in the mouth.

The patient returns in 24 hours for a postoperative checkup. During this time, the denture is to be worn continuously except when it is removed for cleaning. Daily visits continue until initial healing has started and the sutures are removed. This is usually done 48 to 72 hours after surgery. During each visit, the dentist irrigates the area with a mild antiseptic solution and checks the soft tissue for pressure points.

After the sutures have been removed and the dentist and patient are satisfied with the prosthesis, the patient is scheduled for another appointment within a few months.

Overdentures and Implants

Patient satisfaction with a mandibular denture is increased when there are remaining teeth or implants to improve the retention and stability. The surgical phase of the placement of an implant is discussed in Chapter 30.

An overdenture is a complete denture supported by the bony ridge and oral mucosa plus two or more remaining natural teeth. Most often, these remaining teeth are cuspids.

The preparation and placement of the denture for use with implants and for an overdenture are fairly similar and thus are discussed together here.

Overdentures

To permit the denture to fit snugly over the teeth without excessive bulk, the natural teeth are prepared by removing much of their bulk and then protecting the remaining tooth structure with a coping. (A **coping** is a thin cast metal covering fitted over a prepared tooth.)

In the **long coping technique**, only a minimal amount of tooth structure is removed, and the length of tooth remains almost the same as previously. In the **short coping technique**, which is used only on endodontically treated teeth, the tooth structure is greatly reduced and shortened.

The Bar Attachment

The posts from an implant protrude through the gingiva much like teeth, and a casting is created to fit over the posts. In preparation for a mandibular denture, these castings are connected by a bar to provide stability. This forms the "male" portion of the appliance.

The denture is prepared with a recessed "sleeve" in the anterior of the prosthesis, which serves as the **receptor** attachment. This is the "female" portion of the appliance. The denture is snapped over the bar and stabilized in alignment with the opposing arch (see Fig. 30–23).

The in-office steps in the fabrication of this special denture are similar to those for a normal denture.

Relining of a Complete or Partial Denture

The purpose of relining a denture is to have it accommodate the changes in the supporting tissues so that the appliance again fits properly. Relining is accomplished by placing a new layer of denture resin over the tissue surface of the appliance.

Impression for Laboratory Relining

At the preliminary appointment, when it is agreed that relining is necessary, the patient is warned that he will be without his denture for at least 8 to 24 hours while it is being processed in the laboratory.

The impression is taken with the present (loose) denture used as the impression tray. The dentist pours a mix of zinc oxide–eugenol (ZOE) impression paste or an elastomeric impression material into the tissue side of the denture.

The denture is placed on the alveolar ridge, and the patient is instructed to close in normal occlusion and to hold the denture in place until the impression paste reaches a final set.

The denture is removed from the mouth and disinfected. The denture and written prescription are sent to the laboratory technician for relining.

Delivery of a Laboratory-Relined Denture

When the relined denture is returned from the laboratory, it is disinfected before being returned to the patient's mouth. Rarely is there any need to adjust the relined denture, because the only alteration upon the original prosthesis is the addition of material within the tissue side of the denture.

If necessary, minor trimming may be accomplished with an acrylic bur in a straight handpiece. Minor polishing may be done on the laboratory lathe with a sterile rag wheel with pumice paste; however, the tissue-bearing surfaces are *never* polished because this would alter the fit of the appliance.

The patient is dismissed and advised to return for a checkup of the tissue and the adaptation of the prosthesis within a time specified by the dentist.

Denture Repairs

A broken acrylic denture can be repaired. Simple repairs are sometimes handled in the dental office laboratory by using cold-cure acrylics. More complicated repairs, particularly those involving the replacement of teeth or the complex fracture of the denture, are usually sent to the dental laboratory technician.

The patient with a broken denture tooth usually leaves the denture at the dental office. In most cases, it is not necessary for the patient to be seen by the dentist at this time. However, if there has been more extensive damage to the denture, it may be necessary for the dentist to see the patient to obtain a new impression.

When the repaired denture is returned, the patient is scheduled for a few minutes with the dentist to make certain that the repair is satisfactory and that the denture fits properly.

Denture Duplicates

Having a functional denture is important to the patient, and because dentures can break or require time for relining, the patient should have a duplicate denture made. Although it is an extra expense, many patients find this to be excellent investment. Should something happen, they will not need to be without their denture.

To prevent warpage while not in use, the spare denture should be stored in a moist, airtight container.

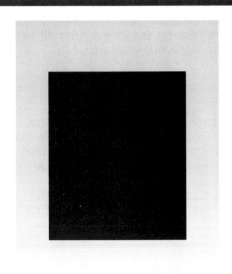

Chapter 33

Business Office Management

Introduction

The business office is the control center, or hub, of the dental practice (Fig. 33–1). Effective management here is the key to efficiently functioning throughout the practice.

This chapter introduces business office functions, including marketing, answering the telephone, patient reception, appointment control, and records management.

Additional topics related to the business aspects of the practice, including accounts receivable and accounts payable, are addressed in Chapters 34 and 35.

Business Office Staff

There are many important responsibilities and roles to be filled in the business office. These duties may include but are not limited to

- Greeting patients and answering the telephone
- Scheduling patient visits
- Managing patient records
- Managing accounts receivable and accounts payable
- Managing the recall and inventory control systems
- Overseeing and monitoring practice marketing activities

Depending upon the size of the practice, these roles may be filled by one or more individuals. In a large practice, these duties may be divided among the receptionist, bookkeeper, appointment clerk, file clerk, insurance clerk, and secretary. A qualified administrative assistant or office manager may be placed in charge of this area.

In a smaller practice, when one individual may handle all of these responsibilities, he or she is known as the administrative or business assistant. In addition to having the specialized skills and basic knowledge of a dental assistant, the administrative assistant must

- Be able to assume responsibility and make decisions without direct supervision
- Possess a mastery of office skills and pay close attention to details

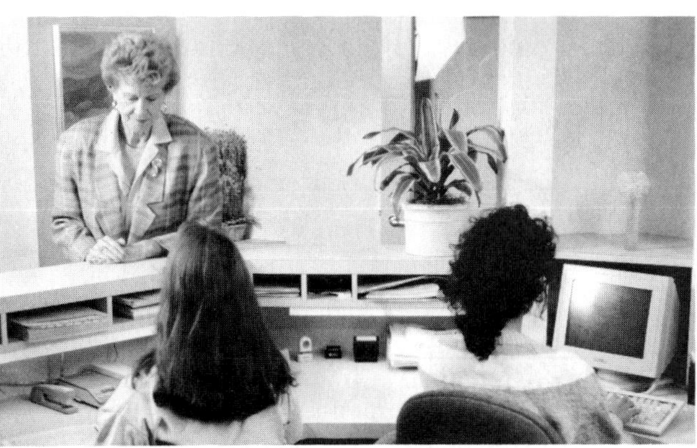

FIGURE 33–1

The assistants working in the business office have a very important role in the dental practice. Shown here, one assistant is greeting a patient while the other is making a computer entry.

- Organize work and be able to carry through on assignments despite numerous interruptions
- Handle multiple tasks simultaneously
- Possess the maturity to respond to patients tactfully —even when they appear to be unreasonable
- Respond calmly, quickly, and appropriately in emergency situations

The many and varied responsibilities of the administrative assistant are described in this chapter and in Chapters 1, 34, and 35.

Importance of an Office Manual

It is essential for a smooth-running dental practice to have an office manual stating, in writing, the policies and procedures that the dentist wants the staff to follow in the practice. Information included in this office manual may include but is not limited to

- Office hours
- Handling of telephone calls
- Billing and insurance procedures
- Ordering of supplies
- Clinical tray setups

PERSONNEL MANUAL

Personnel issues may be included here or covered in a separate personnel manual. Personnel topics include a job description for each employee, pay periods and working hours, and information concerning employee benefits such as paid holidays, vacation, and sick time. It might also include policies on provisional employment, maternity leave, disciplinary measures, and dismissal.

Some practices use a commercially prepared manual, whereas others customize their own. Whichever type is preferred, it is helpful to use a ring binder, which allows for pages to be added or deleted as office policy is updated or information becomes obsolete.

To prevent misunderstandings later on, each new employee should review the office manual during the first weeks of employment. Any areas that are not clear should be addressed during that time.

Marketing

The term *marketing* usually brings to mind large advertising campaigns; however, that is not how this term applies in dentistry. In dentistry, marketing encompasses all activities involved in attracting and retaining satisfied patients in the practice.

Initiating the development of a marketing plan is the responsibility of the dentist; however, for a marketing plan to be successful, *all* members of the dental team should be actively and enthusiastically involved in planning, implementing, and monitoring that plan.

Although this is a team effort, one person (usually the office manager or administrative assistant) may be given the responsibility for ensuring the overall smooth functioning of the marketing program.

Types of Practice Marketing

External marketing activities are those that take place outside of the office and are directed to people who are not patients. These activities include health fairs and presentations to schoolchildren or senior citizens groups.

These external marketing activities may require staff members' participation in the community. If so, they are expected to cooperate in an enthusiastic and fully professional manner. Staff are an extension of the practice at *all* times—especially in public!

Internal marketing strategies are those marketing activities and promotions targeted to current patients of the practice. These too may require staff participation. Such activities may include but are not limited to

- Publishing a practice newsletter
- Developing promotional materials for insertion into monthly statements
- Sending flowers or other appropriate thank-you gifts to those who refer new patients to the practice
- Sending birthday or other special occasion cards to patients
- Sponsoring give-aways, office open house, and other promotional events

The Goal of Practice Marketing

A primary goal of any marketing plan is to create a positive image of the practice as a place where patients receive quality treatment provided in a caring atmosphere.

The positive and cooperative attitudes of *all* staff members are vital to successfully creating this image; however, the administrative assistant is a key person because he or she usually has the all-important first contact with the patient.

A secondary goal is to enroll new patients for the practice. An important part of achieving this goal is to determine the perceived needs of potential patients and seek out ways to meet these needs.

The Logistics of Marketing

The majority of practices that have successful marketing programs attribute this success to good organization, attention to detail, determining a budget, and tracking of the results.

The Plan. For a marketing plan to succeed, written goals and dates must be established. Attention to detail here is essential.

The Marketing Budget. The average amount of investment budgeted by dentists for a practice marketing plan ranges between 3 and 5 percent of the previous year's gross revenues.

Tracking Responses. Determining the success of the marketing plan entails tracking the response to each marketing activity. This may be accomplished by counting the number of new patient referrals that result from a marketing promotion.

For example, "30 new patients entered the practice after (a specific) marketing event" is a measurable response of success.

The Telephone

Most patients make their first contact with the dental office via the telephone. From this first contact, the patient will form his preliminary impression of the dentist, the dental team, and especially of the quality of care provided.

The administrative assistant is responsible for answering the telephone and for making certain that this and every patient contact are positive ones.

Guidelines for Telephone Courtesy

Telephone calls should be governed by the same rules of courtesy that apply to a face-to-face meeting. This courtesy should begin with a prompt and pleasant response to the ring of the telephone and continue until the receiver is gently replaced at the end of the call.

When answering the telephone, you want your voice to convey a warm smile and the message, "I'm glad *you* called!" You do not want to convey that you are tired, angry, preoccupied, or in a hurry or that this telephone call is an unwanted interruption.

- Smile (it shows in your voice).
- Never chew gum, eat, drink, or have a pencil in your mouth while talking on the telephone.
- Speak directly into the transmitter, with your mouth 1 to 2 inches away.
- Speak clearly and slowly, and guard against slurring your words.
- Get the name of the person who is calling, and talk to him, not to the telephone.
- Use the caller's name in the conversation, and give him your complete attention.
- When completing a call, always allow the person originating the call to hang up first.

INCOMING CALLS

The telephone should be answered promptly, preferably after the first ring. Use the wording preferred by the dentist.

- Greet the patient pleasantly.
- Identify the practice and yourself.
- Ask how you may help the caller.

You'll find that the proper identification of yourself at the beginning of the conversation prompts the caller to identify himself, too.

Placing a Caller on Hold. Before placing a caller on hold, ask for the caller's permission, "May I put you on hold for just a moment, Mr. Johnson?" Then wait for his response before pressing the "hold" or "mute" button.

Always be courteous, and do not expect the caller to remain on hold for more than a few moments. If necessary, ask whether you can return the call, and give a specific time when you will do so.

ON-HOLD MESSAGE SYSTEMS

On-hold message systems are recorded messages or music used by the practice to make "on-hold" time educational and more pleasant for callers than a waiting signal. These messages may explain a variety of treatments and services available at the practice.

The messages, or musical interludes, are broken occasionally by professional announcers apologizing for any delay or thanking the caller for waiting.

CALLERS WHO WANT TO SPEAK TO THE DENTIST

Usually the dentist will not be interrupted at chairside to come to the telephone. This is because telephone interruptions (1) reduce productivity and cause treatment delays, (2) are inconsiderate of the seated patient and put the dentist behind schedule, and (3) make it difficult for the dental team to maintain exposure control protocols.

The few most common exceptions when the doctor may come to the phone are to talk to another doctor, the dental laboratory technician, or an immediate family member. It is the business assistant's responsibility to know the dentist's policy on this and to handle all other calls tactfully.

Select your words and phrases with care. If a caller requesting to speak with the doctor does not meet the doctor's specified criteria for interruption, be polite. A statement such as "Dr. Garcia is with a patient now. How may I help you?" is appropriate.

TAKING MESSAGES

Make a written notation of all incoming calls, particularly those that require further action. Many practices use a printed form or a phone log to organize this information.

At the beginning of the conversation, note the caller's name and then ask the appropriate questions. Be sure to record the information completely and accurately. After you take a message, deliver it promptly and accurately. If you promise to follow through on a call, be sure to do just that!

Do not promise that the dentist will call back at a certain time unless you are positive that this is possible and that the dentist is willing to follow through.

When the dentist must return a call in reference to a patient, have the appropriate patient records ready when you deliver the message.

THE ANSWERING SERVICE

When the dental office is closed, some form of telephone coverage must be provided. If an answering service is employed, learn how to use its services properly. In general, it is necessary to call the service and notify them when the office is closing. Relay the following information to the service:

- When the office will reopen
- Whom to contact, and where to contact them, in case of an emergency

When the office reopens, call the service immediately to notify them that you are back and will be taking the incoming calls again.

At this time, the service will give you the messages they have taken during your absence. As the messages are dictated, record them accurately and, as necessary, return calls promptly.

THE ANSWERING MACHINE

The telephone answering machine is a recording device located in the dental office. When the office is closing, the administrative assistant dictates an appropriate message into the machine, giving the following information:

- The identification of the office
- That the telephone is being answered by a recording
- The time when the office will reopen
- Whom to contact, and where to contact them, in case of an emergency
- Instructions on how to leave a message

After you have dictated the message, play it back to check for accuracy and clarity. Remember that even on a recording, you want to create a good impression. Then turn the machine to "on" so that it will answer and record all incoming calls.

When you return to the office, listen to the messages that have been left, note them, and promptly take any necessary follow-through action.

VOICE MAIL

Many dental offices use voice mail to allow the caller to select a variety of options. For example, the call may be forwarded directly to the bookkeeper to answer a question, or the caller may leave a message for the doctor.

OUTGOING CALLS

Telephone calls from the professional office are for business purposes and, although conducted pleasantly, should be handled as efficiently and briefly as possible. If you have questions to ask or supplies to order, have your thoughts organized and your list prepared *before* you place the call.

If you must leave a message, do so with caution. Take care not to reveal any confidential information about a patient, a procedure, or test results. Also, try to avoid leaving messages with small children or others who may confuse the message or fail to deliver it.

Staff members should not make personal calls during office hours. If it is necessary to make or receive such calls, it is best to do so during the lunch hour when the phone lines are free.

THE FAX MACHINE

The fax machine is hooked into the phone system and is used to send and receive written messages electronically. This has many uses, including placing orders with suppliers and relaying and receiving patient consultation information.

When sending a fax, remember that like other forms of written communication, it should be neat and professional in appearance.

Patient Reception

The reception room should be just that: a place where patients are received, but not one where they are required to wait a long time. It should be decorated tastefully and kept neat and orderly at all times, with the furnishings clean and in good repair.

Damage, severe wear, or hazards such as a badly worn carpet should be called to the dentist's attention. The light level in the room should be adequate for reading and preventing accidents as patients move about. Magazines should be kept neat and up-to-date, preferably arranged in a wall organizer to eliminate clutter.

If the reception room has a children's play area, the floor, particularly in the traffic pattern, should be kept clear of toys so that it is not a hazard.

Playthings should be selected for their durability, safety, and play value. They should be kept clean and in good repair and should be replaced when they become worn or damaged.

Patient Amenities

Many practices make a point of providing patients with special amenities to make an office visit more pleasant. (**Amenities** are attractive or desirable features or courteous acts.) Patients appreciate welcoming touches such as

- Complimentary coffee, tea, or juice
- A patient rest room that is easily accessed
- An "easy-listening" or classical music sound system
- A children's play area, video games, and other amusements

Greeting the Patient

The four key words in patient reception are *promptly, pleasantly, properly,* and *politely.* The patient should be welcomed promptly upon his arrival with a warm and pleasant greeting. Be sure to check the appointment book so you will know the name of the next scheduled patient.

Introduce yourself to new patients. If you know the patient, greet him by name; however, take care to use the proper form of address. Adults are always greeted as Mr., Mrs., Miss, or Ms. If an adult wants you to call him by his first name, he will tell you so.

If possible, give the patient an approximate idea as to how long he will have to wait (if at all), and invite him to sit down and make himself comfortable.

If you do not know the waiting individual, ask his name. If he does not have an appointment, determine the reason for his visit. Many dentists have a policy of not seeing walk-in patients. (A **walk-in patient** is a person, with no appointment, who comes to the practice seeking immediate treatment.)

If the walk-in person is a patient of record with a toothache or something he considers to be an emergency, always check with the doctor before making any arrangements.

If the walk-in person is not a patient but someone with an emergency, check to see whether the dentist can see him. If the dentist cannot see him, be courteous and refer him to another dentist.

The doctor will have a policy regarding which sales representatives and other visitors will or will not be seen. If the waiting individual cannot be seen, it is your task to dismiss him *politely.* There is no excuse for ever being curt or rude to anyone in the dental office.

Business Office Systems

There are many separate systems in use in the business office. These include the appointment control system, records management, the accounts receivable bookkeeping system, and the accounts payable bookkeeping system.

The systems described in this chapter may be managed either manually, with the use of one-write or "pegboard" systems, or they may be managed by computer. No matter which format is used, the administrative assistant works with the same types of information and follows through on the same basic steps.

Accounts receivable bookkeeping and the submission of insurance claims are the applications most commonly computerized. These are addressed in Chapters 34 and 35.

Appointment Control

Effective appointment control is vital to the smooth functioning and success of the entire dental practice. With good appointment control,

- Patients are seen on time. (Making patients wait is discourteous and shows a lack of respect for their time.)
- The patient load is well-balanced. (This provides an even pace, and the day is completed without undue tension or hurry.)
- The dentist and staff are able to make good use of their time. (This enables them to maximize their productivity while providing quality care for the patients.)

Appointment control is most effective when *one person* is responsible for all appointment planning and for all entries in the appointment book. This responsibility is usually given to the administrative assistant.

Computerized or Manual Scheduling

Appointment control may be managed with a computerized scheduling system or manually with a traditional appointment book.

Whichever system is used, the basics are the same: the appointment book format must be selected, the days must be outlined, and the patients must be scheduled effectively to make the best possible use of time.

Appointment Book Selection

If the traditional appointment book is used, it must be selected to ensure sufficient space for all necessary entries and to facilitate the efficient scheduling of patients.

- Most appointment books are made to open flat and, when fully open, to show an entire week on the facing pages.
- The space for each day is divided into columns, the most common layout being two columns per day.
- Arrangements with more columns per day are available and are often used in practices in which there are multiple dentists and auxiliaries.

UNITS OF TIME

The basic time increments used in planning appointments are described as units of time. A unit of time may be 10 or 15 minutes, depending upon the doctor's preference. With 10-minute increments, there are six units per hour. With 15-minute increments, there are four units per hour.

Most practices use 10-minute units because they provide greater flexibility in scheduling, which allows the dentist's time to be used more productively. The key is that patients are scheduled according to the time necessary for the procedure, rather than trying to fit all procedures into a standard 30-minute or 1-hour formula.

If a 10-minute time unit is used, when a patient must be scheduled for a procedure that will take 40 minutes to complete, the dentist will request that the patient be given a "four-unit" appointment.

COLUMNS PER DAY

Appointment scheduling for each day may be assigned to separate columns designated specifically for each operator, with each column representing an operatory. (As used here, the term **operator** means one who provides patient care and is scheduled separately. This may be a dentist, a hygienist, or an extended-functions dental assistant [EFDA].)

For example, in a typical solo practice, one column per day is scheduled for the dentist and one for the dental hygienist. If an EFDA is also employed in the practice, a separate column may also be designated for the EFDA.

To make most efficient use of their time, many dentists prefer to use several operatories simultaneously. This preference is reflected in the appointment book by having one column represent each operatory.

In larger practices with many providers, it is necessary to use multiple appointment books or a computerized scheduling system.

Outlining the Appointment Book

The administrative assistant should go through the appointment book for several months in advance and outline basic information (Fig. 33–2).

These entries should be made in pencil, dark enough to be seen but erasable in case of change. The four basic elements to be outlined are (1) times when the office is closed, (2) buffer periods, (3) meetings, and (4) holidays.

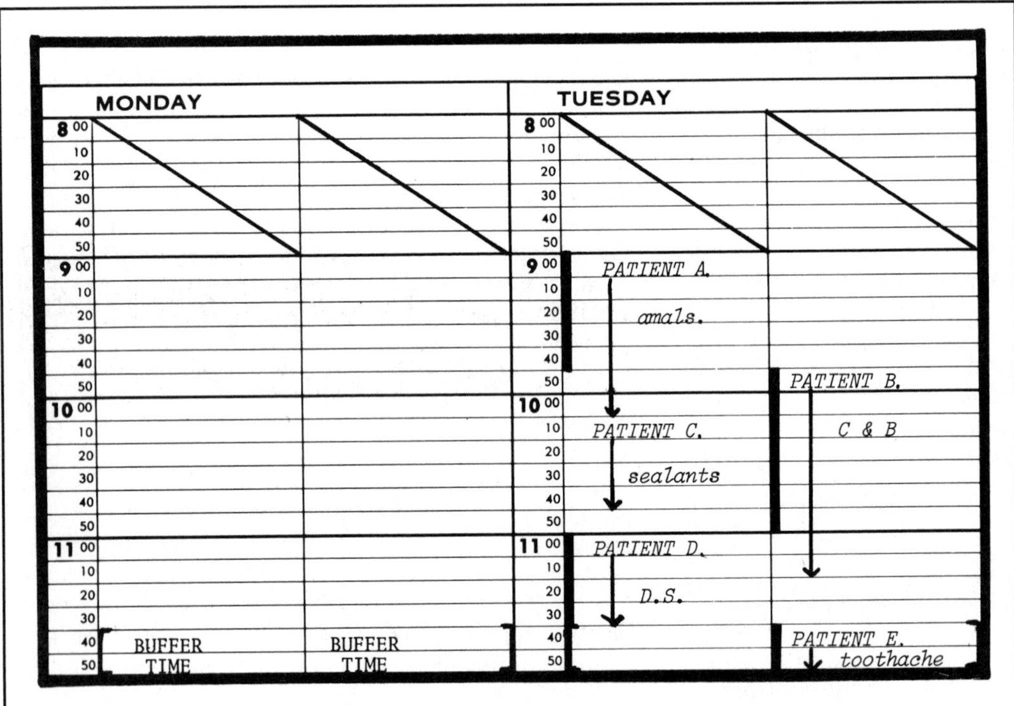

FIGURE 33–2

Outlining the appointment book. The schedule for Monday shows the appointment book outlined with a buffer time reserved late in the morning. The schedule for Tuesday shows scheduling with an extended-function dental assistant (EFDA). The arrow under the patient's name indicates the total length of the appointment. The dark bar on the left side of the column shows when the dentist is scheduled to be with that patient. **Patient A** is scheduled for amalgam restorations. The dentist (with the chairside assistant) will do the preparations and go to patient B while the EFDA completes the restorations for patient A. **Patient B** is scheduled for crown and bridge. After the dentist has completed the preparations and taken the impression, the EFDA will place the temporary coverage. **Patient C** is scheduled for sealants. The EFDA will treat him while the dentist is working on Patient B. **Patient D** is scheduled for denture service, and the entire appointment time is with the dentist. **Patient E** has a toothache and had been scheduled into the buffer time that is reserved for this purpose.

TIMES WHEN THE OFFICE IS CLOSED

These are the hours before opening, after closing, lunch hour, and routine days off. A line is drawn through these time periods to indicate that they are not available for scheduling patients.

BUFFER PERIODS

A buffer period is that time reserved each day for scheduling emergency patients. In many practices there is a buffer period of 20 to 30 minutes scheduled in the late morning and again in the afternoon. These times are bracketed in the appointment book.

Buffer time not needed for emergencies may be used at the last minute for short appointments, such as denture adjustments or suture removal. This time should *not* be filled more than 24 hours in advance.

MEETINGS

Regular meetings that occur during the working day or those that require the dentist to leave the office early should be marked off. The time for staff meetings should also be blocked out well in advance.

HOLIDAYS

Major holidays when the office is closed should also be crossed out. Minor holidays and school vacations, when school is closed but the office is open, should be noted. These times may be more convenient for scheduling schoolchildren and working people.

Making Appointment Book and Appointment Card Entries

All appointment book entries must be **accurate, legible, complete,** and **in pencil** (Fig. 33–3).

- Entries must be clearly written so they are easy to read.
- Entries must be made in pencil, dark enough to be read and light enough to be erased if necessary.
- Entries must be complete and accurate so that it is possible to know exactly who is scheduled and for what treatment.

These entries should be complete but limited to the information directly applicable to the scheduled appointment. Usually the appointment book entry includes (1) the patient's name, (2) the patient's daytime telephone number, and (3) a code for the treatment to be provided.

The proper sequence of making entries in the appointment book is as follows:

1. Make the complete entry in the appointment book.
2. Write the appointment card for the patient.

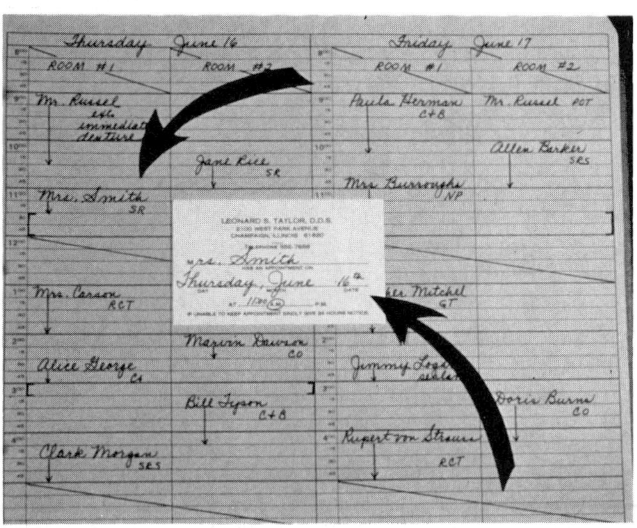

FIGURE 33–3

The information in the appointment book and on the appointment card must be the same. (Courtesy of Colwell Systems, Champaign, IL.)

3. Double-check to see that the information is the same in both places.

When the appointment book entry is complete, the patient is given an appointment card that states the day, date, and time of his appointment (Fig. 33–4). As the administrative assistant hands this to the patient, she orally confirms his understanding of this information.

Unless this sequence is followed and the appointment book entry is made *first,* it is possible to make out the appointment card for the patient and completely forget about making the appointment book entry. Then, at the appointment time, there may be *two* patients rightfully claiming to have appointments for the same time.

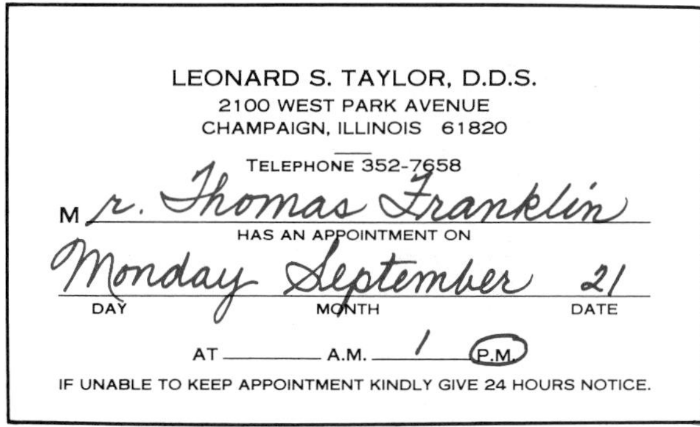

LEONARD S. TAYLOR, D.D.S.
2100 WEST PARK AVENUE
CHAMPAIGN, ILLINOIS 61820

TELEPHONE 352-7658

Mr. Thomas Franklin
HAS AN APPOINTMENT ON
Monday September 21
DAY MONTH DATE

AT ______ A.M. 1 P.M.

IF UNABLE TO KEEP APPOINTMENT KINDLY GIVE 24 HOURS NOTICE.

FIGURE 33–4

Sample completed appointment card. (Courtesy of Colwell Systems, Champaign, IL.)

Scheduling for Maximum Efficiency

SETTING PRODUCTION GOALS

Many efficient practices set production goals to help them maximize chairtime and staff efficiency, and to achieve a stated level of practice earnings. Setting and meeting these goals create a team spirit of cooperation, and in some practices, a bonus system based on these goals may be established as an incentive for the staff.

A major step toward achieving production goals is predetermining, in the appointment book or computer scheduling format, how staff time will be used.

To do this, appointment book outlining includes reserving specific times when extensive procedures, such as crown preparations, will be performed. Reserving these times in advance helps to even out the day's and week's workload. It also aids in ensuring significant production levels.

This time is purposely left unscheduled until a patient in need of this specific type of procedure can be suitably scheduled into this time frame.

SCHEDULING FOR PROCEDURES

Higher stress procedures, such as extensive crown and bridge preparation, implant cases, or molar impactions, require particularly careful scheduling. These types of procedures are often scheduled in the morning when the dentist and staff members are at their highest energy levels.

Scheduling must also be engineered so as to allow efficient use of downtime for greater productivity. For example, during a restorative procedure, the dentist must inject the patient with a local anesthetic and then wait from 3 to 5 minutes for the anesthetic to take effect. (This waiting period is downtime.)

During this downtime, if the doctor's time is well scheduled, he or she may check hygiene patients, make prosthetic adjustments for other patients, return phone calls, or meet with sales representatives.

SCHEDULING AN APPOINTMENT SERIES

Some procedures, such as fabrication of a complete denture or a bridge or quadrant restorations, require a series of appointments. It is usually more efficient to plan all of these at the beginning of treatment. To do this, the administrative assistant must know

- How many appointments will be needed.
- How long (the number of units) each appointment should be.
- How many laboratory working days must be allowed between appointments.

When scheduling a series of appointments, if possible, give the patient the same day of the week and same time of day for each appointment. This makes it easier for the patient to remember his appointments.

SCHEDULING FOR THE DENTAL HYGIENIST

Effective appointment scheduling is also important for the dental hygienist. The administrative assistant must also pay close attention to the time needed for these appointments.

It is best if the hygienist and administrative assistant work out a list of average times required for certain types of hygiene visits: for example, the times needed by the hygienist to see a new adult patient, a new child patient, an adult recall patient, a child recall patient, a child for a fluoride treatment, or pit and fissure sealant treatment.

This list should cover all of the types of procedures commonly performed by the hygienist, and these time estimates should include the time required for the dentist to check the hygiene patient.

On the basis of this information, the administrative assistant can schedule hygiene patients for the correct amount of time so that the hygienist is neither rushed nor wasting time waiting for the next patient.

SCHEDULING FOR AN EFDA

In scheduling for an EFDA, entries in the appointment book are made "by the chair." In order to do this, a separate appointment book column is designated for each operatory.

Appointments must also be planned so that only one patient is scheduled per chair, and per EFDA, at one time.

Before scheduling an appointment, the administrative assistant must know

- What treatment is planned and how much time must be reserved for the entire appointment
- Which units of the visit will be spent with the dentist and which will be solo time for the EFDA before the dentist enters or after the dentist leaves the treatment room.

For example, a patient having teeth prepared for placement of a bridge must first have an alginate impression taken to create a diagnostic cast that can be used in fabricating temporary coverage.

At this patient's visit, the first 10 minutes may be scheduled with the EFDA (or other auxiliary who may legally perform this function) to have the necessary impression completed.

Scheduling Special Patients

NEW PATIENTS

New patients should be scheduled as soon as possible after they call for an appointment—even if it is not an emergency. Some practices accomplish this by reserving a "new patient time" each day.

New patients may be asked to come to the dental office at least 15 minutes before the beginning of their appointment so that they will be able to complete the necessary patient registration forms.

Some practices also send an introductory packet of information to new patients before their first appointment. This packet may contain information that includes

- Practice information such as the doctor's educational and licensure credentials
- Office policies such as payment plans and managing insurance claims
- A map or printed directions to the office (including information about parking facilities if applicable)

RECALL PATIENTS

Recall patients are usually scheduled directly with the hygienist for a prophylaxis, review of home care, and routine radiographs. However, it is also necessary to allow time in this appointment for the dentist to see the patient.

A recall patient must *always* be asked whether there has been any change in his health history, address, or insurance coverage and whether he or she is taking any new or different medications.

YOUNG CHILDREN

Young children are usually at their best in the morning, and most dentists prefer to schedule them early in the day.

Whenever possible, older school children are scheduled after school or at times when school is closed. Having a copy of the school calendar is helpful in planning such appointments.

Sometimes it is necessary to have a child dismissed from school for dental treatment. To minimize the disruption of the school day, it is best to schedule the child either at the beginning of the day (before he goes to school) or near the end of the school day.

EMERGENCY PATIENTS

Emergency patients must be seen as quickly as possible. The buffer period is reserved in the appointment book for this purpose. However, a patient with an acute emergency must be seen immediately. (An **acute emergency** is one in which the patient requires immediate care: for example, a child falls off his bicycle and fractures a tooth.)

An acute emergency may delay the treatment of the regularly scheduled patients. If this happens, the situation should be explained to the waiting patients and their cooperation enlisted. If necessary, the waiting patients should be offered the option of rescheduling.

The Patient in Pain. The patient in pain, who has been seen before in the practice, should be scheduled as soon as possible. The buffer time is reserved for this type of emergency. This caller is known as a "patient of record," and failure to accommodate him could leave the dentist open to charges of abandonment.

Emergency callers who are not patients of record may potentially become regular patients. For this reason, many practices make every effort to accommodate them, too. However, if the schedule is full and such a caller cannot be scheduled, it is helpful to recommend another dentist who will be able to see him sooner.

When you receive a phone call from a patient in pain, gather as much information as possible that will help the doctor; however, do not attempt to diagnose the patient's problem. Helpful information is elicited by the following questions:

- Where is the pain?
- How long has it continued?
- Is there fever or swelling?
- Is the pain constant or on and off?
- Is the pain in response to heat? Cold? Sweets? Chewing? Pressure?
- Has there been recent treatment or injury in the area?

Confirmation of Appointments

One of the greatest obstacles to good appointment control is failure by the patient to keep his appointment. Sometimes these disappointments are unavoidable; however, confirming all appointments by telephone the day before the appointments catches many cancellations far enough in advance to allow the time to be used effectively.

Noting the patient's telephone number next to his name in the appointment book facilitates the task of placing these confirmation calls.

Late Patients

An office that consistently runs late is disrespectful of its patients' time. The dentist will soon find that patients are coming in late for their appointments.

However, if the dentist is usually able to see patients on time, the same courtesy should be expected of the patients. Patients who are chronically late should be tactfully reminded that their tardiness is depriving themselves, and others, of treatment.

Broken Appointments

If a patient has not appeared within 10 minutes of his appointed time, he should be contacted immediately in the hope that he will still be able to use the remainder of the scheduled time. If not, the patient is usually offered another appointment, and every effort is made to schedule another patient into the remainder of the reserved time.

When a patient fails to keep an appointment, the information should be recorded on his treatment record as "B.A." (broken appointment) with the date. This is important clinical data, because in case of a malpractice suit, repeatedly breaking appointments can be considered contributory negligence on the part of the patient.

Short-Notice Appointments

Although filling changed appointments on short notice is not as efficient as careful prior planning, such time can be used to better advantage by maintaining a list of patients who are available to take an appointment on short notice.

Information on such available patients may be placed on file cards or kept as a call list. This listing should include the patient's name, work and home telephone numbers, notes of the treatment to be provided, and those times when the patient is available.

The list should be kept up to date at all times, and the patient's name should be removed when he no longer needs an appointment. A patient who comes in on short notice should be thanked for coming, because he has changed his plans for the convenience of the dental office.

The Daily Schedule

Appointment book information for the next day is transferred to the "Daily Schedule" form (Fig. 33–5). Enough copies of this are produced that a copy may be posted in each treatment room, the laboratory, and the dentist's private office. This list is updated throughout the day as there are changes in the schedule.

On this form, the patient's name and the treatment to be provided are listed next to the appointment time. A check mark is placed to the left of the patient's name when the appointment has been confirmed. A circle around the time indicates that the appointment has not been confirmed (Fig. 33–6).

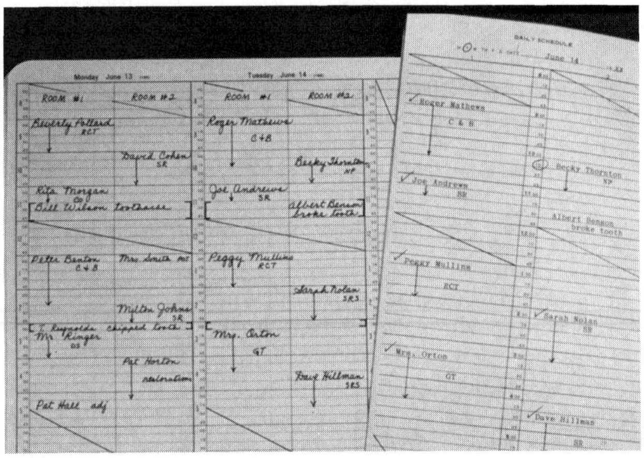

FIGURE 33–5

The daily schedule form is developed directly from the appointment book information. (Courtesy of Colwell Systems, Champaign, IL.)

Prior Appointment Preparations

At the end of the day, there are certain preparations that the administrative assistant must make for the patients who are scheduled to be seen the following day.

The Daily Huddle

Many practices make a point of starting each workday with a team "huddle." This is a brief meeting of 5 to 10 minutes in which the doctor and staff review the daily schedule and any specific treatment procedures or patient concerns. Before the huddle breaks up, a motivational thought or idea is shared by one member of the team to set the tone for the day.

Records Management

The maintenance of adequate records, and their protection against loss, is one of the administrative assistant's most important duties. Maintenance of complete and accurate records is also essential in management of malpractice litigation. (Refer to Chapter 2 for additional information.)

Record Protection and Confidentiality

The destruction or loss of records through fire or other catastrophe could seriously handicap a dental practice. For this reason, it is vital that all records be protected at all times.

Patient records, and all other practice information, are confidential and should be treated with appropriate care. Do not leave records where they can be easily seen. Never discuss any information that you may have seen or overheard.

PROTECTING COMPUTERIZED FILES

If the practice systems are computerized, it is advisable to back up all files at the close of each business day. (**Back up** means to make a copy of the computer files. The back-up file is then available in case there is a problem with the system.)

Many practices keep two sets of back-up files: one in the office and a second in a safe place outside of the office. Thus in the event of fire or other catastrophe, a remaining set of files is available.

PROTECTING PAPER FILES

Never leave records out of their appropriate file space. As you finish using a record, return it to its proper place. When leaving for the day, make certain that all records are protected in file cabinets and that the cabinets are properly closed.

01-11-	DAILY SCHEDULE				Leonard S. Taylor, D.D.S.	
TIME	PATIENT NAME			PROVIDER	REASON FOR VISIT	ACCOUNT
9:00	✓	Dorothy	Hobson	1	Crown & Bridge	23
9:15						
9:30						
9:45						
(10:00)		Lisa	Norman	1	Restorations	50
10:15						
10:30	✓	Ruth	Green	1	Endodontic Treatment	31
10:45						
11:00	✓	Wallace	Pierce	1	Denture Service	66
11:15						
11:30		Faye	Colson	1	Toothache	51
11:45		Lionel	Agnew	1	Post-Op Check	70
12:00						

FIGURE 33–6

Computer-generated daily schedule. A checkmark next to the patient's name indicates that the appointment has been confirmed. A circle around the time indicates that the appointment has not been confirmed.

PROCEDURE: **Preparing for Tomorrow's Patients**

1. Review the treatment to be provided for each patient, and determine that all necessary laboratory work has been returned.
   □ *RATIONALE:* It is embarrassing to the dentist, and a waste of everyone's time, for a patient to come in for a crown cementation only to have the dentist discover that the case has not yet been returned by the laboratory!
2. Confirm all appointments (if this is office policy).
3. Gather pertinent patient records (the patient's chart and radiographs), and store them temporarily in sequential order as the patients are scheduled for that day. (After use, the records are updated and returned to their normal places in the files.)
4. Post the Daily Schedule in the appropriate places.

Precautions should also be taken to prevent cross-contamination when files are moved from the treatment area and returned to the practice business area.

Types of Practice Records and Files

PATIENT RECORD FILES

Maintaining accurate and complete patient records is usually a sign of quality care. The patient records, which are commonly referred to as "the patient chart," are stored together in a file folder or envelope.

This record usually includes the patient registration form, medical and dental history forms, examination findings, diagnosis, treatment plans, and a record of all treatment provided.

In addition, copies of all correspondence and reports regarding the patient are filed as part of the patient's record. Radiographs may be stored with the chart or maintained in a separate file.

PATIENT FINANCIAL RECORDS

Insurance forms and financial information regarding the patient's account do *not* belong in the chart with the clinical information. Instead, these items should be maintained separately as part of the practice business records.

PRACTICE BUSINESS RECORDS

Accurate financial and business records enable the dentist to operate the practice in a well-organized and business-like manner. These records are usually stored through the use of a subject file system; that is, they are filed in categories such as "laboratory expenses" and "business office supplies." Business records include

- Accounts receivable records
- Practice expenses awaiting payment
- Expense records (receipts and paid bills)
- Payroll records
- Business correspondence
- Canceled checks and bank statements
- Records of income and expenses
- Financial statements, tax records, and possibly corporate records
- Computer printouts of practice reports

Guidelines to Efficient Filing

Filing is the act of classifying and arranging records so that they will be preserved safely and can be quickly retrieved when needed. The following are filing guidelines.

Keep the Filing System Simple. The simpler the system, the easier it is to work with. For most practices, alphabetical filing with color coding is the simplest and most efficient system.

Clearly Label Folders. Each file folder should have a neatly typed label showing the patient's full name. This saves having to go through the chart to make certain that you have the right one.

Use an Adequate Number of File Guides. There should be approximately one file guide per every five to ten folders (depending upon the size of the folders). (A **file guide** indicates the letters or numbers of the records that follow it.)

Leave Adequate Working Space in Each File. Papers tightly wedged into the file slow filing, make records hard to find, and may damage filed materials. Leave at least 4 inches of working space on each shelf or drawer.

Label Shelves or Drawers. All files should be clearly, neatly, and accurately labeled as to the contents or other appropriate designation.

Use Outguides. An **outguide** is like a bookmark for the filing system. When a folder is removed from the file, place an outguide to mark its place. This makes it faster to return records to the file and easy to spot where records are missing.

Presort. Presorting folders into approximate order before starting to file will speed the filing process.

Basic Filing Systems

ALPHABETICAL FILING

The alphabetical filing system is by far the easiest and most commonly used system for filing patient records such as charts and ledger cards. In alphabetical filing, all items are filed in straight alphabetical A-B-C order in accordance with the basic rules of indexing. (See Table 33–1.)

Color Coding. Color coding is used to make filing and retrieval of patient records easier and faster (Fig. 33–7). With color coding, tabs that combine colors and letters are used to indicate the first two letters of the patient's last name. In addition to speeding filing and finding, color coding makes it easier to spot a misfiled chart.

NUMERICAL FILING

In numerical filing, each chart or document is assigned a number. In straight numerical filing, all items are filed in strict one-two-three order. Numerical filing is most often used for patient records in a large group practice.

In numerical filing, in order to locate items, it is necessary to maintain a **cross-reference file.** Here each item is listed in alphabetical order, by name, and shows its document number.

Color coding may also be used with numerical filing. Here the color tabs represent the last two numbers of the chart number.

SPECIAL FILES

There are usually several special small filing systems maintained within the dental practice.

TABLE 33–1

Indexing Rules for Alphabetical* Filing

INDEXING† RULES	UNIT 1‡ (CAPTION)§	UNIT 2	UNIT 3	UNIT 4
Names	Brown *(surname)*	John *(first name)*	William *(middle name)*	Senior *(term denoting seniority)*
Married woman	Brown *(surname)*	Mary *(her first name)*	Harris *(her middle name or maiden name)*	Mrs. John W. *(for information only, not an indexing unit)*
Nothing comes before something	Brown			
	Brown	J.		
	Brown	John		
	Brown	John	W.	
	Brown	John	William	
	Brown	John	William	Senior
The prefix is part of surname, not a separate unit	Macdonald	Peter		
(Maintain strict alphabetical order!)	McDonald	Paul		
Abbreviated prefix *(Index as if spelled out)*	St. Andrew *(Saint Andrew)*	Francis	Lee	
Hyphenated names *(Treat as one unit)*	Vaughan-Eames	Henry	David	
Titles are not indexing units	Douglass	James	Richard	Ph.D. *(for information only, not for indexing)*

* **Alphabetizing** is the arrangement of captions and indexing units in strict alphabetical order: A–B–C.

† **Indexing** is the process of selecting a caption under which a paper will be filed. It is also the process of determining the order in which the units of that name are to be considered.

‡ A **unit** is a single important element in a name or subject. Material to be indexed is handled in units. A name can be arranged out of normal order for indexing; however, once it is assigned a unit number, the units are then handled in their normal numerical order.

§ The **caption** is the name or phase under which a paper is filed. This constitutes the first indexing unit.

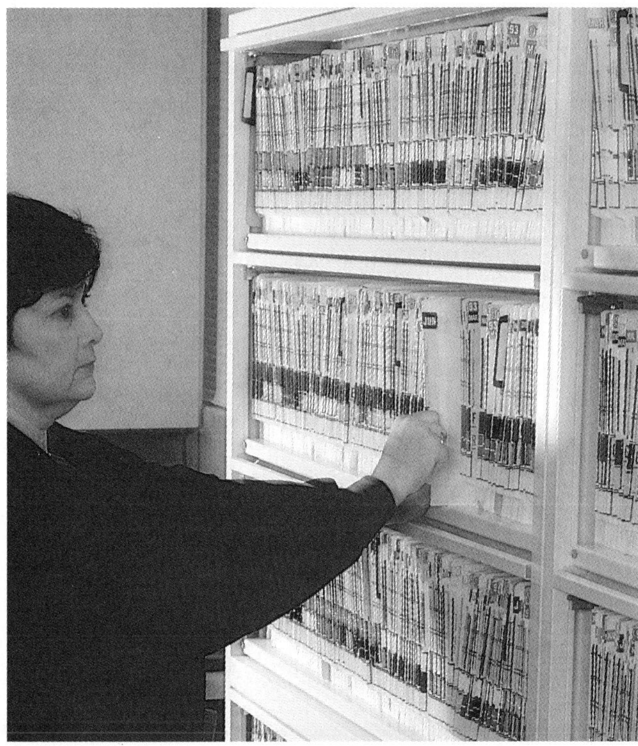

FIGURE 33–7

Color coding files speed filing and retrieval.

A **chronological file** is usually divided into months and may be further subdivided into days of the month. This kind of file may be used for the recall system or as a tickler system for miscellaneous tasks (such as routine maintenance) that should be performed at certain times during the year.

Other special files may be maintained for purposes such as **cross-reference** files, **inventory control** files, and **short-notice appointment** lists.

Active-Inactive Files

Patient records are permanent records. This means that they are never discarded or destroyed without the dentist's specific permission. To reduce the number of charts to be sorted through daily, many practices subdivide patient records into active and inactive files.

Active files are of those patients who have been seen recently (usually within the last 2 to 3 years). These are maintained in the areas of easiest accessibility.

Inactive files, which are not in constant use, are maintained in a less convenient area where they are still accessible if needed.

PURGE TABS

Color-coded purge tabs, which are also known as *aging tabs,* make it easier to sort records into active and inactive categories. This is how they work.

At the patient's first visit in 1995, a red 1995 tag is placed on his folder. At his first visit in 1996, a green 1996 tag is placed over the previous one. When it is time to sort out the charts for all of those patients not seen since 1995, it is easy to go through the file and quickly identify those folders still labeled only with a red 1995 tag.

Preventive Recall Programs

Regularly scheduled preventive care is important for the patient's dental health. The recall system, which is sometimes referred to as the *continuing care program*, is designed to help patients return on time for this treatment. This is an additional service provided for patients by the dentist.

It is the responsibility of the administrative assistant to see that patients are placed on recall and that those who are due to return are notified promptly.

Placing the Patient on Recall

The patient should be placed on recall when he completes his current dental treatment, or upon instruction from the dentist. The most common period of recall is 6 months, and Table 33–2 may be used to calculate when the patient is due to return. However, patients requiring more periodic visits may be placed on 3- or 4-month recall.

All steps necessary to place the patient on recall should be completed before the patient's records are filed after his completion visit. Doing this helps to ensure that the patient's information is placed into the recall system.

TABLE 33–2

Calculating 6-Month Recall Time

Jan. (1)	Feb. (2)	March (3)	April (4)	May (5)	June (6)
July (7)	Aug. (8)	Sept. (9)	Oct. (10)	Nov. (11)	Dec. (12)

From the first half of the year, add 6 to the number of the month.
From the second half of the year, subtract 6 from the number of the month.

Notifying Recall Patients

Recall records may be kept manually or on a computerized system. Whichever system is used, when it is time for patients to return, they may be notified by mail, telephone, or a combination of the two methods.

Types of Recall Systems

CONTINUING APPOINTMENT SYSTEM

This is also known as the *advance or preappointment recall appointment system.* At the time of his last visit in the current series, the patient is given a specific appointment time and date for his recall visit. This is noted in the appointment book, and the patient is given an appointment card.

These appointments are usually coded in the appointment book so that the patient may be sent a reminder 2 weeks before the appointment. These appointments are also confirmed by telephone.

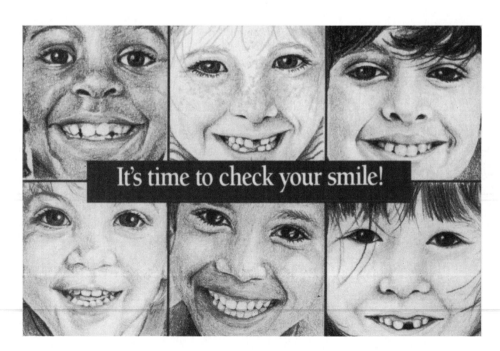

FIGURE 33–8

Sample recall reminder card. (Courtesy of Colwell Systems, Champaign, IL.)

WRITTEN RECALL NOTIFICATION

Many practices send a recall card or postcard to remind the patient to return for continuing care. With a computerized recall system, the cards for each month are quickly prepared by the system (Fig. 33–8).

With a manual system, at the time of his last visit in the current series, the patient may be asked to address a recall card to himself. This card is then filed behind the month of recall.

At the beginning of each month, the administrative assistant removes the cards from the file for that month and mails them to the patients.

RECALL BY TELEPHONE

Another option is to maintain a list of the names and telephone numbers of all patients due to be recalled each month. As time permits, the administrative assistant calls each patient and tries to schedule his recall appointment.

A note is made next to the patient's name as to the results of the call, and the patient's name is crossed out when he has been successfully contacted. Although recall by telephone is time consuming, it is usually more effective than repeatedly sending written reminders.

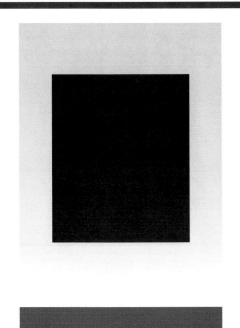

Chapter 34

Accounts Receivable Management

Introduction

There are two types of bookkeeping systems used in a dental practice. One is the **accounts receivable system,** which manages all money *owed to* the practice. The other is the **accounts payable system,** which manages all money *owed by* the practice. (Accounts payable are discussed in Chapter 35.)

Accounts receivable management, which is frequently referred to as *bookkeeping*, involves maintaining financial records regarding all transactions related to collecting fees for professional services provided to patient. (A **transaction** is any charge, payment, or adjustment that is made to a patient account.)

This information must be arranged systematically so that it is accurate at all times and provides data needed to manage these financial matters effectively.

Accounts receivable activities are not difficult; however, in carrying out these activities, the administrative assistant assumes the large responsibility of handling other people's money. In this way, she is responsible for making every effort to keep this money safe, to record it accurately, and to respect the confidence in which all of this information must be held.

The dentist may bond staff members who handle practice funds, such as receiving and banking patient payments or writing checks. (**Bonding** is a special form of insurance that reimburses the employer for a loss resulting from theft of funds by an employee.) Although this insurance will cover a loss, the employee will also be prosecuted under the law for any such theft.

Types of Accounts Receivable Systems

The two most frequently used types of accounts receivable bookkeeping systems in dental practices are a pegboard (manual) system and a computerized system.

Pegboard Accounts Receivable Management

Pegboard accounting, also known as a *one-write* system, is a manual bookkeeping system in which all records are completed with a single entry (Fig. 34–1).

By positioning the daily journal page, ledger card, and a carbonized receipt, all financial records for each patient visit are completed by writing the information just one time. The one-write feature helps to avoid errors by ensuring that the entries have been made and are exactly the same on all records.

Entries for additional records, such as the daily totals and monthly summaries, must be completed manually. The totals must then be calculated and verified for accuracy.

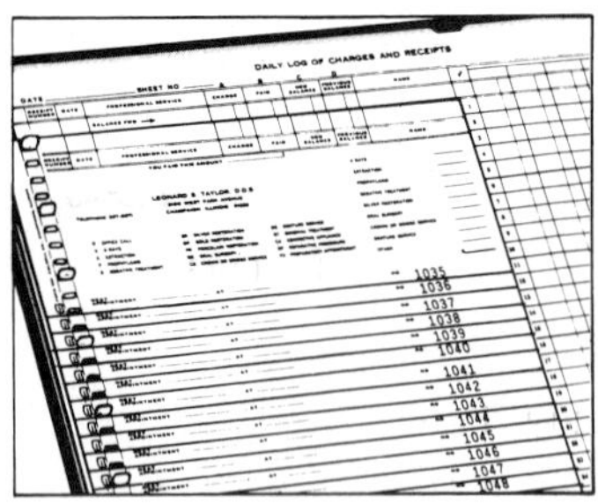

Each morning a DAILY JOURNAL PAGE is placed on the folding pegboard. A series of imprinted, prenumbered and shingled CHARGE/RECEIPT SLIPS are then pegged into position over the journal page.

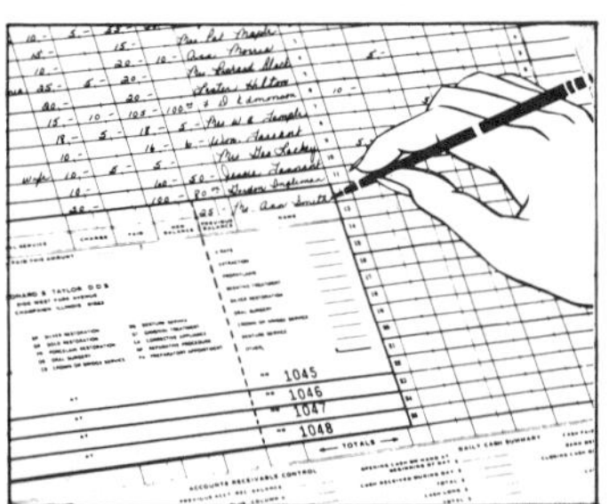

When a patient arrives, the current balance and patient's name and receipt number are entered on the CHARGE SLIP at the next available line on the daily journal page.

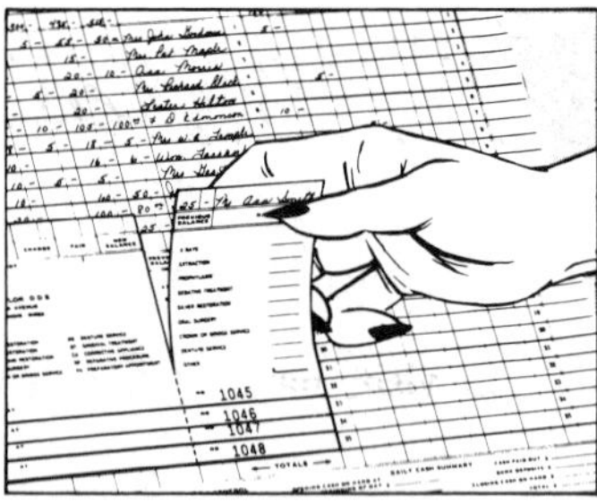

Next, tear off Charge Slip along the perforation and attach to patient's records which are then forwarded to doctor. Thus, the doctor is advised of the current account status before the patient enters. At the conclusion of the visit, the doctor notes fees on the Charge Slip which is returned to the business desk.

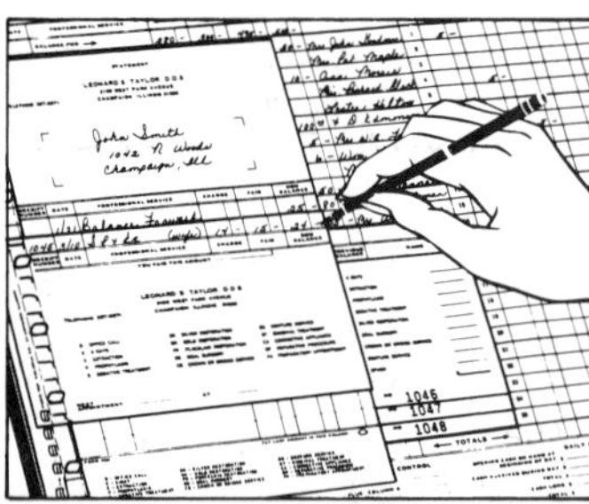

When the Charge Slip is received at the business desk, the patient's Account Record (ledger card) is placed in proper alignment under the correct prenumbered RECEIPT SLIP. The date, services rendered, charge, payment (if any) and new balance data are posted with one writing to THREE records—Receipts, Ledger, and Daily Journal.

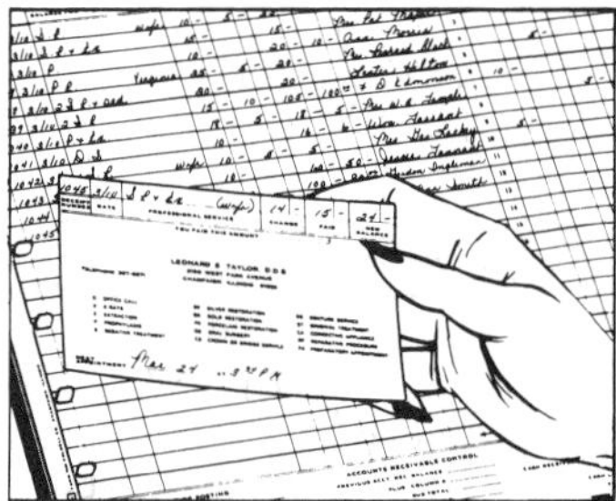

The Receipt Slip is then removed from the pegboard and given to the patient. Space is provided at the bottom of Receipt Slip for scheduling the next appointment.

FIGURE 34–1

Steps in pegboard accounting. (Courtesy of Colwell Systems, Champaign, IL.)

Computerized Accounts Receivable Management

With a computerized accounts receivable system, data entered into the system are used to maintain account histories and practice records (Fig. 34–2).

It is essential that the information be entered into the system accurately, because it is used to generate account totals plus daily and monthly summaries. These and other management reports are automatically calculated and produced by the system.

It is also important that the data stored in the hard drive of the computer be protected by being backed up (copied for safekeeping) at least once daily. An additional set of backups (disks or tapes) should be stored in a safe place outside the office. These records are vital in the event of theft, fire, or other disaster that makes it necessary to reconstruct information that has been lost from the system.

Accounts Receivable Management Basics

Whether the manual or computerized system is used, the same information requirements and organizational format are necessary. Learning to use either system begins with understanding the basics of accounts receivable bookkeeping.

Patient Account Records

Patient account records are organized based on information regarding the responsible party. The **responsible party**, also known as the *guarantor*, is the person who agreed to be responsible for payment of the account. This is *not* always the patient.

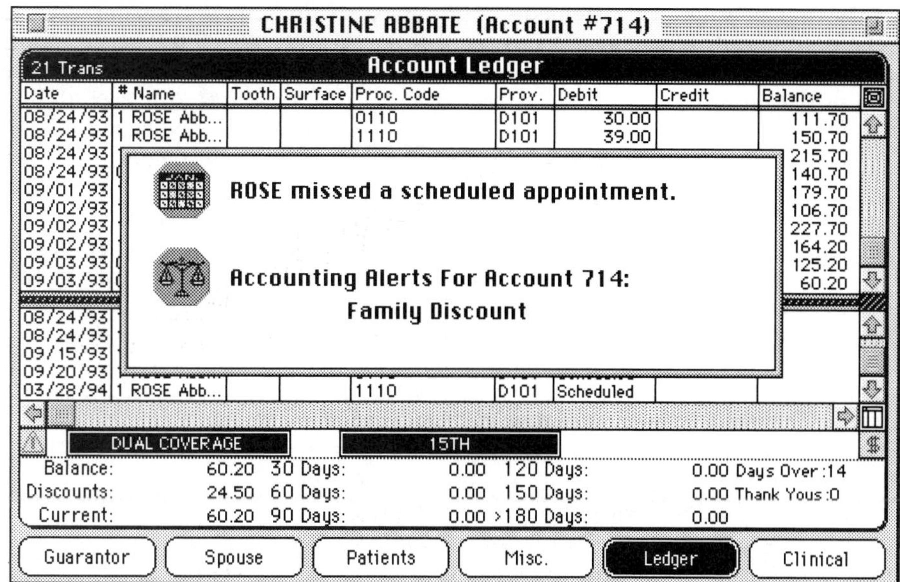

FIGURE 34–2

Computer screen shows patient account history. As shown here, this system also provides reminders concerning a missed appointment and a family discount. (Courtesy of HealthCare Communications, Lincoln, NE.)

These records are usually organized by family, and they include identification information for the responsible party and all family members covered by this account. Gathering this information is discussed further later in this chapter.

The patient account record is used to track all account transactions. A current account balance is maintained at all times, and this information is used to generate statements, insurance claims, and other collection efforts.

In a manual system, the patient account records are maintained on account **ledger cards**. In a computerized system, they are organized as **account histories**.

Encounter Forms

Encounter forms, also known as *charge slips*, are used to transmit financial information between the treatment area and the business office. This form usually shows the current account balance, and if there is an overdue or very large balance, the dentist or office manager may choose to discuss this with the patient.

The encounter form has space for the dentist or assistant to note the treatment provided at each patient visit. The completed encounter form is returned to the business office, and the information is posted (entered) to the accounts receivable system. With a computerized system, an alternative is to enter the data directly from a terminal in the treatment area.

Encounter forms are numbered as part of the audit trail. (An **audit trail** is a method of tracking the accuracy and completeness of bookkeeping records.) There should be an encounter form generated for each patient. At the end of the day, each encounter form must be accounted for by number. This way the dentist knows that all patient visits have been entered into the system.

Daily Journal Page

The daily journal page is the practice record of all transactions for the patients seen each day. This includes the name of each patient seen, plus any charges, payments, and adjustments to that account.

Throughout the day, all transactions are posted to the bookkeeping system. In addition to maintaining the patient account record, this posting generates the daily journal page entry.

A computerized system automatically totals this form and uses the information to generate the other practice reports. With a manual system, it is necessary to total the daily journal page and then carry the totals forward to monthly and annual summaries.

Receipts and Walk-Out Statements

The encounter form is usually printed in duplicate. One copy is used to enter charges and payments into the bookkeeping system. It is then saved as part of the practice records. The other copy is completed and serves as a receipt and/or walk-out statement for the departing patient.

A walk-out statement is similar to a receipt except that it shows the current account balance. A walk-out statement is given to those patients who do not make payment in full. It is presented with a postage-paid reply envelope, and the patient is requested to mail his payment as soon as possible.

The use of walk-out statements improves cash flow because it speeds payments. It also reduces the number of statements that must be prepared and mailed at the end of the month.

Management of Payments Received

CHANGE FUND

The **change fund** is a fixed amount of cash (usually $50 or less) that is maintained in small bills to have change available as needed when a patient pays cash. Each morning this change fund is placed in the cash drawer and used as needed during the day.

At the end of the day, the cash fund is removed and placed in safekeeping. Money from the cash fund does *not* become part of the daily deposit, and the amount in the cash fund at the end of the day must be the same as it was at the beginning of the day.

RECORDING PAYMENTS

All payments must be entered promptly into the bookkeeping system so that they are recorded in the account history and on the daily journal page. Payments received by mail are entered in the same manner as those made in person.

As a safeguard, checks should be stamped immediately with a **restrictive endorsement,** which prevents anyone from cashing a check if it is stolen.

The procedure for recording payments from insurance carriers is explained later in this chapter.

DAILY PROOF OF POSTING

At the end of the day, the listings on the daily journal page are compared with the appointment book to be certain that all patient visits have been entered.

With a manual system, the columns on the daily journal page are then totaled, and the figures are rechecked for accuracy. With a computerized system, these totals are calculated automatically.

The total for receipts must match the amount in the cash drawer minus the change fund. If these two numbers do not match, it is necessary to go back and find the mistake.

BANK DEPOSITS

All receipts should be deposited every day. When the amount of receipts exactly matches the amount of the deposits, the account has met the auditor's critical test to verify bookkeeping accuracy.

A **deposit slip** is an itemized memorandum of the currency and checks taken to the bank to be credited to the practice's account. After the deposit has been made, the date and amount of the deposit should be entered in the practice check register.

- The deposit slip must be imprinted with the practice name, address, and account number.
- The information on the deposit slip must be legible.
- All cash (bills and coins) is listed together under currency.
- Checks are listed separately, usually by the last name and first initial of the person writing the check.
- In many practices, the deposit slip is completed in duplicate so that a copy is retained with the practice records.

Payment Plans

There are several ways in which patients' accounts may be handled. These include payment at the time of treatment, statements, and divided payments. Dental insurance may be considered to be another method of payment, although it must be emphasized that the patient is responsible for the balance not covered by the insurer. Insurance is covered later in this chapter.

Payment at the Time of Treatment

Under this payment policy, patients are asked to make payment, in full, for treatment provided at each visit. This system helps control practice costs by improving cash flow and reducing the cost of sending statements.

Patients must be notified of this payment plan before their first visit. In many practices, this is done during the initial telephone conversation by saying, "In an effort to control the cost of your dental care, we ask that you make payment in full at the time of your visit." Under this plan, cash, checks, and credit cards are accepted as payment.

CASH

Although few patients actually pay for dental treatment in cash, it is necessary to be alert to the needs of cash-paying patients. When accepting payment for service in cash, it is essential to make certain that correct change is available and that it is counted out to the patient.

The patient paying cash must be given a written (or computer-generated) receipt.

CHECK

Many patients pay for dental services by writing a personal check to the dentist or to the name of the professional practice. In some practices, it is office policy to request to see the payor's driver's license number and one other form of identification. The patient paying by check is given a receipt upon request.

CREDIT CARDS

The patient may choose the option of paying for dental services with a credit card. Credit card transactions are listed on the ledger card and on the daily journal page as payments.

Before accepting payment on a patient's credit card, many practices have a policy of calling for account verification and available line of credit (usually when the amount is in excess of $50). While this procedure takes a few extra minutes, it is well worth the peace of mind to verify that the card is valid and that the credit limit has not been exceeded.

The credit card charge form is completed, and a copy is given to the patient. Credit card charges are *not* part of the regular bank deposit. Instead they are managed in accordance with the institution issuing the credit card.

The bank charges a percentage rate as a service fee for handling these transactions. This is sometimes called **discounting**, because at the end of the month the service charge is deducted, or discounted, from these funds. An adjustment entry is made in the checkbook to accommodate this discount as a practice expense. This difference is *not* subtracted from the patient's account.

PROFESSIONAL COURTESY AND DISCOUNTS

Occasionally the dentist extends professional courtesy, in the form of a discount, to professional colleagues or members of their families. In this way, the dentist makes this determination and makes a notation on the chart after completing the treatment for the day.

For example, if the usual fee for a procedure is $50 and the dentist wishes to give a *professional courtesy* of $10, this means that the amount owed for the day's charges is $40.

Discounts are offered by some practices for payment in full before the beginning of planned treatment. For example, if a patient is having a set of complete upper and lower dentures made for the amount of $1,250, the doctor might extend a 5 percent discount ($62.50) for payment in advance. In this case, the patient would pay $1,187.50 in advance, for a saving of 5 percent off the total.

To enter this discount into the bookkeeping system, the total fee of $1,250.00 is posted. Then an adjustment representing the discount is entered for $62.50. This adjustment acts as a credit and leaves an account balance of $1,187.50.

Statements

The monthly statement represents a request for payment of the balance due on the accounts receivable. Under this plan, the patient is expected to pay the balance in full upon receipt of the statement.

With a manual system, this is frequently a photocopy of the ledger card showing the information about charges for treatment provided, payments, and account adjustments. A computer-generated statement shows these data, plus an age analysis of the account balance.

Some practices add a finance charge (usually 1 percent) to those accounts that are not paid within 30 days of receipt of the first statement. When such a charge is made, the patient must be notified of this policy in advance.

CYCLE BILLING

Statements should be routinely mailed at the same time each month. If the statement chore is too large to be handled at one time, the practice may use cycle billing.

In cycle billing, the alphabet is divided into parts, and statements for patients with last names in each part of the alphabet are mailed at specified times during the month.

Divided Payment Plans

Divided payment plans, also known as *budget plans*, are arrangements whereby the patient pays a fixed amount on a regular basis. For example, orthodontic treatment is usually paid for on a divided payment plan.

These arrangements are usually made at the time of the case presentation. After the patient has accepted the proposed treatment plan, the administrative assistant may be asked to work with the patient to develop a divided payment plan. When a divided payment plan is set up, the primary information to be determined is as follows:

- The total fee for services to be rendered
- The balance after deducting the down payment; the resulting number is the amount to be financed
- The annual percentage rate of the finance charge (if there is one)
- The number of payments to be made
- The amount of each payment
- The date on which each payment is due

Once this information has been determined, the payment plan agreement is completed, and both patient and doctor sign it. A copy is given to the patient, and the original is kept in the dental office.

Preventive Account Management

Preventive account management begins with clearly defined financial policies established by the dentist.

Once these guidelines have been determined, it is the responsibility of the administrative assistant to follow through on them.

Basic practice financial policy should cover gathering financial information, presenting the fee, making financial arrangements with the patients, and methods of collecting overdue accounts.

Gathering Financial Information

When the patient calls for an appointment, ask whether he has dental insurance. If he does, request that he bring his identification card and benefits booklet with him. These should be reviewed to determine eligibility and the benefits available.

At the patient's first visit, ask him to complete a registration form. This form gathers all of the basic financial information needed to manage the account history and to complete the patient identification portion of the insurance claim form (Fig. 34–3).

This information includes the following:

1. The name, address, telephone numbers, and place of employment of the person responsible for the account (Fig. 34–4)
2. Information concerning the patient's coverage under a dental insurance plan (Fig. 34–5)
3. Identification information for all individuals included in this account

CREDIT REPORTS

In some practices, a credit report on the responsible party may be requested. If it is the dentist's policy, the responsible party should be informed before the credit report is requested.

Consumer credit reporting agencies, commonly referred to as credit bureaus or agencies, provide a financial profile of the patient. The report covers the record of his paying habits and accounts placed for collection, plus other pertinent information such as lawsuits, judgments, and bankruptcies.

Fee Presentation

Before a case presentation, an estimate must be developed on the basis of the treatment plan to be presented. According to planned treatment information provided by the dentist, this responsibility is usually assigned to the administrative assistant. This estimate is prepared in duplicate: one copy is given to the patient, and the other is retained with the office records.

The fee charged represents a fair return to the dentist for professional treatment provided. It is something that has been earned, and yet for many dentists the hardest part of dental practice is having to discuss fees with their patients. Therefore, after the dentist has completed the case presentation to the patient, the administrative assistant may be asked to handle the discussion of the fees involved.

At that time, the administrative assistant presents the necessary fee information and makes financial arrangements with the patient that are satisfactory to both the dentist and the patient.

Making Financial Arrangements

Financial arrangements must be made for each patient for whom professional services are performed. These arrangements should be made *before* treatment is initiated except in such instances as emergency treatment.

Realistic financial arrangements should be made with the person responsible for the account in a private, unhurried atmosphere. These arrangements are confidential and should be made in a private setting where the discussion cannot be overheard by others.

When making financial arrangements, it is necessary to take into consideration the dentist's stated payment plans and the sound business principles used in the management of the practice. However, it is also necessary to consider the patient's ability to pay, when he gets paid, and his preference in the matter. The resulting arrangements should be equitable to both parties.

The patient must realize that once these arrangements have been made, he is responsible for following through as agreed. All financial agreements should be recorded on the account ledger or in the account history.

The dentist may request that the patient sign a contract for the agreed-upon amount. If a contract is signed, a copy is given to the patient and the original is retained with the office records.

Collections

It is essential that amounts owed to the practice be collected in a timely and organized manner.

Accounts Receivable Report

The accounts receivable report is a valuable management report that shows the total balance due on each account plus an analysis of the "age of the account." This shows how much of the balance is: current (recent charges not yet billed), 30 days old, 31 to 60 days old, 61 to 90 days old, and older. This information is helpful in tracking and taking action on overdue accounts.

A computer can automatically generate this report complete with a breakdown of the account age (Fig. 34–6). Although creation of the report is not automatic with a pegboard system, it is possible to generate one manually.

PATIENT REGISTRATION FORM

Responsible Party James (First Name) A. (Initial) Gridley (Last Name)

Address 670 Northridge Terrace

City Champaign State IL Zip Code 61820

Phone: (Home) 351-4498 (Work) 322-0987

Employer Champion Automotive Supply

Address 9000 Broad Street, Champaign, IL 61820

Name & Address of Nearest Relative (not living with you) ______

______ Phone ______

Referring Physician Dr. Grace Hardy

Family Member Information

Pt. #	First Name	Last Name	Sex	Relationship* I–S–C–O	Birthday
(1)	James	Gridley	M	I	04/05/55
(2)	Ruth	Gridley	F	S	11/30/56
(3)	Lisa	Gridley	F	C	06/20/83
(4)	Ben	Gridley	M	C	10/01/85

Please list additional members on reverse.

*I = Insured, S = Spouse, C = Child, O = Other Dependent

Dental Insurance Information

Subscriber Name James A. Gridley S.S. # 890-49-5381 Pt. # 1

Carrier Name & Address Equitable
2000 Tower Place, New York, NY 10003

Group Name Champion Auto Group Number CH-23000

Does this plan cover all family members? X Yes ___ No

If no specify those NOT Covered.

ASSIGNMENT OF BENEFITS

I authorize payment of dental benefits to myself or the named provider for professional services rendered.

Signed James A. Gridley (Subscriber) Date 1/9/xx

RELEASE OF INFORMATION

I authorize the release of any dental information necessary to process this claim.

Signed James A. Gridley (Patient, or parent if Minor) Date 1/9/xx

FIGURE 34–3

Sample patient registration form. (Courtesy of Colwell Systems, Champaign, IL.)

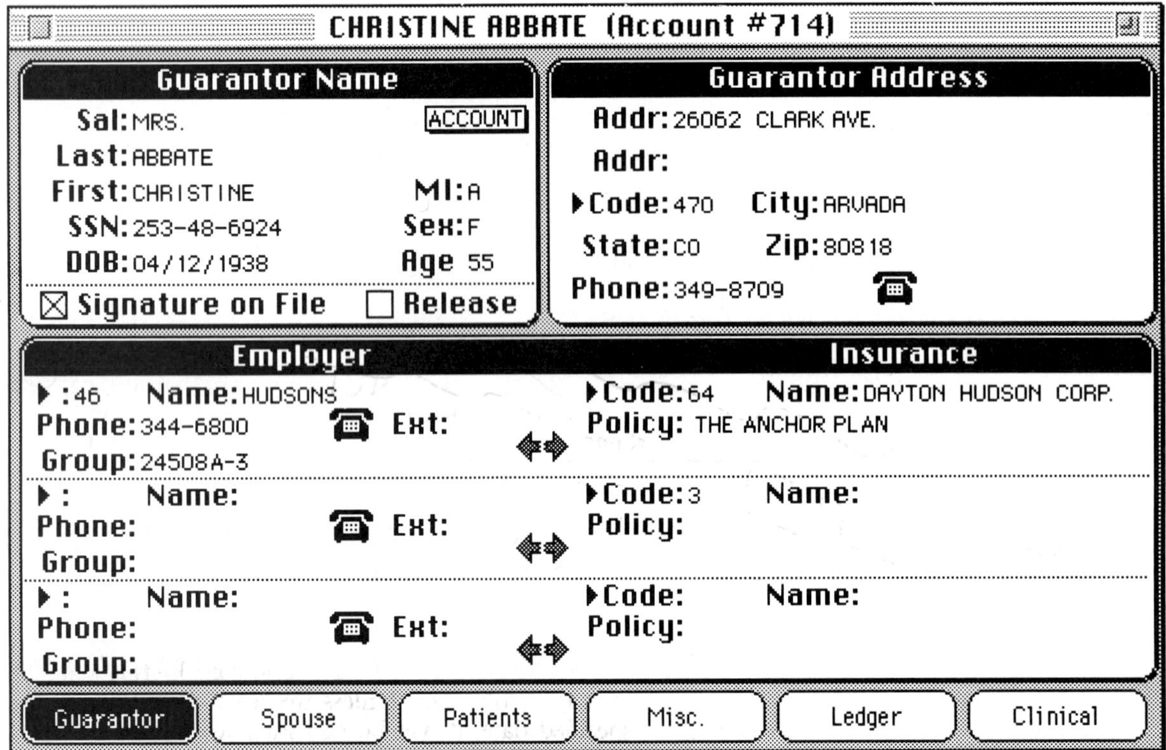
CHRISTINE ABBATE (Account #714)
Guarantor Name
Sal: MRS.
ACCOUNT
Last: ABBATE
First: CHRISTINE
MI: A
SSN: 253-48-6924
Sex: F
DOB: 04/12/1938
Age 55
Signature on File
Release
Guarantor Address
Addr: 26062 CLARK AVE.
Addr:
Code: 470
City: ARVADA
State: CO
Zip: 80818
Phone: 349-8709
Employer
Insurance
:46 Name: HUDSONS
Phone: 344-6800
Ext:
Group: 24508A-3
Code: 64 Name: DAYTON HUDSON CORP.
Policy: THE ANCHOR PLAN
: Name:
Phone:
Ext:
Group:
Code: 3 Name:
Policy:
: Name:
Phone:
Ext:
Group:
Code: Name:
Policy:
Guarantor
Spouse
Patients
Misc.
Ledger
Clinical

FIGURE 34–4

Computer screen shows basic financial information concerning the responsible party. (Courtesy of HealthCare Communications, Lincoln, NE.)

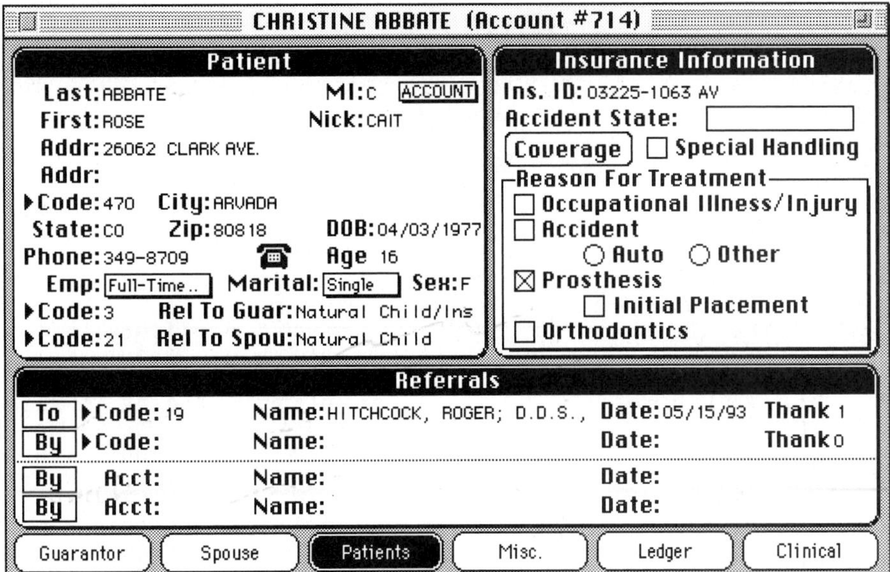

FIGURE 34–5

Computer screen shows patient insurance information. (Courtesy of HealthCare Communications, Lincoln, NE.)

Management of Collection Efforts

All collection efforts must be handled tactfully and in keeping with the dentist's wishes and policies, because the dentist is ultimately responsible for the actions of the employees. The dentist does not want to lose patient good will because of poor collection tactics.

Under the federal **Fair Debt Collection Practice Act,** it is illegal for anyone to

- Telephone the debtor at inconvenient hours (between 5 and 8 P.M. is considered an acceptable time)
- Threaten violence or use obscene language
- Use false pretenses to get information
- Contact the debtor's employer, except to verify employment or residence

Collection Follow-Through

The following is a collection follow-through timetable that is used in many practices:

30 Days. The regular statement, sent at the end of the month, within 30 days, or upon completion of treatment.

60 Days. A second statement, usually with either a sticker containing a mildly worded message or with a handwritten note (a note is much more effective than a printed sticker).

75 Days. The first contact by telephone. The tone of this conversation should be "Is something wrong? How can we help you?"

90 Days. A third statement with a stronger note or a collection letter. Often this letter states that unless payment is made within 10 days, the account will be turned over to a collection agency for action.

105 Days. A second telephone call. In this call, the message should be "Unless the account is paid by the specified date, it will be necessary to turn the account over to a collection agency for action."

120 Days. If no payment has been made and promises have not been kept, the account is turned over to a collection agency for action.

Collection Letters

All collection letters should be phrased in firm, positive, business-like terms that make every effort to persuade the patient to *want* to pay his debt, to help him pay it (if only partially), and to enable him to avoid embarrassment while doing so (Fig. 34–7).

Collection Telephone Calls

Telephone calls are more effective than letters because they are a direct contact with the debtor and therefore are not as easily ignored.

When placing a collection call, be certain to speak *only* to the person responsible for the account. **Important:** Never leave a message that could be misunderstood, could reveal confidential information, or could be considered to be damaging.

Once the proper person has been reached, the administrative assistant should identify himself or herself and wait. The person being called knows what is wanted, and it is best to let him make the first statement.

The debtor may react with anger or hostility. It is important to remember that these are part of his defense mechanisms and not a personal attack. No matter what the debtor says or does, the caller should not become argumentative or defensive with him.

ACCOUNTS RECEIVABLE REPORT
Leonard S. Taylor, D.D.S.

ACCOUNT	NAME	BALANCE	CURRENT	0-30	31-60	61-90	OVER 90
1	Harper	88.00	0.00	88.00	0.00	0.00	0.00
3	Fairchild	177.63	0.00	2.63	175.00	0.00	0.00
6	South	49.00	0.00	49.00	0.00	0.00	0.00
8	Rogers	57.86	0.00	0.86	57.00	0.00	0.00
10	Thompson	306.99	275.00	0.47	0.47	31.05	0.00
12	Martin-Jones	128.78	36.00	1.90	1.88	89.00	0.00
16	Edwards	98.00	0.00	98.00	0.00	0.00	0.00
18	Baker	267.00	149.00	118.00	0.00	0.00	0.00
19	Kilborne	85.26	0.00	1.26	84.00	0.00	0.00
20	Yates	68.00	39.00	29.00	0.00	0.00	0.00
24	Loomis	23.00	0.00	23.00	0.00	0.00	0.00
25	Daniels	257.56	0.00	3.81	3.75	250.00	0.00
27	Miller	117.74	0.00	1.74	116.00	0.00	0.00
29	Greenfield	61.00	0.00	61.00	0.00	0.00	0.00
31	Green	213.00	125.00	88.00	0.00	0.00	0.00
36	Abramson	58.51	7.00	0.76	0.75	50.00	0.00
38	Reed	15.00	0.00	15.00	0.00	0.00	0.00
40	Williams	111.65	0.00	1.65	110.00	0.00	0.00
41	Garrison	128.00	0.00	128.00	0.00	0.00	0.00
42	Parker	77.00	0.00	77.00	0.00	0.00	0.00
45	Yates	197.93	0.00	2.93	195.00	0.00	0.00
47	Blackstone	18.00	0.00	18.00	0.00	0.00	0.00
48	Domber	396.00	125.00	271.00	0.00	0.00	0.00
50	Norman	64.00	64.00	0.00	0.00	0.00	0.00
52	English	82.00	0.00	82.00	0.00	0.00	0.00
55	Nolan	374.00	287.00	87.00	0.00	0.00	0.00
57	Volk	163.04	93.00	1.04	69.00	0.00	0.00
60	Lightner	118.76	0.00	1.76	117.00	0.00	0.00
62	Lawrence	54.00	0.00	54.00	0.00	0.00	0.00
64	Jensen	65.00	0.00	65.00	0.00	0.00	0.00
65	Rockwell	126.00	12.00	114.00	0.00	0.00	0.00
66	Pierce	287.33	287.33	0.00	0.00	0.00	0.00
68	French	40.00	0.00	40.00	0.00	0.00	0.00
70	Agnew	24.45	0.00	0.73	0.72	23.00	0.00
74	Masterson	41.00	0.00	41.00	0.00	0.00	0.00
75	Hardy	115.00	0.00	115.00	0.00	0.00	0.00
77	Clarkson	58.87	0.00	0.87	58.00	0.00	0.00
78	Klein	185.75	0.00	2.75	183.00	0.00	0.00
38 ACCOUNTS		4800.11	1499.33	1686.16	1171.57	443.05	0.00

FIGURE 34–6

Computer-generated accounts receivable report.

Try to be understanding but firm, and never permit yourself to be insulting, no matter what the provocation. Note any agreement made over the telephone on the patient's ledger card. Promises should be followed up carefully, and if they are not kept, the account should be taken to the next step in the collection process.

Final Collection Options

The final decision concerning turning accounts over for collection must be the dentist's, and an account is never turned over without the dentist's specific approval.

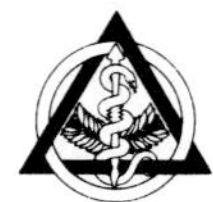

Leonard S. Taylor, D.D.S.
GENERAL DENTISTRY

Today's date

Mr. Marvin Thomas
578 Dogwood Drive
Urbana, IL 61821

Dear Mr. Thomas:

Is something wrong? Our records show that your account of $291 is now more than 60 days overdue.

We want to make certain that there hasn't been a mistake. Please help by checking the appropriate information below and returning this to us in the enclosed envelope.

If you are having a problem paying this account, please telephone me and I will be happy to work out a new payment plan for you.

Thank you.

Sincerely,

Mary Wells

Mary Wells, CDA,
Secretarial Assistant to
Leonard S. Taylor, DDS

- -

____ I paid this amount on __________ with check # _______.

____ My check is enclosed for $291.

____ My check is enclosed for $_______.
I will send the balance by _____________.

__________ (date) ______________________________ (signature)

2100 WEST PARK AVENUE, CHAMPAIGN, ILLINOIS 61820 TELEPHONE 351-5400

FIGURE 34–7

Sample collection letter.

COLLECTION AGENCY

A collection agency makes additional efforts to collect the balance on an overdue account. The agency's charge is a percentage of the amount collected, and this is deducted before the balance is remitted to the dental office.

Some attorneys also attempt to collect overdue accounts in exchange for a percentage of the amount collected.

SMALL CLAIMS COURT

Another option is taking the debtor into small claims court. Sometimes arrangements are made so that the administrative assistant, not the dentist, appears for the hearing.

One difficulty in getting a small claims court judgment is that it is still up to the practice to collect the amount of the judgment.

Dental Insurance Plans

In most practices, reimbursement from dental insurance plans is a major source of practice income. Therefore, it is important that claims be prepared accurately and completely and be filed promptly so that all fees can be collected from the appropriate party in a timely manner.

Dental insurance is designed to make dental care more accessible by reducing the cost to the patient. Although it reduces the cost of care, insurance is not intended to cover all of the expense. Under most plans, the patient remains responsible for any portion of the fee not covered by his insurance.

Beneficiaries

A beneficiary is a person who is entitled to receive benefits under a dental plan. This usually includes the insured, a spouse, and eligible dependents.

- The **insured**, also known as the *subscriber*, is the person who represents the family unit in relation to the dental plan. (This is usually the employee who is earning these benefits.)
- The **spouse** is the wife or husband of the insured.
- A **dependent** is a child who does not exceed the age designated in the contract. Coverage for the child ceases when he passes this age. (This age is usually 18 unless the "child" is still a full-time student.)

Determining Eligibility

Dental plans do not pay for care rendered to patients who are not eligible to receive benefits. When a subscriber starts a new job, there is usually a 30 to 60 day waiting period before coverage comes effective. If a subscriber changes jobs, is laid off, or retires, his coverage is usually terminated within 30 days of the change. If there is any question concerning eligibility, the carrier should be contacted *before* routine dental care commences.

The rules for eligibility under other government programs, such as Medicaid and the Civilian Health and Medical Program of the Uniformed Services (CHAMPUS), vary greatly. There is *no* dental coverage under Medicare.

When working with clients from government programs, the dental assistant must be familiar with the specific form of identification to request to determine eligibility. This is usually an identification card or a proof of eligibility sticker. Because the individual's eligibility may change from month to month, it is essential that this identification be verified at each patient visit.

The Carrier

A carrier is an insurance company that agrees to pay benefits claimed under a dental plan. A single carrier may offer several different dental plans.

The limitations and benefits of these plans are negotiated by the employer, who purchases the coverage as a benefit for his employees. The carrier is responsible for covering *only* the level of treatment that is included in that plan.

Information explaining the coverage under a specific plan is found in the **benefits booklet** that is supplied to the subscriber. The patient is asked to bring this booklet with him to his first visit so that coverage can be reviewed and discussed before the start of treatment.

The two major factors that determine how much the carrier will pay and how much the patient must pay are the **method of payment** and the **limitations** within the plan.

Methods of Payment

Most dental plans are based on the traditional **fee-for-service** concept; that is, the dentist is paid on the basis of services actually rendered. The two most commonly used methods of calculating fee-for-service benefits are "Usual, Customary and Reasonable" (UCR) and "Schedule of Benefits."

USUAL, CUSTOMARY, AND REASONABLE

Usual. The term *usual* refers to the fee that the dentist charges private patients for a given service. These fees are determined by the individual dentist and are routinely charged in the practice.

The dentist files a confidential list of these fees with the carrier. The carrier uses this information, called **prefiled fees**, to determine the customary fee for the area.

Customary. A fee is customary when it is within the *range* of the usual fees charged for the same service by dentists with similar training and experience within the same geographic area (such as a city or county).

Using the information from the prefiled fees, the carrier determines what is customary, on the basis of a **percentile** of the fees charged by dentists within that area. If the carrier uses the 90th percentile, payment is made for any charges at or below that level. For example:

1. There are 100 dentists in the community, and 90 of them charge $150 or less for a given procedure. The other 10 dentists in the community charge $151 or more for the same procedure.
2. The 90th percentile would be $150, and this becomes the "customary" fee for that service in the area.
3. Those dentists who charge $150 or less would be paid their usual fee in full up to the amount of the usual fee. (This means that dentists who normally charge $145 for this service will receive only $145.)
4. Those dentists who charge more than the "customary" amount would be paid only $150, regardless of how much their actual fee may be.

The patient is usually responsible for the difference. However, the limitations of the policy also influence the amount that the dentist receives from the carrier and how much the patient must pay.

Reasonable. A fee is considered "reasonable" if it is justified by special circumstances necessitating extensive or complex treatment. These are the unusual cases for which, because of the problems involved, the dentist would charge more than the usual fee even to a private patient.

A particularly difficult extraction might justify an unusual fee. In these instances, the dentist is able to charge whatever is reasonable for the situation; however, the carrier may request written documentation to explain why the unusual fee was necessary.

SCHEDULE OF BENEFITS

This is also known as a *table of allowances* or a *schedule of allowances.* A schedule of benefits is a list of specified amounts that the carrier will pay toward the cost of covered services. (**Covered services** are those services for which payment is provided under the terms of the dental benefits contract.)

A schedule of benefits is not related in any way to the dentist's actual fee schedule. Under most schedule of benefits plans, the patient is responsible for the difference between what the carrier will pay and what the dentist actually charges.

Under government programs, such as Medicaid, the dentist must accept the amount paid by the carrier as payment in full—and may not bill the patient for the difference.

ALTERNATIVE PAYMENT PLANS

Capitation Programs. Capitation means that the dentist has contracted to provide all or most of the dental services covered under the program to subscribers in payment on a per capita basis.

Under this plan, payment to the dentist is *not* based on services rendered. Instead, the dentist receives a fixed rate per covered member, no matter what services have actually been provided.

Capitation plans are widely used in **Health Maintenance Organizations** (HMOs); in these organizations, dental care may be provided by dentists who are employed by the HMO. An alternative form of capitation is to have services provided by a dentist who has a contract with an HMO. In both situations, the subscriber's choice of dentist is limited to those dentists who are under contract to the HMO.

Direct Reimbursement Plans. A direct reimbursement plan is a self-funded program in which the individual is reimbursed on the basis of a percentage of dollars spent for dental care provided. This type of plan allows beneficiaries to seek treatment from the dentist of their choice.

Under a direct reimbursement plan, no insurance carrier is involved. Instead, the employee pays the dentist, and a portion of this expense is reimbursed by the employer. The amount of reimbursement depends on the benefit design established by the employer.

Individual Practice Associations. An individual practice association (IPA) is an organization formed by groups of dentists or, in some cases, dental societies for the primary purpose of collectively entering into contracts to provide dental services to the enrolled populations. Frequently, services are provided on a capitation basis.

These dentists may practice in their own offices. In addition to treating patients enrolled in the IPA, they may provide care to patients who are not covered by the contract. Treatment of the patients who are not covered is provided on the traditional fee-for-service basis.

Preferred Provider Organizations. A preferred provider organization (PPO) is a formal agreement between a purchaser of a dental benefits program and a defined group of dentists for the delivery of dental services to a specific patient population, in which discounted fees are used for cost savings. This is a variation of fee-for-service practice.

A dentist may join a PPO in the hope of attracting more new patients or in an effort to keep his current patients who are now covered by the PPO plan. These patients are seen in the dentist's own office. The dentist may also continue to see other fee-for-service patients who are not part of the PPO contract. The fee-for-service patients are still charged the dentist's usual fees.

Limitations

In addition to differing methods of payment, other factors also influence the amount of benefits that the beneficiary is entitled to receive under his plan and how much he must pay as his share of these costs.

CO-INSURANCE

Co-insurance is a provision of a dental benefits program by which the beneficiary shares in the cost of covered services, generally on a percentage basis. This percentage is usually expressed in terms of how much the carrier will pay.

For example, the expression "80 percent co-insurance" means that the carrier will pay 80 percent of the cost on the basis of the carrier's method of payment (UCR or schedule of benefits). The patient pays the remaining 20 percent plus any balance not covered by the carrier.

Co-payment is the beneficiary's share of the dentist's fee after the plan benefits have been paid. For example, with 80 percent co-insurance, the patient is responsible for the remaining 20 percent *plus* any difference between what the carrier allows and the dentist's actual fee.

The percentages vary from one plan to another. Under some plans, the carrier pays 100 percent for preventive services (such as a recall prophylaxis and examination), 80 percent for routine or basic services (such as restorations), and 50 percent for major services (such as crown and bridge).

DEDUCTIBLE

A deductible is the specified amount that the insured must pay toward the cost of dental treatment *before* the benefits of the plan go into effect. The amount and type of deductible depend upon the contract.

There may be an **individual deductible.** This means that each family member must meet this amount before he or she becomes eligible for benefits. Or there may be a **family deductible.** Under this plan, the first family member or members meeting the dollar value will satisfy the deductible for the entire family.

EXCLUSIONS

Some policies exclude certain services, such as cosmetic dentistry and orthodontics. In this context, cosmetic dentistry is defined as services provided that are aimed at improving appearance but are not deemed by the carrier to be necessary for the patient's dental health.

This does not mean that the dentist may not provide these services. It simply means that the carrier will not pay for this treatment. The patient may still receive the treatment; however, the patient is responsible for the entire fee.

MAXIMUMS

The carrier may establish a maximum as to the amount that will be paid for dental benefits either as an **annual maximum** or as a **lifetime maximum.**

For example, the plan may include a lifetime maximum of $2,000 for orthodontic treatment. This means that the carrier will not pay more than this amount in orthodontic benefits for this patient no matter how long the treatment takes.

When there is an annual maximum, such as $1,000 annually per patient, the carrier will not pay for any treatment beyond that amount—even if the treatment is a covered service.

LEAST EXPENSIVE ALTERNATIVE TREATMENT

Least expensive alternative treatment (LEAT), also known as an *alternative benefit policy,* is a limitation in a dental plan that allows benefits only for the least expensive treatment.

For example, the patient needs a replacement for a missing tooth. The treatment alternatives are a fixed bridge for $6,000 and a removable partial denture for $1,200. Under LEAT, the carrier will pay benefits only for the partial denture.

The patient may have the bridge placed. However, the carrier will pay benefits only as if he had a partial denture made, and the patient is responsible for the difference in the fee.

PREDETERMINATION OF BENEFITS

Predetermination, also known as a *pre-treatment estimate,* is an administrative procedure that may require the dentist to submit a treatment plan to the third party before treatment begins. The carrier returns the treatment plan indicating the patient's eligibility, covered services, and benefits amounts that are payable. Most commonly, this step is required if the planned treatment exceeds a certain dollar limit.

The request for predetermination should be submitted to the carrier immediately after the patient's first visit. The response from the carrier should be received before the case presentation visit. This way, both the dentist and patient know the amount of benefits that is available to help with the cost of the recommended treatment.

If the carrier requests radiographs with the treatment plan for predetermination, a dual film packet should be used when the x-rays are taken. The extra set of radiographs is then sent to the carrier. If these are not available, the original radiographs are duplicated and the duplicates are submitted to the carrier. Under no circumstances are the original radiographs submitted.

Dual Coverage

If a patient has dental insurance coverage under more than one plan, this is known as dual coverage. When this is the case, it is necessary to take steps to be certain that the appropriate benefits are paid.

DETERMINING PRIMARY AND SECONDARY CARRIERS

When there is dual coverage, it is necessary to determine which carrier is **primary** (and should pay first) and which carrier is **secondary** (and should pay at least a portion of the balance).

The primary carrier is listed at the top right of the claim form. The secondary carrier is listed in answer to questions 11 to 15.

When the patient is the insured, his or her carrier is always primary and the spouse's carrier is secondary. For example, when Mrs. Jamison is the patient, her carrier is primary and Mr. Jamison's carrier is secondary. When Mr. Jamison is the patient, his carrier is primary and Mrs. Jamison's carrier is secondary.

The Birthday Rule. For children with dual coverage, the primary carrier is determined by the birthday rule. This states that the carrier for the parent who has a birthday earlier in the year is primary. This has nothing to do with which parent is older.

If Mrs. Jamison's birthday is in March and Mr. Jamison's is in October, Mrs. Jamison's carrier is primary in providing coverage for the Jamison children. Mr. Jamison's plan is the secondary carrier.

COORDINATION OF BENEFITS

Under coordination of benefits (COB), the patient receives payment from both carriers, but the total received may *not* come to more than 100 percent of the actual dental expenses.

For example, the fee is $250. Benefits from the primary carrier are $175 for this service. No matter what benefits the secondary carrier usually pays for this service, under COB the second carrier will pay only the difference between the fee and the amount paid by the primary carrier. This comes to $75, and the patient has thus been reimbursed for 100 percent of the fee.

NONDUPLICATION OF BENEFITS

Under plans that call for nonduplication of benefits, which is also known as *benefit-less-benefit*, there is a provision relieving the carrier from responsibility for paying for services that are covered under another program. Under these plans, reimbursement is limited to the higher level allowed by the two plans, rather than a total of 100 percent of the charges.

For example, the fee is $250. The primary carrier allows $175 for this service. The secondary carrier allows $190 for this service. In this situation, the primary carrier pays $175. The secondary carrier pays only $15, which is the total of the allowed benefit less the amount that has already been paid. If the primary carrier allowed the higher of the two benefits, the secondary carrier would not pay anything.

The result is that the patient is reimbursed for the higher of the two allowed amounts, but not for 100 percent of the fee.

American Dental Association Procedure Codes

The **Code on Dental Procedures and Nomenclature** was developed by the American Dental Association (ADA) to speed and simplify the reporting of dental procedures. These codes are published in the book **Current Dental Terminology** (CDT), which is published and periodically updated by the ADA.

These codes are *very* specific. The CDT should be reviewed carefully before specific dental treatment is coded. Table 34–1 shows 20 of the most commonly used codes.

In many practices, the encounter forms are preprinted with the codes most commonly used in the practice. To reduce the possibility of coding errors, the dentist notes the treatment for the day and circles the appropriate code.

Submitting Claims

Claims for dental treatment are filed in one of two ways. One is by the submission on a claim form that is mailed to the carrier. The second is by electronic transmission, in which information is submitted electronically to the carrier.

Both types of transmission require the same three primary areas of information: patient and subscriber identification, dentist identification, and details concerning the treatment provided.

TABLE 34–1

Frequently Used Dental Insurance Procedure Codes

CODE	PROCEDURE DESCRIPTION
00110	Initial oral examination
00120	Periodic oral examination
00210	Intraoral: complete series x-rays
02720	Bite-wings, two films
00330	Panoramic film
01110	Prophylaxis, adult
01120	Prophylaxis, child
01201	Topical fluoride, child
02150	Amalgam, two-surface, permanent
02160	Amalgam, three-surface, permanent
02330	Resin, one-surface, anterior
02331	Resin, two-surface, anterior
02386	Resin, two-surface, posterior
02790	Crown: full-cast, high noble metal
02930	Prefabricated stainless steel crown: primary tooth
05110	Complete upper denture
05120	Complete lower denture
06210	Pontic: cast, high noble metal
06790	Bridge retainer crown: full-cast, high noble metal
07110	Extraction, single tooth

CLAIM FORMS

A dental insurance claim form is used either to submit a pre-treatment estimate for planned treatment or to request payment of claims for services that have been rendered.

The "Uniform Report Form" has been approved by the Council on Dental Care Programs of the ADA and is accepted by most dental insurance carriers (Fig. 34–8).

The completed claim form is generated in duplicate. One copy is submitted to the carrier. The other copy is retained with the practice records. Insurance claim forms are financial records; they are *never* stored with the patient's clinical records.

The claim form includes two boxes for patient signatures. These are for the release of information and for the assignment of benefits.

Release of Information. Information regarding the patient's treatment is confidential and may be released only with the patient's written consent. The patient's signature in the "release of information" box gives the dentist permission to reveal information regarding his dental treatment to the insurance carrier.

Assignment of Benefits. Assignment of benefits is a procedure whereby the subscriber authorizes the carrier to make payment of allowable benefits directly to the dentist. If there is no assignment of benefits, the check goes directly to the patient.

To assign the benefits, the subscriber signs the appropriate box on the insurance claim form. If there is no assignment of benefits, financial arrangements are made for the total amount of the fee, just as if the patient did not have dental insurance.

Signature on File. The patient registration form has signature boxes very similar to those on the claim form, and the patient should sign these at the time he completes the form. If the patient is not available to sign the claim form when it is prepared, you may type in "Signature on File."

When claims are submitted electronically, there is no place for a patient signature. Signature on file covers the need to have the patient's information for the release of this information.

ELECTRONIC CLAIMS SUBMISSION

With electronic claims processing, data already stored in the practice's computer are used to generate and submit claims from the practice's computer to the carrier's computer. This has the advantages of speeding claim submission and payment while reducing paperwork and the possibility of errors.

As part of claims preparation on the practice's computer, the system checks each claim for missing information before electronic submission (Fig. 34–9). When the claims have been verified as complete, they are transmitted by modem. This transmission may be directly to the carrier's computer; however, since a practice deals with many carriers, most often the claims are transmitted to a national clearinghouse, which then forwards them to the proper carriers.

Although there is no paper claim generated, the practice must have a record of each claim that was submitted. This record is essential in the event that a claim is lost or disputed and must be submitted again. It is also important in tracking claims for payment.

Preparing Claims

At the end of the patient's visit, all charges are entered into the patient's account history (just as if he did not have insurance). A claim for payment is submitted for these fees.

If this is the patient's first visit, it may also be necessary to file a pre-treatment estimate for planned additional treatment. If so, the pre-treatment estimate is submitted on a separate claim.

Make definite financial arrangements with the patient for payment of his share of the fees.

Tracking Claims in Process

Insurance claims are another form of accounts receivable—that is, money that has been earned and must now be collected. It is important that these claims be handled in a business-like manner.

Most computerized programs generate the reports needed to track these claims. These include reports of

- Claims that have been submitted for predetermination but have not yet been returned
- Claims that have been submitted for payment but have not yet been paid
- Charges for claims that have been generated but have not yet been submitted
- Claims that have been returned for any reason and have not yet been resubmitted

These reports should be printed and reviewed on a regular basis. It is important that you follow up promptly on any claims process that has not been completed in a reasonable period of time.

Payments from Insurance Carriers

Checks received from insurance carriers should be accompanied by an **explanation of benefits** (EOB) explaining what benefits have been paid and what has been denied. This report should be reviewed carefully to determine whether further action is necessary.

The check is entered into the bookkeeping system by patient account with a notation showing the source of the payment. If after this payment the patient owes a balance, he should be notified that his insurance carrier has paid and that he is now responsible for the unpaid balance.

Occasionally it is necessary to make adjustments in the bookkeeping system to write off (deduct) amounts that cannot be collected. The balance of the patient's account is reduced by the amount of the adjustment.

Dental Claim Form

Check one:

☐ **Dentist's pre-treatment estimate**

☒ **Dentist's statement of actual services**

Carrier name and address Delta Dental of Illinois
500 State Plaza
Springfield, IL

PATIENT COVERAGE INFORMATION

1. Patient name — first: Ralph; m.i.: ; last: Henderson
2. Relationship to employee — ☒ self ☐ child ☐ spouse ☐ other
3. Sex — m: x f:
4. Patient birthdate — MM 04 DD 25 YYYY 1960
5. If full time student — school; city
6. Employee/subscriber name and mailing address — 287 Oak Drive, Centerville, IL 61822
7. Employee/subscriber soc. sec. or I.D. number — 543-20-9765
8. Employee/subscriber birthdate — MM 04 DD 25 YYYY 1960
9. Employer (company) name and address — First Bank of Centerville, Centerville, IL
10. Group number — FBOC-333-45
11. Is patient covered by another dental plan? yes (no) If yes, complete 12-a. Is patient covered by a medical plan? yes (no)

12-a. Name and address of carrier(s)

12-b. Group no.(s)

13. Name and address of other employer(s)

14-a. Employee/subscriber name (if different than patient's)

14-b. Employee/subscriber soc. sec. or I.D. number

14-c. Employee/subscriber birthdate MM DD YYYY

15. Relationship to patient ☐ self ☐ parent ☐ spouse ☐ other

I have reviewed the following treatment plan. I authorize release of any information relating to this claim. I understand that I am responsible for all costs of dental treatment.

▶ SIGNATURE ON FILE — 2/1/xx

Signed (Patient, or parent if minor) — Date

I hereby authorize payment of the dental benefits otherwise payable to me directly to the below named dental entity.

▶ SIGNATURE ON FILE — 2/1/xx

Signed (Insured person) — Date

BILLING DENTIST

16. Name of Billing Dentist or Dental Entity — Leonard S. Taylor DDS
17. Address where payment should be remitted — 2100 W. Park Avenue; City, State, Zip — Champaign, IL 61820
18. Dentist Soc. Sec. or T.I.N. — 203-55-9278
19. Dentist license no. — IL-3456
20. Dentist phone no. — 217-351-5400
21. First visit date current series — 1/10/xx
22. Place of treatment — (Office) Hosp. ECF Other
23. Radiographs or models enclosed? No Yes How many?
24. Is treatment result of occupational illness or injury? No: x — If yes, enter brief description and dates.
25. Is treatment result of auto accident? No: x
26. Other accident? No: x
27. If prosthesis, is this initial placement? No: x — (If no, reason for replacement)
28. Date of prior placement
29. Is treatment for orthodontics? No: x — If services already commenced enter: Date appliances placed; Mos. treatment remaining

Identify missing teeth with "x" (FACIAL / LINGUAL; UPPER / LOWER; RIGHT / LEFT; PRIMARY / PERMANENT; teeth 1–32, A–T)

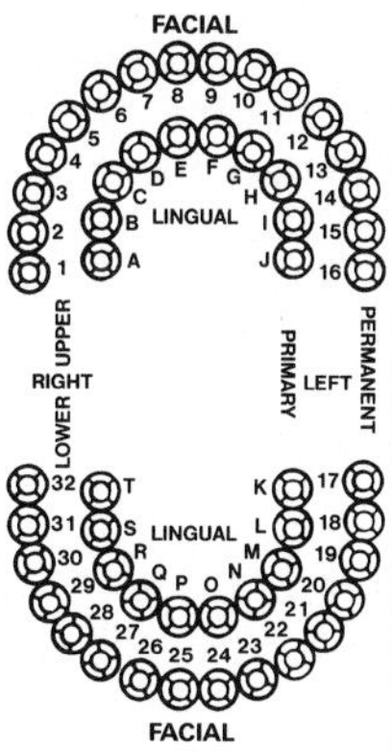

30. Examination and treatment plan—List in order from tooth no. 1 through tooth no. 32—Use charting system shown.

Tooth # or letter	Surface	Description of service (including x-rays, prophylaxis, materials used, etc.)	Date service performed Mo.	Day	Year	Procedure number	Fee
		Initial oral examination	1	10	xx	00110	30 00
		Intraoral – complete series	1	10	xx	00210	55 00
		Prophylaxis – adult	1	10	xx	01110	45 00
		Diagnostic casts	1	10	xx	00470	45 00

For administrative use only

31. Remarks for unusual services

I hereby certify that the procedures as indicated by date have been completed and that the fees submitted are the actual fees I have charged and intend to collect for those procedures.

▶

Signed (Treating Dentist) — License Number — Date

Total Fee Charged	175 00
Max. Allowable	
Deductible	
Carrier %	
Carrier pays	
Patient pays	

Form Approved by the

FIGURE 34–8

The American Dental Association standard claim form. (Courtesy of Colwell Systems, Champaign, IL.)

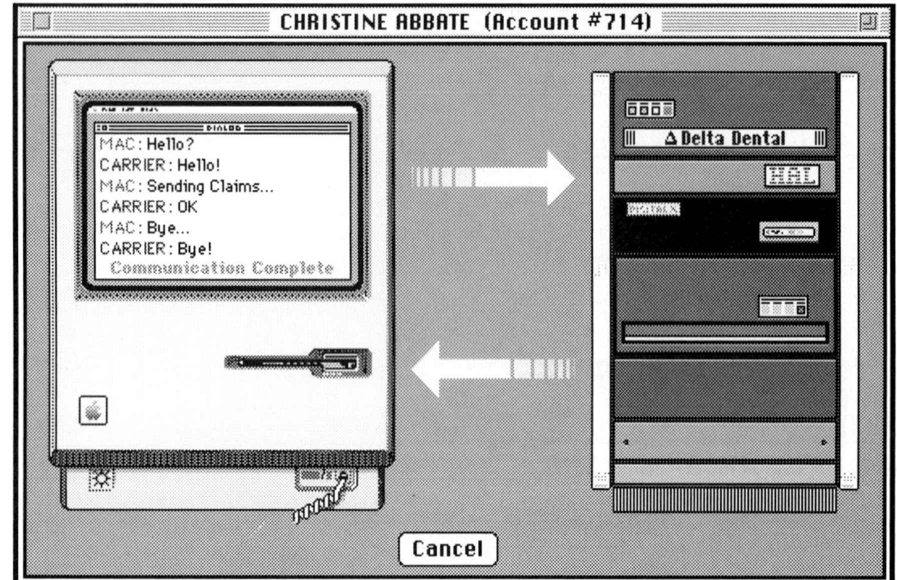

FIGURE 34–9

Electronic claim processing as viewed on the computer screen. (Courtesy of HealthCare Communications, Lincoln, NE.)

HANDLING OVERPAYMENTS

If the patient has paid his account and a check arrives from the insurance carrier, there is a procedure that must be followed to handle the resulting overpayment.

1. Credit the check from the carrier to the patient's account, and deposit it like any other payment on account. Crediting the check to the patient's account will create a credit insurance carriers report to the Internal Revenue Service (IRS) of how much they paid to each dentist, and it is important that the practice records show the receipt of these funds.
2. Write a check from the practice to the patient to refund the amount of the overpayment. This check is from the accounts payable system and shows up as a practice expense.
3. Make an information entry on the account ledger card showing that the check was sent. This will eliminate the credit balance on the account.
4. Because the funds received and the refund check are equal, the total amount of taxable income for the practice is not increased.

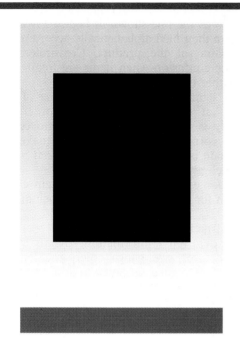

Chapter 35

Accounts Payable Management

Introduction

Expenses and disbursements determine the cost of doing business in the dental practice. **Expenses** are overhead—that is, the actual cost of doing business. As these expenses are incurred, they become **accounts payable. Disbursements** are the payments of the accounts payable. (**Disburse** means to pay out.)

It is the responsibility of the office manager or administrative assistant to ensure accuracy in all accounts payable transactions within the practice.

Dental Office Overhead

Dental office overhead consists of all expenses incurred in the running of the dental practice. These are defined as **fixed overhead** and **variable overhead**. Fee schedules must reflect both of these overhead factors, plus a fair return to the dentist.

FIXED OVERHEAD

Fixed overhead includes those business expenses that continue at all times. These are costs, such as rent or mortgage, utilities, insurance, and salaries, that go on whether or not the dentist is in the office and whether or not professional services are actually being provided.

Note: Not all salaries are part of fixed overhead. Salaries that are not fixed are those of professionals who work as an independent contractor, on a commission basis, or as part-time workers who are employed on an hourly rate "as needed."

VARIABLE OVERHEAD

Variable overhead expenses are those, such as dental and stationery supplies, independent contractors, laboratory fees, and equipment repairs, that change depending upon the type of services rendered.

Gross vs. Net Income

The return the dentist receives for professional services rendered is calculated as **gross income** (the total of *all* professional income received).

Gross income minus payment of all practice-related expenses yields the dentist's **net income** from the practice. Unless the dentist earns an adequate net income, he or she cannot afford to maintain the practice.

A **certified public accountant** (CPA) is often employed on a retainer basis. It is his or her responsibility to handle the major financial records such as annual profit and loss statements, tax returns, and other government reports.

These reports are based on financial information supplied by the dental practice. This information must be accurate, up to date, complete, and in a usable format.

The administrative assistant or office manager is

usually responsible for the management of the day-to-day expenses and disbursements. He or she also helps the accountant by having the required information and records in good order and ready on time.

Supply Inventory, Ordering, and Monitoring

Running out of supplies can create embarrassing situations and unnecessary crises in the dental office. Therefore, an adequate quantity of all necessary dental supplies at all times is essential for the smooth functioning of the practice.

The Inventory System

An inventory system should be simple, readily workable, and kept up to date at all time; it is advisable that one person be responsible for maintaining the inventory control and ordering supplies. However, the cooperation of the entire staff is necessary if the system is to work.

Frequently, the coordinating assistant or chairside assistant is assigned to handle the inventory of treatment area supplies and the administrative assistant to manage inventory of business office supplies.

Of major concern in organizing the inventory system are the expendable and disposable items that are used up in a relatively short time and must be reordered regularly. These include restorative and impression materials, disposable needles, local anesthetic solutions, radiographic film, laboratory supplies, paper products, and business office supplies.

The information concerning these supply items can be organized by making a master file card for each supply item, such as the one shown in Figure 35–1.

These cards are then filed alphabetically according to the common name of the product. Cross-reference cards help reduce confusion when items are frequently referred to by either brand or generic name.

A colored file signal on the upper left corner of the card indicates that the supply is "to be ordered." When the supply is "on order," the tag is moved to the upper right corner. Using these signals makes it easy to differentiate between which supplies need to be ordered and which are already on order.

The file card for each product should contain complete information for ordering that product, including

- The full brand name of the product
- All applicable descriptive information, such as name of the manufacturer, size, gauge, color, grit, length, shank type, fast or regular set, and container size
- The reorder point for that product
- The purchase source, including the name, telephone number, and, if necessary, address of the supplier of that product; it is also helpful to note the name of the contact person who usually handles your order
- Any necessary catalog numbers for that product
- The quantity purchase rates and reorder quantity

REORDER POINT

The reorder point for any given item is the minimum amount that is an adequate reserve for that product. The reorder point, or minimum quantity, should be established for each expendable item used in the practice.

This point, which ensures an adequate supply while the new order is being processed, is based on two factors:

ORDER (ITEM NAME) PATIENT TOWELS **ON ORDER**

ORDER QUANTITY 2000 REORDER POINT 500

ORDER	QTY	REC'D	COST	PREPAID	ON ACCT	ORDER	QTY	REC'D	COST	PREPAID	ON ACCT

INVENTORY COUNT

	JAN	FEB	MAR	APR	MAY	JUNE	JULY	AUG	SEPT	OCT	NOV	DEC
19 ___												
19 ___												

ORDER SOURCE
Acme Dental Supply
1-800-942-8000

UNIT PRICE

FORM 2450 COLWELL CO., CHAMPAIGN, ILLINOIS

FIGURE 35–1

One type of inventory control card. (Courtesy of Colwell Systems, Champaign, IL.)

1. The rate of use of the product on a daily, weekly, or monthly basis (**rate of use** is how many or how much of a product is used within a given time)
2. The **lead time** necessary to order and receive a new supply of that product; this time estimate should include a generous allowance for delays in ordering or shipping or the possibility of back ordering

Marking the Reorder Point. The reorder point for each item should be clearly marked on the supply of that item. This can be done with **reorder tags.** These tags, which are also known as *red flag reorder tags* or *tie tags*, are usually bright red (Fig. 35–2).

The reorder tag is attached to the minimum quantity of the item with a rubber band or tape or by being placed into a stack of a flat product (such as a supply of ledger cards). This tag may be marked with the name of the product only, or it may contain full reordering information. When the reorder point is reached, this tag is removed and immediately processed for reordering.

Automatic Shipments. Many suppliers offer dentists the advantage of bulk quantity pricing with automatic shipments of only a portion of the total order. This ensures the practice a constant supply of the amount of a product necessary to meet the practice's need; it also eliminates bulk storage problems and spreads out the billing over a sequence of monthly or quarterly payments.

Bar Code Reorder System. An automated supply reorder system involves bar coding commonly used dental supplies. The assistant uses a bar code wand to read the product *and* reorder information, which is then transmitted electronically to the supplier (Fig. 35–3).

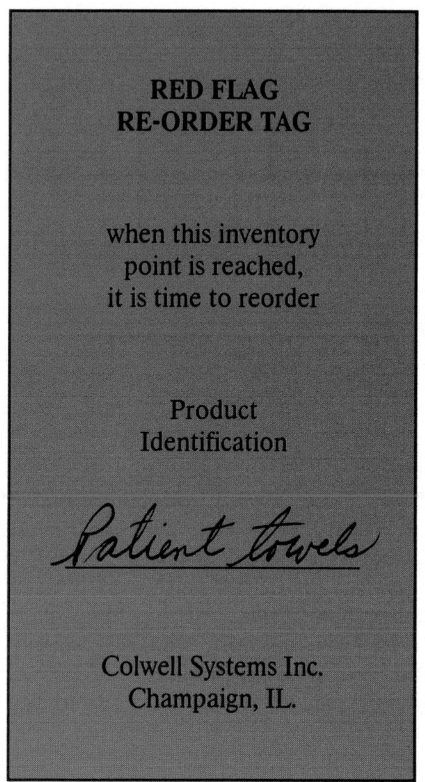

when this inventory

it is time to reorder

FIGURE 35–2

Red flag reorder tag can easily be attached to show the reorder point of a supply. (Courtesy of Colwell Systems, Champaign, IL.)

QUANTITY PURCHASE RATE

The quantity purchase rate is a savings that can be effected by purchasing a product in larger quantities. The **price break** is the point at which the greater savings become effective.

While the office manager takes advantage of the best price per unit on supplies, it is also necessary to take into consideration the available storage space in the office and the rate at which the product is used.

REORDER QUANTITY

Reorder quantity is the *maximum* quantity of a product to be ordered at one time. These should be reviewed periodically and increased or decreased, depending upon changes in these determining factors. The reorder quantity is determined by

- The rate of use
- The shelf life and any storage problems for that product (**shelf life** is the time a product may be stored before it begins to deteriorate and is no longer usable)

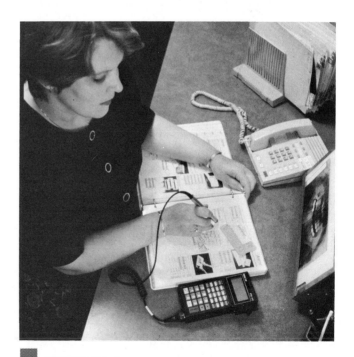

FIGURE 35–3

A bar code wand is used to input a product order. (Courtesy of Patterson Dental Company, Minneapolis, MN.)

PROCEDURE: **Reordering Supplies**

1. When a supply is down to the reorder point, remove the reorder tag to the file box and check the index card for purchasing information for that product.
2. Until the product is ordered, place a color file signal on the *left* corner of the card, and file the reorder tag and card together.
   □ *RATIONALE:* This indicates that this supply is to be ordered as quickly as possible.
3. When the order is placed, move the colored tag to the *right* corner.
   □ *RATIONALE:* This indicates that the product is "on order."
4. When supplies are received and ready to be shelved, remove the color file signal from the inventory card.
5. Attach the reorder tag to mark the minimum quantity, and place the new stock behind any remaining stock.

- Storage problems include bulky items, such as patient bibs, that take up a lot of space; it is also a concern for items such as x-ray film, which is particularly sensitive to heat and light
- The best quantity purchase rate
- The investment involved (purchase of a large quantity of a supply may tie up too much of the practice's cash flow to make it a good buy)

Guidelines for Ordering Dental Supplies

Supplies may be ordered (1) through a dental supply sales representative who calls at the office, or (2) from a catalog via telephone, fax, mail, or bar code scanning.

When ordering and managing dental supplies in the office, it is important to keep all items in one central storage place. This eliminates the need to look through several places in the office to locate a needed product. It also makes treatment room restocking and tray setups more efficient. Many offices make use of alphabetically arranged plastic storage bins to keep supplies neat and organized.

The dentist will specify his or her preference as to the purchase source, quantity, and brand information. When ordering supplies, the assistant should

Be Prepared. Have a want list ready and check with the dentist before the sales representative is due to call. (A **want list** is a list of those supplies to be ordered and questions to be asked of the representative.)

Be Specific. Know *what* is needed and *how much* of it is needed. The assistant should be sure to supply all the necessary information, including the correct catalog or item number, descriptive information, and the quantity desired.

Be Alert. Be on the lookout for "specials" and authentic savings (a special on something that is not needed or used is no bargain). The assistant should plan ahead to take advantage of seasonal savings and convention specials.

Be Informed. Just as the dentist will want to keep abreast of new product information, the assistant also should be alert for new products and ideas that can make business office responsibilities easier to manage.

Journals and catalogs should be reviewed for ideas that can be adapted to the needs of the practice. The assistant should also check regularly with the sales representative and make a point to review the exhibits at dental meetings for new products and ideas.

Back Orders

When an item is not available for delivery with the balance of an order, it is placed on **back order**, to be delivered as soon as it becomes available. A back order

What to Look for When Choosing a Dental Supplier

- Choose a dental supplier with a strong professional reputation and sound track record.
- Choose a supplier with a history of filling orders promptly and accurately.
- Choose a supplier whose goal is customer service satisfaction.
- Choose a supplier who is willing to negotiate on price—especially if your practice is a regular customer.
- Establish a good relationship with your local supplier and request to be placed on the preferred customer mailing list.
- Choose a supplier that is willing to assist your practice in setting up a sound inventory system.
- Do not commit to signing exclusive buying contracts or to making minimum annual supply orders. (Read all supply order contracts very carefully!)
- Order from more than one supplier.

Adapted from Taking stock: how to order, store, and maintain dental supplies. In *AGD Impact—Business Watch*, p 13, Oct. 1992.

notice is usually sent to the dentist to advise him or her of this situation.

If sufficient lead time has been allowed, a back order does not create a major problem. However, if the item is in critical supply, it may be necessary to purchase it elsewhere. In this case, to avoid duplication, the original order must be cancelled.

Order Exchange, Return, or Replacement

Sometimes it is necessary to exchange, return, or replace a product ordered. This may be due to a variety of factors, including

- Wrong item ordered
- Right item ordered, wrong item shipped
- Wrong size, color, or quantity
- Product broken or damaged in shipment

When there is a need to correct the supply order, the office manager must contact the supplier regarding the order and the reason for the exchange, replacement, or request for a credit on account. Until the supplier has made good on the request, a record should be maintained to trace and, if necessary, to follow up on the transaction.

The office manager should keep a record of all exchange, replacement, or refund items until the supplier has made good on the request.

Requisitions and Purchase Orders

In a large group practice, institution, or clinic with a central supply source, dental supplies are requisitioned. (A **requisition** is a formal request for supplies.)

The requisition form is usually completed in duplicate. One copy is submitted to procure the supplies, and the other is retained by the person requesting the supplies.

In institutions with central purchasing, a requisition may be submitted to the purchasing agent, who in turn issues a purchase order. A **purchase order** is a form authorizing the purchase of specific supplies from a specific supplier. These forms are numbered, and when an order is placed, the supplier may refer to the purchase order number.

The Dental Supply Budget

Institutions and well-organized practices operate on a budget. The budget request for dental supplies is based on how much was spent in the previous year and an estimate of the increased rate of use, plus consideration for inflation.

In many practices, the supply budget ranges between 6 and 10 percent of the office overhead expenses. When budgets are established, supplies and equipment are considered in the following terms.

Consumables and Disposables

Consumable supplies are those that are literally "used up" as part of their function: for example, restorative and impression materials.

Disposables are items that are used once and then discarded: for example, a disposable local anesthetic needle, a saliva ejector, and cotton rolls.

Expendables

Expendable items are materials that are relatively small in cost and that are used up in a short time. Minor dental instruments, such as mouth mirrors and burs, are examples of expendable items.

For budget purposes, expendable items may be classified as those items that cost less than a certain amount, such as $50, and are ordered regularly. In some institutions, consumable, disposable, and expendable items are classified together under the heading of expendables.

Nonexpendables

Nonexpendable items are smaller pieces of equipment or instruments that will eventually be replaced as the items wear out or are broken, such as a calculator or a curing light.

Major Equipment

The category includes larger pieces of equipment that are costly to purchase and will depreciate over a 5- to 10-year period. In the treatment area, these include items such as dental chairs, x-ray units, and the air compressor. In the business office, these might include the computer and printer.

Equipment Repairs

The breakdown of dental equipment can cause a major expense, loss of income, and inconvenience for both dentist and patient. The best way to control this situation is through a sound preventive maintenance program.

Equipment Records

When a new piece of equipment is purchased, the following information regarding that equipment should be entered on a service record:

- Date of purchase
- Name of supplier
- Expiration date of manufacturer's warranty
- Model and serial numbers

A **warranty** is a written statement outlining the manufacturer's responsibility for replacement and repair of a piece of equipment over a limited time. A warranty card, which registers this warranty with the manufacturer, is usually enclosed with the instruction manual. This should be completed and mailed promptly.

Instructions for use, care, and cleaning of the equipment should be filed systematically so that they are available for ready reference. The person responsible for the preventive maintenance of that piece of equipment should read the instructions and care manual thoroughly and add this item to the preventive maintenance schedule.

Service Contracts

Some dental equipment is protected under a service contract. Under the terms of this contract, emergency repairs and possibly some routine maintenance are provided on a fixed fee basis. An example would be a service contract for a computer system that guarantees emergency service within a specified period.

The Service Call

The cost of service calls is high because it must be based on mileage, time, expertise of the technician, and the materials and parts involved. Naturally, service calls should be avoided if possible. If the equipment does not work, check these points *before* calling for repair service:

1. Is the equipment properly plugged in and turned on?
2. Did you check the equipment for a blown fuse?
3. Is there a *reset* button that must be pushed?
4. Did someone check the fuse box or circuit breaker to see that the electrical circuit is functioning properly?

If, after you have checked all of these, you must still call for service, be prepared to give complete information so that the service technician may make best use of his or her time and to help avoid the necessity of making a second trip. The information needed includes

- The brand name of the piece of equipment
- The model number and approximate age or year of installation
- A brief description of the problem

Disbursements

The effective management of a dental practice requires organized handling and prompt payment of all bills for practice-related expenses.

The payment of major expenses should be made by check, with records kept up to date and balanced at all times. Minor expenses are handled through petty cash. All expenses should be documented as completely as possible with bills and receipts or canceled checks.

Packing Slips, Invoices, and Statements

A **packing slip** is an itemized listing of the goods shipped that is enclosed with the delivery. However, it does not contain price information, and an invoice or statement is sent separately.

When materials are received, they should be carefully checked against the packing slip to ensure that everything has been received as ordered and is in safe condition. Discrepancies or damage should be reported immediately to the supplier.

An invoice may be included with the shipment or it may be mailed separately. An **invoice** is an itemized list of the goods shipped and usually specifies the prices and terms of the sale. In short, it is a bill. Once an invoice has been verified, unless other arrangements have been made, it should be paid promptly.

A **statement** is a monthly summary of all invoices (charges), payments, credits, and debits for the month.

Organizing Expenditure Records

Statements and invoices that have not yet been paid are placed in the **accounts payable folder**.

As part of the organization of expenditure records, expenses are classified into categories. These usually include groups such as professional supplies, laboratory fees, salaries, rent and upkeep, utilities, and business office supplies.

The category headings, which are determined by the dentist's preference, are used on file folders to store these expense records in an organized manner. At the end of the year, this expense documentation is removed and filed, in these same categories, with other business records for that year.

The same categories are used to organize disbursements in the check register and the budget purposes. If the practice has a computer system that handles disbursements, this information is entered by category and used when disbursements are made and records for the financial management of the practice are maintained.

Payment of Accounts

In the dental office, the accounts payable are routinely paid once or twice a month. Before writing checks to pay these accounts, the administrative assistant removes all invoices and statements from the accounts payable folder.

The statements and invoices are verified by checking the numbers and amounts of the invoices received from each supplier during that period against the monthly statement. It is also necessary to verify that all payments, credits, and returns have been properly entered. To facilitate the handling and storage of records, the invoices are stapled to the statement covering them.

The dentist should review and approve all bills before payment is made. Once these accounts have been approved for payment, the administrative assistant writes the necessary checks. As each statement is paid, the number of the check and the date that payment was made are noted on the statement.

Usually the administrative assistant writes the checks but does not sign them. Instead, the prepared checks are given to the dentist for his or her signature. The office manager, who has been given "limited power of attorney" by the dentist and has proper authorization on file with the bank, may sign checks.

Cash on Delivery

Sometimes goods are shipped C.O.D. **(cash on delivery)**. At the time of delivery, the person receiving the goods must pay the cost of the merchandise plus a C.O.D. handling fee.

Some delivery services handling C.O.D. merchandise accept a check for the exact amount. Others insist on cash. If a check is acceptable, it should be made out to the supplier and not to the delivery service.

The administrative assistant should never accept a C.O.D. package unless it is something that has been ordered and is expected. When paying a C.O.D., the administrative assistant should insist upon a signed receipt for the payment.

Petty Cash

A petty cash fund is kept to meet frequent small expenses, such as postage due, for which cash is needed. The amount in the fund should be large enough to last about a month but not sufficiently large to invite theft.

In most offices, this amount is no more than $50. If more than this is needed within a month, it is likely that the concept of petty cash is being abused.

A **petty cash voucher** must be submitted for all payments made from the fund. Each voucher must include the date, the amount spent, to whom paid, what it was spent for, and who spent it. A receipt should be attached to each voucher.

REPLENISHING PETTY CASH FUNDS

Petty cash should be balanced and replenished on a regular basis, usually at the beginning of the month. Because there is a voucher for each petty cash payment, the sum of all the vouchers plus the cash on hand should always equal the total amount of the petty cash fund.

When these have been balanced, a check is written to refill the fund. If the fund is balanced, the check (which will return the fund to its original amount) should be for a sum equal to that of the vouchers for that month.

The vouchers and attached receipts are stapled together, and the date and total are noted. These are then filed under the "Business Office" expense category.

Writing Checks

CHECK WRITING SYSTEMS

Computerized Check Writing. Some practices have check writing capabilities on their computer systems.

The advantages of computerized check writing are time saving, reduced possibility of error, and ease of storage and retrieval of specific information.

Pegboard Check Writing. Other practices use a manual pegboard check writing system. Like pegboard accounting, it is a *one-write* system in which writing the check and the check register are completed information in a single entry. This saves steps and eliminates the possibility of error in posting this information.

The pegboard check register also has disbursements columns for all of the expenses categories, and posting each expense to the proper category is easily accomplished at the time the check is written.

Smaller practices may use checks that require separate entries to complete the check, the check register, and the expense category record.

No matter what type of system is used, the basic procedures remain the same.

THE TERMINOLOGY OF CHECKS

A **check** is a draft, or an order, upon a specific bank account for payment of a certain sum of money to the payee or to the bearer (Fig. 35–4).

Payment is on demand; that is, when the check is presented to the bank, that amount of money must be paid—provided, of course, that there are sufficient funds in the account to cover the amount of the check.

The **payee** is the person named on the check as the intended recipient of the amount shown. The payee's name is written after the words "Pay to the order of." The name of the payee should be written out in full; however, titles such as Mr. or Mrs. are best omitted. It is preferable to make a check out to "Mary Jones" rather than to "Mrs. John Jones."

The **maker** of the check is the one from whose account the amount of the check will be withdrawn. The maker of the check, or his authorized agent, must sign the check on the signature line.

The **check register** is a record of all checks issued and deposits made to the account. The check register entry should be made *before* the check is written. It should include

- The date (a check should be dated for the day it is written and never be predated or postdated)
- The number of the check
- The name of the payee
- The amount and purpose of the check

Whether a manual or computerized system is used to process check writing, the utmost care should be taken in stating the amount of the check in both figures and words and in making certain that the amount stated agrees in the following three places:

1. On the check register
2. In numbers on the right side of the check close to the dollar sign
3. Written out in words on the line before the word *dollars;* the number of cents is usually written as a fraction so that there can be no mistake about the placement of the decimal point

Checks that are written carelessly or with conflicting numbers can be raised or otherwise altered. A **raised check** is one on which extra numbers have been added, perhaps changing the check from $100.00 to $1000.00. Having the amount listed in both words and numbers is one way of safeguarding against this.

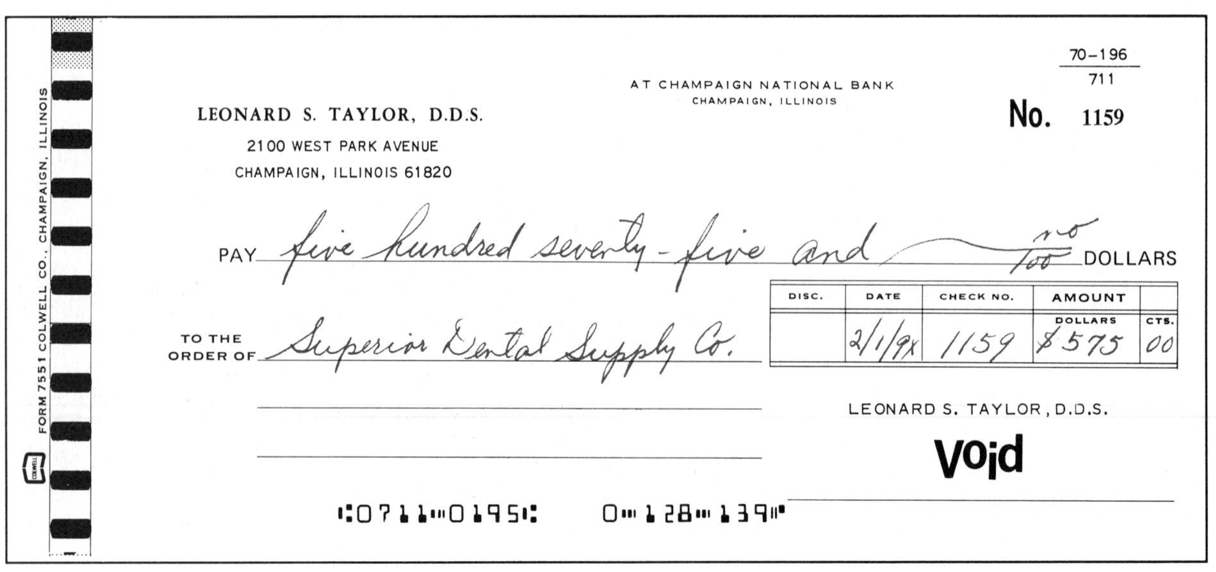

FORM 7551 COLWELL CO., CHAMPAIGN, ILLINOIS

AT CHAMPAIGN NATIONAL BANK
CHAMPAIGN, ILLINOIS

70–196
711

LEONARD S. TAYLOR, D.D.S.
2100 WEST PARK AVENUE
CHAMPAIGN, ILLINOIS 61820

No. 1159

PAY five hundred seventy-five and no/100 DOLLARS

DISC.	DATE	CHECK NO.	AMOUNT DOLLARS	CTS.
	2/1/9x	1159	$575	00

TO THE ORDER OF Superior Dental Supply Co.

LEONARD S. TAYLOR, D.D.S.

Void

⑆0711⑈0195⑆ 0⑈128⑈139⑈

FIGURE 35–4

Sample pegboard check. One entry completes both check and check register. (Courtesy of Colwell Systems, Champaign, IL.)

PROCEDURE: **Writing Pegboard Checks**

1. Select the next available check number, and position the check over the check register.
2. Enter the date and the name of the payee.
3. Write the amount in numbers. Do not leave any blank spaces.
4. Starting at the extreme left of the space, write the amount in words. Draw a wavy line to fill in any blank spaces.
5. If a mistake is made in writing the check, write the word **void** through the check register entry and the check, and then write a new check. The voided check is usually retained with practice records so that it is possible to account for every check number.
6. When the check is complete, also note the amount in the appropriate expense column.

Check Endorsement

Before the payee can receive the cash for his check, he must endorse (sign) it. Endorsement is made on the back, left end, of the check and must match the name shown on the face of the check.

A check signed in this manner has a **blanket endorsement** (is ready to be cashed), and anyone holding that check may cash it (including someone who may have stolen it).

With a **restrictive endorsement,** which may read, "For deposit only to the account of (*the name of the payee*)," the check can only be deposited to the account of that individual. This type of endorsement makes the check **nonnegotiable;** that is, it can be deposited only to that account and, if stolen, cannot be cashed.

A rubber stamp with the appropriate restrictive phrase, and the payee's name, may be used in place of the payee's signature. As a safeguard, such a restrictive endorsement should be placed on all checks as soon as they are received.

Stop Payment Order

If the maker of a check wishes to stop payment of a check he has written, he may request that the bank issue a stop payment order for that check.

The stop payment order must give all the necessary information such as the number of the check, date issued, name of payee, amount of the check, and the reason for stopping payment.

The written stop payment order must reach the bank bookkeeper before the check is presented for payment. These orders are usually in force for 90 days, and the bank makes a charge for this service.

Nonsufficient Funds

A check written for more than the amount in the maker's account will be refused when presented for payment. The check will then be returned to the payee marked N.S.F.

This means there is not enough money in the account to cover the check, and the payee cannot collect any of the amount due him. A check that has been returned for this reason is known as a **returned item;** however, it is commonly referred to as having "bounced"—that is, come back.

The bank makes a charge against the account of the person having written an N.S.F. check; however, there is not usually a charge to the person who received the check.

When a check from a patient is returned, the amount of that check must be "charged back" against the patient's account. Do this by making an entry in the account history (or on the ledger card), noting the date the check was returned. Then make an adjustment that acts like a charge and increases the account balance by the amount of the returned check.

It is also necessary to make a check register entry. Here the amount of the returned check is subtracted from the checking account balance.

Frequently, a telephone call to the maker will resolve the problem, and the check may be redeposited.

A check that must be redeposited should be listed on a separate deposit slip and clearly marked so that it is not credited twice to income.

When the check is redeposited, this should be noted on the account history and the amount of the check should again be subtracted from the balance.

If a returned check cannot be redeposited, there is now an outstanding balance on the account that requires immediate attention.

Reconciling a Bank Statement

A **bank statement** is a record issued by the bank showing all transactions for that account during the period covered. The statement includes the beginning and closing balances plus a record of deposits, canceled checks, and debits against the account through the closing date.

Deposits are those amounts put into the bank and credited to the account. **Deposits in transit** are those deposits that have been made but are not yet credited to the account at the time of the statement.

The term **canceled checks** refers to those checks enclosed in the envelope with the statement. An **outstanding check** is one that has been written but that has not been paid by the bank at the time the statement was prepared.

Debits are items other than canceled checks that have been deducted directly from the account. They include the bank service charge, returned items, or other charges. **Credits** are items such as deposits and earned interest that have been added to the account.

The statement and checkbook should be reconciled (balanced) promptly upon receipt of the statement. The balance as per the check register *must* agree with the bank balance adjusted through these calculations. Errors must be found and corrected. Any bank error must be reported immediately to the bank.

A worksheet form is usually provided on the back of the bank statement. This form may be used to perform the necessary calculations. Before you begin, the check register balance should be current.

IF THE ACCOUNT DOES NOT BALANCE

If the account does not balance, the following is a checklist of points to be reviewed in looking for the error:

PROCEDURE: **Reconciling a Bank Statement**

1. Examine the debit items and canceled checks against those listed on the statement.
   □ *RATIONALE:* There should be a canceled check, or an explained debit item, for each charge listed on the statement.
2. Arrange canceled checks in numerical order, and compare these checks against the check register. Ensure that the amount of the check is the same as that shown on the check register. Place a check mark against the number of each canceled check.
3. Circle the number of each outstanding check and list that check on the worksheet by number and amount.
4. Enter all debits, and their explanations, on the check register. Subtract these charges from the balance. If the account earned interest, enter this in the deposit column.
5. Verify the practice record of deposits made against those listed on the bank statement. If necessary, note and make appropriate adjustments for any corrections in deposits.
6. Note any deposits in transit, and list them on the worksheet by date and amount.
7. Update the account balance, and perform the necessary calculations on the worksheet.
   □ *RATIONALE:* After these calculations, the balance on the check register should match the amount of the bank statement.
8. Place the canceled checks and bank statement together and store them for safekeeping.
   □ *RATIONALE:* These are valuable records and should be maintained in good order and protected with other important records.

NAME Patricia Andrews, CDA	Soc. Sec. Number 123-45-6789			Record of Pay Rate Changes	
				DATE	RATE
STREET 305 Oak Drive	Phone Number 933-0111	No. of Exempt. 1		7/1/9X	9.00
				1/1/9X	10.00
CITY Centerville, NJ 08511	Date Started 7/1/9X Date Left	M	F X		

DATE	HOURS reg	HOURS over	GROSS AMOUNT	DEDUCTIONS Social Sec.	Fed. Inc. Tax	State Inc. Tax				NET AMOUNT
1/8/9X	40		400.00	33.20	40.00	8.50				381.30
1/15/9X	40		400.00	33.20	40.00	8.50				381.30
1/22/9X	40		400.00	33.20	40.00	8.50				381.30
1/29/9X	40		400.00	33.20	40.00	8.50				381.30
GROSS EARNINGS							NET EARNINGS			
JANUARY TOTALS			1600.00	132.80	160.00	34.00				1273.20
	EMPLOYER MAKES MATCHING CONTRIBUTION									

FIGURE 35–5

Sample payroll record form. These hypothetical earnings are included here only to show how deductions are subtracted from gross income. (Courtesy of Colwell Systems, Champaign, IL.)

- Have you correctly entered the amount of each check on your check register?
- Are the amounts of your deposits entered in the check register the same as shown on your bank statement?
- Have all checks written been entered in the check register?
- Have all checks been deducted (subtracted) accurately from the check register?
- Have you reviewed all addition and subtraction in your check register?
- Have you performed all worksheet calculations correctly?

Business Summaries

All checks must be accounted for in a specific expense category. With a computerized system, posting to the appropriate category is part of the check writing process. With pegboard check writing, expenses are posted into categories at the time the check is written. With other manual systems, the expense information is transferred from the check register into the expense categories. This is usually done once a month to create a monthly summary.

Totals from monthly summaries are carried forward to an annual summary. Through the keeping of these records, the dentist and the accountant can at any time quickly tell what the practice expenses have been to date. This is important information for management, budgeting, and tax purposes.

Payroll

Federal regulations require that an employer make certain deductions from an employee's pay and that the employer also pay certain payroll taxes. These federal requirements are explained in the **Circular E** booklet issued by the Internal Revenue Service. Most states also publish similar booklets explaining the requirements within those states.

The administrative assistant who is responsible for handling payroll should study these booklets carefully and ask questions about any point that is not clear. It is better to ask questions first than to make an expensive mistake that can be corrected only with great difficulty.

The government requires that each employer keep records of the hours worked, the amount paid, and the amounts deducted for tax purposes. Complete and accurate employee records must be kept at all times, and back records should be stored with other important financial papers. A separate payroll sheet should be maintained for each employee (Fig. 35–5). The headings of this form show the employee's full name (spelled correctly), social security number, address, and number of exemptions claimed.

The gross (total pretax) pay for each pay period is entered on this form, as are each of the deductions and the net pay (gross pay minus all deductions).

Net pay plus deductions must equal the earned gross pay. A withholding statement must be included with each payroll check. This provides the employee information as to the gross pay and the amount and reason for each deduction.

Payroll Deductions

INCOME TAX WITHHOLDING

All employees must file a federal income tax return before April 15 of each year. A portion of the estimated tax is withheld directly from each paycheck during the year.

The amount withheld by the end of the year is supposed to approximate the annual tax that the employee will owe. Amounts withheld are determined from a schedule in Circular E. These are based on earnings and the number of exemptions claimed. It is the responsibility of the employer to withhold this tax and to remit it to an authorized bank or directly to the Internal Revenue Service.

Each employee must complete an **employee's withholding exemption certificate** (W-4 form): (1) upon beginning of employment; (2) within 10 days of any change of status (such as marriage); and (3) before December 1, for the following year.

This form authorizes the employer to deduct the tax and indicates the number of exemptions that the employee is claiming. These completed forms must be kept with other payroll records.

FICA

Under the **Federal Insurance Contributions Act** (FICA), commonly known as *social security*, the employer is required to deduct a certain percentage of the employee's gross pay. This is a fixed amount regardless of the number of exemptions.

The employer is also required to make a matching contribution. Thus for each FICA dollar withheld from the employee's wages, the employer also contributes a dollar. Both contributions are forwarded quarterly to the federal government to be credited to the employee's account.

So that FICA earnings may be properly credited, it is important to keep the Social Security Administration informed of any change of name. Also, at least once every 3 years, the employee should request a *Statement of Earnings* from the Social Security Administration.

This is a written record of the amount "credited" to the employee's account. Should there be an error here, it must be reported and corrected within 3 years of the time that the error is made.

OTHER DEDUCTIONS

Additional federal, state, and local taxes may also be withheld from the employee's pay. The person in charge of payroll computations is responsible for having current information about the regulations governing these deductions.

Personal deductions, such as the employee's contribution to health or life insurance coverage, an automatic personal savings plan, or pretax retirement contributions, may also be taken directly from the employee's earnings.

The employer must pay additional payroll taxes such as **Workers' Compensation, Federal Unemployment Taxes** (FUTA), and **State Unemployment Insurance** (SUI). These amounts *are not* deducted from the employee's earnings, except in those states where a portion of the SUI tax is paid by the employee.

Remittance to the Government

All government reports must be completed accurately and neatly (preferably typewritten or computer-generated) and filed *on time*. Stiff penalties are issued for late reports.

All employers are required to file an "Employer's Quarterly Federal Tax Return." This is a report of all taxable wages paid during the quarter. Withheld taxes and FICA contributions must be deposited regularly; the frequency of these deposits depends upon the total amount owed.

Within 30 days of the end of the calendar year, or upon termination of employment, the employee must be furnished with a statement of total earnings and taxes withheld for that year (W-2 form).

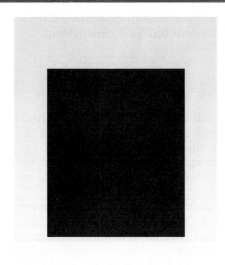

Chapter 36

Employment

Introduction

As you complete your dental assistant education, you naturally think about securing employment. However, before you can actively begin to job hunt, you should begin to plan the best employment situation for *you.* There are three factors to consider:

1. You want to feel physically, psychologically, and socially comfortable in your work environment. You must also be able to work well with everyone on the dental health team.
2. You want to select an employer whom you respect and whose philosophy of practice parallels your beliefs.
3. You also want to find the type of employment situation that will be the most stimulating, interesting, and rewarding for you—one that will provide professional and personal growth.

The decision about what employment situation would be best for you should be based on these general considerations: What do you have to offer? And what are you looking for?

What Do You Have to Offer?

You have many resources to offer a potential employer. One of the most important is *yourself* as an educationally qualified assistant. You should also have a neat and professional appearance and a pleasant professional attitude that will reflect positively both on yourself and on your employer. In addition, you should have enthusiasm for your profession, a willingness to learn, and the ability to work well with others.

What Are You Looking For?

What type of employment situation would be best for you? Given your training and the many roles open within dental assisting, you have a wide range of choices as to the situation in which to utilize your skills. (Refer to Chapter 1 for additional information on specific types of employment in dentistry.)

Types of Dental Practices

General (Solo) Practice

Of the approximately 130,000 dentists in the United States, the majority are in solo private practices. These practitioners provide a wide range of professional services for their patients. A solo practitioner may employ one or more assistants and a hygienist. The practice may also employ additional dentists as associates. (An associate is hired under a contractual agreement.)

Partnerships and Shared Expenses

A **partnership** is a legal arrangement between two or more persons. Partners have equal rights and duties. Each dentist in the partnership is legally liable for the indebtedness incurred by the partners; however, each dentist is responsible for any malpractice that he or she or employees of the partnership have committed.

Partnerships often grow out of **associateships**, in which a "junior dentist" (often recently graduated and licensed) works in the practice on a contractual arrangement for a specified time. After this introductory period, an associate may become a partner in the practice.

In an **expense-sharing relationship**, two or more dentists share the expenses of a shared facility. Each dentist maintains a solo practice as a legal entity and usually has employees of that practice. Sometimes the salary of one employee, such as a receptionist, is a shared expense.

Specialty Dental Practice

A specialty practice enables the assistant to use basic skills plus additional ones required for employment in that specialty. (See Chapter 1.) Like general practice, a specialty practice may consist of an individual dentist or of two or more dentists working together.

Group Practice

A group practice may be composed of almost any number and variety of general practitioners and specialists working together in a shared facility. The benefits of being employed in a larger group include

- Opportunities to develop more specialized skills
- Professional stimulation and sociability of working with many other auxiliaries
- Greater opportunity for advancement
- Potential for a more extensive program of employee benefits than can be offered by a solo practitioner

Professional Corporations

A solo practitioner or a group may form a **professional corporation** (PC) or **professional association** (PA). By law, this status must be identified on all practice letterheads and other printed materials. This will appear as "PC" or "PA" after the name of the dentist or group.

In an incorporated practice, the dentist or dentists become employees of the corporation. As employees, they draw a salary and receive benefits, just as the other employees do. Likewise, they are also subject to Occupational Safety and Health Administration–(OSHA-) required protective measures.

Most professional corporations offer a retirement plan that becomes available to employees after a certain number of years of full-time employment.

Public Health/Government Clinic

Public health and other government-supported dental clinics function at the federal, state, and county levels. Dental auxiliaries may be employed in programs in which dental services are provided at no cost or minimal cost to patients who are eligible to receive care.

These settings sometimes also collect data and report statistics on specific public health issues and services, such as fluoridation, acquired immunodeficiency syndrome (AIDS) incidence, and care for the elderly or specific population groups, including American Indians and migrant workers.

Military Dental Services

Some military installations and veterans' hospitals employ civilian dental auxiliaries under the Civil Service Act. An assistant interested in working in such a position should contact the area Civil Service office to determine when and where the appropriate pre-employment examinations are given.

Dental Schools

Educationally qualified and experienced dental assistants are employed by dental schools to work in clinical settings to provide the dental students with experience in four-handed dentistry.

Employment here provides the assistant with the stimulation of working in an educational setting with faculty, students, and patients.

Teaching Programs

Employment as an **instructor** in an accredited dental assisting program is a challenging and rewarding career option for the ambitious dental assistant. Each school and state has requirements for teacher certification. These vary and may include prescribed college courses in educational methodology, at least a bachelor's degree, and certification or registration as a dental assistant.

An assistant who might enjoy teaching could continue to take college courses in related sciences and teacher training on a part-time basis while simultaneously gaining valuable work experience in the dental office.

The Job Search

Accessing Employment Opportunities

Once you have determined the type of employment situation that would be best for you, the next step is to secure such a position. Information about opportunities comes from many sources.

NEWSPAPER CLASSIFIED ADVERTISEMENTS

Newspaper classified advertisements are an excellent job source. Frequently dentists place advertisements describing the position open and listing a box number rather than a telephone number. This is done for two reasons: first, to protect the office routine from being disrupted by phone calls of inquiry and, second, to give the dentist an opportunity to screen the letters of application before contacting any of the applicants for an interview.

TELEPHONE DIRECTORY PAGES

A sometimes overlooked source for potential employment as a dental assistant is the "business" or "yellow" pages of the telephone directory. Here there are listings of dentists in general and specialty practices. By reviewing this information, you can determine the number of dentists and scope of employment potential within the area.

CAMPUS PLACEMENT SERVICES

If you are attending a formal dental assisting training program, the school probably offers a placement service, and area dentists frequently call the school first when they need an assistant. Long after you have graduated, it is usually possible for you to continue to use the school placement service as a source of employment referral.

EMPLOYMENT AGENCIES

Federal and state governments provide Human Resources Development services and employment opportunity information free of charge.

Private employment agencies charge a fee if they find you a position. You are responsible for paying this fee unless, by special prearrangement, your new employer agrees to pay it. In some cases, you may make an agreement with the employer to split the fee.

DENTAL SUPPLY HOUSES

The sales representatives who call on dental offices in the area frequently know when a dentist is looking for a qualified assistant. When seeking employment, let the salesperson know that you are looking and the type of employment you prefer.

PROFESSIONAL ORGANIZATIONS

Your local dental assistants' society and the local dental society frequently serve as informal employment information centers. Many local dental societies publish monthly news bulletins in which it may be possible to place a classified advertisement at minimal expense.

The First Contact

TELEPHONE

If the advertisement includes a telephone number, your first contact should be by telephone. When you call, identify yourself and your reasons for calling.

The first impression over the telephone is an all-important one, because if you do not make a good impression here, you may not get a second chance to prove yourself in an interview.

It is unlikely that you will be able to speak to the dentist at this time; however, the administrative assistant or office manager usually handles calls of inquiry and sets up an interview appointment. You may be asked to submit a completed application or a résumé before the interview.

LETTER OF APPLICATION

Most frequently, initial contact is made through a letter of application, and the appearance and content of your letter create that all-important first impression of you (Fig. 36–1). Your letter should be brief, business-like, well written, and neatly typed on white paper. If you generate the letter on a computer, use a printer that produces professional-looking output.

Do not include personal information in the letter because this is contained in your résumé, which should be enclosed with your letter of application. However, you may want to include in the letter just enough information to create interest—for example, that you are a certified dental assistant.

RÉSUMÉ

A résumé is a neatly organized statement of pertinent personal and professional information about you. A good résumé goes a long way in helping you make a good impression (Fig. 36–2).

Like your letter of application, your résumé should be typed and well organized to create an impression of neatness and orderliness. A sloppy résumé that contains careless erasures and misspelled words is inexcusable and may instantly rule out your chances for a position in the practice.

Space can be used to isolate important points to which you want to draw attention. Also, sufficient spacing between all elements helps to create a clean, inviting impression. Information to be included is as follows:

Mary Jones, CDA
212 Pleasant Drive
Midville, US 27740

June 16, 19XX

Box 782
Area Tribune
Midville, US 27740

Dear Doctor:

In response to your advertisement in the June 15th Area Tribune, I would like to apply for the position of chairside assistant in your dental practice.

I am a Certified Dental Assistant and a graduate of the Area Accredited School of Dental Assisting. Enclosed is a copy of my resume, which provides additional information about my background and experience in the dental field.

I would appreciate the opportunity to schedule an interview with you and your staff at a time of your convenience. I can be reached at 965-1255 every day after 5:00 P.M. Thank you for your consideration.

Sincerely,

Mary Jones, CDA

Mary Jones, CDA

Enc.

FIGURE 36–1

Sample letter of application.

Your Personal Directory. This is a simple listing of your name, address, and telephone number.

Your Employment Objective. State clearly your job objective. For example, "To work as a chairside assistant in either a general dentistry or a pediatric dental practice."

It is important that you be clear regarding your employment objective (the kind of job you want); however, an objective that is too specific may limit your job opportunities.

Work Experience. Dates should be given along with the company address and a brief description of your work. Your job listing should be in reverse order, beginning with the most recent job you held.

Education. Usually only schools from which you have graduated and dates of graduation are listed; for example, high school and dental assisting school. If you took special courses that may be of interest to your potential employer, however, you may want to make note of them on your résumé.

Other Activities and Special Honors. If you are active as a volunteer in community and school organizations or have received special honors that may relate to your potential as an employee, you may include them

Mary Jones, CDA
212 Pleasant Drive
Midville, US 27740

Employment Objective:
- Chairside assistant in either a pediatric or general dental practice.

Work Experience:
- Student intern in the practice of Dr. Janice Davison.
- Part-time employment as a chairside assistant with Dr. Davison from March 19XX to the present.
- Circulating assistant for Dr. Harold Randolph during the summer of 19XX.

Education:
- Area Accredited School of Dental Assisting, Sept. 19XX–June 19XX. Graduated on the Dean's List.
- Midville High School, 19XX–19XX.

Other Activities:
- Currently Certified Dental Assistant.
- Have applied to be a Registered Dental Assistant.
- Treasurer of local Dental Assistants Society.

Additional Resources:
- Currently American Heart Association–certified in CPR.
- Excellent public speaking skills.

References:
- References and additional information available upon request.

FIGURE 36–2

Sample résumé.

in a special category, or you may list them with the appropriate groups. For example, school honors and achievement awards could be listed with education.

Personal Data. This section includes your present address and telephone number, as well as your social security number. By law you are *not* required to give your race, religion, date of birth, marital status, number of children, gender (if name is ambiguous), existing disabilities, or state of health.

Under **Federal Equal Employment Opportunity (EEO) regulations,** employers may *not* ask questions regarding race, color, religion, gender, national origin, marital status, and child care arrangements, unless they relate to **bona fide occupational qualifications** (BFOQ). However, you may be required to submit verification of citizenship or appropriate alien status.

If you are under 19, age may be a BFOQ question because of certain occupational hazards such as exposure to radiation. Although you are not required to supply this information, you may do so voluntarily.

Omit References. Instead of listing references, note "References and further data available on request." (You should be prepared to supply these to an interested employer at the time of your interview.)

References related to your work experience are preferred to those of social acquaintances. Relatives are never used as references. A former employer and/or an instructor from your dental assisting program may be included if he or she knows you well. It is courteous to receive a person's permission before using his or her name as a reference.

Resources. Some job candidates choose to include a

section, space permitting, that lists resources of interest to a prospective employer, such as "nonsmoker" or "good problem solver."

The Interview

The employment interview is an all-important exchange of information and impressions. This is when you gather information to help you determine whether you would be happy working for this dentist, with this staff, and in this practice. At the same time, the dentist is trying to determine whether you are the right employee for this position.

If you do not send a letter of application, take an extra copy of your résumé along when you go to the interview, and leave it with the interviewer.

APPEARANCE AND PREPARATION

Your appearance is very important. In selecting your clothes, remember that you are looking for employment, not going to a ball game or a party. You want your appearance to reflect the fact that you are a neat, well-organized, and competent professional.

Do not wear your dental assisting uniform to an interview. It is best to wear conservative business attire. Keep jewelry to a minimum; however, a wedding band or engagement ring and a watch are acceptable.

PRESENT YOURSELF PROFESSIONALLY

You should plan to arrive 10 to 15 minutes before the scheduled time of the interview. This will give you plenty of time to find a parking place and freshen up before the first contact. If the interview is scheduled in a geographic area with which you are unfamiliar, it is advisable to take a "dry run" to find the office before the interview.

WHAT IS DISCUSSED DURING THE INTERVIEW

The first 10 minutes of your interview are the most critical, because in this time both you and the interviewer will have formed your first impressions. You will probably be nervous, but try to relax and be natural.

A *warm handshake* and *good eye contact* are essential to create a positive and professional impression (Fig. 36–3). Many questions will be asked and answered on both sides. However, first you may be asked to complete an application form. This will serve as the initial basis of your conversation with the interviewer.

In completing this form, be sure that you *follow directions exactly* and that the information you give is accurate, complete, and neat. You may also be requested to take a standard pencil and paper personnel test or some form of manual dexterity test. Again, remain calm and *follow directions exactly.*

The interviewer will have many questions for you. Try to answer all of them courteously, completely, and honestly. Remember that your attitude and motivation during the interview are an important determining factor. You want to convey a positive attitude without overselling yourself.

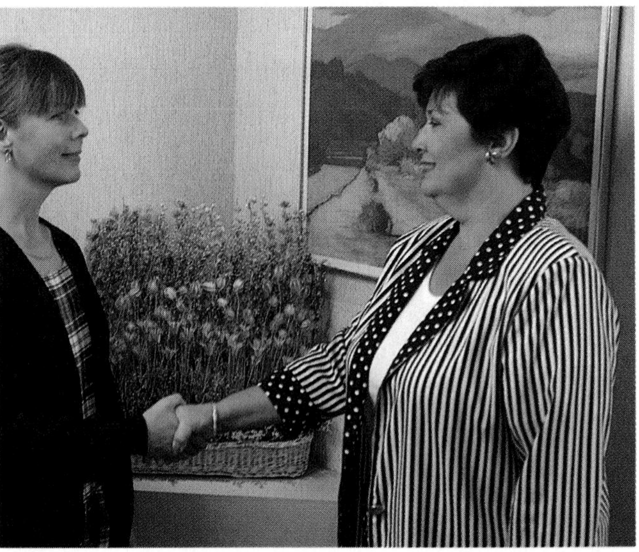

FIGURE 36–3

A warm handshake and good eye contact are essential for creating a positive and professional impression.

You must also be prepared for surprise questions such as "What can I do for you?" or "Tell me about yourself." Feel free to ask questions and, if it seems to be a convenient time, ask to be shown around the office and to meet the other staff members.

Usually the last item to be discussed is "What do you expect in terms of salary and benefits?" If you have a definite and realistic idea, by all means state it. If you are uncertain, however, you may phrase your response along the lines of, "To be fair to everybody, it is open to negotiation," and then wait for an offer to be made.

Although salary should not be the first question in your mind, it is an important factor and should be discussed openly. This is also an excellent opportunity to ask about frequency of reviews, increases, and opportunity to advance with the practice.

AFTER THE INTERVIEW

Let the prospective employer (or office manager) conclude the interview. Do not assume that the interview is over, simply because of a temporary lapse in conversation.

If you feel the interview has concluded, you could say, "Do you have any other questions you'd like to ask at this time?" Usually the interviewer stands up to signal the conclusion of the interview. Make sure to extend your hand for a final handshake and maintain good eye contact when dismissing yourself.

Within the first week after the interview, you will have developed some intuition of how the interview went, as well as whether the office is one in which you would like to pursue employment.

Good business etiquette practice encourages the writing of a follow-up thank-you letter to the interviewer. Make sure that in closing the letter, you restate your desire for employment in the practice and where you can be reached should any additional information be requested (Fig. 36–4).

The Employment Agreement

Before you accept a position, there are several topics that you and the dentist, or office manager, need to explore. These should be organized into a written employment agreement (Fig. 36–5).

An employment agreement is a written document, prepared in duplicate and signed by both employer and employee. One copy is retained in the personnel file, and the other is given to the employee for his or her records.

Reaching a clear understanding of the following topics is important, for it can prevent later misunderstandings.

Duties and Responsibilities. You need to know exactly what your employment duties will be. The dentist or office manager should provide you with a written job description that includes a list of your specific responsibilities.

Working Hours. You need to know what hours and days of the week you are routinely expected to work. It is also important to know how far in advance these are scheduled and how overtime is handled.

Salary and Benefits. Although salary should have already been discussed, you also need to know what provisions are made for performance reviews, salary increases, and benefits.

Mary Jones, CDA
212 Pleasant Drive
Midville, US 27740

June 23, 19XX

Dr. A. Blank and Staff
123 Main Street
Midville, US 27740

Dear Dr. Blank and Staff:

Thank you for the opportunity to interview with you last Tuesday, June 15th. It was delightful to meet with you to discuss the position of chairside assistant.

I also enjoyed being shown around the office and was impressed with your efficient patient-flow system.

As we had discussed at the time of the interview, I am interested in the position and am available at 965-1255 if you have further questions. Again, it was a pleasure meeting you.

Sincerely,

Mary Jones, CDA

Mary Jones, CDA

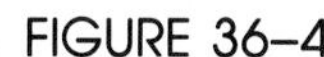

FIGURE 36–4

Sample interview follow-up letter.

EMPLOYMENT AGREEMENT
(Complete form in duplicate: one copy for the employer; one copy for the employee.)

EMPLOYEE'S NAME Debbie Quigley, CDA

Date 11/08/XX Full time/Part Time fulltime

JOB TITLE Chairside assistant to Dr. Hernandez
See attached list for details of duties and responsibilities:

PRACTICE WORK SCHEDULE
(Your hours will be scheduled within these times.)

Usual days per week: S ____ M ✓ T ✓ W 1/2 Th ✓ F ✓ S 1/2

Usual working hours : 8:30 to 5:30 ; lunch 1 hr ; breaks ____ .

Work schedules are posted: two weeks in advance. Assigned hours may vary

SALARY AND BENEFITS

Pay days: every other Friday Starting rate: $XX. per hour

Basis for increases: review at 6 months, then annually

Vacation days: 5 ; Sick days: 5 ; Personal time: 2 .

Additional benefits: group insurance is available
retirement plan after 3 years

TERMINATION

For each new employee, the first 6 weeks are a provisional period of employment.
During this time, the new employee may leave or be dismissed without notice.

After this period, the employee is expected to give 2 weeks notice.

If dismissed, the employee will receive 2 weeks notice or the equivalent in severance pay.

In the event of fraud, theft, illegal drug use, or unprofessional duct, the employee may be dismissed without notice or severance pay.

Debbie Quigley, CDA — Employee's signature

J. Hernandez, DDS — Employer's signature

FIGURE 36–5

Sample employment agreement.

Uniform Requirements. Personal protective equipment (PPE) required by OSHA must be provided and maintained by the employer. If there are other uniform requirements, you need to know who is responsible for supplying and maintaining uniforms and whether there is a uniform allowance.

Provisional Employment. Most employers routinely consider the first several weeks to 90 days as a provisional period during which either party may terminate the relationship without notice.

Continuing Education. Determine what continuing education is provided and who is expected to pay for it. Costs for registration and certification renewal, as well as payment of professional dues and publications, should also be addressed.

Termination. You should be aware of how much notice you are expected to give, or to receive, should you or the dentist terminate your employment after the provisional period.

The Americans with Disabilities Act

The Americans with Disabilities Act (ADA) was made law July 1992. While it is most commonly thought that this law applies to handicapped patients seeking access to public accommodations and health care, the act also applies to job applicants and current employees.

Title I of the Act specifically makes it illegal for the employer to discriminate against prospective job applicants on the basis of handicap or disability.

Under the law, the employer does not legally have to offer a position to the *most* qualified applicant—only to one who presents as qualified *to meet the requirements of the position.*

It also makes it illegal for the employer to discriminate against employees of the practice who *may become disabled.* If a dental staff member becomes disabled while in the employment of the dentist, the law requires that the employer make reasonable accommodation (take action within reason) to continue employment of that person at the same rate of pay. The dentist may not discharge an employee on the basis of disability without the employee's consent.

As of July 1994, this law applies to companies who employ at least 15 people and not to smaller businesses. Thus this law may very well not apply to the practice for which you work.

Maintaining Employment

Maintaining employment is a two-sided situation. There are responsibilities on the part of the employees. There are also responsibilities on the part of the dentist as the employer.

Before accepting employment, try to determine, through observation and by talking to other employees, whether the dentist does indeed carry out the responsibilities of an ethical employer. If it is apparent that the dentist does not, then perhaps you should seek employment elsewhere.

The Dental Assistant's Responsibilities

Following are some, but not necessarily all, of the responsibilities of the dental assistant as an employee of the practice:

- To be a motivated, punctual, cooperative, and responsible worker who performs regularly assigned duties cheerfully and competently and helps other team members as needed
- To be always neat and appropriately uniformed during working hours
- To be pleasant, respectful, and cooperative, yet professional, with *all* patients
- To be able to accept and act upon constructive criticism, and to continually upgrade and update professional skills and knowledge through continuing education
- To maintain high personal, professional, and ethical standards

The Dentist's Responsibilities

Following are some, but not necessarily all, of the dentist's responsibilities as an employer:

- To establish and maintain fair employee policies and practices (these should be in a written format in an office procedures manual available to all employees)
- To treat all employees with professional and personal dignity and respect
- To organize and maintain the practice to provide safe, pleasant working conditions for all
- To encourage employees to give their best performances through praise, encouragement, and other more tangible indications that their efforts have been noticed and appreciated

Physical Well-Being

Physical well-being that comes from proper nutrition, regular exercise, and sufficient rest is an important part of maintaining employment.

General Health

Good nutrition, which involves eating the proper food in the proper quantities, is the basis of good general health (see Chapter 6).

Exercise is an important key to physical and mental well-being. Although you are active at work, you should also engage regularly in a pleasurable form of general exercise such as walking, yoga, jogging, swimming, or participating in sports.

Lack of adequate rest can adversely affect your health and your work. Therefore, it is important to get *sufficient* sleep on a *regular* basis. For most people, this means between 6 and 8 hours of sleep every night.

You should take all the necessary preventive care steps to preserve your physical well-being. This includes keeping your immunizations up to date.

Dental Health

A dental assistant's smile is an ambassador of the practice in which he or she works. The first thing patients may notice about you is your smile.

Therefore, your dental health is particularly important. You must believe in, and carry through, a good program of preventive dental care, which includes having regular dental examinations and completing of any necessary treatment.

Personal and Professional Grooming

As a healthcare professional, you are expected to be a role model of health consciousness as a reflection of your position in the practice. Your first impression with patients casts a high-impact reflection upon the quality of care provided in your practice.

Skin Care and Hair Style

Healthy skin is an important barrier against infection. Proper diet, adequate exercise, and a skin care program, such as the use of protective hand lotion, all aid in maintaining healthy skin.

A suitable hairstyle that is professional in appearance is one that is neat, clean, and easily controlled so it does not fall in your face or the patient's. In many practices, surgical type head covering is worn as part of personal protective equipment to prevent cross-contamination through touching or fussing with hair.

Professional Uniforms and Business-Like Appearance

Clinical personnel do not wear their uniforms out of the office. Instead, street clothes should be worn to the office and when leaving the office for lunch or at the end of the work day. OSHA regulations for protective garb are discussed in Chapters 12 and 13.

For nonclinical personnel, such as the administrative assistant, the dentist may make recommendations regarding clothing to be worn to achieve a business-like appearance. If a specific style is required, the dentist may give an annual uniform allowance or supply the uniform.

For all personnel, the uniform selected should be comfortable without being baggy or sloppy. It should allow for adequate body motion without binding or restricting, yet maintain appropriate modesty when you are sitting or standing.

Because you will be on your feet a lot, well-fitted shoes that offer adequate support are essential. Lightweight support hose are also helpful in preventing aching legs.

Fingernails must be kept short and clean. No nail polish, other than clear, should be worn.

The Legal Aspects of Sexual Harassment

In 1980 the **Equal Employment Opportunity Commission** (EEOC) published its official definition of sexual harassment in the workplace as "Unwelcome sexual advances, requests for sexual favors, and other verbal or physical conduct of a sexual nature, when: submission to such conduct is made either explicitly or implicitly a term or condition of an individual's employment; submission to or rejection of such conduct is used as the basis for decisions affecting an individual's employment status; such conduct has the purpose or effect of substantially interfering with an individual's performance on the job."

This definition has served as a baseline for litigation involving sexual harassment. Because the minimum number of employees in the practice may have a bearing on sexual harassment guideline enforcement, it is wise to check with the local EEOC office for interpretation.

Avoiding Sexual Harassment

The dental assistant who may find himself or herself the object of unwanted or unwelcome sexual advances in the practice may take a number of steps.

1. Inform the perpetrator that advances or remarks of a sexual nature are unwanted and will not be tolerated.
2. Ensure that another person is always present when the alleged perpetrator is in the same room.
3. *Optional:* If repeated advances are made, leave the employment situation and file a complaint with the local branch of the EEOC.

Termination

If it becomes necessary to terminate employment, it should be done in keeping with the terms of the employment agreement. If leaving under friendly conditions, the assistant should give adequate notice and may help to select and train a replacement.

If leaving under other circumstances, the assistant may be asked to leave immediately. Unless specified in an employment agreement, the dentist is not required to provide severance pay.

Summary Dismissal

Summary dismissal is termination without notice or severance pay. The causes for summary dismissal include stealing, use of drugs, and any other form of unprofessional behavior.

Employment laws now make provision for **unlawful discharge** (firing for unjust cause), for which an employer may be taken to court for dismissing an employee without **due cause** (probable or justifiable reason).

To avoid potential legal entanglements later on, both the assistant and the employer should keep written documentation of job performance evaluations.

Glossary

Abandonment: Discontinuation of care after treatment has commenced but before it has been completed.

Abrasion: Pathological wearing away of dental hard tissue by friction.

Abrasive agent: A substance used to remove stain and to polish natural teeth, prosthetic appliances, restorations, and castings.

Abscess, periapical: A localized area of pus formed at the apex of the root tip.

Abscess, periodontal: A localized area of pus formed in periodontal tissue.

Abutment: A tooth, a root, or an implant used for the retention of a fixed or removable prosthesis. Also known as a *retainer.*

Acid attack: The action of acids from plaque upon the enamel.

Acid etch technique: A bonding technique in which tooth structure is etched to create the rough surface necessary for mechanical and micromechanical bonding.

Acquired pellicle: A colorless, translucent film composed of complex sugar-protein molecules. It forms normally on the teeth within minutes of cleaning.

Acrylic: An organic resin from which various types of dental restorations, prostheses, and appliances are constructed.

Active life: The length of time that a solution or material will remain effective after it has been put into use.

Age fog: Fogging on outdated radiographic film.

ALARA: In radiography, an acronym standing for "As Low As Reasonably Achievable."

Alginate: See Hydrocolloid, irreversible.

Alloy: A substance consisting of two or more metals.

Alternative benefit: Contract provision that authorizes the third party to determine the amount of benefits payable, giving consideration to professionally acceptable alternative procedures that may be performed to accomplish the desired result.

Alveolar bone: That part of the alveolar process that lines the bony sockets into which the roots of the teeth are embedded.

Alveolar crest: The highest point of the alveolar process.

Alveolar mucosa: The mucous membrane that covers the alveolar process and continues to form the lining of the cheeks and the floor of the mouth.

Alveolar process: The extension of the maxilla and mandible that surrounds and supports the teeth to form the dental arches. Also known as the *alveolar ridge.*

Alveolar ridge: See Alveolar process.

Alveolar ridge, residual: The bony ridge remaining after the teeth have been extracted.

Alveolar socket: See Alveolus.

Alveolitis: Inflammation and infection associated with a disturbance of the blood clot after tooth extraction. Also known as a *dry socket* or *osteitis.*

Alveoloplasty: Surgical reduction and reshaping of the alveolar ridge.

Alveolus: The cavity within the alveolar process in which the root of the tooth is held in position.

Amalgam: An alloy in which mercury is one of the metals.

Amalgam carrier: A dental hand instrument used to carry and place freshly mixed amalgam into a cavity preparation.

Amalgamation: See Trituration.

Amalgamator: A device used to mix mercury with the amalgam alloy. Also used to mix some cements.

Analgesics: Medications that dull the perception of pain without producing unconsciousness.

Anchor tooth: In dental dam application, the tooth that holds the clamp. See also Key punch hole.

Anchorage: The resistance of teeth and their supporting structures to displacement by mechanical forces.

Anesthesia: The temporary loss of feeling or sensation.

Anesthetic: A drug that produces the temporary loss of feeling or sensation.

Angle former: A dental hand instrument used to accentuate line and point angles in the internal outline and retention form of a cavity preparation.

Angulation: In radiography, the direction or angle at which the central ray position indicating device is aimed at the teeth.

Ankylosis: Abnormal fusion (joining together) of cementum and alveolar bone.

Anodontia: The congenital absence of teeth.

Antagonists: Teeth in opposing arches that normally contact each other in occlusion.

Anterior: Toward the front.

Anterior teeth: The maxillary and mandibular incisors and cuspids.

Antiseptic: An agent that prevents the growth or action of microorganisms; is applied on living tissue.

Apex: The anatomic area at the end of the tooth root.

Apexification: The process in which an environment is created within the root canal and periapical tissues after death of the pulp, which allows a calcified barrier to form across the open apex.

Apexogenesis: The normal development of the apex of a root of a tooth. Also, the treatment of a vital pulp by pulp capping or pulpotomy to permit continued closure of the open apex.

Apical curettage: Surgical removal of infectious material surrounding the apex of a tooth root.

Apicoectomy: The surgical removal of the apical portion of the tooth through a surgical opening made in the overlying bone and gingival tissues.

Apposition: The process of laying down new bone. Also, the deposition of the matrix for the hard dental structures.

Articular disc: A cushion of tough specialized connective tissue within the temporomandibular joint.

Articulate: To come together; to place teeth into occlusion.

Articulation: The contact relationship of upper and lower teeth as they move against each other.

Articulator: A dental laboratory device that simulates the movements of the mandible and the temporomandibular joint when casts of the dental arches are attached to it.

Artifact: A structure or appearance that is produced by artificial means and is not normally present in a radiograph.

Aspirate: To draw back or to draw within; also, to swallow or inhale.

Astringent: An agent applied topically to control moderate bleeding by causing capillaries to contract.

Asymmetrical: Divided into two halves that should be, but are not, mirror images of each other.

Attrition: Loss of tooth structure as a result of wear.

Autogenous bone graft: A bone graft obtained from another area of the same patient and used to induce new bone formation in the defect.

Autogenous: Self-produced.

Avulsed: Torn away; extracted by force.

Axial wall: The vertical portion of a tooth located near the pulpal area and parallel with the long axis of the tooth.

Bar: See Connector.

Bar, overdenture: A "male" portion of the appliance that provides stability and is attached to another tooth in the same dental arch.

Base: The layer of cement that acts as an insulator and protective barrier under a dental restoration. Also known as an *insulating base* or an *intermediary base.*

Base, denture: That portion of the denture, composed of the saddle and gingival area, that is designed to fit over the alveolar ridge.

Baseplate: A rigid, preformed shape used during the fitting of a complete denture to temporarily represent the base of the denture.

Beneficiary: The person entitled to receive benefits under a specific insurance plan.

Benefit: The amount payable by the third party toward the fee charged for various covered dental services.

Bevel: A slanting edge. May be of an instrument, a local anesthetic needle, the enamel margins of a tooth preparation, or the edges of a cast restoration.

Bicuspid: See Premolar.

Bifurcation: The anatomic area in a two-rooted tooth where the roots divide.

Bilateral: Of, or pertaining to, both sides.

Bimanually: Examination style involving the use of both hands simultaneously.

Binangle: An instrument having two off-setting angles in its shank.

Bioburden: Any visible organic debris; in dentistry, most often blood or saliva.

Biopsy: The removal of a tissue specimen for diagnostic purposes.

Bisecting angle technique: A radiographic technique in which the central ray bisects the right angle formed by the long axis of the tooth and film packet.

Bite-block: A device used to hold the mouth open during operative and oral surgery procedures. Also, a holder for radiographic film. Also known as a *mouth prop.*

Bite plane: A fixed appliance made of acrylic used to correct crossbites.
Bite registration: See Occlusal registration.
Bite rims: See Occlusal rims.
Bite-wing radiographs: Intraoral films that show only the coronal portions of opposing teeth in the biting position on the same film.
Bleaching: The use of chemical oxidizing agents to lighten discolored teeth.
Bleeding index: Assessment of the presence or absence of bleeding made by inserting a periodontal probe into the sulcus.
Bloodborne: Disease transmission through contact with blood or body fluids that are contaminated with blood.
Bolus: The mass of food that passes from the mouth into the pharynx.
Bonding: The force by which a substance is secured in intimate contact with another substance. Also, a special form of insurance that reimburses the employer for a loss resulting from theft of funds by an employee.
Bonding, dentin: Establishment of a micromechanical bond between cut dentin and the bonding agent.
Bonding, enamel: Establishment of a mechanical bond between etched enamel and the resin restorative or luting material.
Border-molding: Using the fingers to achieve closer adaptation of the edges of an impression.
Bracket: A small device attached to the teeth that holds the arch wire to the teeth.
Bridge: A fixed prosthetic device consisting of artificial teeth (pontics) that are supported by attaching them to abutment teeth.
Bristle brush: An attachment to the handpiece to remove stain from occlusal surfaces of the teeth.
Broach, barbed: An endodontic instrument with barbs protruding from a metal shaft that is used to remove pulpal tissue.
Bruxism: The involuntary grinding or clenching of the teeth that damages both tooth surface and periodontal tissues.
Buccal: Of, or pertaining to, the cheek.
Buccal tube: A tube to hold an arch wire placed on the buccal side of an orthodontic band.
Buccal wall: Cavity wall nearest the cheek.
Bur, friction-grip: A rotary cutting instrument with a smooth shank to hold it in the high-speed handpiece.
Bur, latch-type: A bur with a notched shank that fits into a latch-type contra-angle handpiece.
Burnisher: A dental hand instrument used to smooth the edges at the margin of a metal restoration and the tooth surface.
Calcification: The process by which organic tissue becomes hardened by the deposit of calcium and other mineral salts.
Calculus: A hard mineralized deposit attached to the teeth.
Canine: See Cuspid.
Cannula: A hollow tube commonly used to aid in the placement of an instrument such as a laser handpiece.
Capitation: A payment plan under which the dentist has contracted to provide all or most of the dental services covered under the program to subscribers in payment on a per capita basis.
Capsule: A fibrous sac that encloses a joint and limits its action. Also, a gelatinous structure that surrounds some bacteria.
Caries: Dental decay. An infectious disease that progressively destroys tooth substance.
Caries, arrested: A carious lesion that does not show any marked tendency for further progression.
Caries, recurrent: Decay occurring beneath the margin of an existing dental restoration.
Carrier: An individual who harbors disease organisms without obvious symptoms and is capable of transmitting this disease to others. Also, the party to a dental contract that may collect premiums, assume financial risk, pay claims, and/or provide administrative services; also known as *third party.*
Carver: An instrument used to shape restorative materials.
Cassette: A light-proof container with intensifying screens in which extraoral radiographic films are placed for exposure to radiation. Also, a specialized container used to organize instruments during use, cleaning, sterilization, and storage.
Catalyst: A material that initiates a chemical reaction.
Cavity: A decay lesion or hole in a tooth.
Cavity liner: The material placed over the pulpal area of the preparation to soothe irritated or sensitive pulp.
Cavity varnish, copal: Cavity varnish with organic component. Applied under amalgam but not compatible with composite resin restorative materials.
Cavity wall: A side of the cavity preparation that aids in enclosing restorative material.
Cavosurface angle: An angle in a cavity preparation formed by the junction of the cavity wall with the exterior tooth surface. Also known as the *cavosurface margin.*
Cavosurface bevel: The bevel found at the cavosurface angle of the cavity preparation.
Cavosurface margin: See Cavosurface angle.
Cementoenamel junction: The junction of the enamel of the crown and the cementum of the root at the cervix of the tooth.
Cementum: The substance covering the root surface of the tooth.
Centers for Disease Control and Prevention: A federal agency that monitors infectious diseases and issues reports, recommendations, and guidelines about diseases.
Central ray: The theoretical center of the x-ray beam as it leaves the tube head; the most direct line of radiation.
Centric occlusion: Closing of the jaws in a position that produces maximum stable contact between the oc-

cluding surfaces of the maxillary and mandibular teeth.

Cephalometric: An extraoral radiographic study of the bones and tissues of the head.

Certified Dental Assistant: One who has passed the Dental Assisting National Board (DANB) examination in chairside assisting.

Cervical erosion: The wearing away of cementum that has been exposed as a result of gingival recession.

Cervix: Neck. The neck of a tooth at the cementoenamel junction.

Chamfer: The tapered finish line or margin at the cervical area of a tooth preparation. Frequently used with metal crown margins.

Cheilosis: Fissuring, drying, and scaling of the vermilion surface of the lips and angles of the mouth.

Chelation: The decalcification and removal of tooth structure by chemical means.

Chisel: A dental hand instrument for cutting or cleaving tooth structure in a cavity preparation.

Chlorhexidine: A disinfectant with broad antibacterial action.

Chlorhexidine stain: An extrinsic stain caused by using a mouthwash containing chlorhexidine.

Cingulum: A prominence of enamel found on the cervical third of the lingual surface of an anterior tooth.

Circumferential: An adjective describing the boundary line of a circle.

Clasp: See Retainer.

Cleoid: A dental hand carving instrument with a blade shaped like a pointed spade. Also, claw-like.

Coagulant: An agent that promotes blood clotting.

Co-insurance: A provision of a dental benefits program by which the beneficiary shares in the cost of covered services, generally on a percentage basis.

Collimation: The elimination of peripheral radiation.

Colloid: A suspension of particles in a dispersion medium such as water. Its two phases are sol (liquid) and gel (solid).

Commissures: The corners of the mouth.

Composite: Resins used for tooth-colored dental restorations.

Composite resin veneer: A veneer of composite resin that is bonded to the tooth surface.

Compressive stress: The stress that occurs when an applied force pushes against a material.

Concentration: In microbiology, the number of pathogens present.

Condensation: The insertion and compression of a dental material into a prepared cavity. Also, the process by which liquid is removed from vapor.

Condenser: A dental hand instrument used to pack plastic-type restorative material into a cavity preparation.

Cone cutting: Failure to center the x-ray beam on the film, leading to unexposed areas on the processed radiograph.

Connector: The bar that joins the right and left quadrant framework of the partial denture.

Consumables: Supply items that are "used up" as part of their function; for example, restorative materials.

Contact: The point on the proximal surface of a tooth where it touches a neighboring tooth.

Contact angle: A measure that describes the wetting ability of a substance.

Contaminated: Not sterile. Potentially capable of spreading disease through indirect contact.

Contour: The shape, form, or surface configuration of an object.

Contra-angle: Having two or more off-setting angles. See also Handpiece.

Contrast: The differences in densities between adjacent areas on the radiograph.

Control tooth: A healthy tooth used as a standard to compare questionable teeth of similar size and structure during pulp vitality testing.

Convenience form: The methods and space needed to gain access to the cavity preparation to insert and finish the restorative material.

Coordination of benefits: A method of integrating benefits payable under more than one group dental insurance plan so that the insured's benefits from all sources do not exceed 100 percent of his allowable dental expenses.

Copal cavity varnish: See Cavity varnish, copal.

Copayment: The beneficiary's share of the dentist's fee after the benefits plan has paid the dentist.

Coping: A thin metal covering or cap placed over a prepared tooth.

Core: The central part. In a post and core restoration, the core is the portion that extends above the gingiva.

Coronal polishing: A procedure in which plaque and extrinsic stains are removed from the coronal portion of the teeth.

Cortical plate: The compact bone covering the alveolar process.

Crevicular fluid: See Sulcular fluid.

Crossbite: Malocclusion in which the facial aspects of the maxillary teeth are located labial to the mandibular teeth.

Cross-contamination: The spread of disease through contact with contaminated items such as handles, food, instruments, or surfaces.

Crown, anatomic: The portion of the tooth covered with enamel.

Crown, cast: A cast restoration that covers the entire anatomic crown of the tooth.

Crown, clinical: That portion of the tooth visible in the mouth above the gingiva.

Cure, dual: Hardening of a material brought about by both self-curing and light-curing.

Cure, light: Hardening of a material in response to exposure to a curing light.

Cure, self: Hardening of a material in response to mixing two chemicals together.

Cure stage: Stage at which an impression material hardens and may give off heat.

Curettage: Scraping or cleaning with a curette.

Curette: A periodontal hand instrument with sharp cutting edges and a rounded toe, used for scaling and root planing.

Curing: The act of polymerization of a chemical compound.

Curve of Spee: The slightly anterior-to-posterior curve of the occlusal surfaces of the posterior teeth.

Curve of Wilson: The cross-arch curvature of the posterior occlusal plane.

Cusp: A pointed or rounded eminence on the surface of a tooth.

Cusp of Carabelli: The fifth cusp located on the lingual surface of many maxillary first molars.

Cuspid: An anterior tooth with a long, thick root. Also known as a *canine.*

Decalcification: The loss of calcium salts from the enamel. The first step in the decay process.

Decay: See Caries.

Deductible: A stipulated sum that the covered person must pay toward the cost of dental treatment before the benefits of the program go into effect.

Deglutition: The act of swallowing.

Dehiscence: Exposure of the root of the tooth through the mucosa and alveolus that extends the full length of the root.

Demineralization: The removal of mineral components from mineralized tissues.

Dental hygienist: A licensed preventive oral health professional who provides educational, clinical, and therapeutic patient services.

Dental implants: Artificial teeth attached to anchors that have been surgically embedded into the bone.

Dentin: The material forming the main inner portion of the tooth structure.

Dentin, peritubular: See Dentin, tertiary.

Dentin, primary: Dentin formed before the eruption of the tooth.

Dentin, reparative: See Dentin, tertiary.

Dentin, sclerotic: See Dentin, tertiary.

Dentin, secondary: Dentin formed after the eruption of the tooth.

Dentin, tertiary: A protective layer of dentin that is formed by the tooth over the pulpal area in response to irritation or injury. Also known as *peritubular dentin, reparative dentin,* and *sclerotic dentin.*

Dentin wall: The portion of a cavity wall that consists of dentin.

Dentinocemental junction: The line of union of the cementum and dentin of the tooth.

Dentition: Natural teeth in the dental arch.

Denture: A prosthesis to replace missing teeth within the same arch. May be complete (full) or partial.

Denture, duplicate: A second denture intended to be a copy of the original.

Dependents: In general, the spouse and children of an insured individual.

Deposition: The process of laying down new bone.

Desiccate: To make excessively dry.

Developer: The chemical solution used first in processing the exposed radiograph.

Diagnostic casts: Replicas of the tissues of the maxillary and mandibular arches made from impressions.

Diastema: An abnormal space between two adjacent teeth in the same arch, usually found between the maxillary central incisors.

Die: An accurate replica of the prepared portion of a tooth used in the laboratory during the fabrication of a cast restoration.

Digitally: Examination style involving the use of the finger and thumb.

Dimensional distortion: Deviation of a radiographic image from the true shape of an object or structure.

Direct technique: See Technique, direct.

Direct Reimbursement Plan: A self-funded program in which the individual is reimbursed on the basis of a percentage of dollars spend for dental care provided. This type of plan allows beneficiaries to seek treatment from the dentist of their choice.

Disc: Rotary instruments of abrasive materials.

Disclosing solution: A coloring agent applied to the teeth to reveal dental plaque.

Discoid: A spoon-shaped dental hand instrument with a cutting edge around the total periphery.

Disinfectant: An agent used to kill pathogenic microorganisms without necessarily sterilizing the material.

Disinfection: The process of killing pathogenic agents by chemical or physical means. It does not include the destruction of spores and resistant viruses.

Disposables: Items that are used once and then discarded.

Distal: Away from the midline.

Distal wall: Cavity wall in the restorative process nearest the distal surface of the tooth.

Dorsum: Top; the upper surface of the tongue.

Dovetail: A fan-shaped detail of the cavity preparation designed to increase the retention of the restoration.

Drift: The lateral movement of a tooth into a space left by a missing adjacent tooth.

Droplet infection: The type of infection transmitted by droplets of moisture, such as from sneezing or from handpiece spray.

Dry socket: See Alveolitis.

Dual coverage: Coverage under more than one insurance plan.

Ductility: The ability of a material to withstand permanent deformation under tensile stress without fracture.

Due care: A legal term meaning just, proper, and sufficient care, or the absence of negligence.

Due cause: A legal term requiring the employer to demonstrate justifiable reason for an action, such as terminating an employee.

Edentulous: Without teeth. Usually meaning having lost all natural teeth.

Edgewise bracket: An orthodontic bracket used to attach the arch wire to the tooth.

Elastic limit: The maximum stress that a structure or material can withstand without being permanently deformed. Also known as the *yield strength.*

Elastic modulus: A measure of the rigidity or stiffness of a material at stresses below its elastic limit.

Elasticity: The ability of a body that has been changed or deformed under stress to resume its original shape when the stress is removed.

Electronic apex locator: A device used during endodontic treatment to determine the location of the apex of the tooth.

Electronic pulp tester: A diagnostic device used to determine tooth vitality.

Elongation: The distortion on a radiograph that results in lengthening of the image in one dimension.

Embrasure: A V-shaped space in a gingival direction between the proximal surfaces of two adjoining teeth in contact.

Enamel: The hard tissue that covers the anatomic crown of the tooth.

Endogenous stain: An intrinsic type of stain, caused during tooth development.

Endosteal implant: An implant that is surgically embedded *into* the bone.

Environmental Protection Agency: A division of the federal government that monitors and regulates environmental issues.

Epinephrine: A substance that causes blood vessels to constrict; a vasoconstrictor.

Equilibration: The act of putting the mandible in a state of balance with the maxilla.

Erosion: The superficial wearing away of tooth substance, not involving bacteria.

Eruption: The migration of a tooth into functional position in the oral cavity.

Esthetic: Pleasing to the eye.

Etch: Treating enamel with phosphoric acid to provide retention for resin sealants, restorative materials, or orthodontic brackets.

Etchant: The acid solution or gel used to etch tooth structure.

Ethics: That part of philosophy that deals with moral conduct, duty, and judgment.

Evulsed: See Avulsed.

Excavator, spoon: A dental hand instrument with a sharp, bowl-shaped edge used to remove carious dentin.

Excision: Cutting away or taking out.

Excursion: Movement of the mandible from the centric position to a lateral or protrusive position.

Exfoliation: The normal process by which primary teeth are shed.

Exodontics: The science and practice of removing teeth.

Exogenous stain: An intrinsic type stain acquired after the tooth has formed and erupted.

Exostosis: A benign growth on the surface of a bone.

Exothermic: Giving off heat during a chemical reaction.

Expendables: Supply items relatively low in cost that are used up in a short period of time; for example, mouth mirrors.

Explorer: A dental hand instrument with a fine tip that is used to detect caries and rough areas on the tooth surface.

Exposure: Being subjected to infectious materials. Also, uncovering the dental pulp. Also, the use of ionizing radiation to produce radiography.

Exposure incident: Contact—specifically parenterally or through the eye, mouth, other mucous membrane, or nonintact skin—with blood or other potentially infectious material (including saliva) that results from the performance of an employee's duties (as in a needlestick injury).

Exposure time: The time, in seconds or fractions of seconds, during which x-radiation is produced by the x-ray machine.

Extraoral films: Radiographs taken with the film outside the patient's mouth.

Extrinsic stain: A stain that can be removed from tooth surfaces by polishing.

Extrusion: Teeth displaced in the socket as a result of an injury. Also, the movement of a tooth beyond its normal occlusal plane in the absence of opposing occlusal force.

Facial: Of, or pertaining to, both the labial and buccal surfaces of the teeth.

Facial wall: The collective reference to the buccal and labial walls in cavity preparation for restorative materials.

Fenestration: Loss of supporting bone structure so that only the marginal bone is intact.

Festooning: Trimming, shaping. In a denture, shaping to simulate normal tissue appearance.

File, chronological: Storage of records by date sequence.

File, cross-reference: A listing that makes it easy to find numerical files by alphabetical reference.

File, Hedström: An endodontic instrument used to enlarge root canals.

File, K-type: An endodontic instrument used to smooth, shape, and enlarge root canals.

Film speed: Radiographic film's sensitivity to radiation. This determines the amount of x-radiation required to produce a diagnostic quality film.

Film thickness: The thickness of an adhesive film.

Filter, aluminum: Removes low-energy, long-wavelength x-rays that are not necessary for producing a diagnostic quality radiograph.

Finger rest: See Fulcrum.

Finish line: The point where the cavity preparation meets the external surface of the tooth.

Fissure: A deep groove or cleft, commonly the result of the imperfect fusion of the enamel.

Fixed appliances: Orthodontic appliances, attached to the teeth, that are removed only by the practitioner.

Fixed overhead: Business expenses that continue at all times.

Flange: The parts of the complete or partial denture base that extend from the cervical areas of the teeth to the border of the denture.

Flap: A loose section of tissue separated from that surrounding it except at the base.

Flash: The excess material that extrudes beyond the intended margins of a restoration or a mold.

Fluorides, systemic: Fluorides ingested into the body in water, food, beverages, or supplements.

Fluorides, topical: Fluorides applied in direct contact with the teeth through mouth rinses, fluoridated toothpaste, and topical fluoride applications.

Fluorosis: Mottled enamel caused by excessive fluoride intake.

Focal-film distance: The distance from the focal spot (target) on the anode of the x-ray tube to the film.

Focal spot: The area of the anode or target bombarded by the electron stream when the tube is in action.

Foreshortening: The distortion of an object on a radiograph in which the image appears shorter than the actual object.

Framework: The metal skeleton of the removable partial denture.

Frenum: A fold of mucous membrane attaching the cheeks and lips to the upper and lower arches, in some instances limiting the motions of the lips and cheeks. (Plural, *frena* or *frenula.*)

Fulcrum: Placement of the fingers used to stabilize the wrist and arm of the operator during use of an instrument. Also, the point or support on which a lever turns. Also known as a *finger rest.*

Furcation: The anatomic area of a multi-rooted tooth where the roots divide.

Gag reflex: Protective mechanism located in the posterior of the mouth. Contact with this area causes gagging, retching, or vomiting.

Galvanism: The small electrical current created whenever two dissimilar metals are present in the oral cavity.

Gates-Glidden burs: Elliptically shaped burs with very long shanks, used in endodontic treatment.

Geometric teeth: See Nonanatomic posterior teeth.

Germicide: A solution capable of killing all microorganisms except spores.

Gingiva: The mucous membrane tissue that immediately surrounds a tooth. (Plural, *gingivae.*)

Gingiva, attached: The portion of the gingiva extending from the gingival margin to the alveolar mucosa.

Gingiva, free: The part of the gingiva that surrounds the tooth and is not directly attached to the tooth surface.

Gingival curettage: The removal of soft tissue that makes up the pocket wall (sulcular or crevicular epithelium) by scraping with periodontal instruments.

Gingival margin: The most coronal portion of the gingiva surrounding the tooth.

Gingival margin trimmer: A dental hand instrument designed to bevel the cervical cavosurface walls of the cavity preparation.

Gingival sulcus: The shallow furrow formed where the gingival tip meets the tooth enamel.

Gingival wall: The wall of a preparation that is nearest the gingiva. This wall is at a right angle to the other cavity walls.

Gingivectomy: The surgical removal of gingival tissue. Most commonly, this is the tissue wall of a periodontal pocket.

Gingivitis: Inflammation of the gingiva characterized clinically by changes in color, gingival form, position, and surface appearance and the presence of bleeding and/or exudate. Also known as Type I periodontal disease.

Gingivoplasty: A surgical procedure to correct gingival deformities, particularly enlargements. It is performed when there are no periodontal pockets present.

Glutaraldehyde: A high-level disinfectant.

Gutta-percha: A plastic type of filling material used in endodontic treatment.

Hand-cutting instruments: Instruments used under hand direction, as opposed to motor-driven instruments.

Handpiece: An instrument to hold rotary instruments in a dental engine connecting them with the power source.

Handpiece, contra-angle: An extension attached to a low-speed handpiece to form an offset angle.

Handpiece, high-speed: A dental handpiece that rotates at a speed up to 450,000 rpm.

Handpiece, laboratory: A dental handpiece designed for use in the laboratory, not in the mouth. Rotates at a speed up to 20,000 rpm.

Handpiece, laser: Delivery system for fiber optic cables on a laser unit.

Handpiece, low-speed: A dental handpiece that rotates at a speed of 25,000 rpm.

Handpiece, prophylaxis: A right-angle attachment to the straight handpiece to hold polishing cups and brushes.

Handpiece, right-angle: An extension attached to a low-speed handpiece to form a right angle.

Handpiece, slow-speed: See Handpiece, low-speed.

Handpiece, sonic: A specialized handpiece operating on the principle of sonic-level vibrations used in endodontic treatment.

Handpiece, straight: A low-speed handpiece that may be used to hold rotary instruments most commonly used in the dental laboratory.

Handpiece, surgical: A specialized handpiece for surgical procedures.

Hardness: The ability of a material to resist permanent indentation or scratching.

Height of contour: The bulge, or widest point, in the facial and lingual contours of the tooth.

Hemisection: The surgical separation of a multi-rooted tooth through the furcation area.

Hemostatic: Controlling bleeding.

Holding solution: A disinfecting solution used to cover contaminated instruments before they are processed for sterilization.

Homogenous: Having a uniform quality and consistency throughout.

Host resistance: The ability of an individual to resist a pathogen.

Hydrocolloid: A colloidal solution in which water is

used as the dispersing medium. Also, a type of dental impression material.

Hydrocolloid, irreversible: A hydrocolloid that once it forms a solid will not return to the liquid phase; alginate impression materials. In dentistry, alginate impression materials.

Hydrocolloid, reversible: A hydrocolloid that may repeatedly be taken from the sol to gel phase.

Hydrophilic: Having an affinity for absorbing water.

Hydrophobic: Antagonistic to or shedding water.

Imbibition: Absorbing water.

Immediate use: Within the 8 hours of a work shift.

Impaction: Remaining unerupted in the alveolus beyond the time at which a tooth should normally be erupted.

Impaction, bony: A tooth that is blocked by both bone and tissue.

Impaction, soft tissue: A tooth that is blocked from eruption only by gingival tissue.

Implant: See Dental implants.

Implant scalers: Scalers with plastic tips used to scale dental implants.

Implosion: Bursting inward; the opposite of an explosion.

Incisal: Of, or pertaining to, the biting edge of an anterior tooth.

Incisal wall: Cavity wall in the restorative process located toward the incisal edge of an anterior tooth. It is at a right angle to the other cavity walls.

Incisor: An anterior tooth with a thin and sharp cutting edge.

Indirect fabrication: Creation of a restoration in the dental laboratory.

Infiltration: Technique of depositing anesthetic solution into the area immediately surrounding the tooth or teeth.

Infrabony pocket: A periodontal pocket that extends apically to the level of the adjacent alveolar bone.

Initiation: The beginning development of a tooth.

Inlay: A cast restoration designed to restore one, two, or three surfaces of the prepared tooth.

Insured: The person, usually the employee, who earns insurance benefits.

Interocclusal registration: See Occlusal registration.

Interproximal: Between the proximal surfaces of adjacent teeth.

Interproximal radiograph: See Bite-wing radiograph.

Intrinsic stain: A stain that cannot be removed from tooth surfaces by polishing; discoloration within the enamel.

Invert: To turn inward or to turn under.

Iodophor: Disinfectant used in differing strengths as a surgical scrub and as a surface disinfectant.

Ionizing radiation: Radiation, including x-rays, that produces ions when interacting with matter and is capable of harming living tissues.

Jurisprudence, dental: Law as it applies to dentistry.

Key punch hole: In dental dam application, the hole that covers the anchor tooth. (See also Anchor tooth.)

Keyway slots: Marks made in the dentin next to the canal space to prevent the rotation and loosening of a post in the canal.

Labial: Of, or pertaining to, the lip.

Labial wall: Cavity wall in the restorative process that is nearest the lips.

Labioversion: Abnormal protrusion of the maxillary incisors toward the lips.

Lamina dura: Thin, compact bone lining the alveolar socket.

Lamina propria: A layer of connective tissue that lies just under the epithelium of the mucous membrane.

Laser: An acronym for "Light Amplification by Simulated Emission of Radiation."

Latent image: An image on film, produced by exposure to x-rays, that is not visible until the film has been processed.

Lateral: Toward the side.

Lateral excursion: A sliding position of the mandible to the left or right of the centric position, in relation to the maxilla.

Latex sensitivity: An allergic-type reaction resulting from contact with latex products, such as gloves and dental dam.

Lentulo spiral: A fine, flexible, needle-like instrument capable of being inserted into a small hole.

Lesion: A broad term to describe tissue damage caused by either injury or disease.

Libel: A written or spoken statement that gives an unfavorable impression of a person, or a statement that could injure a person's reputation.

Licensure: Having a license to practice in a specific state.

Ligature: Cord, thread, or stainless steel wire used to bind teeth together or to hold structures in place. Also, to stabilize a dental dam application.

Limitations: Maximum benefits that an insurance plan covers.

Line angle: In the preparation of a cavity, this is the junction of two walls or tooth surfaces.

Lingual: Of, or pertaining to, the tongue.

Lingual wall: Cavity wall in the restorative process located toward the lingual surface of an anterior or posterior tooth.

Linguoversion: In centric occlusion, the abnormal positioning of the maxillary incisors in back of the mandibular incisors.

Local anesthesia: The temporary loss of sensation of a specific area through the administration of a drug that blocks nerve conduction.

Luting: Bonding or cementing two unlike substances together.

Luxate: To dislocate, bend, or put out of joint.

Malleability: The ability of a material to withstand permanent deformation under compressive stress without rupture.

Malocclusion: An occlusion and positioning of the teeth that is not in accordance with the usual rules of anatomic form.

Malposed: Not in a normal position within the dental arch.

Malpractice: Professional negligence.

Mamelon: A rounded eminence on the incisal edge of a newly erupted incisor.

Mandibular arch: The teeth in position in the alveolar process of the mandible. Also known as the lower jaw.

Mandibular subperiosteal implant: Metal frame implants that are surgically placed *on top* of the mandibular ridge.

Mandrel: A mounting device with a screw and a threaded end or a snap-on attachment to hold the disc in a dental handpiece.

Master cast: Cast created from the secondary impression used in the construction of the baseplates, bite rims, wax setups, and finished prostheses. Also known as a *working cast.*

Mastication: The act of chewing.

Material Safety Data Sheets: Information sheets required by the Occupational Safety and Health Administration on all hazardous substances kept or used in the office.

Matrix: A metal or plastic band used to replace the missing wall of a tooth during placement of the restorative material.

Maxillary arch: The teeth in position in the alveolar process of the maxillae. Also known as the upper jaw.

Mechanical retention: See Retention, mechanical.

Medically compromised: Having an illness or physical condition that may influence proposed dental treatment.

Mesial: Toward the midline.

Mesial wall: Cavity wall in the restorative process nearest the mesial surface of the tooth.

Microleakage: A microscopically small opening between the tooth and restoration that allows fluids and debris to seep downward into the tooth and cause recurrent decay and damage to the pulp.

Microretention: Mechanical retention in which the bonds created are extremely small.

Midline: A plane that divides the body into equal left and right halves.

Mobility: Movement of a tooth within its socket.

Model: See Diagnostic cast.

Molar: A posterior tooth with a broad occlusal surface for chewing.

Mousse: In dentistry, a term used to describe the smooth consistency of impression material used to obtain an occlusal registration.

Mouth guard: A removable appliance used to protect teeth from injury during athletic activities.

Mouth prop: See Bite-block.

Muscle trimming: The process in which the patient makes facial and swallowing movements to develop the base and muscular extensions at the margins of the impression tray.

Nasion: The midpoint between the eyes just below the eyebrows.

Nasmyth's membrane: The enamel cuticle partially remaining on a tooth surface after tooth eruption.

Needlestick injury: See Exposure incident.

Negligence: Failure to use due care, or the lack of care.

Nib: The working end of a dental hand instrument, with a smooth or serrated surface.

Noble metals: Metals that are highly resistant to oxidation, tarnish, and corrosion. The noble metals used in dentistry are gold (Au), palladium (Pd), and platinum (Pt).

Nonduplication of benefits: A provision relieving the carrier from responsibility for paying for services that are covered under another program. Also known as *benefit-less-benefit.*

Nonresponders: Individuals who have been vaccinated against hepatitis B but do not develop antibodies to the virus.

Object-film distance: The distance between the film and the object being radiographed.

Obturation: The process of filling the root canal in endodontic therapy.

Obturator: A prosthesis for closing an opening in the palate.

Occlusal: Of, or pertaining to, the chewing surfaces of the posterior teeth.

Occlusal equilibration: The removal of all occlusal interferences on the teeth.

Occlusal interference: An area on a tooth that prevents the teeth from occluding properly.

Occlusal registration: Normal relationship between the maxillary and mandibular dental arches in occlusion as represented by an impression material. Also known as a *bite registration* or an *interocclusal registration* (IOR).

Occlusal rims: Rims built on the baseplate to register vertical dimension and the occlusal relationship of the mandibular and maxillary arches. Also referred to as *bite rims.*

Occlusion: The contact between the maxillary and mandibular teeth in all mandibular positions and movements.

Occlusion, centric: See Centric occlusion.

Onlay: A cast restoration designed to restore the occlusal and some proximal surfaces of a posterior tooth.

Opaquer: A material placed under a restoration to prevent the discoloration of the tooth from showing through.

Opportunistic disease: One that normally would be controlled by the immune system but cannot be controlled because that system is not functioning properly.

Optimal focal distance: The best, least stressful distance from the operator's eyes to the patient's mouth.

Order of use: The sequence in which the dentist uses a series of instruments. Also known as *sequence of use.*

Orthodontics, interceptive: Procedures designed to intercept orthodontic problems that may worsen if left untreated.

Orthodontics, preventive: Procedures designed to prevent or minimize the degree of severity of future orthodontic problems.

Osseointegration: The attachment of healthy bone to the dental implant.

Osseous surgery: Surgical procedures involving the alveolar bone.

Osteitis: See Alveolitis.

Outline form: The curved shape and border of the restoration and tooth surface.

Overbite: Vertical projection of upper teeth over the lowers.

Overhang: Excess restorative material projecting over the cavity margin.

Overjet: Horizontal projection of upper teeth over the lowers.

Overlapping: In a radiograph, superimposition of the image of one tooth over part of another.

Palatal: Of, or pertaining to, the palate or roof of the mouth.

Palate, hard: The bony anterior portion of the roof of the mouth.

Palate, primary: During early development, the union of the medial nasal process and the lateral nasal processes to form the premaxilla.

Palate, soft: The posterior tissue portion of the roof of the mouth.

Palliative: Affording relief of pain but not a cure.

Palpate: To feel with the fingers.

Palpation: An examination technique of the soft tissues with the examiner's hand or finger tip.

Papilla: Gingiva filling the interproximal spaces between adjacent teeth; projections located on the dorsum of the tongue that contain receptors for the sense of taste. (Plural, *papillae*).

Paralleling technique: In radiography, a technique consisting of placing the film packet parallel to the longitudinal axis of the tooth and directing the central ray perpendicular to the tooth and film packet.

Paresthesia: A condition in which the numbness of a local anesthetic lingers after the effects should have worn off.

Partial denture: A prosthetic device containing artificial teeth supported on a framework and attached to natural teeth with retainers and rests.

Path of insertion: The direction or path that permits a cast restoration or partial denture to be seated.

Percussion: An examination technique that uses sharp, short blows to the involved tooth with a finger or instrument to determine vitality.

Periapical: Surrounding the apex of the root of the tooth.

Periapical abscess: See Abscess, periapical.

Periapical radiograph: An intraoral film that shows the entire tooth and surrounding anatomy.

Peri-implant area: Gingival sulcus surrounding the implant, where it protrudes through the gingiva.

Periodontal abscess: See Abscess, periodontal.

Periodontal dressing: Packs used for the protection of periodontal surgical wounds.

Periodontal ligament: The tissues that support and anchor the tooth in its socket.

Periodontal pocket: A pathological formation created when the depth of the gingival sulcus exceeds 3 mm.

Periodontal scaling and root planing: See Root planing. Also see Sealing.

Periradicular: Surrounding the root of the tooth.

Personal protective equipment: Garments, eyewear, masks, and gloves worn to protect healthcare workers from occupational exposure to potentially infectious material.

Pesso file: A long shank bur used in endodontic treatment primarily for parallel post preparations.

Pit and fissure: Faults that are the result of noncoalescence of enamel during tooth formation.

Plaque: A soft deposit on the teeth consisting of bacteria and bacteria products.

Point angle: An angle in cavity preparation formed by the junction of three walls.

Polymerization: The process of curing a material to change it from a plastic to a rigid form.

Pontic: An artificial tooth that replaces a missing natural tooth.

Porcelain veneer: An indirect veneer made of porcelain and bonded to the tooth surface.

Position indicating device: In radiography, a device used to limit the beam of radiation.

Post: A metal support fitted into the root canal of an endodontically treated tooth to improve the retention of a cast restoration.

Post dam: A seal at the posterior of a full or partial denture that holds it in place. Also known as a *posterior palatal seal.*

Posterior: Toward the back.

Posterior palatal seal: See Post dam.

Posterior teeth: The maxillary and mandibular premolars and molars.

Potentially infectious material: Any item, equipment, or device that may be contaminated. PIMs must be handled with exceptional care to prevent cross-contamination of diseases in the dental office.

Predetermination: An administrative procedure whereby a dentist submits the treatment plan to the third party carrier before treatment begins. Also known as *pre-treatment estimate.*

Premolar: A posterior tooth with points and cusps for grasping, tearing, and chewing. Also known as a *bicuspid.*

Pre-treatment estimate: See Predetermination.

Primary radiation: The stream of radiation emitted from the x-ray unit tubehead.

Prophylaxis, dental: A procedure, performed by a dentist or a registered dental hygienist, for the complete removal of calculus, debris, stains, and plaque from the teeth. Also known as a *prophy.*

Prosthesis: A replacement for a missing body part. (Plural, *prostheses.*)

Protocol: A series of specific steps that must be followed.

Protrusion: The condition of being thrust forward; a position of the mandible placed forward as related to the maxilla.

Proximal: Nearest or adjacent to.

Proximal walls: The tooth surface, mesial or distal, that is nearest to the adjacent tooth. Also, the mesial and distal walls in cavity preparation.

Pulp: The vital tissues of the tooth consisting of nerves, blood vessels, and connective tissue.

Pulp capping: Application of a material to a cavity

preparation that has exposed or nearly exposed the dental pulp.

Pulp vitality testing: A diagnostic test to determine whether the pulp of a tooth is vital (alive) or non-vital (dead).

Pulpal floor: See Pulpal wall.

Pulpal wall: The floor of the cavity preparation overlying the pulp. Located at a right angle to the other cavity walls. Also referred to as the *pulpal floor.*

Pulpectomy: The surgical removal of a vital pulp from a tooth.

Pulpitis: Inflammation of the dental pulp.

Pulpitis, irreversible: Inflammation of the dental pulp in which the pulp will not recover and will require endodontic treatment.

Pulpitis, reversible: Inflammation of the dental pulp in which the pulp will recover.

Pulpotomy: The partial excision of the dental pulp limited to the coronal horns within the pulp chamber.

Pumice: Ground volcanic ash that is used for polishing.

Quadrant: One of the four sections, or quarters, of the mouth.

Radiolucent: A substance that allows radiant energy to pass through it, producing black areas on radiographs.

Radiopaque: A substance that does not allow radiant energy to pass through it, producing light areas on radiographs.

Recapping: Replacing the protective needle guard (sheath) over the exposed end of a used local anesthetic needle. Also known as *resheathing.*

Recession: Loss of part or all of the gingiva over the root of a tooth.

Reimplant: Replacing a lost or extracted tooth into the alveolar process (socket).

Relative analgesia: The use of nitrous oxide and oxygen gases to achieve a state of patient sedation.

Release of information form: The patient's written consent to release information regarding his dental care and related conditions.

Remineralization: The process of restoring minerals to a mineralized tissue that has been demineralized.

Remodeling: Growth and changes in existing bone.

Removable appliance: Orthodontic appliance designed to be placed and removed by the patient.

Resheathing: See Recapping.

Resistance form: Shaping the remaining enamel and dentin to strengthen the tooth and restoration.

Resorption: The body's process of removing existing bone or hard tissue tooth structure.

Rest: In the removable partial denture, a metal projection on or near the retainer of the partial denture.

Retainer: A device used to hold something in place; the attachment or abutments of a fixed or removable prosthesis; an appliance for maintaining the positions of the teeth and jaws immediately after the completion of orthodontic treatment. Also see Abutment.

Retention: The result of adhesion, mechanical locking, or both.

Retention form: The shaping of the cavity walls to aid in retaining the restoration.

Retention grooves: Markings in the surfaces of the tooth that enhance placement and retention of the restoration.

Retention, mechanical: The bonding (locking together) of tooth structure and the bonding agent or restorative material.

Retraction: To draw back in or to draw away from.

Retraction, gingival: A procedure in which temporary tissue displacement is used to widen the gingival sulcus before taking an impression.

Retrusion: A position of the mandible as far posterior as possible from the centric position, as related to the maxilla.

Rheostat: A foot control used to control the high- and low-speed handpieces on the dental unit.

Root planing: The removal of plaque, embedded calculus, and altered cementum from the roots of teeth.

Rotation: The force of moving a tooth to the left or right in its socket.

Rugae: Folds in the mucosal tissue found on the roof of the mouth and in the stomach. (Singular, *ruga.*)

Saddle: The portion of the removable appliance that rests on the mucosa covering the alveolar ridge and retains the artificial teeth.

Safelight: A light that provides illumination while not affecting the emulsion of undeveloped radiographic films.

Scaling: The removal of plaque and calculus from the crown and root surfaces of the teeth with the use of curettes and scalers.

Scattered radiation: Radiation that has been deviated in direction during passage through matter. It is one form of secondary radiation.

Schedule of benefits: A list of covered services that assigns each service a sum that represents the total obligation of the plan with respect to payment for such service. Also known as the *table of allowances.*

Sealant: Resin material used to seal pits and fissures to protect against caries.

Seating: In dentistry, the final placement of a restoration or fixed prosthesis. Also, placement of a removable prosthesis.

Seating lug: Component of an orthodontic band placed on the lingual surface and used as an aid while seating the band.

Secondary radiation: Radiation produced from any substance being struck by primary radiation.

Selective polishing: Polishing only those teeth affected with stain or plaque. Also, polishing limited to certain teeth before a procedure.

Sequence of use: See Order of use.

Serial extraction: The elective extraction of the first premolar in each quadrant.

Serrated: Notched or toothlike edge or surface.

Sextants: The division of the dentition into six parts: maxillary right, maxillary anterior, maxillary left, mandibular right, mandibular anterior, and mandibular left.

Sharps: A term used to describe sharp or pointed objects that may puncture the skin or oral mucosa and must be discarded in a sharps container.

Shelf life: The time a product may be stored before it begins to deteriorate.

Slurry: In dentistry, a mixture of pumice and water used to remove plaque and debris from the crown of the tooth.

Smear layer: Very thin (5 to 10 microns) organic film of organic debris that adheres to dentin as a result of cavity preparation.

Smile line: The level at which the lip covers the teeth when the patient smiles.

Sodium hypochlorite: Common household bleach. Used in various concentrations for disinfection.

Source individual: Any individual whose blood or other potentially infectious materials may be a source of occupational exposure.

Source-film distance: The distance from the radiation source to the dental film.

Space maintainer: Appliance used after the loss of a primary tooth to maintain the space in the arch until the permanent tooth erupts.

Splinting: A support process whereby the teeth are bound together to share the stresses placed on them.

State Board of Dental Examiners: The administrative board designated to interpret and implement regulations under the state dental practice act.

State Dental Practice Act: The law that contains the legal restrictions and controls on the dentist, dental auxiliaries, and the practice of dentistry within each state.

Sterilization: The process by which all forms of life are completely destroyed within a circumscribed area.

Stippling: A textured effect to simulate the normal gingival tissue.

Stones: Mounted rotary instruments used for polishing and refining restorations.

Stops: Small, round, sterile pieces of rubber or plastic that are placed on endodontic instruments to mark the working length. Also, raised areas placed in an impression tray to ensure adequate depth for the impression material.

Strain: The distortion or change produced in a body as the result of stress.

Stress: The internal reaction, or resistance, within a body to an externally applied force.

Stress-breaker: A device in a removable partial denture that relieves the abutment teeth from excessive stress.

Subgingival calculus: Mineralized bacterial plaque below the crest of the marginal gingiva.

Subsupine: Positioned on the back, face upward, with the head slightly lower the knees.

Succedaneous: That which follows; the permanent teeth that replace the primary teeth.

Sulcular fluid: Tissue fluid that seeps into the gingival sulcus through the wall of the sulcus. Also known as *crevicular fluid.*

Sulcus: A groove or depression. (Plural, *sulci.*) See also Gingival sulcus.

Supine: Lying on the back.

Suprabony pocket: A periodontal pocket that extends coronally to the level of the adjacent alveolar bone.

Supragingival calculus: Mineralized bacterial plaque above the crest of the marginal gingiva.

Surfactant: A surface tension releasing or separating agent.

Surgical stent: A clear acrylic template that is placed over the alveolar ridge to assist in locating the proper placement for dental implants.

Surgical template: A clear plastic tray that represents the alveolus as it should appear *after* the teeth have been extracted.

Synthetic phenols: Compounds with broad-spectrum disinfecting action.

Systemic fluorides: See Fluorides, systemic.

Table of Allowances: See Schedule of Benefits.

Tactile: Referring to the sense of touch.

Technique, direct: Shaping a wax pattern in the mouth on the prepared tooth.

Technique, indirect: In the laboratory, the shaping of a wax pattern on a model of a prepared tooth.

Tensile strength: Stress required to rupture a material when it is pulled apart.

Tensile stresses: Force per unit area that tends to stretch, or elongate, an object.

Tension side: The side of the tooth away from the direction in which the tooth is being moved.

Thermal conductivity: The quantity of heat transferred per second across a unit area.

Thermal tests: The application of heat and cold to determine pulpal vitality.

Thermoplastic: The property of becoming softer on heating and harder on cooling; the process being reversible.

Tipping: Moving a tooth into a more upright position.

Tofflemire: A matrix retainer and band system used to replace the missing wall of a tooth while the restoration is being placed.

Tongue thrust swallow pattern: A swallow pattern in which the tongue is pushed forcefully against the anterior teeth.

Topical fluorides: See Fluorides, topical.

Torque: A rotational force; force applied to a tooth to produce rotation during orthodontic treatment.

Torus mandibularis: An exostosis on the medial surface of the mandible. (Plural, *tori.*)

Torus palatinus: An exostosis on the surface of the hard palate. (Plural, *tori.*)

Tragus: The cartilaginous projection anterior to the external opening of the ear.

Transillumination: The process of reflecting high-intensity light through anterior teeth to locate fractures.

Trauma: Injury.

Trifurcation: The areas in a three-rooted tooth where the roots divide.

Trituration: To mix together; the process of mixing the alloy with mercury to form an amalgam paste. Also referred to as *amalgamation.*

Ultimate strength: Maximum stress that a material sustains before it fractures.

Ultrasonic scaling: The use of an ultrasonic scaler to remove mineralized deposits from the tooth surfaces.

Undercut: The portion of a tooth that lies between the height of contour and the gingiva. Also, recessed areas in the surface of the cast.

Unit: Each single component of the fixed bridge; a segment of scheduled time; a piece of dental equipment.

Universal numbering system: Identification of the teeth: the permanent teeth are numbered 1 to 32; primary teeth are lettered A to T.

Universal precautions: A set of precautions designed to prevent transmission of human immunodeficiency virus (HIV), hepatitis B virus (HBV), and other blood-borne pathogens in a healthcare setting.

Varnish: Resin surface coating formed by evaporation of a solvent.

Vasoconstrictor: A substance that causes blood vessels to narrow and stimulates the heart.

Vasodilator: A substance that causes blood vessels to expand.

Veneer: A layer of tooth-colored material (composite or porcelain) that is bonded or cemented to the prepared tooth surface.

Ventral: Refers to the front or belly side of the body.

Vertical angulation: In radiography, the angle made between the x-ray beam and a line parallel to the floor.

Vertical dimension: A measurement of the face at the midline with the teeth in occlusion. Also, the space provided by the height of the teeth in normal occlusion.

Vestibule: The tissues of the mandibular and maxillary mucobuccal folds.

Virulence: The relative capacity of a pathogen to overcome body defenses.

Viscosity: The property of a liquid that causes it *not* to flow easily.

Washed field technique: Use of a water spray from the dental handpiece as a coolant to protect the tooth from injury due to overheating.

Waste, infectious: Contaminated sharps, teeth, pathological waste, and blood-soaked items. (Environmental Protection Agency definition.)

Waste, regulated: Liquid or semiliquid blood or other potentially infectious materials; items that would release blood or other potentially infectious materials if compressed. (Occupational Safety and Health Administration definition.)

Wavelength: In radiography, the distance from the crest of one wave to the crest of the next wave. The energy produced is determined by the length of the wave, with shorter wavelengths (such as x-rays) producing higher energies.

Wax, beading: Soft, pliable wax in a ropelike shape used to modify impression trays.

Wax, boxing: Utility wax strips used to form matrix around impressions before pouring.

Workers' compensation: A payroll tax that the employer is required to pay to cover the cost of insurance in case an employee is injured on the job.

Working cast: See Master cast.

Yield strength: See Elastic limit.

Young's frame: A U-shaped metal or plastic frame used to hold dental dam in place.

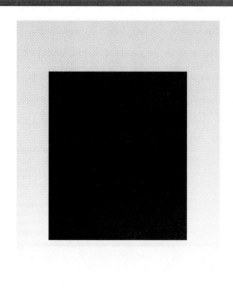

References

A Century of Service to Dentistry, 1844–1944. Philadelphia, The SS White Dental Manufacturing Co., 1944.

A review of procedures available for plaque control. In *Dent. Prod. Report, 26*(8):22–78, 1992.

A symposium: the oral manifestations of gingival hyperplasia. In *Compend. Contin. Educ. Dentistry,* Suppl 14, 1990.

Abbas, A.K., Lichtman, A.H., and Pober, J.S.: Cellular and Molecular Immunology. Philadelphia, W.B. Saunders Co., 1991.

Ackerman, V., and Dunk-Richards, G.: Microbiology. Philadelphia, W.B. Saunders Co., 1991.

ADAA Principles of Ethics and Code of Professional Conduct. Chicago, American Dental Assistants Association, 1980.

Albers, H.: Temporary Crown & Bridge Fabrication, 5th ed. Santa Rosa, CA, Alto Books, 1992.

Allen, C.M.: Diagnosing and managing oral candidiasis. In *J.A.D.A., 123*:77–81, 1992.

Anderson, M.H., Bales, D.J., and Omnell, K.: Modern management of dental caries. In *J.A.D.A., 124*:37–44, 1993.

Applications for dental dam. In *Dent. Prod. Report, 27*(5):86–111, 1993.

Arey, L.B.: Developmental Anatomy, 7th ed. Philadelphia, W.B. Saunders Co., 1974.

Arthur, R.: Manual of Diseases of the Teeth. Philadelphia, Lindsay & Blakiston, 1846.

Ash, M.M.: Wheeler's Dental Anatomy, Physiology, and Occlusion, 7th ed. Philadelphia, W.B. Saunders Co., 1993.

Ash, M.M., Ward, M.L.: Kerr and Ash's Oral Pathology, 5th ed. Philadelphia, Lea & Febiger, 1986.

Avery, J.K.: Oral Development and Histology. Baltimore, Williams & Wilkins, 1987.

Babbush, C.A.: Dental Implants: Principles and Practice. Philadelphia, W.B. Saunders Co., 1991.

Banting, D.W.: The future of fluoride. In *J.A.D.A., 123*:86–91, 1991.

Barbakow, F., et al.: Enamel remineralizations: how to explain it to patients. In *Quintessence International, 22*(5):341–347, 1991.

Baum, L., Phillips, R.W., and Lund, M.R.: Textbook of Operative Dentistry, 2nd ed. Philadelphia, W.B. Saunders Co., 1985.

Beard, J.: Developing a comprehensive maltreatment intervention program. In *Dent. Assist., 62*(1):16–19, 1993.

Beemsterboer, P., and Perry, D.A.: Techniques and Theories of Periodontal Instrumentation. Philadelphia, W.B. Saunders Co., 1990.

Beirle, J.W.: Dental operatory water lines. In *C.D.A.J., 21*(2):13–15, 1993.

Bennett, C.R.: Monheim's Local Anesthesia and Pain Control in Dental Practice, 7th ed. St. Louis, C.V. Mosby Co., 1984.

Black, G.V.: Operative Dentistry, vols. I to IV. Chicago, Medico-Dental Publishing Co., 1908.

Black, H.C.: Black's Law Dictionary, 5th ed. St. Paul, MN, West Publishing Co., 1980.

Boo-Chai, K.: An ancient Chinese text on a cleft lip. In *Plast. Reconstr. Surg., 38*:39, 1966 (as quoted by Hudson, N.C.: In *J.A.D.A., 84*:933, 1972).

Bowen, R.F., and Marjenhoff, W.A.: Adhesion of composites to dentin and enamel. In *C.D.A.J., 21*(6):19–22, 1993.

Bremner, M.D.K.: The Story of Dentistry, 2nd ed. Brooklyn, NY, Dental Items of Interest Publishing Co., 1946.

Bressman, J.K.: Risk management for the '90s. In *J.A.D.A., 124*:63–67, 1993.

Brody, H.A.: UCSF: the fearful dental patient—a challenge and an opportunity. In *J.C.D.A., 21*(3):31–35, 1993.

Cariostatic Mechanisms of Fluoride. Princeton, NJ, Princeton Dental Resource Center, 1990.

Carl, W.: Local radiation and systemic chemotherapy. In *J.A.D.A., 124*:119–123, 1993.

Carlsson, D.S.: Craniofacial Growth Theory and Orthodontic Treatment. Ann Arbor, MI, The Center for Human Growth and Development, University of Michigan, 1990.

Carranza, F.A. Jr.: Glickman's Clinical Periodontology, 7th ed. Philadelphia, W.B. Saunders Co., 1990.

Carranza, F.A., and Perry, D.A.: Clinical Periodontology for the Dental Hygienist. Philadelphia, W.B. Saunders Co., 1986.

Chasteen, J.: A computer database approach for dental practice. In *J.A.D.A., 123*:27–33, 1992.

Chasteen, J.E.: Essentials of Clinical Dental Assisting, 4th ed. St. Louis, C.V. Mosby Co., 1989.

Chernega, J.B.: Emergency Guide for Dental Auxiliaries. Albany, NY, Delmar Publishers, 1987.

Chohayeb, A.A.: Hepatitis B and C: what you should know. In *Compend. Contin. Educ. Dentistry, 13*(9):776–781, 1992.

Christensen, G.J.: Complex fixed and implant prosthodontics: making nearly foolproof impressions. In *J.A.D.A., 123*:69–70, 1992.

Christensen, G.J.: Keeping interocclusal records: how to solve a common problem. In *J.A.D.A., 124*:93–94, 1993.

Christensen, G.J.: Removable prosthodontic impressions. In *J.A.D.A., 124*:112–113, 1993.

Cochran, M.A., Miller, C.H., and Sheldrake, M.A.: The efficacy of the rubber dam as a barrier to the spread of microorganisms during dental treatment. In *J.A.D.A., 119*:141–144, 1989.

Computers in the Dental Office. Chicago, Council on Dental Practice, American Dental Association, 1992.

Council on Dental Materials, Instruments and Equipment: Choosing intracoronal restorative materials. In *J.A.D.A., 125*:102–103, 1994.

Craig, R., O'Brien, W., and Powers, J.: Dental Materials: Properties and Manipulation, 5th ed. St. Louis, C.V. Mosby Co., 1992.

Craig, R.G., et al.: Restorative Dentistry Materials, 9th ed. St. Louis, C.V. Mosby Co., 1993.

Crispin, B. J.: Expanding the application of facial ceramic veneers. In *C.D.A.J., 21*(6):43–54, 1993.

Current Dental Chemotherapeutics. Princeton, NJ, Princeton Dental Resource Center, 1990.

Davis, WL: Oral Histology: Cell Structure and Function. Philadelphia, W.B. Saunders Co., 1986.

Dental Dam Procedures, 9th ed. Akron, OH, Hygienic Corp., 1992.

Dental Implants: Are They Right For You? Chicago, The American Academy of Periodontology, 1989.

Diagnostic and Statistical Manual of Mental Disorders, 3rd ed. Washington, DC, American Psychiatric Association, 1987.

Diet and Caries. Princeton, NJ, Princeton Dental Resource Center, 1990.

Dionne, R.A.: Preventing and treating postoperative pain. In *J.A.D.A., 123*:27–34, 1992.

Dorland's Illustrated Medical Dictionary, 27th ed., Philadelphia, W.B. Saunders Co., 1988.

Dunn, S.M., and Kantor, M.L.: Facts and fictions on digital radiology. In *J.A.D.A., 124*:39–47, 1993.

Dykema, R.W., Goodacre, C.J., and Phillips, R.W.: Johnstone's Modern Practice in Fixed Prosthodontics, 4th ed. Philadelphia, W.B. Saunders Co., 1986.

Ebersold, L.A.: Malpractice: Risk Management for Dentists. Tulsa, OK, PennWell Books, 1986.

Ehrlich, A.: Business Administration for the Dental Assistant, 4th ed. Champaign, IL, Colwell Systems, 1991.

Ehrlich, A.: Ethics, Jurisprudence and Risk Management. Champaign, IL, Colwell Systems, 1994.

Ehrlich, A.: Medical Terminology for Health Professions, 2nd ed. Albany, NY, Delmar Publishers, 1992.

Ehrlich, A.: Nutrition and Dental Health, 2nd ed. Albany, NY, Delmar Publishers, 1994.

Ehrlich, A., and Torres, H.O.: Essentials of Dental Assisting. Philadelphia, W.B. Saunders Co., 1992.

Eklund, K.J., and Bednarsh, H.: Interact Training Systems, Brunswick, ME, 1993.

Employee Training Manual, Volume 2: Introduction to OSHA, the Bloodborne Pathogens Standard and How Infectious Diseases are Transmitted. Health Safe Systems, 1992.

Employee Training Manual, Volume 2: Exposure (Infection) Control Practices. Health Safe Systems, 1992.

Faecher, B.S., Thomas, J.E., and Bender, B.S.: Tuberculosis: a growing concern for dentistry? In *J.A.D.A., 124*:94–104, 1993.

Fauchard, P.: Le Chirurgien Dentiste. (Translated by L. Lindsay.) Pound Ridge, NY, Milford House, 1969.

Fenn, H.R.B., Liddelow, K., Gimson, A., and MacGregor, A.R.: Clinical Dental Prosthetics, 3rd ed. London, Wright of Butterworth Scientific Publications, 1989.

Finkbeiner, B.L., and Patt, J.C.: Practice Management for the Dental Team, 3rd ed. St. Louis, C.V. Mosby Co., 1991.

Finkelman, R.D.: Growth factors in bones and teeth. In *C.D.A.J., 20*(12):3–28, 1992.

Flight, M.R.: Law, Liability, and Ethics. Albany, NY, Delmar Publishers, 1988.

Fluoride: dentistry's hero for nearly 50 years. In *Dent. Prod. Report, 27*(3):18–82, 1993.

Fluoride Products: An Update for the 1990's. Princeton, NJ, Princeton Dental Resource Center, 1990.

Foster, T.D.: A Textbook of Orthodontics. London, Blackwell Scientific Publications, 1990.

Frommer, H.: Radiology for Dental Auxiliaries, 5th ed. St. Louis, C.V. Mosby Co., 1992.

Garretson, J.E.: A System of Oral Surgery, 6th ed. Philadelphia, J.B. Lippincott Co., 1898.

Gatchel, R.J.: Managing anxiety and pain during dental treatment. In *J.A.D.A., 123*:37–41, 1992.

Gerber, A., Steinhardt: Dental Occlusion and the Temporomandibular Joint. Chicago, Quintessence Publishing Co., 1990.

Gobetti, J.P.: Controlling dental pain. In *J.A.D.A., 123*:47–52, 1992.

Gomolka K.: Disinfectant update 1993. In *Dent. Prod. Report, 27*(4):82–100, 1993.

Gomolka K.: Operatory prep. In *Dent. Prod. Report, 27*(2):82–120, 1993.

Gomolka, K.: Oral manifestations of AIDS. In *Dent. Prod. Reports, 27*(6):62–74, 1993.

Goodman, H.S., Ickrath, M.C., and Niessen, L.C.: Managing patients with Alzheimer's disease. In *J.A.D.A., 124*:77–80, 1993.

Grant, D.A., Stern, I.B., and Everett, F.G.: Periodontics in the Tradition of Gottlieb and Orban, 6th ed. St. Louis, C.V. Mosby Co., 1988.

Greene, C.S.: Managing TMD patients. In *J.A.D.A., 123*:43–45, 1991.

Greenspan, D., and Greenspan, J.: Management of the oral lesion of HIV infection. In *J.A.D.A., 122*:26–31, 1991.

Grembowski, D, et al.: How fluoridation affects adult dental caries. In *J.A.D.A.*, 123:49–54, 1992.

Guerini, V.: A History of Dentistry from the Most Ancient Times Until the End of the 18th Century. Philadelphia, Lea & Febiger, 1909.

Gundelach, J., and Lee J.: Schedule your way to improved efficiency. In *Dent. Econ., 83*(6):67–73, 1992.

Haring, J.I., and Lind, L.J.: Radiographic Interpretation for the Dental Hygienist. Philadelphia, W.B. Saunders Co., 1993.

Harris, C.A.: The Principles and Practice of Dental Surgery. Philadelphia, Lindsay & Blakiston, 1845.

Hartnett, A.C., and Shiloah, J.: The treatment of acute necrotizing ulcerative gingivitis. *Quintessence International, 22*(2):95–99, 1991.

Haywood, V.B.: History, safety, and effectiveness of current bleaching techniques. *Quintessence International, 23*(7):471–488, 1992.

Helgeson, B.: 1924–1974: American dental assistants commemorate 50th anniversary. In *J.A.D.A., 89*:539–544, 1974.

Henry, R.J.: Assessing environmental health concerns associated with nitrous oxide. In *J.A.D.A., 123*:41–47, 1992.

Heymann, H.O.: Current concepts in dentin bonding. In *J.A.D.A., 124*:27–36, 1993.

History of the American Dental Assistants Association. Chicago, American Dental Assistants Association, 1970.

Holli, B.B., and Calabrese, RJ.: Communication and Education Skills: The Dietician's Guide, 2nd ed. Philadelphia, Lea & Febiger, 1991.

Holroyd, S.V., Wynn, R.L., and Requa-Clark, B.: Clinical Pharmacology in Dental Practice, 4th ed. St. Louis, C.V. Mosby Co., 1988.

Houston, W.J.B., and Stephens, CD.: A Textbook of Orthodontics. Santa Rosa, CA, Redwood Press, 1992.

Hughes, T.: Electronic claims filing shows dramatic growth. In *Dent. Econ., 82*(2):80–83, 1992.

Ibsen, O.A., and Phelan, J.A.: Oral Pathology for the Dental Hygienist. Philadelphia, W.B. Saunders Co., 1992.

Infection control in dentistry guidelines. *Office Sterilization & Asepsis Procedures Research Foundation Newsletter,* May 1992.

Infection Control in Modern Dental Practice. Rochester, NY, Eastman Kodak Co., 1992.

Infection Control Guidelines for Dental Radiographic Procedures. *Newsletter Am. Acad. Oral Maxillofac. Radiol., 17*(1):10–11, 1990.

Infection Control Recommendations for the Dental Office and the Dental Laboratory. Chicago, American Dental Association, August 1992.

Intraoral Radiography with Rinn XCP/BAI Instruments. Elgin, IL., Rinn Corp., 1993.

Jacob, J.A.: New technology can remineralize teeth. In *A.D.A. News, 23*(18):27, 1992.

Jacob, S.W., and Francone, C.A.: Elements of Anatomy and Physiology, 2nd ed. Philadelphia, W.B. Saunders Co., 1989.

Jacobsen P., Carpenter W., and Cuny, E: Bloodborne exposure incidents: complying with OSHA regulations. In *C.D.A.J., 20*:8, 1992.

Jastak, J.T.: Pharmacosedation. In *C.D.A.J., 21*(2):27–32, 1993.

Jepsen, C.: Neutralizing dental fear. In *C.D.A.J., 21*(3):13–14, 1993.

Kasle, M.J.: An Atlas of Radiographic Anatomy, 3rd ed. Philadelphia, W.B. Saunders Co., 1989.

Keith, D.A.: Atlas of Oral and Maxillofacial Surgery. Philadelphia, W.B. Saunders Co., 1992.

Kells, C.E.: The Dentist's Own Book. St. Louis, C.V. Mosby Co., 1925.

Kells, C.E.: Three Score Years and Nine. New Orleans, published privately, 1926.

Kidd, E.A.M., and Smith, B.A.N.: Pickard's Manual of Operative Dentistry, 6th ed. Oxford, England, Oxford University Press, 1990.

Klineberg, I.: Occlusion: Principles and Assessment. Oxford, England, Wright, Butterworth, Heinemann Publishing Limited, 1991.

Koch, C.R.D.: History of Dental Surgery, Vol. 1. Chicago, National Art Publishing Co., 1909.

Koch, C.R.D.: History of Dental Surgery, Vol. 3. Fort Wayne, IN, National Art Publishing Co., 1910.

Kodak Dental Radiography Tips. Rochester, NY, Eastman Kodak, 1993.

Kodak Recommended Dental Films & Intensifying Screens. Rochester, NY, Eastman Kodak Co., 1993.

Kumar, V., Cotran, R.S., and Robbins, S.F.: Basic Pathology, 5th ed. Philadelphia, W.B. Saunders Co., 1992.

Legal aspects of computerized patient records. In *Dent. Prod. Reports, 27*:4:40–114, 1993.

Leinfelder, K.F.: Changing restorative traditions. In *J.A.D.A.*, 125:65–67, 1994.

Leinfelder, K.F.: Current developments in dentin bonding systems. In *J.A.D.A.*, 124:40–42, 1993.

Levine, N.: Current Treatment in Dental Practice. Philadelphia, W.B. Saunders Co., 1986.

Lewis, D.L., Arens M., Stanton S.A., et al.: Cross contamination potential with dental equipment. *Lancet, 340*:1252–1254, 1992.

Liebgott, B.: The Anatomical Basis of Dentistry. Philadelphia, W.B. Saunders Co., 1982.

Mahan, L.K., Arlin, M.: Krause's Food, Nutrition and Diet Therapy, 8th ed. Philadelphia, W.B. Saunders Co., 1992.

Maier, C.: Save the children. In *Dent. Teamwork, 5*(3):20–22, 1992.

Malamed, S.F.: Managing medical emergencies. In *J.A.D.A., 124*:40–52, 1993.

Malamed, S.F.: Pain and anxiety control in dentistry. In *C.D.A.J., 21*(10):35–41, 1993.

Malamed, S.F., and Sheppard, G.A.: Handbook of Emergencies in the Dental Office, 3rd ed. St. Louis, C.V. Mosby Co., 1987.

Materials update: new generation glass ionomers. In *GP, 1*(5):65–70, 1992.

Matschek, C.: What message are you sending? In *Dent. Econ., 83*(11):63–73, Nov. 1992.

Mazey, K., and Mito, R.: Multidisciplinary Treatment of Dental Phobia. In *C.D.A.J., 21*(3):17–25, March 1993.

McCann, D.: Conquering dental fear. In *J.A.D.A., 119*:20–22, Nov. 1989.

McCann, D.: Nerve disorder eludes diagnosis. In *ADA News, 24*(7):40–41, 1993.

McCarthy, F.M.: Essentials of Safe Dentistry for the Medically Compromised Patient. Philadelphia, W.B. Saunders Co., 1989.

McCarthy, F.M.: Malpractice: prevention and claims. In *C.D.A.J., 15*(25):27, 1987.

McCormick, J. T., Anthony S. J., Dial, M. L., et al.: Wettability of elastomeric impression materials, effects of selected surfactants. In *Int. J. Prosthodontics, 2*:413, 1989.

McDowell, J., Kassebaum, K., and Stromboe, S.: Recognizing and reporting victims of domestic violence. In *J.A.D.A., 123*(9):20–22, 1992.

Melfi, R.C.: Permar's Oral Embryology and Microscopic Anatomy, 8th ed. Philadelphia, Lea & Febiger, 1988.

Menczer, L.F., Mittlemen, M., and Wildsmith, J.A.W.: Horace Wells. In *J.A.D.A., 110*:773–776, 1985.

Miles, D.A., VanDis, M.L., Jensen, C.W., and Ferretti, A.: Radiographic Imaging for Dental Auxiliaries, 2nd ed. Philadelphia, W.B. Saunders Co., 1994.

Miller C.: Cleaning, sterilization and disinfection: basics of microbial killing for infection control. In *J.A.D.A.*, 124:48–56, 1993.

Miller C.: Employers required to supply workers with protective gear. *RDH*, pp 22–23, May 1992.

Mjor, I.A., and Fejerkov, O.: Human Oral Embryology and Histology. Copenhagen, Munksgaard, 1986.

Molinari, J.: Education and communication: a professional response. In *C.D.A.J., 20*(10):19, 1992.

Molinari, J.A., Cottone, J.A., and Gleason, MJ.: Hepatitis B and available vaccines. In *C.D.A.J., 20*(10):43–45, 1992.

Moore, K.L.: The Developing Human: Clinically Oriented Embryology, 4th ed. Philadelphia, W.B. Saunders Co., 1988.

Morris, A.L., Bohannan, H.M., and Casullo, D.P.: The Dental Specialties in General Practice. Philadelphia, W.B. Saunders Co., 1983.

Moss-Salentijn, L., and Hendricks-Klyvert, M.: Dental and Oral Tissues, 3nd ed. Philadelphia, Lea & Febiger, 1990.

Murray, J.J., Rugg-Gunn, A.J., and Jenkins, G.N.: Fluorides in Caries Prevention. Oxford, England, Wright, 1991.

Nanda, R., and Burstone, C.J.: Retention and Stability in Orthodontics. Philadelphia, W.B. Saunders, 1993.

Nester, E.W., Roberts, C.E., Lindstrom, M.E., Pearsall, N.M., and Nester, M.T.: Microbiology, 3rd ed. Philadelphia, W.B. Saunders Co., 1983.

Newbrun, E.: Preventing dental caries: current and prospective strategies. In *J.A.D.A., 123*:68–73, 1992.

Newman, M.G., and Nisengard, R.: Oral Microbiology and Immunology. Philadelphia, W.B. Saunders, 1988.

Niessen, L.C., Mash, L.K., and Gibseon, G.: Practice management considerations for an aging population. In *J.A.D.A., 124*:55–59, 1993.

Nitrous oxide scavenging doesn't eliminate harmful effects of exposure. In *GP, 2*(1):1–4, 1993.

Nizel, A.E., and Papas, E.S.: Nutrition in Clinical Dentistry, 3rd ed. Philadelphia, W.B. Saunders Co., 1989.

Oberbreckling, P.J.: The components of quality dental records. In *Dent. Econ., 85*(5):29–38, 1993.

O'Keson, J.P.: Management of Temporomandibular Disorders and Occlusion, 3rd ed. St. Louis, Mosby Year Book, 1993.

Pallasch, T.J.: How to use antibiotics effectively. In *C.D.A.J., 21*(2):46–50, 1993.

Pansky, P.: Review of Gross Anatomy, 5th ed. New York, Macmillan Publishing Co., 1984.

Paré, A.: Collected Works of Ambroise Paré. Pound Ridge, NY, Milford House, 1969.

Pedersen, G.W.: Oral Surgery. Philadelphia, W.B. Saunders, 1988.

Periodontal Screening and Recording System. Chicago, American Dental Association, 1993; Chicago, American Academy of Periodontology, 1993.

Perry, D.A., Beemsterboer, P., and Carranza, F.A.: Techniques and Theory of Periodontal Instrumentation. Philadelphia, W.B. Saunders, 1990.

Pharmacology expert updates GPs on use of pain relievers. In *GP, 2*(1):1–6, 1993.

Phillips, R.W.: Skinner's Science of Dental Materials, 9th ed. Philadelphia, W.B. Saunders Co., 1991.

Phillips, R.W., and Moore, B.K.: Elements of Dental Materials for Dental Hygienists and Dental Assistants, 5th ed. Philadelphia, W.B. Saunders Co., 1994.

Pindborg, J.J.: Atlas of Diseases of the Oral Mucosa, 5th ed. Philadelphia, W.B. Saunders, 1993.

Pinkham, J.R., Casamassimo, P.S., Fields, H.W., et al.: Pediatric Dentistry: Infancy Through Adolescence. Philadelphia, W.B. Saunders Co., 1988.

Pollack, R.: Cultivating a winning team. In *J.A.D.A.*, *124*:47–49, 1993.

Pontecorvo, D.A.: Expanded duties: Results of ADAA's nationwide survey. In *Dent. Assist.* *57*(9):13, 1988.

Practical barrier technique for infection control in dental radiography. In *Compend. Contin. Educ. Dentistry, 13*:11, 1992.

Prevention and early detection: key to oral cancer. In *J.A.D.A.*, 124:81–82, 1993.

Principles of ethics and code of professional conduct. In *J.A.D.A.*, *123*(9):98–110, 1992.

Prinz, H.: Dental Chronology. Philadelphia, Lea & Febiger, 1945.

Proffitt, W.R.: Contemporary Orthodontics. St. Louis, Mosby–Year Book, 1993.

Proskauer, C., and Witt, F.H.: Pictorial History of Dentistry. Cologne, Verlag M. Dumont Schauberg, 1962.

Radiation Safety in Dental Radiography. Rochester, NY, Eastman Kodak Co., 1993.

Reactions to latex in health care settings. In *J.A.D.A.*, *124*:91–92, 1993.

Reed, G.M., and Sheppard, V.F.: Basic Structures of the Head and Neck. Philadelphia, W.B. Saunders Co., 1976.

Regezi, J.A., and Sciubba, J.J.: Oral Pathology. Philadelphia, W.B. Saunders Co., 1989.

Reis, D.: Dental professionals and the disabled: a new partnership. In *Dent. Prod. Report, 26*(9):14–122, 1992.

Reis, J.J.: High-tech trends: the impact of modern technology on dentistry. In *Dent. Prod. Report, 27*(3):110–117, 1993.

Reis-Schmidt, D.: High-tech trends: the impact of modern technology on dentistry. In *Dent. Prod. Report, 27*(1):26, 1993.

Rice, D.: OSHA checklist for dental practices. In *Dent. Prod. Report, 27*(5):21–103, 1993.

Rightful vs. wrongful termination of dental employees. *C.D.A.J., 18*:8, 1990.

Ring, M.E.: Dentistry: An Illustrated History. St. Louis, Mosby–Year Book, 1985.

Rodu, B., and Mattingly, G.: Oral mucosal ulcers. In *J.A.D.A.*, *123*:83–86, 1992.

Runnells, R.: Countering the concerns: how to reinforce dental practice safety. In *J.A.D.A.*, *124*:65–73, 1993.

Runnells, R: Managing infection control and OSHA. In *Dentistry Today,* pp 31–33, 1992.

Sandoval, S.D.: Supervised nightguard vital bleaching. In *Dent. Assist., 62*(1):21–25, 1993.

Sarnat, B.G., and Laskin, D.M.: The Temporomandibular Joint: A Biological Basis for Clinical Practice, 4th ed. Philadelphia, W.B. Saunders Co., 1992.

Scherman, A., Jacobsen, P.L.: Managing dentin hypersensitivity. In *J.A.D.A.*, *123*:57–61, 1992.

Schonenberger, M.A.: Precision Fixed Prosthodontics: Clinical Laboratory Aspects. Chicago, Quintessence Books, 1990.

Seltzer, S.: Online: computers in dentistry: electronic spread sheets. In *Compend. Contin. Educ. Dentistry, 13*(9):716–720, 1992.

Sheets, C.G., and Taniguchi, T.: Advantages and limitations in the use of porcelain veneer restorations. In *J. Prosthet. Dentistry, 64*:406–412, 1990.

Sherer, J.: Taking stock: How to order, store and maintain dental supplies. In *ADG Impact—Business Watch,* pp 12–14, 1992.

Shrout, M., Comer, R., Powell, B., et al.: Treating the pregnant patient: four basic rules addressed. In *J.A.D.A.*, *123*(5):75–80, 1992.

Silverman, S.: A look at oral cancer lesions. In *Dent. Teamwork, 6*(2):31–32, 1993.

Slavkin, H.C.: Incidence of cleft lips, palates rising. In *J.A.D.A.*, *123*:61–63, 1992.

Smith, C.M., and Reynard, A.M.: Textbook of Pharmacology. Philadelphia, W.B. Saunders Co., 1992.

Sprouls, L.: Dealing with dental phobias. In *Dent. Teamwork,* pp 14–18, November–December 1992.

Steri-Oss Dental Implant System. Anaheim, CA, A Denar Affiliates, 1993.

Sturdevant, C.M., Barton, R.E., Sockwell, C.L., and Strickland, W.D.: The Art and Science of Operative Dentistry, 2nd ed. St. Louis, C.V. Mosby Co., 1985.

Successful Intraoral Radiography. Rochester, NY, Eastman Kodak Co., 1993.

Taylor, L.H.: The mixed blessing of being first. *J.A.D.A.*, 117: 443, 1988.

TenCate, A.R.: Oral Histology: Development, Structure and Function, 2nd ed. St. Louis, C.V. Mosby Co., 1985.

The American Dental Association Regulatory Compliance Manual. Chicago, American Dental Association, 1990 (with updates).

The American National Red Cross: Community First Aid & Safety. St. Louis, Mosby Lifeline, 1993.

The Merck Manual, 16th ed. Rahway, NJ, Merck Research Laboratory, 1992.

Thomson, H.: Occlusion, 2nd ed. London, Wright of Butterworth Scientific Publications, undated.

Thorpe, B. (ed): History of Dental Surgery, vol. 2. Chicago, The National Art Publishing Co., 1909.

Tuberculosis: A ticking time bomb. In *Mayo Clin. Health Letter, 11*(4):1–3, 1992.

Tylenda, C.A., Roberts, M.W., et al.: Bulimia nervosa. In *J.A.D.A.*, *122*:37–41, 1991.

Walton, R.E., and Torabinejad, J.: Principles and Practice of Endodontics. Philadelphia, W.B. Saunders, 1989.

Watson, C.M., and Whitehouse, R.L.S.: Possibility of cross-contamination between dental patients by means of the saliva ejector. In *J.A.D.A.*, *124*:77–80, 1993.

Weinberger, B.W.: An Introduction to the History of Dentistry, Vols. 1 and 2. St. Louis, C.V. Mosby Co., 1948.

Weinberger, B.W.: Pierre Fauchard, Surgeon Dentist. Minneapolis, Pierre Fauchard Academy, 1941.

Weisman, G.: Care for a lifetime. In *Dent. Prod. Report, 26*(2):58–59, 1992.

White, S.N.: Adhesive cements and cementation. In *C.D.A.J., 21*(6):30–36, 1993.

White, S.N.: Adhesive restorative dentistry: introduction. Many new adhesive materials can offer improved clinical results. In *C.D.A.J., 21*(6):17–18, 1993.

Whitehouse, R.L.S., Peters, E., et al.: Influence of biofilms on microbial contamination in dental unit water. In *J. Dent., 1985*:290–295, 1991.

Wilkins, E.M.: Clinical Practice of the Dental Hygienist, 6th ed. Philadelphia, Lea & Febiger, 1989.

Woelfel, J.B.: Permar's Outline for Dental Anatomy, 2nd ed. Philadelphia, Lea & Febiger, 1979.

Woodall, I.R.: Comprehensive Dental Hygiene Care, 4th ed. St. Louis, C.V. Mosby Co., 1993.

Wright, W.F., Yang, L., and Davarpanah, M.: Soft tissue management. In *C.D.A.J., 4*:65–72, 1989.

Young, J.M.: Maintaining dental equipment. In *J.A.D.A.*, *122*:83, 1991.

Your Teeth Can Be Saved by Endodontic Treatment. Chicago, American Dental Association, Division of Communications, 1992.

Yu, X.Y., Joynt, R.B., et al.: Adhesion to dentin. In *C.D.A.J., 21*(6):23–28, 1993.

Zernik, J.H., and Minken, C.: Genetic control of bone remodeling. In *C.D.A.J., 20*(12):14–19, 1992.

Index

Note: Page numbers in *italics* refer to illustrations; page numbers followed by t refer to tables.

B

C

D

E

F

G

I

J

K

L

M

N

O

S

T

U

V

X

Y

Z